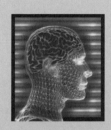

Encyclopedia of the

Human Brain

VOLUME 2

Col–Mem

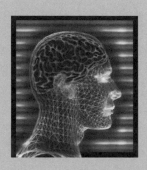

Encyclopedia of the
Human Brain

EDITOR-IN-CHIEF

V. S. RAMACHANDRAN

University of California, San Diego
La Jolla, California

VOLUME 2
Col–Mem

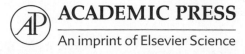

ACADEMIC PRESS
An imprint of Elsevier Science

Amsterdam   Boston   London   New York   Oxford   Paris   San Diego   San Francisco   Singapore   Sydney   Tokyo

This book is printed on acid-free paper. ⊗

Copyright 2002, Elsevier Science (USA).

All Rights Reserved.
No part of this publication may be reproduced or transmitted in any form or by any means, electronic or
mechanical, including photocopy, recording, or any information storage and retrieval system, without
permission in writing from the publisher.

Requests for permission to make copies of any part of the work should be mailed to:
Permissions Department, Academic Press, 6277 Sea Harbor Drive,
Orlando, Florida 32887-6777

Academic Press
An imprint of Elsevier Science
525 B Street, Suite 1900, San Diego, California 92101-4495, USA
http://www.academicpress.com

Academic Press
84 Theobalds Road, London WC1X 8RR, UK
http://www.academicpress.com

Library of Congress Catalog Card Number: 2001093327

International Standard Book Number: 0-12-227210-2 (set)
International Standard Book Number: 0-12-227211-0 (volume 1)
International Standard Book Number: 0-12-227212-9 (volume 2)
International Standard Book Number: 0-12-227213-7 (volume 3)
International Standard Book Number: 0-12-227214-5 (volume 4)

Typeset by Macmillan India Limited, Bangalore, India.

PRINTED IN THE UNITED STATES OF AMERICA
02   03   04   05   06   07   MM   9   8   7   6   5   4   3   2   1

$600.00 (4 VOL.)

CONTENTS

VOLUME 2

C

D

VOLUME 3

N

O

CONTRIBUTORS

CATHERINE ABBADIE
Endorphins and Their Receptors
Memorial Sloan–Kettering Cancer Center

JOHN R. ABSHER
Cerebrovascular Disease
Absher Neurology and Wake Forest University
Baptist Medical Center

CRISTIAN ACHIM
Neural Transplantation
University of Pittsburgh

RALPH ADOLPHS
Emotion
University of Iowa College of Medicine

BO AHRÉN
Neuropeptides and Islet Function
Lund University

JEFFRY R. ALGER
Magnetic Resonance Imaging (MRI)
University of California, Los Angeles

LAURA S. ALLEN
Sex Differences in the Human Brain
University of California, Los Angeles

KAREN E. ANDERSON
Violence and the Brain
University of Maryland

JAY B. ANGEVINE, JR.
Nervous System, Organization of
The University of Arizona, Tucson

KEN W. S. ASHWELL
Chemical Neuroanatomy
University of New South Wales

JAMES R. AVERILL
Anger
University of Massachusetts, Amherst

CLAUDIA AVINA
Sexual Dysfunction
University of Nevada, Reno

PAUL BACH-Y-RITA
Brain Damage, Recovery from
University of Wisconsin, Madison

DAVID T. BADRE
Memory, Neuroimaging
University of Michigan

JANICE I. BALDWIN
Sexual Behavior
University of California, Santa Barbara

JOHN D. BALDWIN
Sexual Behavior
University of California, Santa Barbara

EDWIN J. BAREA-RODRIGUEZ
Information Processing
University of Texas, San Antonio

MICHAEL A. BARRY
Taste
Seton Hall University

JEFFREY T. BARTH
Mild Head Injury
University of Virginia School of Medicine

MICHEL BAUDRY
Synapses and Synaptic Transmission and Integration
University of Southern California

NICOLE A. BAUMANN
Astrocytes
INSERM Unit 495 and University Pierre and Marie Curie, Paris, France

DAPHNE BAVELIER
Neuroplasticity, Developmental
University of Rochester

KATHLEEN BAYNES
Corpus Callosum
University of California, Davis

LORI L. BEASON-HELD
Aging Brain
National Institute of Aging

PELAGIE M. BEESON
Agraphia
University of Arizona, Tucson

MARLENE BEHRMANN
Agnosia
Carnegie Mellon University

MARIO BERTINI
Dreaming
University of Rome

BRENT R. BEUTTER
Motion Processing
NASA Ames Research Center

PETER BLACK
Hydrocephalus
Children's Hospital/Brigham & Women's Hospital, Boston

WILLIAM W. BLESSING
Brain Stem
Flinders University, Adelaide, Australia

JONATHAN BLUMENTHAL
Adolescent Brain Maturation
National Institute of Mental Health

ERIC M. BOWMAN
Alertness
University of St. Andrews, Scotland

J. DOUGLAS BREMNER
Anxiety
Yale University

THOMAS BRIESE
Borna Disease Virus
University of California, Irvine

BETH S. BRODSKY
Suicide
New York State Psychatric Institute and Columbia University College of Physicians and Surgeons

MATTHEW A. BRODSKY
Parkinson's Disease
Mount Sinai Medical Center—New York University

NILS BROSE
Synaptogenesis
Max Planck Institute for Experimental Medicine, Göttingen, Germany

DONNA K. BROSHEK
Mild Head Injury
University of Virginia School of Medicine

ANGUS M. BROWN
Neuroglia, Overview
University of Washington School of Medicine

RICHARD J. BROWN
Conversion Disorders and Somatoform Disorders
Institute of Neurology and National Hospital for Neurology and Neurosurgery, United Kingdom

VERITY J. BROWN
Alertness
University of St. Andrews, Scotland

CHARLES J. BRUCE
Eye Movements
Yale University School of Medicine

JOHN F. BRUGGE
Hearing
University of Wisconsin

JOHN P. BRUNO
Vigilance
Ohio State University

HENRY A. BUCHTEL
Auditory Agnosia
Temporal Lobes
University of Michigan and VA Healthcare System,
Ann Arbor

LAUREN BURHANS
Cingulate Cortex
University of Illinois

ANN B. BUTLER
Cranial Nerves
George Mason University

DANIEL CAGGIANO
Mental Workload
Catholic University of America

SERGE CAMPEAU
Psychoneuroendocrinology
University of Colorado

DAVID CAPLAN
Language Disorders
Language, Neural Basis of
Massachusetts General Hospital

J. PATRICK CARD
Hypothalamus
University of Pittsburgh

ESTEBAN V. CARDEMIL
Depression
Brown University School of Medicine and
Rhode Island Hospital

THOMAS H. CARR
Inhibition
Michigan State University

V. A. CASAGRANDE
Visual System Development and Neural Activity
Vanderbilt University School of Medicine

B. J. CASEY
Anterior Cingulate Cortex
Weill Medical College of Cornell University

DAVID F. CECHETTO
Cerebral Cortex
University of Western Ontario

DANIEL T. CERUTTI
Reinforcement, Reward, and Punishment
Duke University

DENNIS S. CHARNEY
Anxiety
Yale University

ERAN CHEMERINSKI
Mood Disorders
University of Iowa College of Medicine

ROBERT E. CLARK
Classical Conditioning
University of California, San Diego

IRUN R. COHEN
Autoimmune Diseases
Weizmann Institute of Science, Rehovot, Israel

TIMOTHY J. COLLIER
Transplantation
Rush Presbyterian–St. Luke's Medical Center

LISA TABOR CONNOR
Anomia
Washington University School of Medicine and
Boston University School of Medicine

STANLEY COREN
Left-Handedness
University of British Columbia

H. BRANCH COSLETT
Dyslexia
University of Pennsylvania School of Medicine

ERIC COURCHESNE
Autism
University of California, San Diego and Children's
Hospital Research Center

DANIEL E. COUTURE
Cerebral Circulation
University of Virginia, Charlottesville

A. D. CRAIG
Pain
Barrow Neurological Institute, Phoenix

MICHELLE CRANK
Broca's Area
University of Texas Health Science Center,
San Antonio

IAN CREESE
Dopamine
Rutgers University

JULIE K. CREMEANS-SMITH
Behavioral Neuroimmunology
   Kent State University

BRUCE CROSSON
Basal Ganglia
   University of Florida Health Science Center and
   VA Medical Center, Gainesville

WIM E. CRUSIO
Behavioral Neurogenetics
   Brudnick Neuropsychiatric Research Institute

HAYAN DAYOUB
Cerebral Circulation
   University of Virginia, Charlottesville

ECO DE GEUS
Behavioral Neurogenetics
   Vrije Universiteit, The Netherlands

EDWARD H. F. DE HAAN
Prosopagnosia
   Utrecht University

DOUGLAS L. DELAHANTY
Behavioral Neuroimmunology
   Kent State University

SERGIO DELLA SALA
Working Memory
   University of Aberdeen, Scotland

KAREN K. DE VALOIS
Spatial Vision
   University of California, Berkeley

RUSSELL L. DE VALOIS
Spatial Vision
   University of California, Berkeley

PETER B. DEWS
Behavioral Pharmacology
   New England Regional Primate Research Center

EDGAR A. DEYOE
Occipital Lobe
   Medical College of Wisconsin

SEYMOUR DIAMOND
Headaches
   Diamond Headache Clinic and Finch University of
   Health Sciences, Chicago, Illinois

RICHARD L. DOTY
Olfaction
   University of Pennsylvania

JOHN E. DOWLING
Retina
   Harvard University

CANDICE DROUIN
Norepinephrine
   Collège de France, Paris

AARON S. DUMONT
Cerebral Circulation
   University of Virginia, Charlottesville

VALSAMMA EAPEN
*Tourette Syndrome and Obsessive–Compulsive
   Disorder*
   United Arab Emirates University and Royal Free
   and University College Medical School, London

DILANTHA B. ELLEGALA
Cerebral Circulation
   University of Virginia, Charlottesville

MARK H. ELLISMAN
Neuron
   University of California, San Diego School of
   Medicine

JANE EPSTEIN
Hallucinations
   Weill Medical College of Cornell University

PETER S. ERIKSSON
Nerve Cells and Memory
   Sahlgrenska University Hospital

JAMES R. EVANS
Neurofeedback
   University of South Carolina

ROBERT G. FELDMAN
Neurobehavioral Toxicology
   Boston University Schools of Medicine and Public
   Health and Harvard Medical School

DANIEL J. FELLEMAN
Area V2
   University of Texas, Houston Medical School

DAVID L. FELTEN
Psychoneuroimmunology
   Loma Linda University School of Medicine

BRENT A. FIELD
Arousal
   University of Oregon

CHRISTOPHER M. FILLEY
Cerebral White Matter Disorders
Neuroanatomy
    University of Colorado School of Medicine and
    Denver VA Medical Center

LEIF H. FINKEL
Salience
    University of Pennsylvania

DAVID FISHBAIN
Pain and Psychopathology
    University of Miami School of Medicine

J. RANDALL FLANAGAN
Hand Movements
    Queen's University, Canada

MARTHA FLANDERS
Movement Regulation
    University of Minnesota

HERTA FLOR
Phantom Limb Pain
    University of Heidelberg

NANCY G. FORGER
Sexual Differentiation, Hormones and
    University of Massachusetts

JOHN FOSSELLA
Anterior Cingulate Cortex
    Rockefeller University and Weill Medical College of
    Cornell University

PETER T. FOX
Broca's Area
    University of Texas Health Science Center,
    San Antonio

RICHARD S. J. FRACKOWIAK
Imaging: Brain Mapping Methods
    University College, London

MARION E. FRANK
Taste
    University of Connecticut Health Center

JASON R. FREEMAN
Mild Head Injury
    University of Virginia School of Medicine

JENNIFER J. FREYD
Recovered Memories
    University of Oregon

ARNOLD J. FRIEDHOFF
Catecholamines
    New York University Medical Center (deceased)

HARRIET R. FRIEDMAN
Eye Movements
    Yale University School of Medicine

RHONDA B. FRIEDMAN
Alexia
    Georgetown University Medical Center

CHARLES A. FULLER
Circadian Rhythms
    University of California, Davis

PATRICK M. FULLER
Circadian Rhythms
    University of California, Davis

MICHAEL GABRIEL
Cingulate Cortex
    University of Illinois

GIORGIO GANIS
Neuroimaging
    Harvard University

MICHAEL S. GAZZANIGA
Consciousness
    Dartmouth College

JOHN S. GEORGE
Event-Related Electromagnetic Responses
    Los Alamos National Laboratory

MARK S. GEORGE
Sexual Function
    Medical University of South Carolina and
    Ralph H. Johnson Veterans Hospital

RICHARD GEVIRTZ
Biofeedback
    CSSP Alliant International University, California

JAY N. GIEDD
Adolescent Brain Maturation
    National Institute of Mental Health

JOEL C. GLOVER
Hindbrain
University of Oslo

GEORG GOLDENBERG
Body Perception Disorders
Krankenhaus München Bogenhausen, Germany

LESLIE J. GONZALEZ-ROTHI
Apraxia
University of Florida College of Medicine

ROGER A. GORSKI
Sex Differences in the Human Brain
University of California, Los Angeles

PETER GOURAS
Color Processing and Color Processing Disorders
Columbia University College of Physicans and
Surgeons

LAURA GRANDE
Basal Ganglia
University of Florida Health Science Center

IGOR GRANT
HIV Infection, Neurocognitive Complications of
University of California, San Diego and
VA San Diego Healthcare System

MANETH GRAVELL
Glial Cell Types
National Institute of Neurological Disorders and
Stroke

JENNIFER M. GROH
Visual and Auditory Integration
Dartmouth College

MURRAY GROSSMAN
Semantic Memory
University of Pennsylvania

DEBORAH L. HARRINGTON
Time Passage, Neural Substrates
Albuquerque VA Medical Center and University of
New Mexico

LAWRENCE C. HARTLAGE
Neuropsychological Assessment, Pediatric
Augusta Neuropsychology Center, Georgia

STEPHEN A. K. HARVEY
Information Processing
University of Texas, San Antonio

ELIOT HAZELTINE
Motor Skill
NASA—Ames Research Center

ANDREA S. HEBERLEIN
Emotion
University of Iowa College of Medicine

KENNETH M. HEILMAN
Apraxia
Unilateral Neglect
University of Florida College of Medicine

JOSEPH B. HELLIGE
Laterality
University of Southern California

AVISHAI HENIK
Inhibition
Ben Gurion University of the Negev, Israel

RALPH HERTWIG
Heuristics
Max Planck Institute for Human Development,
Berlin

STEPHEN R. HOOPER
Mental Retardation
University of North Carolina at Chapel Hill

MADY HORNIG
Borna Disease Virus
University of California, Irvine

BARRY HORWITZ
Aging Brain
National Institute of Aging

JEAN HOU
Glial Cell Types
National Institute of Neurological Disorders and
Stroke

MATTHEW A. HOWARD
Hearing
University of Iowa

KHALEDA ISLAM
Brain Development
University of Dhaka, Bangladesh

RICHARD IVRY
Motor Skill
University of California, Berkeley

GERALD H. JACOBS
Color Vision
University of California, Santa Barbara

LILY Y. JAN
Ion Channels
University of California, San Francisco

NAZILA JANABI
Glial Cell Types
National Institute of Neurological Disorders and Stroke

SEBASTIAN JANDER
Microglia
Heinrich Heine University, Germany

JOHN A. JANE, JR.
Cerebral Circulation
University of Virginia, Charlottesville

HARRY J. JERISON
Evolution of the Brain
University of California, Los Angeles

DILIP V. JESTE
Schizophrenia
University of California, San Diego and VA San Diego Healthcare System

ROLAND S. JOHANSSON
Hand Movements
Umeå University, Sweden

DOUGLAS C. JOHNSON
Respiration
Harvard Medical School and Massachusetts General Hospital

PHILIP N. JOHNSON-LAIRD
Logic and Reasoning
Princeton University

R. D. JONES
Visual Disorders
University of Iowa College of Medicine

JOHN JONIDES
Memory, Neuroimaging
University of Michigan

JON H. KAAS
Motor Cortex
Neocortex
Vanderbilt University

RICHARD F. KAPLAN
Lyme Encephalopathy
University of Connecticut School of Medicine

NEAL F. KASSELL
Cerebral Circulation
University of Virginia, Charlottesville

ALFRED W. KASZNIAK
Dementia
University of Arizona

JAMES C. KAUFMAN
Intelligence
Yale University

HOMAYOUN KAZEMI
Respiration
Harvard Medical School and Massachusetts General Hospital

MATTHIAS KEIDEL
Brain Lesions
District Hospital of Bayreuth

LADA A. KEMENOFF
Frontal Lobe
University of California, San Francisco

ANDREW KERTESZ
Pick's Disease and Frontotemporal Dementia
St. Joseph's Hospital, University of Western Ontario

RAYMOND P. KESNER
Memory Neurobiology
University of Utah

JOHN F. KIHLSTROM
Cognitive Psychology, Overview
Unconscious, The
University of California, Berkeley

SOFIE R. KLEPPNER
GABA
University of California, Los Angeles Brain Research Institute

KEITH R. KLUENDER
Speech
University of Wisconsin

CLIFFORD M. KNAPP
Opiates
  Boston University School of Medicine and Boston
  VA Health Care System

BARBARA J. KNOWLTON
Categorization
  University of California, Los Angeles

PHYLLIS L. KOENIG
Semantic Memory
  University of Pennsylvania

STEPHANIE A. KOLAKOWSKY-HAYNER
Cognitive Rehabilitation
  Virginia Commonwealth University

DOUGLAS KONDZIOLKA
Neural Transplantation
  University of Pittsburgh

STEPHEN M. KOSSLYN
Neuroimaging
  Harvard University

YURI KOUTCHEROV
Chemical Neuroanatomy
  University of New South Wales

WILMA KOUTSTAAL
Priming
  University of Reading

JOEL H. KRAMER
Frontal Lobe
  University of California, San Francisco

ANDREI V. KRASSIOUKOV
Peripheral Nervous System
  University of Toronto

HANS A. KRETZSCHMAR
Prion Diseases
  Ludwig-Maximilians-Universität, München

JEFFREY S. KREUTZER
Cognitive Rehabilitation
  Virginia Commonwealth University

CLETE A. KUSHIDA
Sleep Disorders
  Stanford University School of Medicine

BARBARA LANDAU
Spatial Cognition
  Johns Hopkins University

HELMUT L. LAURER
Modeling Brain Injury/Trauma
  University of Pennsylvania

PAUL LAURIENTI
Multisensory Integration
  Wake Forest University School of Medicine

DAVID S. LIEBESKIND
Cerebral Edema
  University of California, Los Angeles

W. IAN LIPKIN
Borna Disease Virus
  University of California, Irvine

PIERRE-MARIE LLEDO
Homeostatic Mechanisms
  Pasteur Institute

LORRI J. LOBECK
Multiple Sclerosis
  Medical College of Wisconsin

ROBERT H. LOGIE
Working Memory
  University of Aberdeen, Scotland

CHRISTOPHER R. LONG
Anger
  University of Massachusetts, Amherst

FERNANDO H. LOPES DA SILVA
Electrical Potentials
  University of Amsterdam and Dutch Epilepsy
  Clinic Foundation

JEFFREY P. LORBERBAUM
Sexual Function
  Medical University of South Carolina and
  Ralph H. Johnson Veterans Hospital

JOHN A. LUCAS
Memory, Overview
  Mayo Clinic

STEVEN J. LUCK
Attention
  University of Iowa

SONIA LUPIEN
Stress: Hormonal and Neural Aspects
McGill University

DAVID LYKKEN
Psychophysiology
University of Minnesota

MALCOLM MACMILLAN
Phineas Gage
Deakin University, Australia

MARY E. MAIDA
Psychoneuroimmunology
University of Rochester Medical Center

KENNETH MAIESE
Brain Disease, Organic
Wayne State University School of Medicine

EUGENE O. MAJOR
Glial Cell Types
National Institute of Neurological Disorders
and Stroke

J. JOHN MANN
Suicide
New York State Psychiatric Institute and Columbia
University College of Physicians and Surgeons

VIRGINIA A. MANN
Reading Disorders, Developmental
University of California, Irvine

SUSAN S. MARGULIES
Modeling Brain Injury/Trauma
University of Pennsylvania

LEEZA MARON
Basal Ganglia
University of Florida Health Science Center

JONATHAN J. MAROTTA
Agnosia
Carnegie Mellon University

RICHARD T. MARROCCO
Arousal
University of Oregon

LEE J. MARTIN
Neurodegenerative Disorders
Peptides, Hormones, and the Brain and Spinal Cord
Johns Hopkins University School of Medicine

RANDI C. MARTIN
Language and Lexical Processing
Rice University

ADRIA E. MARTINEZ
Information Processing
University of Texas, San Antonio

JOE L. MARTINEZ, JR.
Information Processing
University of Texas, San Antonio

MARYANN E. MARTONE
Neuron
University of California, San Diego School
of Medicine

RICHARD E. MAYER
Problem Solving
University of California, Santa Barbara

ANDREW R. MAYES
Memory Disorders, Organic
Liverpool University

JOHN C. MAZZIOTTA
Imaging: Brain Mapping Methods
University of California, Los Angeles School
of Medicine

KATHLEEN B. MCDERMOTT
Memory, Explicit and Implicit
Washington University, St. Louis

BRUCE MCEWEN
Stress: Hormonal and Neural Aspects
Rockefeller University

TRACY K. MCINTOSH
Modeling Brain Injury/Trauma
University of Pennsylvania

DAVID F. MEANEY
Modeling Brain Injury/Trauma
University of Pennsylvania

LORNE M. MENDELL
Nociceptors
State University of New York, Stony Brook

CONRAD A. MESSAM
Glial Cell Types
National Institute of Neurological Disorders
and Stroke

M.-MARSEL MESULAM
Brain Anatomy and Networks
Northwestern University Medical School

CHRISTINA A. MEYERS
Cancer Patients, Cognitive Function
University of Texas M. D. Anderson Cancer Center

BRUCE L. MILLER
Frontal Lobe
University of California, San Francisco

MARCO MOLINARI
Cerebellum
Rehabilitation Hospital and Research Institute, Santa Lucia Foundation, Rome

ELIZABETH A. MOLLOY
Adolescent Brain Maturation
National Institute of Mental Health

MARIA CHIARA MONACO
Glial Cell Types
National Institute of Neurological Disorders and Stroke

ANNA B. MOORE
Basal Ganglia
University of Florida Health Science Center and VA Medical Center, Gainesville

FELIX MOR
Autoimmune Diseases
Weizmann Institute of Science, Rehovot, Israel

ROBERT J. MORECRAFT
Prefrontal Cortex
University of South Dakota School of Medicine

ROBIN G. MORRIS
Alzheimer's Disease, Neuropsychology of
Institute of Psychiatry, London, UK

DAVID G. MUNOZ
Pick's Disease and Frontotemporal Dementia
Hospital Universitario "Doce de Octubre," Madrid

ROBERT J. NAYLOR
Nausea and Vomiting
University of Bradford

AARON P. NELSON
Neuropsychological Assessment
Harvard Medical School

CHARLES B. NEMEROFF
Stress
Emory University School of Medicine

HELEN NEVILLE
Neuroplasticity, Developmental
University of Oregon

D. JEFFREY NEWPORT
Stress
Emory University School of Medicine

MARY R. NEWSOME
Language and Lexical Processing
Rice University

PAUL L. NUNEZ
Electroencephalography (EEG)
Tulane University

LORAINE K. OBLER
Anomia
City University of New York and Boston University School of Medicine

WILLIAM O'DONOHUE
Sexual Dysfunction
University of Nevada, Reno

CHIMA OHAEGBULAM
Hydrocephalus
Children's Hospital/Brigham & Women's Hospital, Boston

CHIHIRO OHYE
Thalamus and Thalamic Damage
Hidaka Hospital

DOUGLAS L. OLIVER
Midbrain
University of Connecticut Health Center

JOHN W. OLNEY
Alcohol Damage to the Brain
Washington University, St. Louis, School of Medicine

RAJA PARASURAMAN
Mental Workload
Catholic University of America

LILLIAN PARK
Cognitive Psychology, Overview
University of California, Berkeley

DEREK PARTRIDGE
Artificial Intelligence
University of Exeter, United Kingdom

GAVRIL W. PASTERNAK
Endorphins and Their Receptors
Memorial Sloan–Kettering Cancer Center

GEORGE PAXINOS
Chemical Neuroanatomy
University of New South Wales

DAVID W. PERRY
Music and the Brain
University of California, San Francisco

DANIELLE PHAM-DINH
Astrocytes
INSERM Unit 546 and University Pierre and
Marie Curie, Paris, France

KAREN PIERCE
Autism
University of California, San Diego

MARTHA POPE
Mental Retardation
Goldsboro Middle School and Wayne County
Schools

DAVID E. PRESTI
Psychoactive Drugs
University of California, Berkeley

DONALD L. PRICE
Motor Neuron Disease
Johns Hopkins University School of Medicine

JOSEPH L. PRICE
Limbic System
Washington University School of Medicine,
St. Louis

LUIS PUELLES
Forebrain
University of Murcia, Spain

BRUCE R. RANSOM
Neuroglia, Overview
University of Washington School of Medicine

RAJESH P. N. RAO
Receptive Field
University of Washington

STEPHEN M. RAO
Time Passage, Neural Substrates
Medical College of Wisconsin

STEVEN Z. RAPCSAK
Agraphia
University of Arizona and VA Medical Center,
Tucson

MARCIA HILLARY RATNER
Neurobehavioral Toxicology
Boston University School of Medicine

JOSEF P. RAUSCHECKER
Sensory Deprivation
Georgetown University Medical Center

NAFTALI RAZ
Cognitive Aging
Wayne State University

SANDRA CLUETT REDDEN
Mental Retardation
University of North Carolina at Chapel Hill and
Glenwood Children's Resource Center

CATHERINE L. REED
Tactile Perception
University of Denver

LISA REGEV
Sexual Dysfunction
University of Nevada, Reno

LINDA RINAMAN
Hypothalamus
University of Pittsburgh

MARY M. ROBERTSON
*Tourette Syndrome and Obsessive–Compulsive
Disorder*
University College, London

ROBERT G. ROBINSON
Mood Disorders
University of Iowa College of Medicine

KATHLEEN S. ROCKLAND
Axon
Brain Science Institute, RIKEN, Saitama, Japan

MARIA A. RON
Conversion Disorders and Somatoform Disorders
Institute of Neurology and National Hospital for
Neurology and Neurosurgery, United Kingdom

MARCELLO G. P. ROSA
Visual Cortex
Monash University

ANGELA ROSENBERG
Cerebral Palsy
University of North Carolina, Chapel Hill

JEFFERY ROTHSTEIN
Motor Neuron Disease
Johns Hopkins University School of Medicine

JOHN RUBENSTEIN
Forebrain
University of California, San Francisco

NAVA RUBIN
Vision: Brain Mechanisms
New York University

MARK A. RUNCO
Creativity
California State University, Fullerton and
University of Hawaii, Hilo

ELEANOR M. SAFFRAN
Wernicke's Area
Temple University School of Medicine

PAUL SAJDA
Neural Networks
Columbia University

MARGARITA SANCHEZ DEL RIO
Migraine
Thomas Jefferson University Hospital

MARTHA TAYLOR SARNO
Aphasia
New York University School of Medicine

MARTIN SARTER
Vigilance
Ohio State University

JEFFREY L. SAVER
Aggression
University of California, Los Angeles

ROBERT L. SAVOY
Functional Magnetic Resonance Imaging (fMRI)
MGH/MIT/HST Athinoula A. Martinos Center

PAIGE SCALF
Cingulate Cortex
University of Illinois

BETTINA SCHMITZ
Epilepsy
Humboldt University, Berlin

JONATHAN SCHOOLER
Recovered Memories
University of Pittsburgh

MICHAEL SCHROETER
Microglia
Heinrich Heine University, Germany

JAMES H. SCHWARTZ
Neurotransmitters
Columbia University

DAVID E. SCOTT
Ventricular System
Eastern Virginia Medical School

MEGHAN M. SEARL
Neuropsychological Assessment
Boston University

REZA SHADMEHR
Motor Control
Johns Hopkins University

ROBERT SHAPLEY
Vision: Brain Mechanisms
New York University

STEPHEN SILBERSTEIN
Migraine
Thomas Jefferson University Hospital

DAVID SILBERSWEIG
Hallucinations
Weill Medical College of Cornell University

RAUL SILVA
Catecholamines
New York University Medical Center

JONATHAN M. SILVER
Violence and the Brain
Lenox Hill Hospital

HEIDI SIVERS
Recovered Memories
Stanford University

JOHN R. SLADEK, JR.
Transplantation
University of Colorado Health Sciences Center

FRANS SLUYTER
Behavioral Neurogenetics
Institute of Psychiatry, UK

JOHN F. SOECHTING
Movement Regulation
University of Minnesota

TERRENCE R. STANFORD
Multisensory Integration
Superior Colliculus
Wake Forest University School of Medicine

BARRY E. STEIN
Multisensory Integration
Superior Colliculus
Wake Forest University School of Medicine

IWONA STEPNIEWSKA
Motor Cortex
Vanderbilt University

EMILY STERN
Hallucinations
Weill Medical College of Cornell University

ROBERT J. STERNBERG
Intelligence
Yale University

GUIDO STOLL
Microglia
Heinrich Heine University and Julius Maximilians University, Germany

PHILIPP STUDE
Brain Lesions
University of Essen

HELEN TAGER-FLUSBERG
Language Acquisition
Boston University School of Medicine

ANDREW TALK
Cingulate Cortex
University of Illinois

JEAN-POL TASSIN
Norepinephrine
Collège de France, Paris

EDWARD H. TAYLOR
Manic–Depressive Illness
University of Minnesota

LISA A. TAYLOR
Dopamine
Rutgers University

ALLAN J. TOBIN
GABA
University of California, Los Angeles Brain Research Institute

PETER M. TODD
Heuristics
Max Planck Institute for Human Development, Berlin

JANE C. TOPOLOVEC
Cerebral Cortex
University of Western Ontario

D. TRANEL
Visual Disorders
University of Iowa College of Medicine

ELIZABETH TYLER-KABARA
Neural Transplantation
University of Pittsburgh

GEORGE J. URBAN
Headaches
Diamond Headache Clinic and Finch University of Health Sciences, Chicago, Illinois

WILLIAM R. UTTAL
Pattern Recognition
Arizona State University

JYOTSNA VAID
Bilingualism
Humor and Laughter
Texas A&M University

GIUSEPPE VALLAR
Short-Term Memory
Università degli Studi di Milano-Bicocca and IRCCS Fondazione S. Lucia, Roma

GILLES VAN LUIJTELAAR
Behavioral Neurogenetics
University of Nijmegen, The Netherlands

FREDERIQUE VAROQUEAUX
Synaptogenesis
Max Planck Institute for Experimental Medicine, Göttingen, Germany

SHAUN P. VECERA
Attention
University of Iowa

PREETI VERGHESE
Motion Processing
Smith Kettlewell Eye Research Institute

ABOUT THE EDITOR-IN-CHIEF

V. S. RAMACHANDRAN is Director of the Center for Brain and Cognition and professor of neuroscience and psychology at the University of California, San Diego. He is additionally an adjunct professor of biology at the Salk Institute. He obtained an M.D. from Stanley Medical College and a Ph.D. from Trinity College at the University of Cambridge, where he was elected a senior Rouse Ball Scholar.

He has received many honors and awards, including a fellowship from All Souls College, Oxford, an honorary doctorate from Connecticut College, a Gold Medal from the Australian National University, and the Ariens Kappers Medal from the Royal Nederlands Academy of Sciences for landmark contributions in neuroscience.

Dr. Ramachandran's early research was on visual perception, but he is best known for his work in neurology. In 1995 he gave the Decade of the Brain Lecture at the 25th annual (Silver Jubilee) meeting of the Society for Neuroscience. More recently he gave the inaugural keynote lecture at the Decade of the Brain Conference held by the National Institute of Mental Health at the Library of Congress. He also gave the first Hans Lucas Teuber lecture at MIT, the Rudel-Moses lecture at Columbia, the Dorcas Cumming (inaugural keynote) lecture at Cold Spring Harbor, the Raymond Adams lecture at Massachusetts General Hospital, Harvard, and the presidential keynote lecture at the annual meeting of the American Academy of Neurology.

Dr. Ramachandran has published over 120 papers in scientific journals, including three invited review articles in *Scientific American*, and is editor-in-chief of Academic Press' acclaimed *Encyclopedia of Human Behavior*. His work is featured frequently in the major news media, and *Newsweek* magazine recently named him a member of "the century club": one of the hundred most prominent people to watch in this century.

ABOUT THE ADVISORY BOARD

Antonio R. Damasio, the Van Allen Professor and Head of Neurology at the University of Iowa, and Adjunct Professor at the Salk Institute, has had a major influence on our understanding of the neural basis of decision-making, emotion, language and memory, and consciousness. He elucidates critical problems in the fundamental neuroscience of mind and behavior at the level of large-scale systems in humans, although his investigations have also encompassed parkinsonism and Alzheimer's disease. The laboratories that he and Hanna Damasio (a distinguished neurologist who is independently recognized for her achievements in neuroimaging and neuroanatomy) created at the University of Iowa are a leading center for the investigation of cognition using both the lesion method and functional imaging.

Dr. Damasio is a member of the Institute of Medicine of the National Academy of Sciences, a Fellow of the American Academy of Arts and Sciences, a member of the Neurosciences Research Program, a Fellow of the American Academy of Neurology, a member of the European Academy of Sciences and

Arts and of the Royal Academy of Medicine in Belgium, a member of the American Neurological Association and of the Association of American Physicians, and a board member of leading neuroscience journals. He has received numerous scientific prizes and delivered some of the most prestigious lectures in the United States and in Europe. His book *Descartes' Error: Emotion, Reason and the Human Brain* (Putnam, 1994) is taught in universities worldwide. His new book *The Feeling of What Happens: Body, Emotion, and the Making of Consciousness*, published by Harcourt, has received several awards and has been translated into 18 languages.

Martha J. Farah is the Bob and Arlene Kogod Professor of Psychology and the Director of the Center for Cognitive Neuroscience at the University of Pennsylvania. She is known for her work on the neural bases of human perception and cognition, described in over a hundred research publications as well as in five books. Her current interests are in emotion–cognition interaction and development. Dr. Farah's work has been honored with a number of awards, including the American Psychological Association Distinguished Scientific Award for an Early Career Contribution, the National Academy of Sciences Troland Research Award, and a Guggenheim Fellowship.

Michael F. Huerta received both his B.A. in zoology and his Ph.D. in anatomy from the University of Wisconsin in Madison. He was a postdoctoral fellow at Vanderbilt University, served on the faculty of the University of Connecticut Health Center, and was a guest researcher in the intramural program of the National Institute of Mental Health at the National Institutes of Health. Most of Dr. Huerta's research publications concern sensorimotor integration at the systems level of analysis. He is currently Associate Director of the Division of Neuroscience and Basic Behavioral Research and Director of the Office of Translational Research and Scientific Technology at the National Institute of Mental Health.

Dr. Huerta's research efforts are focused on integrating the many disciplines, perspectives, and approaches that comprise neuroscience. He also has significant interest in advancing the research and development of technologies useful to brain researchers, particularly informatics tools. Dr. Huerta has received numerous awards for his leadership in areas including neuroscience, imaging, informatics, and bioengineering. He continues to review manuscripts for journals, edits scientific books, and serves as an editor on the new journal *Neuroinformatics*.

Sue Iversen is professor of experimental psychology and Pro-Vice-Chancellor for Planning and Resource Allocation at the University of Oxford. She studied for her undergraduate degree and Ph.D. at Cambridge, then spent her postdoctoral years in the United States at the National Institutes of Health and at Harvard Medical School. She was formerly Research Director at the U.S. pharmaceutical company Merck & Co., where she was involved in establishing the largest commercial Neuroscience Research Centre in the United Kingdom, based at Harlow in Essex, and has previously held research posts at Cambridge University.

Dr. Iversen's research and publications focus on disorders of brain function, particularly schizophrenia and Alzheimer's disease with particular reference to the biological bases of these disorders, their clinical presentation, and treatment. She has published 307 papers, edited 24 volumes, and is co-author with L. L. Iversen of *Behavioural Pharmacology*. Until recently she was Editor-in-Chief of *Neuropsychologia* and has held senior office in a number of professional psychological and neuroscience societies.

Edward G. Jones received his Medical Degree from the University of Otago, New Zealand, and his Ph.D. from Oxford University. He is an authority on brain anatomy and is recognized as a leading researcher of the central nervous system. He was a leading figure in introducing molecular biology methodology to systems neuroscience, and has done groundbreaking work on schizophrenia, focusing on how changes at the molecular and cellular level are associated with the disorder. Dr. Jones also belongs to a group of scientists who are working on the U.S. Human Brain Project, which supports the development of databases on the brain and development of technologies to manage and share neuroscience information. He was a founding member of the Frontier Research Program in Brain Mechanisms of Mind and Behavior at Riken, Japan.

Dr. Jones' many awards include the Cajal medal for excellence in research and Krieg Cortical Discoverer (1989), the Henry Gray Award, American Association of Anatomists (2001), and the Karl Spencer Lashley Award, American Philosophical Society (2001). He has served as the President of the Society for Neuroscience, is a Fellow of the American Association for the Advancement of Science, and is an original member of the Thomson Scientific ISI Highly-Cited

Researchers. He is currently the Director of the Center for Neuroscience at the University of California, Davis.

Jon H. Kaas is a Distinguished, Centennial Professor of Psychology at Vanderbilt University, where he is also professor of cell biology. He is an elected member of the National Academy of Sciences, the American Academy of Arts and Sciences, and the Society of Experimental Psychologists. He has received the Sutherland Prize for Achievement in Research, the Javits Neuroscience Investigator Award, the Krieg Cortical Discoverer Award, and the American Psychological Association Distinguished Scientific Contribution Award.

One of Dr. Kaas' major research interests is how sensory-perceptual and motor systems are organized in mammalian brains, especially those of primates. This interest has led to comparative studies of primate brains and efforts to infer the course of human brain evolution. Related research efforts have revealed aspects of brain specializations in mammals with unusual adaptations such as moles and bats. Another research focus has been the plasticity of developing and mature sensory and motor systems with efforts to determine mechanisms of brain reorganization and recovery after sensory loss.

Raja Parasuraman is Director of the Cognitive Science Laboratory, and professor of psychology at The Catholic University of America in Washington, D.C. He received a B.Sc. (1st Class Honors) in electrical engineering from Imperial College, University of London, UK (1972) and an M.Sc. in applied psychology (1973) and a Ph.D. in psychology (1976) from the University of Aston, Birmingham, UK. Dr. Parasuraman has carried out research on attention, automation, aging and Alzheimer's disease, event-related brain potentials, functional brain imaging, signal detection, vigilance, and workload. His books include *The Psychology of Vigilance* (Academic Press, 1982), *Varieties of Attention* (Academic Press, 1984), *Event-Related Brain Potentials* (Oxford University Press, 1990), *Automation and Human Performance* (Erlbaum, 1996), and *The Attentive Brain* (MIT Press, 1998).

Dr. Parasuraman served as a member of the Human Development and Aging Study Section of the National Institutes of Health from 1992 to 1995, and was a member of the National Research Council's Panel on Human Factors in Air-Traffic Control Automation from 1994 to 1998. He is currently Chair of the National Research Council Panel on Human Factors. He is also on the editorial board of several journals, including *Neuropsychology* and *Human Factors.* Dr. Parasuraman was elected a Fellow of the American Association for the Advancement of Science (1994), the American Psychological Association (1991), the American Psychological Society (1991), and the Human Factors and Ergonomics Society (1994).

Michael I. Posner is Professor Emeritus at the University of Oregon and is currently Director of the Sackler Institute for Development Psychobiology at the Weill Medical College of Cornell University in New York. Since the mid-1960s, Dr. Posner has been involved in the effort to measure human thought and to understand its physical basis. His 1978 book *Chronometric Explorations of Mind* was selected as one of the most influential books in cognitive science. Dr. Posner joined with Marcus Raichle at Washington University in neuroimaging studies that served to localize brain networks of cognitive processes in normal subjects. Their book in this field, *Images of Mind*, received the 1996 Williams James award for the most outstanding volume in the field of psychology. They jointly received awards from the Dana Foundation and the American Philosophical Society, and received the Pasarow and Grawenmeyer awards for research contributions to understanding mental processes. Currently Dr. Posner is working with many colleagues at the Sackler Institute and the University of Oregon to examine the anatomy and circuitry of attention and self regulation in infants and children.

Henry C. Powell is a graduate of University College Dublin and the National University of Ireland (M.B., B.Ch., B.A.O., 1970). He was awarded the degrees of M.D. (1985) and D.Sc. (1994) based on published work in pathology. Dr. Powell is also a Fellow of the Royal College of Pathologists (UK). He interned in pathology and medicine at Philadelphia General Hospital (1970–1971) and completed residency training in Anatomic and Clinical Pathology at the University of California, San Diego from 1971 to 1975. He held a fellowship in neuropathology at Massachusetts General Hospital (1975–1976), prior to being appointed assistant professor of pathology at the University of California, San Diego. Currently he is professor and interim chairman of the department of pathology and head of the division of neuropathology and electron microscopy.

Dr. Powell's research interests are focused on metabolic, inflammatory, and degenerative diseases of the nervous system, with emphasis on the pathogenesis of peripheral neuropathies in diabetes. He and his collaborators study experimentally induced neuropathy in diabetic rats as well as the nervous system effects of spontaneously occurring diabetes in feline and human disease.

John Smythies is a graduate of the University of British Columbia, where he was awarded an M.Sc. in neuroanatomy, philosophy, and anthropology, and of Cambridge University, where he was awarded the degrees of M.Sc. in psychology and M.D. He is currently Director of the Division of Neurochemistry at the Center for Brain and Cognition as well as a research scientist in the department of psychology at the University of California, San Diego. He is also a senior research fellow at the Institute of Neurology at National Hospital in London and a visiting professor in the department of psychiatry at Harvard University.

Dr. Smythies is a member of numerous scientific societies and editorial boards in neuroscience and neuropsychiatry. He has authored 244 publications in neuroscience and medicine and has written 12 books. His main research interests are the neurochemistry of schizophrenia, redox mechanisms in the brain, the biochemical basis of synaptic plasticity, and the mind-brain problem.

Elizabeth Warrington has been associated with London University since 1951. She was awarded a B.Sc. in 1954, a Ph.D. in 1960 and a D.Sc. in 1975. She joined the staff of the Institute of Neurology in 1954 in a research capacity. In 1972 Dr. Warrington was appointed head of the department of clinical neuropsychology, a post she held until she retired in 1996. In addition to her clinical duties she has pursued an active research career with special interests in perception, memory, and language disorders.

Dr. Warrington was elected to the Fellowship of the Royal Society in 1986, and she has been awarded honorary degrees from the Universities of Bologna, Italy, and York, UK. At present she is an honorary consultant neuropsychologist to the Dementia Research Group where she is engaged in active research.

Jeremy M. Wolfe became interested in vision research during the course of a summer job at Bell Labs in New Jersey after his senior year in high school. He graduated summa cum laude from Princeton in 1977 with a degree in psychology and went on to obtain his Ph.D. in 1981 from MIT, studying with Richard Held. His Ph.D. thesis was entitled "On Binocular Single Vision." Dr. Wolfe remained at MIT as a lecturer, assistant professor, and associate professor until 1991. During that period, he published papers on binocular rivalry, visual aftereffects, and accommodation. In the late 1980s, the focus of the lab shifted to visual attention—a transition marked most clearly by the publication of the first version of Dr. Wolfe's "Guided Search" model of visual search in 1989. Since that time, he has published numerous articles on visual search and visual attention.

In 1991, Dr. Wolfe moved to Brigham and Women's Hospital and Harvard Medical School, where he remains to the present day. He continues to teach in the MIT Concourse Program. Dr. Wolfe has served in editorial capacities for a number of journals, currently as Associate Editor of *Perception and Psychophysics*. He is member of the National Institutes of Health VIS-B Study Section, and is President of the Eastern Psychological Association. Dr. Wolfe won the Baker Memorial Prize for teaching at MIT in 1989. He is a Fellow of the American Psychological Association and a member of the Society for Experimental Psychologists.

PREFACE

The functions of the human brain are the last major challenge to science. Despite having made rapid strides in understanding the cosmos, subatomic particles, molecular biology, and genetics, we still know very little about the organ that made these discoveries possible. How does the activity of 100 billion nerve cells—mere wisps of protoplasm that constitute the brain—give rise to the broad spectrum of abilities that we call consciousness, mind, and human nature?

There is now, more than ever before, a real need for a standard reference source covering all aspects of the human brain and nervous system, and the *Encyclopedia of the Human Brain* is the most up-to-date and comprehensive coverage to date. It is a compendium of articles contributed by many of the world's leading experts in neuroscience and psychology. These essays will be of interest to a wide range of individuals in the behavioral and health sciences.

Written in an engaging, accessible style, the encyclopedia not only is an important major reference work but also can be browsed informally by anyone who seeks answers about the activities and effects of the brain, such as why and how we dream, what parts of the brain are involved in memory, how we recognize human faces and other objects, what are the brain mechanisms involved in cognition and language, what causes phantom limb pain, what are the implications of left-handedness, or what current treatments are available for Parkinson's disease. Here in the *Encyclopedia of the Human Brain* will be found brief yet comprehensive summaries on all of these topics and some 200 more.

Many of the articles will appeal equally to a student preparing an essay for class, a novice researcher looking for new fields to conquer, a clinician wanting to become up-to-date on recent research in his or her field, or even an interested lay reader.

Each of the articles has been through a long process of author nomination, peer review, revision, and copyediting. Most of the entries were written by acknowledged experts in the field. Given the nature and scope of this enterprise, a degree of overlap among the articles was not only inevitable but also desirable, since our goal was to ensure that each article was a self-contained summary of one specific aspect of the human brain. Given space limitations, each author was encouraged to provide a broad overview of an area of research rather than an exhaustive review. The result is a stimulating and informative compilation of material.

The eighties were dubbed the "decade of the brain," an apt term given the subsequent progress made in understanding the structure, function, and development of this mysterious organ. This encyclopedia should prove to be an invaluable resource on this fascinating subject and would not have been possible without the dedicated efforts of more than 350 authors, 12 associate editors, 150 peer reviewers, and the following Academic Press personnel: Nikki Levy, Barbara Makinster, Christopher Morris, Carolan Gladden, Joanna Dinsmore, and Jocelyn Lofstrom.

V. S. Ramachandran
Editor-in-Chief
University of California, San Diego

GUIDE TO THE ENCYCLOPEDIA

The *Encyclopedia of the Human Brain* is organized to provide the maximum ease of use for its readers. Each article in the encyclopedia provides an overview of the selected topic to inform a broad spectrum of readers, from researchers to students to the interested general public. In order that you, the reader, will derive the maximum benefit from the *Encyclopedia of the Human Brain*, we have provided this guide. It explains how the book is organized and how the information within its pages can be located.

Subject Areas

The *Encyclopedia of the Human Brain* presents 224 separate articles on the entire range of human brain research. Articles in the encyclopedia are arranged alphabetically. So that they can be more easily identified, article titles begin with the key word or phrase indicating the topic, with any descriptive terms following this.

Article Format

Each article contains an outline, a glossary, an introductory paragraph that defines the topic being discussed and summarizes the content of the article, cross-references, and a list of suggested readings. The outline allows a quick scan of the major areas discussed within each article. The glossary contains terms that may be unfamiliar to the reader, with each term defined in the context of its use in that article. Thus, a term may appear defined in a slightly different manner or subtle nuance specific to that article. For clarity, we have allowed these differences in definition to remain.

The articles have been cross-referenced to other related articles in the encyclopedia. Cross-references will appear at the end of an article. The cross-references are listed in alphabetical order by title. We encourage readers to use the cross-references to locate other encyclopedia articles that will provide additional information about a subject.

The suggested readings at the close of each article list recent secondary sources to aid the reader in locating more detailed or technical information. Review articles and research articles that are considered of primary importance to the understanding of a given subject area are also listed. This section is not intended to provide a full reference listing of all material covered in the context of a given article, but is provided as a guide to further reading.

Subject Index

A comprehensive user-friendly index is provided to make this work amenable to all levels of readers. Within the subject index entry for a given topic, references to general coverage of the topic appear first, such as a complete article on the subject. References to more specific aspects of the topic then appear below this in an indented list. A particular topic that may appear not to have coverage may be subsumed under a broader entry. The index, rather than the table of contents, should be used as the primary road to accessing information.

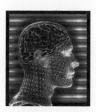

Color Processing and Color Processing Disorders

PETER GOURAS
Columbia University College of Physicians and Surgeons

GLOSSARY

achromatic contrast Gradients of energy in an image resulting in black–white vision.

achromats Subjects who have either only short-wave-sensitive or no cones; they have no color vision.

chromatic contrast Gradients of wavelength in an image responsible for color vision.

color opponency Colors that cancel each other when mixed, such as red and green or blue and yellow.

cone opponency Signals from two spectrally different cones that have opposite effects on the same neuron (i.e., one cone signal excites and the other inhibits the neuron).

deuteranopes Subjects who lack middle-wave-sensitive cones; their color vision is also divariant (about 1% of males).

opsins Proteins in photoreceptors that absorb light and trigger a neural response.

protanopes Subjects who lack longwave sensitive cones; their color vision depends on two variables and is divariant (about 1% of males).

successive color contrast Enhancement of a color appearing just after another color disappears (i.e., red is redder when it appears just after green goes off).

simultaneous color contrast Enhancement of a color when next to another color (i.e., reds are redder when surrounded by green).

tritanopes Subjects who lack short-wave-sensitive cones; they are also divariant but extremely rare.

trivariance The fact that normal human color depends on only three variable—the three different types of cones.

Color vision is a neural process occurring in our brain that depends on a comparison of responses of at least two, but normally three, spectrally different cone photoreceptors. The brain uses these cone systems to detect achromatic and chromatic contrasts. Achromatic contrasts depend on light energy gradients across an image; chromatic contrasts depend on wavelength gradients of light across an image. Achromatic contrast is detected by the two longer but not by the short-wave-sensitive cones; in the fovea, achromatic contrast can resolve the dimensions of neighboring cones (about 1 μm on the retina). Chromatic contrasts are detected using all three types of cones and is done by comparing their responses to the same object. From an evolutionary perspective, the first comparison was between the short- and the longer wavelength-sensitive cones creating blue/yellow color vision. This still occurs in most mammals and in about 2% of human males. In this case, if an object affects the short-wave more than long-wave cones, it appears blue. The converse appears yellow. If the object affects both cone systems equally, it appears white, gray, or black. In the Land color vision model this comparison between cone signals occurs after each cone system's response is normalized over visual space. The second comparison evolved in primates when the longer wave cones were split into long- and middle-wave cones; this created red/green color vision. If an object affects the long-wave more than the middle wave-sensitive cones, it appears red. The converse appears green. If an object affects both of these cones equally, it appears yellow, white, or bluish depending on the former comparison. Color vision compares responses of groups of cones rather than single neighboring cones; it has a lower spatial resolution than achromatic vision. The neural processing responsible for color perception occurs in visual cortex. The retina and the lateral geniculate nucleus provide the signals from each cone mechanism in a form that allows the comparisons necessary for color vision. Our brain combines cues from both chromatic and achromatic contrast to perceive a particular color. There are several different mechanisms involved. One depends on the blue/yellow and red/green comparison signals and is most related to the hue of a color, reflected by the words red, green, etc. The second is related to the amount of white, gray, or black that is mixed with the previous signal. This confers a quality called saturation of a color; it distinguishes pinks from reds. The third depends on the achromatic system to establish the lightness or darkness of a color. Together these separate operations provide us with about 1 million different colors. All these operations, which involve both achromatic and chromatic contrast detection, provide cues to the form of an object. Although we can mentally separate the form of an object from its color, it is not known where in cerebral cortex this separation of form from color occurs.

I. COLOR VISION

Light has several independent properties, including its energy and its wavelength or frequency of vibration. Color vision takes advantage of both of these properties, allowing us to detect objects and navigate in the external world. Wavelength and energy contrasts vary independently in a visual image and therefore require different neural circuits for their analysis. The secret of color vision is to understand how the brain distinguishes wavelength from energy contrasts. The addition of wavelength contrasts to energy contrasts

greatly increases the potential cues to the visual universe. In addition, energy contrasts depend on both the surface properties of an object and its position relative to its illuminant, sunlight for our past evolutionary history. Positional variations can lead to highlights and shading that can obscure the identity or existence of objects. The wavelength reflectance of an object is relatively independent of such effects and therefore a more reliable identifier. For this reason, wavelength contrast and derivative, color vision, have been important to survival. In man it has added an aesthetic dimension that far exceeds the value for survival in modern society.

Figure 1 shows a colorful Renaissance painting, which has been decomposed into its wavelength (chromatic) and achromatic (black-and-white) contrasts. When these two operations are combined in our brain, the picture is seen in color. Energy contrast leads to the perception of achromatic forms of different brightness (white, gray, or black). Wavelength contrast leads to the perception of forms that have a new dimension (color). Energy contrast provides finer detail than wavelength contrast, but the latter adds a new dimension to vision. The combination of both forms of contrast is what we normally experience as color vision.

II. NEURAL BASIS OF COLOR VISION

A. The Photoreceptors

Vision starts in the photoreceptor cells of the retina and their outermost organelle that contains specialized protein molecules, called opsins (from the Greek word "to see"), which absorb and amplify light energy. In the human retina, there are four types of photoreceptors, defined primarily by the opsin they contain. Usually one type of cone contains only one type of opsin. Each type of opsin absorbs a particular waveband of light in the visible spectrum. The wavelength selectivity, defined by an absorption spectrum, is related to the opsin's amino acid sequence interacting with a specific isomer of vitamin A.

One set of photoreceptors, called rods because of the shape of their long outer segments, function only at dim light levels. Their extraordinarily high sensitivity to light drives them into saturation at daylight levels. Rods are very sensitive and numerous in our retina but only work well in moonlight and play little to no role in

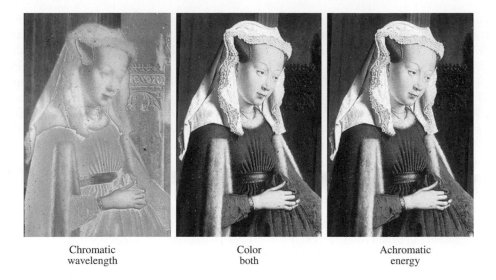

Chromatic
wavelength

Color
both

Achromatic
energy

Figure 1 A segment of a painting by Jan van Eyck (1434) in which the luminance information has been removed (left) rendering an image based on chromatic contrasts alone. (Right) The chromatic contrast has been removed, rendering an achromatic black-and-white image of the same scene; the latter has more fine detail. In the middle and fusion of these two different forms of contrast produces color vision. (See color insert in Volume 1).

color vision. Rod vision is without color and has become vestigial in modern society.

Color vision is mediated by the other three photoreceptors called cones, which require broad daylight to work well. Figure 2 shows the absorption spectra of the three cones of human vision. Cones are much more important to human vision than rods because if they are lost or fail to function, one is legally blind. The absence of rod function, on the other hand, is only a minor inconvenience. Cones' tolerance of high levels of illumination depends in great part on their ability to adapt to light. As light levels increase, cones reduce their sensitivity and speed up their responses, making them almost impossible to saturate. For color vision, the responses of the three types of cones are compared. Figure 2 shows the spectral colors that result from these comparisons. The colors we see in the spectrum are not near the peak absorption of the cone opsins because they depend on sophisticated neural comparisons.

B. Long-Wavelength Cone System

Long-wavelength-sensitive cones dominate the primate retina, comprising 90% of all the cones. The short-wavelength-sensitive or S cones comprise only 10% of the cones and are absent from the central fovea, the area of highest visual resolution. The long-

wave cones are composed of two types of cones, with similar opsins. Both absorb best in the long wave or yellow half of the spectrum. One type, M or "green" cones, absorbs slightly better in the middle or green part of the spectrum, and the other, L or "red" cones, absorbs slightly better in the long or red part of the spectrum (Fig. 2). These L and M cones seem to be

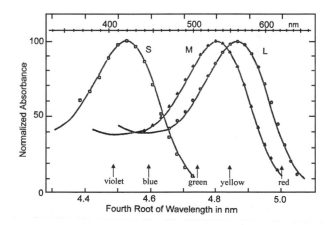

Figure 2 Normalized absorption spectra of the three cone mechanisms of human vision plotted against the fourth root of wavelength, which tends to make these curves independent of their position on the abscissa. An equivalent wavelength abscissa is shown above. Short-wave- (S), middle (M), and long-wavelength (L)-sensitive cones. The colors perceived at different points in the spectrum are shown below.

organized in an identical way, although there may be slightly more L than M cones. The central fovea contains only L and M and no S cones. L and M cones in the fovea are slender, optimizing their ability to sample small areas of visual space.

Each L and M cone synapses with at least two different bipolar cells. One is an on bipolar that is excited (depolarized) whenever its cone or cones absorb light; the other is an off bipolar, which is excited (depolarized) whenever light absorption by its cone or cones decreases (Fig. 3). This is a push–pull system that provides excitatory signals for increments (lightness) in one channel and excitatory signals for decrements (darkness) of light energy in a parallel channel. These signals are used in visual cortex to sense both energy (achromatic) and wavelength (chromatic) contrasts.

In the fovea, each L and M cone on and off bipolar synapses with a single cone (Fig. 3, left). Each single bipolar cell synapses with a single on or off ganglion cell. This is the so-called "midget cell" system discovered by Stephen Polyak. The signals from single L or M cones are transmitted by relay cells in the parvo cellular layers of the lateral geniculate nucleus of the thalamus to striate cortex mediating the high visual resolution of the fovea.

Away from the fovea, the midget arrangement ceases and several L and/or M cones synapse with single on or off bipolar cells. The breakdown of the midget system creates a problem for transmitting information about both energy and wavelength con-

trast in the same neural channel. For energy contrast, it is best to minimize the area within which the cones are selected. Therefore, selecting both L and M cones would be preferable (Fig. 3, right). For wavelength contrast it is best to select only L or only M cones in any one area. This tends to expand the area from which cones were selected and therefore decrease spatial resolution. It is not clear how this situation is handled.

1. The Parvo System: L and M Cone Antagonism

The selectivity for either an L or M cone input (Fig. 3) exposes antagonistic cone interaction in these retinal ganglion cells that depends on the wavelength of stimulation and is mediated by amacrine and horizontal cell interneurons. Ganglion cells transmitting signals of L cones are antagonized by stimuli that affect M cones and vice versa. This antagonism enhances both achromatic and chromatic contrast.

It enhances achromatic spatial contrast by reducing a ganglion cell's response to large but not small stimuli covering the center of the receptive field of the ganglion cell. It enhances chromatic contrast by reducing a ganglion cell's spectral response to green light if it is transmitting signals of L cones or reducing the cell's response to red light if it is transmitting the signals of M cones. It also enhances successive chromatic contrast, which occurs when a stimulus moves over the retina. The removal of green (antagonizing) light as red light enters the receptive field of an on ganglion cell transmitting the signals of L cones will enhance its response to the following red light. The removal of red (antagonizing) light as green light enters the receptive field of an on ganglion cell transmitting the signals of M cones will enhance its response to the green light. Off cells will also exhibit successive color contrast in the opposite way.

Retinal ganglion cells showing this behavior, called "cone or color opponency," are a system of small cells relatively concentrated at the fovea, including the "midget system." These cells transmit their signals to the parvocellular layers of the lateral geniculate nucleus of the thalamus. This system seems to be involved in both achromatic and chromatic contrast and is responsible for the high spatial resolution of the fovea. These cells receive no input from S cones.

2. The Magno System: L and M Cone Synergism

There is a parallel system of on- and off-bipolars and ganglion cells transmitting signals from L and M cones to striate cortex via relay cells in the magnocellular

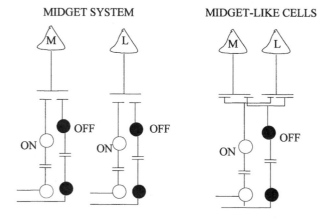

Figure 3 The retinal circuitry of the parvocellular L and M cone system. The midget system on the left is characteristic of the fovea, where each L and M cone has a private on and off bipolar and ganglion cell. Away from the fovea, this private line breaks down. Some cells, midget-like, are thought to preserve the selectivity for only one type of cone, a prerequisite for chromatic contrast.

layers of the lateral geniculate nucleus. These are larger cells, which have faster conduction velocities and respond phasically to maintained stimuli. They mix synergistic signals of L and M cones. They are only involved in achromatic contrast, showing no color opponency (Fig. 4). This phasic magnocellular system is relayed to layer 4C alpha of striate cortex. The system is not as foveally oriented as the parvosystem. It is not involved in high spatial resolution and color vision; it receives no input from S cones. It seems to play a role in the detection of movement and body orientation and perhaps brightness perception.

C. Short-Wavelength Cone System

The S cones are only involved in chromatic contrast, which has a lower spatial resolution than achromatic contrast. Chromatic aberration makes the short wavelength image out of focus when the image that the long-wave cone system sees is in focus. Therefore, the S cones have been excluded from high-resolution achromatic vision and the central fovea. S cones transmit their signals to the brain by a unique system of retinal ganglion cells. S cones synapse on S cone-specific on bipolars, which excite a bistratified ganglion cell that is also excited by L and M cone off bipolars (Fig. 5). Such a ganglion cell cannot mediate energy contrasts, being excited by both increments and decrements of light energy. It is designed for successive chromatic contrast, being excited when short wavelengths enter and long wavelengths leave its receptive field. The S cone channel is transmitted by relay cells in the parvo and/

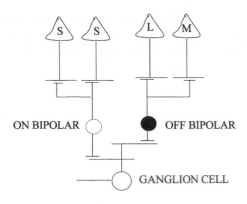

Figure 5 The retinal circuitry of the S cone channel. There are two inputs to a bistratified retinal ganglion cell. One is from on bipolars from S cones and the other is from off bipolars from L and M cones. Both bipolars excite the ganglion cell. The S cones excite their bipolars when there is an increment and the L and M cones excite their bipolar when there is a decrement of light absorption in the corresponding cone. The existence of an antagonistic amacrine cell that interacts off with on bipolars can explain transient tritanopia, a phenomenon of S cone vision.

or the intercalated layers of the lateral geniculate nucleus of the thalamus to striate cortex, layer 4C beta, where it is used to distinguish chromatic contrasts.

There is agreement that this S cone channel, consisting of an on–off ganglion cell, is a major route, possibly the only route for information from S cones to reach striate cortex and visual perception. This channel exhibits relatively little cone opponent behavior. Both white and blue lights excite this cell. Long wavelengths excite the cell when they go off, producing strong responses to successive color contrast. It responds best to white or blue after yellow. This cell informs the brain that the S cone system is or is not absorbing significant light in a particular area of visual space.

Whether there is also an S cone off channel is unclear. Few investigators have detected it. The strongest evidence for its existence comes from measurements with stimuli changing along the tritanopic axis of color space. It is possible that some of the more numerous tonic L and M cone opponent cells could also respond uniquely to such a stimulus. Because S cones are not involved in achromatic contrast, an off channel may not be necessary. Evidence suggesting the absence of an S cone off channel is the subjective phenomenon of transient titanopia, which involves a brief weakening of the appearance of blue whenever a long-wavelength field is turned off. There is no corresponding weakening of yellow when a

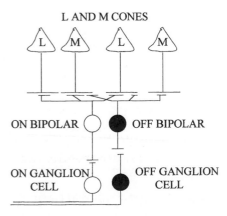

Figure 4 The retinal circuitry of the magnocellular L and M cone system. Here, the L and M cone act synergistically on both on and off channels.

short-wavelength field is turned off. S cones appear to lack the ability to antagonize the other cone channels at the retinal level, presumably because their image is so out of focus that it would interfere with achromatic vision.

III. ACHROMATIC VERSUS CHROMATIC CONTRAST

Achromatic contrast detects spatial differences, which depend on the distribution of light energy in the retinal image. For daylight vision, it is mediated by the two longer wavelength-sensitive cones. It is well developed in the fovea, mediating our highest spatial resolution, and represented in relatively large areas of visual cortex. The foveal area of striate cortex is about 36 times larger than that of striate cortex serving peripheral vision. In the fovea, the responses of neighboring cones are compared for achromatic contrast (Fig. 6). Extrafoveally, spatial resolution is reduced because ganglion cells collect synergistic signals from more than one cone. Achromatic contrasts establish local lightness and darkness, which input orientation-selective neurons in striate cortex and undoubtedly contribute to form perception. Lightness or darkness is determined entirely by simultaneous contrast. Absolute values of light energy are discarded by antagonistic interactions between neurons representing different areas of visual space. An object is light or dark depending entirely on its background.

Chromatic (wavelength) contrast is established by eliminating the effects of energy contrast. It compares the responses of one set of cones to those of another in the same area of space (Fig. 6) and then compares this with comparisons obtained in neighboring areas of space (Fig. 7). Chromatic contrast depends on the difference between cone responses in a unit area of chromatic visual space and not on the absolute responses of the cones. Chromatic contrast does not resolve the detail offered by a single cone because a cone cannot provide an unambiguous clue to wavelength contrast as it can to energy contrast.

A cone's response depends on the energy absorbed, regardless of wavelength. Wavelength determines the probability with which a quantum is absorbed. A response to any wavelength can be reproduced by any other wavelength by varying energy. A mosaic of at least two different types of cones must be sampled to distinguish wavelength contrast. Wavelength contrast needs a double comparison. First, the responses of two different sets of cones in one area of visual space must be compared, and then this comparison must be compared with other areas of visual space to establish spatial contrast based on gradients of wavelength. If one compared only two neighboring cones, a gradient of energy contrast would create an ambiguous signal. For this reason, a unit area of chromatic space is larger than that of achromatic space. The lower spatial resolution of chromatic contrast has been demonstrated psychophysically. The spatial resolution of chromatic contrast for all three cone mechanisms appears to be identical. Figure 8 shows the difference between the spatial resolution of chromatic and achromatic

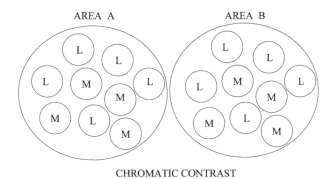

AREA A   AREA B

CHROMATIC CONTRAST

1. COMPARE L TO M RESPONSES IN EACH AREA
2. COMPARE THIS VALUE IN AREA A WITH AREA B

UNIT AREA OF   UNIT AREAS OF
CHROMATIC SPACE   ACHROMATIC SPACE

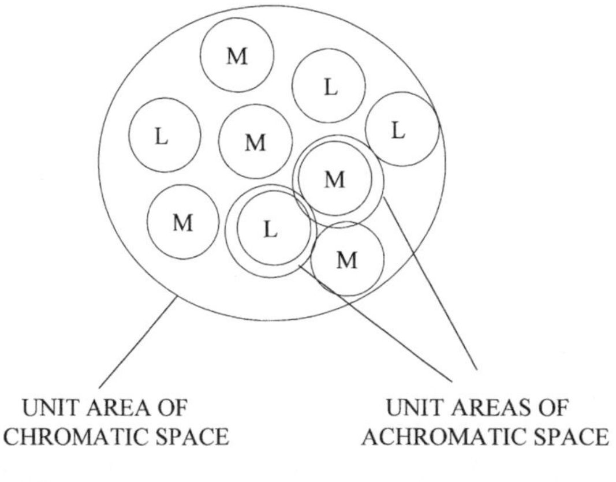

Figure 6 This figure illustrates that the unit areas of chromatic and achromatic space differ because of the nature of the neural comparison. For chromatic contrast, the responses of a group of L cones must be compared with the responses of a neighboring group of M cones in the same area of visual space. For achromatic contrast a single cone can be compared with a neighboring L or M cone.

Figure 7 In order to establish chromatic contrast, a unit area of chromatic space must be compared with a neighboring area of chromatic space. Two neighboring L and M cones cannot be compared because a border of any wavelength could create ambiguity.

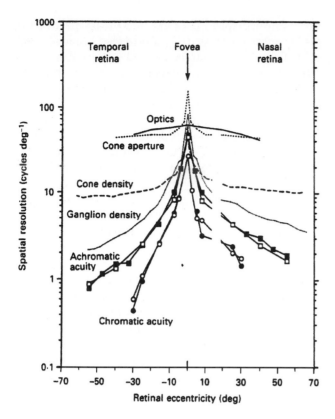

Figure 8 The degree of spatial resolution of the achromatic and chromatic systems of human vision and their distribution across the retina. The symbols represent the data of two normal subjects. They are shown in relationship to the optical properties of the eye and the filtering characteristics of the cones and ganglion cells of the retina (reprinted with permission of Cambridge University Press).

contrast across the human retina. Everywhere the former is lower than the latter, and this increases with eccentricity. Chromatic vision is relatively more developed centrally than achromatic vision.

IV. PSYCHOLOGY OF COLOR VISION

A. Trivariance

In the 1850s, Maxwell in England demonstrated that all human color perception depends on three variables, which he assumed reflected three different types of cones. In Germany, Helmholtz was arriving at a similar conclusion, led by the intuitive insights of Grassmann. The ability to define color by measured amounts of three physically defined variables led to colorimetry. Any color can now be defined by three international standards. The spectral properties of the

three-cone mechanisms of human color vision were first derived psychophysically by Stiles in England in the 1950s. Subsequently, microspectrophotometry of single human cones confirmed these measurements. Defining the absorption spectra of the cones is the starting point for understanding human color vision (Fig. 2).

B. Hering Theory of Color Vision

Ewald Hering, a German physiologist, proposed a unique theory of color vision that went beyond trivariance in its insights into how the nervous system compares cone signals to perceive color. He proposed the existence of antagonism between certain pairs of colors, such as blue and yellow and red and green. The brain could not perceive a blue–yellow or a red–green color, whereas it could perceive red–yellow, green–yellow, red–blue, or green–blue colors. Blue and yellow cancel each other so that one cannot perceive bluish-yellow. Similarly, red and green cancel each other so that one cannot perceive reddish-green. This cancellation of one color impression by another was thought to represent neural antagonism. This was a major insight into how the brain compares the three cones in two pairs in order to perceive color.

Hering's theory was based on subjective experience. The discovery of antagonism between cone responses in single neurons of fish retina led to a renaissance of his theory. Linking the physiology of retinal neurons with subjective colors has proven to be difficult, however. The major reason for the difficulty is that color does not appear to be determined at the retinal or geniculate level but depends on additional operations that occur in visual cortex. Antagonism between cones, which occurs in the retina, is not equivalent to antagonism between colors, which occurs in the cortex.

1. Blue–Yellow Opponency

A scheme that combines physiology and Hering's color opponency is shown in Fig. 9. The operations occurring at the retinal and geniculate level are separated from those thought to be occurring in visual cortex. For blue–yellow color vision, the brain combines excitatory signals from S cone on bipolars with excitatory signals from long-wave cone off bipolars at the retinal level. This on–off–S cone channel excites a cell in the cortex that signals blue; this cell also receives antagonistic (inhibitory) signal from L and M

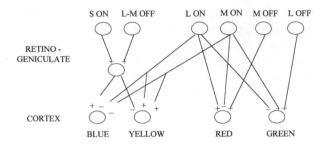

Figure 9 Circuitry that logically organizes the retinogeniculate inputs from the parvocellular system to establish cells responsive to opponent colors in local areas of visual space. (Right) The circuitry of blue–yellow opponent colors in which two different cortical cells receive inputs from the retinal S cone channel, on the one hand, and the long-wavelength tonic system, on the otherhand. The latter excites and the former inhibits the cell detecting "yellow." The converse arrangement affects the cell detecting "blue." If neither cell is excited, achromatic vision determines the color as white, gray, or black. (Left) The circuitry of red–green opponent colors. L cone on and M cone off signals excite and L cone off and M cone on signals inhibit a cell detecting "red"; the converse arrangement detects "green."

cones. This on–off–S cone channel also antagonizes (inhibits) a cell in cortex that signals yellow; this same cell receives an excitatory signal from the L and M cone on-system. These two cells form a blue–yellow opponent system.

If the S cone on-system and the L–M cone on system are excited, the blue and yellow cells are both silent (inhibited) and the system defaults to black-and-white (achromatic) vision. If the S cone on system is excited and the L–M cone on system is not excited (its off system is excited), the color is blue (and dark). If the S cone on system is not excited and the L–M cone on system is, the color is yellow. If both the S cone and the L–M cone on systems are not excited, the color is black (and dark). Whether white and yellow are dark (i.e., gray or brown) is determined by achromatic simultaneous brightness contrast. Humans share this prototypical blue–yellow color vision system, with many other mammals.

The scheme as it stands, however, is deficient in not addressing simultaneous color contrast and in disregarding a fundamental principle in the Land model of color vision, which requires that each cone's system's response be normalized over the visual scene before a comparsion is made for color.

2. Red–Green Opponency

In primates, a second comparison arose with the evolution of two different long-wavelength-sensitive

opsins, which split the bright and yellow part of the visible spectrum in two. This provided a new dimension of chromatic contrast (i.e., red–green) (Figs. 9 and 10). The M on and L off channels are not brought together in the same retinal neuron as is the case for the S cone system, presumably because the L and M systems mediate achromatic as well as chromatic contrast. At the cortical level, where many more neurons are available, these systems are brought together in an opponent manner to form cells that respond uniquely to color (i.e., red or green). Again, this scheme disregards simultaneous chromatic contrast as well as the requirement required in the Land model of color vision for normalization of the responses of each cone mechanism over space before color is determined.

This model has another weakness in disregarding a role for the S cone system in determining redness. There is evidence for trivariant interactions in the perception of red–green opponent colors, and this has not been incorporated into this scheme.

There is another controversy in neural modeling of the red–green opponent system. There are two competing models that have been proposed to mediate red–green opponent responses as depicted in Fig. 9. One theory employs all the midget cells of the fovea as well as hypothetical midget-like cells in the parafovea. This is attractive because these cells are very numerous and they possess an essential requirement for transmitting signals for color to the brain. They isolate in one neural channel the signals of one spectral type of cone. However, they have an inappropriate retinal receptive field for a cell mediating color vision. These cells receive excitatory signals from one cone mechanism in

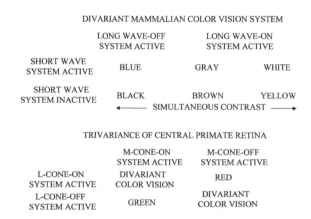

Figure 10 A comparison of the divariant color vision of most mammals and about 2% of human males with that of trivariant color vision.

the center and antagonistic signals from the opponent cone mechanism in the surrounding receptive field. It would be more appropriate to receive the antagonism from the same area of visual space (i.e., its receptive field center rather than from surrounding retina). Nevertheless, this drawback has been disregarded in most models of color vision, which routinely employ this variety of retinal cell. It has been intuitively assumed that visual cortex can correct this deficiency by assembling groups of these cells that subserve coextensive areas of visual space.

A second complexity involved in using the midget system to transmit information about color is that it is also transmitting information about achromatic contrast. Therefore, the brain needs two different detectors to extract the achromatic from the chromatic information from the same neural channel. A scheme suggesting how chromatic and achromatic information, "multiplexed," in a single neural channel is demultiplexed by the brain is shown in Fig. 11. In this scheme synergistic signals from L on and M off channels become logical ways to facilitate the perception of red; similar ones from M on and L off channels are logical to facilitate the perception of green. On the other hand, neurons receiving synergistic inputs from either L on or M on would lose their advantage for chromatic contrast detection but could function to detect achromatic lightness. Similarly, L off and M off channels could function to detect achromatic darkness. By disregarding the source of the cone input achromatic contrast can exploit the fine pixel grain of the fovea. This model does not solve how midget cells

with concentric cone opponent fields compare cone responses over coextensive areas of visual space.

A different model has been proposed by Rodieck, who assumes that the midget system does not mediate chromatic contrast. Instead, he postulates a much smaller group of retinal ganglion cells that receive coextensive inputs from L and M cones. These cells would be similar to the S cone retinal channel and perhaps also involve bistratified retinal ganglion cells. There is no anatomical evidence that such retinal cells exist; however, there is physiological evidence that such cells do exist. Further research is required to distinguish which of these two models is correct.

3. Simultaneous Color Contrast

Simultaneous chromatic contrast is not as strong as simultaneous brightness contrast, probably because the comparison of cones in the same area of visual space provides a unique local signal not present in achromatic contrast. Cells sensitive to simultaneous chromatic contrast are first found in visual cortex. Such cells respond best to a red area surrounded by green or the converse. The logical way to establish such cells is to have similar color comparison in one area of space inhibit a similar comparison in neighboring areas or have dissimilar comparisons excite each other (Fig. 12). Cells organized in this manner are first encountered in striate cortex but have also been detected in higher visual areas.

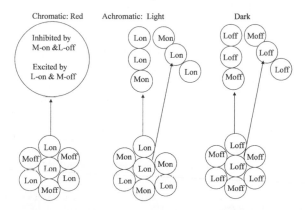

Figure 11 A scheme showing how the same signals from the midget cell system are processed by different sets of parallel circuits, which extract a chromatic signal on the left and an achromatic signal on the right. The chromatic detector mixes synergistic signals from L-on and M-off cells. The achromatic detectors mix only on or only off signals but from either L or M cones.

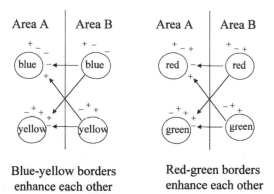

Figure 12 For simultaneous color contrast, the logical arrangement is to have cells responsive to a particular color (in this case "red" or "green" in one area of space) inhibit the same type of neuron in a neighboring area of space. In addition, a cell detecting one color should excite cells detecting the opponent color in neighboring areas of space. In this way, red/green or yellow/blue borders can be enhanced.

C. Land's Retinex Model

Edwin Land emphasized the importance of global influences in color vision. He demonstrated that objects stimulating the retina identically could have totally different colors depending on their surrounding spectral illumination. He proposed a model to handle such global effects called the Retinex model, implying that it depended on both the retina and the cerebral cortex. The model corrects for changes in the spectral characteristics of the illuminant and therefore facilitates color constancy. Color constancy allows us to see a green plant as green in sunlight or artificial light, usually tungsten light, which emits many more long wavelengths than sunlight. The key element in his model is that the signals from each cone mechanism have to be normalized across the visual scene before being compared with another cone mechanism to establish color. It implies that Hering's paired comparisons occur after a stage in which each cone mechanism's response is normalized over a large part of the visual field. Such wide field interactions are quite possible in visual cortex as or before the paired comparisons of cone signals occur.

V. FORM AND COLOR

The most difficult problem in color vision and vision as a whole is to understand how form perception occurs and how once an object's form is determined its color is appended. A reasonable explanation for form perception is Marr's idea of arrays of orientation-selective detectors coding for an object's configuration based on a retinotopic order. The initial detectors of contrast are retinogeniculate neurons with a center-surround receptive field organization based on energy contrast. The mathematical descriptions of such detectors are best represented by a difference of two-dimensional Gaussian-shaped fields. The central field is smaller and overlapped by a larger antagonistic field. The interaction of such detectors can lead to orientation-selective units that detect edges of contrast based on achromatic contrast. The neural machinery for doing this is highly developed in areas of visual cortex serving the fovea. Most of the neurons encountered in striate cortex of primates are sensitive to achromatic (energy) contrast and not selective for color. A smaller amount of neural machinery appears to be devoted to chromatic contrast and color vision in any one area of visual cortex, probably due to its lower spatial resolution.

It is reasonable to assume that chromatic detectors of contrast contribute to form perception in a similar way as achromatic detectors but as a parallel system. Here, wavelength rather than energy contrast determines the activation of the detectors established by cone opponent interactions as independent systems. One system detects blue–yellow chromatic contrasts and the other red–green contrasts. In general, the cues produced by energy contrasts are reinforced by chromatic contrast in detecting the same object. If there are ambiguities, the brain must make a decision favoring one or the other, perhaps favoring chromatic contrast because of its relative independence from shading. Other properties of an object, such as well-defined borders or texture, would be better determined by the achromatic system. In this scheme, three parallel systems for contrast detection are envisaged—one for achromatic (black–white–gray), one for blue–yellow, and one for red–green chromatic contrasts, each arranged with its own retinotopic order. Whether all three systems converge on a single neuron to determine the fused sense of color is unclear. For colors such as magenta, such interactions may occur. In addition, there seem to be neurons that respond to both chromatic and achromatic signals to perform neural functions but are not involved in the perception of color.

A clue to the cortical processing of vision comes from observations of multiple areas of prestriate cortex where the entire visual field is re-represented. These areas send and receive signals from each other. Working together they create a unified and presumably richer impression of the visual world. The actual role of each subarea is poorly understood.

Zeki proposed that one of these subareas, visual area 4, is unique for color processing. He argued that in this area cells correct for color constancy and respond to true color. At earlier stages cells may respond to wavelength contrast but not to color. It has been difficult to prove this hypothesis. Single neuron recordings from most visual areas reveal cells selective for chromatic contrast and color vision but usually in the minority. Visual area 4 has been reported to have a larger proportion of color-selective cells but there is no universal agreement about this.

There is little doubt that the cortex works by dividing different aspects of visual function into anatomically distinct areas and that perception of a unified image depends on the multiple physiological linking of these separate subareas. A critical element in this reasoning is the question of retinotopic order, which seems to be the backbone of form perception.

The integration of form must be based on linking inputs labeled by retinal coordinates. Chromatic contrasts must be handled in a similar way as achromatic contrasts, each with its own retinal co-ordinates. Does the lower spatial resolving chromatic contrast system get funneled into a separate cortical area for color vision even though color vision depends as much on achromatic contrast as on chromatic contrast? It seems more likely that chromatic and achromatic processing occurs in all the areas to which the parvocellular system projects, and color discrimination as well as color constancy improve as increasingly more visual areas are involved in the processing.

Color discrimination continues to improve with the size of the object being judged. Surfaces subtending 20° and more of visual angle significantly improve color discrimination when compared with those subtending only a few degrees. Color discrimination can integrate over very large areas of visual space and consequently striate cortex. One of the characteristics of neurons in higher visual areas is the relatively large size of their receptive fields. They require inputs from large areas of the retina before deciding to respond. The larger size of visual stimuli activates more antagonistic interactions and therefore could increase the variety of experience. If one is judging a small object, he or she may not be using as much of his or her brain. If the object is enlarged, it begins to activate more cells in higher visual areas and its recognition is improved. This operation may depend on all subareas working in concert through feedback rather than a serial progression from lower to higher areas.

VI. DISORDERS OF COLOR PROCESSING

A. Genetic Defects

The major abnormalities of color vision are due to genetic defects (Table I). The most common involve red–green color vision and are due to defects in the genes for L and M cone opsins located on the X chromosome. Therefore, they occur mainly in males. In the most severe cases, both genes fail to function. This leads to achromatopsia, loss of all color vision. Such subjects have only S cones and rods and are called S cone achromats. With only one class of cones, color vision is impossible. Such subjects may experience a primitive form of color vision that depends on a comparison between S cones and rods. Without L and M cones, they also lack high spatial resolution and are

Table I
Classification and Incidence of Color Vision Defects

Type	% Males
Congenital	
Trivariants (three cones present)	
Normal	91.2
Anomalous	
Protanomaly (L cone opsin abnormal)	1.3
Deuteranomaly (M cone opsin abnormal)	5
Tritanomaly (S cone opsin abnormal)	0.001
Divariants (Two cones present)	
Protanopia (L cones absent)	1.3
Deuteranopia (M cones absent)	1.2
Tritanopia (S cones absent)	0.001
Achromats	
Complete achromat (all cones absent)	0.00001
S cone achromat (L and M cones absent)	0.000001
Acquired	
Tritanopia (outer or peripheral retinal disease)	0.01
Protan deuteranopia (inner or central retinal disease)	0.01
Cerebral achromatopsia (brain disease)	0.0000001

legally blind. A second form of achromatopsia is due to a gene defect on chromosome 2 for an ion channel exclusive to cones. These subjects only have functional rods.

In less severe defects, only an L or an M cone gene is functional. Such subjects have blue–yellow color vision obtained by comparing S cones with the remaining long-wave cone mechanism. Subjects who lack L cones are called protanopes. They are insensitive to the long wave end of the spectrum (the red end). Subjects who lack M cones are called deuteranopes. They are sensitive to the entire spectrum. Both protanopes and deuteranopes cannot distinguish reds from greens and have only blue–yellow color vision. They all have high spatial resolution.

In milder defects, both L and M cone opsins are transcribed but the absorption spectrum of one is shifted closer to the other, diminishing the potential for chromatic contrast. Such subjects are called deuteranomalous if the M cone opsin is abnormal and protanomalous if the L cone opsin is abnormal. They have reduced red–green but normal blue–yellow color vision. They all have high spatial resolution. The similarities of colors vary in different ways for each color deficiency (Fig. 13).

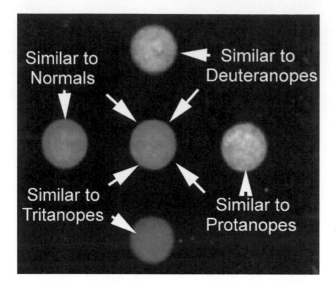

Figure 13 These spots of color appear different to subjects with color deficiencies. Normal subjects see the spot on the left most similar to the central spot. Deuteranopes see the upper, protanopes the right, and tritanopes the lower spot as most similar to the central spot.

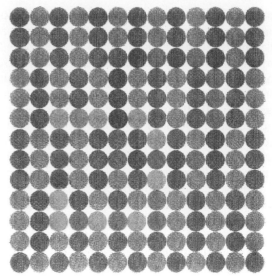

Deuteranopes, protanopes and tritanopes
don't see the blue square

Figure 14 A pseudoisochromatic plate that detects protanopes, deuteranopes, and tritanopes, who fail to see the blue square at the upper right side. (See color insert in Volume 1).

Such color deficiences can also be detected by the use of plates in which spots of different colors that confuse defective subjects are arranged in different sizes so that a figure can be seen by normal subjects but not by defective ones and sometimes vice versa. One that detects both red–green and blue–yellow defective vision is shown in Fig. 14.

Defects in the S cone opsin located on chromosome 7 are rare. They are usually autosomal-dominant mutations. Such subjects are called tritanopes and have only red–green color vision. They retain high spatial resolution. A pseudoisochromatic plate that detects tritanopia is shown in Fig. 15.

Interestingly, there is no gene defect that produces achromatopsia without decreasing acuity, but the converse frequently occurs, including virtually all disorders of the macula.

B. Color Vision Defects Associated with Other Diseases

There is a group of retinal degenerations, primarily genetic in origin such as retinitis pigmentosa, that destroy peripheral vision first and in general slowly progress toward the fovea. These diseases tend to produce tritanopia. This may reflect the possibility that blue–yellow color vision extends further into peripheral retina and therefore is more vulnerable to this disease process. It may also reflect the possibility that S cones are more susceptible to the degeneration than L and M cones.

There is a second class of diseases that tend to affect central vision and are due to defects in either the optic nerve or the macula area of the retina. These can be

Pseudo-isochromatic color plate

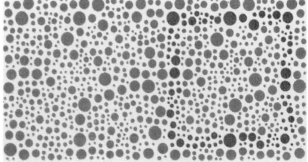

Tritanopes do not see the green square

Figure 15 A pseudoisochromatic plate that detects tritanopes, who fail to see the pattern on the right.

associated with red–green color vision defects but they are always accompanied by a diminution in acuity. The vulnerability of red–green defects in these diseases may reflect the possibility that red–green color vision is more developed centrally than blue–yellow vision.

There is a class of autoimmune diseases that arise from cancers that express antigens, which are also expressed by photoreceptors. The immune system detects these antigens and reacts to them both on the cancer cells and on the photoreceptors. This class of diseases has been called cancer-related retinopathies. Some of these diseases are highly specific, involving only cones and not rods. Such subjects can lose all cone vision and consequently color vision. Recently, we found a subject who lost only L and M cones but not S cones or rods. These are examples of acquired achromatopsia.

C. Abnormalities of Acuity and Color Vision

In general, abnormalities of central vision, such as those involving the macula, reduce spatial resolution but have little or no effect on color vision. A remarkable example is "oligocone trichromasy." These subjects have very few cones and greatly reduced acuity but retain normal color vision. This must reflect the fact that color vision integrates over larger areas of the visual field and is disconnected from the high spatial resolution discrimination mediated by achromatic contrast and the "midget" system. This does not mean that the midget system does not mediate chromatic contrast and consequently color vision; it must mean that there is considerable overlap in the integration of these midget cell signals that are used for chromatic contrast. There is an alternative view that there are specific ganglion cells divorced entirely from the midget system.

D. Cerebral Achromatopsia

There are rare exceptions to the tolerance of color discrimination despite large losses in acuity. An occasional subject loses color vision but maintains normal visual acuity after acquired damage of visual cortex. The cases that have been studied most completely with the entire gamut of color testing methods confirm major but not complete loss of color discrimination. They appear to be able to use wavelength contrast to detect objects but are unable to perceive colors from these cues. Such a subject can distinguish the shape and achromatic brightness differences of traffic lights but cannot see them as red, green, or yellow. They appear as washed-out objects of white and gray. Testing reveals a greater tendency for a blue–yellow (tritanopic) than a red–green deficiency. In general, the recovery from damage to visual cortex will usually include a stage in which white and grays are seen first before colors return. The first color to return is usually red. Increasing the size of the stimulus also tends to improve color perception. Nevertheless, such subjects are indeed very deficient in color vision and retain normal acuity.

These clinical findings imply that there is a significant anatomical separation of chromatic and achromatic contrast processing in the cerebral cortex. This is consistent with a cortical area devoted exclusively to the perception of color, but it is not proof. All of these patients invariably have prosopagnosia, the inability to recognize faces, and a scotomatous area, usually in their superior visual field. There are no reports of isolated acquired achromatopsia without other concurrent visual deficits. It is possible that the perception of color requires feedback from prestriate to striate cortex that facilitates the fusion of chromatic contrast with achromatic contrast perception. This feedback may be more important for incorporating the relatively sparse chromatic processing centers in striate cortex into visual perception.

VII. THE FUTURE OF COLOR VISION

Color vision offers a valuable insight into how the cerebral cortex works because it is a well-defined process that depends on three retinal variables serving each area of visual space and is intimately associated with form vision. Many of the logical operations necessary for color vision, which are performed by circuits of nerve cells, are relatively well understood. The major impasse in our understanding of the process is how its clues to contrast are unified into the recognition of form. It is our poor understanding of form vision that makes the final stage of understanding color vision difficult. Understanding how nature interweaves clues from chromatic and achromatic contrast into those for form perception using arrays of neurons and neuronal interactions should lead to a better understanding of not only color vision but also the cerebral cortex in general. The problem of researching this topic, however, has been that the tools to study it have been and still are too crude. It is necessary to monitor large numbers of single neurons performing their operations within a fraction of a second and to continue doing so during long-term experiments. Such techniques are just beginning to evolve.

See Also the Following Articles

SPATIAL VISION • VISION: BRAIN MECHANISMS • VISUAL CORTEX • VISUAL DISORDERS • VISUAL SYSTEM DEVELOPMENT AND NEURAL ACTIVITY

Suggested Reading

Dacey, D. M. (1999). Origins of spectral opponency in primate retina. In *The Retinal Basis of Vision* (J. I. Toyoda, M. Murakami, A. Kaneko, and T. Saito, Eds.). Elsevier, Amsterdam.

Ehrlich, P., Sadowski, B., and Zrenner, E. (1997). "Oligocone" trichromasy, a rare form of incomplete achromatopsia. *Ophthalmology* **94**, 801–806.

Hubel, D. H. (1988). Eye, brain, and vision, Scientific American Library Series No. 22.

Hurvich, L. (1981). *Color Vision*. Sinauer, Sunderland, MA.

Land, E. H. (1986). Recent advances in retinex theory. *Vision Res.* **26**, 7–21.

Marr, D. (1982). *Vision*. Freeman, San Francisco.

Mullen, K. T. (1990). The chromatic coding of space. In *Vision: Coding and Efficiency* (C. Blakemore, Ed.). Cambridge Univ. Press, Cambridge, UK.

Pokorny, J., Smith, V. C., Verriest, V. G., and Pinckers, A. J. L. G. (1979). *Congenital and Acquired Color Vision Defects*. Grune & Stratton, New York.

Rattner, A., Sun, H., and Nathans, J. (1999). Molecular genetics of human retinal disease. *Annu. Rev. Genet.* **33**, 89–131.

Rizzzo, M., Smith, V., Pokorny, J., and Damasio, A. R. (1993). Color perception profiles in central achromatopsia. *Neurology* **43**, 995–1001.

Rodieck, R. W. (1991). Which cells code for color? In *From Pigments to Perception* (A. Valberg and B. B. Lee, Eds.), pp. 83–93. Plenum, New York.

Stiles, W. S. (1978). *Mechanisms of Color Vision*. Academic Press, New York.

Walsh, V. (1999). How does the cortex construct color? *Proc. Natl. Acad. Sci. USA* **96**, 13594–13596.

Zeki, S. (1993). *A Vision of the Brain*. Blackwell, Oxford.

Zollinger, H. (1999). *Color: A Multidisciplinary Approach*. Wiley–VCH Verlag Helvetica Chimica Acta, Weinheim, Zurich.

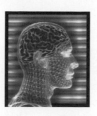

Color Vision

GERALD H. JACOBS

University of California, Santa Barbara

GLOSSARY

cones The retinal receptor cells that underlie vision for daylight conditions; there are three classes of cone in retinas of individuals having normal color vision.

metamers Lights of different wavelength compositions that appear identical.

opponent colors Pairs of colors that are perceptually mutually exclusive (e.g., red–green and yellow–blue).

opsin genes Genes specifying the protein component of photopigment molecules; variations in these genes can be mapped directly into variations in color vision.

photopigments Molecules located in photoreceptors that absorb energy from light and initiate the visual process.

principle of univariance Encompasses the observation that the responses of photoreceptors are proportional to the number of photons absorbed by the photopigment they contain independent of the wavelength of the light.

spectrally opponent cells Nerve cells that transmit information useful for the production of color vision; these cells combine excitatory and inhibitory inputs reflecting the activation of different classes of cone.

trichromatic The formal characterization of normal human color vision; derived from the results of experiments in which it is shown that three primary lights can be combined to match the appearance of any other spectral light.

Color vision is the neural process that provides one of the important and dramatic aspects of the brain's interpretation of the visual world. This process is initiated by variation in the spectral distribution of light reaching the eye and culminates in the rich range of human color experience. Fundamental features of color vision are described in this article, including a summary of human capacities to perceive and discriminate color, an outline of the principal biological mechanisms underlying color vision, and a description of variations in color vision among people.

I. THE PERCEPTION AND DISCRIMINATION OF COLOR

At least for simple viewing situations, color experience has been traditionally ordered along three principal perceptual dimensions—brightness, hue, and saturation. The first is considered to be part of both achromatic and chromatic features of color, whereas the latter two are chromatic features. In terms of everyday experience, brightness is that aspect of a percept most closely associated with changes in the intensity of a light yielding visual experience along a dimension that encompasses verbal descriptions running from dim to bright to dazzling. Hue is primarily correlated with the wavelength of light and is typically designated through the use of common color terms—red, green, blue, and so on. Saturation is the degree to which a chromatic sensation differs from an achromatic sensation of the same brightness—for example, yielding sensory experiences that are situated on a continuum changing from white (achromatic) to light pink and to a deep red.

Many aspects of color have been conveniently summarized in geometric configurations. The three perceptual dimensions of color just described are often represented in a so-called color solid. In this color solid, hues are positioned around the circumference of a circle where they are placed in the order in which they are perceived in a spectrum. The ends of the spectrum (reds and blues) are connected through a series of purple hues. White is located at the center of the hue circle and saturation is then represented as increasing along lines drawn from the center to the various hues located on the circle circumference. The plane surface thus formed encompasses chromatic variation at a single brightness level; increases and decreases in brightness from this level are plotted along a third dimension that runs perpendicular to the plane. Within this color solid any particular color experience can be conceived as representing a location in the three-dimensional space.

A. Environmental Signals

A basic problem for students of color vision is to relate the perceptual dimensions of color to physical features of the environment. Common experience suggests that color is an inherent property of objects: Apples are red; grass is green, and so on. However, is that the case, or is it rather that color is produced by active processes in a perceiver that are initiated by light? Philosophers and others have long debated these alternatives and their arguments continue to reverberate today. Most vision scientists, however, incline to some version of the second alternative and, in so doing, follow the lead of Isaac Newton, the great English scientist whose 16th-century observations caused him to conclude that "the Rays to speak properly are not coloured. In them there is nothing else than a certain Power and Disposition to stir up a Sensation of this or that Colour."

Light reaching the eye from any location in space can vary in intensity (number of photons per unit time) and wavelength. People are sensitive to a narrow band of wavelengths, extending from about 400 to 700 nm (1 nm$=10^{-9}$ m). For most ordinary viewing, the distribution of wavelengths and intensities reaching a viewer depends jointly on characteristics of the source of illumination, on the surface reflectance properties of an illuminated object, and on the geometric relationship between the object and the viewer (Fig. 1). For instance, a snowfield seen in full sunlight yields a very

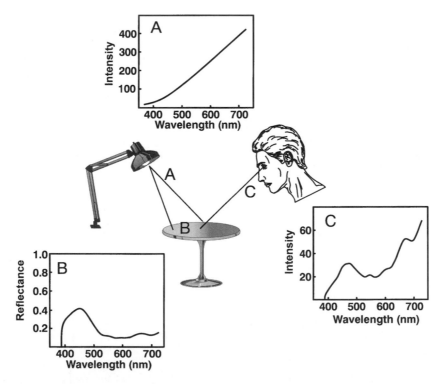

Figure 1 Light reaching a viewer is dependent on the nature of the light source and on the reflectance properties of the object being viewed. In this illustration the spectral distribution of energy emerging from a light source (A) is indicated at the top. The spectral reflectance properties of the surface of the table (B) are given on the left. The spectral distribution of light reaching the viewer (C) that is shown on the right is the product of the spectral distribution of the illuminant and the reflectance property of the object.

different array of wavelengths and intensities for analysis from that provided by an expanse of lawn seen at twilight. Viewed across natural scenes there are usually substantial local variations in the wavelength and the intensity of light, and the number of possible combinations of the two is virtually infinite. All species with sight can exploit intensity variations as an aid to the discrimination of the form, location, and movement of objects. However, only those that also have a capacity for color vision can disentangle the effects of joint variations in wavelength and intensity and in so doing yield the experience of color.

B. The Dimensionality of Color Vision

Color vision has been frequently studied in laboratories by asking observers to judge whether pairs of stimuli—typically viewed as the respective halves of a small, illuminated circle (Fig. 2)—appear the same ("match") or are different. If the two halves are identical in wavelength and intensity content, they of course match. Differences in color appearance may be introduced by changing the intensity or wavelength content of one half or by changing both these features. A change in the intensity of the light in one half of the circle yields a mainly achromatic difference between the two; one side becomes brighter than the other. Changes in the wavelength content of one half may yield a complex of change, in hue and saturation principally but also possibly in brightness. If the observer is then allowed to adjust the relative intensity so as to remove any brightness difference, the two sides will have a pure chromatic difference. It is from this basis that color vision is often studied.

Special cases of this viewing arrangement are those in which the two sides of the small circle differ in wavelength content but have identical color appearances. Pairs of stimuli that differ physically but appear the same are said to be metameric. The occurrence of such metameric matches defines a fundamental feature of human color vision—its limited dimensionality. To better understand this feature, consider color matches obtained when separate lights having fixed spectral content are superimposed on one half of the matching field (Fig. 2). Each of these separate lights is called a primary (P), and the task given to a viewer is to adjust the relative intensity (e) of each of the primaries so as to make that half of the field appear identical to the other half (in turn, traditionally called the test light). The test light can be composed of any fixed combination of wavelengths and intensities. The important result is that most human observers can match the appearance of all test lights by simply adjusting the relative intensities of only three primary lights. Some matches are possible with only one or two primaries, and more than three will work, but three is the minimum needed to complete all matches. Humans are thus said to have trichromatic color vision. There are some qualifications to this conclusion; (i) there are restrictions on the wavelengths that can be employed as primaries, and (ii) for some test lights one of the primaries must be added to the side containing the test light. In any case, the ability of humans to complete matches using only three independent variables means that any color can be represented in a three-dimensional space where the location in that space is specified by the proportions of the three primaries required to capture the appearance of the color. Such spaces are highly useful in the many practical uses of color (e.g., the specification of colored

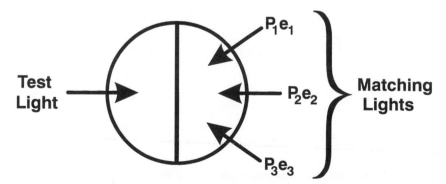

Figure 2 Schematic representation of the color matching test. In this test a subject views a small circular field. The two halves of the field are independently illuminated from different light sources. As shown here, a light of some fixed wavelength and intensity content (a test light) is projected onto the left half of the field. Lights from three separate sources are superimposed on the left. These are primary lights (P_1–P_3) that differ in wavelength. The task of the subject is to adjust the intensities of the three lights (e_1–e_3) until the two halves of the field appear identical. Illustrated is a trichromatic match where combinations of three primary lights are required to complete the match.

signal lights or of the color of a commercial logo) and so have been intensively evaluated.

The mixing of lights reveals another surprising feature of color perception. Many pairs of lights can be added together to yield an achromatic percept. Such pairs are called complementary colors and their occurrence is counterintuitive in that the perceived colors associated with the two wavelengths viewed separately utterly disappear when they are mixed together. In the color solid described previously, complementary colors are placed on opposite sides of the hue circle such that a line drawn between them passes through the location of white. The facts of color mixing make clear that the visual system is not a simple wavelength analyzer. From the viewpoint of the biology of color vision, the fact that people are trichromatic has long been taken to predict the nature of the transformations occurring in the visual system.

Indeed, more than two centuries ago it was hypothesized that the fundamental facts of human color perception imply that there must be three kinds of physiological mechanisms in the eye responsible for processing those aspects of light that lead to color. This turned out to be an inspired prediction.

C. Color Discrimination Indices

One way to characterize human color vision is to ask how good we are at making color discriminations. Figure 3 summarizes results from four different tests of human color vision. Just as it does for all other animals, the sensitivity of humans to light varies as a function of the wavelength of the light. The results shown in Fig. 3A illustrate this point. The continuous line is called a spectral sensitivity function and it plots

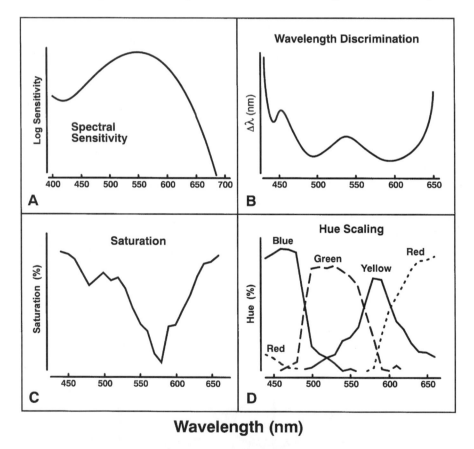

Figure 3 Four measurements of human color discrimination abilities. (A) Spectral sensitivity function. The continuous line plots the reciprocal of the intensity of spectral lights required for detection under daylight test conditions. (B) Wavelength discrimination function. Plotted is a measure of how much wavelength has to be changed in nanometers at each spectral location in order to yield a perceptible color difference. Higher values indicate poorer discrimination. (C) Spectral saturation. The continuous line shows the variation in the saturation of spectral lights as a function of the wavelength of the light. High values indicate greater degrees of saturation. (D) Spectral hues. Plotted as a function of spectral wavelength are the percentages of cases in which each of four separate hue categories (blue, green, yellow, and red) was employed to describe the colors of various lights.

the inverse of the intensity of light required for detection under daylight test conditions. This is a measure of the degree of achromatic variation across the spectrum. The sensitivity variations shown in Fig. 3A predict that colors produced by lights of different wavelengths but equal intensities vary greatly in brightness, and so they do. This characteristic feature of the visual system is so important that a standard spectral sensitivity curve representing the averaged values for many subjects has been derived. This curve has come to be used to provide another specification of the brightness dimension—a metric referred to as luminance. Because luminance has formal properties that brightness does not possess (e.g., luminance units can be additively combined, whereas units of brightness cannot), vision scientists typically prefer luminance as a means of specifying the visual effectiveness of lights.

As noted previously, color depends centrally on the wavelength of light. Figure 3B illustrates how sensitive humans are to changes in wavelength. Plotted is a measure of the size of the wavelength difference ($\Delta\lambda$) required to yield a discriminable change in the appearance of a light for all locations across the spectrum. This result is sometimes called a hue discrimination function, although in fact wavelength change may induce both hue and saturation differences. Note that people are exquisitely sensitive to wavelength changes in two parts of the spectrum. Indeed, under stringent test conditions humans can reliably discriminate some wavelength differences that amount to no more than fractions of a single nanometer. Saturation can be measured in several ways, but they all indicate that spectral lights differ greatly in the degree to which they yield a saturated color. As illustrated in Fig. 3C, lights of both long and short wavelength (usually having an appearance of red and blue, respectively) are seen as highly saturated; lights of about 570–580 nm (seen as yellow) are very unsaturated. The results shown in Figs. 3A–3C imply that people are acutely attuned to detecting differences in several color dimensions when these dimensions are probed separately. However, how good are we at detecting differences when all three perceptual dimensions can vary as they do in normal viewing? One way to appreciate human color vision is to ask how many different colors people can see. A recent estimate suggests that those of us with normal color vision can discern in excess of 2 million different surface colors. Clearly, the human color palette is very extensive.

The results of Figs. 3A–3C are discrimination measures in which people were asked to operate as instruments solely designed to detect differences, entirely ignoring how these lights actually appear. In our ordinary experience with color the rich medium of language is most often employed to give objects color names. It turns out that people can apply color names to lights varying in wavelength and intensity in a sufficiently systematic fashion to generate very reliable indications of color appearance. Figure 3D shows the results from a so-called hue-scaling experiment in which people were asked to name the colors of lights varying in wavelength. They were allowed to use only four different color names (red, yellow, green, and blue), either singly or in pairs; the latter being the case in which one of the four names could be used to modify another (e.g., yellowish red). Not only can people do this reliably but also, perhaps surprising, there is very high consistency of the use of hue names among individuals. There are two important aspects of these results. First, note that in some parts of the spectrum hue changes rapidly with changes in wavelength (i.e., there are well-defined transitions between the color names used by the subjects). Not surprisingly, these regions are those where wavelength discrimination is most acute. Therefore, for example, at approximately 580 nm there are abrupt changes in the hue names given to lights of different wavelengths and this coincides with one of the locations where wavelength discrimination is most acute (compare Fig. 3D with Fig. 3B). Second, there are apparently mutually exclusive categories of hue appearance: A light may be seen to yield both red and yellow components (i.e., reddish yellow or yellowish red) or green and yellow components, but people almost never describe lights as containing both red and green components. The same conclusion holds for yellow and blue. This mutually exclusive pairing of color sensations has long been known and traditionally interpreted as reflecting mutually antagonistic interactions between color processing mechanisms somewhere in the visual system. The antagonistic hue pairs (red/green and yellow/blue) are usually called opponent colors.

The utilization of names to group colors into coherent categories seems universal across all human populations. Results from a survey conducted by Berlin and Kay in 1969, involving an analysis of more than 100 languages, indicated that there are only 11 basic color terms (the English equivalents are white, black, red, yellow, green, brown, purple, pink, orange, and gray). The survey further suggested that these basic color terms have "evolved" among human populations in a reasonably predictable sequence in the sense that rules can be established to specify which names are present in languages that do not contain the full set of color terms. For example, languages that contain only two basic color terms have black and white, and those with three color terms have black, white, and red. These observations have been taken to imply that basic color terms could reflect universal properties of the organization of the human nervous system. This conclusion has not escaped criticism, particularly from professional linguists, and although attempts have been made to connect these universal color categories to features of visual system physiology, no completely compelling linkages have been established.

D. Context and Constancy

Those aspects of color vision summarized previously were measured with small illuminated spots of specified wavelength and intensity presented in otherwise featureless, usually achromatic, visual fields or with small, carefully calibrated colored papers viewed against an achromatic background. Although ideal for examining human color vision in rigidly controlled circumstances, these conditions are quite unlike everyday visual worlds that are most often rich with both spatial and temporal variegation. From many laboratory studies of the influence of spatial and temporal variables it is clear that perceived color depends not only on the wavelength and intensity of the light reaching the eye from some point in a scene but also on a host of contextual features.

Color context effects have long been appreciated and often exploited for visual effect by painters, tapestry makers, and dyers. For example, the reddishness of a region in a visual scene can be much enhanced if adjoined by a region that appears green. Similarly, surrounding a yellow spot with an expanse of blue can increase the perceived yellowness significantly. These are examples of simultaneous color contrast. Analogous effects on perceived color operate along a timescale. Thus, exposing the eye to a red surface causes a subsequently viewed white surface to take on a greenish cast. Note that these successive contrast effects are similar to the spatial effects in that they tend to enhance the perception of colors that are complementary to those inducing the effect: Yellows enhance blueness; greens enhance redness, and so on. In this sense, they support the idea of a mutual exclusivity of some color sensations similar to that noted previously for the naming of colors.

Seemingly opposed to such contrast effects are instances of what has been called color assimilation. Assimilation occurs when a background color and an interlaced region tend to take on the same color rather than that of a contrast color. For example, consider a white hatched pattern that periodically interrupts a continuous red field. On the grounds of simultaneous color contrast one might expect the white region to take on a greenish appearance, but instead it looks red. It is as if the predominant color has spread into these neighboring regions. The conditions that determine whether contrast or assimilation occurs are incompletely understood, but the relative sizes and configurations of the spatially opposed regions are certainly factors. In any case, both contrast and assimilation effects make it clear that the visual system constructs a color world that is not solely based on the array of wavelengths and intensities coming from each individual region in the scene.

As Fig. 1 illustrated, light reaching the eye from an object depends jointly on surface reflectance of the object and on the nature of the illumination. Surface reflectance is an intrinsic property of objects, but the nature of the illumination is changeable and, consequently, the light reflected from any particular object can vary significantly. For example, the spectral distribution of light reflected from a clump of grass will change drastically as the sun moves from its overhead position to one on the horizon. If color depended solely on the distribution of wavelengths and intensity reaching the eye, one might expect the color of the grass would also change during this period of time. In fact, for the most part, the grass appears to remain resolutely green in appearance. The ability of the visual system to maintain a reasonably consistent object color in the face of these variations in illumination is called color constancy. The occurrence of color constancy implies that somehow the visual system is able to register the nature of the changes in illumination and then to substantially discount these changes. Although the mechanisms in the nervous system that allow this are not well understood, color constancy is supremely important in enhancing stability in our perceptual representations of the color world.

II. COLOR VISION AND THE RETINA

The processing of information that leads to color vision begins in the retina. The retina is an exquisitely organized portion of the nervous system lining the interior of the back surface of the eye. Each human retina is made up of approximately 115 million cells that act in concert to extract information from the optical image formed on the retinal surface. Our understanding of the processing of color information in the retina and the rest of the visual nervous system is drawn mainly from studies of humans and from our close relatives, the Old World monkeys.

A. Cone Photopigments

There are two classes of photoreceptor—rods and cones. Rods are involved in supporting vision under low-light conditions (technically called scotopic vision). Cones subserve color vision and other characteristic features of daylight vision (photopic vision), such as high spatial and temporal sensitivity. The conversion of energy from light into nerve signals is accomplished in the photoreceptors. The initial step in this transduction process involves the absorption of photon energy by photopigments. Molecules of cone pigment are densely packed in a series of parallel membranes making up one end of the photoreceptor, a physical arrangement that is particularly effective in trapping incoming light. The pigment molecule has two essential components—a protein called opsin and a covalently linked chromophore, the latter being a derivative of vitamin A. Absorption of energy from a photon of light causes the chromophore to undergo a conformational change, an isomerization. This change is virtually instantaneous, complete in no more than 200 fsec (fsec=10^{-15} sec). It serves as a first step in a cascade of molecular changes that produce a modulation in the flow of ionic current across the photoreceptor membrane. This induced electrical change spreads along the length of the photoreceptor and in turn alters the rate of release of neurotransmitter to second-order cells in the retina and thereby communicates a signal onward into the retinal network.

The efficiency with which photopigments absorb light varies continuously as a function of the wavelength of the light. Figure 4 illustrates the absorption spectra for the three classes of cone pigment found in the retinas of people with normal color vision. When properly scaled the shapes of absorption spectra for all photopigments are similar, and thus they can be economically specified by using one number, the wavelength to which they are maximally sensitivity (λ_{max}). The human cone pigments have λ_{max} values at about 420, 530, and 560 nm. The shape and width of

the absorption spectrum for the photopigment are dependent on features of the chromophore, whereas the spectral positioning of the pigment along the wavelength axis depends on structural features of the opsin. Note that there is a significant amount of overlap in the wavelengths of light absorbed by these pigments. This is important because it is the comparison of the amount of light absorbed by different pigments that constitutes the basis for the nerve signals that lead to color vision. Among vision scientists, the receptors containing these three pigments are usually termed S, M, and L cones, respectively (shorthand for short-, middle-, and long-wavelength sensitive). The three classes of cone are unequally represented in the retina, having an overall ratio of 1S:3M:6L, with some significant individual variations. As discussed later, this fact is important in understanding some features of human color vision.

A fundamental feature of the operation of pigments is that their response to light is proportional to the number of photons they absorb independent of the wavelength of these photons so that, once absorbed, each photon contributes equally to any generated signal. This means that the signal provided by a given type of receptor contains no information about the wavelength of the light that was absorbed. The blindness of a single type of photopigment to wavelength differences is formally called the principle of univariance. An important functional consequence of pigment univariance is that a retina having only a single type of photopigment could not support any color vision capacity. This is one reason why colors disappear under scotopic conditions when only a single (rod) pigment is operational.

Color matching behavior can be traced directly to the univariant property of the cone pigments. Thus, in a color match of the sort described previously, the subject is actually adjusting the amounts of the primary lights so that the three types of cone will absorb equal numbers of photons from the primary lights and from the test light. A consequence is that color matches are very sensitive to the relative spectral positions of the cone pigments. Indeed, other things being equal, the retinas of two individuals who set different color matches must contain photopigments that differ in their spectral positioning. This single fact constitutes one of the earliest and still most persuasive examples of a compulsive linkage between behavior and nervous system organization. Most humans have trichromatic color vision because their retinas contain three classes of cone pigment, each of which behaves univariantly. It is obvious from the absorption spectra

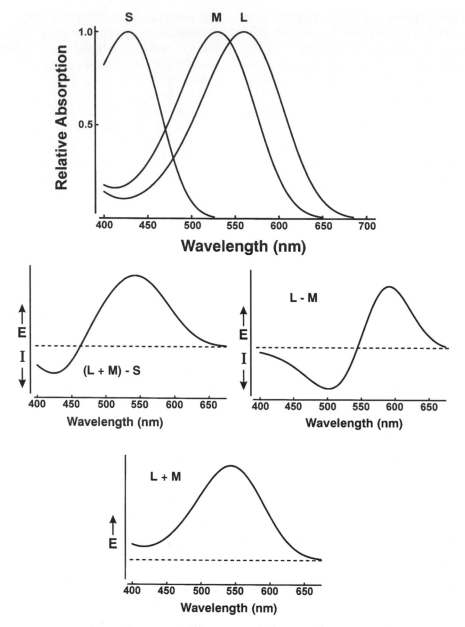

Figure 4 Response properties of photopigments and nerve cells. (Top) The absorption curves for the three classes of cone found in the eyes of people with normal color vision. The peak sensitivities of the three cone types are at 430 nm (S), 530 nm (M), and 560 nm (L). The three graphs at the bottom illustrate the responses of nerves cells in the visual pathway that combine inputs from the three cone types. (Middle) Spectrally opponent cells that show additive and subtractive combinations of cone signals. The inputs are indicated. E, excitation; I, inhibition. (Bottom) Response property of a nonopponent cell that additively combines signals from M and L cones.

of Fig. 4 that S cones absorb very little light from the middle- to long-wavelength portion of the spectrum. A consequence of this is that only two primary lights are required to complete color matches in this part of the spectrum (i.e., over those wavelengths, three-variable, trichromatic color vision gives way to two-variable, dichromatic color vision).

B. Genes and Photopigments

Single genes specify the opsins of each of the types of cone pigment. The human opsin genes were first isolated and sequenced in 1986. As long predicted from observations about the inheritance of color vision defects, the genes for the M and L pigments are located on the q-arm of the X chromosome where they lie in a head-to-tail tandem array. Each of the X chromosome genes specifies an opsin composed of 364 amino acids, and the two are so similar in structure that the amino acid sequences for M and L pigments are 96% identical. Most individuals (at least 75% of the population) have more than one copy of the M cone pigment gene, although the functional significance of these "extra" genes remains debatable. The S cone opsin gene is autosomal, located on chromosome 7. It specifies a photopigment opsin containing 348 amino acids. The sequence of this gene differs from the other two enough to produce an S cone opsin that is 40–45% identical to that of the M and L cone pigments.

The close physical proximity on the X chromosome of the M and L opsin genes and their great sequence similarities makes them particularly susceptible to unequal recombination during meiosis. Such recombination events can result in the loss or the gain of complete copies of the opsin genes, or they can produce novel genes through recombination of partial sequences drawn from the original M and L genes. All of these changes will have an impact on the nature of the photopigments that get produced and hence they will alter significantly the details of color vision in that individual. For example, a loss of either the M or the L pigment gene reduces the retina so that it contains two, not three, types of cone pigment and consequently limits the individual to a dichromatic form of color vision.

C. Evolution of Human Color Vision

In recent years, the study of color vision in nonhuman species has expanded greatly, as has our view of the nature of opsin genes and photopigments in a host of different species. This has begun to allow an understanding of the evolution of human color vision. Comparison of opsin gene sequences indicates that visual pigments have an ancient origin and that there is evidence for the presence of two separate cone pigments very early in vertebrate history (perhaps as long as 400 million years ago). This arrangement would have provided the necessary basis for a dichromatic color vision system, although there is currently no way of knowing if that potential was actually realized. The nature of color vision and the physiology that allows for color vision vary significantly among present-day vertebrates. As previously mentioned, humans normally have three classes of cone pigment

and trichromatic color vision. The retinas of many fishes, reptiles, and birds contain at least four classes of cone pigment, and there is evidence to support the conclusion that these may well provide a four-variable form of color vision—a tetrachromacy. On the other hand, the retinas of most mammals (e.g., domestic dogs and cats) contain only two types of cone pigment allowing a basic dichromacy. This difference has led to the hypothesis that the potential for a sophisticated form of color vision was lost sometime early in mammalian history. Among mammals, the presence of three types of cone pigment and trichromatic color vision is restricted to primates. From this fact, it can be concluded that our exceptional color vision sense appeared during the evolution of primates.

Comparison of opsin genes and color vision in Old World primates (in particular, Old World monkeys, apes, and humans) and in New World monkeys indicates that the essential change from a basically dichromatic form of color vision to uniform trichromatic color vision occurred shortly after the divergence of Old World and New World primates approximately 30–40 million years ago. The means for accomplishing this was an X chromosome opsin gene duplication that yielded two separate M and L genes. Whether that duplication arose from identical X chromosome genes that eventually diverged in structure or whether it was built from the baseline of a polymorphism at a single gene site is not clear. In any case, the origins of human trichromacy can be traced to changes that first appeared in the retinas of our early primate ancestors. An important consequence of this is that human color vision is very similar in its detail to the color vision enjoyed by all contemporary Old World monkeys and apes.

D. Neural Mechanisms for Color Vision in the Retina

As noted previously, the human retina contains multiple types of cone photopigment. Multiple cone types are a necessary but not sufficient basis to support a color vision capacity. In addition, there must also be an appropriately organized nervous system. The extraction of information that allows for color vision begins in the neural networks of the retina.

In addition to the photoreceptors, there are four other major classes of nerve cell in the retina: bipolar, ganglion, horizontal, and amacrine cells. These form intricately organized vertical and horizontal possessing networks arrayed through the thickness of the retina with bipolar and ganglion cells serving as the principal vertical pathway and the other two types providing a rich array of horizontally organized connections. Each of the four types of cell in turn consists of discrete subtypes. Currently, a majority of the latter are poorly defined, both structurally and functionally, but it is believed that it will eventually be possible to characterize as many as 50 distinct types of cells in the primate retina. The main business of the networks formed by these cells is to perform the first stages in the processing of the retinal image. These tasks include the analysis of local spatial and temporal variations and the regulation of visual sensitivity. The processing of color information proceeds in the context of all these other analyses.

Because each cone type behaves univariantly, the extraction of color information requires the comparison of the signals from cone types containing different photopigments. There are two principal ways in which cone signal information is combined in the nervous system: additively (spectrally nonopponent) or subtractively (spectrally opponent). Cells of the former type sum signals from the L and M cone types (L + M). Because they do not respond differentially to wavelength differences irrespective of the relative intensity, cells so wired cannot transmit information useful for the production of color vision. The response properties of spectrally opponent cells are produced by convergence of excitatory and inhibitory signals onto recipient nerve cells. The cone signal combinations are classified into two main groups: L−M and (L + M)−S (for each of these types the signs can be reversed, i.e., there are both L−M and M−L types). Response profiles for opponent and nonopponent cells are shown in Fig. 4. It can be seen that, unlike the nonopponent cells, spectrally opponent cells will yield different responses to different wavelengths of light irrespective of the relative intensities of those lights. They thus can transmit information that may be useful for supporting color vision. With regard to color information, the output cells of the retina (the ganglion cells) are classified into three groups: those that transmit nonopponent information into the central nervous system, those carrying M−L information, and those whose response patterns are (M + L)−S (Fig. 4). Much is known about the anatomy of such cells and the input pathways that yield these different response patterns.

Several structural and functional properties of the retina map are directly mapped into the quality of human color vision. For example, S cones are sparsely distributed across the retina and are absent entirely from its very central portion (the fovea). A consequence is that the color information contributed from S cone signal pathways is lost for stimuli that are very small (i.e., trichromacy gives way to dichromacy under such viewing conditions). The connection pathways from the L and M cones also vary across the retina. Although the picture is still somewhat controversial, in general there is an observed decrease in the relative potency of L/M spectrally opponent signals toward the peripheral parts of the retina. This decrease is presumed to be a factor in the gradual decline in sensitivity of red/green color vision for stimuli located away from the direction of gaze. Finally, due to variations in the neural circuitry, there are significant differences in the spatial and temporal sensitivities of the different types of retinal cells. One consequence of this is that our color vision becomes progressively more restricted for regions in the visual scene that are very small and/or are changing very rapidly. Thus, human color vision is trichromatic only for relatively large and slowly changing stimuli, giving way to dichromatic color vision as the space/time components of the stimulus are increased and, eventually, one can lose color vision entirely (i.e., become monochromatic) for very small and/or very rapidly changing stimuli.

III. THE CENTRAL VISUAL SYSTEM AND COLOR

Behavioral studies of vision have led to a consensus view that the facts of human color vision can best be understood as reflecting the operation of three separate mechanisms. These mechanisms are conceived as implying the presence of three parallel channels of information in the central visual system. Two of these are opponent channels reflecting, respectively, the mutual antagonisms of red and green and of yellow and blue. The third is a nonopponent channel that provides achromatic information (the luminance mechanism). The spectrally opponent and nonopponent cells of the type described previously were first recorded approximately 40 years ago not in the retina but in the lateral geniculate nucleus (LGN), which is a large thalamic structure that serves as a relay site situated in the central visual pathway between the retina and the visual cortex. Following the discovery of these cells it was immediately recognized that there is a compelling analogy between the physiological results and the behavioral conception of the color mechanisms. Thus, the L−M cells and the (L + M)−S cells

(Fig. 4) have many characteristic features that appear to be like those of the behaviorally defined red/green and yellow/blue color channels. Similarly, the $L+M$ cells have the appropriate spectral sensitivity as well as many other features that appear to make them ideal candidates to serve as the luminance mechanism.

Over time, however, closer examination of the relationships between the standard behavioral model and the physiological results has revealed a lack of complete correspondence between the two, and this forced a reevaluation of the idea that the spectrally opponent cells of the retina and LGN directly represent the color mechanisms documented in behavioral experiments. To note just one problem, consider the perceptual observation that the spectrum takes on a distinctly reddish appearance in the short wavelengths (this can be seen in the hue naming results of Fig. 3C). Among color vision theorists, the conventional explanation for this fact is that the red/green color mechanism must receive some signals from the S cones. However, electrophysiological studies indicate that the $L-M$ cells do not have an S cone input so they cannot directly account for this feature of red/green color vision. Many other disparities between the behavioral aspects of human color vision and the physiology of cells located early in the visual pathway have also been enumerated. The inevitable conclusion is that although the spectrally opponent cells clearly transmit the information necessary for color vision, the response properties of these cells cannot directly account for many features of human color vision. This means that there must be some further transformations of the signals provided by spectrally opponent cells and those transformations are assumed to take place somewhere in the visual cortex.

The picture of how color information is processed and elaborated in the visual cortex is still very sketchy. Researchers have tried to understand how color information is encoded by cortical neurons, and they have pursued the hypothesis that color processing might be localized to particular component regions of the cortex. Analysis of the response properties of single cortical cells has been avidly pursued. Unfortunately, the results have led to conflicting views as to how cortical cells encode color information. This is understandable since the task is far from simple. Much of the difficulty arises from the fact that although the responses of cells in the retina and in the LGN are only modestly dependent on the spatial and temporal features of the stimulus, the responses of cortical cells are very much conditioned by these properties. The consequence is that studies utilizing differing spatio-temporal stimulus features have often reached quite different conclusions about the nature of cortical color coding. What is known, both from single cell studies conducted on monkeys and imaging studies of human brains, is that color-selective responses can indeed be recorded in primary visual cortex (area V-1) and at other locations in the extrastriate cortex. Studies also make clear that transformations of the spectrally opponent responses of LGN cells do occur in V-1 and that such transformations arise, at least in part, from dynamic interactions between cortical cells. For example, neural feedback circuits may significantly amplify contributions from signals originating in S cones relative to those S cone signals recorded at more peripheral locations. Such a change brings the physiological picture more in line with behavioral measures of color vision. Similarly, at least some cells in V-1 are known to combine signals from the two classes of LGN spectrally opponent cells. This too brings the physiology closer to the coding scheme inferred from behavioral studies of color vision. Although the relationships between cortical codes for color and psychophysical models of color coding are not clear, significant progress is being made toward their rationalization.

For years it has been argued that the processing of color information can be localized in the extrastriate visual cortex. From studies of both monkey and human brains, regions in the lingual and fusiform gyrus (sometimes characterized as area V-4) have been identified as particularly important for color. In humans this area responds robustly to the presentation of stimuli designed to specifically probe color vision, and it has been reported that cells in monkey area V-4 exhibit some forms of color constancy. Providing additional support for the idea of localized cortical representation of color are clinical descriptions of patients who have suffered a loss of color vision as a result of cortical damage (cerebral achromatopsia). The nature of the color vision loss in cerebral achromatopsia is complex and beyond the scope of this article. For our purposes, the important fact is that although the locus of damage that results in cerebral achromatopsia varies significantly among described cases, it most often does include area V-4.

IV. VARIATIONS IN HUMAN COLOR VISION

In 1794, John Dalton, the celebrated chemist, offered a series of astute observations about his own color perceptions. He noted, for instance, that the spectrum appeared to him to contain just three colors (yellow, blue, and purple) and that flowers that appeared pink to others seemed to him "an exact sky blue." Dalton eventually discovered that many other individuals shared his atypical color perceptions and he was led to offer a hypothesis to explain the condition based on the presumed presence of some unusual intraocular filter. Retrospective analysis shows that Dalton suffered from deuteranopia, a common congenital color vision defect that affects about 1% of all males. Dalton was not the first to learn of defective color vision among humans, and his explanation of the source of the defect was wrong, but his detailed descriptions were very instrumental in initiating a long series of examinations of color defect that continue to the present day. Studies of color vision defects, and of other individual variations in color vision, have provided significant insights into the biology of color vision. In addition to the congenital color vision defects, color vision change may be acquired through a wide variety of visual system pathologies as well as senescent changes occurring in the visual system.

A. Congenital Color Vision Defects

There are many distinct types of congenital color defect and each yields a characteristic pattern of results on behavioral tests of color vision (these include both laboratory tests of the kinds described previously and the familiar plate tests used for the clinical screening of color vision). Those most severely impacted have dichromatic color vision, like that of John Dalton. When tested in color matching experiments of the sort described previously, such individuals require only two primary lights to complete all the color matches. The number of discrete color discriminations that can be made is also severely reduced. For instance, in the wavelength discrimination test (Fig. 3B), dichromats basically fail to discriminate among wavelengths in the middle to long wavelengths while retaining an ability to discriminate wavelengths shorter than approximately 490–500 nm from wavelengths longer than that value. As a result, they are commonly characterized as "red/green color blind." This is a somewhat misleading description since dichromats are not blind to color in this part of the spectrum: Rather, they simply fail to discriminate among these colors. The full gamut of saturations that dichromats see is also significantly smaller than that seen by people with normal trichro-

matic color vision. There are two major types of congenital dichromacy, protanopia and deuteranopia. Individuals of the two types differ both in the details of color discriminations they can make and in their spectral sensitivity.

In addition to the dichromacies, there are also trichromatic individuals whose color vision nevertheless differs significantly from normal trichromacy. These people are said to have anomalous trichromatic color vision and, like the dichromats, their color vision defects can be detected by color discrimination tests. Anomalous trichromats are of major two types: protanomalous and deuteranomalous. An essential difference between the two types emerges from a simple color matching task in which an individual is asked to complete a color match by adding green and red lights in proportion to match a yellow test light. Dichromats so tested fail to set a reliable match since they cannot discriminate among colors in this part of the spectrum. All trichromatic individuals can make such matches. Relative to the normal, the protanomalous observer will require additional red light to complete the match, whereas the deuteranomalous individual needs additional green light. A wide range of other discrimination tests can be similarly used to distinguish among the trichromatic subtypes. Although the trichromatic anomalies are usually classified as color vision defects, it is important to note that in fact many anomalous trichromats have quite acute color vision.

Individuals with these congenital defects thus differ significantly from those with normal color vision in their discrimination abilities. What do they actually see? This intriguing question has not been easy to answer. Growing up as a minority in a color-coded world, most color defectives acquire a rich vocabulary of color names that they learn to use in a discerning fashion. They can do this because there are many secondary cues to allow one to apply color names in accord with the majority view (e.g., familiar objects are often characteristically colored and objects of different color often have systematic brightness differences). It is only when these secondary cues become scarce or disappear entirely (as they do in formal tests of color vision) that color defect become readily apparent. Some insights into the color world of the color defective come from examination of the occasional individual who has defective color vision in one eye and normal color vision in the other. Similarly, inferences can be drawn from comparison of the discrimination abilities of the normal and the color defective. These pieces of evidence suggest that the two major types of dichromat view the world in what to the normal would be varying shades of only two hues—blues and yellows. Furthermore, there are significant losses in the saturation of lights so that the perceptual world of the dichromat is distinctly pallid relative to that of the normal. Recently, computer algorithms have been developed that allow one to transform a digitized colored image to obtain a perceptual prediction of the dichromatic world. Although defective color vision is often treated as a benign condition, there is documented evidence to indicate that those who have defective color vision find that it provides a real barrier in many aspects of normal life—from things as mundane as making judgments about the ripeness of a piece of fruit to issues as far reaching as a choice of a profession.

A vast majority of those with defective color vision are male. The incidence of defective color vision among males is given in Table I. In total, approximately 8% of the in Western Europe and in the United States can be classified into one or another of these diagnostic categories with 5% of all males having deuteranomalous color vision. The incidence of red/green defective color vision is low in females, being approximately the square of the frequency of the corresponding male color vision defects.

There are also rare congenital color vision defects that arise from change or alteration in the ability to discriminate among short-wavelength lights (tritanopia and tritanomaly). The incidences of these defects do not differ for male and females. Finally, in addition to dichromats and anomalous trichromats, a relatively few individuals lack color vision completely (are monochromatic) or only show an ability to discriminate color in very restricted test circumstances.

B. The Biology of Congenital Color Defects

Protanopia, deuteranopia, protanomaly, and deuteranomaly all arise from changes in the X chromosome opsin genes. As noted previously, unequal recombination events that occur during meiosis can lead to additions and losses of genes from the X chromosome as well as to the production of novel genes (Fig. 5). Thus, a loss of the L cone opsin produces a protanopic dichromacy; loss of the M opsin yields deuteranopia. On the other hand, the anomalous trichromacies reflect the genomic presence of atypical opsin genes. In these cases, a new pigment replaces either the normal M pigment (in cases of deuteranomaly) or the normal L pigment (in protanomaly). The spectrum of

Table I
Incidence of Congenital Defective Color Vision among Caucasian Males[a]

Diagnostic category	%
Protanopia	1.0
Deuteranopia	1.1
Tritanopia	0.001
Protanomaly	1.0
Deuteranomaly	4.9
Monochromacy	0.003

[a]The incidence values are based on large-scale surveys of defective color vision and should be considered approximate.

this new pigment is shifted so as to be closer to that of the other (normal) M or L pigment. Depending on which of several atypical genes is present, the spectral separation of the M and L pigments is made either greater or smaller and severity of the color vision defect is correspondingly more or less. Only females that are homozygous for these defective X chromosome opsin genes show classical indications of these red/green color defects, thus explaining why the frequency of defective color vision in females is low. Pedigrees of color vision defects have long indicated that in the usual case sons inherit a color defect from mothers who carry a defective gene but who have normal color vision. The tritan defects similarly result from changes in S opsin genes. Since these represent changes in autosomal genes, the incidences of these defects do not differ for males and females. The biology underlying the complete loss of color vision is not straightforward and, in different cases, is apparently traceable to either photopigment or nervous system alterations.

Surveys indicate that the incidence of defective color vision varies significantly among different population groups. The highest frequencies are found in the United States and Western Europe, where approximately 7–9% of all males show a form of red/green color vision defect. Elsewhere, the incidence is often lower. For instance, several populations have been reported to show comparable defects in only about 1% of the males. These regional/ethnic differences have received various interpretations, perhaps the most popular being that the higher rates of defect are found in those populations in which there has been a relaxation of natural selection pressure against color vision defects. According to this view, those societies that are least altered from their hunter/gatherer origins should have the lowest incidences of defective color

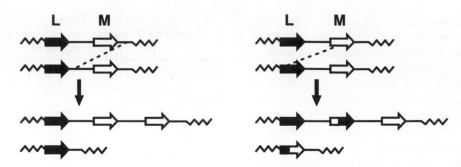

Figure 5 X chromosome gene combinations leading to defective color vision. Arrows represent genes for M and L cone opsins. Illustrated are two examples of unequal recombinations that yield new gene arrays. The dashed lines indicate where crossing over occurs during meiosis. (Left) The unequal crossover yields two new gene arrays, one with an L opsin gene and two copies of the M opsin gene. This genotype is common in individuals having normal color vision. The second result is a deletion of the M cone opsin gene. A male with this genotype would have dichromatic color vision. (Right) The crossovers occur within the gene. This produces new genes whose pigment products will differ from those of the normal M and L opsin genes, and depending on the resultant combination of genes the effects on color vision can be subtle or drastic.

vision. There is no compelling evidence to support this idea, but neither can it be flatly rejected.

C. Subtle Variations in Human Color Vision

The differences in color vision between normal trichromats and various color defectives are major and dramatic, but there are also reliable differences in color vision among individuals within each of these groups and study of these small variations can provide a useful tool for understanding the biological basis of color vision. One particular example comes from the study of variations in the color matching among normal trichromats. In a standard version of the color-matching task, people are asked to adjust the proportions of red and green primaries to match a yellow test light (with lights drawn from this part of the spectrum, trichromats make dichromatic matches). Color discrimination is particularly acute for lights from this part of the spectrum and, consequently, subjects make extremely reliable matches. It has long been known that individual matches may differ in that some people consistently require relatively more red light to complete the match, and others need relatively more green light. As previously explained, differences in color matches mostly arise from differences in the spectral positioning of the retinal photopigments, so an implication is that individuals who make different color matches must have different photopigments.

In recent years, the biological basis of this small variation in color matching has been uncovered. As predicted, it reflects the fact that normal human trichromats show small variations in the spectral positioning of their photopigments. Unexpectedly

however, the variation is not continuously distributed in the population but rather appears to have a discrete character. This variation has been shown to result principally from a polymorphism in the gene specifying the L cone opsin. This polymorphism, involving a difference of only a single nucleotide, in turn causes a variation in a single amino acid in the photopigment molecule and thus there are two forms of the L cone pigment. This variation allows the L cone pigment to occupy either one of two spectral positions, with the two varying in their λ_{max} values by about 4 nm. A male who has the longer of the two pigment versions will require systematically less red light in the color match than will a male who has the shorter of the two pigments. These two polymorphic variants of the L cone opsin gene are nearly equally represented in the population. It is remarkable that this very small genetic variation sorts individuals of normal color vision into groups that go through life experiencing the colors of the world as biased to appear either slightly redder or slightly greener.

See Also the Following Articles

EYE MOVEMENTS • MULTISENSORY INTEGRATION • SENSORY DEPRIVATION • SPATIAL VISION • VISION: BRAIN MECHANISMS • VISUAL DISORDERS • VISUAL SYSTEM DEVELOPMENT AND NEURAL ACTIVITY

Suggested Reading

Abramov, I., and Gordon, J. (1994). Color appearance: On seeing red—or yellow, or green, or blue. *Annu. Rev. Psychol.* **45**, 451–485.

Backhaus, W. G. K., Kliegl, R., and Werner, J. S. (Eds.) (1998). *Color Vision—Perspectives from Different Disciplines.* de Gruyter, Berlin.

Dacey, D. M. (1999). Primate retina: Cell types, circuits and color opponency. *Prog. Ret. Eye Res.* **18,** 737–763.

Foster, D. H. (Ed.) (1991). *Inherited and Acquired Colour Vision Deficiencies.* Macmillan, London.

Gegenfurtner, K. R., and Sharpe, L. T. (Eds.) (1999). *Color Vision: From Genes to Perception.* Cambridge Univ. Press, Cambridge, UK.

Gouras, P. (Ed.) (1991). *The Perception of Color.* CRC Press, Boca Raton, FL.

Jacobs, G. H. (1993). The distribution and nature of colour vision among the mammals. *Biol. Rev.* **68,** 413–471.

Kaiser, P. K., and Boynton, R. M. (1996). *Human Color Vision,* 2nd ed. Optical Society of America, Washington, DC.

Komatsu, H. (1998). Mechanisms of central color vision. *Curr. Opin. Neurobiol.* **8,** 503–508.

Lamb, R., and Bourriau, J. (Eds.) (1995). *Colour: Art & Science.* Cambridge Univer. Press, Cambridge, UK.

Martin, P. R. (1998). Colour processing in the retina: Recent progress. *J. Physiol.* **513,** 631–638.

Nathans, J. (1999). The evolution and physiology of human color vision: Insights from molecular genetic studies of visual pigments. *Neuron* **24,** 299–312.

Neitz, M., and Neitz, J. (2000). Molecular genetics of color vision and color vision defects. *Arch. Ophthalmol.* **118,** 691–700.

Wandell, B. A. (1995). *Foundations of Vision.* Sinauer, Sunderland, MA.

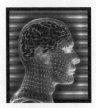

Consciousness

MICHAEL S. GAZZANIGA
Dartmouth College

I. The "Interpreter"

II. Anosagnosia and Paramnesia

III. Creating Our Autobiography

Just what is consciousness? The answer, I believe, is that consciousness is an instinct—a built-in property of brains. Like all instincts, it is just there. You do not learn to be conscious and you cannot unlearn the reality of conscious experience. Someday we will achieve a more mechanistic understanding of its operation, but I warn you now: That won't be especially fulfilling on a personal level. We have to shed our expectation that a scientific understanding of consciousness will sweep away our sense of strangeness, like finding out how ships get in bottles. Take our reproductive instinct. Does it help our sense of desire to understand the role of testosterone when we see a shapely figure across the room? Or take the human instinct for language. Does it help us to enjoy language if we understand that grammar is a universal built-in reflex but that our lexicon is learned? Understanding the problem of consciousness may be essential to our ultimate ability to deal with some mental disorders. Disorders of conscious experience, whether autism or schizophrenia or dementia, will be illuminated by a mechanistic understanding of personal conscious experience.

My own thinking on this topic started early, in Roger Sperry's laboratory at the California Institute of Technology on an afternoon almost 40 years ago, when I first tested a split-brain patient. It seemed that,

whatever consciousness was, you could have two of them after the surgical severy of the corpus callosum connecting the two cerebral hemispheres. Mind Left did not appear to know about Mind Right and vice versa. Those first impressions, which still endure, nevertheless left much to be desired as a sophisticated perspective on the question of consciousness. My plight as a researcher echoed Tom Wolfe's admonition to practice writing for 20 years before you seek a publisher.

Classic split-brain research highlighted how the left brain and the right brain serve distinctive functions and led us to believe that the brain is a collection of modules. The left brain (or hemisphere) is specialized not only for language and speech but also for intelligent behavior. After the human cerebral hemispheres are disconnected, the patient's verbal IQ remains intact and his problem-solving capacity (as observed in hypothesis formation tasks) remains unchanged for the left hemisphere. Indeed, that hemisphere seems to remain unchanged from its presurgical capacity. Yet the largely disconnected right hemisphere, which is the same size as the left, becomes seriously impoverished for many cognitive tasks. While it remains superior to the left hemisphere in certain activities (in recognizing upright faces, having better skills in paying attention, and perhaps in expressing emotions), it is poorer after separation at problem solving and many other mental activities.

Apparently the left brain has modules specialized for higher cognitive functions, while the right has modules specialized for other functions. Visuospatial function, for example, is generally more acute in the right hemisphere, but left hemisphere integration may be needed to perform higher order tasks. The use of

This article is reproduced from Gazzaniga, M. S. (1999). The interpreter within: The glue of conscious experience. *Cerebrum* **1**(1). with permission of the Dana Foundation.

tactile information to build spatial representations of abstract shapes appears to be better developed in the right hemisphere, but tasks such as the Block Design test, which are typically associated with the right parietal lobe, appear to require integration between the hemispheres in some patients. Furthermore, even though the right hemisphere is better able to analyze unfamiliar facial information than is the left hemisphere, and the left is better able to generate voluntary facial expressions, both hemispheres can generate facial expression when spontaneous emotions are expressed.

In addition to the skills named previously, our big human brains have hundreds if not thousands more individual capacities. Our uniquely human skills may well be produced by minute, circumscribed neuronal networks, sometimes referred to as "modules," but our highly modularized brain generates a feeling in all of us that we are integrated and unified. If we are merely a collection of specialized modules, how does that powerful, almost self-evident feeling come about?

I. THE "INTERPRETER"

The answer appears to be that we have a specialized left hemisphere system that my colleagues and I call the "interpreter." This interpreter is a device (or system or mechanism) that seeks explanations for why events occur. The advantage of having such a system is obvious. By going beyond simply observing contiguous events to asking why they happened, a brain can cope with such events more effectively should they happen again.

We revealed the interpreter in an experiment using a "simultaneous concept test." The split-brain patient is shown two pictures, one presented exclusively to his left hemisphere, one exclusively to his right. He is then asked to choose from an array of pictures the ones he associates with the pictures that were presented (or "lateralized") to his left brain and his right brain. In one example of this, a picture of a chicken claw was flashed to the left hemisphere and a picture of a snow scene to the right. Of the array of pictures then placed in front of the subject, the obviously correct association was a chicken for the chicken claw and a shovel for the snow scene. Split-brain subject case 1 did respond by choosing the shovel with his left hand and the chicken with his right. Thus each hemisphere picked the correct answer.

Now the experimenter asked the left-speaking hemisphere why those objects were picked. (Remember, it would only know why the left hemisphere had picked the shovel; it would not know why the disconnected right brain had picked the shovel.) His left hemisphere replied, "Oh, that's simple. The chicken claw goes with the chicken, and you need a shovel to clean out the chicken shed." In other words, the left brain, observing the left hand's response, interprets the response in a context consistent with its own sphere of knowledge —one that does not include information about the snow scene presented to the other side of the brain.

One can influence the left-brain interpreter in many ways. As I mentioned, we wanted to know whether the emotional response to stimuli presented to half of the brain would influence the emotional tone of the other half. Using an optical computer system that detects the slightest eye movement, we projected an emotion-laden movie to the right hemisphere. (If the patient tried to cheat and move the eye toward the movie, it was electronically shut off.)

When we did this experiment with case 2, the movie that her right hemisphere saw was about a vicious man pushing another off a balcony and then throwing a firebomb on top of him. The movie then showed other men trying to put the fire out. When V. P. was first tested on this problem, she could not access speech from her right hemisphere. She was able to speak only out of her left brain. When asked what she had seen, her left brain (the half brain that had not actually seen the movie) replied, "I don't really know what I saw. I think just a white flash." When I asked, "Were there people in it?" case 2, replied, "I don't think so. Maybe just some trees, red trees like in the fall." I asked, "Did it make you feel any emotion?" and V. P. answered, "I don't really know why, but I'm kind of scared. I feel jumpy. I think maybe I don't like this room, or maybe it's you; you're getting me nervous." She turned to one of the research assistants and said, "I know I like Dr. Gazzaniga, but right now I'm scared of him for some reason."

This kind of effect is common to all of us. A mental system that is operating outside the conscious realm of the left hemisphere's interpreter generates a mood that alters the general physiology of the brain. Because the alteration in brain physiology is general, the interpreter is able to note the mood and immediately attributes some cause to it. This is a powerful mechanism; once clearly seen, it makes one wonder how often we are victims of spurious emotional/cognitive correlations.

Our recent investigations have looked further at the properties of the interpreter and how it influences mental skills. For example, there are hemisphere-specific changes in the accuracy of memory processes. Specifically, the predilection of the left hemisphere to interpret events has an impact on the accuracy of memory. When subjects are presented with pictures representing common events (e.g., getting up in the morning or making cookies) and several hours later asked to say if pictures in another series appeared in the first, both hemispheres are equally accurate in recognizing the previously viewed pictures and rejecting the unrelated ones. Only the right hemisphere, however, correctly rejects pictures in the second set that were not previously viewed but were related to pictures previously viewed. The left hemisphere incorrectly "recalls" significantly more of these related pictures as having occurred in the first set, presumably because they fit into the schema it has constructed. This finding is consistent with the hypothesis that a left hemisphere interpreter constructs theories to assimilate perceived information into a comprehensible whole. In doing so, however, the process of elaborating (story making) has a deleterious effect on the accuracy of perceptual recognition. This result has been shown with verbal as well as visual material.

A recent example of the interpreter can be found in studies of case 3, a split-brain patient who can speak out of his right hemisphere as well as his left. His naming of stimuli in the left field seems to be increasing at a rapid rate. Although there is no convincing evidence of any genuine visual transfer between the hemispheres, during trials when J. W. was certain of the name of the stimulus, he maintained that he saw it well. On trials when he was not certain of the name of the stimulus, he maintained that he did not see it well. This is consistent with the view that the left hemisphere interpreter actively constructs a mental portrait of past experience, even though that experience did not directly occur in that hemisphere. This experience was probably caused by the left hemisphere's interpreter giving meaning to right hemisphere spoken responses, possibly by activating the left hemisphere mental imagery systems.

The left hemisphere's capacity for continual interpretation may mean that it is always looking for order and reason, even where there is none. This came out dramatically in a study by George Wolford and me. On a simple test that requires one to guess if a light is going to appear on the top or the bottom of a computer screen, we humans perform in an inventive way. The experiment manipulates the stimulus to appear on the top 80% of the time. While it quickly becomes evident that the top button is being illuminated more often, we keep trying to figure out the whole sequence—and

deeply believe that we can. We persist even if, by adopting this strategy, we are rewarded only 68% of the time (whereas if we guessed "top" repeatedly, by rote, we would be rewarded 80% of the time). Rats and other animals are more likely to learn to maximize their score by pressing only the top button! Our right hemisphere behaves more like the rats. It does not try to interpret its experience to find the deeper meaning; it lives only in the thin moment of the present. But when the left brain is asked to explain why it is attempting to psych out the whole sequence, it always comes up with a theory, however spurious.

II. ANOSAGNOSIA AND PARAMNESIA

Neurology yields weird examples of how the interpreter can work, and understanding the interpreter increases our insight into some bizarre syndromes. Take, for example, a malady called "anosagnosia," in which a person denies awareness of a problem he has. People who suffer from right parietal lesions that render them hemiplegic and blind on their left side frequently deny that they have any problem. The left half of their body, they insist, is simply not theirs. They see their paralyzed left hand but maintain that it has nothing to do with them. How could this be?

Consider what may happen as a result of a lesion in a person's optic tract. If the lesion is in a nerve that carries information about vision to the visual cortex, the damaged nerve ceases to carry that information; the patient complains that he is blind in part of his visual field. For example, such a patient might have a huge blind spot to the left of the center of his visual field. He rightly complains. If another patient, however, has a lesion not in the optic tract but in the visual cortex, creating a blind spot of the same size and in the same place, he does not complain at all. The reason is that the cortical lesion is in the place in his brain that represents that exact part of the visual world, the place that ordinarily would ask, "What is going on to the left of visual center?" In the case of the lesion on the optic nerve, this brain area was functioning; when it could not get any information from the nerve, it put up a squawk—something is wrong. When that same brain area is itself lesioned, the patient's brain no longer cares about what is going on in that part of the visual field; there is no squawk at all. The patient with the central lesion does not have a complaint because the part of the brain that might complain has been incapacitated, and no other can take over.

As we move farther into the brain's processing centers, we see the same pattern, but now the problem is with the interpretive function. The parietal cortex is where the brain represents how an arm is functioning, constantly seeking information on the arm's whereabouts, its position in three-dimensional space. The parietal cortex monitors the arm's existence in relation to everything else. If there is a lesion to sensory nerves that bring information to the brain about where the arm is, what is in its hand, or whether it is in pain or feels hot or cold, the brain communicates that something is wrong: "I am not getting input." But if the lesion is in the parietal cortex, that monitoring function is gone and no squawk is raised, though the squawker is damaged.

Now let us consider our case of anosagnosia, and the disowned left hand. A patient with a right parietal lesion suffers damage to the area that represents the left half of the body. The brain area cannot feel the state of the left hand. When a neurologist holds a patient's left hand up to the patient's face, the patient gives a reasonable response: "That's not my hand, pal." The interpreter, which is intact and working, cannot get news from the parietal lobe since the flow of information has been disrupted by the lesion. For the interpreter, the left hand simply does not exist anymore, just as seeing behind the head is not something the interpreter is supposed to worry about. It is true, then, that the hand held in front of him cannot be his. What is the mystery?

An even more fascinating syndrome is called "reduplicative paramnesia." In one such case studied by the author, the patient was a women who, although she was being examined in my office at New York Hospital, claimed we were in her home in Freeport, Maine. The standard interpretation of this syndrome is that the patient has made a duplicate copy of a place (or person) and insists that there are two.

This woman was intelligent; before the interview she was biding her time reading the *New York Times*. I started with the "so, where are you?" question. "I am in Freeport, Maine. I know you don't believe it. Dr. Posner told me this morning when he came to see me that I was in Memorial Sloan–Kettering Hospital and that when the residents come on rounds to say that to them. Well, that is fine, but I know I am in my house on Main Street in Freeport, Maine!" I asked, "Well, if you are in Freeport and in your house, how come there are elevators outside the door here?" The grand lady peered at me and calmly responded, "Doctor, do you know how much it cost me to have those put in?"

This patient has a perfectly fine interpreter working away trying to make sense of what she knows and feels and does. Because of her lesion, the part of the brain that represents locality is overactive and sending out an erroneous message about her location. The interpreter is only as good as the information it receives, and in this instance it is getting a wacky piece of information. Yet the interpreter still has to field questions and make sense of other incoming information—information that to the interpreter is self-evident. The result? It creates a lot of imaginative stories.

III. CREATING OUR AUTOBIOGRAPHY

The interpreter's talents can be viewed on a larger canvas. I began this article by observing our deep belief that we can attain not only a neuroscience of consciousness but also a neuroscience of human consciousness. It is as if something wonderfully new and complex happens as the brain enlarges to its full human form. Whatever happens (and I think it is the emergence of the interpreter module), it triggers our capacity for self-reflection and all that goes with it. How do we account for this?

I would like to make a simple, three-step suggestion. First, focus on what we mean when we talk about "conscious experience." I believe this is merely the awareness we have of our capacities as a species—awareness not of the capacities themselves but of our experience of exercising them and our feelings about them. The brain is clearly not a general-purpose computing device; it is a collection of circuits devoted to these specific capacities. This is true for all brains, but what is amazing about the human brain is the sheer number of capacities. We have more than the chimp, which has more than the monkey, which has more than the cat, which runs circles around the rat. Because we have so many specialized systems, and because they may sometimes operate in ways that are difficult to assign to a given system or group of them, it may seem as though our brains have a single, general computing device. But they do not. Step one is to recognize that we are a collection of adaptive brain systems and, further, to recognize the distinction between a species' capacities and how it experiences them.

Now consider step two. Can there be any doubt that a rat at the moment of copulation is as sensorially fulfilled as a human? Of course it is. Do you think a cat does not enjoy a good piece of cod? Of course it does.

Or a monkey does not enjoy a spectacular swing? Again, it has to be true. Each species is aware of its special capacities. So what is human consciousness? It is awareness of the very same kind, except that we can be aware of so much more, so many wonderful things. A circuit, perhaps a single system or one duplicated again and again, is associated with each brain capacity. The more systems a brain possesses, the greater our awareness of capacities.

Think of the variations in capacity within our own species; they are not unlike the vast differences between species. Years of split-brain research have shown that the left hemisphere has many more mental capacities than the right. The left is capable of logical feats that the right cannot manage. Even with both our hemispheres, however, the limits to human capacity are everywhere in the population. No one need be offended to realize that some people with normal intelligence can understand Ohm's law, while others, such as yours truly, are clueless about hundreds of mathematical concepts. I do not understand them and never will; the circuits that would enable me to understand them are not in my brain.

When we realize that specialized brain circuits arose through natural selection, we understand that the brain is not a unified neural net that supports a general problem-solving device. If we accept this, we can concentrate on the possibility that smaller, more manageable circuits produce awareness of a species' capacities. By contrast, holding fast to the notion of a unified neural net forces us to try to understand human conscious experience by figuring out the interactions of billions of neurons. That task is hopeless. My scheme is not.

Hence step three. The same split-brain research that exposed startling differences between the two hemispheres revealed as well that the human left hemisphere harbors our interpreter. Its job is to interpret our responses—cognitive or emotional—to what we encounter in our environment. The interpreter sustains a running narrative of our actions, emotions, thoughts, and dreams. The interpreter is the glue that keeps our story unified and creates our sense of being a coherent, rational agent. To our bag of individual instincts, it brings theories about our life.

These narratives of our past behavior seep into our awareness; they give us an autobiography. Insertion of an interpreter into an otherwise functioning brain creates many by-products. A device that begins by asking how one thing relates to another, a device that asks about an infinite number of things, in fact, and that can get productive answers to its questions, cannot help giving birth to the concept of self. Surely one question the device would ask is "Who is solving all these problems?" "Let's call it me"—and away it goes! A device with rules for figuring out how one thing relates to another will quickly be reinforced for having that capacity, just as an ant's solving where to have its evening meal reinforces the ant's food-seeking devices. In other words, once mutational events in the history of our species had brought the interpreter into existence, there would be no getting rid of it.

Our brains are automatic because physical tissue carries out what we do. How could it be otherwise? Our brains are operating before our conceptual self knows it. But the conceptual self emerges and grows until it is able to find interesting—but not disheartening—the biological fact that our brain does things before we are consciously aware of them. The interpretation of things that we encounter has liberated us from a sense of being determined by our environment; it has created the wonderful sense that our self is in charge of our destiny. All of our everyday success at reasoning through life's data convinces us of this. And because of the interpreter within us, we can drive our automatic brains to greater accomplishment and enjoyment of life.

See Also the Following Articles

EMOTION • EVOLUTION OF THE BRAIN • UNCONSCIOUS, THE

Suggested Reading

Crick, F., and Koch, C. (1998). Consciousness and neuroscience. *Cerebral Cortex* **8**(2), 97–107.
Dennett, D. (1991). *Consciousness Explained*. Little, Brown, Boston.
Gazzaniga, M. S. (1998). *The Mind's Past*. Univ. of California Press, Berkeley.
Searle, J. (1984). *Minds, brains, and science*. Harvard University Press, Cambridge.
Tononi, G., and Edelman, G. M. (1998). Consciousness and complexity. *Science* **282**, 1856–1851.

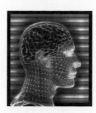

Conversion Disorders and Somatoform Disorders

RICHARD J. BROWN and MARIA A. RON

Institute of Neurology and National Hospital for Neurology and Neurosurgery, United Kingdom

GLOSSARY

conversion Putative psychological process whereby emotional distress is converted into physical symptoms to resolve internal conflict.

conversion disorder Disorder characterized by the presence of at least one unexplained neurological symptom thought to be caused by the process of conversion.

dissociation Putative psychological process whereby normally integrated aspects of memory become separated.

dissociative disorder Disorder characterized by at least one unexplained neurological symptom thought to be caused by the process of dissociation.

factitious illness Deliberate simulation of physical symptoms and/or signs to obtain medical attention.

hysteria Label traditionally used to describe either a condition characterized by unexplained physical symptoms or a type of personality characterized by overdramatic expression (i.e., hysterical personality disorder).

malingering Deliberate simulation of physical symptoms for personal gain.

somatization Tendency to experience or express psychological distress as physical symptoms.

somatization disorder A severe, chronic form of somatoform disorder involving multiple unexplained physical symptoms across several bodily systems.

somatoform disorder A group of disorders characterized by the presence of disabling unexplained physical symptoms for which there is no medical explanation.

Individuals who report physical symptoms for which no organic explanation can be found are commonly encountered by medical practice. Such symptoms are often associated with high levels of disability, distress, and medical resource utilization and are attributed to psychological factors. This article addresses the nature of "unexplained" physical symptoms, how they are diagnosed and treated, and current ideas concerning the mechanisms involved in their pathogenesis.

I. NOSOLOGY

Attempts to identify the mechanisms involved in the pathogenesis of unexplained physical symptoms extend as far back as ancient Egyptian times, when the prevailing view attributed their origin to a "hysterical" process involving abnormal movements of the uterus within the sufferer's body (the ancient Greek *hysteron*="uterus"). Although the so-called "wandering womb" hypothesis lost favor almost 2000 years ago, the term *hysteria* continued to be used as a generic label for the occurrence of medically unexplained symptoms until 1980, when the terms *hysteria* and *hysterical* were eliminated from the third edition of the *Diagnostic and Statistical Manual of Mental Disorders* (*DSM-III*) and two new superordinate categories, subsequently refined in *DSM-IV*, were created to capture the basic elements of the hysteria concept (Table I). The *somatoform disorders* category encompasses a range of complaints characterized by the symptoms of somatic illness (e.g., pain, fatigue, and nausea) in the absence of underlying physical pathology. Broadly speaking, *DSM-IV* categorizes somatoform complaints according to the nature, number, and duration of the unexplained symptoms in question. The *somatization disorder* category corresponds to the traditional conception of hysteria as a syndrome characterized by large numbers of unexplained symptoms across multiple bodily systems (also known as *Briquet's syndrome*). A *DSM-IV* diagnosis of somatization disorder (onset before the age of 30) requires a history of unexplained pain in at least four different bodily sites, at least two unexplained gastrointestinal symptoms, at least one unexplained sexual or reproductive symptom, and at least one unexplained neurological symptom. The *undifferentiated somatoform disorder* category includes less severe cases, in which unexplained symptoms have persisted for at least 6 months but are fewer in number and may be less disabling. Similar unexplained symptoms of a shorter duration are categorized as instances of *somatoform disorder not otherwise specified*. Each of the latter categories encompasses all possible physical symptoms, with the exception of unexplained neurological phenomena, which are categorized separately as

conversion disorders. In addition, the term *pain disorder* is reserved for syndromes specifically characterized by the occurrence of persistent unexplained pain. In all cases, symptoms are classified as unexplained if adequate medical investigation has failed to identify a plausible physical cause for their occurrence; they must also cause clinically significant functional disability or distress to meet diagnostic criteria. Moreover, the symptoms should not be attributable to hypochondriasis or other forms of overt psychopathology, such as anxiety, depression, or psychosis. In addition, *DSM-IV* assumes that somatoform symptoms are not produced intentionally by the person. Rather, "unexplained" symptoms that are intentionally produced in order to obtain medical attention (e.g., as in Münchausen's disorder) are classified within the *factitious illness* category; symptoms that are intentionally produced for personal gain (e.g., in the context of a litigation claim or to avoid military service) are labeled as instances of *malingering*.

The *DSM-IV dissociative disorders* category includes unexplained symptoms involving an apparent disruption of consciousness, such as instances of amnesia and the alteration of personal identity (encompassing *dissociative amnesia, dissociative fugue*, and *dissociative identity disorder*). *Depersonalization disorder*, characterized by persistent and unpleasant feelings of detachment from the self or the world, is also placed within this category. Although, strictly speaking, the dissociative disorders should be viewed as one dimension of the hysteria concept, they are not typically regarded as medically unexplained symptoms and we will not consider them in detail in this article.

The nosological status of medically unexplained symptoms continues to provoke controversy. First, there is very little evidence to suggest that there are natural boundaries between the different categories of somatoform illness. Indeed, evidence suggests that the different somatoform categories should be regarded as points on a continuum of severity, with somatization disorder at the pathological extreme. Second, the persistence and stability of many cases of somatoform illness suggest that these conditions could be more appropriately viewed as a form of personality disorder rather than an acute psychiatric condition in their own right.

II. TERMINOLOGY

Despite being abandoned as a nosological entity, hysteria is still commonly used as a generic label for the

Table I

Classification of Somatoform and Dissociative Disorders in *DSM-IV*

Somatoform disorders	Dissociative disorders
Somatization disorder	Dissociative amnesia
Undifferentiated somatoform disorder	Dissociative fugue
Conversion disorder	Dissociative identity disorder
Pain disorder	Depersonalization disorder
Somatoform disorder not otherwise specified	Dissociative disorder not otherwise specified
Hypochondriasis	
Body dysmorphic disorder	

occurrence of medically unexplained symptoms. The continuing popularity of the term is viewed with regret by many. First, it implies that medically unexplained symptoms are an exclusively female phenomenon, despite the fact that somatoform illness is observed in both men and women (although much more commonly in the latter). Second, the terms *hysteria* and *hysterical* have acquired different and pejorative meanings in popular parlance that no longer apply to medically unexplained symptoms. Not surprisingly, many individuals suffering from such symptoms strongly object to the use of the hysterical label.

In addition to hysteria and the diagnostic labels provided in *DSM*, many other terms have been used in relation to medically unexplained symptoms, including *functional*, *nonorganic*, *psychosomatic*, and *psychogenic*, each of which is ambiguous or has unfortunate connotations. For the sake of neutrality and descriptive ease, we use *somatoform illness* and *unexplained medical symptoms* as labels encompassing the range of phenomena described in the somatoform disorder category; we use *unexplained neurological symptoms* as a label for those phenomena specifically included in the conversion disorder category. We use the term *somatization* to refer to the process underlying the generation of unexplained medical symptoms.

III. PRESENTATION

A. Clinical Features

Unexplained symptoms may be related to any bodily system. Indeed, every branch of medicine has its own syndrome characterized by the presence of such symptoms. Pain, fatigue, dizziness, shortness of breath, and general malaise are the most commonly observed symptoms in primary care, although gastrointestinal and sexual/reproductive symptoms are frequently found. Within the neurological domain, the most common symptoms are limb weakness, gait disturbances, abnormal movements, sensory disturbances, amnesia, and cognitive impairment. Contrary to popular belief, somatoform symptoms are subjectively real to the patient—that is, their experience is "as if" they have the symptoms of organic illness.

In some cases, a somatoform diagnosis may be suspected on the basis of the inconsistency or medical implausibility of the symptoms in question, although in other cases they may closely resemble symptoms of organic disease. Symptoms are often internally inconsistent. For example, a patient may have a preserved ability to cough (requiring intact vocal chord function) despite being unable to speak or whisper, or a patient may display weakness for some movements and not others involving the same muscle groups. Other symptoms may not fit with recognized disease patterns (e.g., asynchronous generalized tonic–clonic seizures) and may even be physiologically impossible (e.g., triplopia). Often, symptoms correspond more closely to what the patient believes about the body and illness than to actual physical processes. Indeed, the role of beliefs in determining the nature of somatoform phenomena has been widely recognized since the time of Charcot. It is well evidenced by the fact that individuals prone to the development of somatoform illness often develop symptoms that mirror those observed in others. It is also reflected in the varying prevalence of different unexplained symptoms across cultures. Burning hands or feet, for example, are more common in African and Asian cultures than in North America, reflecting local concerns about health and illness. A core set of somatoform symptoms is nevertheless observed across all cultures (e.g., pain, fatigue, pseudoseizures, and paralysis). A history of other unexplained medical symptoms is also frequently found in these patients.

B. Comorbidity

Comorbid psychopathology is extremely common in somatoform illness, with as many as 75% of these patients meeting criteria for an additional psychiatric disorder. Almost all forms of psychiatric illness are more prevalent in these patients compared to primary care patient averages, with elevated levels of depression and anxiety being particularly common. Psychiatric comorbidity studies suggest that between 40 and 80% of patients with somatoform illness meet diagnostic criteria for an affective disorder, whereas between 15 and 90% meet criteria for an anxiety disorder (particularly panic, phobic, and obsessive–compulsive disorders). Such variations in comorbidity estimates are a function of several factors, including the study sample used and somatoform illness severity. Studies conducted on psychiatric populations, for example, are likely to yield disproportionately high rates of psychiatric comorbidity compared to community, primary care, or other specialist samples. Similarly, patients meeting criteria for somatization disorder are considerably more likely to report psychiatric symptoms than are patients with fewer unexplained symptoms.

The comorbidity between somatoform illness and personality disorders is also much higher than that in patients with other psychiatric diagnoses. About 60% of patients with somatoform illness meet criteria for at least one personality disorder; of these, a significant proportion are likely to meet criteria for two or more such diagnoses. Contrary to historical belief, there is no particular association between medically unexplained symptoms and histrionic (i.e., hysterical) personality disorder. Indeed, evidence suggests that the most common personality disturbances in these patients are of the avoidant, dependent, paranoid, and obsessive–compulsive types. Similarly, there is little evidence in support of the traditional view that antisocial personality disorder is a common concomitant of unexplained medical symptoms.

Somatoform illness is also commonly found in the context of physical illness. In such cases, a somatoform diagnosis is made on the grounds that identifiable pathology is unable to account for the range of symptoms and degree of disability exhibited by the patient. In the neurological setting, as many as 60% of patients diagnosed with somatoform illness have comorbid organic diagnoses, although there is no consistent pattern to the type of neurological pathology found in these patients. In contrast, physical comorbidity is often less than 5% within the general psychiatric setting. Such findings indicate that neurological dysfunction plays an important role in the development of somatoform illness. However, many of these patients have extracerebral comorbid neurological disease, which contradicts the view that altered cerebral function provides a fertile soil for the development of conversion disorder. Rather, it is more likely that exposure to neurological illness provides a model for the development of symptoms and an environment in which illness behavior is rewarded.

IV. DIAGNOSTIC ISSUES

Diagnosing somatoform illness is important in order to offer relevant psychiatric treatment and to avoid unnecessary medical intervention. A much-quoted study by Eliot Slater in the 1960s suggested that the rate of misdiagnosis was very high and questioned the validity of hysteria as a diagnostic entity. Recently, the advent of noninvasive investigative techniques (e.g., brain imaging and video telemetry) and the better characterization of neurological disease patterns have made the exclusion of organic pathology easier and more reliable. Indeed, recent studies of patients with both acute and chronic unexplained symptoms suggest that neurological illness is rarely missed in these patients.

Currently, the gold standard for the diagnosis of somatoform illness involves a combination of careful history taking, the judicious use of investigations to rule out significant organic disease, and the assessment of psychiatric morbidity. The exclusion of organic pathology is essential, although it is often difficult to establish the right balance between the benefits and dangers of further investigations. Moreover, the presence of organic disease does not exclude the possibility of somatization; it is therefore important to assess all patients for unexplained symptoms or disability. The clinical history may reveal many features that support a positive diagnosis of somatoform illness, including the inconsistency and implausibility of symptoms, a previous history of unexplained symptoms, and psychosocial stressors preceding the development of symptoms. The successful alleviation of symptoms in response to placebo, suggestions, or psychological treatment also supports a positive somatoform diagnosis.

In some cases, symptoms are consistent and plausible and there may be few or no additional diagnostic features in evidence. For example, although *DSM-IV* explicitly requires the presence of psychosocial stressors for a firm diagnosis of both conversion and somatoform pain disorder, obvious stressors are absent in many cases. Even when present, establishing a causal link between such stressors and physical symptoms can be extremely difficult and involves considerable subjectivity. Other clinical features previously thought to be characteristic of somatoform illness have been found to have little or no diagnostic validity. For example, historically it has been thought that patients suffering from unexplained symptoms display an unusual lack of concern over the condition, so-called *la belle indifférence*. However, research indicates that patients with somatoform illness show no more indifference to their physical condition than do patients with organic illness. The traditional notion that unexplained medical symptoms are exclusive to individuals of low socioeconomic status has also been disputed.

Even in cases in which positive somatoform features are present, many physicians are reluctant to diagnose somatoform illness for fear of missing an underlying physical illness. However, in the clear absence of pathology following appropriate investigation, and particularly if positive signs are present, a diagnosis of somatoform illness can be safely made. In cases in which somatoform illness is suspected but an organic explanation cannot be ruled out unequivocally, careful follow-up is often the best diagnostic tool.

V. EPIDEMIOLOGY

Somatoform illness is a ubiquitous phenomenon, representing one of the most common categories of illness encountered within the health care system. Precise prevalence estimates vary enormously due to the different diagnostic criteria employed across studies. In general, prevalence estimates decrease as symptoms become more severe, chronic, and greater in number. Recent evidence suggests that approximately 25% of patients attending primary care have a history of four or more unexplained symptoms. In contrast, studies have estimated the prevalence of *DSM-IV* somatization disorder (defined as a history of eight symptoms across multiple bodily sites) to be between 3 and 5% of primary care attenders. Within the neurological domain, evidence suggests that between 20 and 60% of new inpatient admissions have symptoms that cannot be fully accounted for by organic factors.

The understandable reluctance of many physicians to make formal somatoform diagnoses suggests that current data may underestimate the true prevalence of unexplained medical symptoms. In addition, many patients with diagnoses such as chronic fatigue syndrome, fibromyalgia, and noncardiac chest pain may be more appropriately viewed as having somatoform illness.

VI. RESOURCE UTILIZATION

The health service costs associated with somatoform illness are considerable and are not simply attributable to the ubiquity of these conditions. Rather, patients with somatoform illness often consume a disproportionate amount of resources compared to other service users. Indeed, it has been estimated that the health care costs of patients meeting criteria for somatization disorder are nine times the U.S. national average. The bulk of resource utilization by these patients is on diagnostic tests rather than psychiatric services. The frequency of general practitioner and emergency room visits, as well as the number and length of hospital admissions, also tends to be elevated in these patients. In general, the level of resource use increases with the severity and chronicity of unexplained symptoms. Improved physician recognition of these conditions and the limitation of needless investigations could significantly reduce the health care costs of this group of patients.

VII. MANAGEMENT AND TREATMENT

A. Presenting the Diagnosis

The way in which a diagnosis of conversion or somatoform illness is presented can have a considerable effect on the doctor–patient relationship; it may also be an important factor in whether the patient cooperates with the management plan. Coming to terms with a diagnosis of conversion or somatization is difficult for many patients, who often believe that their suffering is being dismissed as "all in the mind" or, worse, deliberately faked. Understandably, many patients find it difficult to accept that their debilitating symptoms may be caused by psychological rather than physical processes, particularly if they have no obvious psychological symptoms, such as anxiety or depression.

Where somatoform illness is suspected, considerable effort should be made to establish a strong therapeutic alliance between physician and patient while necessary physical investigations are being conducted. This prepares the groundwork for the later exploration of possible psychological factors that may be contributing to the presentation of unexplained symptoms and reduces resistance if a formal somatoform diagnosis is being considered. At all times, it is essential to explicitly acknowledge that the patient's symptoms are subjectively real and that they cause significant distress and disability. Such an approach allows the patient to feel that he or she is taken seriously, thereby reducing the likelihood of subsequent doctor shopping. At the appropriate point, the patient should be reassured that all necessary investigations have been done, that no sinister cause for their symptoms has been identified, and that they are not suffering from a serious physical illness. It should be emphasized that further physical investigation would be of no benefit, that certain physical treatments will not be prescribed, and that current medications might need to be withdrawn. Patients may then be gently introduced to the notion that psychological factors may be important in causing their symptoms. It should be emphasized that such an interpretation does not mean that their symptoms are faked or all in the mind and that they are not insane or crazy; the words hysteria and hysterical should be avoided. It is also common to introduce the idea that their symptoms may be caused by psychological events of which they are unaware, giving everyday examples demonstrating the close link between psychological processes (e.g., anxiety) and physical symptoms (e.g., tremor and dizziness).

Many practitioners believe that it is unnecessary to label patients with a formal diagnosis of conversion or somatoform illness, preferring to describe their symptoms simply as "medically unexplained." Indeed, if it is possible to make therapeutic progress without psychological referral, the use of an explicit diagnosis may be unnecessary and potentially damaging to the doctor–patient relationship. Many patients with acute symptoms respond to simple measures, such as reassurance and physiotherapy; a greater therapeutic challenge is presented by patients with chronic symptoms, where an explicit diagnosis can help ensure patient cooperation with the management plan. The development of new symptoms, a refusal to accept reassurance, and/or demands for further physical investigation may also necessitate the use of a formal diagnosis. To many people, a diagnosis of "medically unexplained symptoms" implies that further physical investigation could eventually yield a medical explanation for their suffering—a belief that ultimately undermines the appropriate management of somatoform conditions. Indeed, without a firm diagnosis, many patients persist in the belief that "the doctor couldn't find what was wrong with me"—a belief that simply serves to intensify their perceived need for further physical investigation. In contrast, use of the somatoform or conversion label serves to legitimize the patient's complaint, firmly identifying it as a recognizable condition that is commonly encountered within medical care. Where psychological referral is indicated, it may be more appropriate to leave diagnostic labeling to the psychiatrist or psychologist.

B. General Management Principles

The general practitioner plays a central role in the management of somatoform illness, with the often difficult task of controlling the patient's access to further investigation and hospitalization. Referrals should only be made when clearly indicated by the clinical picture, paying particular attention to the signs rather than the symptoms of illness. It is important to remember, however, that individuals with somatoform disorders are no less likely to suffer from physical illness than are other patients; it should not be

assumed, therefore, that any new complaints are necessarily somatoform. When further investigations are indicated, their purpose and results should be clearly explained to the patient.

Investigating and treating physicians should liaise with the general practitioner and make him or her aware of any explanation and advice given to the patient. A consistent approach should be adopted where possible, aimed at ensuring that the patient does not receive mixed messages. For this reason, the patient should be strongly discouraged from doctor shopping. One useful approach within primary practice is to schedule regular, time-limited appointments for the patient every 4–6 weeks. Such an approach allows the patient to feel that he or she is being taken seriously and that his or her physical health is being monitored; this is particularly useful for patients who are reluctant to accept a psychological interpretation of their symptoms. It is also preferable to a "return-as-needed" approach, which can encourage the development of new symptoms in order for the patient to obtain physician contact.

It is also important to screen for psychiatric problems such as anxiety and depression, which can prove difficult with this patient group. Often, the patient will deny being anxious or depressed, despite exhibiting clear physiological indicators to the contrary (e.g., sleep and appetite disturbance in depression and palpitations and dizziness in anxiety). Rather than directly asking the patient whether he or she is anxious or depressed, it is useful to question the patient about his or her psychological reaction to his or her symptoms. Such an indirect approach often elicits useful information concerning the patient's mental state while maintaining a strong therapeutic alliance.

C. Treatment

The way in which somatoform illness is treated depends largely on the nature of the individual and his or her symptoms. Where appropriate, efforts are made to resolve any psychosocial problems that may have provoked the presenting symptoms. Symptomatic treatments, such as physiotherapy, orthopedic treatment, occupational therapy, and speech therapy, are often used to reduce loss of function and disability and to prevent secondary damage. Other approaches, such as pain management techniques, are used to ameliorate the distress caused by symptoms. Where appropriate, depression and anxiety are treated using medication. Often, the use of these and other techniques, combined with a careful management approach, is sufficient to provide the patient with lasting symptomatic relief. In some cases, however, more specific psychological treatment is necessary. In such cases, cognitive-behavioral therapy is most commonly used, typically targeting maladaptive beliefs about health and illness, behavioral patterns that maintain symptoms, and social factors that reinforce them. Cognitive-educational therapy, typically aimed at informing patients about the relationship between symptoms and psychological processes, is also sometimes used, often in a group context. Insight-oriented psychotherapy may be used in cases in which emotional issues appear to be a significant pathogenic factor. In terms of efficacy, evidence suggests that a cognitive approach is often effective in the treatment of somatoform illness; however, very few data exist on the efficacy of psychotherapy in these conditions.

In cases in which symptomatic and psychological interventions fail to provide complete resolution of the patients' symptoms, it may be necessary to adjust the therapeutic goal from curing the patients to simply caring for them. Accordingly, management should aim to contain the patients' symptoms and distress, limit their health care utilization, and prevent iatrogenic damage.

VIII. OUTCOME

The majority of studies addressing outcome in somatoform illness have concentrated either on conversion disorder or on somatization disorder, and research explicitly addressing other forms of somatoform illness is rare. It is nevertheless likely that studies investigating the outcome of conditions such as chronic fatigue syndrome, fibromyalgia, irritable bowel syndrome, and chronic pain conditions are implicitly addressing other aspects of somatoform illness. A review of the substantial literature concerning these conditions is beyond the scope of this article.

One of the earliest follow-up studies of unexplained symptoms was conducted in the mid-19th century by Paul Briquet, who studied 430 patients with a variety of symptoms over a period of 10 years. In about half of these patients, symptoms followed a course of progressive, chronic deterioration and recurrent episodes were common; in other cases, recovery occurred after 3–6 months. Briquet identified many factors associated with outcome in these patients. For example, onset

during adolescence carried a poor prognosis, whereas a favorable change in social circumstances was associated with a positive outcome.

Several recent studies have provided information concerning outcome in adult patients with unexplained neurological symptoms and identified many prognostic indicators. Given the heterogeneity of the samples studied, it is not surprising that reported remission rates vary considerably; that notwithstanding, a relatively good prognosis has been found in most studies. On average, complete recovery of the index symptom is observed in about two-thirds of acute cases, whereas little or no improvement is observed in up to 20%. The chances of recovery in acute patients are increased in cases in which symptoms have been precipitated by traumatic events. Evidence suggests that between one-fourth and one-third of patients with chronic neurological symptoms receiving inpatient treatment show complete remission of the index symptom; moreover, between 20 and 60% show some improvement at follow-up. Evidence suggests that patients are most likely to recover during the period of hospital admission; after this time, recovery is much less likely. The findings of such outcome studies should be interpreted with caution, however. Most studies conducted in this domain report improvement for the index symptom only; information concerning other symptoms and subsequent referral patterns is rarely provided.

Younger patients tend to have a better prognosis than older patients; indeed, children with unexplained neurological symptoms of recent onset have a particularly favorable outcome. Other factors predicting outcome include the presence of comorbid psychopathology and personality disorders. The presence of comorbid personality disorder typically carries a poor prognosis, although there is no apparent association between outcome and any specific personality type. Conversely, the presence of comorbid anxiety and depression are associated with a good prognosis.

Outcome is broadly similar across the range of unexplained symptoms; the same prognostic factors (e.g., duration of symptoms) are relevant in all cases.

IX. PSYCHOPATHOLOGICAL MECHANISMS

Current theorizing concerning the psychopathological mechanisms of somatoform illness is dominated by the concepts of dissociation, conversion, and somatization; these models, and the evidence cited in their support, are described here. Currently, no one model provides a completely satisfactory explanation of how it is possible for the symptoms of illness to be experienced in the absence of organic pathology. Although current models have shed light on many aspects of somatoform illness, they are conceptually underspecified and, in certain respects, not well supported by empirical research. Although it is likely that a complete account of unexplained medical symptoms will incorporate aspects of the dissociation, conversion, and somatization models, the development of such an account ultimately requires a more detailed examination of psychological and neuroscientific concepts not currently considered in this domain.

A. Dissociation and Conversion

The term *dissociation* originated in the 19th-century work of Pierre Janet, who proposed one of the earliest systematic accounts of the psychopathological mechanisms underlying somatoform phenomena. Although more than a century old, many of Janet's ideas concerning the organization of mental processes remain popular (albeit implicitly) within contemporary cognitive psychology. According to Janet, personal knowledge is represented by an integrated network of associated memories, which are accessible to consciousness through the operation of attention. This process of attentional selection is responsible for synthesizing the contents of conscious experience by which the execution of volitional actions is coordinated (Fig. 1). In this view, the synthetic functions of attention are disrupted in hysterical patients, rendering them susceptible to a breakdown in psychological

integration in the face of extreme trauma. Traumatic experience initiates the separation or *dissociation* of memories from the main body of knowledge by an amnesic barrier. Although these dissociated memories or "fixed ideas" are prevented from entering consciousness by the amnesic barrier, they may be automatically activated by external events. The activation of dissociated memories in this way is responsible for the generation of hysterical symptoms (Fig. 2) that, because they are produced without conscious control, are essentially nonvolitional phenomena. According to Janet, this automatic activation of fixed ideas is a process of suggestion, with the underlying deficit in attention being akin to a state of hypnosis.

Shortly after the publication of Janet's account of hysteria, the dissociation model was extended by Josef Breuer and Sigmund Freud with the introduction of the *conversion* concept. According to Breuer and Freud, the process of dissociation occurs when the subject attempts to regulate his or her experience of negative affect by defensively suppressing (or *repressing*) the conscious recall of memories associated with personal trauma. In the conversion model, this repression of negative affect serves as the primary determining factor in the generation of hysterical symptoms rather than the dissociation of memories *per se*. According to Breuer and Freud, emotions are associated with high levels of neural energy that must be discharged if the energetic balance of the brain is to be preserved. By avoiding negative affect through the repression of traumatic memories, however, this discharge of neural energy is prevented. In order for it to occur, negative affect is transformed or "converted" into a somatic (i.e., hysterical) symptom, which allows the individual to discharge emotional energy without recalling the traumatic memories

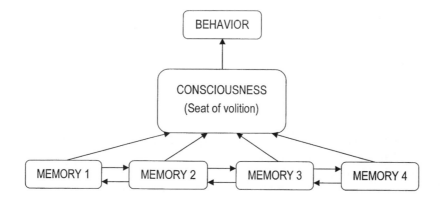

Figure 1   Organization of the cognitive system as described by Janet (1924).

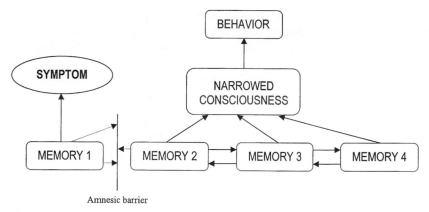

Figure 2 Generation of an unexplained symptom through the dissociation of a memory from consciousness.

giving rise to it. By this account, therefore, hysterical symptoms serve an important psychological purpose (i.e., defense), with the discharge of emotional energy representing the *primary gain* from symptoms. In this model, symptoms generated by the process of conversion correspond to sensations present at the time of the underlying trauma, or they are a symbolic representation of it.

Although more than a century old, the theoretical analyses of hysteria offered by Janet, Breuer, and Freud continue to influence nosology, theory, and clinical practice concerning medically unexplained symptoms. Several lines of evidence provide information concerning the validity of the dissociation and conversion models.

1. Attention

Many theoretical models have endorsed Janet's idea that somatoform illness involves an alteration in attention that prevents processed information from entering conscious awareness. Recent electrophysiological research indicating that conversion disorder is associated with normal early evoked potentials but a deficit in the later P300 component provides strong support for such a view. Several cognitive and psychophysiological studies have also found evidence for a diffuse attentional deficit in individuals with conversion symptoms, with patients showing decrements on tasks assessing vigilance, habituation, cognitive flexibility, set shifting, and mental transformation. However, the precise nature of the attentional deficit underlying conversion remains unclear; further research is required if it is to be described in greater detail.

2. Hypnosis

Janet's proposal that hysterical and hypnotic phenomena share similar psychological mechanisms also continues to attract support. In line with this hypothesis, many studies have shown that individuals with somatoform and conversion illness tend to exhibit high levels of suggestibility. Moreover, recent imaging studies using positron emission tomography have provided limited evidence indicating that similar neuroanatomical substrates may be involved in both conversion and hypnotic paralysis. Currently, however, the link between hypnosis and somatoform illness is still largely theoretical; further empirical evidence based on larger sample sizes is required before firm conclusions can be drawn in this regard.

3. Psychological Trauma

The view that unexplained symptoms are related to traumatic experiences, central to both the dissociation and the conversion models, has also been widely adopted. Indeed, current diagnostic criteria require that clear psychosocial precipitants be present for a diagnosis of conversion disorder or somatoform pain disorder. Although there is substantial evidence to suggest that many instances of somatoform illness are either preceded by psychosocial precipitants or associated with significant early trauma, it is clear that traumatic precipitants are absent in many cases. Moreover, many traumatized individuals with somatoform illness have not experienced amnesia for their trauma, and symptom resolution is not guaranteed by the recovery of previously forgotten traumatic memories. As such, trauma cannot play the primary pathogenic role in the generation of medically unexplained symptoms suggested by Janet, Breuer, and Freud, although it is clearly relevant in many instances.

4. Alexithymia

Although the concept of emotionally derived neural energies has long since been abandoned, the work of Freud and Breuer still remains influential. The notion that a reduction in anxiety is the primary gain associated with unexplained symptoms is largely responsible for the continuing popularity of *la belle indifférence* as a diagnostic indicator of somatoform illness. As noted previously, however, patients with somatoform illness show no more indifference to their condition than do patients with comparable physical illnesses. Moreover, it is clear that many individuals with somatoform illness show high levels of anxiety, demonstrating that any conversion process that is occurring is far from effective in controlling this emotion. However, there is evidence that somatoform illness is associated with an inability to identify and report on one's emotional states (so-called *alexithymia*). Such evidence could be interpreted as indicating that the process of conversion occurs as a means of discharging unexpressed emotion. These findings must be interpreted with caution, however, because there is evidence that existing measures of alexithymia are confounded by psychopathology in general.

5. Symptom Laterality

The Freudian view that unexplained symptoms are the expression of unconscious emotional conflict has led many to conclude that the right cerebral hemisphere (traditionally viewed as one of the neural sites responsible for emotion) plays an important role in the pathogenesis of unexplained symptoms. Several studies have provided evidence suggesting that unexplained symptoms are more common on the left than the right, apparently providing support for this hypothesis. However, recent research has shown that left- and right-sided symptoms are equally common; bilateral symptoms are also frequently found.

B. Somatization

Dissociation and conversion represent the main theoretical precursors to contemporary accounts of the somatoform disorders based on the concept of *somatization*. The term somatization originated in the psychoanalytic literature of the early 19th century as a label for the hypothetical process whereby bodily dysfunction (i.e., unexplained symptoms) was generated by "unconscious neurosis." Since the 1960s, however, the work of Zbigniew Lipowski has encouraged many within the field to adopt a more descriptive usage of the term. According to this approach, somatization may be broadly defined as the tendency to experience or express psychological distress as the symptoms of physical illness. Unlike previous approaches, which attempted to identify neuropsychological processes underlying the occurrence of medically unexplained symptoms, the somatization model places explanatory emphasis on the entire biopsychosocial context surrounding the experience of physical and mental illness. In this respect, the somatization model is influenced by the concept of "illness behavior"—that is, the way in which we perceive, evaluate, and react to our physical and psychological states in relation to socially sanctioned models of health and illness (the so-called "sick role"). According to this model, individuals suffering from somatoform illness are said to display *abnormal* illness behavior—that is, a tendency to adopt the sick role that is inappropriate given the absence of identifiable physical pathology. Many features of somatoform illness have been identified as instances of abnormal illness behavior. For example, many somatoform disorder patients dispute the diagnoses they have been given, refuse to accept that they have been investigated adequately, or fail to comply with treatment. Indeed, many such patients are perceived as "difficult" by the treating physician, and the doctor–patient relationship is often less than satisfactory.

The somatization model views the development of abnormal illness behavior as a multifactorial process in which social, cultural, cognitive, perceptual, personality, and physiological factors are all implicated.

1. Sociocultural Factors

Research and theory suggest that abnormal illness behaviors may pass from generation to generation through early social learning within the familial context. Disproportionate parental concern over a child's physical symptoms, the misattribution of normal sensations to pathological causes, and inappropriate help-seeking behavior have all been linked to subsequent bodily preoccupation, which may serve as a risk factor for the development of somatoform illness. Moreover, some studies have shown that children exposed to abnormally high amounts of family illness are more likely to experience somatoform illness as adults. Early exposure to pathology may reinforce illness behavior and provide a model for the subsequent development of symptoms. In addition, repeated exposure to illness provides misleading information concerning illness base rates, leading those that are exposed to overestimate the likelihood of certain forms of pathology.

The dynamic relationship between illness behavior and culture in general may also play an important role in the development of somatization. In most cultures, there is a stigma attached to mental illness that is not associated with physical forms of infirmity; as such, expressing emotional distress somatically offers a socially acceptable way of gaining support via the sick role. Cultural factors pertaining to the health care system are also likely to be influential in shaping the nature and occurrence of somatization. Some studies, for example, have implicated iatrogenic factors in the maintenance of many medically unexplained symptoms, often involving physical misdiagnoses that could serve to perpetuate symptoms by legitimizing the individual's somatic interpretation of their condition. Moreover, the biological emphasis of modern health care systems encourages individuals to communicate nonspecific distress somatically rather than psychologically.

2. Perceptual and Cognitive Factors

What we know and believe about bodily states is inextricably bound with our experience of physical sensations as well as our behavioral response to them. For example, some studies have suggested that the acquisition of maladaptive beliefs about health and illness may be related to the development of somatization. Thus, the somatizing individual may hold the mistaken belief that health is a state devoid of physical symptoms, and that symptoms necessarily imply the presence of disease. Recently, Arthur Barsky and colleagues argued that such beliefs lead the somatizing individual to develop a preoccupation with his or her bodily states and a tendency to misinterpret them as pathological. Once symptoms are attributed to illness, further attention may be directed toward the body, with subsequent physical events being perceived as evidence in support of a pathological interpretation. Evidence demonstrating that hypochondriasis is associated with body-focused attention provides support for this model, as do several studies indicating that self-

focused attention is positively related to somatic symptom reports in nonclinical populations. Clinical experience strongly suggests that body-focused attention is also a central aspect of somatoform illness.

3. Personality Factors

It is likely that cognitive and perceptual factors precipitate and maintain somatization by maximizing the degree to which physical states are experienced as aversive. Research suggests that the tendency to experience physical and psychological states as aversive is also related to the personality dimension of negative affectivity (NA), characterized by a negative self-concept and a trait-like tendency to experience distress and dissatisfaction. Indeed, subjective symptom reports consistently correlate with NA, despite there being no correlation between NA and objective health markers. Individuals high in trait NA are hypervigilant about their bodies and have a lower threshold for perceiving physical sensations, so-called somatic amplification. Such individuals are also more likely to interpret physical symptoms as the signs of serious disease and seek medical attention accordingly.

4. Physiological Factors

Unlike previous theories, the somatization model embraces the idea that normal physical processes (e.g., the physical component of an emotional state) and minor pathological events may contribute to the development of unexplained symptoms. For example, anxiety is typically associated with increased autonomic arousal that may result in physical changes such as shaking, sweating, and tachycardia; moreover, fear-related hyperventilation can produce symptoms such as breathlessness, chest pain, and fatigue. Similarly, the sleep problems and physical inactivity often associated with depression may give rise to fatigue, pain, and the feeling that increased effort is required to execute everyday tasks. Other physical processes unrelated to emotional states may also contribute to the development of medically unexplained symptoms. For example, muscle wasting resulting from illness-related inactivity may produce fatigue that perpetuates itself by preventing the resumption of physical exercise after illness remission.

A recent model of the interaction between these different factors has been described by Lawrence Kirmayer and colleagues (Fig. 3). According to this model, illness, emotional arousal, and everyday physiological processes produce bodily sensations that capture the individual's attention to varying degrees. These sensations may be interpreted as indicators of disease, an attribution that can serve to generate illness worry, catastrophizing, and demoralization. As a result, individual may adopt the sick role by pursuing assessment and treatment for his or her putative condition, thereby exposing himself or herself to social forces that may reinforce their illness behavior and experience. This process may be moderated by many situational and dispositional factors, including previous illness experience, environmental contingencies that reward illness behavior, the response of significant others to illness worry, and individual differences in personality, attentional set, coping behavior, and autonomic reactivity.

Despite their obvious explanatory power, there are certain problems with models based on the concept of somatization. First, such models obscure potentially important differences between the various forms of medically unexplained symptoms, such as those that are the physical concomitants of conditions such as anxiety and depression, normal physical sensations or minor pathological events that are mistakenly attributed to serious illness through hypochondriacal misinterpretation, and those characteristic of the conversion and somatoform disorders. Although there is considerable overlap between these conditions in clinical practice, these different forms of somatization can be distinguished both conceptually and empirically. Although the somatization model offers a powerful account of the medically unexplained symptoms associated with depression, anxiety, and hypochondriasis, it fails to provide an adequate account of the mechanisms underlying conversion and somatoform symptoms. Arguably, a proper understanding of

somatoform illness requires a theoretical approach that is specific to this form of somatization—an approach that is inherent to dissociation and conversion models.

Second, the model of somatization described here assumes that medically unexplained symptoms are necessarily the product of physiological processes, such as the physical components of emotional states, and minor pathological events. Although such processes might play an important role in the generation of certain somatoform symptoms, it is difficult to understand how unexplained neurological (i.e., conversion) symptoms can be explained in this way.

Third, as with theories based on the concepts of conversion and dissociation, the somatization model assumes that unexplained symptoms are necessarily the expression of psychological distress. Although this may be true in many cases, particularly those associated with anxiety, depression, or hypochondriasis, it is apparent that such an assumption may be inappropriate in many other cases.

Finally, it may be misleading (and, indeed, pejorative) to identify somatoform illness as necessarily involving "abnormal" illness behavior. In our view, seeking help for subjectively compelling and debilitating symptoms is more appropriately regarded as *normal* illness behavior, regardless of whether an underlying pathophysiological basis for those symptoms can be found. Similarly, it is unclear what constitutes a "normal" illness response to repeatedly negative physical investigations despite the persistence of symptoms, particularly when disability is high (e.g., as in paralysis). As such, it may be more appropriate to reserve the concept of abnormal illness behavior for those cases in which the problem appears to involve more than just a poor doctor–patient relationship or the presentation of unexplained symptoms *per se.*

X. SUMMARY

In summary, the following points should be noted:

1. Somatoform illness is one of the most common forms of psychiatric disorder encountered within the health care system and is associated with high levels of resource utilization.
2. Almost every symptom of organic illness has an "unexplained" (i.e., somatoform or conversion) counterpart.
3. In some cases, unexplained medical symptoms have positive features (e.g., internal inconsistency) that

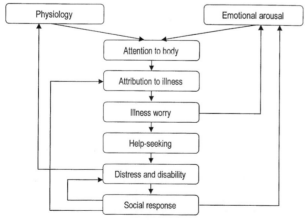

Figure 3 A multifactorial model of somatization (based on Kirmayer and Taillefer (1997)).

are indicative of a somatoform diagnosis; however, other somatoform symptoms closely resemble the symptoms of organic disease.

4. Comorbid psychopathology, particularly depression, anxiety, and personality disorders, is extremely common in patients with unexplained medical symptoms; comorbid organic pathology is also common in these patients.

5. The diagnosis of somatoform illness involves careful history taking, the exclusion of physical illness through appropriate investigation, and the assessment of psychiatric morbidity.

6. Management of somatoform illness involves containing the patient's symptoms and distress, limiting their access to investigations and hospitalizations, and preventing iatrogenic damage; careful consideration must be given to whether a formal diagnosis of somatoform illness should be used and, if so, how such a diagnosis should be presented.

7. A typical therapeutic approach involves the use of reassurance, symptomatic treatments and, where necessary, psychological intervention; the prognosis of somatoform illness is quite good, with acute symptoms being more responsive to treatment than chronic symptoms.

8. Current theorizing concerning unexplained medical symptoms is dominated by the concepts of dissociation, conversion, and somatization. Although there is limited evidence in support of these concepts, they fail to provide a complete account of the psychopathological mechanisms underlying these conditions.

See Also the Following Articles

ANXIETY • ATTENTION • DEPRESSION • NEUROPSYCHOLOGICAL ASSESSMENT • PAIN AND PSYCHOPATHOLOGY

Suggested Reading

Barsky, A. J. (1979). Patients who amplify bodily symptoms. *Ann. Internal Med.* **91,** 63–70.

Breuer, J., and Freud, S.(1893–1895/1955). Studies on hysteria. In *The Standard Edition of the Complete Psychological Works of Sigmund Freud* (J., Strachey and A., Strachey, Eds.), Vol. 2. Hogarth Press/Institute of Psycho-Analysis, London, (English translation, 1955).

Brown, R. J., and Trimble, M. R. (2000). Dissociative psychopathology, non-epileptic seizures and neurology. *J. Neurol. Neurosurg. Psychiatr.* **69,** 285–291.

Crimlisk, H. L., and Ron, M. A. (1999). Conversion hysteria: History, diagnostic issues and clinical practice. *Cognitive Neuropsychiatr.* **4,** 165–180.

Crimlisk, H. L., Bhatia, K., Cope, H., David, A., Marsden, C. D., and Ron, M. A. (1998). Slater revisited: 6 year follow up of patients with medically unexplained motor symptoms. *Br. Med. J.* **316,** 582–586.

Iezzi, A., and Adams, H. E. (1993). Somatoform and factitious disorders. In *Comprehensive Handbook of Psychopathology* (P. B. Sutker and H. E. Adams, Eds.), pp. 167–201. Plenum, New York.

Janet, P. (1924). *The Major Symptoms of Hysteria,* 2nd ed. Macmillan, New York.

Kirmayer, L. J., and Robbins, J. M. (Eds.) (1991). *Current Concepts of Somatization: Research and Clinical Perspectives.* American Psychiatric Press, Washington, DC.

Kirmayer, L. J., and Taillefer, S. (1997). Somatoform disorders. In *Adult Psychopathology and Diagnosis* (S. M. Turner and M. Hersen, Eds.), 3rd ed. pp. 333–383. Wiley, New York.

Lipowski, Z. J. (1988). Somatization: The concept and its clinical application. *Am. J. Psychiatr.* **145,** 1358–1368.

Ludwig, A. M. (1972). Hysteria: A neurobiological theory. *Arch. Gen. Psychiatr.* **27,** 771–777.

Martin, R. L., and Yutzy, S. H. (1999). Somatoform disorders. In *The American Psychiatric Press Textbook of Psychiatry* (R. E. Hales, S. C. Yudofsky, and J. A. Talbot, Eds.), 3rd ed. pp. 663–694. American Psychiatric Press, Washington, DC.

Mayou, R., Bass, C., and Sharpe, M. (Eds.) (1995). *Treatment of Functional Somatic Syndromes.* Oxford Univ. Press, Oxford.

Pilowsky, I. (1978). A general classification of abnormal illness behaviours. *Br. J. Med. Psychol.* **51,** 131–137.

Ron, M. (1994). Somatisation in neurological practice. *J. Neurol. Neurosurg. Psychiatr.* **57,** 1161–1164.

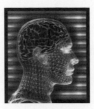

Corpus Callosum

KATHLEEN BAYNES

University of California, Davis

GLOSSARY

agenesis of the corpus callosum A chronic condition in which the corpus callosum fails to develop. The condition has been increasingly recognized due to the widespread use of imaging techniques that reveal the distinctive ventricular pattern that occurs when this major fiber tract fails to develop. Persons with this condition may be cognitively normal but show increased interhemispheric transfer times on a variety of tests.

alien (anarchic) hand sign A condition in which one hand performs complex motor acts outside of the person's conscious control. It can occur in either the dominant or nondominant hand. One form of anarchic hand is thought to occur following a callosal lesion. The other type occurs after disruption of the motor system due to medial frontal lobe damage. Both types are usually intermittent and transitory.

anterior commissure A fiber bundle that connects the two hemispheres. It is inferior to the corpus callosum, near the rostrum. It is thought to connect the anterior temporal lobes, but in humans it may carry fibers from more widely distributed areas.

body of the corpus callosum The central fibers of the corpus callosum. The fibers lie between the genu and the isthmus.

callosotomy The surgical section of the corpus callosum. It is usually accomplished in two stages. The anterior two-thirds of the callosum is sectioned first, followed by the section of the splenium if

satisfactory seizure control has not been achieved. In humans, this procedure is only used in the treatment of intractable epilepsy.

commissurotomy The surgical section of the corpus callosum, the anterior commissure, and the hippocampal commissure. This more radical procedure was introduced when the first callosotomies appeared to be ineffective. It remains an alternative to the callosotomy.

contralateral This term refers to the hand, visual field, etc. that is on the opposite side from the structure under discussion. The left hemisphere controls the right or contralateral hand.

fiber tract A group of axons that follows the same path through the brain.

genu The anterior fibers of the corpus callosum that appear to bend like a knee in sagittal section before becoming the more horizontal body of the corpus callosum.

hippocampal commissure One of the fiber tracts inferior and dorsal to the callosum that is usually cut during the posterior section of the callosum. It carries fibers from the hippocampus, a structure important in forming new memories.

homonomous hemianopsia Cortical blindness in one complete visual field. It commonly results from destruction of the right or left occipital lobe, causing blindness in the contralateral visual field.

ipsilateral This term refers to the hand, visual field, etc. that is on the same side as the structure under discussion. The left hemisphere does not control the left or ipsilateral fingers well, although it can participate in ipsilateral limb movement.

isthmus The portion of the corpus callosum just anterior to the splenium.

laterality This term refers to the tendency for one hemisphere to perform a particular cognitive or motor task better than the other.

rostrum The most anterior portion of the corpus callosum.

splenium The most posterior portion of the corpus callosum. It conveys visual information between the hemispheres.

split-brain A term used to refer to a person who has undergone either commissurotomy or callosotomy for the treatment of intractable epilepsy.

The corpus callosum is one of the most anatomically prominent structures in the human brain. It is composed of approximately 200 million fibers that course across the brain's midline to connect the two cerebral hemispheres. Despite its structural prominence, which led early investigators to believe it played an important role in cognition and behavior, identifying the role of callosal connections in modifying behavior has proven difficult. This article discusses the anatomy of the callosum, the changing view of its role in behavior, the effects of surgical and other lesions on different aspects of behavior, studies of callosal transfer times, and theories of the role of the callosum in human laterality, cognition, and consciousness.

I. ANATOMY

The corpus callosum is composed of millions of nerve fibers that connect the two halves of the brain. These fibers traveling together from one cerebral hemisphere to the other form a brain structure easily visible to the beginning student of neuroanatomy. Figure 1 shows a saggital section of the brain, which is a slice that runs from front to back on a vertical plane. This slice passes through the midline. The large curved structure in the middle of the brain is the corpus callosum.

Although there is considerable variability in the size and shape of the corpus callosum in humans, it is known that it contains approximately 200 million fibers that carry neural signals from one side of the brain to the other. Although most of these fibers are thought to be excitatory, their effect may be inhibitory due to the activity of inhibitory interneurons. Approximately half of these fibers are small and unmyelinated. These fibers transmit information more slowly than the larger myelinated axons, which are capable of extremely rapid transmission of information. Some of the fibers connect to similar areas in the right and left hemispheres; other fibers go to areas in the contralateral hemisphere that are analogous to areas that have dense ipsilateral connections with their area of origin. A final group of fibers are diffusely connected to the contralateral hemisphere. If there is an analogy in the human brain with findings reported in the animal literature, some neurons may cross the callosum and descend to the subcortical structures before terminating.

Fibers from different areas of the cortex cross the callosum in discrete locations. To understand this phenomenon, it is necessary to examine the divisions of

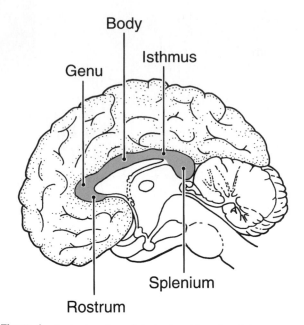

Figure 1 Sagittal section of the brain with major divisions of the corpus callosum labeled.

the corpus callosum (Fig. 1). The most anterior part of the callosum is the rostrum. Just behind the rostrum, the callosum bends to form the genu (or knee) and then extends posteriorly in the body. The body constricts slightly to become the isthmus and finally terminates in the slightly bulbous splenium. There is a great deal of individual variation in the shape and thickness of the different parts of the callosum. There have been attempts to understand differences in the anatomy of the right and left hemispheres and in the lateralization of function with regard to the morphology of the corpus callosum. As behavioral claims regarding the contributions of different areas of the callosum become more precise, it will become more crucial to be able to carefully define the areas of the callosum in which particular fibers cross. Currently, however, the areas are conventionally defined as proportions of the length of the callosum. There seems to be minimal difference whether the curvature of the callosum is taken into account or simply maximum anterior and posterior extension is used for the partition. The anterior one-fourth of the callosum is considered the genu. The rostral body begins directly behind the genu, extending back to include the anterior one-third of the callosum. The center one-third of the callosum is split into two equal sections, the anterior and posterior midbody. The isthmus extends from the posterior one-third to the posterior one-fifth of the callosum. Finally, the most posterior one-fifth is considered the splenium.

Because these definitions are arbitrary, they may differ in detail from investigator to investigator, depending on the investigator's emphasis.

Generally, however, it is believed that the fibers that pass through the different regions of the corpus callosum represent the anterior-to-posterior organization of the cerebral cortex (Fig. 2). Deepak Pandya and Benjamin Seltzer demonstrated an anterior-to-posterior organization of the callosal fibers of passage in the rhesus monkey. Prefrontal cortex and premotor cortex axons cross in the rostrum and genu. Motor and somatosensory axons are found primarily in the body. Auditory and association areas are represented in the isthmus and visual areas in the splenium. Stephen Lomber and colleagues document a similar arrangement in the corpus callosum of the cat, although auditory fibers are found throughout the body and dorsal splenium, largely overlapping with limbic and visual fibers except in the very ventral sections of the splenium, which are entirely visual. The same anterior-to-posterior organization has been demonstrated by Marie Christine de Lacoste and colleagues in the

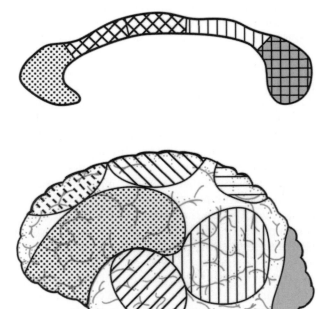

Figure 2 Areas of the cortex where fibers of the corpus callosum originate are coded to match the section of the corpus callosum where those fibers cross to the other hemisphere (adapted from M. C. DeLacoste, J. B. Kirkpatrick, and A. D. Ross, Topography of the human corpus callosum, *J. Neuropathol. Exp. Neurol.* **44**, 578–591, 1985).

human brain. That is, the right and left prefrontal, orbital–frontal, and frontal language areas are connected in the rostrum and the genu. The anterior part of the body carries fibers from the sensory and motor regions that abut the central sulcus. It appears that fibers from the area around the Sylvian fissure, associated with language function in the left hemisphere, cross in the posterior part of the body or isthmus. Finally, the splenium carries fibers connecting the visual areas of the occipital lobe.

Although it is now known that there are distinctive behavioral deficits associated with lesions to some regions of the callosum, contributions of the corpus callosum to behavior have not been easy to observe and understand. Some scientists have argued that evolutionary evidence suggests that the corpus callosum plays a distinctive role in human behavior. The callosum is not present in some primitive marsupials and takes on greatly increased prominence in the human species. The prominence of the corpus callosum appears to increase as lateralization increases, but this relationship is currently very speculative. In fact, James Rilling and Thomas Insel argue that, based on studies of 11 primate species, only the size of the splenium increases in proportion to increasing brain size, whereas the size of the corpus callosum as well as that of the anterior commissure are actually reduced relative to the size of other structures in higher primates. This observation suggests that any changes in the callosum related to human evolution are specific to particular areas of the callosum such as the splenium.

Developmentally, the callosum is a small structure in the neonatal brain that increases in size and prominence as the fibers myelinate (Fig. 3). At approximately 7 weeks of gestation, the lamina terminalis begins to thicken forming the commissural plate. By approximately 9 weeks cells begin to form the massa commissurelis, which supports the growth of the first commissural fibers at approximately 12 weeks. The basic structure of the callosum is present by 20 weeks and it continues to thicken and develop until birth, with development of the genu and body occurring before that of the splenium and rostrum. The myelinization of the corpus callosum is not believed to be complete until puberty, and recent evidence suggests that it reaches its maximum size at approximately age 25. It has been argued that the distinctive evolutionary and developmental patterns suggest a special role for the callosum in human behavior. Sandra Witelson has argued strongly that the anatomy of the callosum may be key to

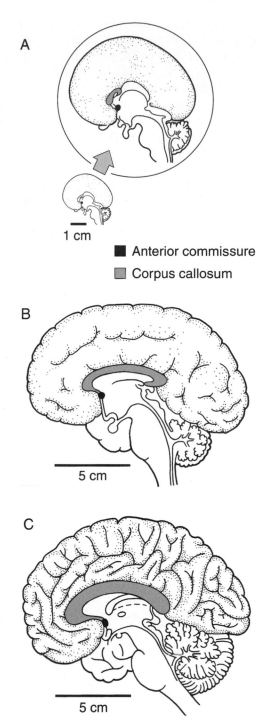

1 cm

■ Anterior commissure
▨ Corpus callosum

5 cm

5 cm

Figure 3   Relative size of the corpus callosum is seen in at 16 weeks (A), 40 weeks (B), and at adulthood (C) (adapted from S. P. Springer and G. Deutsch, *Left Brain, Right Brain: Perspectives from Cognitive Neuroscience*. p. 260. Freeman, New York, 1997).

understanding developmental issues of lateralization and hemispheric specialization. Deliniating that role has proven difficult.

II. HISTORY

The previously mentioned observations, specifically that of the sheer size of the fiber tract and its position as a unique midline structure, were important in suggesting to early scientists that it would be crucial to understand the callosum's role in behavior to fully understand the organization of the brain. In the early literature, it even competed with the pineal gland as a potential seat of the soul. Responding to an increasing belief that the corpus callosum played a major role in the integration of brain activities, Thomas Huxley called the corpus callosum "the greatest leap forward anywhere made by Nature in her brain work."

However, in the 20th century, studies of the callosum suggested that it was of much less interest than its prominent anatomy might indicate. Work in Pavlov's laboratory by Konstantin Bykov and Aleksei Speransky demonstrated that the transfer of conditioned learning from one side of the body to the other in dogs was abolished after section of the corpus callosum. However, this interesting work failed to gain significant recognition and was overshadowed by other animal work that did not document an important role for the corpus callosum in behavior. In the 1940s, William Van Wagenen and Robert Herren resected the callosum in a series of patients as treatment for epilepsy. These patients were extensively tested for psychological and behavioral changes. Although some patients improved, there did not appear to be consistent benefits in control of epilepsy nor consistent changes in their cognitive ability as a result of the severing of this enormous band of fibers. This series of surgeries did not continue and the interest in callosal function waned. Psychologist Karl Lashley was so unimpressed with the effect of severing the corpus callosum that he concluded that the corpus callosum played only a minimal role in psychological function.

It was the remarkable developments in animal research in the 1950s that paved the way for a greater understanding of the function of the corpus callosum in humans. Roger Sperry and Ronald Meyers, after splitting both the corpus callosum and the optic chiasm in the cat, showed that if one eye of the cat was covered while it learned a task, when that eye was covered and the other eye uncovered the animal acted as if it had no knowledge of the task. When exposed to the same learning trials, it had to learn again from scratch with no significant benefit from the prior exposure. In this case, the hemisphere of the brain that had not been able to see the task being learned had to complete the task and showed no evidence of having learned it previously. The important principle that their approach uncovered was that care had to be taken to introduce information only to one hemisphere of the brain and to test that hemisphere independently as well. For the first time, the discovery that learning of a task could occur independently in the separate hemispheres of the brain was widely appreciated.

In the 1960s, Norman Geschwind published his influential review of disconnection syndromes. Disconnection syndromes are patterns of behavior that occur when the fibers that connect areas of the brain responsible for different aspects of a task are damaged, preventing communication needed to complete complex behaviors. Perhaps the most striking of these syndromes is alexia without agraphia—that is, the ability to write in the absence of the ability to read. Patients with this striking disorder can write words and sentences spontaneously or to dictation, but they are unable to read what they have written. All reading is severely impaired in this group due to a disruption of the fibers that carry visual information to the area of the left hemisphere that decodes words into sound and meaning. However, that decoding area is intact and, hence, the ability to write and spell is intact. The existence of such syndromes suggested that a complete section of the corpus callosum should produce other dramatic behavioral changes.

Geshwind's comprehensive review of the animal and human literature emphasized the importance of the corpus callosum and other fiber tracts in producing complex behaviors. The corpus callosum was obviously the largest of the known fiber tracts and Geshwind's review suggested that it played an important role in transmitting information between the two hemispheres of the brain, despite the discouraging results from the series of split-brain surgeries performed by Van Wagenen. Pursuing this idea, Geschwind and colleague Edith Kaplan were among the first to observe disconnection symptoms in a patient with a naturally occurring lesion of the corpus callosum.

Meanwhile, physicians continued to consider a possible role for the corpus callosum in the spread of epileptic seizures. After a careful review of the Van Wagenen series and with the new observations of Geschwind in mind, Philip Vogel and Joseph Bogen decided once again to attempt to resect the corpus callosum as a treatment for epilepsy, but with some differences in procedure. The corpus callosum is not the only fiber tract that connects the left and right hemispheres. Many smaller tracts, the anterior commissure in particular, that were not severed in the Van

Wagenen series also cross the midline and could serve as an alternative route to spread seizure activity. Bogen and Vogel suspected that some of the original surgeries had not alleviated the epilepsy because these alternate tracts served to spread the seizure activity in the absence of the callosum. Hence, they initiated a new series of surgeries that resected not just the corpus callosum but also additional tracts, including the anterior commissure.

Guided by the exciting observations made in the Sperry laboratory with cats and by the renewed interest in disconnection syndromes, plans were made for a more intensive study of the disconnection effects in humans after commissurotomy. A team consisting of Joseph Bogen, Roger Sperry, and Michael Gazzaniga assembled the tasks and methods of response they thought would be necessary to demonstrate the effect of split-brain surgery in humans. To understand their approach and observations, some knowledge of functional anatomy is necessary.

The most crucial problem the researchers faced was that the left hemisphere in most people is the only one that controls speech. Hence, if only a verbal response to a task is accepted, the mute right hemisphere will not be able to respond and may appear unable to do simple tasks. They realized that if right hemisphere skills were to be probed, a manual response was required. Tasks had to be designed to allow a button press response or some other tactile response.

Second, because there is some ipsilateral control of motor output, knowledge being tested had to somehow be isolated in one hemisphere or the other to prevent interference between the two hemispheres in controlling a tactile response. Because of the unique anatomy of the visual system in humans, it was possible to isolate visual words and pictures to one hemisphere but only under very special conditions. Figure 4 shows the organization of the visual system. Information from the right side of space first reaches the cortex in the back of the left side of the brain or occipital lobe and vice versa. Unlike in the cat in the earlier Sperry experiments, covering one eye does not isolate information to one hemisphere, so more elaborate procedures are necessary. In most people, the information about the two sides of space is quickly woven together into a seamless visual world through the neural transmission across the callosum. Once these fibers are severed, information in one visual field is isolated in the contralateral hemisphere. This only holds true, however, if the eyes remain focussed on a single central location or fixation point. In everyday life, though, our eyes are always in motion and are

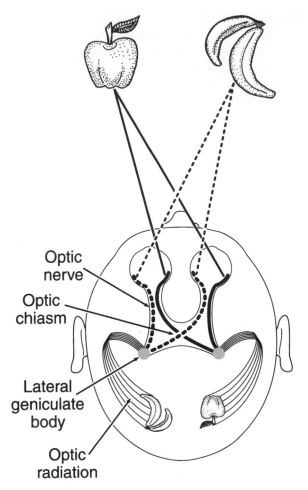

Optic
nerve

Optic
chiasm

Lateral
geniculate
body

Optic
radiation

Figure 4 After the corpus callosum is cut, the unique anatomy of the human visual system displays material presented on one side of space only to the contralateral hemisphere. When the callosum is intact, this visual information is shared between the hemispheres via the fibers of the splenium.

drawn quickly to changes in the visual environment. Hence, to an investigator who wishes to have visual information presented in the left visual field seen only in the right hemisphere, this reflexive orienting movement presents a challenge. To prevent cyc motion from interfering with lateralization, words or pictures had to be presented for 150 msec or less so that there was not time for the eyes to move from the fixation point to the stimulus display. The early devise used to ensure brief presentations was known as a tachistoscope, but today many investigators control the length of the stimulus display with a computer.

Although the visual system provides clean lateralization of information in a split-brain subject, the auditory system does not. Fibers from the auditory system of one ear reach both hemispheres of the brain, with about 60% of the pathway arriving in the

contralateral hemisphere and 40% in the ipsilateral hemisphere. In order to test auditory comprehension separately in the left and right hemispheres, an auditory stimulus had to be compared with some completely lateralized visual stimulus.

One other neural pathway, although it has some ipsilateral representation, provides relative isolation of information to the contralateral hemisphere. Somatosensory information from the hands is predominently transferred to the contralateral hemisphere. Hence, when real objects are placed in the hands and palpated to aid in identification, the somatosensory information about the object remains in one hemisphere. The ipsilateral fibers do provide the ipsilateral hemisphere with some basic perceptual information but do not generally provide enough cues for identification of the object.

Bogen, Sperry, and Gazzaniga used these basic facts about the anatomy of the nervous system to guide their investigations of the changes that follow section of the corpus callosum. By carefully isolating the hemispheres via these methods, they were able for the first time to map the profound changes that do occur after callosotomy. They examined the subjects in this new series before and after surgery and were able to confirm one of the early observations: These patients appear quite normal after surgery. To the casual observer, there appears to be very little difference in the presentation of the person before and after surgery. After the initial few weeks following surgery in which there may be symptoms such as mutism and inter-manual conflict, the split-brain subjects experience the world as unified and converse and interact normally. The subjective response to what might be expected to be a radical and frightening change in one's inner world appears to be minimal. Gazzaniga observed, "Indeed, one would miss the departure of a good friend more, apparently, than the left hemisphere misses the right."

However, when observations were made under conditions that allowed only one hemisphere access to information and gave the mute right hemisphere a means of response, the now well-known hemispheric disconnection syndrome was elicited. The researchers gave patients objects to palpate in one hand at a laboratory table that screened the hand and the item from the subject's view. When an item was palpated by the right hand, there was no difference from normal behavior. The patient was easily able to name the item because all the tactile information from the right hand was available to the speaking left hemisphere. In contrast, when the same common objects were placed in the left hand (and kept out of view), the talking left hemisphere was not able to identify the item and could not name it. The subject appeared to be anomic. However, despite being unable to name the object being grasped, the left hand of the subject could often demonstrate how the object was used or identify it from a group of objects. The somatosensory information from the left hand allowed the right hemisphere to identify but not to name the object. Because the information about the object could not be transmitted across the callosum, the talking left hemisphere could not help and supply the spoken name of the item. This was a vivid demonstration of what is now generally accepted about lateralization of function in right-handed people. The right hemisphere may possess knowledge about objects and their use in the world, but it lacks knowledge of how to produce the spoken name. This information is represented only in the left hemisphere, and once the callosum is cut the right hemisphere is left mute.

Another way to demonstrate the inability to transfer somatosensory information between the hemispheres in the absence of the callosum is to lightly touch different points on the patient's hand when it is out of view. If the right hand is touched in different positions, the right thumb can accurately point to each of the stimulated positions, but if the patient is asked to respond to the right-sided touch on the homologous area of the left hand, the task is impossible. This is equally true in reverse. The left hand can point to stimulated areas on the left hand but cannot transfer this information to the right hand. This task is trivial for people with an intact callosum, and if you are in doubt, try it. With your eyes closed, have a friend tap different areas on the palm and fingers of each hand. You will be able to respond easily with either the ipsilateral or the contralateral hand to the light touches.

Perhaps the most striking change demonstrated by Gazzaniga and Sperry was the inability to transfer visual information between the hemispheres. When two visual stimuli, either words or pictures, were lateralized one to each hemisphere, simple same/different judgments were performed at chance levels. That is, the patients could not accurately decide if the two words or pictures were identical or different when one was seen by the right hemisphere and one by the left hemisphere. However, within a hemisphere, both the right and the left hemispheres not only were able to decide if two stimuli were identical but also to match words and pictures. The ability to match words and pictures within the right hemisphere was particularly

exciting because it showed that the isolated right hemisphere was able to read for meaning at least at the single word level (although it could not say the words out loud).

These basic observations ignited a period of rapid and productive investigation of the capacities of the two hemispheres. In the following sections, only the work that bears on a closer examination of the functional significance of the callosum will be presented.

III. ANATOMY AND BEHAVIOR

As the resurgence of interest in the results of callosotomy helped to elucidate the functional capacities of each hemisphere, questions arose regarding the specificity of callosal function. In an early review of the literature on callosal organization, Georgio Innocenti offered some general principles regarding the topography of callosal fibers. He considered the organization of the callosum in humans to be an interesting question because of the demonstration by Sidtis, Gazzaniga, and colleagues in the human split-brain subject that semantic and sensory aspects of visual stimuli were transferred in different parts of the callosum. The Gazzaniga laboratory and others have continued to report very specific limitations on transfer after partial lesions to the callosum.

Nonetheless, Francisco Abolitz and Eran Zaidel argue that there is great equipotentiality across the callosum. There is other anatomical support for this view. The de Lacoste work demonstrates substantial overlap between temporal lobe and superior frontal lobe fibers in the body of the callosum. The superior parietal lobe, temporal parietal junction, and occipital lobe all have some fibers passing in the splenium. Behaviorally, inconsistencies reported later suggest minimally that there may be notable individual differences.

One factor that can make the specific role of the callosum difficult to isolate is the myriad of additional interhemispheric tracts and other interactions that occur in the midbrain and brain stem. There are numerous other commissures not routinely part of split-brain surgery in humans, including the posterior commissure, the habenular commissure, the commissures of the inferior and superior colliculi and the massa intermedia, and the thalamic commissure (which is not present in all brains). As fibers descend into the brain stem, there is much less segregation and many pathways may share information across the midline. These commissures are so deep in the brain that they are never severed during split-brain surgery in humans because of the devastating effects this would have on life-sustaining behavior. Hence, when an unexpected transfer of information occurs, the possibility that there is some subcortical communication that accounts for it is often raised.

Nonetheless, there are consistent deficits after complete section of the corpus callosum. Joseph Bogen outlined the principal deficits associated with lesions of the corpus callosum. He enumerated 10 symptoms that should be tested to confirm cases of callosal disconnection in normally lateralized right-handed subjects. In all cases, information is isolated in one hemisphere due to the loss of callosal fibers, resulting in the following symptoms:

1. Unilateral "verbal anosia": If an odor is presented unilaterally to the right nostril, it cannot be named, although the left hand can pick out the item associated with the odor.

2. Double hemianopsia: If responses are permitted from one hand at the time, the patient will appear to have a homonomous hemianopsia (i.e., an apparent blindness for one-half of space) in the field ipsilateral to the response hand. When responses are required from the opposite hand, the side of the "blind" field will change.

3. Hemialexia: If words are presented rapidly in one visual field, the ipsilateral hemisphere cannot give any sign that it has read or even seen the words.

4. Auditory suppression: Information presented from one ear is suppressed or extinguished by the ipsilateral hemisphere.

5. Unilateral (left) ideomotor apraxia: Because the left hemisphere is dominant not just for language but also generally for motor planning, the left hand is unable to carry out actions to command. It is essential to demonstrate that the deficit is not due to weakness or problems with coordination or ataxia.

6. Unilateral (left) agraphia: Most right-handed people have some ability to write with their left hand, although the letters may be less fluent and well formed than those made by their dominant hand. After callosal disconnection, the left hand loses this ability.

7. Unilateral (left) tactile anomia: Objects placed in the left hand but not seen cannot be named. Often, the function of the object can be demonstrated or a related object can be selected.

8. Unilateral (right) constructional apraxia: Because the right hemisphere is better at visual–spatial problems, the right hand will have difficulty executing complex drawings or manipulating three-dimensional objects or puzzles. However, it should be noted that the Gazzaniga laboratory has observed bilateral constructional apraxia in several patients. Gazzaniga has argued that these skills depend on interhemispheric integration in some patients, and therefore can be observed to decline for either hand after callosal section in these patients.

9. Spatial acalculia: The degree of visual–spatial impairment may be sufficiently great that patients are more successful at solving verbal arithmetic problems mentally than at writing them down with paper and pencil due to the distortion introduced by the act of writing. However, observation of this symptom may vary in the same way that it does for constructional apraxia.

10. Inability to transfer somesthetic information: As discussed previously, sensory and position information cannot be passed from hand to hand after callosotomy.

These distinctive sequelae of the disruption of cortical fibers had been noticed in part by the great 19th-century neurologists who laid the groundwork for our modern understanding of brain function. Sadly, many of their insights were lost or obscured by later experiments that failed due to shortcomings in observational techniques.

IV. SPECIFICITY

Here, we examine evidence from partial split-brain surgery, agenesis of the corpus callosum, and callosal lesions caused by stroke to better understand if different portions of the corpus callosum can be associated with different symptoms. After complete callosotomy, the whole range of symptoms discussed by Bogen should be found, with exceptions due to individual differences in lateralization. However, partial lesions may result in a subset of symptoms occurring, and these natural lesions provide another window into callosal function.

The discoveries of the Sperry, Gazzaniga, and Bogen group led to the identification of a new syndrome, alien (or anarchic) hand syndrome, by the French neurologists Serge Brion and C. P. Jedynak. They recognized that the unusual behaviors of a series of patients were related to naturally occurring callosal lesions. These lesions were the result of cerebrovascular disease or tumor. The patients shared a partial lesion of the corpus callosum and the experience of a left or nondominant hand that appeared to be completing complex motor behaviors outside of the control of the dominant left hemisphere. Although Gary Goldberg subsequently showed that medial frontal lobe damage can result in anarchic hand sign that has both a dominant and a nondominant form, patients with no evidence of frontal damage represent what Todd Feinberg terms the callosal type of anarchic hand syndrome. Comparison of the symptoms and lesion location of patients with callosal anarchic hand sign provides another window into the location of the information that transfers in the callosum.

First, we review the observations made based on partial callosotomies, and then we use reports from patients with natural lesions of the callosum to refine these observations regarding specific transfer of information. We know from the differences observed in spilt-brain patients who had either anterior or posterior section of the callosum first that the splenium or posterior callosum is important in the transfer of visual information. This is expected given the function of the occipital lobes and the preservation of the anterior/posterior cortical organization of the cortex in the position of the callosal fibers.

Gail Risse and colleagues examined the transfer of visual, somatosensory, kinesthetic, auditory, and motor information in seven patients with section of the anterior callosum sparing the splenium and varying amounts of the posterior section of the body. By comparing transfer ability across these patients, they were able to confirm that intact splenial fibers permitted transfer of visual information for both naming and same/different judgments. However, patients that had only splenial fibers intact were unable to name objects palpated by the left hand. This suggests that the information transferred in the splenium is specifically visual and does not include higher order information synthesized from sensory information in another modality (i.e., it is generally observed that the right hemisphere is able to identify objects palpated by the left hand). If palpated objects cannot be identified by name in subjects with an intact splenium, it suggests that the tactile information necessary to build a semantic representation cannot cross to the left hemisphere in the splenium and neither can higher order information representing the semantic identification. In contrast, patients with the posterior one-third to one-fifth of the body of the callosum intact were able to name these objects relatively well. Generally, this patient group could also match limb position across hemispheres and could complete tests of apraxia with

both the right and the left hand. Some difficulty with intermanual point localization was observed. A suppression of left ear auditory stimuli under dichotic conditions was noted for all but one subject. Although prior work indicates a role for the anterior callosum in praxis (due most likely to an interruption in the pathway necessary to carry the left hemisphere to "translation" of verbal commands for the right hemisphere to perform), there was little evidence of limb apraxia in this study except in the patients with sections that extended to the splenium. Another point made by Risse is that the left suppression on dichotic listening tasks in patients with good somatosensory function suggests that auditory fibers may be crossing anterior to somatosensory fibers, contrary to the results of Deepak Pandya and Benjamin Seltzer.

Although many sources confirm the importance of the splenium in the transfer of visual information, there may be even more specific function within the splenium. One of the patients investigated by the Gazzaniga laboratory, V.P., has shown some very specific transfer abilities. Margaret Funnell, Paul Corballis, and Michael Gazzaniga demonstrated that although V.P. is unable to transfer information about color, size, or shape across these spared fibers, she does show evidence of some access to words displayed to either hemisphere in the other, despite MRI confirmation of her status as a "complete" split. This remarkable specificity is supported by the work of Kyoko Suzuki and colleagues, who studied a young man with a small ventroposterior lesion to the callosum who could not read words in the left visual field. He could name pictures, however, suggesting that the anterior to middle section transfers picture information and the ventroposterior region is specific to letter transfer. Such precise lesions are rare but are revealing when carefully investigated. Of course, further work to confirm these observations is required, but they suggest that we are moving toward a much more specific understanding of the nature and location of the information transmitted in the callosum.

There remains disagreement regarding the relation between somatosensory and auditory fibers. A patient with a very discrete callosal lesion following a head injury showed increased suppression of left ear stimuli in dichotic testing when investigated by Michael Alexander and colleagues. His lesion appears to coincide with the posterior one-third to one-fourth of the body observed to be intact in some of Risse's patients. However, Risse found no auditory suppression in patients with good somatosensory function, suggesting auditory fibers were crossing anteriorly.

This was not true of Alexander's patient, who showed mildly impaired praxis and somatosensory function. (Unfortunately, transfer could not be tested because there were too many errors within a single hand to make it possible to observe decline in transfer.)

Early dichotic studies were in agreement that the portion of the callosum that caused greater left ear suppression was anterior to the splenium and was made up of the posterior one-half or one-third of the body of the callosum or was in the area of the isthmus. This was consistent with anatomical observations that indicated superior temporal lobe fibers crossed the callosum in this position. However, Sugushita and colleagues' careful examination of six patients with varied abnormalities of the corpus callosum suggested that damage to the splenium and posterior trunk leads to chronic left ear suppression. The patients in this study often had tumors that resulted in partial callosal resections, so there may have been some reorganization of function in response to tumor growth.

Given the individual differences in gyri, it may be that splenial fibers might better be defined by a common point of origin or by functional criteria rather than by a mathematically defined proportion. One paradox is that although some very precise disruptions in callosal transfer have been documented, there is significant variation in the areas where this transfer occurs. If this represents individual differences in the organization of the callosum, mathematical precision in separating the sections may not be helpful. In the meantime, the Risse observation remains difficult to reconcile with our current understanding of anatomy, and further observations will be necessary to understand the nature of the differences.

Another important function of the callosum is the transfer of information about an item identified either visually or tactilely in the right hemisphere to the left for oral naming. In a systematic investigation of the clinical signs associated with callosal transfer during a 12-month review of 282 new cases of cerebral infarction, Giroud and Dumas noted only 1 case of tactile anomia, and this patient had the most posterior callosal lesion, including the anterior one-third of the splenium. A patient investigated by Kathleen Baynes, Mark Tramo, and Michael Gazzaniga corroborates the observation that the anterior one-third of the splenium may be crucial for naming of items palpated by the left hand. This may represent transfer of word information as in the patient V.P., discussed previously.

However, all these observations await a better method for defining the regions of the callosum and tracing the origin and destination of fiber tracts than is currently available in order to be adequately confirmed or denied. It is also necessary to consider differences between right-to-left and left-to-right transmission because there are consistent behavioral advantages associated with direction of transfer.

V. CALLOSAL TRANSFER

Many research groups have been predominantly concerned with the speed and direction of callosal transfer or interhemispheric transfer time (IHTT). Perhaps the oldest method of estimation was developed by Albert Poffenberger in the early 19th century. He used lateralized visual displays to compare reaction time to material in the fields ipsilateral and contralateral to each response hand. Material in the contralateral field should be processed in the same hemisphere that initiates the manual response without need for callosal transfer. In contrast, ipsilateral displays must be processed in the opposite hemisphere and the signal must be transferred into the responding hemisphere. He subtracted crossed from uncrossed reaction times to yield a crossed–uncrossed difference as an estimate of how much time was required for this transfer. His results yielded an estimate of 2 or 3 msec for healthy adults. Such short transfer times are thought to implicate the large myelinated fibers of the callosum.

The advent of averaged evoked potentials to measure electrophysiological responses of populations of neurons provided another way of measuring IHTT. By comparing the time course of ipsilateral and contralateral peaks to lateralized visual or somatosensory stimulation, another estimate of IHTT has been obtained. Clifford Saron and Richard Davidson found about a 12-msec IHTT to visual stimuli. In contrast, somatosensory stimulation yielded estimates from 8 to 26 msec. The differences in even these simple stimulus-response IHTTs suggest to some that there is more than one route of callosal transfer, which would be expected if different sources of information indeed cross in different sections of the callosum. However, anatomical evidence of widespread callosal distribution of fibers from particular cortical loci also presents the possibility of multiple routes of crossing for specific types of information.

There have been many studies of callosal transfer that suggest that this transfer of information may not be symmetric. Carlo Marzi performed a meta-analysis that indicated that for right-handed people, responses to displays in the left visual field with the right hand are faster than the converse. One implication of this finding is that the right hemisphere transfers information to the left hemisphere more rapidly than the left hemisphere transfers it to the right hemisphere. Because this advantage does not appear in left-handed people (although determination of hemispheric dominance is more problematic in this population), it may not mark a consistent or important principle of brain organization. It is nonetheless interesting to note that the nondominant hemisphere appears to be more adept at "reporting" to the dominant hemisphere, at least in simple reaction time tasks.

VI. CORPUS CALLOSUM AND COGNITION

Despite the remarkably normal presentation of split-brain subjects, profound changes can be observed when the appropriate experimental controls are in place to observe them. However, there remain many claims regarding the role of the corpus callosum in normal and abnormal behavior that are intriguing but require further study to determine if they have merit. Such diverse mental characteristics as lateralization of language, disposition of attention, mnemonic processing, conscious behavior, disorders of learning, and schizophrenia have all been linked to callosal changes.

The relatively large size of the corpus callosum in humans compared with other primates and the prominent cerebral lateralization in humans suggest that corpus callosum may play a role in the development or maintenance of lateralized behaviors. The first premise has been challenged, but despite increasing evidence of some lateralization of function in other species, it remains true that the lateralization of language in the human is one of the most striking examples of cerebral specialization. In a twist on this logic, Sandra Witelson suggested that within the human species, greater lateralization of function may lead to decreased callosal size because fewer fibers are necessary to connect bilateral areas with similar functions. Therefore, if right-handed people are more clearly lateralized than left-handed people, as data from examinations to determine lateralization of language and memory prior to brain surgery indicate, one would expect to see greater relative size of the corpus callosum in left-handed people. Likewise, there have been claims that males are more clearly lateralized than females, so females should as a group have larger callosums. Moreover, because language is the most clearly lateralized cognitive skill, and the axons

from the language areas cross the midline primarily in the isthmus of the callosum, that structure is most likely to vary with relatively strong and weak lateralization.

With the advent of magnetic resonance imaging (MRI), visualization of the corpus callosum and measurement of its relative size in the living brain have become more straightforward. This has stimulated many attempts to test hypotheses regarding relative callosal size in right- and left-handed people, males and females, etc. The conclusions remain far from clear, although Witelson's work found a strong relationship between the site of the isthmus and handedness in men. Jeffrey Clark and Eran Zaidel, among others, have reported greater isthmus size in right-handed males compared to left-handed males. This effect is not found in females, although it is not known why handedness should have a different effect on lateralization and isthmus size in females. The Clark and Zaidel laboratories have performed many studies attempting to link behavioral measures to the size of the isthmus, with some success.

Although split-brain patients do not display the profound memory deficits associated with amnestic disorders, there do appear to be changes in the ability to integrate new memories in both laboratory and real-life settings. Most researchers with a long history of investigating these patients would agree that they exhibit a stereotypical conversational pattern that repeatedly returns to the same stories and episodes. This repertoire can expand to include information about things that happened postsurgically (unlike the dense memory deficits associated with hippocampal damage), but there is a lack of richness in the quality of reminiscence. These are, of course, subjective observations, and a more systematic evaluation of the clarity and accuracy of the pre- and postsurgical memory for life events in this population has yet to be completed.

There is evidence that clinical measures of memory show declines in some patients. Dahlia Zaidel observed declines on memory scales postsurgery, but this does not appear to be the case for all of the split-brain patients examined by the Gazzaniga laboratory. Elizabeth Phelps observed that memory scores decline after the posterior but not the anterior section of the corpus callosum, suggesting that perhaps inadvertent damage to the hippocampal commissure during surgery may contribute to the decline in memory skills. Amishi Jha and colleagues found that split-brain patients have difficulty "binding" both visual and verbal memory traces perhaps due to the dependence of some lateralized aspects of the memory trace formation on interhemispheric communication. Hence, it seems likely that some combination of extracallosal damage as well as the resection may result in some decline in memory function that implicates the callosum in the formation of a complete memory trace.

Work in the laboratories of Marie Banich and Jacqueline Liederman has indicated that greater task difficulty leads to a greater advantage for bilateral presentations. The conclusion is that for tasks that are easy, one hemisphere is able to accomplish them with the same speed and accuracy as two. When tasks become more difficult, bilateral presentations can be more advantageous. Banich employed many cleverly designed and careful experiments to demonstrate the complexity of such interactions, with the corpus callosum providing a crucial mechanism for the division of labor across the hemispheres. Essentially, attention is a resource that depends at least partially on the corpus callosum for allocation. Since most tasks can be accomplished by either hemisphere, there must be a flexible neural mechanism for determining whether a single hemisphere or both are necessary under different task demands. Liederman stressed the corpus callosum as a mechanism to "shield" incompatible neural processes. Although it is clear that the corpus callosum plays some role in attentional processing because deficits in both selective and sustained attention have been observed in split-brain subjects, a detailed model for this role remains a goal for the future.

A theoretical model that depends heavily on callosal inhibition as a mechanism for some aspects of lateralized behavior has been proposed by Norman Cook. Although it is generally agreed that most callosal fibers are excitatory, their effect can be inhibitory via interneurons. Cook stresses the inhibitory processes in describing the process of homotopic callosal inhibition. Excitation of an area in one hemisphere leads to inhibition of the analogous area in the other hemisphere and excitation of immediately surrounding areas in a sort of center-surround arrangement. He also posits a bilateral neural semantic net such that when an item such as "farm" is excited in one hemisphere, the analogous item in the opposite hemisphere is inhibited. Immediately related items (tractor, pig, cow, sheep, and plow in one of his examples) are excited via center-surround mechanisms. This arrangement is the underlying cause of the denotative language capacity of the left hemisphere and the connotative language of the right hemisphere. He presumes this mirror-symmetric activation pattern

to be a general mechanism, applicable to more than semantics. As Joseph Hellige rightly points out, the best evidence for interhemispheric inhibition is at the cellular level, whereas Cook often appears to be talking about a more functional role. Moreover, as his model stands, it would seem as if the hemispheric activation patterns could be easily reversed. This does not appear to be the case, at least for language functions. Despite the current lack of empirical support, this remains an interesting model of callosal function.

Despite many attempts to link morphological callosal differences to sex differences in lateralization, learning disabilities, and schizophrenia, definitive work in these areas remains elusive, and they will not be discussed here. The possibilities are intriguing, but the problems at this point contain too many degrees of freedom. The callosum appears to be a lever that could unlock our knowledge of brain function, but choosing the correct place to stand to use that leverage remains a problem.

VII. CORPUS CALLOSUM AND CONSCIOUSNESS

The study of split-brain patients during the past 40 years has helped change our understanding of the nature of consciousness. It has offered a prime example of the modularization of cognitive processes and documented the distinctions between a dominant and nondominant hemisphere. It has raised the question of whether the callosum may have played a unique role in the development of human consciousness. One of the key observations made regarding the Vogel and Bogen series of commissurotomies was that severing the callosum seemed to yield two separate conscious entities with the ability to respond independently. The idea of a "dual consciousness" was embraced by some scientists such as Pucetti, who hypothesized that the human condition was always made up of dual-consciousnesses that were only revealed after the section of the callosum. Others rejected the status of the right hemisphere as conscious. Daniel Dennett concluded that the right hemisphere had, at best, a "rudimentary self."

Michael Gazzaniga, Paul Corballis, and Margaret Funnell, recently proposed a new role for the corpus callosum as "the prime enabler for the human condition." They suggest the corpus callosum allows the brain to be more efficient, allowing hemispheric specialization but permitting integration of specialized functions as needed. In their view, lateral specialization reflects the emergence of new skills and the retention of others. An advantageous mutation that changes the function of one hemisphere can be maintained and flourish while established functions continue without disruption. The callosum permits a reduction of redundant function and the easier acquisition of new skills. They suggest that the corpus callosum facilitated the development of a "theory of mind," the skills that support the ability to understand the point of view of another creature, by permitting "this extended capacity [to arise] within a limited cortical space."

The best examples of behavior that appear to represent a separate consciousness in the right hemisphere come from split-brain patients with at least some language capacity. The newest completely split patient with normal intelligence, V.J., is anomalous in that she controls written and spoken output with different hemispheres. She is also unique in another way. She is the first split in my experience who is frequently dismayed by the independent performance of her right and left hands. She is discomforted by the fluent writing of her left hand to unseen stimuli and distressed by the inability of her right hand to write words she can read out loud and spell. In the myriad of articles discussing duality of consciousness, consciousness is sometimes considered as arising from the need for a single serial channel for motor output. In normally lateralized persons, the left hemisphere maintains control of output of both speech and writing. In V.J., there are two centers of control of the motor output of language, one partially disabled but still functional. One problem of this view point is that some split-brain patients, notably J.W. and V.P., also have some control of motor speech from either hemisphere. However, in both of these cases, the control of spoken language developed after the surgical intervention and this sequence of events may have different consequences for the conscious experience of it. If serial control of output is an important determinant of the function experienced as consciousness and the fluent shifting of control of output from one system to another is a part of that function, we may still have a good deal to learn from the split-brain model.

VIII. FUTURE DIRECTIONS

Giorgio Innocenti suggests that the complexity of callosal connections promises that these functional problems will remain fascinating but frustrating for some time. He points out that there is not yet an adequate understanding of the neural parameters that contribute to differences in size and shape of the callosum, including the number and size of axons that make up the callosum, the proportion of those axons that are myelinated, the thickness of the myelin sheath, and the number and size of blood vessels and other supporting elements. Although work in numerous laboratories is focused on answering some of these questions, until they are answered, studies correlating the size of the callosum or any of its sections to behavior are likely to continue to be frustrating.

Many of the fascinating but unproven hypotheses discussed previously could be more clearly addressed or ruled out if we had a better understanding of the neurophysiology of the human corpus callosum. Relatively little work has been done on the human callosum, although there is a large body of correlative data on differences in the morphology of the callosum derived from MRI and various aspects of behavior. However, there is still a very limited understanding of the anatomy of the callosum, where the crossing fibers originate and terminate, and the differences in the proportion of large and small fibers in different areas. Little is known about the connectivity of interneurons and how it affects the nature of the information transferred.

The advent of MRI led to a major increase in the number of studies examining gross correlations between anatomy and behavior, but the lack of a better understanding of the anatomy of callosal fibers and the basic mechanisms of transmission allowed too much freedom of interpretation. Hence, many of these studies reached inconsistent or conflicting conclusions.

A new method of image analysis known as diffusion tensor weighting is allowing researchers to examine the direction of movement in individual fiber tracts during different cognitive tasks. As this method is refined, and if it can be combined with a more explicit knowledge of callosal anatomy, the plethora of theories regarding the function of the callosum and its contribution to cognition may at last be open to more satisfying investigation.

See Also the Following Articles

ANTERIOR CINGULATE CORTEX • EPILEPSY • NEUROANATOMY

Suggested Reading

Beaton, A. A. (1997). The relation of planum temporale asymmetry and morphology of the corpus callosum to handedness, gender, and dyslexia: A review of the evidence. *Brain Language* **60,** 255–322.

Bogen, J. E. (1993). *The callosal syndromes.* In *Clinical neuropsychology* (K. M. Heilman and E. Valenstein, Eds.), 3rd ed. pp. 337–407. Oxford Univ. Press, New York.

Clarke, J. M., McCann, C. M., and Zaidel, E. (1998). *The corpus callosum and language: Anatomical–behavioral relationships.* In *Right Hemisphere Language Comprehension: Perspectives from Cognitive Neuroscience* (M. Beeman and C. Chiarello, Eds.), pp. 27–50. Erlbaum, Mahweh, NJ.

Cook, N. D. (1986). *The brain Code: Mechanisms of Information Transfer and the Role of the Corpus Callosum.* Methuen, London.

Gazzaniga, M. S. (1970). *The Bisected Brain.* Appleton–Century–Crofts, New York.

Gazzaniga, M. S. (2000). Cerebral specialization and interhemispheric communication Does the corpus callosum enable the human condition? *Brain* **123,** 1293–1326.

Harris, L. J. (1995). *The corpus callosum and historic communication: An historical survey of theory and research.* In *Hemispheric Communication: Mechanisms and Models* (F. L. Kitterle, Ed.), pp. 1–59. Erlbaum, Hillsdale, NJ.

Hellige, J. (1993). *Hemispheric Asymmetry: What's Right and What's Left.* Harvard Univ. Press, Cambridge, MA.

Hoptman, M. J., and Davidson, R. J. (1994). How and why do the two cerebral hemispheres interact? *Psychol. Bull.* **116,** 195–219.

Innocenti, G. M. (1994). Some new trends in the study of the corpus callosum. *Behav. Brain Res.* **64,** 1–8.

Reeves, A. G., and Roberts, D. W. (Eds.) (1995). *Epilepsy and the Corpus Callosum 2.* Plenum, New York.

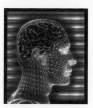

Cranial Nerves

ANN B. BUTLER

George Mason University

GLOSSARY

branchial arches The third and several additional visceral arches (usually five in all), which in fishes are in the region of the gills.

epimere The dorsal portion of the mesodermal layer in the developing body wall and head; also called paraxial mesoderm. It forms a segmental, rostrocaudal series of mesodermal masses called somites in the body and the caudal part of the developing head. Further rostrally in the head, it forms incompletely divided, segmental masses called somitomeres.

hypomere The ventral portion of the mesodermal layer in the developing body wall; also called lateral plate mesoderm. It gives rise to the smooth muscle of the gut and to the cardiac muscle of the heart.

mesomere The middle portion of the mesodermal layer in the developing body wall; also called the nephric ridge. It gives rise to the kidneys and gonads.

neural crest Ectodermally derived cells initially located at the lateral edge of the invaginating neural tube that subsequently migrate and contribute to numerous parts of the developing nervous system and body, including some of the bipolar neurons that lie in the ganglia of most sensory cranial nerves, all of the bipolar neurons of the sensory spinal nerve ganglia, the postganglionic neurons of the autonomic nervous system, most of the cranium, and the visceral arches.

neurogenic placodes Thickened regions of the epidermis that give rise to many of the bipolar neurons that lie in the ganglia of most of the sensory cranial nerves. Placodes occur only in the developing head region.

somites The segmental, mesodermal masses of the developing body wall and caudal head that are derived from epimere. In the body, somites give rise to the striated skeletal muscle of the body wall and limbs. In the caudal head, the somites give rise to most of the branchial arch muscles of the palate, pharynx, and larynx (innervated by cranial nerve X) and to the hypobranchial muscles of the tongue (innervated by cranial nerve XII).

somitomeres The incompletely divided, mesodermal masses of the developing head that are derived from epimere. They give rise to the striated muscles of the eyes (innervated by cranial nerves III, IV, and VI) and of the first three visceral arches (innervated by cranial nerves V, VII, and IX).

visceral arches A series of skeletal arches that occur in the region of the jaw and throat (pharynx) in mammals; they include the mandibular arch that forms the jaw, the hyoid arch, and the branchial arches. Most of the tissues of these arches are in fact somatic rather than visceral in developmental origin and function.

The cranial nerves provide the sensory and motor interfaces between the brain and the structures of the head. They supply the sensory inputs from our more than five senses and the motor (effector) innervation of muscles and glands. Like spinal nerves, the cranial nerves have sensory, or afferent, components that innervate structures in the head as well as the viscera of the thorax and abdomen and motor, or efferent, components that innervate muscles and glands in the head and the viscera. Three additional "special" components of cranial nerves are commonly recognized that spinal nerves lack; however, insights into the embryological derivation of sensory structures and muscles in the head allow us to discard this special category. Considering the sensory cranial nerves, humans arguably have at least 13 different senses, but even so we lack some additional senses that are present in other vertebrates. Some tetrapods, including most mammals, have an accessory olfactory (vomeronasal) system, for example, that is present in humans only

Copyright 2002, Elsevier Science (USA).
All rights reserved.

transiently during embryological development, and humans (along with other mammals) entirely lack the lateral line mechanoreceptive and electroreceptive systems of most aquatic vertebrates. We do not possess the infrared-receptive system of snakes or the independently evolved electroreceptive and mechanoreceptive systems via the trigeminal nerve that platypuses have. With regard to these other systems, we are, as William Wordsworth wrote, "creature[s] moving about in worlds not realized." Nevertheless, our set of sensory and motor, cranial and spinal nerves is the essential and only connection that the human central nervous system has with the external world. Via these nerves, all the sensory stimuli that one can detect are brought into the brain, and all the motor actions that one makes are commanded.

I. INTRODUCTION

Some of the cranial nerves are purely sensory, others are purely motor, and the rest have both sensory and motor components. Twelve cranial nerves have traditionally been recognized in humans, which are designated by Roman numerals as well as by descriptive names (Table I). The first two cranial nerves, the olfactory nerve (I) and the optic nerve (II), are purely sensory and innervate the nasal mucosa for the sense of smell (olfaction) and the eye for the sense of sight (vision), respectively. The 10 cranial nerves of the midbrain and hindbrain collectively comprise 23 individual, traditionally recognized components.

Table I
Traditional 12 Cranial Nerves

Nerve	Name
I	Olfactory
II	Optic
III	Oculomotor
IV	Trochlear
V	Trigeminal
VI	Abducens
VII	Facial
VIII	Vestibulocochlear (or statoacoustic)
IX	Glossopharyngeal
X	Vagus
XI	Spinal accessory
XII	Hypoglossal

Three purely motor nerves that innervate the muscles of the eye are collectively called oculomotor nerves and comprise the oculomotor nerve (III), the trochlear nerve (IV), and the abducens nerve (VI). The 4 nerves with both sensory and motor components that innervate the jaws, face, throat, and the thoracic and abdominal viscera are the trigeminal nerve (V), the facial nerve (VII), the glossopharyngeal nerve (IX), and the vagus nerve (X). Cranial nerve VIII, the vestibulocochlear (or statoacoustic) nerve, innervates the inner ear organs for the auditory and vestibular senses. Cranial nerves XI, the spinal accessory nerve, and XII, the hypoglossal nerve, are purely motor and innervate the muscles of the neck that are used to turn the head (the sternocleidomastoid and upper part of the trapezius) and the muscles of the tongue, respectively.

Most of the sensory cranial nerves are formed by the processes of bipolar (or pseudounipolar) neurons whose cell bodies lie within one or two sensory ganglia located on the nerve in the peripheral part of the nervous system. The sensory neurons each have a distal portion that either innervates a separate receptor cell or has a modified ending that itself is the receptor. Sensory transduction—the translation of the sensory stimulus into neuronal activity—involves a variety of physical and chemical mechanisms. The proximal portions of the bipolar sensory neurons project to a group of multipolar neurons that lie within nuclei in the central nervous system and in turn project to other groups of multipolar neurons in the sensory pathway. For each sensory system pathway, the bipolar-receptive, multipolar neurons are referred to here as first-order multipolar neurons since they are the first of several groups of multipolar neurons in the pathway. The sensory nuclei that contain the first-order multipolar neurons are named for the name of their major cranial nerve input (vestibular, cochlear, and trigeminal nuclei), the particular sensory system (gustatory nucleus), or for their appearance (solitary nucleus).

The motor cranial nerves innervate either muscles or glands. Most of the nerves that innervate muscles have cell bodies within their respective nuclei in the brain stem; their axons exit the brain in the cranial nerve and terminate directly on the particular muscle. Most of the nuclei of these nerve components have the same name as the nerve (oculomotor, trochlear, trigeminal motor, abducens, facial motor, and hypoglossal nuclei) or arise from a nucleus named for its indistinct appearance (nucleus ambiguus). Glands are innervated via a two-neuron chain of neurons that belong to the parasympathetic division of the autonomic nervous system. The cell bodies of the first neurons in the chain, called preganglionic parasympathetic neurons, lie within nuclei in the brain stem, and their axons exit the brain in the cranial nerve. These axons terminate on a second set of neurons that lie in a ganglion located close to the target organ and are called postganglionic parasympathetic neurons in reference to their axons, which exit the ganglion and innervate the gland. Three small muscles within the eye are also innervated by the autonomic nervous system. Two of these intraocular muscles (for pupillary constriction and control of the shape of the lens) are innervated by the axons of postganglionic parasympathetic neurons, whereas the third (for pupillary dilation) is innervated by postganglionic axons that are part of the sympathetic division of the autonomic nervous system, which arises from neurons located within thoracic and upper lumbar spinal cord segments. The parasympathetic cell groups of the brain stem have a variety of names, including the eponymic Edinger–Westphal nucleus, the superior and inferior salivatory nuclei, the dorsal motor nucleus of X, and some of the neurons in nucleus ambiguus.

The motor nuclei of the brain stem all receive a variety of inputs from other neuron cell groups in the brain. These inputs include relatively local connections with reticular formation neurons and long, descending projections from motor regions of neocortex. Since the latter connections arise from neurons located above (rostral to) the cranial nerve nuclei, they are referred to as supranuclear connections. The majority of supranuclear inputs to cranial nerve nuclei are bilateral.

II. TRADITIONAL FUNCTIONAL COMPONENTS

Each of the various components of most of the cranial nerves has traditionally been classified as somatic (referring to body wall structures) or visceral (referring to internal organs), afferent (sensory) or efferent (motor), and general or special. The latter pair of terms are used in reference to earlier beliefs concerning the embryological derivation of some of the sensory structures and muscles in the head. Recent new information will allow us to discard these categories later in this article, but their current widespread use necessitates discussing them here.

The first two pairs of classification terms for cranial nerves correspond to the four components of spinal nerves. Sensory nerve components are thus either somatic afferent or visceral afferent, and motor

components are likewise either somatic efferent or visceral efferent. Spinal nerve components and some cranial nerve components are additionally classified as general, so they are designated general somatic afferent (GSA), general visceral afferent (GVA), general somatic efferent (GSE), and general visceral efferent (GVE). The sensory GSA components innervate the skin of the face and position sense (proprioception) receptors in head musculature, whereas GVA components innervate the viscera of the thorax and abdomen and a few structures in the head and neck, such as the mucous membranes of the oral cavity. The motor GSE components innervate extraocular eye muscles and the muscles of the tongue, whereas GVE components supply parasympathetic innervation to the thoracic and abdominal viscera and to glands and intraocular muscles in the head.

Two sensory cranial nerve components are categorized as special and thus designated special somatic afferent (SSA) and special visceral afferent (SVA). The SSA category is applied to the auditory and vestibular senses, whereas the SVA category is applied to the sense of taste (gustation). The two most rostral cranial nerves of the traditional 12, for olfaction and vision, are frequently not categorized at all. One cranial nerve motor category is also designated as special—the special visceral efferent (SVE) components of cranial nerves V, VII, IX, and X. Cranial nerve XI is sometimes not categorized but can be included in this traditional SVE category as well. SVE components of cranial nerves innervate muscles of the face, the mandibular and hyoid arches, the throat, and the neck, which all develop embryologically from muscles of the visceral arches that include the mandibular arch for the jaw, the hyoid arch, and a series of branchial arches. The latter give rise to the gill region in fishes and to components of the throat in tetrapods. The variously recognized traditional components of the midbrain and hindbrain cranial nerves are summarized in Table II, whereas the newer, revised classification is presented in Table III.

In the spinal cord, the two sensory afferent and two motor efferent components of the spinal nerves have their central cell groups organized in a dorsal to ventral order of GSA, GVA, GVE, and GSE. These rostrocaudally running functional columns extend into the brain stem so that the central cell groups of the cranial nerves in the hindbrain and midbrain lie in a similar topographic order. Due to the geometry of the brain's ventricular system, these cell columns lie in a lateral to medial order of GSA, GVA, GVE, and GSE. The two additional "special" sensory components of the cranial

Table II
Traditionally Recognized Components of Midbrain and Hindbrain Cranial Nerves[a]

Cranial nerve	Component	Sensory ganglion or motor ganglion and/or nucleus
Oculomotor (III)	GSE	Oculomotor nucleus
	GVE	Edinger–Westphal and anterior medial nuclei/ciliary ganglion
Trochlear (IV)	GSE	Trochlear nucleus
Trigeminal (V)	GSA	Trigeminal ganglion
	SVE	Trigeminal motor nucleus
Abducens (VI)	GSE	Abducens nucleus
Facial (VII)	GSA	Geniculate ganglion
	SVA	Geniculate ganglion
	GVE	Superior salivatory nucleus/pterygopalatine and submandibular ganglia
	SVE	Facial motor nucleus
Vestibulocochlear (VIII)	SSA	Spiral and vestibular ganglia
Glossopharyngeal (IX)	GSA	Superior (jugular) ganglion
	GVA	Inferior (petrosal) ganglion
	SVA	Inferior (petrosal) ganglion
	GVE	Inferior salivatory nucleus/otic ganglion
	SVE	Nucleus ambiguus
Vagus (X)	GSA	Superior (jugular) ganglion
	GVA	Inferior (nodose) ganglion
	SVA	Inferior (nodose) ganglion
	GVE	Dorsal motor nucleus of X and nucleus ambiguus/parasympathetic ganglia of thoracic and abdominal viscera and heart
	SVE	Nucleus ambiguus
Spinal accessory (XI)	SVE	Cervical anterior horn cells
Hypoglossal (XII)	GSE	Hypoglossal nucleus

[a]Abbreviations used: GSA, general somatic afferent; GVA, general visceral afferent; SSA, special somatic afferent; SVA, special visceral afferent; GSE, general somatic efferent; GVE, general visceral efferent; SVE, special visceral efferent.

nerves (SSA and SVA) have central cell groups that lie near the GSA nuclei. The SVE cell column lies in a more displaced, ventrolateral position, which is a legacy of its early evolutionary origin. The SVE cranial nerves and the visceral arch muscles that they supply evolved in the earliest vertebrates before the GSE column and its associated set of muscles were gained.

A. Cranial Nerves of the Medulla

Four of the cranial nerves are present in the medulla: the hypoglossal nerve (XII), the spinal accessory nerve (XI), the vagus nerve (X), and the glossopharyngeal nerve (IX). Cranial nerves XII and XI are simple nerves that have only a single component, which is motor. Cranial nerves X and IX are the two most complex cranial nerves, each with five traditional functional components.

1. Hypoglossal Nerve

Cranial nerve XII innervates the muscles of the tongue. A fleshy tongue and thus a distinct hypoglossal nucleus and nerve are present only in tetrapods. The tongue develops embryologically from hypobranchial musculature that lies ventral to the visceral arches of the pharyngeal region. The only component present in the hypoglossal nerve is the GSE. The nerve arises from motor neurons in the hypoglossal nucleus, which lies in a medial position in the dorsal part of the medulla and is the caudalmost portion of the GSE column in the brain stem. Hypoglossal nerve fibers run ventrally from the hypoglossal nucleus and exit the medulla on its ventral surface between the medially lying pyramidal (corticospinal) tract and the more laterally lying inferior olivary nucleus. Hypoglossal innervation of the tongue is ipsilateral.

Damage to the ventromedial medulla may thus result in the syndrome called inferior alternating hemiplegia, which is motor impairment on the contralateral side of the body (due to damage to the pyramidal tract) combined with weakness of tongue muscles on the ipsilateral (i.e., alternate) side due to a lower motor neuron lesion of the nerve. When protruded, the tongue deviates toward the side of the lesion. Supranuclear innervation of the hypoglossal nucleus is bilateral, so lesions that interrupt this input result only in mild weakness of the tongue musculature on the side opposite to the lesion. During normal usage, the pattern of tongue movements is modulated by inputs to the hypoglossal nucleus relayed from other cranial nerve nuclei, including those of V for

Table III
New Classification of Cranial Nerve Components in Humans[a]

Cranial nerve	Traditional classification	New classification	Embryological derivation or site of innervation
Terminal	—	SA	Olfactory placode
I	—	SA	Olfactory placode
II	—	NTA	Neural tube
Epiphyseal	—	NTA	Neural tube
III	GSE	SE	Epimeric muscles
	GVE	VE	Ciliary ganglion
IV	GSE	SE	Epimeric muscle
V	GSA	SA	Neural crest and trigeminal placode
	SVE	SE: branchial motor	Epimeric muscle
VI	GSE	SE	Epimeric muscle
VII	GSA	SA	Neural crest and/or ventrolateral placode
	SVA	VA	Neural crest and/or ventrolateral placode
	GVE	VE	Neural crest
	SVE	SE: branchial motor	Epimeric muscles
VIII	SSA	SA	Dorsolateral placode
IX	GSA	SA	Neural crest and/or ventrolateral placode
	GVA	VA	Neural crest and/or ventrolateral placode
	SVA	VA	Neural crest and/or ventrolateral placode
	GVE	VE	Neural crest
	SVE	SE: branchial motor	Epimeric muscle
X	GSA	SA	Neural crest and/or ventrolateral placode
	GVA	VA	Neural crest and/or ventrolateral placode
	SVA	VA	Neural crest and/or ventrolateral placode
	GVE	VE	Neural crest
	SVE	SE: branchial motor	Epimeric muscles
XI	SVE	SE: branchial motor	Epimeric muscles
XII	GSE	SE	Epimeric muscles

[a]Abbreviations used: GSA, general somatic afferent; GVA, general visceral afferent; SSA, special somatic afferent; SVA, special visceral afferent; GSE, general somatic efferent; GVE, general visceral efferent; NTA, neural tube afferent; SVE, special visceral efferent; SA, somatic afferent; VA, visceral afferent; SE, somatic efferent; VE, visceral efferent.

proprioception and IX and X for stimuli from the mucosal lining of the oral cavity.

2. Spinal Accessory Nerve

Cranial nerve XI (the accessory nerve) has traditionally been considered to comprise two parts, a cranial part that arises from neuron cell bodies in the caudal part of nucleus ambiguus (which lies in the lateral region of the medulla) and a spinal part that arises from neuron cell bodies located in the lateral part of the gray matter within upper segments of the cervical spinal cord. The laterally displaced position of the latter cell group is similar to that of the corresponding cell column in the brain stem. The so-called cranial part of XI (not included in Table II) is in fact merely the more caudal part of the vagus nerve. It supplies innervation to the intrinsic muscles of the larynx on the ipsilateral side. The spinal part of XI innervates the ipsilateral sternocleidomastoid muscle and the upper parts of the trapezius muscle. Contraction of the sternocleidomastoid muscle on one side causes the mastoid process (which lies behind the ear) to approach the sternum and medial part of the clavicle ("cleido"), thus causing the head to turn toward the contralateral side. Innervation of the spinal nucleus of XI from motor cortex appears to be predominantly ipsilateral. Damage to the spinal accessory nerve results in weakness of the ipsilateral muscles, which is revealed when trying to turn the head toward the opposite side against resistance.

The accessory nerve is sometimes unclassified, but it is a branchial motor nerve and belongs in the traditional category of SVE. The sternocleidomastoid and trapezius muscles evolved from the levator muscles of the branchial arches.

3. Vagus Nerve

Cranial nerve X has five components and by this measure joins cranial nerve IX in the distinction of being most complex. It has three sensory components GSA, SVA, and GVA and two motor components GVE and SVE. The GSA component is a minor one; its fibers innervate the region of the external auditory meatus and the tympanic membrane. These GSA fibers have cell bodies located in the superior (jugular) ganglion of X and enter the brain stem via the vagus nerve. They terminate in a rostrocaudally elongated group of first-order multipolar neurons that receive most of their input from GSA fibers of the trigeminal nerve. This group of neurons is called the spinal, or descending, nucleus of V since it extends from the pontine levels caudally into the upper part of the spinal cord, ending at the level of the second cervical segment. The ascending sensory pathway that arises from the spinal nucleus of V is discussed later.

The GVA and SVA sensory components of the vagus nerve are more substantial than the GSA component. The GVA component has its bipolar neurons located in the inferior (nodose) ganglion of X and provides sensory innervation to the viscera of the thorax and abdomen as well as to mucous membranes lining the pharynx, larynx, trachea, and esophagus. In the brain stem, these GVA axons enter a fiber bundle that is surrounded by its nucleus and thereby appears to be isolated from neighboring structures. This bundle is called tractus solitarius, and its nucleus, which contains the first-order multipolar neurons that receive the visceral sensory input, is called nucleus solitarius (the nucleus of the solitary tract). Nucleus solitarius projects to multiple brain stem sites, including the dorsal motor nucleus of X and nucleus ambiguus.

Additional visceral sensory innervation is via afferent fibers that traverse sympathetic and parasympa-

thetic nerves and then terminate on spinal cord dorsal horn neurons, which in turn project to the dorsal thalamus (ventral posterolateral and intralaminar nuclei). This information is then relayed to the neocortex. This ascending system accounts for most of the sensations from thoracic, abdominal, and pelvic viscera that are consciously experienced. Since the same pool of dorsal horn neurons also receives inputs from the somatic part of the body at each segmental level, this pattern of innervation is responsible for the phenomenon of "referred pain," in which visceral sensations are perceived as originating from the body wall.

The SVA component of the vagus nerve has bipolar neurons located in the inferior (nodose) ganglion of X. The cell group that receives taste afferents via this SVA component of the vagus nerve (and the SVA components of the glossopharyngeal and facial nerves as well) has previously been viewed as the rostral part of nucleus solitarius but is now recognized as a distinct and separate entity, the gustatory nucleus. The first-order multipolar neurons located in this nucleus receive taste sensation via the superior laryngeal branch of the vagus nerve from taste buds located on the epiglottis and esophagus. An ascending pathway originates from the gustatory nucleus and projects to a nucleus in the dorsal thalamus, specifically the parvicellular portion of the ventral posteromedial nucleus (VPMpc), which in turn projects to two neocortical gustatory regions, one in the insular region and the other in parietal opercular cortex. The gustatory nucleus has other projections, including those to nucleus ambiguus and to the hypoglossal and salivatory nuclei for throat, lingual, and secretory reflexes.

The two motor components of the vagus nerve are both traditionally classified as visceral components. The GVE component provides innervation to the parasympathetic ganglia that supply the viscera of the thorax and abdomen. (The parasympathetic ganglia for pelvic viscera receive their parasympathetic innervation from preganglionic neurons located in the sacral spinal cord.) Preganglionic parasympathetic GVE neurons are mostly located in the dorsal motor nucleus of X, which lies immediately dorsolateral to the hypoglossal nucleus. Some GVE neurons also lie within nucleus ambiguus and specifically supply additional parasympathetic innervation to the heart. The vagus nerve exits the lateral surface of the medulla, and its GVE fibers distribute to parasympathetic ganglia for the esophagus, trachea and lungs, heart, and most of the abdominal viscera. Parasympathetic activity results in decreased heart rate, bronchial constriction, increased blood flow to the gut, and increased peristalsis and secretion.

The SVE, branchial motor component of the vagus nerve arises from neurons in nucleus ambiguus and innervates muscles of the palate, pharynx, and larynx. These muscles are embryologically derived from muscles associated with the branchial arches. Nucleus ambiguus receives bilateral corticobulbar input and input from other cranial nerve nuclei for coordination of movements involved in reflex actions (such as coughing or vomiting) and for phonation and swallowing. The latter, for example, is a complex action that also involves motor neurons of the trigeminal (V), facial (VII), and hypoglossal (XII) nerves.

Damage to nucleus ambiguus or to the fibers of the vagus nerve results in reduction of the arch of the palate on the ipsilateral side, difficulty in swallowing, and hoarseness. Hoarseness is one of the manifestations of Parkinson's disease. It is due to supranuclear effects on the function of SVE vagal neurons. Hoarseness can also result from a lung tumor on the left side that involves the left recurrent laryngeal nerve; the latter arises from the vagus nerve in the upper part of the thorax, an anatomical relationship that does not occur on the right due to a higher origin of the recurrent nerve.

4. Glossopharyngeal Nerve

Like the vagus nerve, cranial nerve IX has five components, three of which are sensory and two of which are motor. The GSA component is a minor one, which innervates a small region of skin behind the ear. The GSA fibers of the glossopharyngeal nerve have cell bodies located in the superior (jugular) ganglion of IX, and they traverse the spinal tract of V to terminate in the spinal nucleus of V with similar GSA afferents from cranial nerves X, VII, and V. The GVA component of IX has a much more restricted distribution than the GVA component of X. Glossopharyngeal GVA fibers innervate the mucosal membranes that line the internal surface of the middle ear and cover the posterior third of the tongue, the tonsils, the posterior and upper surfaces of the pharynx, and the Eustachian tube. These GVA fibers have cell bodies in the inferior (petrosal) ganglion of IX. They enter the tractus solitarius and terminate in its nucleus. The latter projects to sites that include nucleus ambiguus (for throat reflexes), the dorsal motor nucleus of X, and the reticular formation. The carotid sinus reflex depends on some additional glossopharyngeal GVA fibers that innervate the carotid sinus (which is located at the bifurcation of the internal and external carotid arteries) and are stimulated by increases in arterial blood pressure. These fibers terminate on solitary nucleus neurons that project to the dorsal motor nucleus of X, which, via its projection to the parasympathetic ganglia of the heart, decreases heart rate and the arterial blood pressure. The SVA component of IX innervates taste buds located on the posterior third of the tongue. These fibers have cell bodies located in the inferior (petrosal) ganglion of IX and project to first-order multipolar neurons in the gustatory nucleus, which, as discussed previously, projects to VPMpc in the dorsal thalamus for relay to gustatory cortical areas.

The glossopharyngeal nerve has two efferent components, GVE and SVE. In the latter, branchial motor fibers arise from neurons in nucleus ambiguus and innervate the stylopharyngeus muscle (which arises from part of the styloid process on the inferior surface of the temporal bone of the skull and inserts along the side of the pharynx and part of the thyroid cartilage). The stylopharyngeus muscle is embryologically derived from the muscles of the branchial arches. The GVE component of IX arises from a nucleus that lies rostral to the dorsal motor nucleus of X but is displaced laterally away from the ventricular surface; it is called the inferior salivatory nucleus. As its name implies, its neurons give rise to preganglionic parasympathetic fibers that project via the tympanic and lesser superficial petrosal nerves to the otic ganglion, which in turn gives rise to postganglionic parasympathetic fibers that innervate the largest of the salivary glands—the parotid gland. Parasympathetic stimulation increases the secretory activity of the parotid gland. The glossopharyngeal nerve is rarely involved clinically in isolation, and deficits are predominantly sensory. Damage to cranial nerve IX results in loss of the pharyngeal (gag) reflex due to loss of the sensory input, a similar loss of the carotid sinus reflex for blood pressure regulation, and loss of taste to the posterior third of the tongue. Loss of salivatory activity by the parotid gland results from damage to the glossopharyngeal GVE component.

B. Cranial Nerves of the Pons

Four cranial nerves are present at pontine levels: the vestibulocochlear nerve (VIII), the facial nerve (VII), the abducens nerve (VI), and the trigeminal nerve (V). Cranial nerve VIII has a single sensory component that comprises two divisions, and cranial nerve VI has only a single motor component. Cranial nerve VII is second in complexity only to the vagus and glossopharyngeal nerves, with four traditionally recognized functional components, whereas cranial nerve V is a mixed nerve with two components, one sensory and one motor.

1. Vestibulocochlear Nerve

The eighth cranial nerve traditionally has been classified in one of the special categories, SSA. It comprises the two senses of audition and the relative position and motion of the head in space. The eighth nerve innervates the inner ear organs—the spiral-shaped cochlea, which transduces auditory stimuli via vibration of its perilymphatic fluid, and the vestibular labyrinth, which transduces the effects of gravity and acceleration on its receptor apparatus.

a. Cochlear Division The bipolar neurons of the cochlear division of VIII innervate the hair cells of the cochlear organ of Corti. The apical surfaces of the hair cells are studded with stereocilia and border the inner chamber of the cochlea, the scala media, which is filled with endolymph. A tectorial membrane overlies the stereocilia. An outer chamber, formed by the scala vestibuli and scala tympani, contains perilymph, and the scala tympani portion is separated from the organ of Corti by a basilar membrane. Sound waves cause vibration of the perilymph and resultant displacement of the basilar membrane, which in turn pushes the stereocilia against the tectorial membrane, bending them and opening ion channels. Influx of potassium from the endolymph through the opened channels causes depolarization of the receptor cell. The frequency of the auditory stimuli is tonotopically mapped along the length of the cochlear spiral, with best responses to high frequencies occurring at its base and those to lower frequencies at more apical locations. The bipolar neurons preserve the tonotopic map for relay to the cochlear nuclei and then throughout the ascending auditory pathway. They also encode intensity by their discharge rate.

Cell bodies of cochlear bipolar neurons lie within the spiral ganglion, named for the shape of the cochlea. Their central processes enter the lateral aspect of the brain stem at a caudal pontine level and terminate in the dorsal and ventral cochlear nuclei. The cochlear nuclei project to multiple sites, including the superior olivary nuclear complex in the pons and the inferior

colliculus in the midbrain roof. The superior olivary complex (SO) receives bilateral input mainly from the so-called bushy cells of the ventral cochlear nucleus; SO neurons are coincidence detectors that utilize the time delay between the inputs from the two sides in order to compute the location in space of the sound source. The ascending auditory projections predominantly originate from pyramidal neurons within the dorsal cochlear nucleus and from the superior olivary complex and pass via the lateral lemniscus to the inferior colliculus, which in turn projects to the medial geniculate body of the dorsal thalamus. The latter projects to auditory cortex in the temporal lobe. Damage to the cochlear division of VIII results in dysfunction (such as experiencing a buzzing sound) and/or deafness.

b. Vestibular Division The bipolar neurons of the vestibular division of VIII innervate hair cells within several parts of the vestibular labyrinth. The fluid-filled labyrinth consists of three semicircular canals that transduce rotational movements (angular acceleration) of the head and two chambers, the saccule and utricle, that constitute the otolith organ and transduce linear acceleration and gravitational force. The three semicircular canals are arranged at right angles to each other for responses in the various planes of space, and each contains a dilated area, the ampulla, that contains a ridge, the crista ampullaris. Vestibular hair cells on the surface of the crista have stereocilia and a longer kinocillium that are displaced by movement of an overlying gelatinous cupula, which moves due to fluid displacement within the canal caused by rotational motion. Similarly, the saccule and utricle contain hair cells in an area called the macula. The cilia of these hair cells are displaced by movement of an overlying gelatinous mass, the otolith membrane, that contains the otoliths (or otoconia), which are small particles of calcium carbonate that are denser than the surrounding fluid and are displaced by gravity when the head is tilted or during linear acceleration.

Cell bodies of vestibular bipolar neurons lie within the vestibular (Scarpa's) ganglion. The central processes of these neurons enter the lateral aspect of the pons along with the cochlear nerve fibers; most terminate in the superior, inferior, medial, and lateral vestibular nuclei, which lie in the floor of the fourth ventricle. A small number of vestibular afferent fibers bypass the vestibular nuclei and project directly to the cerebellar cortex, particularly within its flocculonodular lobe, which is concerned with the maintenance of posture, balance, and equilibrium. The vestibular nuclei also receive a substantial input from the cerebellum via its deep nuclei.

Descending projections from the vestibular nuclei form the medial and lateral vestibulospinal tracts that innervate spinal cord neurons for extensor muscles involved in postural maintenance and related reflexes. Unlike other brain stem nuclei that give rise to descending spinal projections, the vestibular nuclei do not receive any direct input from the cerebral cortex. Other major vestibular connections are with the oculomotor nuclei of cranial nerves III, IV, and VI via the medial longitudinal fasciculus for the vestibuloocular reflex—the stabilization of eye fixation on a target while the head is moving—and other vestibular–oculomotor interactions. The ascending pathway for conscious perception of vestibular stimuli arises from neurons in the superior, lateral, and inferior vestibular nuclei and terminates in several dorsal thalamic nuclei, including part of the ventral posterolateral (VPLc) nucleus and the ventral posteroinferior (VPI) nucleus. Thalamocortical vestibular projections are to ventrally lying parietal cortical areas (designated 2v and 3a), which are adjacent to the head representation of somatosensory and motor cortices, respectively. Damage to the vestibular division of VIII results in dizziness, pathologic nystagmus (an involuntary, repeated eye movement pattern consisting of conjugate movement of the eyes to one side followed by a rapid return to the original position), nausea and vomiting, vertigo (the sensation of rotation in the absence of actual movement), and other related symptoms.

2. Facial Nerve

Cranial nerve VII contains four of the five components present in the vagal and glossopharyngeal nerves, namely, GSA, SVA, GVE, and SVE. The seventh nerve can be divided into two parts—the intermediate nerve (of Wrisberg), which comprises the GSA, SVA, and GVE components, and the facial branchial motor nerve, which is the SVE component. The two sensory components of VII both have cell bodies located in the geniculate ganglion. As is also the case for cranial nerves IX and X, the GSA component of VII is minor, innervating a small area of skin behind the ear and the external auditory meatus. The GSA fibers terminate in the spinal nucleus of V, for which the ascending sensory pathway is discussed later. Facial SVA fibers innervate taste buds that lie on the anterior two-thirds of the tongue via the chorda

tympani nerve. These neurons project to the gustatory nucleus, which, as discussed previously, projects to VPMpc in the dorsal thalamus for relay to gustatory cortical areas.

Special visceral efferent fibers arise in the branchial motor nucleus of VII, which lies ventrolateral to the abducens (VI) nucleus in the pons. The axons of motor VII initially follow a dorsomedial course within the pons and then turn laterally and curve over the dorsal surface of the abducens nucleus, forming the internal genu of the nerve. This course is due to ventrolateral migration of the neuron cell bodies during embryological development. The facial motor fibers then traverse the pons in a ventrolateral direction to exit on its lateral surface near the junction of the pons with the medulla. The facial branchial motor nerve innervates muscles embryologically derived from the muscles of the branchial arches, including the platysma (a superficial muscle of the skin of the neck), buccinator (which forms the cheek), stapedius (which inserts on the stapes bone within the middle ear), auricular and occipital muscles, and the muscles of facial expression. An additional component supplies efferent innervation to the inner ear. The branchial motor nucleus of VII receives afferent input from structures that include the spinal nucleus of V for corneal and other trigeminofacial reflexes, auditory input from the superior olivary complex for facial reflexes to loud noise (including closing the eyes and the stapedius reflex to damp sound transmission through the middle ear ossicles), and corticobulbar input, which is bilateral to the facial motor neurons for the forehead and upper face but predominantly contralateral for the lower face and mouth region.

The GVE component of the facial nerve arises from neurons in the superior salivatory nucleus. Some preganglionic parasympathetic fibers project via the greater petrosal nerve to the pterygopalatine ganglion for innervation of the lacrimal gland. Other preganglionic fibers project via the chorda tympani nerve to the submandibular ganglion for innervation of the sublingual and submandibular salivary glands. Damage to cranial nerve VII results in deficits according to the location of the lesion and the components involved. Sensory loss of taste to the anterior two-thirds of the tongue occurs with involvement of the SVA component, and loss of production of tears from the lacrimal gland and saliva from the sublingual and submandibular salivary glands occurs with involvement of the GVE component. Damage to the nucleus or nerve for the SVE motor VII component results in paralysis of all the muscles of the ipsilateral face, whereas a supranuclear lesion affecting corticobulbar input results in paralysis of only the lower part of the face on the contralateral side. Motor VII damage also results in sounds being abnormally loud due to loss of the stapedius reflex.

3. Abducens Nerve

Cranial nerve VI is one of the set of three ocular motor (oculomotor) nerves (III, IV, and VI) and innervates one of the six extraocular muscles of the eye, the lateral rectus muscle. The abducens nerve is a purely motor nerve with only a GSE component. The nerve arises from motor neurons in the abducens nucleus, which lies in a medial position in the dorsal pons and, along with the other oculomotor nuclei and the hypoglossal nucleus, forms the GSE column of the brain stem. Abducens nerve fibers run ventrally from the nucleus and exit the brain stem on its ventral surface at the junction of the pons with the medulla. The abducens nerve runs forward along the side of the brain stem, traverses the cavernous sinus, and passes through the superior orbital fissure (along with the other oculomotor nerves) to innervate the ipsilateral lateral rectus muscle. Contraction of the lateral rectus causes abduction (lateral movement) of the eye. Damage to the ventral region of the brain stem at the level of the abducens nerve may result in the syndrome called middle alternating hemiplegia, which is motor impairment on the contralateral side of the body (due to damage to the corticospinal tract) combined with medial deviation of the eye on the ipislateral (i.e., alternate) side due to a lower motor neuron lesion of the abducens nerve. In this situation, the eye deviates medially due to the unopposed contraction of the medial rectus muscle, which is innervated by cranial nerve III. Supranuclear innervation of the oculomotor nuclei derives from the superior colliculus and from cortical eye fields in the frontal and parietal lobes, and it is relayed to the oculomotor nuclei via gaze centers in the brain stem.

Connections from the gaze centers and vestibular nuclei and among the oculomotor nuclei via the medial longitudinal fasciculus serve to coordinate the actions of the extraocular muscles so that, for example, when a person moves both eyes to the right, the right lateral rectus contracts to move the right eye laterally, the right medial rectus does not oppose the action, and the actions of the medial and lateral recti of the left eye are similarly coordinated to produce the conjugate movement. Damage to the medial longitudinal fasciculus results in internuclear ophthalmoplegia; this condition

is characterized by weakness in adduction of the eye on the side ipsilateral to the lesion during attempted conjugate eye movements toward the opposite side accompanied by nystagmus in the contralateral, abducting eye. Bilateral internuclear ophthalmoplegia can occur due to multiple sclerosis.

4. Trigeminal Nerve

Cranial nerve V has only two components, GSA and SVE. The trigeminal nerve is named for its three divisions: The ophthalmic division provides sensory innervation to the upper face, including the forehead, upper eyelid, and cornea; the maxillary division to the region of the upper jaw, including the upper lip, jaw, and cheek, parts of the nose, and upper teeth; and the mandibular division to the region of the lower jaw, including the lower lip, jaw, cheek, lower teeth, and anterior two-thirds of the tongue. The mandibular division also provides motor innervation to the muscles of the jaw used for mastication (chewing). The trigeminal nerve emerges from the lateral aspect of the brain stem at a midpontine level.

The GSA fibers of the trigeminal nerve have most of their cell bodies located within the trigeminal ganglion and innervate the face and upper head region for fine (discriminative) touch, position sense, vibratory sense, pain, and temperature. GSA fibers for the modalities of fine touch, vibration, and position enter the brain stem and terminate in the principal sensory nucleus of V in the lateral part of the pons, which in turn projects to the ventral posteromedial nucleus (VPM) in the dorsal thalamus. The latter projects to the face representation within somatosensory cortex. GSA fibers for pain and temperature enter the brain stem and distribute to the spinal (or descending) nucleus of V, which also receives inputs from the GSA components of the facial (VII), glossopharyngeal (IX), and vagus (X) nerves. Like the principal sensory nucleus of V, the spinal nucleus projects to VPM for relay of its inputs to somatosensory cortex. (Trigeminal innervation of the mucous membranes of the nose and anterior tongue region has traditionally been lumped with the GSA components, but since these membranes are embryologically derived from endoderm, this component is technically general visceral afferent.)

A third trigeminal sensory nucleus, the mesencephalic nucleus of V, is present along the lateral border of the central gray matter encircling the upper part of the fourth ventricle and the cerebral aqueduct of the midbrain. This nucleus comprises bipolar neurons that lie within the central nervous system rather than in the cranial nerve ganglion. The neurons' peripheral processes form the mesencephalic tract of V and carry pressure and position information from structures including the teeth, the palate, and the muscles of mastication. The mesencephalic V neurons project to multiple sites, including the motor nucleus of V for reflexive control of jaw position.

SVE, branchial motor fibers arise in the motor nucleus of V, which lies medial to the principal sensory nucleus and receives bilateral corticobulbar input. The axons exit the brain stem on its lateral surface in the trigeminal nerve head and distribute via the mandibular division to the jaw muscles used in mastication—the temporalis and masseter muscles and the medial and lateral pterygoids, which are embryologically derived from the muscles of the branchial arches. Additional branchial arch-derived muscles innervated by the branchial motor component of V are the tensor veli palatini muscle of the palate, the tensor tympani muscle of the middle ear (which inserts on the malleus), and two suprahyoid muscles, the anterior belly of the digastric and mylohyoid.

Damage to the GSA components of cranial nerve V results in sensory loss to the face and loss of many reflexes due to lack of the sensory part of the reflex arc, including the corneal reflex (closing the eyes in response to light touch to the cornea) via the facial motor nucleus (via the reticular formation), the tearing reflex via the superior salivatory nucleus, the sneezing reflex via nucleus ambiguus, the vomiting reflex via vagal nuclei, salivatory reflexes via the superior and inferior salivatory nuclei, and the jaw-jerk reflex via the mesencephalic nucleus of V. The sensation for hot pepper (capseisin) on the anterior two-thirds of the tongue is also lost. Damage to the SVE component of V results in paralysis of the jaw muscles on the ipsilateral side, whereas a supranuclear lesion produces only moderate weakness due to the bilaterality of the supranuclear input. Changes in the loudness of sounds can also result from loss of innervation to the tensor tympani muscle.

C. Cranial Nerves of the Midbrain

Only two cranial nerves are present in the midbrain: the trochlear nerve (IV) and the oculomotor nerve (III). Cranial nerve IV has only a single component, which is motor. Cranial nerve III has two motor components.

1. Trochlear Nerve

Cranial nerve IV is one of the set of three oculomotor nerves (III, IV, and VI) and innervates one of the six extraocular muscles of the eye, the superior oblique muscle. The trochlear nerve is a purely motor nerve with only a GSE component. The nerve arises from motor neurons in the trochlear nucleus, which lies in a medial position in the dorsal part of the caudal half of the midbrain tegmentum. The trochlear nerve is unique among cranial nerves in that it decussates to the contralateral side (through the superior medullary velum that forms the roof of the fourth ventricle), and its point of exit is through the dorsal surface of the brain. The trochlear nerve thus innervates the superior oblique muscle of the contralateral eye.

The superior oblique muscle arises from the dorsomedial surface of the orbit and ends in a tendon that bends through a connective tissue pulley and then passes laterally to insert on the dorsal part of the eye bulb lateral to its center. Contraction of the superior oblique muscle causes intorsion (rotation of the eyeball around a horizontal, anteroposterior axis through the pupil such that the top moves medially), depression, and abduction. Deviation of the eye due to isolated damage to the trochlear nucleus or nerve is not readily apparent due to the actions of the other extraocular muscles, which mask most of the deficit. Supranuclear innervation of the trochlear nucleus is via the gaze centers in the brain stem, and the gaze centers, the three oculomotor nuclei, and vestibular nuclei are interconnected via the medial longitudinal fasciculus.

2. Oculomotor Nerve

Cranial nerve III innervates four of the six extraocular muscles of the eye as well as the levator palpebrae superioris muscle of the eyelid and, via projections to the ciliary ganglion, the small intraocular muscles that control the constriction of the pupil and the shape of the lens. Unlike the other two oculomotor nerves—the abducens nerve, which innervates the lateral rectus muscle, and the trochlear nerve, which innervates the superior oblique muscle—the oculomotor nerve has more than one functional component. It contains a GSE component for innervation of the extraocular and levator palpebrae superioris muscles and a GVE parasympathetic component for innervation of the ganglion that in turn innervates the intraocular muscles. The oculomotor nerve fibers traverse the tegmentum and exit the brain in the interpeduncular fossa medial to the crus cerebri and then pass rostrally to the orbit with the other oculomotor nerves.

The GSE component of cranial nerve III arises from motor neurons in the oculomotor nucleus proper, which lies in the dorsomedial part of the rostral half of the midbrain tegmentum. This component innervates four muscles that insert on the globe of the eye: the inferior oblique muscle, which extorts, elevates, and abducts the eye; the medial rectus muscle, which adducts the eye; the inferior rectus muscle, which depresses, extorts, and adducts the eye; and the superior rectus muscle, which elevates, intorts, and adducts the eye. (Extorsion is rotation of the eyeball around a horizontal, anteroposterior axis through the pupil such that the bottom moves medially; intorsion is rotation in the opposite direction.)

The oculomotor nuclear complex comprises several nuclei in addition to the GSE main nucleus, including the Edinger–Westphal nucleus and several accessory oculomotor nuclei—the nucleus of Darkschewitsch, the interstitial nucleus of Cajal, and the nuclei of the posterior commissure. These accessory nuclei receive inputs from a variety of visual- and vestibular-related sources and contribute to vertical and smooth-pursuit movements of the eyes directed by the GSE component. The Edinger–Westphal nucleus and a more rostral anterior median nucleus contain preganglionic parasympathetic neurons (GVE) that project via the oculomotor nerve to the ipsilateral ciliary ganglion, which lies deep to the posterior boundary of the eye. Postganglionic parasympathetic fibers from the ciliary ganglion supply the ciliary muscle, which affects the shape of the lens for focusing on near objects, and the sphincter (or constrictor) pupillae muscle. The consensual pupillary light reflex of evoking bilateral constriction of the pupils when light is shined in one eye depends on a pathway from the retina to the olivary pretectal nucleus, which in turn projects bilaterally via the posterior commissure to the anterior median and Edinger–Westphal parasympathetic nuclei. In this context, it should be noted that dilation of the pupil is accomplished by the action of sympathetic innervation that arises from preganglionic neurons in the intermediolateral column of the spinal cord and affects the dilator pupillae muscle fibers via postganglionic neurons of the superior cervical ganglion.

Damage to the ventral region of the midbrain may result in the syndrome called superior alternating hemiplegia, which is motor impairment on the contralateral side of the body (due to damage to the corticospinal fibers in the crus cerebri) combined with lateral and downward deviation of the eye on the ipsilateral (i.e., alternate) side due to a lower motor neuron lesion of the oculomotor nerve. In this situation, the eye deviates laterally due to the unopposed contraction of the lateral rectus muscle, which is innervated by cranial nerve VI. Supranuclear innervation of the oculomotor nuclei is mediated by cortical eye fields and the superior colliculus via gaze centers in the brain stem and is coordinated among the oculomotor, trochlear, and abducens nuclei and the vestibular system via the medial longitudinal fasciculus. Damage to the oculomotor nuclear complex or nerve also results in drooping of the eyelid (ptosis) and pupillary dilation.

D. Cranial Nerves of the Forebrain

Two of the traditionally recognized cranial nerves are present in the forebrain: the optic nerve (II) and the olfactory nerve (I). Both of these nerves are purely sensory, but they are usually left unclassified according to the traditional scheme.

1. Optic Nerve

Cranial nerve II is composed of the distal parts of the axonal processes of retinal ganglion cells. These axons course caudally and medially from the retina to the optic chiasm, where some decussate (cross over) to the opposite side. The proximal parts of these same axons are then called the optic tract as they continue caudally and laterally from the chiasm to sites in the diencephalon and midbrain.

The retinal ganglion cells receive input from retinal bipolar cells, which in turn receive input from the receptor cells of the retina (rods and cones). Rods are predominantly located in the peripheral parts of the retina, whereas cones are densely packed in the central part of the retina, particularly within the fovea. Rods transduce light stimuli of a broad range of wavelengths, whereas cones are of three types for color vision, each transducing a different part of the spectrum. The transduction process is a complex series of biochemical events initiated by the absorption of a photon by pigment within the receptor cells. The visual world topologically maps in precise order onto the retina, and this map is preserved throughout the system.

The retinal bipolar neurons correspond to the bipolar neurons that lie within the ganglia of other sensory cranial nerve components in terms of their relative position in the sensory pathway. The retinal ganglion cells are the first-order multipolar neurons of the pathway. At the optic chiasm, optic nerve fibers that arise from retinal ganglion cells in the nasal (medial) retina decussate, whereas axons from retinal ganglion cells in the temporal (lateral) retina do not. The net result is that the axons in the optic tract on the right side, for example, receive input that initiates from stimuli in the left half of the visual world. Thus, the right brain "sees" the left visual world and vice versa.

The optic tract projects to multiple sites in the diencephalon and midbrain. The major visual pathway for conscious vision is to neocortex via the dorsal lateral geniculate nucleus in the dorsal thalamus. This nucleus contains two large-celled (magnocellular) layers; they receive input relayed from rods via ganglion cells in the peripheral parts of the retina that conveys the general location of stimuli and their motion. It also contains four small-celled (parvicellular) layers that receive fine form and color input from cones. The dorsal lateral geniculate nucleus projects to primary (striate) cortex, which lies in the caudal and medial part of the occipital lobe. The spatial information from retinal ganglion cells via the magnocellular layers of the dorsal lateral geniculate nucleus is relayed from striate cortex via multiple synapses predominantly to posterior parietal cortex, which is involved in spatial cortical functions, whereas the form and color information via the parvicellular geniculate layers is likewise relayed predominantly to inferotemporal cortex, which is involved in numerous complex functions including the visual recognition of objects and individuals.

Midbrain visual projections are to the superficial layers of the rostral part of the midbrain roof, the superior colliculus, in which visual information is mapped in register with similar maps of somatosensory and auditory space that are projected into its deeper layers. The superior colliculus visual input is relayed to part of the pulvinar in the dorsal thalamus, which in turn projects to extrastriate visual cortical areas, which border the primary visual cortex in the occipital lobe. The midbrain visual pathway is concerned with the spatial orientation of the visual world.

Damage to the retina or optic pathway causes loss of vision in part or all of visual space (the visual field) depending on the location and extent of the lesion. Although damage to the retina or optic nerve results in blindness for the eye on the same side, damage located in the thalamocortical part of the pathway causes a deficit for the visual field on the opposite side. Damage to the central part of the optic chiasm, as can occur with a pituitary gland tumor in that region, causes "tunnel vision"—loss of the peripheral parts of the visual field on both sides.

2. Olfactory Nerve

Cranial nerve I is composed of the set of axonal processes that arise from the olfactory bipolar cells that lie within the nasal mucosa. These sensory cells lie in a sheet-like formation across the mucosal surface rather than being condensed into a ganglion as is the case for other peripheral nerves. Unlike the situation with the visual, vestibulocochlear, and gustatory systems, there are no separate receptor cells for the olfactory system. The distal ends of the olfactory bipolar cells have the molecular machinery to bind oderant molecules and transduce the signal via various complex biochemical events. These bipolar neurons terminate on first-order multipolar neurons called mitral cells that are located within the olfactory bulbs, which lie ventral to the frontal lobes.

The bipolar cell axons form complex synaptic contacts with the mitral cell processes in a series of spherical structures called glomeruli. The glomeruli form a layer superficial to the layer of mitral cell bodies in the olfactory bulb. Different oderant molecules stimulate different sets of glomeruli, but a simple oderant "map" across the region of different oderant molecules has not been found. The mitral cells project via the olfactory tract to multiple sites in the ventral region of the telencephalon collectively referred to as the olfactory cortex. An olfactory pathway to part of neocortex is via a relay from olfactory cortex to the mediodorsal nucleus of the dorsal thalamus and then to prefrontal cortex, which occupies a large portion of the frontal lobe and is concerned with a multitude of complex, higher cognitive functions.

Damage to the olfactory system results in the loss of the sense of smell. The appreciation of the sensation of the flavors of food is also impaired since flavor is a complex sensation based on olfactory and gustatory interactions at the cortical level. In some cases of epilepsy caused by lesions involving the ventral, olfactory-related regions of the cerebral hemispheres (particularly a structure called the uncus), an aura involving an olfactory hallucination may preceed seizure activity.

III. NEW INSIGHTS FROM EMBRYOLOGY AND NEW CLASSIFICATION OF THE CRANIAL NERVE COMPONENTS

Studies of embryological development, most within the past decade and including the work of LeDouarin, Gilland and Baker, Noden and colleagues, Northcutt, Gans, and others, require several changes to our treatment of cranial nerves. Two additional cranial nerves need to be recognized in humans—a terminal nerve (T) and an epiphyseal nerve (E)—and the two diencephalic cranial nerves (E and II) can be classified as neural tube afferent (NTA). The traditional classification of cranial nerve components needs to be revised and simplified. The distinctions between the "general" and "special" categories can now be eliminated, and the components of spinal nerves and most cranial nerves can be reduced to the four simple categories of somatic afferent (SA), visceral afferent (VA), somatic efferent (SE), and visceral efferent (VE). The branchial motor nerves form a subset of the SE column since the branchial muscles are derived from the same mesodermal source as are the extraocular muscles and the muscles of the tongue.

A. Terminal Nerve

The terminal nerve is arguably the most rostral cranial nerve. Its bipolar neurons have free nerve endings that are located in the nasal mucosa, but their modality (possibly chemosensory) has not been established. These neurons project to several sites in the ventral and medial regions of the forebrain, including the septum, olfactory tubercle, and preoptic area. The terminal nerve neurons contain the reproductive hormone, luteinizing hormone-releasing hormone, and may be involved in the regulation of reproductive behavior.

B. Sensory Cranial Nerves Derived from the Neural Tube

The optic nerve (II) and neural retina develop as an outgrowth from the diencephalon. The optic nerve is thus in fact not a true cranial nerve but rather a tract of the central nervous system. Unlike most sensory cranial nerves that have receptors and/or bipolar neurons in the peripheral nervous system, the receptor rods and cones of the retina and the retinal bipolar cells are within the central nervous system. Nevertheless, the optic nerve is so firmly and universally considered to be a cranial nerve that eliminating it from the list is not an option. A second, similar tract of the central nervous system that innervates a diencephalic outgrowth, the epiphyseal nerve, thus also needs to be included in the list of cranial nerves for completeness.

The epiphysis forms from the roof plate of the diencephalon and comprises a variety of structures in various vertebrates, including a frontal organ and pineal gland in frogs, a parietal eye and pineal gland in lizards, and a pineal gland in mammals. The pineal gland does not receive light directly, as do the neural retina and the parietal eye, but it is influenced by light via a pathway from the suprachiasmatic nucleus of the hypothalamus to the sympathetic intermediolateral column of the spinal cord and then via postganglionic sympathetic fibers that arise from the superior cervical ganglion and travel on branches of the internal carotid artery to reach the pineal gland, where the sympathetic input inhibits the conversion of serotonin to melatonin. In mammals, the pineal gland contains neurons that project to the medial habenular nucleus and part of the pretectum. Pineal projections to other brain sites are minor in humans, but recognition of an epiphyseal cranial nerve is justified based on its similarities of development and organization with the optic nerve. Neither the optic nerve nor the epiphyseal nerve can be categorized as somatic or visceral sensory, however. Since both derive from the neural tube, they can be classified as NTA. They are unique among the cranial nerves in this regard.

C. Afferent Components

Components of six cranial nerves could arguably be assigned to the traditional category of special afferent. The facial (VII), glossopharyngeal (IX), and vagus (X) nerves have SVA components for taste sensation. The olfactory nerve (I) is sometimes classified as SVA, and the terminal nerve could be provisionally included in this category as well. The vestibulocochlear nerve (VIII) is traditionally classified as SSA. Of the nondiencephalic sensory cranial nerves, only the trigeminal nerve (V) and small components of VII, IX, and X have been classified as GSA. The fourth traditional afferent category of GVA has been assigned to the neurons of the glossopharyngeal and vagus nerves that predominantly innervate the visceral structures of the body cavities. What all these sensory cranial nerve components have in common is that their bipolar neurons are embryologically derived from the same two tissues: neural crest and/or placodes.

1. Neural Crest and Placodes

During embryological development, the neural tube forms by a process of invagination of the ectoderm along the dorsal midline of the body and the head. At the edges of the invaginating neural tube tissue, a population of neural crest cells arises from the dorsomedial wall of the neural folds and migrates laterally and ventrally to contribute to many different structures of the adult, including the dorsal root ganglion cells (bipolar neurons) for all the spinal cord sensory nerves. In the head region, neural crest cells likewise migrate away from the region of the neural tube and give rise to multiple structures. A second tissue present only in the head region is a set of neurogenic placodes, which are thickened patches of ectodermal cells. The bipolar sensory neurons for all the cranial nerves except II and the epiphyseal are derived from the neurogenic placodes and/or neural crest tissues.

In the region of the nose, an olfactory placode forms that gives rise to the bipolar neurons of the olfactory and terminal nerves, and additional sets of placodes form along the sides of the head. Neural crest and/or placodally derived cells give rise to the bipolar neurons for the sensory ganglia of the trigeminal (V), facial (VII), vestibulocochlear (VIII), glossopharyngeal (IX), and vagus (X) nerves. A trigeminal placode contributes neurons to the trigeminal ganglion. The sensory neurons within the vestibular and spiral ganglia for the vestibulocochlear nerve arise from a dorsolateral, otic placode; this is a much simpler situation than in fishes, in which a series of dorsolateral placodes gives rise to the vestibulocochlear nerve and to the set of mechanoreceptive and electroreceptive lateral line nerves. The receptor hair cells for the vestibulocochlear system likewise are derived from this dorsolateral placode.

The gustatory system is more variable across vertebrates in terms of both its peripheral and its central components. Mammals have a relatively limited gustatory system. A set of ventrolateral, or epibranchial, placodes contributes sensory neurons to ganglia of cranial nerves VII, IX, and X, but, unlike the situation in the vestibulocochlear system, the taste receptor cells of the taste buds are all derived locally from the pharyngeal endoderm in the oral cavity. This system thus is classified here as visceral. Fishes, in comparison, have much more elaborate taste systems than mammals, and in some groups, such as catfishes, the taste receptor cells are distributed over the entire body surface. The gustatory afferent fibers project into elaborate, laminated lobes in the brain stem and preserve a topographic map of the inputs.

2. Somatic Afferent and Visceral Afferent Cranial Nerve Components

Due to these recent findings on the embryological derivation of these cranial nerve components, their former classification into four separate categories of SVA (I the terminal nerve, and the components of VII, IX, and X for taste sensation), SSA (VIII), GSA (V, VII, IX, and X), and GVA (IX and X) can be revised (Table III). Since the bipolar sensory neurons for all these nerves are derived from the same embryonic source (i.e., neural crest and/or placodes), the "special" versus "general" distinction is not warrented. We are thus left with the resolution of classifying most of the cranial nerve sensory components (i.e., the traditional GSA and SSA components plus I and the terminal nerve) simply as somatic afferent (SA). Due to the derivation of the receptor cells from endoderm, the taste components of VII, IX, and X are assigned to the simple category of visceral afferent (VA). The remaining sensory category of GVA for innervation of the thoracic and abdominal viscera and pharyngeal region by the vagus nerve and of the tongue and pharyngeal region by the glossopharyngeal nerve can likewise be revised to the VA category.

D. Efferent Components

Some of the motor components of four cranial nerves have traditionally been assigned to the category of SVE—the trigeminal (V), facial (VII), glossopharyngeal (IX), vagus (X), and spinal accessory (XI) nerve components that innervate muscles derived from the branchial arches. Four purely motor cranial nerves classified as GSE—III, IV, VI, and XII—innervate eye and tongue muscles. Recent embryological findings, particularly from the work of Noden and collaborators, have shown that the nerve components of the SVE and GSE categories both innervate striated skeletal muscles that are all derived from the same embryonic muscle masses in the developing head and neck regions. Components of the third efferent category, GVE, are present in cranial nerves III, VII, IX, and X and give rise to preganglionic parasympathetic fibers for innervation of the ganglia that supply glands in the head and the viscera of the thorax and abdomen.

1. Epimere versus Hypomere and the Development of Striated Muscles in the Head

To appreciate the resolution of the problem of head musculature and its innervation, one must consider it in the context of the pattern of development of the muscular components of the body. The body is essentially a tube with three layers—an outer layer of ectoderm that forms the central nervous system, the neural crest, the epidermis, and other tissues; an inner layer of endoderm that forms the lining of the gut and related organs; and an intermediate layer of mesoderm that forms the bones, muscles, blood vessels, dermis, and other structures of the body. The mesoderm has three dorsal-to-ventral components. The epimere (or paraxial mesoderm), the most dorsal component, forms somites, which are segmental mesodermal masses that give rise to the striated, skeletal muscles of the body wall and the limbs. The intermediate component, mesomere (or nephric ridge), gives rise to the kidneys and gonads, whereas the ventral component, hypomere (or lateral plate mesoderm), gives rise to the smooth, visceral muscles of the gut as well as to the cardiac muscle of the heart.

In the head, the embryological derivation of the various groups of muscles was until recently incorrectly understood, particularly concerning the pharyngeal region. In addition to giving rise to multiple components of the peripheral nervous system and to most of the skull, neural crest cells give rise to mesenchymal tissue that forms the so-called "visceral" arches of the pharynx. The muscles of this region were long thought to arise from a rostral continuation of hypomeric muscle—the ventral part of the mesodermal tissue that in the body gives rise to the smooth muscle of the gut. Muscles derived from the visceral arch region, which in mammals are the muscles of the mandibular arch (lower jaw muscles innervated by the trigeminal nerve), hyoid arch (facial and other muscles innervated by the facial nerve), and the several branchial arches (throat and larynx muscles innervated by the glossopharyngeal and vagus nerves), were thus presumed to be visceral muscles. In conflict with this view was the resemblance of the visceral arch

muscles to the striated, skeletal muscle of the body wall and of the tongue and extraocular muscles. The histological structure of the visceral arch muscles and their single-motor neuron innervation pattern are both markedly different from the histological structure and two-neuron chain, parasympathetic innervation pattern of the smooth muscle of the gut. The designation of "special" acknowledged these differences.

Recent work by Gilland, Noden, Northcutt, and others has revealed a different embryological source for the muscles of the visceral arches and has resolved the previous confusion. Rather than being derived from hypomere, the muscles of the visceral arches are in fact derived from the epimeric muscle of the head, the caudal continuation of which gives rise to the striated, skeletal muscles of the body wall. Somites and somitomeres, which are incompletely separated somites, form in the head region and give rise to the extraocular muscles, the muscles of the visceral arches, and the muscles of the tongue. Thus, none of the visceral arch muscles are actually visceral, and there is nothing special about them. They are embryologically derived and innervated in the same manner (by neural tube-derived motor neurons) as the extraocular and tongue muscles. The visceral arch muscles probably evolved before the extraocular muscles were acquired by early vertebrates, however, and long before the muscular tongue was gained by tetrapods, and this difference in history may account for the different position within the brain stem of the two columns of motor neurons that innervate them.

2. Somatic Efferent and Visceral Efferent Cranial Nerve Components

Due to these recent findings on the embryological derivation of the visceral arch muscles, the former classification of their motor cranial nerve components of SVE can be revised. These components can be classified as somatic, just like those that supply the extraocular muscles and the tongue. Since the classification of visceral is invalid, the distinction of special (for V, VII, IX, X, and XI) versus general (for III, IV, VI, and XII) is also moot. All these motor components are simply somatic efferents (Table III). For the remaining motor category, GVE, the parasympathetic components of cranial nerves III, VII, IX, and X are indeed visceral efferents, and with the elimination of the special visceral category the use of the term general is not needed here. These parasympathetic components can simply be classified as visceral efferents.

See Also the Following Articles

BRAIN ANATOMY AND NETWORKS • NERVOUS SYSTEM, ORGANIZATION OF • NEUROANATOMY • PERIPHERAL NERVOUS SYSTEM

Suggested Reading

Butler, A. B., and Hodos, W. (1996). *Comparative Vertebrate Neuroanatomy: Evolution and Adaptation.* Wiley–Liss, New York.

Gilland, E., and Baker, R. (1993). Conservation of neuroepithelial and mesodermal segments in the embryonic vertebrate head. *Acta Anat.* **148,** 110–123.

Haines, D. E. (1997). *Fundamental Neuroscience.* Churchill–Livingstone, New York.

Liem, K. F., Bemis, W. E., Walker, W.F., Jr., and Grande, L. (2001). *Functional Anatomy of the Vertebrates: An Evolutionary Perspective,* 3rd ed. Harcourt, Fort Worth, TX.

Nieuwenhuys, R., Ten Donkelaar, H. J., and Nicholson, C. (1998). *The Central Nervous System of Vertebrates.* Springer, Berlin.

Noden, D. M. (1991). Vertebrate craniofacial development: The relation between ontogenetic process and morphological outcome. *Brain Behav. Evol.* **38,** 190–225.

Noden, D. M. (1993). Spatial integration among cells forming the cranial peripheral nervous system. *J. Neurobiol.* **24,** 248–261.

Northcutt, R. G. (1993). A reassessment of Goodrich's model of cranial nerve phylogeny. *Acta Anat.* **148,** 150–159.

Northcutt, R. G. (1996). The origin of craniates: Neural crest, neurogenic placodes, and homeobox genes. *Israel J. Zool.* **42,** S273–S313.

Northcutt, R. G., and Gans, C. (1983). The genesis of neural crest and epidermal placodes: A reinterpretation of vertebrate origins. *Q. Rev. Biol.* **58,** 1–28.

Parent, A. (1996). *Carpenter's Human Neuroanatomy,* 9th ed. Williams & Wilkins, Baltimore.

Webb, J. F., and Noden, D. M. (1993). Ectodermal placodes: Contributions to the development of the vertebrate head. *Am. Zool.* **33,** 434–447.

Young, P. A., and Young, P. H. (1997). *Basic Clinical Neuroanatomy.* Williams & Wilkins, Baltimore.

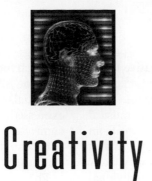

Creativity

MARK A. RUNCO

California State University, Fullerton, and University of Hawaii, Hilo

GLOSSARY

alexithemia Lack of affect; low emotionality. This often characterizes the individual with a "split brain" and seems to inhibit his or her creativity.

creativity complex Influences on creativity reflect personality, attitude, affect, cognition, and metacognition. Creativity is not unidimensional or tied to a single domain.

divergent thinking Problem solving and ideation which moves in different directions rather than converging on one correct or conventional idea or answer.

intrinsic motivation The personal interests that often lead to creative work and are independent of extrinsic influences, such as rewards and incentives.

range of reaction Genetic potential delimits the range of potential; environmental influences determine where within that range the individual performs.

split brain Lay term for the result of a commisurotomy, which surgically separates the two hemispheres of the brain.

Creativity is important, and probably vital, for innovation, technological progress, and societal evolution. It may be more important now than ever before because it plays a role in adaptations. Creativity also benefits the individual, providing coping skills and a means for self-expression. Very likely the creativity of individuals determines the creative potential of society. Just as likely, the creative potentials of individuals is dependent on brain structure and process.

I. INTRODUCTION

The brain and creativity are typically studied from very different perspectives. Simplifying, the human brain is a topic for the hard sciences, including neurology and medicine. Creativity, on the other hand, is traditionally studied by social and behavioral scientists. This makes it more difficult to bring the two topics together and may explain why there is not more literature on the brain and creativity. Efforts are being made, especially very recently, to bridge the two topics. In fact, researchers are discovering advantages to this kind of cross-disciplinary investigation.

One advantage is conceptual. Useful concepts and ideas can be borrowed from one field and applied to the other. Consider the concept of a range of reaction. This was originally proposed in the hard sciences (genetics) but is vital for our understanding of virtually all behavior (psychology), including creative behavior. As is the case with the biological contributions to other human characteristics, biology contributes to creativity by providing a range of possible expressions. This range delimits our potential, but it guarantees nothing. The environment determines how much of that potential we fulfill. Family experiences seem to influence the fulfillment of creative potentials, just to name one example of how experience interacts with biology.

Encyclopedia of the Human Brain
Volume 2

The range of potential delimits the levels of performance in simple terms, the amount of creative talent the individual will express but also the domain of expression. This is an important point because creativity in the visual arts is very different from musical creativity, and both of these are very different from mathematical creative talent. There are many domains and possible areas of expression, and each very likely has particular biological underpinnings. An individual may inherit the potential to excel in music but not mathematics or to excel in languages but not the performing arts. It is quite possible that the different domains of creative expression are associated with different brain structures.

Such domain specificity further complicates matters, especially for investigations focused on creativity. This is because creativity is often a kind of self-expression, and it is frequently maximal when the individual is intrinsically motivated. This simply means that the individual is expressing himself or herself in an original fashion or putting the effort into solving a problem in a creative manner, not because of incentive or reward (both of which are extrinsic) but because of personal interests. However, what if those interests do not fit well with the biological potentials? What if the individual is intrinsically motivated to study music but biologically predisposed to excel in a field that involves very different talents, such as science? We can hope that most persons inherent a potential to be interested in the same domain in which they have inherited the potential for relevant skills, but we should also accept the strong likelihood that some persons have unfulfilled creative potentials. This is all the more reason to examine the brain and creativity.

Creativity is multifaceted. There are cognitive skills involved in all creative acts, but these are also attitudes that can facilitate or inhibit creative performance. Personality has long been recognized as an important determinant, and increasingly more is being done with the emotions that play significant roles in creative work. Creativity is often operationalized for research or practice (e.g., education or organizational efficacy) in a fairly simplistic fashion, with an emphasis on divergent thinking or the production of original ideas. However, definitions that focus on one or two traits or abilities do not do justice to the creative efforts that have literally changed each of our lives through technological innovation or the artistic perspective. Often, in the research creativity is called a syndrome or complex because of its multifaceted nature. We must keep this in mind as we discuss the specific research

findings on the brain and creativity. Most of the research focuses on one kind of creativity or one of the relevant skills. I previously noted that biological potentials do not guarantee that the talent will be expressed, and the same thing must be said about any connection we discover between the brain and a particular facet of the creativity complex: That is no guarantee of actual creative performance.

The creativity complex comprises cognitive, attitudinal, and emotional components. These are described in this article and tied to brain structure and function.

II. SPLIT BRAIN

Probably the best known research on the brain and creativity is that of Roger Sperry. He was awarded the Nobel prize for his research with individuals who had commisurotomies (i.e., the corpus callosum is cut, thereby functionally disconnecting the two hemispheres of the brain). Sperry did not administer any tests of creativity per se to the commisurotomy patients, but his research is very relevant because he found that certain important alogical and simultaneous processes tended to be controlled by the right hemisphere. Logical and linguistic processes seemed to be controlled by the left hemisphere. This is quite telling, although we must be careful not to make the mistake that is made in the popular press.

Sperry studied more than two dozen individuals, and not all of them demonstrated the dramatic differences between the right and left hemispheres. Additionally, Sperry worked with epileptic individuals who had the surgery because of this disease. It was an attempt to reduce the number of grand mal seizures. Surely epileptic persons have atypical nervous systems. They also had commissurotomies, further precluding generalizations from Sperry's research. Finally, it is simplistic and inappropriate to view creativity as a solely right hemisphere function. Clearly, individuals cannot use one hemisphere or the other. None of us can do that, unless of course you are one of Sperry's patients and have had a commissurotomy. Nor should we try to rely on one hemisphere: Creativity involves both logic and imagination, divergent and convergent thinking.

Sperry's patients have been studied many times. Klaus Hoppe, for example, reported what may be some of the most relevant findings about individuals with split brains—namely, that they often have trouble understanding their own emotional reactions, if they have them. In "Dual Brain, Creativity, and Health," he and Neville Kyle referred to this as alexithymia. It is especially significant because creativity so often involves enthusiasm, excitement, and the like.

Hoppe and Kyle's interpretation focuses on the corpus callosum. They described how

commisurotomy patients, in comparison with normal controls, use significantly fewer affect laden words, a higher percentage of auxiliary verbs, and applied adjectives sparsely revealing a speech that was dull, uninvolved, flat, and lacking color and expressiveness. ... Commissurotomy patients tended not to fantasize about, imagine, or interpret the symbols, and they tended to describe the circumstances surrounding events, as opposed to describing their own feelings about these events. ... Commisurotomy patients, in comparison with normal controls, symbolized in a discursive, logically articulate structure, using mainly a secondary process, as opposed to a presentational structure as an expression of a predominantly prominent process. They also showed a concreteness of symbolization, emphasizing low rather than creative capacity... showed a relatively impoverish fantasy life, and tended not to be able and convey symbolic meanings.

III. ELECTROENCEPHALOGRAM PATTERNS

Electroencephalogram (EEG) data were also collected. These indicated that the subjects had low activity in the right temporal area (T4) when listening to music and viewing an emotionally stimulating film. They also had low levels of activity in the left hemisphere, particularly in Broca and Wernickes' areas (F3 and T3). Hoppe and Kyle believed that this suggested a lack of inner speech. The same patients had high levels of activity in the left parietal area (P3).

Perhaps most important was the fact that the patients had what Hoppe called a high coherence between the left parietal area (P3) and the right frontal area (F4). This was interpreted as "a possible inter-hemispheric aspect of inhibition of expression." The control subjects who were more emotional and expressive, in contrast, had coherence between the left temporal (T3) and the right frontal (F4) areas, which suggested "a possible mechanism facilitating the transformation of the effective understanding in the

right hemisphere into verbal expression of the lower left hemisphere."

Hoppe and Kyle believe strongly that communication between the hemispheres is necessary for creative thinking. Earlier, Salvatore Arieti described "a magic synthesis," the title of his 1976 book, and Arthur Koestler proposed in his book *The Art of Creation* that creativity could be understood as bisociation. Both of them were pointing to the need for communication between and collaboration by the two hemispheres of the brain. There are other relevant data. Most, however, involve indirect measurement.

For example, there are studies of handedness, which is supposedly an indication of hemispheric dominance and preference. Yet other studies use dichotic listening tasks wherein particular messages are played to one ear or the other, and thereby presented to one hemisphere or the other. In a 1999 review of this research, Albert Katz indicated that the findings were not all that convincing, although they were in the direction in what would be expected with a right hemisphere contribution to creative thinking. It is very likely that such indirect measures will not be used very frequently or very much longer, given new technologies for brain imaging and the like. Importantly, Katz, like Hoppe and others, concluded that

creative activity cannot be localized as a special function unique to one to the cerebral hemispheres. Rather, productive thought involves the integration coordination of processes subserved by both hemispheres. ... There appears to be privileged role in creativity to the cognitive functions associated with the right hemisphere. ... There is some evidence that different creative tasks may differentially call on cognitive resources for which the two hemispheres were specialized. ... Finally, there is some evidence that creativity related hemispheric asymmetries can be found both online (as the person performs a task) and as a consequence of habitual patterns of behavior.

IV. STAGES OF THE CREATIVE PROCESS

Colin Martindale, like Hoppe, employed EEGs. Martindale examined particular brain wave patterns and their association with specific stages within the problem-solving process. Findings indicated that EEG patterns vary as a function of stage of the creative process, at least in creative individuals. These phases are usually labeled preparation, incubation, illumination (or inspiration), and verification. Creative individuals have higher alpha during the inspirational phase of creative work than during elaboration phases. There are no differences in basal alpha. EEG was measured at right posterior temporal areas.

Another technique for the study of the biology of creativity involves individuals who have had accidental trauma to the nervous system. In his 1982 book, *Art, Mind, and Brain*, Howard Gardner tells how through use of this technique he was able to infer much about processes that are very important for creativity, such as the use of metaphor. This kind of research is useful because it identifies particular parts of the brain. However, the locations studied are not chosen by the researchers but of course are the result of various unfortunate accidents.

V. MAGNETIC IMAGING

We probably need not look to accidents much longer. We now have systematic techniques, such as magnetic imaging. In a 1995 investigation, Thomas Albert, Christo Pantey, Christian Wiendruch, Bridget Rockstroh, and Edward Taub found that the cortical representation of the digits of the left hand of string players was larger than that in controls. The effect was smallest for the left thumb and no such differences were observed for representations of the right hand digits. The amount of cortical reorganization in the representation of the fingering digits was correlated with the age at which the person had begun to play. These results suggested that the representation of different parts of the body and the primary somatosensory cortex of humans depends on use and changes to conform to the current needs and experiences of the individual.

Recall the idea introduced earlier in this article, that performance often reflects both biological potential and experience. Note also the fact that this research focused on individuals within a very specific domain of performance (stringed instruments). Generalizations cannot be applied to other instruments, let alone other kinds of musical creativity or other kinds of art. Finally, it is critical to keep in mind that although the participants of this study were musicians, their actual creativity was not assessed. Music may be an unambiguously creative domain, but it would be interesting to know the actual level of creative skill of the individuals and to correlate that with the size of the cortical representations.

VI. EINSTEIN'S BRAIN

Given the complexity of creativity and the diversity of definitions that have been proposed, some scholars prefer to focus on unambiguously creative persons. The advantage of this approach is that the creativity of the research subjects (e.g., Darwin, Picasso, and Einstein) is beyond question.

This approach is often used in the psychological research but has also been employed in physiological research, such as the 1985 study of the brain of Albert Einstein by Marian Diamond, Arnold Scheibel, Greer Murphy, and Thomas Harvey. These authors found that Einstein's brain had a significantly smaller mean ratio of neuron to glial cells (connections) in "area 39" of the left hemisphere than did control scientists. This was not the case in three other areas. It was not true of the right hemisphere. The interpretation focused on the "metabolic need" of Einstein's cortex and the role of the cortex in associative thinking. Diamond and his colleagues concluded that the exceptionality of Einstein's brain may have given him outstanding "conceptual power."

VII. CONCLUSIONS

One area of the brain may be involved in creativity but has received little attention. More than one theorist has pointed to the prefontal lobes. Salvatore Arieti did so long ago, and others have echoed it, often citing tendencies involved in creativity and controlled by the prefrontal lobes. Elliott, for example, argued that creative behavior is a product of the human capacity to will. He believed that this implies that the prefrontal lobe must be engaged, "thereby facilitating the harmonious functioning of the entire brain (left–right, top–bottom, front–back) and thus regulating all psychological functions associated with the creative process." In 2000, Torsten Norlander came to a similar conclusion but drew from what is known about the prefrontal dysfunction and hypofrontality of schizophrenic patients. (Data include the cerebral regional blood flow of schizophrenic patients.) Although largely inferential, this line of thought is noteworthy in part because it is consistent with the idea of balanced processes contributing to creative thinking. The balance may require communication between the left and right hemispheres of the brain, and between logic and imagination (the magic synthesis), but it may also benefit from collaboration with the prefrontal lobes.

Empirical research on the prefrontal lobes and their role in creative thinking is needed. Fortunately, we can expect a great deal of progress to be made in the very near future. There are two reasons for this. First, the field of creative studies in growing explosively. The implications of creativity for health and learning are now widely recognized, as is the role of creativity in innovation, business, and technological advancement. Even more important may be the technological advances that are being made in medicine. These provide sophisticated methods for studying the brain. Soon, we should understand how the different parts and processes of the human brain correspond to the various components of the creativity complex.

See Also the Following Articles

ARTIFICIAL INTELLIGENCE • CONSCIOUSNESS • EMOTION • HUMOR AND LAUGHTER • INTELLIGENCE • LANGUAGE ACQUISITION • LOGIC AND REASONING • MUSIC AND THE BRAIN • PROBLEM SOLVING • UNCONSCIOUS, THE

Suggested Reading

Albert, T., Pantey, C., Wiendruch, C., Rockstroh, B., and Taub, E. (1995). Increased cortical representation of the fingers of the left hand in string players. *Science* **270,** 305–307.

Arieti, S. (1976). *The Magic Synthesis*. Basic Books, New York.

Diamond, M. C., Schiebel, A. B., Murphy, G. M., and Harvey, T. (1985). On the brain of a scientist: Albert Einstein. *Exp. Neurol.* **88,** 198–204.

Elliott, P. C. (1986). Right (or left) brain cognition, wrong metaphor for creative behavior: It is prefrontal lobe volition that makes the (human/humane) difference in release of creative potential. *J. Creative Behav.* **20,** 202–214.

Hoppe, K. D., and Kyle, N. L. (1990). Dual brain, creativity, and health. *Creativity Res. J.* **3,** 150–157.

Katz, A. (1997). *Creativity in the cerebral hemispheres*. In *Creativity Research Handbook* (M. A. Runco, Ed.), pp. 203–226. Hampton Press, Cresskill, NJ.

Martindale, C., and Hasenfus, N. (1978). EEG differences as a function of creativity, stage of the creative process, and effort to be original. *Biol. Psychol.* **6,** 157–167.

Runco, M. A., and Albert, R. S. (2001). *Theories of Creativity*, 2nd ed. Hampton Press, Cresskill, NJ.

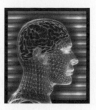

Dementia

ALFRED W. KASZNIAK

University of Arizona

neuropsychological assessment An approach to the evaluation of dementia and other neurobehavioral disorders involving structured interviewing, behavioral observation, and the administration of standardized tests of cognitive and emotional functions.

perseveration Persistence in a particular action or thought after task demands have changed and the action or thought is no longer appropriate.

prosopagnosia Deficit in the ability to recognize familiar faces.

verbal fluency Ability to quickly generate words from within a particular semantic category (e.g., animal names, items that can be found in a grocery store) or beginning with a particular letter of the alphabet.

GLOSSARY

aphasia Impairment in the expression and/or comprehension of language.

cognitive functions Distinct domains of intellectual ability, including memory, language, visuospatial ability, judgment, and abstraction, among others.

depression A clinical disorder characterized by at least five of the following nine symptoms present during at least a 2-week period: depressed mood, markedly diminished interest in activities, significant weight loss or gain, difficulty sleeping or excessive sleeping, agitation or slowing of thought and action, fatigue or loss of energy, feelings of worthlessness or guilt, diminished ability to think or concentrate, and suicidal ideation.

executive functions That subgroup of cognitive functions necessary to plan and carry out complex, goal-oriented behavior. Executive functions include planning, organizing, sequencing, and abstracting abilities.

neuroimaging Technologies available for the detailed visualization of brain structure and/or function. These technologies include computerized tomography (CT), magnetic resonance imaging (MRI), functional magnetic resonance imaging (fMRI), positron emission tomography (PET), and single photon emission computed tomography (SPECT).

The clinical syndrome of dementia is characterized by impairment of multiple cognitive functions (e.g., memory, language, visuospatial abilities, judgment), typically due to chronic or progressive brain disease. The cognitive impairments are frequently accompanied by personality changes, including deficits in motivation and emotional control. Several different illnesses can cause the dementia syndrome, and the pattern of cognitive deficits and personality changes may differ by the type of illness as well as by the specific brain structures and systems most affected. This article will present an overview of the more common dementia syndromes, emphasizing their epidemiology, clinical presentation, and pattern of neuropsychological deficits. Neuropathological characteristics and neurobiological research concerning causes and treatments are mentioned only briefly because these aspects are specifically reviewed in other articles (e.g., Alzheimer's Disease) within this volume.

I. CHARACTERISTICS AND EPIDEMIOLOGY OF DEMENTIA

Most diagnostic criteria for the dementia syndrome stipulate that two or more cognitive functions must be sufficiently impaired so as to interfere with social and/ or occupational functioning and that there must not be clouding of consciousness. Clouding of consciousness, particularly in the context of a sudden onset of confusion, disorientation, hallucinations, disturbance in attention, or marked behavior change, is typically indicative of delirium (also termed acute confusional state). Delirium may be caused by an acute or chronic systemic illness (e.g., bacterial infection, hypoglycemia), adverse effects of medication, or serious neurological event requiring immediate medical attention. Untreated, these illnesses may result in death or irreversible impairment.

The risk of developing dementia increases markedly with age in later adulthood and is the single most prevalent category of mental illness for older persons. Worldwide, between 10 and 15% of persons over the age of 65 show at least mild dementia and approximately 6% show severe dementia. After age 65, dementia prevalence doubles approximately every 5 years. Overall, dementia is somewhat more common among women and may be more common in community-dwelling older black Americans. Prevalence for other nonwhite ethnic and racial groups is difficult to estimate due to the small number of adequate epidemiological studies. Annual incidence of new cases of dementia is also age-related, estimated to steadily increase from 0.33% at age 65 to 8.68% for those 95 years of age and older. A family history is a risk factor for dementia, increasing with the number of first-degree relatives similarly affected. Low educational background or low lifetime occupational attainment also increases the risk of dementia diagnosis. Studies have suggested that higher levels of education and higher levels of linguistic ability in early adulthood may be protective against the development of dementia, although controversy concerning this conclusion still remains.

A. Prevalence of Specific Dementia Types

More than 50 different illnesses can produce the symptoms of dementia. Available studies indicate that, on average, 5% of all causes of dementia are reversible and 11% have some specific treatment available, although not typically resulting in symptom reversal. Among the more common potentially reversible causes are those due to prescription and nonprescription drug toxicity, metabolic disorder, brain tumors, subdural hematoma (a collection of blood under the outermost meningeal covering of the brain), and depression. The more common dementia types that are presently irreversible include Alzheimer's disease, Parkinson's disease, dementia with Lewy bodies, Huntington's disease, frontotemporal dementias, vascular dementia, and traumatic brain injury.

Autopsy studies have varied in their estimates of the relative proportion of all dementia cases accounted for by each of these causes or types, although all agree that Alzheimer's disease (AD) is the most common. The neuropathological characteristics of AD consist primarily of neuritic plaques and neurofibrillary tangles, as well as neuronal loss. The neuropathology appears to be focused in the medial temporal lobe regions (including the hippocampus, entorhinal cortex, and subiculum) early in the illness course, with progression to the frontal, temporal, and parietal association cortices. Neuronal loss is also seen within the subcortical neurons of the nucleus basalis of Meynert (a major source of cholinergic neurotransmitter input to widespread cortical areas) and in the locus ceruleus (a major source of widespread noradrenergic neurotransmitter projections). Eventually, diffuse neuronal loss results in gross cerebral atrophy, which can easily be seen in autopsied brains, and in structural neuroimaging evidence of ventricular and sulcal enlargement, such as that provided by computerized tomography (CT) and magnetic resonance imaging (MRI; see Fig. 1). Across several studies, AD alone has been found to account for between 53 and 66% of total dementia cases and may be present in combination with the neuropathology of other diseases in as many as 87%. Vascular disease, typically in the form of multiple infarctions of blood vessels (blockages, with resultant tissue death in the area supplied by the vessel), had previously been thought to be the second most frequent cause. However, more recent studies suggest that multiple infarctions alone may account for less than 2% of all dementias, although contributing to dementia severity, along with coexistent AD, in approximately 13%.

Lewy body disease has only relatively recently been recognized as a significant cause of dementia, and earlier autopsy studies typically did not include it. Lewy bodies are microscopic intracellular abnormalities seen in the brain stem structures of patients with Parkinson's disease but are also found distributed

Enlarged Lateral Ventricles

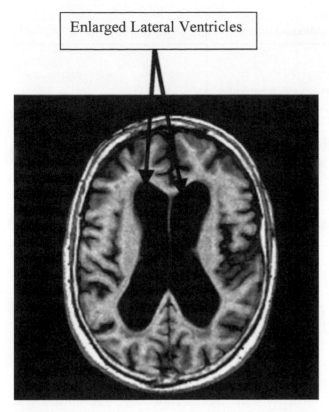

Figure 1 Magnetic resonance image (MRI) showing the greatly enlarged lateral ventricles characteristic of cerebral atrophy in later stage Alzheimer's disease.

diffusely throughout the cortex and subcortex when associated with dementia. Autopsy studies have suggested that dementia with Lewy bodies (DLB) might account for 15–30% of all cases of dementia, which would make it the second largest subgroup after AD.

The frontotemporal dementias (FTD) include both Pick's disease and non-Pick's neuropathology and account for about 3.5% of all dementia cases. Pick's disease is characterized by Pick's cells (enlarged neurons with displaced nuclei) and Pick's inclusion bodies (round inclusions within the neuron cell body) in frontal and temporal cortical areas. Non-Pick's neuropathology of FTD includes microvacuolation (small holes or vacuoles) or spongiosus (spongelike softening), predominantly in the frontal cortex.

Other causes, including Huntington's disease, Parkinson's disease, corticobasal degeneration (all considered among the frontal–subcortical dementias), depression, and several very rare causes, account for the remaining percentage of dementia cases. Within the following sections, the clinical and neuropsychological features characterizing the major dementia types will be described.

II. ALZHEIMER'S DISEASE

Alzheimer's disease (AD) is a chronic, progressive degenerative brain disease. The most striking behavioral changes of AD include increasing difficulty in learning and retaining new information, handling complex tasks, reasoning, spatial ability and orientation, language, and social behavior. In 1984, a task force assembled by the United States Department of Health and Human Services developed the diagnostic criteria for AD shown in Table I. These criteria now form the basis for standard AD diagnosis in research and have been incorporated into widely used clinical diagnostic criteria (e.g., those of the *American Psychiatric Association Diagnostic and Statistical Manual of Mental Disorders*, 4th ed.). These criteria have been shown to achieve good sensitivity (against the criterion of neuropathological confirmation), although more limited specificity, in the clinical diagnosis of AD.

Early in the course of AD, the most sensitive indicators of cognitive impairment are standardized tests of memory (particularly delayed recall) for recently presented verbal or nonverbal information. This is not surprising given that neuropathology in hippocampal and entorhinal cortices appears early in the illness course and that rapid forgetting is the hallmark of focal damage to these structures in both human and nonhuman animal studies. Several studies now provide evidence that AD has a long, preclinical (i.e., prior to the time when the patient meets standard diagnostic criteria) course, during which subtle memory changes occur. Mild memory impairments, measurable with sensitive neuropsychological tests, thus have been documented in apparently well-functioning persons several years prior to their diagnosis of AD. Similar memory impairments are seen in those presently healthy persons at genetic risk (i.e., showing the apolipoprotein e4 gene allele, a known risk for AD). Of persons demonstrating mild cognitive impairment (MCI), typically defined as standardized memory test performance that is one standard deviation below age- and education-specific normative expectations, between 6 and 25% per year progress to meet diagnostic criteria for dementia (most typically AD). However, preclinical AD is not the only cause, because those with MCI also show higher rates of overall poorer health, cerebrovascular disease, and disability and are more often depressed than those with normal memory functioning.

Also relatively early in the course of AD, individuals tend to show decreased verbal fluency, best documented by an ability to produce words within a given

Table I
Alzheimer's Disease (AD) Diagnostic Criteria

A clinical diagnosis of *probable* AD is made when:

  (1) Dementia is established by clinical examination and documented by performance on a standardized mental status examination, *and*

  (2) confirmed by neuropsychological testing, documenting deficits in two or more areas of cognition, *and*

  (3) characterized by a history of progressive worsening of memory and other cognitive deficits, *with*

  (4) no disturbance in level of consciousness, *and*

  (5) symptom onset between the ages of 40 and 90 years, most typically after age 65, *and*

  (6) there is an absence of systemic disorders or other brain diseases that of themselves could account for the progressive deficits.

  The diagnosis of probable AD is further supported by evidence (i.e., from neuropsychological reexamination) of progressive deterioration of specific cognitive functions, impairment in activities of daily living (ADLs), a family history of similar disorders, and results of particular laboratory tests (e.g., a normal lumbar puncture, normal pattern or nonspecific changes in the electroencephalogram, and evidence of cerebral atrophy on structural neuroimaging).

The clinical diagnosis of *possible* AD is made when:

  (1) the syndrome of dementia is present, *and*

  (2) there is an absence of other neurologic, psychiatric, or systemic disorders sufficient to cause the dementia, *but*

  (3) variations are present from criteria for probable AD in the onset, presentation, or clinical course. Possible AD may also be diagnosed when a systemic brain disease sufficient to produce a dementia is present but (for various reasons) is not considered to be the cause of the patient's dementia.

semantic category (e.g., names of animals or items that can be found in a supermarket) that is significantly below normative expectation. With disease progression, difficulties in spatial orientation and visuospatial abilities (e.g., ability to accurately draw a clock face), facial recognition, and language comprehension all occur. These impairments appear to reflect increasing neurofibrillary tangle and neuritic plaque involvement of the parietal and temporal association cortices. In addition, increasing problems with focusing and shifting attention and "executive functions" are seen with disease progression. Executive functions refer to those various abilities (including volition, planning, organizing, sequencing, abstracting, and performance self-monitoring) that contribute to the capacity to plan and carry out complex, goal-oriented behavior. Apathy, difficulty in shifting behavioral set to accommodate new task demands, impaired abstract reasoning, difficulty in the correct sequencing of behavior, and poor awareness of cognitive deficits are all aspects of executive dysfunction and are also correlated with the degree of behavioral disinhibition and agitation among AD patients. The increasing difficulties in attention and executive functioning appear to reflect the frontal cortex neuritic plaque and neurofibrillary tangle density increase that occurs with AD progression.

Apathy and other aspects of executive dysfunction have been found to correlate with functional neuroimaging measures (see Fig. 2) documenting decreased blood flow in the anterior cingulate, dorsolateral frontal, orbitofrontal, and anterior temporal cortical regions. In general, functional neuroimaging [e.g., positron emission tomography (PET)] studies have shown that, in AD patients with mild dementia (relatively early in the illness course), cerebral metabolism is decreased in temporal and parietal cortices, with progression to metabolic decreases in the frontal cortex as dementia severity worsens. There is also evidence for heterogeneity in the relative severity of various cognitive deficits among persons with AD. If we equate for overall severity of dementia, those who show the greatest visuospatial impairments demonstrate the lowest right-hemispheric metabolism, and those with the greatest language impairments have the lowest left-hemispheric metabolism. By the late stage of severe dementia in AD, only sensory and motor cortical areas show preserved metabolic rates.

III. FRONTAL–SUBCORTICAL DEMENTIAS

The most common clinical features of the frontal–subcortical dementias are bradyphrenia (a slowing of thought processes and information processing speed), memory problems, impairment of executive functions, mood changes, and sometimes visuospatial deficits.

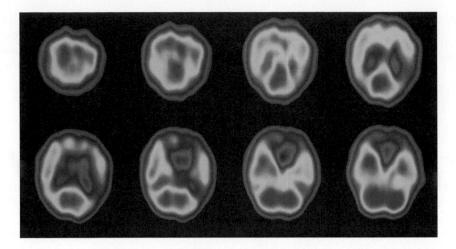

Figure 2 Single photon emission computed tomographic (SPECT) image of the brain of an individual with Alzheimer's disease, showing decreased blood flow (darker areas) in frontal regions as well as in temporal–parietal association cortices.

Those diseases that can cause this dementia syndrome include progressive supranuclear palsy (PSP), Huntington's disease (HD), Parkinson's disease (PD), dementia with Lewy bodies (DLB), and corticobasal degeneration (CBD). Damage to the rostral brain stem, thalamus, basal ganglia, and/or reciprocal connections between these subcortical regions and frontal cortical areas appears to be the common factor in these dementias. These structures all participate in several distinct, semi-closed-loop-circuits that subserve particular motor, cognitive executive, and emotional functions.

A. Progressive Supranuclear Palsy (PSP)

PSP is also known as Steele–Richardson–Olszewski syndrome. It is a degenerative disorder of subcortical nuclei, including the subthalamic nucleus, substantia nigra, globus pallidus, caudate, putamen, and periaqueductal gray. Clinically, persons with PSP show paralysis involving motor neurons of the eye, leading to impaired downward ocular gaze and other ocular symptoms. Clinical diagnosis requires documentation of at least two of the following signs: axial dystonia (abnormal pattern of muscle tonus in the axial musculature) and rigidity (especially of the neck), pseudobulbar palsy (manifested as sudden crying or laughing without apparent cause or accompanying experienced emotion), bradykinesia (slowness in the initiation of movement), signs of frontal lobe dysfunction (e.g., motor perseveration, difficulty in behavioral

set-shifting in response to changing task demands), postural instability with backward falling, and sometimes dysarthria (difficulty in the motor aspects of speech). Cognitive deficits, documented by neuropsychological testing, include memory loss, slowed information processing speed, apathy and depression, irritability, and executive function deficits.

B. Huntington's Disease (HD)

HD is an autosomal-dominant genetic disorder marked by initial abnormal choreiform (dancelike) movements, slowed voluntary movements, depressive and manic emotional disturbances, and eventual dementia. HD manifests in an insidious onset, usually in young to middle adulthood. The dementia of HD is characterized neuropsychologically by impaired attention and concentration, executive function deficits, and impaired encoding and retrieval of new information. However, if care is taken to make sure that the person with HD adequately encodes the information (e.g., by having the individual semantically categorize it) and procedures are used that do not require effortful retrieval strategies (e.g., recognition memory rather than a free recall task), then it can be shown that the retention of new information is more intact in HD than in AD patients with comparable overall dementia severity. The neuropathology of HD includes cell loss and atrophy that begins in the medial caudate nucleus and eventually includes the entire caudate and putamen. Some degree of cortical atrophy is also typically seen in the brains of persons with HD at autopsy.

C. Parkinson's Disease (PD)

PD is primarily a progressive, extrapyramidal (involving motor systems of the basal ganglia rather than the pyramidal tract) disorder with clinical motor features of stooped posture, bradykinesia (slowing of movement initiation), tremor (when the affected limb is at rest, but typically not during movement), cogwheel rigidity (i.e., rigidity that seems to catch and release, much like a cogwheel, when the clinician attempts to passively move the patient's limb), and festinating gait. Dementia has been estimated to occur in approximately 35–40% of persons with PD. The neuropsychological impairments manifested in the dementia of PD include psychomotor slowing, impaired cognitive tracking and set-shifting flexibility, visuospatial deficits, diminished learning and retrieval (although, as with HD, often there is evidence of more intact information retention shown by recognition memory tasks), decreased verbal fluency, and abstract reasoning impairment. Neuronal degeneration (with Lewy bodies; see later discussion) occurs primarily in pigmented cells of the substantia nigra (particularly the pars compacta region) and other brain stem structures (e.g., locus ceruleus, dorsal vagal nucleus). The substantia nigra degeneration causes a severe reduction in dopamine neurotransmitter projections to the striatum, responsible for the observed extrapyramidal motor disorder and contributing to the cognitive impairments.

D. Dementia with Lewy Bodies (DLB)

In addition to occurring in brain stem structures in persons with PD, Lewy bodies are the neuropathological characteristic of DLB, where they appear diffusely distributed throughout the neocortex, diencephalon, brain stem, and basal ganglia. Because of the brain structures involved, DLB is sometimes considered to be among the frontal–subcortical dementias. The core clinical features of DLB are the presence of dementia, gait–balance disorder, prominent hallucinations and delusions, sensitivity to neuroleptic antipsychotic drugs, and fluctuating alertness. A consensus has been reached concerning the clinical criteria for diagnosing DLB (see Table II). These criteria have demonstrated high specificity, although relatively low sensitivity, against neuropathological findings.

Illness progression in DLB is often rapid, with severe dementia and the motor features of PD present

Table II
Criteria for Dementia with Lewy Bodies (DLB)

The central required feature is progressive cognitive decline of sufficient magnitude to interfere with normal social or occupational function.

    (1) Prominent or persistent memory impairment may not necessarily occur in early stages but usually is evident with progression.

    (2) Deficits on tests of attention, frontal–subcortical functions, and visuospatial abilities may be especially prominent.

Core features (two required for probable DLB and one for possible):

    (3) Fluctuating cognition with pronounced variations in attention and alertness.

    (4) Recurrent visual hallucinations that are typically well-formed and detailed.

    (5) Spontaneous motor features of parkinsonism.

Features supportive of the diagnosis:

    (6) Repeated falls

    (7) Syncope

    (8) Transient loss of consciousness

    (9) Neuroleptic drug sensitivity

    (10) Systematized delusions

    (11) Hallucinations in other modalities

Diagnosis of DLB is less likely in the presence of:

    (12) Evidence of stroke from focal neurological signs or brain imaging.

    (13) Evidence of any physical illness or other brain disorder sufficient to account for the clinical features.

within 1–5 years of diagnosis. It has been suggested that a diagnosis of DLB should require that cognitive dysfunction occur within 12 months of the onset of parkinsonian motor features. Patients with PD who develop dementia more than 12 months after the onset of their motor signs are diagnosed as having PD with dementia. The neuropsychological test profiles of persons with DLB show marked deficits in attention and visual–constructive skills (e.g., ability to copy a geometric pattern with blocks), frequently with relative sparing of memory. However, neuropsychological testing has not been able to reliably differentiate DLB from either AD or vascular dementia, given the clinical variability and overlap of the cognitive impairments in these dementia types. Structural neuroimaging (CT or MRI) also has not been successful in differentiating DLB from AD.

E. Lewy Body Variant (LBV) of AD

The Lewy body variant of AD (sometimes also referred to as "common" DLB, in contrast to "pure" DLB) is characterized by the typical neuritic plaques and neurofibrillary tangles of AD, the subcortical changes of PD, and the presence of diffusely distributed cortical Lewy bodies. Persons with the LBV of AD, compared to persons with "pure" AD, show a greater proportion of mild parkinsonian or other extrapyramidal motor findings, a typically fluctuating cognitive impairment, visual or auditory hallucinations, and frequent unexplained falls.

F. Corticobasal Degeneration (CBD)

CBD is a rare disorder that presents clinically as an asymmetric, akinetic rigid syndrome with apraxia (impaired voluntary execution of symbolic movements and gestures), myoclonus, and sometimes dementia. When dementia is present, the pattern of neuropsychological test performance resembles that of PSP, except that apraxia is typically more severe in CBD. Symptoms of cortical sensory loss (e.g., impaired visual or tactile discrimination) are also common early in CBD. Persons with CBD often show the "alien limb" syndrome, in which the individual reports that their limb is moving without their volitional control, and often are mildly depressed. CBD is associated with markedly asymmetric patterns of cortical metabolism

alteration (as measured by PET). Cortical metabolism contralateral to the affected limb is typically lower in inferior parietal, lateral temporal, and sensory motor cortices than that seen in PSP.

IV. FRONTOTEMPORAL DEMENTIAS

FTD includes both Pick's disease and non-Pick's frontotemporal dementia (also called frontal lobe dementia, FLD), motor neuron disease, and progressive subcortical gliosis. Although estimates of the prevalence of FTD remain somewhat controversial, some investigators think that these disorders have been underestimated and could account for 10–19% of all demented cases. The usual age of onset is between 45 and 65 years, with equal sex incidence. A family history of the illness is present in approximately 50% of persons with FTD. FTD includes subtypes of semantic dementia, primary progressive aphasia, and progressive prosopagnosia, as described later.

Pick's disease is characterized by Pick's cells (enlarged neurons with displaced nuclei) and Pick's inclusion bodies (round intraneuronal cellular inclusions) in frontal and temporal cortical areas. In Pick's disease, marked atrophy (termed "knife edge" due to the extreme thinning of the cortical gyri) is found in the frontal and anterior temporal lobes, with some patients also showing atrophy in the basal ganglia and caudate nucleus. The gross neuropathology of non-Pick's FTD is similar to that of Pick's, with atrophy primarily affecting the frontal lobes. However, those with non-Pick's FTD do not typically show Pick's cells and bodies. Some show microvacuolation or spongiosus (often termed the frontal lobe dementia type, FLD). Degeneration of bulbar cranial nerve nuclei and anterior horn cells may also be present in some persons with FTD. Chromosome 17 abnormality with τ protein aggregation and decreased τ binding to neuronal cell microtubules has been found in the brains of persons who died with FTD.

Personality and behavioral changes, executive dysfunction, and language disturbances are predominant early signs of FTD. Language deficits are progressive in nature and may eventually lead to mutism. Neurological signs including akinesia, rigidity, masked facies (markedly decreased spontaneous facial expression), gait disturbance, dysarthria, dysphagia (swallowing difficulty), and tremor are present throughout the disease for some patients and only in advanced disease for others.

A. Behavioral and Emotional Characteristics of FTD

The most common behavioral changes that accompany FTD are loss of social awareness and insight, personal neglect, disinhibition, impulsivity, impersistence, inertia, aspontaneity, mental rigidity and inflexibility, motor and verbal perseveration, stereotyped activities and rituals, utilization behavior (tendency to compulsively use whatever object is placed before the individual), and hyperorality (tendency to frequently mouth objects). Emotional changes of FTD include unconcern, apathy, emotional shallowness and lability, loss of empathy and sympathy, and a fatuous jocularity. Consensus clinical criteria, based on these behavioral and emotional characteristics, have been developed for FTD (see Table III). However, as yet there is insufficient research comparing these criteria to neuropathological findings, preventing adequate assessment of sensitivity and specificity.

Neuropsychological testing of persons with FTD typically reveals deficits in verbal fluency, abstraction ability, and other areas of executive functioning. However, because some AD patients also demonstrate substantial executive function deficits, this pattern of neuropsychological test performance cannot be considered specific to FTD.

B. Semantic Dementia

Semantic dementia is a subtype of FTD characterized by fluent, anomic aphasia (marked difficulty with word-finding and naming), with impaired verbal comprehension and loss of semantic knowledge. The neuropathology in semantic dementia is typically most marked in the left (or bilateral) temporal pole and inferolateral cortex.

C. Progressive Nonfluent Aphasia

Another subtype of FTD, known as progressive nonfluent aphasia, is characterized by nonfluent, hesitant, distorted speech with preserved verbal comprehension. The neuropathology is typically most marked in the left perisylvian cortical area.

D. Progressive Prosopagnosia

The progressive prosopagnosia subtype of FTD is characterized by impaired identification of familiar faces, followed by loss of person knowledge. The neuropathology is typically most marked in the right temporal pole and inferolateral cortex.

V. VASCULAR DEMENTIA

In the presence of cerebrovascular disease, dementia may be observed when there are multiple infarctions within both cerebral hemispheres. The clinical features that accompany multiple infarctions of relatively large cerebral blood vessels (termed multi-infarct dementia, MID) depend upon the particular brain regions

Table III
Criteria for Frontotemporal Dementia (FTD)

Core diagnostic features:
  (1) Insidious onset with gradual progression
  (2) Early decline in interpersonal conduct
  (3) Early impairment in the regulation of personal conduct
  (4) Early emotional blunting
  (5) Early loss of insight
Supportive diagnostic features:
  (6) Behavioral disorder, including decline in personal hygiene and grooming; mental rigidity and inflexibility; distractibility and impersistence; hyperorality and dietary changes; perseverative and stereotyped behavior; and/or utilization behavior.
  (7) Speech impairment, including altered speech output (either aspontaneity and economy of speech or press of speech); stereotype of speech; echolalia; perseveration; and/or mutism.
  (8) Physical signs, including primitive reflexes; incontinence; akinesia, rigidity, and tremor; and/or low and labile blood pressure.
  (9) Investigations, including significant impairment on neuropsychological tests of executive functioning in the absence of severe amnesia, aphasia, or visuospatial disorder; normal electroencephalogram despite clinically evident dementia; and brain imaging (structural and/or functional) showing predominant frontal and/or anterior temporal abnormality.

affected. Dementia may also be the result of multiple small subcortical (termed lacunar) infarctions. As previously noted in this article, although vascular disease was earlier thought to be the second most frequent cause of dementia, more recent autopsy studies have indicated that dementia most typically occurs when both multiple infarctions and the neuropathology of AD or Lewy bodies are present. Consensus criteria for the diagnosis of VAD have been proposed (see Table IV). Evaluation of these criteria against neuropathological findings has shown relatively high specificity, but low sensitivity.

In studies of neuropsychological test performance, persons with pure VAD (i.e., those without coexistent AD pathology or Lewy bodies) show less memory impairment than persons with AD matched for overall dementia severity. In contrast, persons with VAD may be relatively more impaired that those with AD on tests of executive functioning. However, the considerable variability of the neuropsychological test performance in both VAD and AD limits the specificity of these features for differential diagnosis.

VI. DEMENTIA ASSOCIATED WITH DEPRESSION

Depression in older age has been given increasing clinical and research attention. Although the preva-lence of depression (according to standard diagnostic criteria) is not higher for older than for younger adults, older persons with depressive symptoms have health care costs about 50% higher than those without depressive symptoms. These increased costs are not accounted for by mental health service utilization. Depression frequently coexists with neurological disorders among older adults (e.g., stroke, AD, PD) and is often underdiagnosed in older persons, especially when physical illness is present.

Further complicating both accurate diagnosis and treatment is the fact that various prescription and nonprescription medications (and their interactions) can cause, aggravate, or mimic depression symptoms. In addition, persons with depression show impairment on a range of neuropsychological measures of cognitive functioning, particularly on speeded tasks, vigilance tasks, and tasks with pleasant or neutral (in contrast with unpleasant) content. The magnitude of cognitive impairment tends to increase with older age, severity of depression, and history of electroconvulsive treatment (ECT). Previously, the term "pseudo-dementia" was often used to describe persons with depression and cognitive impairment, reflecting the expectation that the cognitive deficits would reverse along with effective treatment of the depression. However, this term is no longer used because several

Table IV
Criteria for Vascular Dementia (VAD)

The clinical diagnosis of *probable* VAD is made when:

(1) Dementia is present, defined by (a) cognitive decline from a previously higher level of functioning; (b) impairment of memory and two or more other cognitive domains (preferably established by clinical examination and documented by neuropsychological testing); (c) sufficient severity as to interfere with activities of daily living; and (d) not due to the sensorimotor effects of stroke alone, *and*

(2) the patient does *not* show disturbance of consciousness, delirium, psychosis, severe aphasia, sensorimotor impairment sufficient to preclude neuropsychological testing, systemic disorders, or other brain diseases (e.g., AD) that could account for the cognitive deficits, *and*

(3) cerebrovascular disease is present, defined by (a) the presence of focal neurologic signs (e.g., hemiparesis, sensory deficit, hemianopsia, Babinski sign, etc.); (b) evidence of relevant features consistent with cerebrovascular disease on brain imaging (CT or MRI), *and*

(4) a relationship is established between the dementia and the cerebrovascular disease inferred by one or more of the following: (a) onset of dementia within 3 months following a recognized stroke; (b) abrupt deterioration in cognitive functioning; or (c) fluctuating, stepwise progression of cognitive deficits.

The diagnosis of probable VAD is further supported by (a) the early presence of a gait disturbance; (b) a history of unsteadiness and frequent falls; (c) early urinary urgency, frequency, and other urinary symptoms not explained by urologic disease; (d) pseudobulbar palsy; and (e) mood and personality changes, psychomotor retardation, and abnormal executive function.

The clinical diagnosis of *possible* VAD is made when:

(1) The patient meets criteria for dementia with focal neurologic signs, *but*

(2) brain imaging studies to confirm cerebrovascular disease are missing, *or*

(3) when there is absence of a clear temporal relationship between dementia and stroke, *or*

(4) in patients with subtle onset and variable course (improvement or plateau) of cognitive deficits and evidence of relevant cerebrovascular disease.

studies have indicated that substantial numbers of these individuals show progressive dementia that does not reverse with depression treatment. Such studies have indicated the need for both caution and persistent follow-up in any attempts to clinically differentiate dementia associated with depression from that due to AD or other dementia syndromes.

Although the severity of cognitive impairment in depression is typically less than that in dementia syndromes such as AD or VAD, differential diagnosis can sometimes be difficult. Depression can coexist with AD, VAD, and other dementia types, complicating differential diagnosis when dementia severity in these disorders is relatively mild. Further, research has shown that those with a first onset of depression in older age (in contrast to older persons with depression onset earlier in life) often show clinical and/or structural neuroimaging evidence of cerebrovascular damage. Persons with later-age-of-onset depression and MRI evidence consistent with relatively large areas of cerebrovascular damage in the subcortical white matter are also more likely to show executive function deficits on neuropsychological testing and are less responsive to antidepressant pharmacotherapy than older adults with depression onset in younger adulthood.

Research comparing the neuropsychological test performance of persons with depression to those with AD has suggested that the following features can be helpful in differential diagnosis. First, as already noted, the cognitive deficits of depression tend to be less severe and extensive than in AD. Second, consistent impairment across various memory tests (particularly involving delayed recall and recognition memory) is more consistent with AD than with depression. Persons with depression are also less likely than those with AD to show impaired naming ability, verbal fluency, and visuospatial ability. Finally, those with depression may appear to exert less effort than those with AD in the performance of various neuropsychological tests and may complain more about their cognitive difficulties (even when testing does not document significant deficits).

VII. NEUROPSYCHOLOGICAL ASSESSMENT IN DEMENTIA DIAGNOSIS

Accurate diagnosis of dementing illness often necessitates the efforts of multidisciplinary teams of physicians (particularly neurologists and psychiatrists), neuropsychologists, and other mental health professionals (e.g., social workers). As noted throughout the previous sections, neuropsychological assessment, utilizing standardized tests of cognitive and emotional functioning, makes an important contribution to the clinical identification of the dementia syndrome and the differentiation of various dementia types.

Brief mental status questionnaires can provide a quick and valid documentation of the presence of dementia. However, such questionnaires generally are not sufficiently sensitive to detect very mild dementia, particularly in persons with high premorbid intellectual functioning. This limitation in sensitivity reflects the fact that these questionnaires are composed of relatively easy questions and memory items. In addition, they lack the specificity to assist in differential diagnosis of dementia types. In comparison, standardized neuropsychological tests typically contain a range of task difficulty, so that test scores approximate a normal distribution when administered to individuals in the general population. This can provide for greater sensitivity to mild or subtle cognitive deficits than what is possible through the use of mental status questionnaires, for which normative performance distributions are markedly skewed due to most individuals achieving near-perfect scores.

Appropriate neuropsychological tests thus may reveal subtle and circumscribed cognitive impairments in patients who show no evidence of cognitive deficit on commonly employed mental status questionnaires. The ability of neuropsychological test batteries to examine the pattern of performance across different, reliably measured domains of cognitive functioning may be particularly important in assessing persons with high premorbid intellectual functioning. This is due to the fact that the different dementia types do not manifest with equivalent impairment across all cognitive functions. Thus, performance on those cognitive tests that are likely to be affected can be compared to those that are likely to remain intact as an aid in improving detection of relatively circumscribed cognitive decline.

In selecting, administering, and interpreting neuropsychological tests, several factors need to be considered. First, specific tests should be selected on the basis of adequate standardization, including demonstrated reliability and normative data appropriate to the age, educational background, and other demographic characteristics of the person being examined. In addition, the tests should have demonstrated sensitivity and specificity for the diagnostic possibilities to be differentiated. Fortunately, there is a growing empirical literature that allows for a comparison of the expected test performance of persons with differing dementia types. In addition to test standardization, sensitivity, and specificity, the impact of various patient characteristics must be considered. Age-related sensory acuity changes and response slowing can influence test performance, as can the physical limitations of such prevalent illnesses as arthritis.

In addition to a diagnostic role, neuropsychological assessment provides a foundation for the accurate provision of information to patients, family members, and health care providers concerning specific strengths and deficits. Accurate information can reduce ambiguity and anxiety (for both patients and their caregivers), and the identification of relatively intact areas of functioning facilitates the maximizing of patient independence. Identification of intact functioning helps in developing plans for sharing daily responsibilities between the patient and others in his or her environment, directing caregivers to areas in which the patient will require additional supervision or assistance. Early identification of dementia and accurate feedback to the patient and family members allows time for them to make future plans (e.g., disposition of estate, medical and long-term care wishes) while the patient is still able to communicate his or her wishes. Neuropsychological tests are also a critical component in the assessment of treatment effects or disease progression, and they provide guidance for treatment and management of cognitive and behavior problems. Tracking of disease progression, through periodic reexamination, is important for guiding caregivers and adjusting the goals of clinical management. Research has also shown that feedback to patients, based on neuropsychological test performance, results in the improved utilization of coping strategies in persons with preserved awareness of their cognitive deficits.

Evaluation of behavior problems, utilizing standardized and validated informant questionnaire and behavioral observation instruments, can be particularly helpful in efforts to assist the caregivers of dementia patients. Apathy, agitation, depression, delusions, and diurnal rhythm disturbance (e.g., wandering and agitation at night and somnolence during the day) are common in persons with AD and other dementias. These behavior problems are associated with increased caregiver distress, higher rate of nursing home placement, and more rapid disease progression. Once identified and accurately described by careful assessment, family members and other caregivers can be instructed in approaches to minimizing the occurrence and frequency of these behavior problems.

VIII. TREATMENT AND CLINICAL MANAGEMENT OF DEMENTIA

Pharmacological treatment options for the dementias presently are limited, although numerous experimental treatments are being evaluated. The one well-validated approach to symptomatic treatment of AD is based upon the documented deficit in acetylcholine neurotransmitter levels, due to the loss of cholinergic projecting neurons within the nucleus basalis of Meynert. It has been shown that this deficit can be partially compensated for by interfering with the action of that enzyme (cholinesterase), which breaks down acetylcholine after it enters the synaptic junction, allowing the constituent molecules to be taken back into the presynaptic neuron to synthesize additional acetylcholine. There are four such cholinesterase inhibitors that have been approved by the U.S. Food and Drug Administration: Tacrine, Donepezil, Rivastigmine, and Galantamine. These drugs have all been shown to result in some temporary improvement of function in at least some AD patients. However, none of these drugs interrupts the progression of the illness, and the search continues for treatments that can alter the fundamental neuropathological processes of AD. Vitamin E (α-tocopherol) has been shown to delay the time to institutionalization and the loss of ability in common activities of daily living in moderately severe AD patients; thus, it is often prescribed along with cholinesterase inhibitors.

Some of the behavioral problems of dementia (e.g., aggression) may be treated with antipsychotic drugs (e.g., Risperidone, Haloperidol). However, caution must be exercised because those with DLB may be excessively sensitive to such neuroleptic drugs, and several deaths have been reported within weeks of starting such drugs in these patients. Antidepressant drugs (e.g., tricyclics, monoamine oxidase inhibitors, selective serotonin re-uptake inhibitors) may also be useful in the treatment of depression in persons with dementia.

In addition to pharmacological treatment, behavior management strategies can assist in minimizing the consequences of cognitive deficits and managing the behavior problems of dementia. Memory aids and household memory cues (e.g., reminders posted on the refrigerator or above the toilet) can partially compensate for memory deficits. There are also interventions available to reduce behavioral problems in dementia. Small-scale empirical studies of various behavior management procedures have shown some efficacy in reducing select behavior problems (e.g., aggressiveness, agitation, incontinence). A larger scale study has documented the effectiveness of a behavioral therapy taught to caregivers in reducing coexistent depression in AD. Other research has shown that intensive, long-term education and support services for caregivers can delay the time to nursing home placement for AD patients. Even short-term programs that educate family caregivers about AD may improve caregiver morale and satisfaction. Finally, education about AD and other dementias for the staff of nursing homes and other long-term care facilities may help to reduce the use of unnecessary antipsychotic medications.

Thus, although there is no available treatment capable of reversing or arresting the progression of dementia, both symptomatic treatment and interventions to reduce behavior problems are available. The vigor with which experimental treatments are being evaluated creates hope for a future in which the dementias can be more effectively treated, and someday perhaps even cured.

See Also the Following Articles

AGING BRAIN • AGNOSIA • ALZHEIMER'S DISEASE, NEUROPSYCHOLOGY OF • APHASIA • CEREBRAL WHITE MATTER DISORDERS • COGNITIVE REHABILITATION • DEPRESSION • HIV INFECTION, NEUROCOGNITIVE COMPLICATIONS OF • LANGUAGE, NEURAL BASIS OF • NEUROPSYCHOLOGICAL ASSESSMENT • PARKINSON'S DISEASE • PICK'S DISEASE AND FRONTOTEMPORAL DEMENTIA

Suggested Reading

Bondi, M. W., Salmon, D. P., and Kaszniak, A. W. (1996). The neuropsychology of dementia. In *Neuropsychological Assessment of Neuropsychiatric Disorders* (I. Grant and K. H. Adams, Eds.), 2nd ed., pp. 164–199. Oxford University Press, New York.

Christensen, H., Griffiths, K., Mackinnon, A., and Jacomb, P. (1997). A quantitative review of cognitive deficits in depression and Alzheimer-type dementia. *J. Int. Neuropsychol. Soc.* **3**, 631–651.

Cummings, J. L., and Benson, D. F. (1992). *Dementia: A Clinical Approach*, 2nd ed. Butterworth-Heinemann, Boston.

Doody, R. S., Stevens, J. C., Beck, C., Dubinsky, R. M., Kaye, J. A., Gwyther, L., Mohs, R. C., Thal, L. J., Whitehouse, P. J., DeKosky, S. T., and Cummings, J. L. (2001). Practice parameter: Management of dementia (an evidence-based review). *Neurology* **56**, 1154–1166.

Duke, L. M., and Kaszniak, A. W. (2000). Executive control functions in degenerative dementias: A comparative review. *Neuropsychol. Rev.* **10**, 75–99.

Green, J. (2000). *Neuropsychological Evaluation of the Older Adult: A Clinician's Guidebook*. Academic Press, San Diego, CA.

Kaszniak, A. W. (1996). Techniques and instruments for assessment of the elderly. In *A guide to Psychotherapy and Aging* (S. H. Zarit and B. G. Knight, Eds.), pp. 163–219. American Psychological Association, Washington, DC.

Khachaturian, Z. S., and Radebaugh, T. S. (Eds.). (1996). *Alzheimer's Disease: Cause(s), Diagnosis, Treatment, and Care.* CRC Press, Boca Raton, LA.

Knopman, D. S., DeKosky, S. T., Cummings, J. L., Chui, H., Corey-Bloom, J., Relkin, N., Small, G. W., Miller, B., and Stevens, J. C. (2001). Practice parameter: Diagnosis of dementia (an evidence-based review). *Neurology* **56**, 1143–1153.

Nussbaum, P. D. (Ed.). (1997). *Handbook of Neuropsychology and Aging*. Plenum, New York.

O'Brien, J., Ames, D., and Burns, A. (Eds.). (2000). *Dementia*, 2nd ed. Arnold, London.

Petersen, R. C., Stevens, J. C., Ganguli, M., Tangalos, E. G., Cummings, J. L., and DeKosky, S. T. (2001). Practice parameter early detection of dementia: Mild cognitive impairment (an evidence-based review). *Neurology* **56**, 1133–1142.

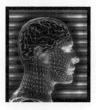

Depression

ESTEBAN V. CARDEMIL

Brown University School of Medicine and Rhode Island Hospital

GLOSSARY

anhedonia One of the core symptoms of depression; defined as the loss of interest in, and inability to derive pleasure from, activities that were previously considered interesting and pleasurable.

catecholamine A group of neurotransmitters that includes norepinephrine, epinephrine, and dopamine.

concordance rates The proportion of twins in a sample that both possess the disorder of interest.

heritability The proportion of the variance of a disorder in the population that is due to genetic factors.

indoleamines A group of neurotransmitters that includes serotonin and histamine.

lifetime prevalence The proportion of individuals in an epidemiological sample that have ever experienced a disorder at some point in their lives.

Depression is a psychiatric disorder with emotional, cognitive, physiological, and behavioral symptoms. This article presents both biological and psychological theories and treatments of depression.

I. SYMPTOMS OF DEPRESSION

Depression is a disorder characterized by emotional, cognitive, physiological, and behavioral symptoms.

The primary emotional symptom is a profound sense of sadness and low mood. Irritability, frustration, and anger often accompany this low mood. Cognitive symptoms include a sense of hopelessness and helplessness, worthlessness, and guilt. Depressed individuals often have difficulty concentrating or making simple decisions. Physiological symptoms include changes in appetite and sleep, fatigue, and concerns about aches and pains. Diminished sexual interest is also commonly reported in depressed individuals. Behavioral symptoms include decreased activity, often the result of anhedonia, which is the loss of interest in and an inability to derive pleasure from activities that previously were interesting and pleasurable.

Depression tends to be classified into two major categories: major depressive disorder and dysthymic disorder. The principal differences between major depressive disorder and dysthymic disorder are severity and chronicity. Major depressive disorder is more severe and characterized by discrete major depressive episodes, whereas dysthymic disorder is less severe and characterized by a more chronic course. These disorders are not mutually exclusive; a major depressive episode superimposed on a chronic course of dysthymic disorder is conceptualized as double depression.

The American Psychiatric Association, in its *Diagnostic and Statistical Manual of Mental Disorders (DSM-IV)*, defined the symptomatic criteria for a major depressive episode (Table I). Once the criteria for a major depressive episode have been met, and the appropriate diagnostic rule-outs have been made (e.g., other psychiatric disorder and general medical condition causing the depressive episode), a diagnosis of major depressive disorder can be made.

Table I

DSM-IV **Criteria of a Major Depressive Episode**

Five or more of the following symptoms must be present during the same 2-week period and represent a change from previous functioning. At least one of the symptoms must be either depressed mood or loss of interest or pleasure.

1. Depressed mood most of the day, nearly every day

2. Markedly diminished interest or pleasure in all, or almost all, activities most of the day, nearly every day (anhedonia)

3. Significant weight loss when not dieting or weight gain (e.g., a change of more than 5% of body weight in 1 month) or decrease or increase in appetite nearly every day

4. Insomnia or hypersomnia nearly every day

5. Psychomotor agitation or retardation nearly every day (noticeable by others)

6. Fatigue or loss of energy nearly every day

7. Feelings of worthlessness or retardation nearly every day (noticeable by others)

8. Diminished ability to think or concentration, or indecisiveness, nearly every day

9. Recurrent thoughts of death (not just fear of dying), recurrent suicidal ideation without a specific plan, or a suicide attempt, or a specific plan for committing suicide

A. Subtypes of Depression

DSM-IV distinguishes among several subtypes of depression in order to capture some of the different patterns of depressive symptoms with which individuals present. Melancholic depression is characterized by a loss of interest or pleasure in all, or almost all, activities. Individuals with melancholic depression do not show reactivity to normally pleasurable stimuli and do not show even temporary improvements in mood following good events. In addition, at least three of the following symptoms are present: the sensation that depression is worse in the morning than in the evening, significant weight loss or loss of appetite, insomnia characterized by early morning awakening, psychomotor agitation, and excessive or inappropriate guilt.

In contrast, individuals with atypical depression show mood changes in response to actual life events. Their mood might temporarily brighten with the development of good news, for example. In addition, individuals also demonstrate two or more of the following symptoms: significant weight gain or appetite increase, hypersomnia, feelings of heaviness in the limbs, and a long-standing pattern of sensitivity to interpersonal rejection.

Individuals who display a characteristic onset and remission of depressive episodes at specific times of the year are given the specifier "with seasonal pattern." Most cases of depression with seasonal pattern occur in the winter months and tend to be found in locations where winter seasons are long and accompanied by days with short exposure to sun. The symptoms include increased fatigue, hypersomnia, weight gain, and a craving for carbohydrates.

Women who develop a major depressive episode within 4 weeks of giving birth are given the specifier "with postpartum onset." The symptoms do not seem to differ from nonpostpartum depressive episodes but may be more fluctuating in course. Often, the focus of the depression is related to the newborn and can be accompanied by obsessional thoughts of harming the child, suicidal ideation, and psychomotor agitation. Researchers currently disagree about the extent to which depression with postpartum onset is actually distinctive enough to warrant a separate category.

II. EPIDEMIOLOGY OF DEPRESSION

Up to 17% of the general population in the United States will meet criteria for a major depressive episode at some time. The lifetime prevalence for dysthymia is approximately 6%, and that of depression with a seasonal pattern is approximately 0.4%. Also, many more people will have some experience with lower, subclinical levels of depressive symptoms. Children and adolescents also experience depression and its associated symptoms: Estimates of the number of children who will experience a depressive episode by the end of high school range as high as 20%.

The annual economic consequences of depression in the United States have been estimated at $44 billion (e.g., medical expenses and lost work hours). In addition to the financial burdens to society associated with depression, there are tremendous psychological and emotional consequences of depression. Almost 75% of individuals who reported a lifetime history of depression also reported experience with one or more other psychiatric disorders, including anxiety disorders (58%) and substance use disorders (39%). Up to 15% of individuals with severe major depressive disorder will attempt to commit suicide.

A. Demographic Risk Factors for Depression

The prevalence rates of depression are approximately twice as high in women as in men. At some point during their lives, as many as 20% of women will experience a major depressive episode. Prevalence rates of depression range from 0.4 to 2.5% in children and are between 0.4 and 8.3% in adolescents. Epidemiological studies in the United States have consistently found lower lifetime prevalence rates of major depression among African Americans than among Caucasians and similar lifetime prevalence rates between Latinos and Caucasians. Although comparable rates of depression have been found in many non-Western cultures, there is evidence that depression may be more prevalent in Western societies. In particular, it appears that the increased prevalence of depression in women may be more characteristic of Western cultures.

Other demographic risk factors that have been consistently associated with depression include a family history of depression, low socioeconomic status, and specific stressful life events (including assaults and robberies, serious marital problems, divorce, loss of employment, serious illness, and significant financial problems). Research on the role of stressful life events has also found that specific buffers may protect against the development of depression. Some of the buffers include the existence of supportive relationships, the presence of three or fewer children, employment, self-identification with a religion, and the possession of clear roles in life.

B. Course of Depression

Major depression can begin at almost any age, but the average age of onset is in the mid-20s, although data are emerging that suggest that the average age of onset is steadily dropping. Once they begin, depressive symptoms can develop over the course of days or weeks. An untreated depressive episode usually lasts between 6 and 10 months and is often followed by a

return to normal functioning with the complete absence of symptoms. However, in a significant minority of cases (20–30%), depression either does not abate at all or significant symptoms persist that continue to interfere with normal functioning. After 2 years, approximately 20% of patients will continue to meet criteria for depression, 12% will meet criteria at 5 years, and 7% will continue to meet criteria 10 years after the onset of the episode. Currently, there are few diagnostic predictors that can distinguish among individuals who return to functioning and those who experience a more chronic course of depression.

Depression is also a recurring disorder: Recent estimates have found that approximately 50–85% of individuals who meet criteria for a depressive episode will experience multiple episodes, and between 25 and 40% of patients will have a second depressive episode within 2 years of their first. Moreover, the risk for relapse appears to increase as time goes on; in some studies the rate increases to 60% and higher after 5 years. Given this high risk for relapse, depression is now more commonly understood as a recurrent and potentially lifelong disorder.

III. BIOLOGICAL THEORIES OF DEPRESSION

Depression can be caused by specific biological conditions, including strokes, nutritional deficiencies, and infections. In these cases, the diagnosis mood disorder due to a general medical condition is given. Depression can also be the result of alcohol or substance abuse, often associated with the symptoms of withdrawal and intoxication. In these cases, the diagnosis substance-induced mood disorder is appropriate. Apart from these two categories, however, the role of biological causes in the development of depression is less definitive. Researchers view the role of biology as contributing one important element to the development of depression.

A. Genetic Theories

To date, researchers have been unable to identify specific genes, acting singly or in combination, that account for the expression of depression. As such, the evidence that has supported the proposition that depression is a heritable disorder comes from family studies, twin studies, and adoption studies. Unfortunately, this research has been unable to definitively separate the respective contribution of genetics and environment.

For example, depression is up to three times more common in first-degree biological relatives of persons with the disorder than among the general population, and it is almost twice as common in first-degree biological relatives of persons with bipolar disorder. Moreover, children of parents with other psychiatric disorders, including anxiety and substance use disorders, are more than twice as likely to develop depression than are children of parents without psychiatric disorders. However, this support for a genetic contribution to depression is confounded with the increased likelihood of shared environment of first-degree biological relatives.

Twin studies have found mixed evidence for heritability in depression. Concordance rates of depression in identical twins tend to be up to twice as high as the concordance rates in fraternal twins, suggesting a genetic component. However, with heritability estimates only reaching 50%, the genetic contribution must also be considered in the context of environmental factors. Adoption studies have yielded similarly equivocal findings with respect to the heritability of depression. One large-scale study reported that biological relatives of individuals with depression have up to eight times the risk of adoptive relatives, but two other studies did not replicate these findings.

Taken together, the evidence suggests that genetic factors play a contributory role in the etiology of depression, but nowhere near as primary a role as in some other psychiatric disorders (e.g., bipolar disorder and schizophrenia).

B. Neuroanatomical Theories

Early neuroanatomical conceptualizations of depression focused on the limbic system, given its predominant role in normal mood and affect regulation. These early conceptualizations have been bolstered by recent functional imaging studies, which are conducted while depressed patients perform a variety of cognitive tasks. The functional imaging research has generally found abnormal patterns of limbic activity in depressed patients when compared to normal controls, although no coherent pattern has emerged across studies. For instance, some research has noted decreased activation in the midcingulate gyrus; other studies have found reduced activity in the inferior frontal gyrus. Researchers have also reported decreased cerebral blood flow in brain structures other than the limbic system,

including the frontal and prefrontal lobes, the cerebrum, and the cerebellum. This hypometabolism is often in direct proportion to the severity of the depressive symptoms.

Given both the correlational nature of this neuroanatomical research and the fact that it is still in its relative infancy, researchers have been unable to determine the extent to which these neuroanatomical dysfunctions are the result or the cause of depression. One recent study found intriguing similarities between depressed and remitted (previously depressed) patients in that both groups displayed decreased prefrontal and limbic activation compared with normal controls. This finding raises the possibility that a neuroanatomical dysregulation may produce a vulnerability to depression and/or relapse.

Taken as a whole, neuroanatomical theories of depression have yet to produce reliable and specific insights into the causes and treatment of depression. However, given the power of functional imaging research, it is likely only a matter of time before researchers begin to clarify the neuroanatomical substrates of depression.

C. Neurotransmitter Theories

Most of the biological research on depression has focused on the role of dysregulation of neurotransmitters and has progressed in step with the development of antidepressant medications that affect these neurotransmitters. The two primary classes of neurotransmitters that have been implicated in depression are the catecholamines (primarily norepinephrine) and the indoleamines (primarily serotonin).

The observation that medications with depressive side effects depleted norepinephrine (NE) in the brain led researchers to hypothesize that catecholamines played a primary role in depression. Reserpine, a medication prescribed for hypertension in the 1950s, was found to produce depression in a significant minority of cases and subsequently found to reduce NE levels in the brain. Moreover, medications that increased the availability of NE, including amphetamines, produced antidepressant effects. These discoveries led to the catecholamine theory of depression, which posits that deficits in NE are the cause of depression. This theory led to the development of antidepressant medications that increased the availability of NE in the brain: the tricyclic antidepressants (TCAs) and the monoamine oxidase inhibitors (MAOIs).

Researchers soon noted that in addition to affecting NE, both TCAs and MAOIs appeared to also increase the availability of serotonin (5-HT) in the brain. This discovery led to the indoleamine theory of depression, which hypothesized that deficits in 5-HT were the root cause of depression. As a result, researchers soon developed a class of drugs that primarily increased the availability of 5-HT: the selective serotonin reuptake inhibitors (SSRIs). More than 14 subtypes of 5-HT receptors have been subsequently identified, and evidence is emerging that has linked 5-HT_{1A} and 5-HT_2 receptors with mood. Given that the definition of depression includes a combination of cognitive, physiological, and behavioral symptoms, future research is likely to identify more 5-HT receptor subtypes that play a significant role in depression.

Neither the catecholamine nor the indoleamine theories of depression account for some important clinical observations, however. For example, the biochemical action of antidepressant medication (in particular the TCAs) occurs quickly, whereas the clinical response takes several weeks to develop. That is, the increased availability of both NE and 5-HT precedes the amelioration of depressive symptoms by several weeks. In addition, TCAs vary in their ability to increase the availability of NE and 5-HT, and SSRIs vary in the extent to which they increase the availability of 5-HT, but all antidepressants have generally the same effectiveness. These observations, among others, have led researchers to doubt that simple deficits in either NE or 5-HT can explain the development of depressive symptoms. Instead, researchers are considering more complicated models that involve the dysregulation of one or more neurotransmitter systems and the various interactions across neurotransmitter systems to explain the development of depression.

D. Neuroendocrine Theories

Approximately 40–60% of depressed individuals produce and secrete excessive amounts of cortisol, primarily during the afternoon and evening. In these patients, cortisol secretion returns to normal levels after the depressive episode remits. This excessive cortisol is thought to be due to the overproduction by the hypothalamus of corticotropin-releasing hormone (CTRH), a compound that is stimulated by norepinephrine and acetylcholine, leading some to believe that CTRH and the noradrenergic system may be interconnected. Administration of dexamethasone, a chemical that temporarily suppresses the production of cortisol in nondepressed adults, was at one point believed to be a useful tool in the diagnosis of depression since many depressed individuals did not demonstrate this cortisol suppression. Recent evidence has indicated that many nondepressed psychiatric patients also fail to display a response to the dexamethasone suppression test, thus limiting its utility in the diagnosis of depression.

IV. PSYCHOLOGICAL THEORIES OF DEPRESSION

Despite the prominent role of biological theories of depression, psychological theories continue to play a significant role in understanding depression. There exist many different psychological approaches to understanding depression that can be considered to emerge from three primary theoretical orientations. Psychoanalytic and psychodynamic theories postulate that depression is the result of unconscious developmental processes that lead to anger being turned inwards. Behavioral theories maintain that depression is the result of excessive behaviors and activities that contribute to low mood. Cognitive theories of depression posit that maladaptive thinking puts individuals at greater risk for developing a depressive episode when faced with negative life events.

A. Psychoanalytic and Psychodynamic Theories

Sigmund Freud and his followers developed the first psychological theories of depression. According to Freud, depression (or melancholia) was comparable to normal grief following the loss of a loved one. Depression, however, would occur in certain people who experienced a loss or disappointment at an early age. These individuals would actually feel rage at the lost loved object, but since part of their personality had become identified with this lost loved object, the individuals would then direct this rage at the self. Often, this redirected self-hatred was safer than rage at the lost loved object. Thus, according to the psychoanalytic model, depression is actually anger turned inwards toward the self. This "anger turned inwards" is the source of low self-esteem, feelings of guilt and worthlessness, and sense of deserving punishment, and it may ultimately lead to suicide.

The psychoanalytic model was not originally developed to explain the development of discrete psychological disorders. Rather, it was developed as a comprehensive model of human personality and development. As such, until recently its relationship to the development of depression was not the subject of much empirical investigation; therefore, few data exist to support its perspective.

Modern psychodynamic theories of depression, while tied to the original psychoanalytic theories, tend to emphasize the role of maladaptive social relationships in the development of depression. In general, these maladaptive relationships mirror significant early childhood relationships. Some theorists, including John Bowlby and Harry Stack Sullivan, have argued that the quality of young children's attachments to their mothers will influence the development of future relationships. Some empirical evidence exists, including some animal data, to support the role of maladaptive relationships in depression. The extent to which these early maladaptive relationships play a primary causal role is disputed, however.

B. Behavioral Theories

Behavioral theories of depression focus on the links between behaviors and mood. These dysfunctional connections lead to an excess of behaviors and activities that produce depressed mood and a deficit in behaviors and activities that produce positive mood. This disconnect between behavior and positive mood can occur because of insufficient engagement in pleasurable activities (e.g., living in an impoverished environment) and/or deficiencies in interpersonal skills (e.g., excessive shyness). Depressed individuals thus find themselves engaging in fewer activities and relationships that promote positive mood. This withdrawal and avoidance of pleasurable activities results in increased depressed mood, which then contributes to a cycle of continued lack of engagement and skill deficits.

C. Cognitive Theories

Cognitive theories of depression emphasize the role of accessible cognitive processes in the development and maintenance of depression. Maladaptive cognitions contribute to the etiology of depression by making individuals susceptible to depression in the face of significant negative life events. Moreover, these maladaptive cognitions and behaviors play a critical role in the maintenance of the depressive state by preventing depressed individuals from considering any alternatives to the pervasive hopelessness that dominates their thinking.

Two influential cognitive theories of depression are Aaron T. Beck's negative cognitive triad and Martin E. P. Seligman's learned helplessness theory.

1. Beck's Negative Cognitive Triad

In his 1967 book, *Depression: Causes and Treatments*, Beck first proposed that depression was the result of the activation of overly negative views (or schemas) of oneself, one's world, and one's future. A negative view of oneself would produce low self-esteem, a negative view of the world could produce helplessness, and a negative view of the future would lead to hopelessness. These depressive schemas begin to develop in childhood as individuals begin to form beliefs about their place in the world. They are maintained and reinforced through a system of cognitive distortions, whereby individuals lend excessive credence to evidence that supports their negative beliefs and selectively ignore evidence that contradicts these beliefs.

Extensive research supports the presence of negative schemas and cognitive distortions in depressed individuals. The extent to which these negative cognitions precede and cause the development of depression is less clear. Some researchers argue that negative cognitions should be considered symptoms of depression rather than causes.

2. Seligman's Learned Helplessness Model

The learned helplessness model posits that individuals become depressed and helpless if they experienced a disconnect between their behavior and life outcomes. This experience with uncontrollable outcomes leads to expected noncontingencies between future responses and outcomes. This theoretical model evolved from animal research in which dogs that were exposed to inescapable shock demonstrated helplessness deficits when they were later exposed to escapable shock. This learned helplessness, which included motivational and emotional symptoms, appeared to mimic many of the motivational, emotional, and cognitive deficits found in individuals experiencing depression.

In 1978, Lyn Abramson, Martin Seligman, and John Teasdale reformulated the original learned helplessness model because the theory was unable to explain why not everyone who was exposed to uncontrollable negative life events would become helpless and depressed. The reformulated learned helplessness model proposed that individuals have habitual ways of explaining the stressors that occur in their lives. This tendency to explain stressors in a characteristic manner was termed attributional or explanatory style. There are three dimensions along which explanatory style can be measured: internality, stability, and globality. Internality refers to the extent to which the cause of an event is due to something about the individual or something outside of the individual (e.g., other people or luck). Stability refers to the extent to which the cause of the event will remain stable over time or is more transient in nature. Globality refers to the extent to which the cause of the event affects many different life domains or those most immediately related to the stressor. A pessimistic explanatory style is the tendency to explain negative life events with internal, stable, and global causes, and according to the reformulated learned helplessness model it puts individuals at risk for developing depression when exposed to uncontrollable life events.

Considerable evidence exists to support the role of a pessimistic explanatory style in depression, both in children and in adults. In particular, the role of a pessimistic explanatory style as a psychological risk factor for depression in the face of negative life events has received much support.

V. BIOLOGICAL TREATMENTS FOR DEPRESSION

The primary forms of biological treatments for depression are the antidepressant medications. Electroconvulsive therapy (ECT) is generally used with only severely depressed individuals. Alternative biological treatments (e.g., herbal supplements) are also discussed.

A. Antidepressant Medication

Given the emphasis on neurotransmitter theories of depression, the primary biological treatments of depression are antidepressant medications, all of which appear to effectively treat depression in approximately 60–70% of individuals. Antidepressants typically improve mood, energy, and sleep and reduce anhedonia, and they generally accomplish these changes by increasing the availability to the brain of norepinephrine and serotonin. More recent antidepressants also increase dopamine levels in the brain. Because research has not been able to definitively identify the relationship between antidepressant chemical structure and function, antidepressants tend to be classified by their action on neurotransmitters. As such, antidepressants can be categorized into three primary classes: those that inhibit the reuptake of neurotransmitter, those that inhibit the degradation of neurotransmitter, and those that act at specific receptor sites to induce greater production of neurotransmitter (Table II).

1. Reuptake Inhibitors

There exist four types of reuptake inhibitors. The first antidepressants to be identified were the tricyclic antidepressants that inhibited the reuptake of both serotonin and norepinephrine (serotonin–norepinephrine reuptake inhibitors). A second generation of tricyclic antidepressants was developed that predominately inhibited the reuptake of norepinephrine (selective norepinephrine reuptake inhibitors). By interfering with the normal reuptake process by which the synapse cleanses itself of excess neurotransmitter, the tricyclic antidepressants increased the availability of norepinephrine and serotonin in the synapse. Both sets of tricyclic antidepressants interact with other neurotransmitter system receptor sites, including histamine, acetylcholine, and epinephrine, producing a wide range of unwanted side effects (e.g., dry mouth, dizziness, blurred vision, constipation, orthostatic hypotension, and cardiovascular effects). In addition, given tricyclics' high solubility in lipid tissue, and subsequent difficult extraction in emergency, risk of death from overdose remains a serious concern.

The effort to develop effective antidepressants that produced fewer and less serious side effects than the tricyclics led researchers to those that selectively inhibit the reuptake of serotonin (e.g., the SSRIs). SSRIs are well tolerated, provide safety from overdose, and do not appear to increase the risk for seizures. The most common side effects associated with SSRIs include some anxiety and agitation, nausea, sleep disruption, sexual dysfunction, gastrointestinal cramps, diarrhea, and headache. SSRIs are currently the most commonly prescribed antidepressant medication.

Recently, researchers have developed several new classes of antidepressants. Venlafaxine is a serotonin–norepinephrine reuptake inhibitor, similar to the first generation of tricyclic antidepressants, but it does not affect the other neurotransmitter systems and thus has significantly fewer side effects. Buproprion is a novel antidepressant that inhibits the reuptake of norepinephrine and dopamine while having no effect on

Table II
Antidepressant Medications

Class	Mechanism of action	Example drugs	Common side effects
Tricyclic antidepressants I	Block reuptake of both norepinephrine and serotonin	Amitryptaline (Elavil), doxepin (Sinequan), imipramine (Tofranil)	Dry mouth, dizziness, blurred vision, constipation, orthostatic
Tricyclic antidepressants II	Selectively block reuptake of norepinephrine	Desipramine (Norpramin), nortryptaline (Pamelor), protriptyline (Vivactil)	Hypotension and cardiovascular effects
Monoamine oxidase inhibitors	Inhibit degradation of norepinephrine, serotonin, and dopamine	Phenelzine (Nardil), tranylcypromine (Parnate)	Dizziness, sleep disturbances, sedation, fatigue, general weakness, hyperreflexia, dry mouth, and gastrointestinal disturbances; important to avoid food rich in tyramine to avoid hypertensive crises or seizures
Selective serotonin reuptake inhibitors	Block reuptake of serotonin by interfering with the serotonin transport system	Citaprolam (Celexa), fluoxetine (Prozac), fluvoxamine (Luvox), paroxetine (Paxil), sertraline (Zolaft)	Some anxiety and agitation, nausea, sleep disruption, sexual dysfunction, GI cramps, diarrhea, headache
Non-tricyclic serotonin–norepinephrine reuptake inhibitor	Block reuptake of serotonin and norepinephrine	Venlafaxine (Effexor)	Nausea, dizziness, drowsiness, possible sexual dysfunction; at high doses, risk for hypertension, sweating, and tremors
Norepinephrine–dopamine reuptake inhibitor	Block reuptake of norepinephrine and some dopamine	Buproprion (Wellbutrin)	Dry mouth, dizziness, constipation, nausea/vomiting, blurred vision, agitation, seizure risk at high doses (0.4%)
Serotonin antagonist and reuptake inhibitors	Block 5-HT2a receptor and block reuptake of serotonin	Trazodone (Desyrel), nefazodone (Serzone)	Dry mouth, drowsiness, dizziness or lightheadedness, nausea/vomiting, constipation, blurred vision, priapism (1 in 15,000) with Trazodone
Norepinephrine antagonist and serotonin antagonist	Block α_2-adrenoreceptor and 5-HT_2 and 5-HT_3 receptors which leads to increased norepinephrine and specific serotonin production	Mirtazapine (Remeron)	Drowsiness, increased appetite, weight gain

serotonin. Our current understanding of the role of dopamine in depression is poor.

2. Monoamine Oxidase Inhibitors

The antidepressants that inhibit the degradation of neurotransmitter act by interfering with the enzyme monoamine oxidase, which destroys excess norepinephrine, serotonin, and dopamine in the synapse and the presynaptic terminal. Like the tricyclics, MAOIs have unpleasant side effects, including dizziness, sleep disturbances, sedation, fatigue, general weakness, hyperreflexia, dry mouth, and gastrointestinal disturbances. More serious is the fact that MAOIs can interact with tyramine (a protein building block for norepinephrine that is found in many common foods) and produce lethal hypertension. As such, individuals taking MAOIs must adhere to a tyramine-free diet, avoiding such foods as cheese, smoked meats, wine and beer, and yeast.

3. Serotonin and Norepinephrine Antagonists

Mirtazapine (Remeron) is a novel antidepressant that appears to produce antidepressant effects by blocking both the α_2-adrenoreceptor and two postsynaptic serotonin receptors, 5-HT2 and 5-HT3, which increases norepinephrine activity and specific serotonin activity in the brain. Common side effects of mirtazapine include drowsiness, increased appetite, and weight gain.

Currently, practice guidelines recommend SSRIs and some of the newer antidepressants (e.g., buprorion, nefazodone, and venlafaxine) as first choice antidepressants given their relatively modest side effect profile. For nonresponders to the first choice antidepressant, current guidelines suggest consideration of tricyclic antidepressants followed by MAOIs.

B. Electroconvulsive Treatment

ECT is the second form of biological treatment for depression and is currently used predominately with individuals experiencing severe and/or intractable depression that has not responded to antidepressant medications and psychotherapy. ECT involves the induction of a general seizure via the application of a brief electrical stimulus through electrodes that are placed on the scalp. Individuals are placed under general anesthesia and given a muscle relaxant in order to prevent discomfort and injury resulting from the seizure.

It is the seizure that is believed to produce the antidepressant effect, although the mechanism of action remains unclear. Animal studies suggest that ECT exerts its effects via the enhancement of norepinephrine and serotonin systems, paralleling the effects of antidepressant medications. In addition, ECT appears to affect the dopaminergic, cholinergic, GABA, and opioid systems.

Considerable research has supported the short-term efficacy of ECT in alleviating depressive symptoms, particularly those that are accompanied by psychotic symptoms: ECT produces significant improvement in approximately 80–90% of individuals with severe depression. Research has shown that both the dosage of the electrical current and the placement of the electrodes (unilateral or bilateral) are related to the alleviation of depressive symptoms and the production of unwanted side effects (mostly short-term memory loss and other cognitive impairments, including mild disorientation). Bilateral stimulation produces greater and more rapid improvement from depressive symptoms than does unilateral stimulation; however, bilateral stimulation also produces greater short-term disorientation and retrograde amnesia. High-dose unilateral stimulation, while producing fewer side effects than bilateral stimulation, appears to improve depressive symptoms more than low-dose unilateral stimulation, although not to the extent of bilateral stimulation.

C. Alternative Treatments

Little research exists to support the efficacy or mechanism of action of alternative biological treatments, generally in the form of herbal supplements. For example, St. John's Wort, a popular herbal supplement, appears to inhibit the reuptake of serotonin, norepinephrine, and dopamine. Several studies have shown it to be relatively effective in alleviating mild to moderate depression; however, given the significant methodological flaws present in these studies, no general consensus currently exists regarding the effectiveness of this or any other particular supplement.

D. Limitations of Biological Treatments

Although considerable evidence exists demonstrating the effectiveness of antidepressant medication in the alleviation of depressive symptoms, antidepressant medications are not a panacea. Approximately 30–40% of individuals with depression will not respond to antidepressants. In addition, no empirical data exist to guide practitioners in the selection of specific antidepressants, or even classes of antidepressants, over another. Practice guidelines suggest that failure to respond to an antidepressant in one class will likely predict failure to respond to other antidepressants of the same class, but no empirical data exist to conclusively support this proposition.

Furthermore, the relapse rates are very high for individuals who have been treated exclusively with biological treatments. Approximately 40–60% of individuals will relapse if antidepressant medication is discontinued within the first few months of a response. Up to 60% of individuals treated with ECT will relapse in the following year, particularly if they do not continue on antidepressant medication after the ECT regimen. Given the increasingly accepted conception of depression as a chronic, relapsing disorder, practitioners have begun moving toward prescribing biological treatments over many years, often beyond the length of the original depressive episode.

Research on the use of antidepressant medication with children and adolescents remains sparse, and the few well-designed experiments that have been conducted have not shown that antidepressants are more effective than placebo. There also exists little research that has investigated the safety of these medications with pregnant women or women who are breast-feeding.

VI. PSYCHOLOGICAL TREATMENTS FOR DEPRESSION

There currently exist many different psychological treatments with varying levels of empirical support for their efficacy in treating depression in adults and a few that have been evaluated with children and adolescents. Although each has been developed and studied in its pure form, most psychotherapy available in the community incorporates some elements from more than one theoretical orientation.

A. Psychodynamic Psychotherapy

Psychodynamic psychotherapies evolved from psychoanalytic therapies, and as such they were originally designed to assist patients in the modification of their personality. This task occurs via the uncovering and bringing to awareness of unconscious conflicts that interfere with functioning. Recent adaptations of psychodynamic psychotherapies that have focused on depression emphasize more active approaches while continuing to uncover unconscious conflicts. Psychodynamic psychotherapies tend to emphasize the development of a therapeutic alliance that can increase patients' self-efficacy with respect to problem solving. Once the therapeutic alliance is developed, patients are then better able to gain insight into their problems by learning more about their relationship patterns, which then leads to increased potential for change. Some of this insight is developed via an exploration of the therapist–patient relationship and an examination of the ways in which this relationship mirrors the patients' real-world relationships.

When compared with other forms of psychotherapy for adults, psychodynamic psychotherapy tends to perform equivalently. Unfortunately, few studies have successfully compared psychodynamic psychotherapy with placebo conditions; therefore, the extent to which psychodynamic psychotherapy offers benefits that are particular to the psychoanalytic orientation remains in dispute.

B. Interpersonal Therapy

Interpersonal therapy (IPT) attempts to reduce depressive symptoms by focusing on current interpersonal problems. Specifically, IPT examines grief, role conflicts in relationships, role transitions, and social deficits, all in the context of problematic relationships. Depressed individuals are asked to pay close attention to all of their social interactions and social disappointments. By carefully examining their own role, patients become better able to reconstruct (or construct new) relationships more productively.

Empirical support exists for the efficacy of IPT in the treatment of depression in adults, and preliminary evidence suggests that it may be useful with adolescents. Several studies have found that it consistently outperforms control conditions and produces results at least equivalent to those of cognitive therapy and antidepressant medication.

C. Behavior Therapy

The primary goal of most behavior therapies is to increase the amount of pleasurable activity in patients' lives. Patients learn to monitor the fluctuations in their mood over the course of the week. They are taught to note what events produce positive changes in mood and what events bring about negative changes in mood. The therapist and patient then attempt to institute changes in the patient's life that would bring about more positive mood states. In situations in which the patient lacks the skills necessary to bring about changes in behavior, the therapist and the patient work together to enhance these skill deficits. Social skill training, relaxation skills, and assertiveness training are all examples of skill-building exercises in which patients may engage.

Empirical support exists for the effectiveness of behavior therapy in the treatment of depression in adults, although it has not been as extensively evaluated in clinical populations. Several studies have found results equal to those of other forms of psychotherapy, and one study found that behavior therapy produced comparable results to those of the antidepressant amitriptyline.

D. Cognitive Therapy

Cognitive therapy reduces depressive symptoms by addressing the maladaptive and pessimistic thinking in which depressed individuals engage. Working collaboratively, the individual and therapist attempt to identify and then change those elements of a patient's thinking and behavior that are contributing to the depressive symptoms. Once patients learn about the relationships among life events, thinking, and mood, they are taught to recognize the presence of "negative automatic thoughts" and pessimistic thinking that contribute to the maintenance of their depressed mood. These pessimistic thinking styles are examined together by the therapist and patient in order to consider their validity and utility. Patients learn how to generate alternative explanations for events, search for relevant information, and then decide on the most realistic explanation. Often, the most realistic explanation is less hopeless than the original belief and can lead to behavior change. When the most realistic explanation continues to be depressive, the patient and therapist work together to generate realistic solutions to the problems.

Considerable evidence exists to support the efficacy of cognitive therapy in the treatment of depression in both adults and adolescents, and many researchers consider cognitive therapy to be superior to many other forms of therapy for depression. Researchers are currently investigating the extent to which cognitive therapy can produce results equivalent to or better than those produced by antidepressant medication. Long-term data suggest that cognitive therapy is effective in the prevention of relapse, even more effective than that afforded by antidepressant medication.

E. Alternative Models of Therapy

Although different psychological orientations have led to the development of discrete psychological treatments, alternative models of psychotherapy complement these existing theoretical orientations. For example, cognitive and behavioral therapy techniques are often consolidated into an overarching cognitive–behavioral therapy. Moreover, modern cognitive therapy approaches are beginning to focus more on the therapist–patient relationship in ways that were originally developed by psychodynamic psychotherapies.

In addition to developments in individual-based psychotherapy, alternative models of therapy have also effectively expanded this focus to include multiple participants. For example, research suggests that group psychotherapy for depression can be as effective in treating depression as individual psychotherapy, particularly those group therapies that utilize a cognitive or behavioral approach. Family and marital treatments for depression also have considerable support for their effectiveness in treating depression in adults. In general, both group and family-based approaches work within their respective theoretical orientations to enhance the social support of the participants. Group therapy accomplishes this task by providing a novel social support system, and family-based approaches attempt to modify existing social networks.

F. Limitations of Psychological Treatments

One of the primary limitations of psychological treatments is the difficulty that researchers have in identifying the specific ingredients of the treatment that are most responsible for the alleviation of depressive symptoms. Very few psychological treatments have been compared against "placebo" psychological treatments. This limitation, coupled with the fact that placebo psychological treatments tend to produce some reduction in depressive symptoms, prevents researchers from definitively knowing what aspects of their treatment are acting to reduce depressive symptoms. A second important limitation lies in the differences that exist between the treatment providers in the community and those utilized in treatment studies. The treatment providers in depression treatment research are rigorously trained and supervised while providing the treatment. As such, it is plausible that their skill level is not representative of the skill level of the average community treatment provider, for whom there currently exists a wide range of formal training. A third limitation is the dearth of rigorous, controlled studies evaluating the effectiveness of psychotherapy with children. Although evidence supports the efficacy of cognitive–behavioral treatment with adolescents, less is known about the efficacy of other forms of treatment with adolescents and younger children.

VII. COMBINED BIOLOGICAL AND PSYCHOLOGICAL TREATMENTS

Given the strengths of both the biological and the psychological perspectives on depression, many clinicians and researchers have assumed that combining different forms of treatments would provide individuals with the most benefit. Antidepressant medications could reduce many of the physiological symptoms of depression (e.g., sleep and appetite dysregulation) while psychotherapy could reduce the maladaptive cognitions and behaviors. However, the research evidence supporting the efficacy of combined treatment for depression has produced mixed results. Adding psychological treatments to biological treatments has been shown to reduce relapse rates; however, various studies examining the combination of antidepressant and psychotherapy from the outset of treatment have not found significant advantages of using either antidepressant medication or psychotherapy alone.

At this point, it is unclear to what to attribute this lack of a consistent effect, although some have argued that the modest advantages produced by combined treatment may not yield statistically significant effects in single research studies, and thus more sophisticated research investigations are warranted. For example, analyses that combine results from single studies into a larger meta-analytic study have demonstrated the advantages of combined treatment for depression, particularly for patients with more severe levels.

Thus, researchers have begun to more closely examine patient variables that might contribute to improved response from combined treatment. For example, a recent large-scale study conducted by Martin Keller and associates clearly demonstrated the advantages of combined treatment over single modality treatment for chronic depression. In this study, the researchers examined the efficacy of combining nefazodone and a variant of cognitive–behavioral treatment for patients with chronic depression (defined as having significant depressive symptoms for more than 2 years). Results showed that the combination of treatments was significantly more effective than either treatment alone. Among the 519 subjects who completed the study, the rates of response after 12 weeks (as defined by either a complete remission or a significant reduction in depressive symptoms) were 55% in the nefazodone group, 52% in the cognitive–behavioral group, and 85% in the combined treatment group.

Currently, the evidence is strongest for the proposition that combined treatment is more effective for individuals with more severe and chronic levels of depression. However, there remain considerable gaps in our knowledge of the effects of combined treatment on depression.

VIII. SUMMARY AND FUTURE DIRECTIONS

Depression is a serious disorder with significant economic and social consequences that appears to be increasing in prevalence. Attempts to understand the causes of depression must encompass both biological and psychological perspectives. Treatments of depression offer significant hope: Up to 70% of individuals will respond to antidepressant medication; specific forms of psychotherapy produce similar rates of symptom alleviation. ECT is even more effective: Up to 90% of people will respond to treatment. However, depression appears to be a chronic, relapsing disorder. The risk for relapse remains high in both treated and untreated individuals.

Future research will likely continue to link the biological and psychological nature of depression. Linkage of specific receptor sites with specific symptoms of depression, imaging studies that examine the extent to which psychotherapies produce noticeable biological changes, and more studies that explore the potential for joint biological and psychological treatments are all on the horizon. In addition, more research is needed to better understand the extent to which current theories of depression apply to children and adolescents.

See Also the Following Articles

ALCOHOL DAMAGE TO THE BRAIN • ALZHEIMER'S DISEASE, NEUROPSYCHOLOGY OF • ANGER • APHASIA • BASAL GANGLIA • BEHAVIORAL NEUROGENETICS • COGNITIVE PSYCHOLOGY, OVERVIEW • DEMENTIA • HUMOR AND LAUGHTER • MANIC–DEPRESSIVE ILLNESS • NEUROPSYCHOLOGICAL ASSESSMENT • PSYCHOACTIVE DRUGS • PSYCHONEUROENDO- CRINOLOGY • PSYCHOPHYSIOLOGY • SUICIDE

Suggested Reading

American Psychiatric Association (1994). *Diagnostic and Statistical Manual of Mental Disorders,* 4th ed. American Psychiatric Association, Washington, DC.

Blazer, D. G., Kessler, R. C., McGonagle, K. A., and Swartz, M. S. (1994). The prevalence and distribution of major depression in a national community sample: The National Comorbidity Survey. *Am. J. Psychiatr.* **151,** 979–986.

Consensus Development Panel (1985). Mood disorders: Pharamacologic prevention of recurrences. *Am. J. Psychiatr.* **142,** 469–476.

Consensus Development Panel (1986). Report on the NIMH–NIH Consensus Development Conference on electroconvulsive therapy. *Psychopharmacol. Bull.* **22,** 445–502.

DeRubeis, R. J., and Crits-Cristoph, P. (1998). Empirically supported individual and group psychological treatments for adult mental disorders. *J. Consulting Clin. Psychol.* **66,** 37–52.

Elkin, I., Shea, M. T., Watkins, J. T., Imber, S. D., Sotsky, S. M., Collins, J. F., Glass, D. R., Pilkonis, P. A., Leber, W. R., Docherty, J. P., Fiester, S. J., and Parloff, M. B. (1989). National Institute of Mental Health treatment of depression collaborative research program. *Arch. Gen. Psychiatr.* **46,** 971–982.

Fava, G. A., Rafanelli, C., Grandi, S., Canestrari, R., and Morphy, M. A. (1998). Six-year outcome for cognitive behavioral treatment of residual symptoms in major depression. *Am. J. Psychiatr.* **155,** 1443–1445.

Horst, W. D., and Preskorn, S. H. (1998). Mechanism of action and clinical characteristics of three atypical antidepressants: Venlafaxine, nefazodone, buproprion. *J. Affective Disorders* **51,** 237–254.

Keitner, G. I., and Miller, I. W. (1990). Family functioning and major depression: An overview. *Am. J. Psychiatr.* **147,** 1128–1137.

Keller, M. B., McCullough, J. P., Klein, D. N., Arnow, B., Dunner, D. L., Gelenberg, A. J., Markowitz, J. C., Nemeroff, C. B., Russell, J. M., Thase, M. E., Trivedi, M. H., and Zajecka, J. (2000). A comparison of nefazodone, the cognitive–behavioral–analysis system of psychotherapy, and their combination for the treatment of chronic depression. *N. Engl. J. Med.* **342,** 1462–1470.

Kessler, R. C., Nelson, C. B., McGonagle, K. A., Liu, J., Swartz, M., and Blazer, D. G. (1996). Comorbidity of DSM-III-R major depressive disorder in the general population: Results from the National Comorbidity Survey. *Br. J. Psychiatr.* **168**(Suppl. 30), 17–30.

Luborsky, L., Mark, D., Hole, A. V., Popp, C., Goldsmith, B., and Cacciola, J. (1995). Supportive–expressive dynamic psychotherapy of depression: A time-limited version. In *Dynamic Therapies for Psychiatric Disorders (Axis I)*. (J. Barber and P. Crits-Cristoph, Eds.). Basic Books, New York.

Mesulam, M. M. (2000). *Principles of Behavioral and Cognitive Neurology*, 2nd ed. Oxford Univ. Press, Oxford.

Paykel, E. S., Scott, J., Teasdale, J. D., Johnson, A. L., Garland, A., Moore, R., Jenaway, A., Cornwall, P. L., Hayhurst, H., Abbott, R., and Pope, M. (1999). Prevention of relapse in residual depression by cognitive therapy. *Arch. Gen. Psychiatr.* **56,** 829–835.

Stahl, S. M. (1998). Mechanism of action of serotonin selective reuptake inhibitors: Serotonin receptors and pathways mediate therapeutic effects and side effects. *J. Affective Disorders* **51,** 215–228.

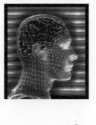

Dopamine

LISA A. TAYLOR and IAN CREESE

Rutgers University

GLOSSARY

avoidance learning A behavioral test in which subjects can avoid a noxious stimulus if a correct response is elicited.

G protein A guanine nucleotide-binding regulatory protein that mediates the interaction between extracellular receptors and intracellular effector molecules. The Gi protein is the inhibitory G protein that reduces subsequent intracellular effects. The Gs protein is the stimulatory G protein that increases subsequent intracellular effects.

intracranial self-stimulation A task in which subjects are rewarded with electrical stimulation to brain areas such as the medial forebrain bundle.

operant task A task in which an animal is rewarded for making a particular motor response such as a bar press.

Dopamine (3-Hydroxytyramine) was initially characterized as a neurotransmitter in the central and peripheral nervous system during the 1950s. Although comprising less than 1% of the neurons in the brain, dopamine mediates a variety of physiological functions and modulates many behavioral states. Given the paucity of noninvasive techniques to study dopamine in the central nervous system (CNS) of humans, most studies characterizing the role of dopamine in the brain have been carried out in experimental animals or tissue

culture expression systems or by extrapolation from human responses to dopaminergic drugs. With the relatively recent development of more sophisticated neuroimaging techniques, however, studies of dopamine function in the human brain are increasing. Since the focus of this encyclopedia is the human brain, studies using humans are emphasized. Data from animal studies or tissue culture expression systems are presented when there is a lack of data from human subjects or when specific examples illuminate the human literature.

I. ANATOMICAL DISTRIBUTION IN THE CENTRAL NERVOUS SYSTEM

There are several dopamine-containing pathways in the CNS. The nigrostriatal dopamine pathway accounts for approximately 70% of the dopamine in the brain. Cells bodies in this pathway are located in the substantia nigra pars compacta and project to the caudate, putamen, and the globus pallidus (Fig. 1). An interesting characteristic of these dopamine neurons is that they contain extensive dendritic trees, which extend ventrally into the substantia nigra pars reticulata. Dopamine release occurs from these dendrites in addition to the axon terminals. Deterioration of the nigrostriatal pathway underlies Parkinson's disease (PD).

The mesocorticolimbic dopaminergic pathway originates in the ventrotegmental area (VTA) and innervates the olfactory tubercle, nucleus accumbens, septum, amygdala, and adjacent cortical structures (medial frontal, anterior cingulate, entorhinal, perirhinal, and piriform cortet pallidus) (Fig. 1).

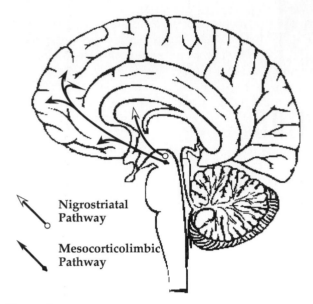

Figure 1 The nigrostriatal and mesocorticolimbic dopamine pathways.

The substantia nigra and VTA dopamine cell bodies are often referred to as the A-9 and A-10 nuclear groups, respectively, following the original designation of Dahlsstrom and Fuxe from their pioneering rodent studies using a novel technique that made dopamine neurons fluorescent. However, more detailed immunohistochemical studies suggest that the A-9 and A-10 nuclear groups are a continuum, with laterally situated cells innervating the striatum and medial cells innervating mesolimbic and mesocortical areas.

The tuberoinfundibular dopamine pathway originates in the arcuate and periventricular nuclei of the hypothalamus and projects to the intermediate lobe of the pituitary and the median eminence. Dopamine released from these neurons is secreted into the hypophysed and portal blood regulates prolactin secretion from the pituitary through inhibitory D_2 receptor on nanotrophic cells.

Other pathways containing dopamine include (i) the incertohypothalamic neurons, which connect the dorsal and posterior hypothalamus with the dorsal anterior hypothalamus and lateral septal nuclei; (ii) the medullary periventricular group, which includes dopamine cells of the dorsal motor nucleus of the vagus nerve, the nucleus tractus solitarius, and the tegmentum radiation in the periaqueductal gray matter; (iii) the interplexiform amacrine-like neurons, which link the inner and outer plexiform layers of the retina; and (iv) the periglomerular dopamine cells in

the olfactory bulb, which link mitral cell dendrites in adjacent glomeruli.

II. SYNAPTIC DOPAMINE

A. Synthesis

In dopamine-secreting cells, the first step in dopamine synthesis is the conversion of dietary tyrosine into L-3,4-dihydroxyphenylalanine (L-DOPA) (Fig. 2). This reaction is catalyzed by the rate-limiting enzyme tyrosine hydroxylase (TH). L-DOPA is then converted to dopamine via the enzyme L-aromatic amino acid decarboxylase.

TH is composed of four identical subunits and contains iron ions, which are required for its activity. The cofactors oxygen and tetrahydrobiopterin are also required for its activity. A single gene encodes TH, although in humans four isoforms have been shown to result from alternative splicing of the primary transcript. TH is present in both soluble (cytoplasmic) and membrane-bound forms.

Under basal conditions TH is nearly saturated by tyrosine. The observation that pharmacological agents

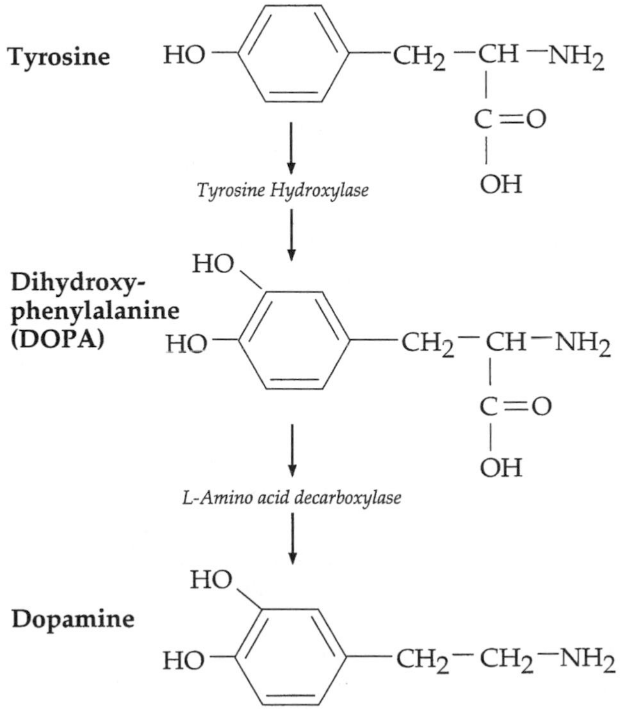

Figure 2 The dopamine synthesis pathway.

known to block TH activity have greater effects on extracellular dopamine levels than agents that block dopa-decarboxylase indicates that the rate-limiting step for dopamine synthesis is tyrosine hydroxylation of tyrosine to L-DOPA by TH. Thus, increasing levels of tyrosine by dietary modifications may also regulate dopamine synthesis.

The conversion of L-DOPA to dopamine by dopamine β-hydroxylase results from the removal of a hydroxyl group and requires pyridoxal 5-phosphate (vitamin B$_6$) as a cofactor.

Dopamine synthesis is regulated in a variety of ways. End product inhibition is the major regulator when dopamine neuronal activity and release are low. In contrast, when dopaminergic fibers are electrically stimulated, TH activity is increased. This increase appears to be a function of enhanced enzyme substrate kinetics, in part caused by TH phosphorylation. This results in a net decrease in affinity of TH for dopamine, which overrides end product inhibition.

B. Storage and Release

There are two release mechanisms for dopamine. The first is calcium-dependent, tetrodotoxin (TTX)-sensitive, vesicular release at the axon terminal that occurs following an action potential. The second is calcium and TTX independent and occurs following the administration of stimulant drugs that reverse the direction of the dopamine transporter (DAT). Under normal, nondrug conditions the DAT carries released dopamine from the extrasynaptic space back into the terminal region.

Pharmacological studies indicate that dopamine exists in three pools or compartments within the axon terminal. Two of these are vesicular dopamine stores, one containing newly synthesized dopamine and the second containing a longer term store of dopamine. A cytoplasmic pool has also been identified, and it consists of dopamine newly taken up by the dopamine transporter.

C. Inactivation

Dopamine inactivation is accomplished by a combination of reuptake and enzymatic catabolism. Dopamine uptake is an energy-dependent process that requires sodium and chloride. Catabolism occurs through two enzymatic pathways (Fig. 3). Although it is not clear how much dopamine is catabolized in each of these

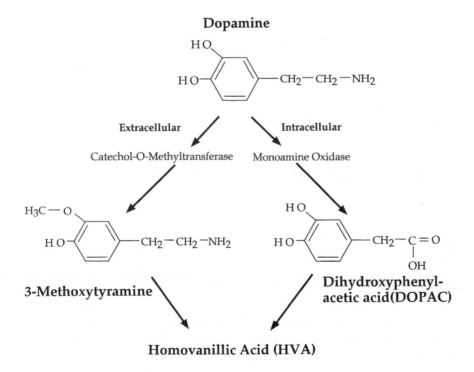

Figure 3 The dopamine metabolic pathway.

pathways in the human brain, almost 90% of catabolism in the rat striatum takes place via the monoamine oxidase (MAO) pathway. In the rat, the level of 3,4-dihydroxylphenylacetic acid is thought to reflect catabolism of intraneuronal dopamine, which includes dopamine that is taken back up by the dopamine transporter, whereas 3-methoxytyramine levels are thought to reflect metabolism of extracellular dopamine. Cerebrospinal fluid (CSF) levels of homovanillic acid (HVA) are often used as an indicator of dopaminergic activity in humans.

III. DOPAMINE RECEPTORS

A. Subtypes

Initial biochemical and pharmacological studies indicated the presence of two dopamine receptor subtypes with differential coupling to G proteins: D1 receptors stimulate adenylate cyclase through Gs protein, and D2 receptors inhibit adenylate cyclase through Gi protein. The recent application of molecular cloning techniques has revealed the existence of five dopamine receptor genes, each encoding a distinct seven-transmembrane spanning receptor. These receptors have been classified according to their structures and divided into two subfamilies, the D2-like receptors (D_2–D_4) and the D1-like receptors (D_1 and D_5). In the case of the D_2 receptor, two isoforms (D_{2L} and D_{2S}), generated by alternative splicing of the primary transcript, have been identified. Given their structural similarity, members of each subfamily exhibit similar pharmacological characteristics.

B. Distribution

The distribution of messenger RNA (mRNA) encoding all five dopamine receptors has been determined in the rat and human brain by *in situ* hybridization. High levels of D_1 mRNA are found in the caudate–putamen, nucleus accumbens, and olfactory tubercle; lower levels are found in lateral septum, olfactory bulb, hypothalamus, and cortex. In contrast, D_5 mRNA is predominantly localized to the hippocampus and the parafascicular nucleus of the thalamus.

The highest concentration of D_2 mRNA is present in the neostriatum, olfactory tubercle, substantia nigra, ventral tegmental area, and the nucleus accumbens. The levels of D_3 and D_4 receptor mRNAs are much lower in the brain relative to the level of D_2 mRNA. D_3 receptor mRNA is predominantly expressed in limbic areas, such as the nucleus accumbens, Islands of Calleja, bed nucleus of the stria terminalis, hippocampus, mammillary nuclei, and the substantia nigra. The areas with the highest levels of D_4 mRNA include the olfactory bulb, hypothalamus, and thalamus, with lower levels present in the hippocampus, cortex, and basal ganglia.

There is evidence in the rat that D_1 and D_2 receptor expression is segregated at the level of the striatum (caudate and putamen in the human). *In situ* hybridization analysis has reported two distinct post synaptic populations of striatal neurons that express D_1 or D_2 receptors: the enkephalinergic striatopallidal neurons, which express D_2 receptors, and the substance P, dynorphin-positive, striatonigral neurons, which express D_1 receptors. However, other groups using different methodologies have reported considerably more overlap in the expression of D_1 and D_2 mRNA in the striatum. They found significant coexpression of D_1 and D_2 mRNAs in the same striatal neurons. These studies suggest that at least a portion of D_1 and D_2 receptors is colocalized in the striatum.

Electrophysiological and neurochemical data suggest that a portion of dopamine receptors are located presynaptically on the axon terminals of striatal dopaminergic neurons where they serve as autoreceptors. These terminal autoreceptors modulate the synthesis and release of dopamine. These activation inhibits production and release of dopamine. These autoreceptors were originally classified as D_2 receptors. However, since D_2 and D_3 mRNA are present in nigral neurons D_3 as well as D_2 receptors are implicated as autoreceptors. Somatodendritic autoreceptors, responding to dendritically released dopamine, have also been observed. Activation of these receptors reduces the firing rate of dopamine neurons.

C. Signal Transduction Pathways

Like other G protein-coupled receptors, dopamine receptors transduce their signals through second messengers regulated by G proteins. In general, D1-like receptors stimulate adenylate cyclase via the Gs, and the D2-like receptors inhibit adenylate cyclase through the Gi. The signaling cascade is initiated by dopamine binding to the extracellular portion of the receptor. The binding of dopamine alters the receptor so that it activates a G protein present on the intracellular face of the neuron cell membrane. Once activated, G proteins modulate adenylate cyclase activity. G proteins bind guanosine triphosphate (GTP) or guanosine diphosphate (GDP). Dopamine binding to its receptor causes GDP to be replaced with GTP. Then, in the case of the D1-like receptors, a GTP–Gs complex is formed and associates with the catalytic subunit of adenylate cyclase, stimulating the conversion of ATP to cyclic (AMP) adenosine monophosphate. The GTP–Gs protein and the catalytic subunit of adenylate cyclase together constitute the active form of adenylate cyclase. The association of the G protein with the catalytic subunit of the cyclase also results in the hydrolysis of GTP to GDP. This hydrolysis causes the G protein to dissociate from the catalytic subunit and to reassociate with the receptor. This reaction terminates the synthesis of cyclic AMP. Therefore, the duration of cyclic AMP synthesis is regulated by GTPase activity. In the case of the D2-like receptors, receptor activation causes GTP binding to Gi, and this complex inhibits cyclase activity.

It should also be noted that several other second messenger systems are involved in D2-like receptor-mediated signal transduction, such as the stimulation of aracadonic acid metabolism and the activation of potassium channels.

D. Regulation

Most studies concerned with the regulation of CNS dopamine receptors *in vivo* have examined the effects of long-term treatment with receptor agonists, antagonists, or denervation induced by 6-hydroxydopamine, a selective neurotoxin for catecholaminergic neurons, on striatal D2-like dopamine receptors.

Studies examining chronic agonist exposure have yielded mixed results. Repeated treatment with amphetamine, which increases synaptic levels of dopamine, both increased and had no effect on the density of D2-like receptors in the striatum, probably depending on dose and timing. Treatment with systemic L-DOPA, which also increases synaptic levels of dopamine, has been reported to decrease the density of D2-like receptors in the striatum.

Treatment with D1-like or D2-like antagonists has been shown to increase the density of D1-like and D2-like receptors, respectively, without changing the affinity of these receptors for dopamine. Similarly, denervation following 6-hydroxydopamine administration also leads to an increased dopamine D2-like, but not D1-like, receptor density as well as an

enhanced behavioral responsiveness to dopamine. Thus, it appears that dopamine D2-like receptors upregulate in response to reduced levels of dopamine. It is not clear, however, if the molecular mechanism responsible for lesion-induced upregulation of dopamine receptors is the same as that underlying the upregulation observed after long-term antagonist treatment. The fact that D1-like receptors upregulate after long-term antagonist treatment, but not after denervation, suggests that the mechanisms must be different, at least for D1-like receptors. In the case of long-term antagonist treatment, it is also possible that the intrinsic properties of the antagonist may play a role in the upregulation of dopamine receptors.

The pathway of protein synthesis, from the initial stage of gene transcription to mRNA splicing, translation, protein processing, and insertion into the membrane, provides a number of potential points of control for the regulation of dopamine receptor number. The rate of receptor removal from the membrane and the recycling or degradation rates are also factors that contribute to the number of receptors available for binding.

It should be noted that the molecular mechanisms underlying dopamine receptor trafficking (another mechanism regulating dopamine receptor expression) are only beginning to be studied.

IV. DOPAMINE AND NEUROPSYCHIATRIC DISORDERS

Many lines of evidence suggest a role for dopamine in neuropsychiatric disorders such as PD, schizophrenia, attention deficit hyperactivity disorder (ADHD), and drug abuse. The first evidence for dopamine's involvement in these disorders came from either postmortem histological/neurochemical studies or the observation that the drugs used to treat these disorders either increased or blocked dopamine neurotransmission in the brain. Since the advent of neuroimaging techniques such as positron emission topography (PET), a majority of the current human studies use this technique to further define the role of dopamine in these disorders.

PET enables the direct measurement of components of dopamine neurotransmission in the living human brain by using radiotracers, which label dopamine receptors, dopamine transporters, and precursors of dopamine or compounds that have specificity for the enzymes that degrade dopamine. Certain types of PET studies also provide information on regional brain metabolism or blood flow, thus, PET can be used to assess the functional consequences of changes in brain dopamine activity.

A. Parkinson's Disease

PD is a neurodegenerative disorder of unknown etiology that is associated with the degeneration of dopamine neurons primarily in the substantia nigra and manifested by disturbances in the motor system. There is evidence for genetic and environmental causes. The symptoms of PD can be classified as positive or negative. The positive symptoms of PD consist of tremor, muscular rigidity, and involuntary movements. Negative symptoms include bradykinesia, postural disturbances, and cognitive impairments. During the early course of the disease, unilateral symptoms may initially appear. Often, the disease begins with a mild tremor and some muscular rigidity. As the disease progresses, the symptoms present bilaterally, the tremor is exacerbated, and bradykinesia appears. During the later stages of the disease patients are incapacitated and are usually confined to a wheelchair.

L-DOPA is probably the single most effective medication for controlling the early symptoms of Parkinson's disease. L-DOPA is transported to the brain and taken up by the remaining dopaminergic cells, where it is converted into dopamine and increases its synaptic availability. L-DOPA therapy is effective in most patients for several years. However, as the loss of nigrostriatal neurons increases, symptoms continue to worsen and the dose of L-DOPA must be increased. As the dose is increased, it is not uncommon for patients to develop adverse effects, which may not be tolerable. In such cases, a MAO inhibitor is sometimes coadministered with a lower dose of L-DOPA to prolong the actions of dopamine at the synapse. Alternatively, direct-acting dopamine agonists, such as bromocriptine and pergolide, can be used to treat PD.

B. Schizophrenia

Schizophrenia is a serious psychiatric disorder affecting approximately 1% of the world population. Symptoms usually appear in late adolescence or early adulthood. This disease has a devastating impact on the lives of patients as well as their families. Positive symptoms include hallucinations and delusions, whereas negative symptoms consist of flattened affect social withdrawal and cognitive deficits. Several lines of evidence emerged in the 1970s that suggested alterations in dopamine transmission might constitute the pathophysiological basis for schizophrenia. Amphetamine and cocaine, which enhance dopamine transmission in the brain, can produce paranoid psychosis similar to that observed in patients with paranoid schizophrenia and exacerbated symptoms in schizophrenics. Also, a significant positive correlation between the clinical potency of neuroleptic drugs and their ability to block D2-like dopamine receptors has been consistently observed.

Although early studies suggested a postsynaptic locus for the disease because increased D2-Like receptors were observed in postmortem studies evaluating dopamine receptors, it seems likely that these results may have been caused by prior neuroleptic drug treatment. Neuroimaging studies also indicate that increased dopaminergic neurotransmission is involved in schizophrenia and is associated with activation of psychotic symptoms. Furthermore, enhanced dopamine transmission is detected in drug-naïve patients experiencing their first episode of the illness and is not detected in patients during remission, suggesting that the hyperdopaminergic state associated with schizophrenia fluctuates over time.

With respect to the negative symptoms of schizophrenia, PET studies evaluating regional brain glucose metabolism in untreated schizophrenic patients have reported reduced rates of glucose metabolism in neocortical areas, although these differences did not always reach statistical significance. Importantly, there may be a tendency toward a more pronounced reduction in metabolism in patients exhibiting negative symptoms. Since the premise underlying these studies is that glucose consumption in nerve cells is directly proportional to the impulse activity of neurons, it was postulated that decreased dopamine transmission in the mesocortical dopaminergic pathway, which is known to modulate the activity of prefrontal cortical neurons, might underlie the negative symptoms observed in schizophrenia. Support for this hypothesis has been obtained from a variety of studies. For example, animal studies have demonstrated that lesions of the prefrontal cortex in nonhuman primates lead to cognitive disturbances and poor social skills that resemble some of the negative symptoms observed in schizophrenic patients. In addition, many patients with primarily negative symptoms exhibit ventricular enlargement suggesting a loss of neurophil.

C. Attention Deficit Hyperactivity Disorder

A role for altered dopamine neurotransmission as the underlying cause of ADHD has been suggested by several observations. First, drugs used to treat ADHD, such as methylphenidate (Ritalin) and amphetamine (Adderal), increase synaptic levels of dopamine in experimental animals and in human subjects. In patients with ADHD, the maximal therapeutic effects of these drugs occur during the absorption phase of the kinetic curve, which parallels the acute release of dopamine into the synaptic cleft. These drugs are said to have "paradoxical" effects in ADHD children because they cause hyperactivity in normal children but have a "calming" or cognitive-focusing effect on ADHD children. Second, molecular genetic studies have identified genes that encode proteins involved in dopamine neurotransmission as candidate genes for ADHD. Third, neuroimaging studies have shown reduced activation in the striatum and frontal cortex of ADHD patients that is reversed by the administration of methylphenidate at least in a subset of children. Recently, functional magnetic resonance imaging studies have demonstrated differences between children with ADHD and normal controls in the degree of corticostriatal activation during a stimulus-controlled go/no-go task and its modulation by methylphenidate. Off drug, ADHD children showed impaired inhibitory control on this task and reduced striatal activation relative to the control subjects. Administration of methylphenidate significantly increased inhibitory control and frontostriatal activation in ADHD patients. These observations indicate that an optimal level of corticostriatal activation is necessary for subjects to display normal inhibitory control. Since methylphenidate increased both corticostriatal activation and inhibitory control, it follows that decreased corticostriatal activation and the poor inhibitory control may be due to reduced dopamine tone in the brain, perhaps in the striatum. However, it is equally likely that the mesolimbic dopamine system may mediate these effects by virtue of its afferent projections to the prefrontal cortex.

D. Psychostimulant Drug Abuse

Amphetamine and cocaine are psychostimulant drugs that are abused by humans because they produce feelings of euphoria. Both of these drugs increase extracellular levels of dopamine. Cocaine blocks the dopamine transporter and amphetamine primarily reverses it. Studies indicate these drugs are also primary reinforcers in animals because they will self-administer these drugs, and their propensity to do so is an excellent predictor of abuse liability in humans.

Many animal studies using a variety of different paradigms to study the role of dopamine in the rewarding properties of the psychostimulant drugs have suggested that dopamine is critically involved in this process in experimental animals. In the case of cocaine, studies carried out in human subjects have also supported the idea that enhanced dopamine transmission is responsible for the euphoric effects of this drug in humans. Dopamine appears to be a critical mediator of reward in the brain.

Dopamine also appears to play a role in craving, which often leads to relapse in abstinent human substance abusers. Brain imaging studies have identified the amygdala and the dopamine-rich nucleus accumbens as putative neuroanatomical substrates for cue-induced craving. Nucleus accumbens dopamine levels increased withdrawn from cocaine when they were exposed to cues that were previously associated with cocaine intake. Studies in humans examining the level of the dopamine metabolite HVA have reported that craving during abstinence is associated with increased HVA.

It also appears that the dopamine D_3 receptor may be involved in cocaine craving. Animal models of cocaine craving have shown that the D_3 selective partial agonist, BP 897, attenuates craving while lacking any intrinsic, primary rewarding effects.

A very interesting aspect of repeated amphetamine or cocaine administration is behavioral sensitization. Behavioral sensitization or reverse tolerance refers to the progressive augmentation of drug affects that are elicited by repeated administration of the drug. Sensitization to psychostimulants was characterized in experimental animals as early as 1932 and in humans in the 1950s. Behavioral sensitization develops when psychostimulant administration is intermittent. Tolerance develops during continuous administration.

V. DOPAMINE AND LEARNING

Animal research shows that dopamine is involved in the acquisition of operant tasks, avoidance learning, and intracranial self-stimulation. It is thought that dopamine in mesolimbic regions (most notably the nucleus accumbens) is involved in both the acquisition and the maintenance of these behaviors. This conclusion was based primarily on results from studies using dopamine-depleting agents and dopaminergic drugs to evaluate their effects on acquisition or maintenance of reinforced behaviors. The results of acquisition studies showed that administration of dopamine antagonists or the dopamine-depleting agent, 6-hydroxydopamine, prevented the acquisition of these tasks. Reinterpretation of studies evaluating the effects of these agents on the maintenance of such behaviors has not been so clear-cut. For example, the acute administration of a dopaminergic antagonist after acquisition of an operant task often has no effect or increases the level of operant responding. This has been interpreted to be the result of a decrease in the perceived "salience" of the reward, whereas chronic administration of these agents blocks these behaviors. Recent *in vivo* voltammetry studies, which directly measure fast changes in dopamine release at the level of the synapse, carried out by Garris, Wightman, and colleagues have shown that evoked dopamine release in the nucleus accumbens is associated with the acquisition but not the maintenance of reinforced behavior, at least in the case of intracranial stimulation.

VI. DOPAMINE AND WORKING MEMORY

The prefrontal cortex receives elaborate dopamine inputs from the VTA and an optimal level of dopamine in the prefrontal cortex appears necessary for cognitive performance in experimental animals. Significant increases in dopamine levels in the dorsolateral prefrontal cortex have been observed in monkeys performing a delayed alternation task. In addition, reduced levels of dopamine in the prefrontal cortex have detrimental effects on spatial working memory tasks. It has also been reported that very large increases in dopamine levels in the prefrontal cortex can cause deficits on spatial working memory tasks. These deficits are ameliorated by the administration of dopamine D1-like drugs. Taken together, the previously mentioned observations support the idea that an optimal level of dopamine is required to perform spatial working memory tasks. If that level is reduced or increased, performance will be negatively affected.

Behavioral studies conducted in humans also indicate a role for prefrontal D1 receptors in working memory modulation in humans, although one study has also shown that the administration of the D2-like antagonist sulpride produced a dose-dependent impairment in spatial working memory.

Studies examining the performance of PD patients on working memory tasks also support the idea that dopamine may be involved in working memory in humans as well as in experimental animals. Imaging studies in PD patients have shown reduced fluorodopa uptake in the caudate nucleus and frontal cortex, which correlates with deficits in working memory as well as attention.

Some studies have also evaluated the effects of dopamine receptors in the ventral hippocampus on working memory tasks in rats. These studies suggest that D2-like but not D1-like receptors in the ventral hippocampus modulate spatial working memory.

See Also the Following Articles

CATECHOLAMINES • CHEMICAL NEUROANATOMY • ENDORPHINS AND THEIR RECEPTORS • MANIC–DEPRESSIVE ILLNESS • NOREPINEPHRINE • PARKINSON'S DISEASE • SCHIZOPHRENIA • WORKING MEMORY

Suggested Reading

Goldman-Rakic, P. S. (1998). The cortical dopamine system: Role in memory and cognition. *Adv. Pharmacol.* **42,** 707–711.

Laruelle, M. (2000). Imaging synaptic neurotransmission with in vivo binding competition techniques: A critical review. *J. Cereb. Blood Flow Metab.* **20**(3), 423–451.

Neer, E. J. (1994). G proteins: Critical control points for transmembrane signals. *Protein Sci.* **3**(1), 3–14.

Schultz, W., Tremblay, L., and Hollerman, J. R. (1998). Reward prediction in primate basal ganglia and frontal cortex. *Neuropharmacology* **37**(4–5), 421–429.

Sibley, D. R., Ventura, A. L., Jiang, D., and Mak, C. (1998). Regulation of the D1 dopamine receptor through cAMP-mediated pathways. *Adv. Pharmacol.* **42,** 447–450.

Spanagel, R., and Weiss, F. (1999). The dopamine hypothesis of reward: Past and current status. *Trends Neurosci.* **22**(11), 521–527.

Tedroff, J. M., (1999). Functional consequences of dopaminergic degeneration in Parkinson's disease. *Adv. Neurol.* **80,** 67–70.

Vallone, D., Picetti, R., and Borrelli, E. (2000). Structure and function of dopamine receptors. *Neurosci. Biobehav. Rev.* **24**(1), 125–132.

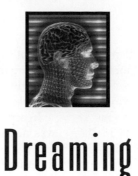

Dreaming

MARIO BERTINI

University of Rome

GLOSSARY

bizarreness The presence of highly unlikely elements in the dream narrative. Improbable events are usually associated with discontinuities of time, place, person, object, and action as well as incongruities of these features.

REM sleep The stage of sleep defined by the concomitant appearance of relatively low-voltage, mixed frequency electroencephalograph activity with episodic rapid eye movement (REM) and low-amplitude electromyogram.

Dreaming is a term interchangeably used to indicate both the function of generating a dream and the dream itself. That is a special kind of sleep mentation usually characterized by visual imagery, bizarreness, and hallucinatory and story-like quality.

I. HISTORICAL BACKGROUND

Dreaming is a complex psychobiological function, that eludes a precise and universally shared definition. Research into this important dimension of the human mind is continually evolving, and despite the fact that much progress has been made, we are still a long way from a satisfactory understanding of its biological and psychological implications.

Given the peculiar methodological limitations of the research in this area, it is worth presenting an overview of our current knowledge in a historical perspective. I hope it will allow the reader to better judge the validity and the possible lines of development of the field.

In the antiquity, sleep had a dual significance. On the one hand, it symbolized death, in the abandonment of the limbs and in shutting oneself away from the experience of the senses (Hesiod's Theogony depicted Sleep and Death as two brothers); on the other hand, sleep was like a door that, through the secret pathways of dreams, led to a dimension beyond intelligence and enabled humans to come into contact with the supernatural.

Even on a philosophical level, there were two somewhat opposite orientations that can still be recognized in some of today's scientific views. Some thinkers viewed sleep as a passive withdrawal from consciousness and dreaming was thus an illusion or a nonsense; according to others, sleep represented the theater of a different form of mental activity and dreams bore meanings.

In *Sleep and Wake* (453 BC), Aristotle defined sleep, and what takes place in it, as a "privation of wakefulness," i.e., as a purely negative concept—a pause in human sensory experience and intellectual functioning. During sleep, either intelligence is silent and everything is dark or it is deceived by a flow of disconnected fleeting images that give rise to dreams.

In *Republic*, Plato discussed the obscure depths of the psyche that are revealed through nocturnal dreams. Not only may the gods reveal themselves to man through dreams but also in the same way man reveals himself to himself. Even Heraclitus seems to hint at a different orientation of the psyche in the transition from wakefulness to sleep: "He who is awake lives in a single world common to all; he who is asleep retires to his own particular world."

Over the centuries, dreaming aroused more the curiosity than the systematic interest of researchers. The views of 19th-century neurophysiologists, strongly influenced by positivistic thought, essentially adhered to the original Aristotelian lines.

As a matter of fact, until recently, states of consciousness were believed to vary along one continuous dimension in parallel with behavioral performance, from deep coma to the opposite extreme of manic excitement. In this view, rational thought appeared as a form of mental activity exclusively belonging to waking states, whereas dreaming was simply the expression of the fragmentation and dissolution of thought, in close relationship with the lowering of vigilance and the deepening of sleep.

Only toward the end of the 19th century were some contributions made that considered dreaming an event deserving direct attention. The observations of two French scholars, the Marquis d'Hervey de Saint-Denis and Alfred Maury, are worth mentioning here, along with those of the initiator of experimental psychology, the German Wilhelm Wundt. However, the contribution that truly catalyzed the attention of contemporary culture was the brainchild of a scholar, Sigmund Freud, who had no real connection with the emerging experimental psychology approaches. Freud pointed out a methodological flaw in the way those who considered dreaming a completely meaningless activity examined the oneiric content. Researchers were trying to understand dreams according to the same register that was used for comprehending "normal" language instead of searching for the appropriate key to decrypt a language that is quite peculiar. According to Freud, this was like expecting to understand a rebus, with its apparently bizarre compositions, by reading it as a common rational message.

Freud's book on the interpretation of dreams, which was published in 1900, is a cornerstone in psychoanalytical theory and a significant historical event in contemporary culture. However, it is well-known that Freudian studies mainly focused on the contents of the phenomenon, whereas the proposed functional explanations suffered from the poor knowledge at the time of the central nervous system's physiology and of the organization of the mind in general, matters brought to the forefront of research by modern neuroscience.

In order to probe the functional basis of dreaming, it was necessary to shed light on objective, measurable aspects, such as the frequency and periodicity of dreaming, its universality, episodic and total duration throughout the night, and especially its neurophysiological regulation. The first step in solving these and other general problems was the discovery of some objective indicators that could reveal the presence of the dream itself.

As sometimes happens in science, the first curtain protecting the mystery of dreaming was lifted almost by chance by a young student working on his doctoral thesis in the early 1950s. Studying attention in children, under the supervision of Nathaniel Kleitman at the University of Chicago, Eugene Aserinsky observed that sometime after the onset of sleep, the subjects' eyes could be observed, under the closed eyelids, moving left and right and up and down while all the major body movements ceased. After several minutes, these eye movements would stop altogether, only to resume again with the same characteristics at more or less regular intervals throughout the night. Since the pattern of eye movements resembled that of an awake subject exploring a visual scene with his or her gaze, the hypothesis was put forward that dreaming occurs in these periods.

To test the hypothesis, the experimenters set out to awaken and question subjects at various times during the night. In most cases, subjects were able to report dream content when awakened during periods of eye movements, whereas they could rarely recall dreams if awakened while their eyes did not move. The results seemed to clearly confirm the conjecture, and Aserinsky's accidental observation took on the proportions of a profound scientific discovery.

II. THE SLEEP AND DREAMING LABORATORIES

Further confirmation of such association was obtained in the Chicago sleep laboratory. By the end of the 1950s, William Dement and Nathaniel Kleitman had obtained vivid, detailed reports of dreams with an incidence of 80% when awakenings occurred during periods of sleep characterized by rapid eye movements (REM sleep), whereas dreams could be reported in only 7% of the cases when subjects were awakened while no rapid eye movements could be observed (non-REM sleep). Various demonstrations of proportionality between objective duration of REM sleep periods and subjective length of dreaming further confirmed the relation between the two events and prompted the hypothesis that dream activity continuously progresses throughout the length of a REM phase.

Beginning in the 1960s, many other sleep and dreaming laboratories were set up throughout the world in which subjects were monitored with electroencephalographic (EEG) and polygraphic recordings throughout their sleep. The observations made in these laboratories offered a convincing picture of the physiological processes accompanying the REM stage of sleep. The term REM soon came to represent a particular sleep stage that appeared to be the privileged place for dreams. Besides rapid eye movements, this phase is characterized by fast EEG activity, resembling that of the wake alert state, contrasted by muscle tone so relaxed that the sleeper is virtually paralyzed. Heart and breathing rate are higher and more irregular than in the other sleep stages. Penis erection in males and vaginal moistening in females have also been highlighted in connection with the REM stage of sleep.

Continuous laboratory monitoring has shown that in adult humans REM phases last, on average, 20–30 min each and reoccur regularly at intervals of approximately 90–100 min throughout sleep. Thus, each subject has an average of four or five REM episodes a night that recur cyclically. These episodes, on the whole, comprise approximately 20–25% of an adult's sleep.

In the words of William Dement, "the discovery of REM sleep was the breakthrough, the discovery that changed the course of sleep research." As a matter of fact, the emphasis attributed to the REM stage has been such that the other four stages of sleep are often defined simply as non-REM sleep. As discussed later, this extreme simplification, including the exclusive attribution of dreaming to REM sleep, was later criticized in various ways.

III. PSYCHOPHYSIOLOGICAL FEATURES OF DREAMING

A. Eye Movements and Dream Imagery

The discovery of characteristic bursts of eye movements in sleep led to the hypothesis of a direct relationship with the oneiric imagery, as some anecdotal reports seem to suggest. For example, one subject—who was awakened after a period 15 min of eye inactivity followed by some large shifts from right to left—reported having dreamed of driving a car while staring at the road ahead of him until, coming to a crossroads, he was struck by the sudden appearance of another car approaching quickly from the left. Some empirical studies, albeit not completely exemplary on a methodological level, seemed to support the hypothesis of a close connection between eye movements and dream images. According to some researchers, rapid eye movements are indeed the result of the actual scanning of the dreamed "scene."

According to other researchers, however, eye movements represent random, inevitable bursts of motor activity. Eye movements could merely be one of a variety of physiological signs of the peculiar pattern of activation processes of the organism that coexist with dreaming. If a correlation between REMs and dream content were to be verified, it would still be unclear whether chaotically generated eye movements forced appropriate dream content or dream content forced appropriate eye movements; correlation is not causation. The study of subjects blind since birth soon appeared to be the most logical approach to test the "scanning hypothesis."

B. Dreaming in the Blind

Blind people do have dreams that include visual imagery, but only if blindness occurs later than 6 or 7 years of age. It has been known, however, that dreams in congenitally blind people are nonvisual, and that their content is mostly linked to other sensory modalities. If the scanning hypothesis were true, then one might argue that subjects who have never had the opportunity to gaze upon their surroundings should not show rapid eye movements while dreaming. Sleep laboratory studies, however, have demonstrated quite the opposite (i.e., the presence of eye movements in the REM sleep of congenitally blind subjects). An even greater difficulty in accepting the hypothesis that eye movements follow dream scenes arises when we consider the dreaming of newborn babies or even animals deprived of the cerebral cortex.

As discussed later, newborn infants (and even prematurely born infants) show the presence of all those physiological features that accompany the subjective phenomenon of dreaming in adults, including eye movements. Furthermore, a persistence of eye movement bursts, although more disorganized, has been found even in decorticated cats and humans. It would certainly be difficult in these cases to postulate their relation to any kind of imaginative activity.

A different interpretation of the phenomenon, which takes into account the apparently contrasting findings, may be considered within a developmental view. Eye movement may be considered as a physiological mechanism included since birth in the constellation of functional characteristics of the REM stage. The overall and experiential maturation of the organism involves a change in these automatic movement bursts along the lines established by the interaction with psychic phenomena as they occur in dreaming processes. After all, the relationships between eye movement and dream imagery may be another example of various physiological functions controlled by lower brain centers that are coordinated in the area of higher brain processes as they mature.

C. Dream Recall

Dreaming in the course of a night takes up a considerably longer amount of time than was previously supposed. Each one of us has 1 or 2 hr per night of REM sleep; however, even those who remember dreams best generally recall only one or at most two fragments per night, and most people remember much less. Even the few dreams that are well remembered after awakening normally fade from memory after a few minutes or a few hours unless special effort is made to keep them in mind. These considerations give rise the following questions: Is it really true that everyone dreams in the proportions reported by the studies carried out in the sleep laboratories? Why are dreams so much more difficult to remember with respect to wake experiences?

An answer to the first question was provided by a study conducted in 1959 at the Downstate Medical Center in New York. Donald Goodenough and coworkers used the EEG technique to record the pattern of brain activity during sleep in two groups of subjects. The first group was composed of people claiming to dream at least once a night, whereas subjects in the second group claimed they dreamed less than once a month or even not at all. These researchers showed that (i) REM periods occurred with the same frequency in both groups; (ii) all subjects, even those who claimed they had never dreamed before, were able to

report at least one dream during the nights spent in the laboratory when awakened during REM sleep; (iii) the so-called "dreamers" reported a significantly higher number of dreams than did "non-dreamers". These findings, widely confirmed in later studies, led to the conclusion that, albeit with considerable individual differences, everyone dreams. The distinction between dreamers and nondreamers should therefore be reformulated as those who remember dreams and those who do not.

This brings to the forefront the question of why there is widespread forgetting of nocturnal dreaming experiences. Even "good dreamers" do not normally remember as many dreams as they do if awakened toward the end of a REM phase. Thus, even taking into account individual differences, the basis for this forgetting should be searched for in some ubiquitous physiological factors. The reasons for the failure of transferring sleep mentation from short- to long-term memory are still not completely clear, and the most popular hypotheses present differences that depend on the stress placed on biological vs psychological factors.

One repeatedly put forward hypothesis, which has little credibility today, maintains that the periods of non-REM sleep that follow REM are responsible for forgetting, as if non-REM sleep contained conditions that were somehow incompatible with the long-term consolidation of dreams. Another biologically oriented theory, which finds greater support, considers the particular biochemical substratum underlying the REM phase as responsible for forgetting. According to Allan Hobson and Robert McCarley of Harvard University, dream amnesia depends on the cutoff during REM sleep of a special class of neurotransmitters (namely, the monoamines noradrenaline and serotonin) that are needed to convert our immediate- or short-term memories into long-term storage. According to this hypothesis, when we awaken from a dream the noradrenergic and serotonergic neurons, located in many subcortical centers and widely projecting to the cerebral cortex, turn on and give our brain a shot of these transmitters. If a dream experience is still encoded in activated networks of neurons, it can be reported, recorded, and remembered.

Researchers oriented more toward analyzing the psychological factors tend to minimize or even to deny a substantial subcortical influence on the production and forgetting of dreams. While rejecting Freud's original censorship theory, most dream scientists in the modern cognitive research area would probably accept the general idea of a relationship between the specific process of dream construction and the easiness of dream forgetting. David Foulkes, for instance, believes that it is the very nature of the dream production process (i.e., the limited presence of the self and the quality of the encoding competence) to make remembering difficult: "When we are dreaming we are not deliberately selecting and organizing the contents of our conscious thoughts and we are not able to reflect on them in a self-conscious way."

Allan Rechtschaffen, another outstanding researcher in the field, has described this peculiarity of our dreaming state as "single-mindedness." While dreaming, there are no alternative lines of thought as in wake, when we are self-reflective and contextually aware; in a sense, our consciousness, functions as a "single channel." A connection can be seen between the tendency to forget and the absence of simultaneous channels to monitor the oneiric mentation and to put it in the more general context of our previous knowledge.

A satisfactory clarification of the reasons why dreams are so easily forgettable will have to wait for a deeper understanding of both the psychological and the biological correlates of sleep and, above all, of their dynamic integrative constraints and interactions.

IV. DEVELOPMENTAL ASPECTS OF DREAMING

A. REM Sleep at the Beginning of Life

The discovery of a sleep stage accompanied by dreaming and characterized by distinct physiological correlates had scientific implications of undoubted significance. It inaugurated investigation of the neurophysiological substratum and functional significance of REM sleep as well its ontogenetic and phylogenetic features.

The developmental aspects of sleep could certainly not be ignored and very soon the sleep and dreaming laboratories started to study newborns and even premature infants. Sleep in these subjects was monitored using the classical polygraphic recording techniques. With some surprise, it was found that the REM phenomenon is clearly present from the beginning of life. However, at variance with what is observed in older children and in adults, REM sleep in the neonate is characterized by the presence of a variety of body movements. In particular, a surprising range of facial expressions can be observed that are not present in the other sleep and wake states. In fact, in the REM state almost all the typical motor components of adult emotional face expressions have been observed since the first days of life. Because of the characteristic presence of facial and body motility, the immature REM sleep of the infant is generally called "active sleep," whereas the rest is known as "quiet sleep." Another characteristic difference from the adult is that the REM phase in the newborn is usually the first stage of sleep. However, perhaps the most relevant difference from adult REM is a quantitative one: whereas adults spend about 20–25% of their total sleep time in the REM stage, and this is reduced to about 15% in people older than 60 years of age, in newborn babies this percentage is about 50%, and it is even higher in prematurity. In various recording experiments, it was found that the proportion of REM to total sleep time reaches 70% in 7-month premature babies. These values are even more impressive if one considers the absolute amount of sleep time of children in the months following birth with respect to that of adults.

B. Do Infants Dream?

The physiological signs that accompany the dreaming experience in the adult are also present in the early months after birth; indeed, they are present in higher proportions. The question of whether infants dream, however, still cannot be answered directly. With regard to subjective characteristics and content, we can make inferences on the basis of indirect evidence whose interpretations, however, vary in relation to the theoretical assumptions and the definition of dreaming adopted by various researchers.

According to David Foulkes, a dream is not a mere analog and pictorial representation of the outside world as perceived by the subject but, rather, a product of psycholinguistic processes that are largely similar to those used in the normal waking state. The peculiar quality of the dream mentation stems from the fact that the cognitive organizing processes are applied to uninhibited memory stores, rather than to the events of the outside world and that such processes occur in the particular situation of loss of voluntary control and of self-regulation induced by sleep, particulary in the REM stage. Thus, dream would be the product of a complex symbolic activity that is not possessed at birth but acquired, in parallel with the development of cognitive–linguistic development. Supported by a longitudinal study conducted in the sleep laboratory, Foulkes claims that "young children may fail to report dreams because they are not having them, rather than because they have forgotten them or are unable to verbalize their contents."

This view is considerably influenced by cognitive approaches oriented more toward studying the mind as an organ of pure cognition. Other researchers place greater emphasis on "sentient" aspects of the mind, and in any case believe it more parsimonious to postulate the ability of dreaming also in the first stages of life. Following this line of reasoning, the researcher is prompted to consider different levels of development of dreaming "skills" and to accept the idea that an infant can experience emotions and fictive visual and kinesthetic sensations. At any rate, the use of narrative as the largely prevalent method to report experiences that may have multimodal origins, though understandable, poses a strong limitation to the interpretation of the data available in the literature.

V. DREAMING IN ANIMALS

Is the REM stage something peculiar to human beings or does it exist in other animal species? After the first successful study carried out in the 1950s by William Dement on cats, research on animals spread rapidly; studies have been carried out on dogs, rats, rabbits, sheep, goats, monkeys, donkeys, chimpanzees, elephants, and even on the opossum (one of the most primitive mammals). Practically all the studied mammals have shown the presence of the REM stage, and its cyclical occurrence is now considered a fundamental feature of sleep in mammals. Apart from mammals, studies seem to indicate the existence of a REM stage, at least in a rudimentary form, in birds but not in reptiles. However, it has been found that at least one reptile, the chameleon, has periods of rapid eye movements when asleep. Phylogenetic considerations therefore lead us to hypothesize that the REM stage appeared for the first time on our planet more than 150 million years ago.

Since it is certain that many animals have recurring periods of REM sleep, is it also reasonable to assume that they dream in the sense that humans do? Anyone with a pet dog, cat, or other animal would swear that their pets dream, judging by the muscle twitches of their limbs, head, and ears that occur ocassionally when asleep. Even Lucretius, in the second century BC, having observed this kind of muscle activity in horses, suggested the possibility that it was linked to their dreaming. According to some, from the developmental

evidence in children we must assume that animals do not dream; according to others, this competence cannot be excluded.

Bearing in mind that, in any case, there is no direct evidence for what takes place in animals' minds, the problem cannot merely imply a straight yes or no answer; even at the purely speculative level, hypotheses for and against dreaming in animals must first specify what is meant by dreaming within the context of the animal species under consideration.

VI. NEUROPHYSIOLOGICAL AND NEUROCHEMICAL MECHANISMS OF DREAMING

The discovery of a REM stage in animals opened up new possibilities of experimental research obviously unfeasible in humans. In the early 1960s, transection studies in cats conducted by the French sleep scientist Michel Jouvet and coworkers pointed to structures in the brain stem as the source of REM sleep. More precisely, these researchers discovered the presence of both a trigger mechanism and a REM sleep clock in the pons. Investigating the pontine reticular formation through the recording microelectrode technique, McCarley and Hobson reported a series of findings that led to the formulation of a "neurochemical" model of the rhythmic appearance of REM sleep. They called this hypothesis the reciprocal interaction model because of its central concept: During REM sleep, aminergic subsets of neurons (the so-called REM-off cells) were inhibited, while cholinergic (REM-on) cells actively discharged. The opposite pattern of neuronal activity was observed during wake.

The relevance of the pontine brain stem in REM sleep generation has been recently confirmed using neuroimaging techniques. Studies based on positron emission tomography (PET), for example, have shown activation of the pontine tegmentum during REM sleep. Significant activations, however, were also seen in many other brain areas, including limbic and paralimbic forebrain regions that are thought to mediate emotion, an important aspect of dreaming. Finally, PET studies have found, during REM sleep, an increase in the activation of unimodal associative visual (Brodmann areas 19 and 37) and auditory (Brodmann area 22) cortices, whereas heteromodal association areas in the frontal and parietal cortex were deactivated. The frontal deactivation could be responsible for another important aspect of dreaming—the bizarreness of dream content. Despite the general deactivation in much of the parietal cortex, an activation of the right parietal operculum, a neural structure that is important for spatial imagery construction, has been reported.

Although in REM sleep the global cerebral metabolism tends to be equal to or greater than that of waking, on the whole these findings suggest that the regional activation during dream mentation is very different from that of waking mentation. In particular, the reduced involvement of the cortical areas devoted to processing sensory information in the waking state, as reported in recent imaging studies, appears to further confirm what was already known—that is, a block against external sensory inputs during REM state and the resorting to systems connected to the internal sphere of emotions and memories.

Having recognized that REM sleep originates in neural structures located in the hindbrain, and not in the forebrain, the following was next question to address: To what extent do these centers control dreaming as well? Evidence in this respect could in theory be gained by studying brain-damaged patients. In fact, if dreaming is caused by neural activity in the brain stem, then brain stem lesions should eliminate both REM and dreaming. The available evidence in this respect is not conclusive, mostly because brain stem lesions that are extensive enough to prevent REM render the patients unconscious. Researchers who do not believe in the causal link between the brain stem and dreaming find indirect support to their claim from evidence in the literature that shows that dreaming is eliminated by forebrain lesions that completely spare the pontine brain stem. However, arguments of this sort rely on an unjustified assumption: They equate the process of dream generation to the process of dream recall and report. Cessation or reduction of dream recall after brain damage may indicate an impairment in any of the processes allowing the production of the dream experience, its recall, and its report and should not be attributed exclusively to the process underlying its production.

The question therefore remains largely unanswered despite major effort. Trying to trace the origin of dreaming to one specific brain area or another may represent too simplistic an approach that does not take into account the complex relationships between higher and lower brain centers. A highly rigid separation between the different sleep and wake phases and between rational thought and the oneiric experience is another source of bias that may have a negative impact on the progress of research. The complex psychophysiological nature of dreaming is increasingly evident, to the point that it has been questioned whether dreaming is a mental experience that can only be linked to sleep.

VII. DOES DREAMING BELONG TO SLEEP?

At the beginning of the 1960s, the interest evoked by the discovery of the REM stage was such that a proposal for calling it "the third state of consciousness" was often advanced. Instead of "wake" and "sleep," it was popular at that time to speak of "wake," "dreaming," and "nondreaming" stages. Meanwhile, the occasional reports of dreaming outside of REM sleep were attributed either to recall of REM material or to the subject's waking confabulations.

Later, however, on the basis of consistent empirical findings of dream-like mentation in non-REM sleep, the notion that thought modalities are completely segregated within the different physiological states was seriously questioned. It was shown that non-REM reports could not be safely ascribed to recall of mental events taking place during REM. A considerable amount of mental activity often indistinguishable from REM dreams was found even at sleep onset (i.e., *before* the first occurrence of a REM phase). The debate between those favoring and those rejecting the hypothesis that dreaming is an exclusive production of REM is ongoing.

It seems clear that some form of mental activity is present in non-REM sleep, although in the past, there was substantial agreement on the fact that REM reports are more frequent, longer, bizarre, and more visually animated and emotional compared to non-REM reports, which appear substantially more mundane and thought-like. Later, however, some researchers challenged this notion, claiming that the special quality of REM imagery largely depends on the greater length of reports due to the stronger and more widespread brain activation present in the REM state; when data are statistically checked for report length, qualitative differences would tend to diminish and often disappear. These findings support the so-called "single dreaming generator" hypothesis—that all sleep mentation derives from a common imagery source that is driven by different levels of brain activation.

Those who oppose such a hypothesis maintain that qualitative differences are not the result of longer report length. On the contrary, report length would depend on the characteristic features of dreaming experiences, which require a greater number of words to explain them, as demonstrated especially by Hunt. If we consider the relations between REM and non-REM stage phenomenology and the neurochemical substrates underlying them, we can see how the debate is not a purely academic one but is quite important in the context of a general psychophysiological theory of dreaming.

On the whole, there is substantial agreement on the fact that when a subject is awakened during the REM stage of sleep, chances of obtaining a more precise report on dream-like mentation are highest. This appears to be the main stage for dreaming activity, but not the exclusive one. Indeed, nobody today would claim that dreaming is absolutely unique to REM sleep. Dream-like mentation, in fact, can be reported in every phase of sleep.

Dream-like mentation has been demonstrated even in certain waking situations. Several years ago, a series of experiments conducted at McGill University in Canada showed that subjects placed in conditions of isolation and sensory deprivation begin, after a certain time, to experience quite vivid pseudohallucinatory-type imagery. An abundance of dream-like mentation was elicited through a so-called "reverie technique" derived from the McGill studies and developed by Mario Bertini, Helen Lewis, and Herman Witkin at the Downstate Medical Center in New York. When put in a particularly monotonous and perceptually destructured environment, awake subjects often experience scattered images and even articulated scenes with a clear dream-like character. Such images, often as complex and bizarre as dreams, seem to appear spontaneously to the subject, sometimes beyond any voluntary effort or control.

Furthermore, this type of imagery can be experienced and reported during wakefulness even without using techniques aimed at facilitating its onset. David Foulkes had subjects lie in laboratory beds during the day and at regular intervals asked them to describe their experience. Most subjects seemed to forget their surroundings and reported vivid and bizarre episodes described as "hallucinatory daydreams" that were so compelling that they were briefly experienced as real. These and other empirical observations justify a growing interest in cutting across the traditional divisions between sleep and waking states and devoting more attention to understanding the functional unifying principles, and organizational coherence, of similar experiences in different states and, specifically, of dream-like experiences through REM, non-REM, and wake states.

VIII. THE FUNCTIONS AND THE MEANING OF DREAMING

Dreaming researchers are usually asked the following fundamental questions: What is the purpose of dreaming? Do dreams have any meaning?

A. The Functions of Dreaming

In answering the first question, today's dream researchers can take advantage of a wealth of precious information available on the physiological characteristics of the stage in which dreaming mainly takes place. This is important information, if only for the opportunity offered from a methodological standpoint, for anyone studying dreaming in a laboratory and from the perspective of one's own specific level of analysis. A problem arises when considering the usefulness of findings at a biological level for understanding the nature and function of dreaming at the mental level. If, as it obviously seems, an accurate description of the psychological sphere of dreaming cannot explain the underlying REM physiology, then the opposite must also be considered true: Finding a physiological basis for dreaming is not the same as explaining it.

While greatly respecting the separate levels of analysis and avoiding any dangerous reductionism toward one side or the other, I believe that a specific analysis of the interface between levels may be useful both for a flexible reformulating of the respective theories and for proposing a general theory of dreaming.

1. Dreaming and Memory Systems

The consistent presence in most dream reports of past memories intermixed with what Freud named "day residues" prompts the commonsense idea that dreaming plays a role in the organization and consolidation of what is experienced during waking.

The hypothesis that memories are consolidated during sleep is a long-standing one. In particular, the diffuse brain activation that characterizes REM sleep could provide the appropriate context for the modifications of synaptic strength within the circuits activated during the wake experience. Such changes are thought to represent the neural basis of memory consolidation.

The evidence in favor of this hypothesis, based mostly on animal experimental models, has been methodologically criticized and is countered by some negative findings. In particular, no damage to memory and learning has occurred after the use of major antidepressant drugs that cause a marked suppression of REM sleep. However, functional brain imaging studies have recently shown that the waking experience influences regional brain activity during subsequent sleep. Specifically, several brain areas that are activated during the execution of a task during wakefulness were significantly more active during REM sleep in subjects previously trained on the task than in nontrained subjects. These results support the hypothesis that memory traces are processed during REM sleep in humans.

Thus, the relation between memory and REM is probably more complex than indicated by the idea of a consolidation function. Special attention to REM state ontogenetic development may offer a first guideline to a better understanding of dreaming function.

2. The Relevance of REM Sleep in the Beginning of Life

As already mentioned, the quantity of REM is particularly high in the early stages of life, in which it is accompanied by the appearance of new behaviors (e.g., facial emotional expressions such as smiling, anger, or fear). The fact that this pattern manifests itself at a time of maximum development of the learning processes leads to a reflection on the role of REM sleep in the structural development of behaviors that are essential for survival.

Howard Roffwarg, Joseph Muzio, and William Dement first proposed that neonate REM sleep provides endogenous nervous system stimulation, which facilitates the maturation and differentiation of sensory and motor brain areas in the absence of external stimuli. Although not above criticism, this view has found credit with many scholars who, albeit with some variations, consider REM sleep to be functional to the general processing and adaptive reprocessing of learning and memory systems.

According to Jouvet, REM sleep would serve the maturation of species-specific basic behavioral patterns at the beginning of life, when there is the highest need for brain programming, as well as the modification and continuous revision of the programs after a certain age, when plasticity in interacting with environment is increasingly required. The shift from the substantial amount of REM sleep in the prenatal and early neonatal period to a sharp downward trend, observed between the second and third postnatal months, should constitute a critical period in the development of interaction between the infant and the environment.

The exchange between what is genetically preordained and rooted in the species' history and what is epigenetic and belonging to the subject's recent and distant past appears to be a suggestive hypothesis for the function of dreaming.

3. REM as a Paradoxical Event

It is possible to deeper into this field of complexity by reflecting on the physiologically peculiar characteristics of the REM stage that have suggested the adjective "paradoxical" for this phase (in fact, this phase appears to be a specific psychophysiological condition in which elevated EEG activity paradoxically coexists with deep muscle atonia and high threshold awakening).

If we monitor an adult human subject's nocturnal sleep by using polygraph recordings, we will find the following sequence of events: Before falling asleep, the EEG signal is mostly composed of low-amplitude, high-frequency waves that are typical of a state of alert activity of the cerebral cortex. Upon sleep onset the signal tends to become increasingly more ample and slower in frequency in direct relation to sleep depth and, therefore, to reduced vigilance. However, with the onset of the REM stage (after approximately 90–100 min) and for the whole duration of it, the EEG trace looks flatter and faster again, with characteristics similar to those of the waking state, even though the subject remains in a state of complete nonresponsiveness.

The paradoxical aspect of the transition from non-REM to REM sleep is that, in parallel with EEG signs of a generalized cortical reactivation, a further "detachment" from the outside world can be clearly observed. A mechanism of presynaptic inhibition originating in the brain stem reduces the input of sensory information from the environment (hence, the heightened awaking thresholds). Furthermore, with the exception of the oculomotor and middle ear muscles, a descending mechanism of postsynaptic inhibition causes a generalized tonic paralysis. Thus, during REM sleep the human organism appears disconnected from the outside world, but brain activity is quite intense, especially in certain regions.

Some researchers view paradoxical sleep and wakefulness as almost identical intrinsic functional states, both able to generate subjective awareness. The difference is in the orientation of the attention. According to Rodolfo Llinas, REM sleep can be considered as a modified attentive state in which attention is turned away from the sensory input and toward memories. The idea of an attentive state of REM sleep receives further support from the similarities between some physiological features of this phase and the classic physiological counterparts of the wake Pavlovian orientation reflex.

Thus, the brain in REM sleep appears to shift to an off-line status where inhibition of the sensory and motor systems corresponds to an activation of limbic and paralimbic regions that neuroimaging studies have shown to be connected with memories and emotions. The subjective experience of dream imagery characteristic of this phase could be the result of such a shift.

The idea of a duality between executive control (i.e., the waking state) oriented toward the outside and a state that favors internal reprocessing (i.e., the sleep state) has prompted several researchers to use the metaphor of the computer, which at times is in the state of executing programs and at other times undergoes reprogramming. To a certain extent, the same concept can be found, in a less prosaic style, in Heraclitus' thinking: "He who is awake lives in a single world common to all; he who is asleep retires to his own particular world."

Some experiments in animals may provide further insight into the processes that take place in the REM phase. Michael Jouvet and subsequently Adrian Morrison obtained some interesting results when certain pontine nuclei known to be responsible for motor paralysis during REM sleep were lesioned in cats. Each time the animal entered REM sleep, it showed an astonishing pattern of highly organized but entirely automatic motor behaviors, such as orienting and exploring its territory, using the cat litter, licking itself, attacking an imaginary prey, and having a fit of rage. The animal seemed to act out basic instinctive and highly species-specific behavioral patterns. These experimental observations reinforced the previously mentioned hypothesis of a role of REM sleep in programming such patterns.

On the whole, psychophysiological data on the ontogenetic development and phenomenological characteristics of REM sleep have opened interpretational scenarios centered on the idea of a privileged function of the REM phase with respect to the adaptive organizing and reorganizing of memory systems. This function does not necessarily imply the subjective experience of dreaming; in principle, it is not necessary for the dream to be recalled in order to accomplish it.

B. Does Dreaming Have Any Meaning?

Everything that has been said so far about the REM stage (i.e., the long philogenetic history and the presence of a physiological mechanism guaranteeing its regular ultradian cycle) amply justifies the recognition of the important biological value attributed to a sleep stage that is also called dreaming stage because of its strong links with dream mentation. Moreover, the hypothesis that this biological function may be linked to processes that are crucial for the development and adaptive functioning of the mind is a reasonable one, even though not all researchers agree with it.

Even the most compelling evidence in favor of a primary role for the REM stage in mammalian physiology would not in itself justify the attribution of meaning to the subjective experience of dreaming. In principle, dreaming could be a mere by-product of a fundamental but still largely unknown biological function.

There is no doubt that all cultures throughout history have posited the meaningfulness of dreams. Modern neurophysiology as well as cognitive neuroscience have focused more on the dreaming process than on its content. In the most entrenched positions of these approaches, a question such as "Is it possible to recognize the presence of a message or the intention to communicate in dreaming?" would normally receive a negative answer.

The activation–synthesis theory supported by Hobson and McCarley, for example, maintains that dreaming is the result of a "bad job" carried out by the cerebral cortex when, intensely activated by random stimulation coming from the brain stem, it tries to provide a plausible narrative context for the stimulation. For more cognitiveley oriented scholars such as Foulkes, the precondition of dreaming is the relinquishment of the voluntary self-regulation and the consequent diffuse activation of mnemonic systems; the organization imposed by a dream production system on the mnemonic units is syntactic in nature, not semantic.

According to both views, dreaming is devoid of any meaningful intention. At the formal level of dream mentation, however, the interpretations differ. Hobson and MacCarley, more anchored to the biological side, believe that the formal aspects of dreams are isomorphic expressions of the peculiar physiological state of REM sleep. According to Foulkes dream mentation is substantially independent from the REM physiology and under the direct control of the same narrative-linguistic generator that controls cognitive processes during wakefulness. In both cases, we are evidently a long way from the Freudian view, whereby the manifest content of dreams conveys a censored deeper latent message to be decoded that strongly points to the dreamer's unconscious problems.

It must be stressed, however, that even in modern neuroscientific literature, there is wide agreement that dreams do convey some sort of meaning and reveal something about the dreamer. The information may be of two types. The first kind concerns the peculiar characteristics of the processes with which the dreamer constructs the dream. This aspect is particularly meaningful for cognitive sciences. Authoritative scholars hold that, applying the same cognitive–linguistic methods of analysis used in waking or stimulus-dependent narrations, the study of self-organizational mechanisms of dreaming may yield information of great value not only concerning dreaming but also on all those forms of stimulus-independent thought occurring spontaneously over the 24-h period. In this sense, although it is true that the application of the cognitive approaches is certainly useful for the study of dreaming, we should not overlook the importance of studying the mind's involuntary organizing system, in REM as well as in other sleep and wake conditions, in order to broaden our knowledge of the overall mental functioning.

A second, generally accepted notion concerns dreams as sources of information on the dreamer's personality. For example, the fact that some people may experience more frequent dreams of certain expressive or conflictual contents rather than others may, with suitable care and attention to context, provide indirect indications of the dreamer's personality. In this view, which implies the possibility of diverse clinical applications, the dream is "informative" and not "intentional" in nature.

Other perspectives that are worth considering view dream not as "random nonsense" but as a different form of intelligence with respect to that expressed in the rational, logical forms more typical of wakefulness (i.e., not alternative but complementary to it). In line with certain anticipatory views expressed by Jung, Harry Hunt summarizes this concept as follows:

A host of contemporary "dream-workers" holds that the emergent sources of dreaming, at least much of the time, are not "primitive" or "disruptive" at all.

Rather, they constitute the spontaneous expressions of a symbolic intelligence alternative to standard representational thought and variously termed "imagistic," "affective," or "presentational". ... I would not want ... to imply an adherence to rigid dual code models of human intelligence, which tend to distinguish an abstract verbal capacity from a more rudimentary imagistic one. Not only is the latter fully capable of its own line of abstract development, as seen in certain dreams, alterations of consciousness, and aesthetics, but each of these "frames" seems capable of endlessly, complex interactions at all levels of their potential unfolding.

IX. CONCLUDING REMARKS

Studies carried out during the past 50 years, particularly those using recent neuroimaging techniques, show that the areas of the central nervous system that seem more active in REM sleep are found in the brain stem, in the limbic system, and in secondary, associative cortical areas, at variance with the alert waking state, during which the frontal lobes and the primary sensory and motor cortices are privileged. Thus, the stage of sleep in which dreaming has its greatest expression appears to be characterized by a prevalent orientation toward the inner world of memories and emotions. In line with this view, the adjective "paradoxical," as applied to the REM stage, may sound improper. Its physiological characteristics, in fact, appear perfectly orthodox if considered as an expression of a positive and qualitative shifting toward a greater resonance of the inner world—a shifting, however, that although paradigmatic for the REM state, may be available throughout the sleep and wake cycle.

As discussed earlier, a variety of findings encourage stepping beyond the Manichean barriers separating the states of wakefulness, REM sleep, and non-REM sleep in order to appreciate the continuity of the mind across these states. For instance, although it may be true that mentation during REM is largely bizarre, systematic demonstrations indicate that REM dream content also shows a heavy reliance on representations of familiar elements from the waking environment. By the same token, if it is true that during the awake state resources are usually employed in relating to the external environment, there are still opportunities for coding operations and processing of internal material. Consider, for instance, the fantasy activity conceived as ongoing information processing. As Jerome Singer states, "the popular notion of a daydream represents only one manifestation of a more general class of phenomena perhaps best described as internally generated diversion from an ongoing motor or cognitive task." There is evidence that some type of coding and restructuring of long-term stored material goes on a great deal of the time while the organism is awake.

The critical point that needs further examination is the psychophysiological significance of this shifting. The first question is whether accessing and activating the previously mentioned brain areas in the REM stage—besides serving a possible, although not yet known, biological function—involves any direct functional value for the mind. Second, the problem arises of the semantic meaning of dream and dream-like mentation; as stated earlier, dreaming activity could in principle produce some objective organizational benefit to the mind, independently from the subjective experiencing of dreaming and from the content of the experienced dream, and that organizational benefit may be augmented by dream recall and interpretation.

An overview of the different positions on these issues shows that scholars in the broader field of dreaming can be divided into approximately two groups. On the one hand are those who, although not rejecting the adaptive hypothesis, from various angles and with different reasoning tend to characterize dream mentation as a degradation of the self-conscious, self-controlled thought of wakefulness. For example, sleep physiologist Giuseppe Moruzzi, while maintaining that sleep has a function coherent with the need to restore the myriad of cerebral neural networks, also believed dreaming to be the expression of an "impoverished conscience." Taking into account the intense activity of the brain in REM sleep, he stated that "the plastic debt accumulated during wakefulness could be paid while the cortical neurons continued to discharge impulses, even if in a different way than usual." Loss of consciousness could thus be the result not of a silence but of the temporary loss of a meaningful dialogue between nerve cells.

On the other hand, there are scholars who view REM sleep as a privileged theater for the type of plastic revision on which the adaptive flexibility of our central nervous system is based. In their view, accessing memory stores may set the potential for creating new associations, rearranging past patterns, and reformulating future plans in accord with experiences of the day. Rather than "temporary loss of a meaningful dialogue," dreaming represents the "temporary emergence of a differently meaningful dialogue." In such a perspective, at least some dreaming would be the expression of an alternative form of "intelligence," common to a variety of thinking modalities leaning toward the imagery and metaphoric side of the human vast symbolic capacity. A "symbolic–presentational" form of intelligence (Susanne Langer's terminology), although semantic and communicative, resists a complete narrative formulation when compared to the "symbolic–representational" intelligence that prevails in the vigilant waking state.

In 1890, William James stated: "Our normal waking consciousness, rational consciousness as we call it, is but one special type of consciousness, whilst all about it, parted from it by the filmiest of screens, there lie potential forms of consciousness entirely different." Thus, even though the age-old dilemma of dreaming has been engaged by modern science, we still remain within the interpretational dualism that has characterized the history of thought on dreaming. The work carried out during the past 50 years, however, seems to justify a certain optimism with respect to a converging of views in the near future.

See Also the Following Articles

COGNITIVE PSYCHOLOGY, OVERVIEW • CONSCIOUSNESS • CREATIVITY • DEMENTIA • HALLUCINATIONS • NEUROIMAGING • SLEEP DISORDERS • UNCONSCIOUS, THE

Suggested Reading

Antrobus, J., and Bertini, M. (Eds.) (1992). *The Neuropsychology of Sleep and Dreaming.* Erlbaum, New York.

Aserinsky, E., and Kleitman, N. (1953). Regularly occurring periods of ocular motility and concomitant phenomena during sleep. *Science* **118**, 1150–1155.

Dement, W., and Kleitman, N. (1957). The relation of eye movements during sleep to dream activity: An objective method for the study of dreaming. *J. Exp. Psychol.* **55**, 339–346.

Foulkes, D. (1985). *Dreaming: a Cognitive–Psychological Analysis.* Erlbaum, New York.

Hobson, A. (1988). *The Dreaming Brain.* Basic Books, New York.

Hunt, H. (1989). *The multiplicity of dreams.* Yale Univ. Press, New Haven, CT.

Sleep and dreaming [Special issue] (2000). *Behav. Brain Sci.* **23**(6).

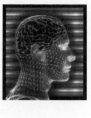

Dyslexia

H. BRANCH COSLETT
University of Pennsylvania School of Medicine

GLOSSARY

central dyslexia A reading disorder caused by impairment of the "deeper" or "higher" reading functions by which letter strings mediate access to meaning or speech production mechanisms.

deep dyslexia A disorder characterized by semantic errors (e.g., "king" read as "prince"), poor reading of abstract compared to concrete words (e.g., "idea" vs "desk"), and an inability to "sound out" words.

peripheral dyslexia A reading disorder attributable to a disruption of the processing of visual aspects of the stimulus that prevents the patient from reliably processing a letter string.

phonologic dyslexia A disorder characterized by a largely preserved ability to read familiar words but an inability to read unfamiliar words or nonword letter strings (e.g., "flig") because of an inability to use a "sounding out" strategy.

surface dyslexia A disorder characterized by reliance on a "sounding out" strategy with the result that words that have atypical print-to-sound correspondences are read incorrectly (e.g., "yacht" read as "yatchet").

Unlike the ability to speak, which has presumably evolved over tens of thousands of years, the ability to read is a relatively recent development that is dependent on both the capacity to process complex visual stimuli and the ability to link the visual stimulus to phonologic, syntactic, and other language capacities. Perhaps as a consequence of the wide range of cognitive operations involved, reading is compromised in many patients with cerebral lesions, particularly those involving the left hemisphere. The resultant reading impairments, or acquired dyslexias, take many different forms, reflecting the breakdown of specific components of the reading process. In this article, I briefly review the history of the study of acquired dyslexia and introduce a model of the processes involved in normal reading. Specific syndromes of acquired dyslexia are discussed. I also briefly discuss connectionist accounts of reading and the anatomic basis of reading as revealed by recent functional imaging studies.

I. HISTORICAL OVERVIEW

Perhaps the most influential early contributions to the understanding of dyslexia were provided in the 1890s by Dejerine, who described two patients with quite different patterns of reading impairment. Dejerine's first patient manifested impaired reading and writing subsequent to an infarction involving the left parietal lobe. Dejerine termed this disorder "alexia with agraphia" and attributed the disturbance to a disruption of the "optical image of words" that he thought to be supported by the left angular gyrus. In an account that in some respects presages contemporary psychological accounts, Dejerine concluded that reading and writing required the activation of these optical images and that the loss of the images resulted in the inability to recognize or write even familiar words.

Dejerine's second patient was quite different. This patient exhibited a right homonymous hemianopia and was unable to read aloud or for comprehension but could write. This disorder, designated "alexia without agraphia" (also known as agnosic alexia and pure alexia), was attributed by Dejerine to a "disconnection" between visual information presented to the right hemisphere and the left angular gyrus that he assumed to be critical for the recognition of words.

After the seminal contributions of Dejerine, the study of acquired dyslexia languished for decades, during which time the relatively few investigations that were reported focused primarily on the anatomic underpinnings of the disorders. The field was revitalized by the elegant and detailed analysis by Marshall and Newcombe that demonstrated that by virtue of a careful investigation of the pattern of reading deficits exhibited by dyslexic subjects, distinctly different and reproducible types of reading deficits could be elucidated. The insights provided by Marshall and Newcombe provided much of the basis for the "dual-route" model of word reading.

II. READING MECHANISMS AND THE CLASSIFICATION OF DYSLEXIAS

Reading is a complicated process that involves many different procedures, including low-level visual processing, accessing meaning and phonology, and motor aspects of speech production. Figure 1 provides a graphic depiction of the relationship between these procedures. This "information processing" model will serve as the basis for the discussion of the mechanisms involved in reading and the specific forms of acquired dyslexia. It must be noted, however, that the dual-route model of reading that will be employed for purposes of exposition is not uncontested. Alternatives to the information processing accounts, such as the triangle model of Plaut, Seidenberg, McClelland, and colleagues, will also be discussed.

Reading requires that the visual system efficiently process a complicated stimulus that, at least for alphabet-based languages, is composed of smaller meaningful units—letters. In part because the number of letters is small in relation to the number of words, there is often a considerable visual similarity between words (e.g., "structure" vs "stricture"). Additionally, the position of letters within the letter string is also critical to word identification (consider "mast" vs

"mats"). In light of these factors, it is perhaps not surprising that reading places a substantial burden on the visual system and that disorders of visual processing or visual attention may substantially disrupt reading.

Normal readers recognize written words so rapidly and seemingly effortlessly that one might suspect that the word is identified as a unit, much as we identify an object from its visual form. At least for normal readers under standard conditions, this does not appear to be the case. Instead, analyses of normal reading suggest that word recognition requires that letters be identified as alphabetic symbols. Support for this claim comes from demonstrations that presenting words in an unfamiliar form—for example, by alternating the case of the letters (e.g., wOrD) or introducing spaces between words (e.g., f o o d)—does not substantially influence reading speed or accuracy. These data argue for a stage of letter identification in which the graphic form (whether printed or written) is transformed into a string of alphabetic characters (W-O-R-D), sometimes referred to as abstract letter identities.

The mechanism by which the position of letters within the stimulus is determined and maintained is not clear. Possibilities include associating the letter in position 1 to the letter in position 2, and so on; binding each letter to a frame that specifies letter position; or labeling each letter with its position in the word. Finally, it should be noted that in normal circumstances letters are not processed in a strictly serial fashion but letter strings are processed in parallel (provided they are not too long). Disorders of reading resulting from impairment in the processing of the visual stimulus or the failure of this visual information to contact stored knowledge appropriate to a letter string are designated as peripheral dyslexias.

In dual-route models of reading, the identity of a letter string may be determined by many distinct procedures. The first is a "lexical" procedure by which the letter string is identified by means of matching the letter string to an entry in a stored catalog of familiar words, or visual word form system. As indicated in Fig. 1 and discussed later, this procedure, which in some respects is similar to looking up a word in a dictionary, provides access to the meaning, phonologic form, and at least some of the syntactic properties of the word. Dual-route models of reading also assume that the letter string can be converted directly to a phonological form by means of the application of a set of learned correspondences between orthography and phonology. On this account, meaning may then be accessed from the phonologic form of the word.

Support for dual-route models of reading comes from a variety of sources. For present purposes, perhaps the most relevant evidence was provided by Marshall and Newcombe's groundbreaking description of "deep" and "surface" dyslexia. These investigators described a patient (GR) who read approximately 50% of concrete nouns (e.g., "table" and "doughnut") but was severely impaired in the reading of abstract nouns (e.g., "destiny" and "truth") and all other parts of speech. The most striking aspect of GR's performance, however, was his tendency to produce errors that appeared to be semantically related to the target word (e.g., "speak" read as "talk"). Marshall and Newcombe designated this disorder deep dyslexia. These investigators also described two patients whose primary deficit appeared to be an inability to reliably apply grapheme–phoneme correspondences. Thus, JC, for example, rarely applied the rule of "e" (which lengthens the preceding vowel in words such as "like") and experienced great difficulties in deriving the appropriate phonology for consonant clusters and vowel digraphs. The disorder characterized by impaired application of print-to-sound correspondences was termed surface dyslexia.

On the basis of these observations, Marshall and Newcombe argued that the meaning of written words could be accessed by two distinct procedures. The first was a direct procedure whereby familiar words activated the appropriate stored representation (or visual word form), which in turn activated meaning directly; reading in deep dyslexia, which was characterized by semantically based errors (of which the patient was often unaware), was assumed to involve this procedure. The second procedure was assumed to be a phonologically based process in which grapheme-to-phoneme or print-to-sound correspondences were employed to derive the appropriate phonology (or "sound out" the word); the reading of surface dyslexics was assumed to be mediated by this nonlexical procedure. Although many of Marshall and Newcombe's specific hypotheses have subsequently been criticized, their argument that reading may be mediated by two distinct procedures has received considerable empirical support.

The information processing model of reading depicted in Fig. 1 provides three distinct procedures for oral reading. Two of these procedures correspond to those described by Marshall and Newcombe. The first (Fig. 1A), involves the activation of a stored entry in the visual word form system and the subsequent access to semantic information and ultimately activation of the stored sound of the word at the level of the

phonologic output lexicon. The second (Fig. 1B), involves the nonlexical grapheme-to-phoneme or print-to-sound translation process; this procedure does not entail access to any stored information about words but, rather, is assumed to be mediated by access to a catalog of correspondences stipulating the pronunciation of phonemes. Many information processing accounts of the language mechanisms subserving reading incorporate a third procedure. This mechanism (Fig. 1C), is lexically based in that it is assumed to involve the activation of the visual word form system and the phonologic output lexicon. The procedure differs from the lexical procedure described previously, however, in that there is no intervening activation of semantic information. This procedure has been called the direct reading mechanism or route. Support for the direct lexical mechanism comes from many sources, including observations that some subjects read aloud words that they do not appear to comprehend. For example, Coslett reported a patient whose inability to read aloud nonwords (e.g., "flig") suggested that she was unable to employ print-to-sound conversion procedures. Additionally, she exhibited semantic errors in writing and repetition and performed poorly on a synonymy judgment task with low imageability words, suggesting that semantic representations were imprecise. Semantic errors and imageability effects were not observed in reading; additionally, she read aloud low imageability words as well as many other words that she appeared to be unable to comprehend. Both observations suggest that her oral reading was not mediated by semantics. We argued that these data provided evidence for a reading mechanism that is independent of semantic representations and does not entail print-to-sound conversion—that is, a direct route from visual word forms to the phonological output representations.

III. PERIPHERAL DYSLEXIAS

A useful starting point in the discussion of acquired dyslexia is the distinction made by Shallice and Warrington between "peripheral" and "central" dyslexias. The former are conditions characterized by a deficit in the processing of visual aspects of the stimulus that prevents the patient from reliably matching a familiar word to its stored visual form or visual word form. In contrast, central dyslexias reflect impairment to the "deeper" or "higher" reading functions by which visual word forms mediate access to meaning to speech production mechanisms. In the

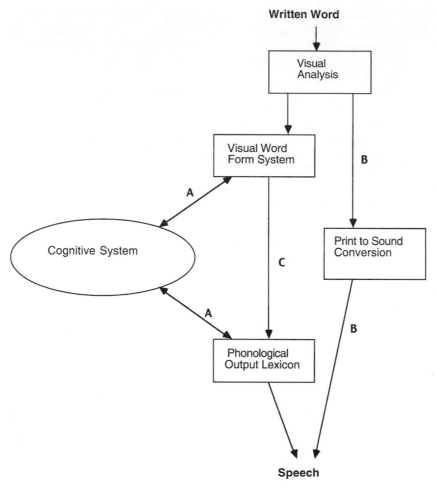

Figure 1   The relationship between the procedures involved in reading.

following sections, I discuss the major types of peripheral dyslexia.

A. Alexia without Agraphia (Pure Alexia; Letter-by-Letter Reading)

This disorder is among the most common of the peripheral reading disturbances. It is associated with a left hemisphere lesion affecting left occipital cortex (responsible for the analysis of visual stimuli on the right side of space) and/or the structures (left lateral geniculate nucleus of the thalamus and white matter, including callosal fibers from the intact right visual cortex) that provide input to this region of the brain. It is likely that the lesion either blocks direct visual input to the mechanisms that process printed words in the left hemisphere or disrupts the visual word form

system. Some of these patients seem to be unable to read at all, whereas others do so slowly and laboriously by means of a process that involves serial letter identification (often termed "letter-by-letter" reading). At first, letter-by-letter readers often pronounce the letter names aloud; in some cases, they misidentify letters, usually on the basis of visual similarity, as in the case of N → M. Their reading is also abnormally slow.

It was long thought that patients with pure alexia were unable to read except letter by letter. There is now evidence that some of them do retain the ability to recognize letter strings, although this does not guarantee that they will be able to read aloud. Several different paradigms have demonstrated the preservation of word recognition. Some patients demonstrate a word superiority effect of superior letter recognition when the letter is part of a word (e.g., the "R" in "WORD") than when it occurs in a string of unrelated letters (e.g., "WKRD"). Second, some of them have been able to perform lexical decision tasks (determining whether a letter string constitutes a real word or not) and semantic categorization tasks (indicating whether or not a word belongs to a category, such as foods or animals) at above chance levels when words are presented too rapidly to support letter-by-letter reading. Brevity of presentation is critical in that longer exposure to the letter string seems to engage the letter-by-letter strategy, which appears to interfere with the ability to perform the covert reading task. In fact, the patient may show better performance on lexical decision at shorter (e.g., 250 msec) than at longer presentations (e.g., 2 sec) that engage the letter-by-letter strategy but do not allow it to proceed to completion. A compelling example comes from a previously reported patient who was given 2 sec to scan the card containing the stimulus. The patient did not take advantage of the full inspection time when he was performing lexical decision and categorization tasks; instead, he glanced at the card briefly and looked away, perhaps to avoid letter-by-letter reading. The capacity for covert reading has also been demonstrated in two pure alexics who were completely unable to employ the letter-by-letter reading strategy. These patients appeared to recognize words but were rarely able to report them, although they sometimes generated descriptions that were related to the word's meaning (e.g., "cookies" → "candy, a cake"). In some cases, patients have shown some recovery of oral reading over time, although this capacity appears to be limited to concrete words.

The mechanisms that underlie implicit or covert reading remain controversial. Dejerine, who provided the first description of pure alexia, suggested that the analysis of visual input in these patients is performed by the right hemisphere as a result of the damage to the visual cortex on the left. It should be noted, however, that not all lesions to the left visual cortex give rise to alexia. A critical feature that supports continued left hemisphere processing is the preservation of callosal input from the visual processing on the right. One possible account is that covert reading reflects printed word recognition on the part of the right hemisphere, which is unable either to articulate the word or (in most cases) to adequately communicate its identity to the language area of the left hemisphere. By this account, letter-by-letter reading is carried out by the left hemisphere using letter information transferred serially and inefficiently from the right. Furthermore, this assumes that when the letter-by-letter strategy is implemented, it may be difficult for the patient to attend to the products of word processing in the right hemisphere. Consequently, performance on lexical decision and categorization tasks declines. Additional evidence supporting the right hemisphere account of reading in pure alexia is presented later.

Alternative accounts of pure alexia have also been proposed. Behrmann and colleagues, for example, proposed that the disorder is attributable to impaired activation of orthographic representations. By this account, reading is assumed to reflect the residual functioning of the same interactive system that supported normal reading premorbidly.

Other investigators have attributed pure dyslexia to a visual impairment that precludes activation of orthographic representations. Chialant and Caramazza, for example, reported a patient, MJ, who processed single, visually presented letters normally and performed well on a variety of tasks assessing the orthographic lexicon with auditorily presented stimuli. In contrast, MJ exhibited significant impairments in the processing of letter strings. The investigators suggest that MJ was unable to transfer information from the intact visual processing system in the right hemisphere to the intact language processing mechanisms of the left hemisphere.

B. Neglect Dyslexia

Parietal lobe lesions can result in a deficit that involves neglect of stimuli on the side of space contralateral to the lesion, a disorder referred to as hemispatial. In most cases, this disturbance arises with damage to the right parietal lobe; therefore, attention to the left side of space is most often affected. The severity of neglect is generally greater when there are stimuli on the right as well as on the left; attention is drawn to the right-sided stimuli at the expense of those on the left—a phenomenon known as "extinction." Typical clinical manifestations include bumping into objects on the left, failure to dress the left side of the body, drawing objects that are incomplete on the left, and reading problems that involve neglect of the left portions of words (i.e., neglect dyslexia).

With respect to neglect dyslexia, it has been found that such patients are more likely to ignore letters in nonwords (e.g., the first two letters in "bruggle") than letters in real words (compare with "snuggle"). This suggests that the problem does not reflect a total failure to process letter information but, rather, an attentional impairment that affects conscious recognition of the letters. Performance often improves when words are presented vertically or spelled aloud. In addition, there is evidence that semantic information can be processed in neglect dyslexia, and that the ability to read words aloud improves when oral reading follows a semantic task.

Neglect dyslexia has also been reported in patients with left hemisphere lesions. In these patients, the deficiency involves the right side of words. Here, visual neglect is usually confined to words and is not ameliorated by presenting words vertically or spelling them aloud. This disorder has therefore been termed a "positional dyslexia," whereas the right hemisphere deficit has been termed a "spatial neglect dyslexia."

C. Attentional Dyslexia

Attentional dyslexia is a disorder characterized by at least relatively preserved reading of single words but impaired reading of words in the context of other words or letters. This infrequently reported disorder was first described by Shallice and Warrington, who reported two patients with brain tumors involving (at least) the left parietal lobe. Both patients exhibited relatively good performance with single letters or words but were significantly impaired in the recognition of the same stimuli when presented as part of an array. For example, both patients read single letters accurately but made significantly more errors naming letters when presented as part of 3×3 or 5×5 arrays. Similarly, both patients correctly read more than 90% of single words but read only approximately 80% of words when presented in the context of three additional words. Although not fully investigated, it is worth noting that the patients were also impaired in recognizing line drawings and silhouettes when presented in an array.

Two additional observations from these patients warrant attention. First, Shallice and Warrington demonstrated that for both patients naming of single black letters was adversely affected by the simultaneous presentation of red flanking stimuli and that flanking letters were more disruptive than numbers. For example, both subjects were more likely to correctly name the black (middle) letter when presented "37L82" compared to "ajGyr." Second, the investigators examined the errors produced in the tasks in which patients were asked to report letters and words in rows of two to four items. They found different error patterns with letters and words. Whereas both patients tended to err in the letter report task by naming letters that appeared in a different

location in the array, patients often named words that were not present in the array. Interestingly, many of these errors were interpretable as letter transpositions between words. Citing the differential effects of letter versus number flankers as well as the absence of findings suggesting a deficit in response selection, these investigators attributed the disorder to a failure of transmission of information from a nonsemantic perceptual stage to a semantic processing stage. Another patient, BAL, was also reported by Warrington and colleagues. BAL was able to read single words but exhibited a substantial impairment in the reading of letters and words in an array. BAL exhibited no evidence of visual disorientation and was able to identify a target letter in an array of "X"s or "O"s. He was impaired, however, in the naming of letters or words when these stimuli were flanked by other members of the same stimulus category. This patient's attentional dyslexia was attributed to an impairment arising after words and letters had processed as units.

Recently, Saffran and Coslett reported a patient, NY, with biopsy-proven Alzheimer's disease that appeared to selectively involve posterior cortical regions who exhibited attentional dyslexia. NY scored within the normal range on verbal subtests of the WAIS-R but was unable to perform any of the performance subtests. He performed normally on the Boston Naming Test but performed quite poorly on a variety of experimental tasks assessing visuospatial processing and visual attention. Despite his visuoperceptual deficits, NY's reading of single words was essentially normal. He read 96% of 200 words presented for 100 msec (unmasked). Like previously reported patients with this disorder, NY exhibited a substantial decline in performance when asked to read two words presented simultaneously. He read both words correctly in only 50% of 385 trials with a 250-msec stimulus exposure. Most errors were omissions of one word. Of greatest interest, however, was the fact that NY produced a substantial number of "blend" errors in which letters from the two words were combined to generate a response that was not present in the display. For example, when shown "flip shot," NY responded "ship." Like the blend errors produced by normal subjects with brief stimulus presentation. NY's blend errors were characterized by the preservation of letter position information; thus, in the preceding example, the letters in the blend response ("ship") retained the same serial position in the incorrect response. NY produced significantly more blend errors than did five controls whose overall level of performance had been matched to NY's by virtue of brief stimulus exposure (range, 17–83 msec). A subsequent experiment demonstrated that for NY, but not for controls, blend errors were encountered significantly less often when the target words differed in case ("desk FEAR").

Saffran and Coslett considered the central deficit in attentional dyslexia to be impaired control of a filtering mechanism that normally serves to suppress input from unattended words or letters in the display. Specifically, they suggested that as a consequence of the patient's inability to effectively deploy the "spotlight" of attention to a particular region of interest (e.g., a single word or a single letter), multiple stimuli fall within the attentional spotlight. Because visual attention may serve to integrate visual feature information, impaired modulation of the spotlight of attention would be expected to generate word blends and other errors reflecting the incorrect concatenation of letters.

Saffran and Coslett also argued that loss of location information also contributed to NY's reading deficit. Several lines of evidence support such a conclusion. First, NY was impaired relative to controls with respect to both accuracy and reaction time on a task in which he was required to indicate if a line was inside or outside a circle. Second, NY exhibited a clear tendency to omit one member of a double-letter pair (e.g., "reed" → "red"). This phenomenon, also demonstrated in normal subjects, has been attributed to the loss of location information that normally helps to differentiate two tokens of the same object. Finally, it should be noted that the well-documented observation that the blend errors of normal subjects and attentional dyslexics preserve letter position is not inconsistent with the claim that impaired location information contributes to attentional dyslexia. Migration or blend errors reflect a failure to link words or letters to a location in space, whereas the letter position constraint reflects the properties of the word processing system. The latter, which is assumed to be at least relatively intact in patients with attentional dyslexia, specifies letter location with respect to the word form rather than space.

D. Other Peripheral Dyslexias

Peripheral dyslexias may be observed in a variety of conditions involving visuoperceptual or attentional deficits. Patients with simultanagnosia, a disorder characterized by an inability to "see" more than one object in an array, are often able to read single words but are incapable of reading text. Other patients with simultanagnosia exhibit substantial problems in reading even single words.

Patients with degenerative conditions involving the posterior cortical regions may also exhibit profound deficits in reading as part of their more general impairment in visuospatial processing. Several patterns of impairment may be observed in these patients. Some patients exhibit attentional dyslexia with letter migration and blend errors, whereas other patients exhibiting deficits that are in certain respects similar do not produce migration or blend errors in reading or illusory conjuctions in visual search tasks. It has been suggested that at least some patients with these disorders suffer from a progressive restriction in the domain to which they can allocate visual attention. As a consequence of this impairment, these patients may exhibit an effect of stimulus size such that they are able to read a word in small print but when shown the same word in large print see only a single letter.

IV. CENTRAL DYSLEXIAS

A. Deep Dyslexia

Deep dyslexia, initially described by Marshall and Newcombe in 1973, is the most extensively investigated of the central dyslexias and, in many respects, the most compelling. Interest in deep dyslexia is due in large part to the intrinsically interesting hallmark of the syndrome—the production of semantic errors. Shown the word "castle," a deep dyslexic may respond "knight"; shown the word "bird," the patient may respond "canary." At least for some deep dyslexics, it is clear that these errors are not circumlocutions. Semantic errors may represent the most frequent error type in some deep dyslexics, whereas in other patients they comprise a small proportion of reading errors. Deep dyslexics also typically produce frequent "visual" errors (e.g., "skate" read as "scale") and morphological errors in which a prefix or suffix is added, deleted, or substituted (e.g., "scolded" read as "scolds" and "governor" read as "government").

Additional features of the syndrome include a greater success in reading words of high compared to low imageability. Thus, words such as "table," "chair," "ceiling," and "buttercup," the referent of which is concrete or imageable, are read more successfully than words such as "fate," "destiny," "wish," and "universal," which denote abstract concepts.

Another characteristic feature of deep dyslexia is a part of speech effect such that nouns are typically read more reliably than modifiers (adjectives and adverbs), which are in turn read more accurately than verbs. Deep dyslexics manifest particular difficulty in the reading of functors (a class of words that includes pronouns, prepositions, conjunctions, and interrogatives including "that," "which," "they," "because," and "under"). The striking nature of the part of speech effect may be illustrated by the patient who correctly read the word "chrysanthemum" but was unable to read the word "the." Most errors to functors involve the substitution of a different functor ("that" read as "which") rather than the production of words of a different class, such as nouns or verbs. Because functors are in general less imageable than nouns, some investigators have claimed that the apparent effect of part of speech is in reality a manifestation of the pervasive imageability effect. There is no consensus on this point because other investigators have suggested that the part of speech effect is observed even if stimuli are matched for imageability.

All deep dyslexics exhibit a substantial impairment in the reading of nonwords. When confronted with letter strings such as "flig" or "churt," deep dyslexics are typically unable to employ print-to-sound correspondences to derive phonology; nonwords frequently elicit "lexicalization" errors (e.g., "flig" read as "flag"), perhaps reflecting a reliance on lexical reading in the absence of access to reliable print-to-sound correspondences.

Finally, it should be noted that the accuracy of oral reading may be determined by context. This is illustrated by the fact that a patient was able to read aloud the word "car" when it was a noun but not when the same letter string was a conjunction. Thus, when presented the sentence "Le car ralentit car le moteur chauffe" ("The car slowed down because the motor overheated"), the patient correctly pronounced only the first instance of "car." Recently, three deep dyslexics were demonstrated to read function and content words better in a sentence context than when presented alone.

How can deep dyslexia be accommodated by the information processing model of reading illustrated in Fig. 1? Several alternative explanations have been proposed. Some investigators have argued that the reading of deep dyslexics is mediated by a damaged form of the left hemisphere-based system employed in normal reading. In such a hypothesis, multiple processing deficits must be hypothesized to accommodate the full range of symptoms characteristic of deep dyslexia.

First, the strikingly impaired performance in reading nonwords and other tasks assessing phonologic function suggests that the print-to-sound conversion procedure is disrupted. Second, the presence of semantic errors and the effects of imageability (a variable thought to influence processing at the level of semantics) suggest that these patients also suffer from a semantic impairment. Lastly, the production of visual errors suggests that these patients suffer from impairment in the visual word form system or in the processes mediating access to the visual word form system.

Other investigators have argued that deep dyslexics' reading is mediated by a system not normally used in reading (i.e., the right hemisphere). Finally, citing evidence from functional imaging studies demonstrating that deep dyslexic subjects exhibit increased activation in both the right hemisphere and non-perisylvian areas of the left hemisphere, other investigators have suggested that deep dyslexia reflects the recruitment of both right and left hemisphere processes.

B. Phonological Dyslexia: Reading without Print-to-Sound Correspondences

First described in 1979, phonologic dyslexia is perhaps the "purest" of the central dyslexias in that, at least by some accounts, the syndrome is attributable to a selective deficit in the procedure mediating the translation from print to sound. Thus, although in many respects less arresting than deep dyslexia, phonological dyslexia is of considerable theoretical interest.

Phonologic dyslexia is a disorder in which reading of real words may be nearly intact or only mildly impaired. Patients with this disorder, for example, correctly read 85–95% of real words. Some patients read all different types of words with equal facility, whereas other patients are relatively impaired in the reading of functors (or "little words"). Unlike patients with surface dyslexia described later, the regularity of print-to-sound correspondences is not relevant to their performance; thus, phonologic dyslexics are as likely to correctly pronounce orthographically irregular words such as "colonel" as words with standard print-to-sound correspondences such as "administer." Most errors in response to real words bear a visual similarity to the target word (e.g., "topple" read as "table").

The striking and theoretically relevant aspect of the performance of phonologic dyslexics is a substantial impairment in the oral reading of nonword letter strings. We have examined patients with this disorder, for example, who read >90% of real words of all types but correctly pronounce only approximately 10% of nonwords. Most errors to nonwords involve the substitution of a visually similar real word (e.g., "phope" read as "phone") or the incorrect application of print-to-sound correspondences [e.g., "stime" read as "stim" (to rhyme with "him")].

Within the context of the reading model depicted in Fig. 1, the account for this disorder is relatively straightforward. Good performance with real words suggests that the processes involved in normal lexical reading (i.e., visual analysis, the visual word form system, semantics, and the phonological output lexicon) are at least relatively preserved. The impairment in nonword reading suggests that the print-to-sound translation procedure is disrupted.

Recent explorations of the processes involved in nonword reading have identified many distinct procedures involved in this task. If these distinct procedures may be selectively impaired by brain injury, one might expect to observe different subtypes of phonologic dyslexia. Although the details are beyond the scope of this article, there is evidence suggesting that different subtypes of phonologic dyslexia may be observed.

Lastly, it should be noted that several investigators have suggested that phonologic dyslexia is not attributable to a disruption of a reading-specific component of the cognitive architecture but, rather, to a more general phonologic deficit. Support for this assertion comes from the observation that the vast majority of phonologic dyslexics are impaired on a wide variety of nonreading tasks assessing phonology.

In certain respects, phonologic dyslexia is similar to deep dyslexia, the critical difference being that semantic errors are not observed in phonologic dyslexia. Citing the similarity of reading performance and the fact that deep dyslexics may evolve into phonologic dyslexics as they improve, it has been argued that deep and phonologic dyslexia are on a continuum of severity.

C. Surface Dyslexia: Reading without Lexical Access

Surface dyslexia, first described by Marshall and Newcombe, is a disorder characterized by the relatively preserved ability to read words with regular or predictable grapheme-to-phoneme correspondences but substantially impaired reading of words with "irregular" or exceptional print-to-sound correspon-

dences. Thus, patients with surface dyslexia typically are able to read words such as "state," "hand," "mosquito," and "abdominal" quite well, whereas they exhibit substantial problems reading words such as "colonel," "yacht," "island," and "borough," the pronunciation of which cannot be derived by sounding out strategies. Errors to irregular words usually consist of "regularizations"; for example, surface dyslexics may read "colonel" as "kollonel." These patients read nonwords (e.g., "blape") quite well. Finally, it should be noted that all surface dyslexics reported to date read at least some irregular words correctly; patients will often read high-frequency irregular words (e.g., "have" and "some") but some surface dyslexics have been reported to read such low-frequency and highly irregular words as "sieve" and "isle."

As noted previously, some accounts of normal reading postulate that familiar words are read aloud by matching the letter string to a stored representation of the word and retrieving the pronunciation by means of a mechanism linked to semantics or by means of a "direct" route. A critical point to note is that because reading involves stored associations of letter strings and sounds, the pronunciation of the word is not computed by rules but is retrieved, and therefore whether the word contains regular or irregular correspondences does not appear to play a major role in performance.

The fact that the nature of the print-to-sound correspondences significantly influences performance in surface dyslexia suggests that the deficit in this syndrome is in the mechanisms mediating lexical reading—that is, in the semantically mediated and "direct" reading mechanisms. Similarly, the preserved ability to read words and nonwords demonstrates that the procedures by which words are sounded out are at least relatively preserved.

In the context of the information processing discussed previously, how would one account for surface dyslexia? Scrutiny of the model depicted in Fig. 1 suggests that at least three different deficits may result in surface dyslexia. First, this disorder may arise from a deficit at the level of the visual word form system that disrupts the processing of words as units. As a consequence of this deficit, subjects may identify "sublexical" units (e.g., graphemes or clusters of graphemes) and identify words on the basis of print-to-sound correspondences. Note that semantics and output processes would be expected to be preserved. The patient JC described by Marshall and Newcombe exhibited at least some of the features of this type of surface dyslexia. For example, in response to the word "listen," JC said "Liston" (a former heavyweight champion boxer) and added "that's the boxer," demonstrating that he was able to derive phonology from print and subsequently access meaning.

In the model depicted in Fig. 1, one might also expect to encounter surface dyslexia with deficits at the level of the output lexicon. Support for such an account comes from patients who comprehend irregular words but regularize these words when asked to read aloud. For example, MK read the word "steak" as "steek" (as in seek) before adding, "nice beef." In this instance, the demonstration that MK was able to provide appropriate semantic information indicates that he was able to access meaning directly from the written word and suggests that the visual word form system and semantics are at least relatively preserved.

In the model depicted in Fig. 1, one might also expect to observe semantic dementia in patients exhibiting semantic loss. Indeed, most patients with surface dyslexia (often in association with surface dysgraphia) exhibit a significant semantic deficit. Surface dyslexia is most frequently observed in the context of semantic dementia, a progressive degenerative condition characterized by a gradual loss of knowledge in the absence of deficits in motor, perceptual, and, in some instances, executive function.

Note, however, that the information processing account of reading depicted in Fig. 1 also incorporates a lexical but nonsemantic reading mechanism by means of which patients with semantic loss would be expected to be able to read even irregular words not accommodated by the grapheme-to-phoneme procedure. Surface dyslexia is assumed to reflect impairment in both the semantic and the lexical but nonsemantic mechanisms. It should be noted that in this context the triangle model of reading developed by Seidenberg and McClelland provides an alternative account of surface dyslexia. In this account, to which I briefly return later, surface dyslexia is assumed to reflect the disruption of semantically mediated reading.

V. READING AND THE RIGHT HEMISPHERE

One important and controversial issue regarding reading concerns the putative reading capacity of the right hemisphere. For many years investigators argued that the right hemisphere was "word blind." In recent years, however, several lines of evidence have suggested that the right hemisphere may possess the capacity to read. Indeed, as previously noted, many investigators have argued that the reading of deep dyslexics is mediated at least in part by the right hemisphere.

One seemingly incontrovertible finding demonstrating that at least some right hemispheres possess the capacity to read comes from the performance of a patient who underwent a left hemispherectomy at age 15 for treatment of seizures caused by Rasmussen's encephalitis. After the hemispherectomy the patient was able to read approximately 30% of single words and exhibited an effect of part of speech; she was unable to use a grapheme-to-phoneme conversion process. Thus, as noted by the authors, this patient's performance was similar in many respects to that of patients with deep dyslexia, a pattern of reading impairment that has been hypothesized to reflect the performance of the right hemisphere.

The performance of some split-brain patients is also consistent with the claim that the right hemisphere is literate. For example, these patients may be able to match printed words presented to the right hemisphere with an appropriate object. Interestingly, the patients are apparently unable to derive sound from the words presented to the right hemisphere; thus, they are unable to determine if a word presented to the right hemisphere rhymes with an auditorally presented word.

Another line of evidence supporting the claim that the right hemisphere is literate comes from the evaluation of the reading of patients with pure alexia and optic aphasia. We reported data, for example, from four patients with pure alexia who performed well above chance on many lexical decision and semantic categorization tasks with briefly presented words that they could not explicitly identify. Three of the patients who regained the ability to explicitly identify rapidly presented words exhibited a pattern of performance consistent with the right hemisphere reading hypothesis. These patients read nouns better than functors and words of high imageability (e.g., "chair") better than words of low imageability (e.g., "destiny"). Additionally, both patients for whom data are available demonstrated a deficit in the reading of suffixed (e.g., "flower") compared to pseudosuffixed (e.g., "flowed") words. These data are consistent with a version of the right hemisphere reading hypothesis postulating that the right hemisphere lexical–semantic system primarily represents high imageability nouns. By this account, functors, affixed words, and low imageability words are not adequately represented in the right hemisphere. An important additional finding is that magnetic stimulation applied to the skull, which disrupts electrical activity in the brain, interfered with the reading performance of a partially recovered pure alexic when it affected the parietooccipital area of the right hemisphere. The same stimulation had no effect when it was applied to the homologous area on the left. Additional data supporting the right hemisphere hypothesis come from the demonstration that the limited whole-word reading of a pure alexic was abolished after a right occipitotemporal stroke.

Although a consensus has not been achieved, there is mounting evidence that, at least for some people, the right hemisphere is not word blind but may support the reading of some types of words. The full extent of this reading capacity and whether it is relevant to normal reading, however, remains unclear.

VI. THE ANATOMIC BASIS OF DYSLEXIA

A variety of experimental techniques, including position emission tomography, functional magnetic resonance imaging (fMRI), and evoked potentials, have been employed to investigate the anatomic basis of reading in normal subjects. Although differences in experimental technique and design inevitably lead to variability in reported sites of activation, there appears to be at least relative agreement regarding the anatomic basis of several components of the reading system.

As previously noted, most accounts of reading postulate that after initial visual processing, familiar words are recognized by comparison to a catalog of stored representations that is often termed the visual word form system. A variety of recent investigations involving visual lexical decision with fMRI, viewing of letter, and direct recording of cortical electrical activity suggests that the visual word form system is supported by inferior occipital or inferior temporooccipital cortex.

Additional evidence for this localization comes from a recent investigation by Cohen et al. of five normal subjects and two patients with posterior callosal lesions. These investigators presented words and nonwords for lexical decision or oral reading to either the right or the left visual fields. They found initial unilateral activation in what was thought to be V4 in the hemisphere to which the stimulus was projected. More importantly, however, for normal subjects activation in the left fusiform gyrus (Talairach coordinates −42, −57, and −6) that was independent of the hemisphere to which the stimulus was presented was observed. The two patients with posterior callosal lesions were impaired in the processing of letter strings presented to the right compared to the left hemisphere;

fMRI in these subjects demonstrated that the region of the fusiform gyrus described previously was activated in the callosal patients only by left hemisphere stimulus presentation. As noted by the investigators, these findings are consistent with the hypothesis that the hemialexia demonstrated by the callosal patients is attributable to a failure to access the visual word form system in the left fusiform gyrus.

Deriving meaning from visually presented words requires access to stored knowledge or semantics. Although the architecture and anatomic bases of semantic knowledge remain controversial, investigations involving semantic access for written words implicate cortex at the junction of the superior and middle temporal gyrus (Brodman areas 21, 22, and 37).

VII. ALTERNATIVE MODELS OF READING

Our discussion has focused on a "box and arrow" information processing account of reading disorders. This account not only has proven useful in terms of explaining data from normal and brain-injured subjects but also has predicted syndromes of acquired dyslexia. One weakness of these models, however, is the fact that the accounts are largely descriptive and underspecified.

In recent years, many investigators have developed models of reading in which the architecture and procedures are fully specified and implemented in a manner that permits an empirical assessment of their performance. One computational account of reading has been developed by Coltheart and colleagues. Their dual-route cascaded model represents a computationally instantiated version of dual-route theory similar to that presented in Fig. 1. This account incorporates a lexical route (similar to C in Fig. 1) as well as a nonlexical route by which the pronunciation of graphemes is computed on the basis of position-specific correspondence rules. The model accommodates a wide range of findings from the literature on normal reading.

A fundamentally different type of reading model was developed by Seidenberg and McClelland and subsequently elaborated by Plaut, Seidenberg, and colleagues. This model belongs to the general class of parallel distributed processing or connectionist models. Sometimes referred to as the triangle model, this approach differs from information processing models in that it does not incorporate word-specific representations (e.g., visual word forms and output phonologic representations). In this approach, subjects are assumed to learn how written words map onto spoken words through repeated exposure to familiar and unfamiliar words. Learning of word pronunciations is achieved by means of the development of a mapping between letters and sounds generated on the basis of experience with many different letter strings. The probabilistic mapping between letters and sounds is assumed to provide the means by which both familiar and unfamiliar words are pronounced. This model not only accommodates an impressive array of the classic findings in the literature on normal reading but also has been "lesioned" in an attempt to reproduce the patterns of reading characteristic of dyslexia. For example, Patterson *et al.* attempted to accommodate surface dyslexia by disrupting the semantically mediated reading, and Plaut and Shallice generated a pattern of performance similar to that of deep dyslexia by lesioning a somewhat different connectionist model.

A full discussion of the relative merits of these models as well as approaches to the understanding of reading and acquired dyslexia is beyond the scope of this article. It appears likely, however, that investigations of acquired dyslexia will help to adjudicate between competing accounts of reading and also that these models will continue to offer critical insights into the interpretation of data from brain-injured subjects.

Acknowledgment

This work was supported by Grant RO1 DC2754 from the National Institute of Deafness and Other Communication Disorders.

See Also the Following Articles

AGRAPHIA • ALEXIA • LANGUAGE ACQUISITION • LANGUAGE AND LEXICAL PROCESSING • LANGUAGE DISORDERS • READING DISORDERS, DEVELOPMENTAL

Suggested Reading

Coltheart, M. (1996). Phonological dyslexia: Past and future issues. *Cognitive Neuropsychol.* **13** (Special issue).

Coltheart, M. (1998). Letter-by-letter reading. *Cognitive Neuropsychol.* **15** (Special issue).

Coltheart, M., and Rastle, K. (1994). Serial processing in reading aloud: Evidence for dual-route models of reading. *J. Exp. Psychol. Hum. Perception Performance* **20**, 1197–1211.

Coltheart, M., Patterson, K., and Marshall, J. C. (Eds.) (1980). *Deep Dyslexia*. Routledge Kegan Paul, London.

Coslett, H. B. (1991). Read but not write "idea": Evidence for a third reading mechanism. *Brain Language* **40**, 425–443.

Coslett, H. B., and Saffran, E. M. (1989). Evidence for preserved reading in "pure alexia". *Brain* **112**, 327–359.

Coslett, H. B., and Saffran, E. M. (1998). *Reading and the right hemisphere: Evidence from acquired dyslexia*. In *Right Hemisphere Language Comprehension* (M. Beeman and C. Chiarello, Eds.), pp. 105–132. Erlbaum, Mahway, NJ.

Fiez, J. A., and Petersen, S. E. (1998). Neuroimaging studies of word reading. *Proc. Natl. Acad. Sci. USA* **95**, 914–921.

Funnell, E. (Ed.) (2000). *Case Studies in the Neuropsychology of Reading*. Psychology Press, Hove, UK.

Marshall, J. C., and Newcombe, F. (1973). Patterns of paralexia: A psycholinguistic approach. *J. Psycholinguistic Res.* **2**, 175–199.

Patterson, K. E., Marshall, J. C., and Coltheart, M. (Eds.) (1985). *Surface Dyslexia*. Routledge Kegan Paul, London.

Patterson, K. E., Plaut, D. C., McClelland, J. L., Seidenberg, M. S., Behrmann, M., and Hodges, J. R. (1997). *Connections and disconnections: A connectionist account of surface dyslexia*. In *Neural Modeling of Cognitive and Brain Disorders* (J. Reggia, R. Berndt, and E. Ruppin, Eds.), World Scientific, New York.

Plaut, D. C., and Shallice, T. (1993). Deep dyslexia: A case study of connectionist neuropsychology. *Cognitive Neuropsychol.* **10**, 377–500.

Plaut, D. C., McClelland, J. L., Seidenberg, M. S., and Patterson, K. (1996). Understanding normal and impaired word reading: Computational principles in quasi-regular domains. *Psychol. Rev.* **103**, 56–115.

Saffran, E. M., and Coslett, H. B. (1996). "Attentional dyslexia" in Alzheimer's disease: A case study. *Cognitive Neuropsychol.* **13**, 205–228.

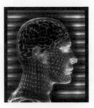

Electrical Potentials

FERNANDO H. LOPES DA SILVA

University of Amsterdam and Dutch Epilepsy Clinic Foundation

GLOSSARY

alpha rhythms Electroencephalogram (EEG)/magnetoencephalogram (MEG) rhythmic activity at 8–13 Hz occurring during wakefulness, mainly over the posterior regions of the head. It is predominant when the subject has closed eyes and is in a state of relaxation. It is attenuated by attention, especially visual, and by mental effort. There are other rhythmic activities within the same frequency range, such as the mu rhythm and the tau or temporal alphoid rhythm, that in MEG recordings have been associated with cortical auditory function, but these are less clear in EEG recordings.

beta/gamma rhythms These rhythmic activities represent frequencies higher than 13 Hz; typically, the beta rhythmic activity ranges from 13 to approximately 30–40 Hz and the gamma extends beyond the latter frequency. Rhythmical beta/gamma activities are encountered mainly over the frontal and central regions and are not uniform phenomena. These rhythmic activities can occur in relation to different behaviors, such as during movements or relaxation after a movement.

desynchronization A state in which neurons are randomly active. Desynchronization is reflected in the absence of a preferred EEG/MEG frequency component. Event-related desynchronization of the ongoing EEG/MEG is a state characterized by a decrease in the power of spectral peaks at specific frequency components, elicited by an event.

electroencephalogram, magnetoencephalogram Electrical potentials or magnetic fields recorded from the brain, directly or through overlying tissues.

excitatory synaptic potential or current An active electrical response of the postsynaptic membrane of a neuron to the release of a neurotransmitter that consists of a local, graded depolarization or of the corresponding ionic current.

event-related potential or field A change in electrical or magnetic activity related to an event, either sensory or motor. The event may precede or follow the event-related potential or field.

evoked potentials or fields A change in electrical or magnetic activity in response to a stimulus. Typically, these transients last tens or hundreds of milliseconds.

inhibitory postsynaptic potential/current Consists of a local, graded hyperpolarization or the corresponding ionic current.

mu or rolandic (central) rhythm Rhythmic activity within the same frequency range as the posterior alpha rhythm but with a topographic distribution that is predominant over the central sensorimotor areas. It is attenuated or blocked by movements.

nonlinear dynamics and brain oscillations Systems with nonlinear elements, such as neuronal networks, may exhibit complex dynamics. Typically, these systems may have different kinds of evolution in time and may switch from one oscillatory mode to another. A qualitative change in the dynamics that occurs as a system's parameter varies is called a bifurcation. Some brain oscillations appear to be generated by systems of this kind, with complex nonlinear dynamics.

sleep or sigma spindles Waxing and waning spindle-like waves occurring during the early stage of sleep at 7–14 Hz within sequences lasting 1 or 2 sec. Sleep spindles typically recur at a slow rhythm of about 0.2–0.5 Hz.

synchronization State in which neurons oscillate in phase as a result of a common input and/or of mutual influences. Event-related synchronization of the ongoing EEG/MEG signals is a state characterized by an increase in power of specific frequency components.

theta rhythms or rhythmical slow activity This term denotes rhythmic activity in the frequency range from 4 to 7 Hz in humans, although macro-osmatic animals show a powerful limbic, and especially hippocampi, rhythm from 3 to 12 Hz that is activated by arousal and motor activity.

The recording of the electrical activity of the brain [i.e., the electroencephalogram (EEG)], either the ongoing activity or the changes of activity related to a given sensory or motor event [the event-related potentials (ERPs)], provides the possibility of studying brain functions with a high time resolution but with a relatively modest spatial resolution. The latter, however, has been improved recently with the development of the magnetoencephalogram (MEG) and more sophisticated source imaging techniques. These new methods allow an analysis of the dynamics of brain activities not only of global brain functions, such as sleep and arousal, but also of cognitive processes, such as perception, motor preparation, and higher cognitive functions. Furthermore, these methods are essential for the characterization of pathophysiological processes, particularly those with a paroxysmal character such as epilepsy. In this article, the possibilities offered by EEG/MEG recordings to analyze brain functions, and particularly the neural basis of cognitive processes, are discussed. In this respect, special attention is given to the basic mechanisms underlying the generation of functional neuronal assemblies (i.e., the processes of synchronization and desynchronization of neuronal activity) and their modulation by exogenous and endogenous factors. Therefore, a brief overview of the neurophysiology of the dynamics of neuronal networks and of the generation of brain oscillations, an account of the phenomenology of EEG/MEG activities, and a discussion of the main aspects of ERPs and/or magnetic fields are presented. The article concludes with a short discussion of the roles that brain oscillations may play in the processing of neural information. In this respect, the need to understand what happens at the level of neuronal elements within brain systems in relation to different types of oscillations is emphasized. Only in this way is it possible to obtain insight into the functional processes that occur in the brain, at the level of information transfer or processing, during the occurrence of brain oscillations and the transition between different states. The relevance of electrophysiological studies of the human brain regarding neurocognitive investigations is also discussed in light of recent advances in brain imaging techniques.

I. THE ELECTROPHYSIOLOGICAL APPROACH VERSUS OTHER APPROACHES OF STUDYING BRAIN FUNCTIONS

In the past decade, the emergence of brain imaging techniques, such as positron emission tomography and functional magnetic resonance (fMRI), has made important contributions to our understanding of basic brain processes underlying neurocognitive functions. Notwithstanding the fact that, in particular, fMRI can provide maps of brain activity with millimeter spatial resolution, its temporal resolution is limited. Indeed, this resolution is on the order of seconds, whereas neurocognitive phenomena may take place within tens of milliseconds. Therefore, it is important to use electrophysiological techniques to achieve the desired temporal resolution in this kind of investigation, although this is done at the cost of spatial resolution. The essential problem of electro/magnetoencephalography is that the sources of neuronal activity cannot be derived in a unique way from the distribution of EEG or MEG activity at the scalp; thus, the inverse problem is an ill-posed problem. However, new possibilities are emerging to solve this problem. A promising solution is to solve the inverse problem by imposing spatial constraints based on anatomical information provided by MRI and additional physiological information from metabolic or hemodynamic signals, derived from fMRI, that are associated with the neuronal activity. The precise nature of this association, however, is not trivial and it is a matter of current investigation. This implies that we may expect that in the near future technical advances in combining fMRI and EEG/MEG measures of brain activity will contribute to a better understanding of neurocognitive and other brain functions.

II. HISTORY OF THE ELECTROPHYSIOLOGY OF THE BRAIN

The existence of the electrical activity of the brain (i.e., the EEG) was discovered more than a century ago by Caton. After the demonstration that the EEG could be recorded from the human scalp by Berger in the 1920s, it was slowly accepted as a method of analysis of brain functions in health and disease. It is interesting to note that acceptance came only after the demonstration by Adrian and Mathews in the 1930s that the EEG, namely the alpha rhythm, was likely generated in the occipital lobes in man. The responsible neuronal sources, however, remained undefined until the 1970s, when it was demonstrated in dog that the alpha rhythm is generated by a dipole layer centered on layers IV and V of the visual cortex. It is not surprising that the mechanisms of generation and the functional significance of the EEG remained controversial for a relatively long time, considering the complexity of the underlying systems of neuronal generators and the involved transfer of signals from the cortical surface to the scalp due to the geometric and electrical properties of the volume conductor (brain, cerebrospinal fluid, skull, and scalp).

The EEG consists essentially of the summed electrical activity of populations of neurons, with a modest contribution of glial cells. Considering that neurons are excitable cells with characteristic intrinsic electrical properties and that interneuronal communication is essentially mediated by electrochemical processes at synapses, it follows that these cells can produce electrical and magnetic fields that may be recorded at a distance from the sources. Thus, these fields may be recorded a short distance from the sources [i.e., the local EEG or local field potentials (LFPs)], from the cortical surface (the electrocorticogram), or even from the scalp (i.e., the EEG in its most common form). The associated MEG is recorded usually by way of sensors placed at a short distance around the scalp.

In order to understand how the electrical and magnetic signals of the brain are generated, it is necessary to examine how the activity of assemblies of neurons is organized both in time and in space and which biophysical laws govern the generation of extracellular field potentials or magnetic fields.

III. THE GENERATION OF ELECTRIC AND MAGNETIC EXTRACELLULAR FIELDS

It is generally assumed that the neuronal events that cause the generation of electric and/or magnetic fields in a neural mass consist of ionic currents that have mainly postsynaptic sources. For these fields to be measurable at a distance from the sources, it is important that the underlying neuronal currents are well organized both in space and in time. The ionic currents in the brain obey Maxwell's and Ohm's laws.

The most important ionic current sources in the brain consist of changes in membrane conductances caused by intrinsic membrane processes and/or by synaptic actions. The net membrane current that results from changes in membrane conductances,

either synaptic or intrinsic, can be either a positive or a negative ionic current directed to the inside of the neuron. These currents are compensated by currents flowing in the surrounding medium since there is no accumulation of electrical charge. Consider as the simplest case that of synaptic activity caused by excitatory postsynaptic currents (EPSCs) or inhibitory postsynaptic currents (IPSCs). Because the direction of the current is defined by the direction along which positive charges are transported, at the level of the synapse there is a net positive inward current in the case of an EPSC and a negative one in the case of an IPSC. Therefore, extracellularly an active current sink is caused by an EPSC and an active current source by an IPSC. Most neurons are elongated cells; thus, along the passive parts of the membrane (i.e., at a distance from the active synapses) a distributed passive source is created in the case of an EPSC and a distributed passive sink in the case of an IPSC. In this way, a dipole configuration is created (Fig. 1). At the macroscopic level, the activation of a set of neurons organized in parallel is capable of creating dipole layers. The following are important conditions that have to be satisfied for this to occur: (i) The neurons should be spatially organized with the dendrites aligned in parallel, forming palisades, and (ii) the synaptic activation of the neuronal population should occur in synchrony.

Lorente de Nó named the type of electric field created in this way an "open field," in contrast to the field generated by neurons with dendrites radially distributed around the soma which form a "closed field." In any case, as a result of synaptic activation, extracellular currents will flow. These may consist of longitudinal or transversal components, the former being those that flow parallel to the main axis of a neuron and the latter flow perpendicular to this axis. In the case of an open field, the longitudinal components will add, whereas the transversal components tend to cancel out. In the case of a closed field, all components will tend to cancel, such that the net result at a distance is zero.

The importance of the spatial organization of neuronal current sources for the generation of electric and/or magnetic fields measurable at a distance can be stated in a paradigmatic way for the cortex. Indeed, the pyramidal neurons of the cortex are lined up perpendicular to the cortical surface, forming layers of neurons in palissade. Their synaptic activation can occur within well-defined layers and in a synchronized way. The resulting electric fields may be quite large if the activity within a population of cells forms a

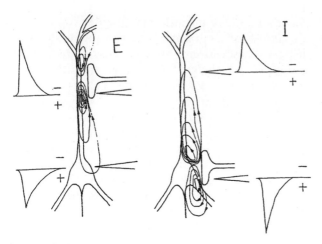

Figure 1 Model cortical pyramidal cell showing the patterns of current flow caused by two modes of synaptic activation at an excitatory (E) and an inhibitory (I) synapse. Typically, the apical dendrites of these cells are oriented toward the cortical surface. E, current flow caused by the activation of an excitatory synapse at the level of the apical dendrite. This causes a depolarization of the postsynaptic membrane (i.e., an EPSP), and the flow of a net positive current (i.e., EPSC). This current flow creates a current sink in the extracellular medium next to the synapse. The extracellularly recorded EPSP is shown on the left. It has a negative polarity at the level of the synapse. At the soma there exists a distributed passive current source resulting in an extracellular potential of positive polarity. I, current flow caused by activation of an inhibitory synapse at the level of the soma. This results in a hyperpolarization of the postsynaptic membrane and in the flow of a negative current. Thus, an active source is created extracellularly at the level of the soma and in passive sinks at the basal and apical dendrites. The extracellularly recorded IPSP at the level of the soma and of the apical dendrites is shown. Note that both cases show a dipolar source–sink configuration, with the same polarity, notwithstanding the fact that the postsynaptic potentials are of opposite polarity (EPSP vs IPSP). This illustrates the fact that not only does the nature of the synaptic potential determine the polarity of the potentials at the cortical surface but also the position of the synaptic sources within the cortex is important (adapted with permission from Niedermeyer and Lopes da Silva, 1999).

coherent domain (i.e., if the activity of the neuronal sources is phase locked). In general, the electric potential generated by a population of neurons represents a spatial and temporal average of the potentials generated by the single neurons within a macrocolumn.

A basic problem in electroencephalography/magnetoencephalography is how to estimate the neuronal sources corresponding to a certain distribution of electrical potentials or of magnetic fields recorded at the scalp. As noted previously, this is called the inverse problem of EEG/MEG. It is an ill-posed problem that has no unique solution. Therefore, one must assume

specific models of the sources and of the volume conductor. The simplest source model is a current dipole. However, it should not be considered that such a model means that somewhere in the brain there exists a discrete dipolar source. It simply means that the best representation of the EEG/MEG scalp distribution is by way of an equivalent dipolar source. In the sense of a best statistical fit, the latter describes the centroid of the dipole layers that are active at a certain moment. The estimation of equivalent dipole models is only meaningful if the scalp field has a focal character and the number of possible active areas can be anticipated with reasonable accuracy. An increase in the number of dipoles can easily lead to complex and ambiguous interpretations. Nevertheless, methods have been developed to obtain estimates of multiple dipoles with only the a priori information that they must be located on the surface of the cortex. An algorithm that performs such an analysis is multiple signal classification (MUSIC), which is illustrated in Fig. 2 for the case of the cortical sources of the alpha rhythm. An alternative approach is to use linear estimation methods applying the minimum norm constraint to estimate the sources within a given surface or volume of the brain. Currently, new approaches are being explored that use combined fMRI and EEG/MEG recordings in order to create more specific spatial constraints to reduce the solution space for the estimation of the underlying neuronal sources. In general, the problems created by the complexity of the volume conductor, including the scalp, skull, layer of cerebrospinal fluid, and brain, are easier to solve in the case of MEG than EEG since these media have conductivities that affect the EEG much more than the MEG. The major advantage of MEG over EEG is the relative ease of source localization with the former. This means that when a dipole source algorithm is used on the basis of MEG recordings, a simple homogeneous sphere model of the volume conductor is usually sufficient to obtain a satisfactory solution. The position of the sources can be integrated in MRI scans of the brain using appropriate algorithms.

IV. DYNAMICS OF NEURONAL ELEMENTS: LOCAL CIRCUITS AND MECHANISMS OF OSCILLATIONS

Here, I discuss the dynamics of the electrical and magnetic fields of the brain, i.e., their time-dependent properties. These properties are determined to a large extent by the dynamical properties of ionic currents.

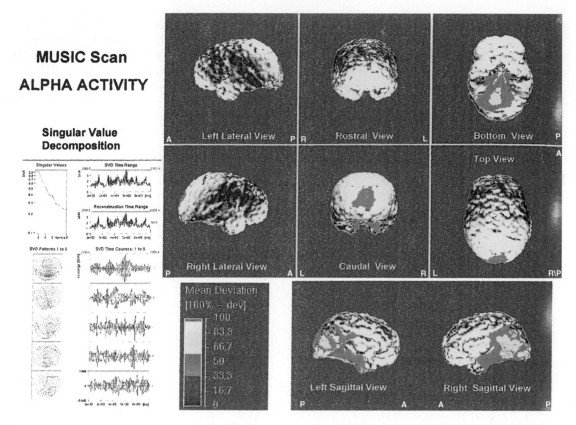

Figure 2   Results of a multiple signal classification analysis (MUSIC) scan of a 5-sec-long epoch of alpha activity recorded using a whole-head 151 MEG system during the eyes-closed condition. A singular value decomposition of the MEG signals yielded four factors. The scale indicates the cortical areas where the most significant sources were estimated (reproduced with permission from Parra *et al.*, *J. Clin. Neurophysiol.* **17**, 212–224, 2000).

The most elementary phenomenon to be taken into account is the passive time constant of the neuronal membrane. This is typically about 5 msec for most cortical pyramidal neurons. Therefore, the activation of a synapse causing an ionic current to flow will generate a postsynaptic potential change that decays passively with such a time constant. However, there are other membrane phenomena that have much longer time constants. Some of these are intrinsic membrane processes, whereas others are postsynaptic. Among the intrinsic membrane phenomena, a multitude of ionic conductances, distributed along both soma and dendrites, enable neurons to display a variety of modes of activity. Among the synaptic phenomena, some present much longer time constants than the membrane passive time constant. This is the case, for example, for the $GABA_B$-mediated inhibition that consists of a K^+ current with slow dynamics. The synaptic actions of amines and neuropeptides, in contrast with those of amino acids such as glutamate and GABA, also have slow dynamics. The effect of acetylcholine (ACh) is mixed since fast and slow actions occur, depending on the type of receptors to which ACh binds. Furthermore, note that the dendrites do not consist of simple passive membranes, as in the classical view; rather, the dendrites also have voltage-gated ion conductances that can contribute actively to the electrical behavior of the whole neuron. Thus, a neuron must be considered as a system of functional nodes, where each node represents a chemical synapse, an active ionic conductance, a metabolic modulated ion channel, or, in some cases, a gap junction (i.e., a direct electrical coupling between adjacent cells through a low-resistance pathway).

The sequence of hyperpolarizations and depolarizations caused by inhibitory and excitatory synaptic activity, respectively, can induce the activation or the removal of inactivation of intrinsic membrane currents. This aspect is difficult to analyze in detail under natural conditions in intact neuronal populations. However, much was learned about this kind of phenomena from studies carried out *in vitro* both in isolated cells and in brain slices. To illustrate this, consider the typical behavior of thalamic neurons that participate in the thalamocortical circuits with feed-forward and feedback connections (Fig. 3). Even in isolation, these cells may show intrinsic oscillatory modes of activity, either in the alpha range of activity (namely, in the form of spindles at 7–14 Hz) or in the delta frequency range (0.5–4 Hz). To understand how

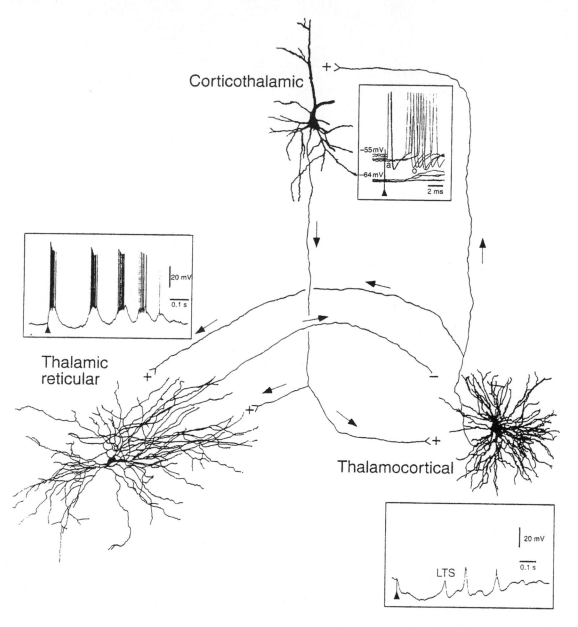

Figure 3 Corticothalamic circuits and different types of neuronal activities. A thalamocortical relay cell is shown on the lower right-hand side, a neuron of the reticular nucleus (GABAergic) is shown on the left, and a cortical pyramidal cell is shown on top. The direction of the flow of action potentials along the axons is indicated by arrows. Positive signs indicate excitatory synapses and negative signs indicate inhibitory synapses. The insets show cellular responses obtained intracellularly. In this case, the activity of the cortical neuron was obtained by electrical stimulation of the intralaminar nucleus of the thalamus. At the membrane potential of −55 mV the response consisted of an antidromic spike (a) followed by a bursts of orthodromic spikes (o). At a more hyperpolarized level (−64 mV), the antidromic response failed but the orthodromic response consisted of a subthreshold EPSP. The responses of the two thalamic neurons were obtained by stimulation of the cortex. The response of the neuron of the reticular nucleus consists of a high-frequency burst of spikes followed by a series of spindle waves on a depolarizing envelope. The response of the thalamocortical neuron consists of a biphasic IPSP that leads to a low-threshold calcium spike (LTS) and a sequence of hyperpolarizing spindle waves (reproduced with permission from Steriade, 1999).

oscillations can take place in these circuits it is important to realize that these cells have, among other kinds of ionic currents, a low-threshold Ca^{2+} conductance (I_T) that contributes to the low-threshold spike. This I_T conductance is de-inactivated by a previous membrane hyperpolarization and causes sufficient depolarization of the cell for the activation of a persistent (non-inactivating) Na+ conductance. These cells also have a nonspecific cation "sag" current (I_h) that has much slower kinetics than I_T and is activated by hyperpolarization. The alpha range oscillatory mode depends essentially on the low-threshold Ca^{2+} current I_T. In addition, other currents contribute to the oscillatory behavior—namely, a fast transient potassium current (I_A) that has a voltage dependence that is similar to that of I_T, a slowly inactivating potassium current, and calcium-dependent potassium currents that need increased intracellular Ca^{2+} concentration for activation—and are mainly responsible for after-hyperpolarizations. In this way, a sequence of hyperpolarizations followed by depolarizations tends to develop. This could be sufficient for such cells to behave as neuronal "pacemakers." Under the *in vitro* conditions in which these basic properties have been studied, the initial hyperpolarization that is necessary for the removal of the inactivation of the Ca^{2+} current is provided artificially by an intracellular injection of current. However, under natural conditions in the intact brain, the oscillatory behavior cannot occur spontaneously (i.e., it is not autonomous). For the de-inactivation of the low-threshold Ca^{2+} current to occur, initially the cell has to be hyperpolarized by a synaptic action mediated by GABAergic synapses that impinge on these cells and stem from the GABAergic neurons of the reticular nucleus of the thalamus. Therefore, the notion that these thalamo-cortical relay cells behave as pacemakers, in the sense of generating pure autonomous oscillations, *in vivo* is only a relative one. Indeed, they need a specific input from outside to set the conditions under which they may oscillate. Thus, *in vivo* the alpha spindle and delta waves result from network interactions. Nevertheless, the intrinsic membrane properties are of importance in setting the frequency response of the cells and of the network to which they belong.

In general terms, it must be considered that neurons, as integrative units, interact with other neurons through local circuits, excitatory as well as inhibitory. In a neuronal circuit feedforward and feedback elements have to be distinguished. In particular, the existence of feedback loops can shape the dynamics of a neuronal network affecting its frequency response and even creating the conditions for the occurrence of resonance phenomena and other forms of oscillatory behavior. Furthermore, note that the transfer of signals in a neuronal network involves time delays and essential nonlinearities. This may lead to the appearance of nonlinear oscillations and possibly even to what is in mathematical terms called chaotic behavior.

In recent years, much has been learned about these issues with the advent of the theory of nonlinear dynamics. This has resulted in the application of nonlinear time series analysis to EEG signals, with the aim of estimating several nonlinear measures to characterize different kinds of EEG signals. This matter is the object of recent interesting studies reported in specialized publications in which the question "chaos in brain?" is discussed. I stress here only that a theoretical framework based on the mathematical notions of complex nonlinear dynamics can be most useful to understanding the dynamics of EEG phenomena. In this context, insight may be obtained into how different types of oscillations may be generated within the same neuronal population and how such a system may switch from one type of oscillatory behavior to another. This occurs, for example, when an EEG/MEG characterized by alpha rhythmic activity suddenly changes into a 3-Hz spike and wave pattern during an absence seizure in epileptic patients. Based on the use of mathematical nonlinear models of neuronal networks, it is possible to formulate hypotheses concerning the mechanisms by means of which a given neuronal network can switch between these qualitatively different types of oscillations. This switching behavior depends on input conditions and on modulating parameters. Accordingly, such a switch can take place depending on subtle changes in one or more parameters. In the theory of complex nonlinear dynamics, this is called a bifurcation. In this respect, the most sensitive parameter is the neuronal membrane potential that in the intact brain is modulated by various synaptic inputs. Typically, the change of oscillation mode may be spectacular, whereas the initial change of a parameter may be minimal.

The frequency of a brain oscillation depends both on the intrinsic membrane properties of the neuronal elements and on the properties of the networks to which they belong. Considerations regarding the membrane conditions that determine which ionic currents can be active at a given time lead to the conclusion that the modulating systems mediated by several neurochemical systems are of utmost importance in setting the initial conditions that determine the activity mode of the network (i.e., whether it will display oscillations or not and at which frequency). Different behavioral states are characterized by the interplay of different chemical neurotransmitter and neuromodulator systems.

A fundamental property of a neuronal network is the capacity of the neurons to work in synchrony. This depends essentially on the way the inputs are organized and on the network interconnectivity. Thus, groups of neurons may work synchronously as a population due to mutual interactions. The experimental and theoretical work of Ad Aetsen and Moshe Abeles showed the existence of precise (within 5 msec) synchrony of individual action potentials among selected groups of neurons in the cortex. These synchronous patterns of activity were associated with the planning and execution of voluntary movements. These researchers noted that during cognitive processes the neurons tend to synchronize their firing without changing the firing rates, whereas in response to external events they synchronize firing rates and modulate the frequency at the same time. In addition, they also showed that the synchronization dynamics are strongly influenced by the level of background activity. This indicates the importance that the ongoing electrical activity can have in setting the activity climate in a given brain system.

A fundamental feature of the cortex is that groups of neurons tend to form local circuits organized in modules with the geometry of cortical columns. The basic cortical spatial module is a vertical cylinder with a 200–300 μm cross-section. There exist different systems of connecting fibers between cortical columns, namely, (i) the collaterals of axons of pyramidal neurons that may spread over distances of approximately 3 mm and are mostly excitatory; (ii) the ramifications of incoming terminal axons that may extend over distances of 6–8 mm along the cortical surface; and (iii) the collaterals of interneurons, an important part of which are inhibitory, that may branch horizontally over 0.5–1 mm within the cortex. These systems range over distances on the order of magnitude of hundreds of micrometers, and this determines the characteristic length of intracortical interactions.

It is not simple to directly relate the dynamic behavior of a neuronal network to the basic parameters of neurons and synapses. In order to construct such relationships, basic physiological and histological data have to be combined like pieces of a puzzle. However, the available knowledge of most neuronal networks in terms of detailed physiological and even histological information is still incomplete. To supplement this lack of specific knowledge, a synthetic approach can be useful. This implies the construction of connectionist models of neuronal networks using all available and relevant data. Such models can be of practical use to obtain a better understanding of the main properties of a network. Indeed, a model offers the possibility of studying the influence of different parameters on the dynamic behavior of the network and of making predictions of unexplored properties of the system, which may lead to new experiments. In this way, EEG signals, particularly local field potentials (LFPs), can also be modeled. Thus, hypotheses concerning the relevance of given neuronal properties to the generation of special EEG features may be tested.

V. MAIN TYPES OF EEG/MEG ACTIVITIES: PHENOMENOLOGY AND FUNCTIONAL SIGNIFICANCE

A. Sleep EEG Phenomena

In the neurophysiology of sleep two classic EEG phenomena have been established: the spindles or waves between 7 and 14 Hz, also called sleep or sigma spindles, which appear at sleep onset, and the delta waves (1–4 Hz), which are paradigmatic of deeper stages of sleep. Recently, the work of Mircea Steriade and coworkers in Quebec described in animals another very slow oscillation (0.6–1 Hz) that is able to modulate the occurrence of different typical EEG sleep events, such as delta waves, sleep spindles, and even short high-frequency bursts. This very slow oscillation was recently revealed in the human EEG by Peter Acherman and A. Borbély and in the MEG by our group.

The basic membrane events that are responsible for the occurrence of sleep spindles and delta waves were described previously. The sleep spindles are generated in the thalamocortical circuits and result from the interplay between intrinsic membrane properties of the thalamocortical relay neurons (TCR) and the GABAergic neurons of the reticular nucleus, and the properties of the circuits to which these neurons belong. It is clear that the spindles are a collective property of the neuronal populations. Experimental evidence has demonstrated that the sleep spindle oscillations are generated in the thalamus since they can be recorded in this brain area after decortication and high brain stem transection. The very slow rhythm (0.6–1 Hz), on the contrary, is generated intracortically since it survives thalamic lesions, but it is disrupted by intracortical lesions. Interestingly, note that the rhythmicity of the very slow oscillation appears to be reflected in that of the typical K complexes of human EEG during non-REM sleep.

How are these oscillations controlled by modulating systems? It is well-known that sleep spindles are under brain stem control. It is a classic neurophysiological phenomenon that electrical stimulation of the brain stem can block thalamocortical oscillations causing the so-called "EEG desynchronization," as shown in studies by Moruzzi and Magoun. This desynchronization is caused by the activation of cholinergic inputs (Fig. 4) arising from the mesopontine cholinergic nuclei, namely, the pedunculopontine tegmental and the laterodorsal tegmental areas. Indeed, both the reticular nucleus and the TCR neurons receive cholinergic muscarinic synapses. Cholinergic activation of the reticular nucleus neurons elicits hyperpolarization with a K^+ conductance increase that is mediated by an increase in a muscarinic-activated potassium current. In contrast, it causes depolarization of TCR neurons.

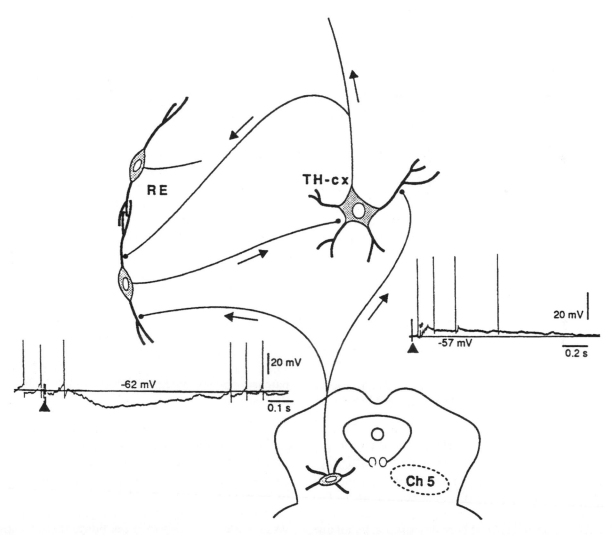

Figure 4 Basic thalamic network responsible for the generation of spindles at 7–14 Hz. A thalamocortical (TH-cx) neuron and two neurons of the reticular nucleus (RE), which are interconnected by mutual inhibitory synapses, are shown. This network is under the modulating influence of mesopontine afferents arising from the cholinergic (Ch5) neurons of the pedunculopontine tegmental nucleus. The stimulation of Ch5 neurons causes depolarization of TH-cx neurons and hyperpolarization of RE neurons. In this way, the occurrence of spindles is blocked (i.e., desynchronization of the corresponding oscillation takes place) (reproduced with permission from Steriade *et al.*, *Electroencephalogr. Clin. Neurophysiol.* **76,** 481–508, 1990).

Furthermore, the reticular nucleus receives inputs from the basal forebrain that may be GABAergic and can also exert a strong inhibition of the reticular neurons leading to the subsequent suppression of spindle oscillations. In addition, monoaminergic inputs from the brain stem, namely those arising at the mesopontine junction (i.e., from the noradrenergic neurons of the locus coeruleus and the serotoninergic neurons of the dorsal raphe nuclei), also modulate the rhythmic activities of the forebrain. These neuronal systems have only a weak thalamic projection but have a diffuse projection to the cortex. Metabotropic glutamate receptors also appear to exert a modulating influence on the activation of thalamic circuits by descending corticothalamic systems.

Because this point is often misunderstood, it is emphasized that slow-wave sleep, characterized by typical EEG delta activity, does not correspond to a state in which cortical neurons are inactive. On the contrary, in this sleep state cortical neurons can display mean rates of firing similar to those during wakefulness and/or REM sleep. Regarding the neuronal firing patterns, the main difference between delta sleep and wakefulness and REM sleep is that in the former the neurons tend to display long bursts of spikes with relatively prolonged interburst periods of silence, whereas in the latter the firing pattern is more continuous. The functional meaning of these peculiar firing pattern of delta sleep has not been determined.

In general, EEG signals covary strongly with different levels of arousal and consciousness. The changes of EEG with increasing levels of anesthesia are typical examples of this property.

B. Alpha Rhythms of Thalamus and Neocortex

Alpha rhythms recorded from the occipital areas occur in relaxed awake animals and show a typical reactivity to eye closure. Although the frequency range of alpha rhythms overlaps that of sleep spindles, these two phenomena differ in many aspects. Namely, the behavioral state in which both types of oscillations occur is quite different, and their distribution over the cortex and thalamus also differs considerably. The basic mechanisms responsible for alpha oscillations at the cellular level have not been described in detail due to the inherent difficulty in studying a phenomenon that by definition occurs in the state of relaxed wakefulness under conditions that allow measuring the underlying membrane currents under anesthesia, or, optimally, in slice preparations *in vitro*. To over-

come this difficulty, some researchers assumed that spindles occurring under barbiturate anesthesia were analogous to alpha rhythms. However, this analogy was challenged on experimental grounds because a comparative investigation of alpha rhythms, obtained during restful awakeness at eye closure, and spindles induced by barbiturates, recorded from the same sites over the visual cortex and lateral geniculate nuclei in dog, presented differences in frequency, spindle duration, topographic distribution, and amount of coherence among different cortical and thalamic sites. Investigations using multiple electrode arrays placed on the cortical surface, depth intracortical profiles, and intrathalamic recordings from several thalamic nuclei elucidated many elementary properties of alpha rhythms:

- In the visual cortex, alpha waves are generated by a current dipole layer centered at the level of the somata and basal dendrites of the pyramidal neurons of layers IV and V.
- The coherence between alpha waves recorded from neighboring cortical sites is greater than any thalamocortical coherence.
- The influence of alpha signals recorded from the pulvinar on cortical rhythms can be conspicuously large, depending on cortical area, but intercortical factors play a significant role in establishing cortical domains of alpha activity.

These experimental findings led to the conclusion that in addition to the influence of some thalamic nuclei, mainly the pulvinar, on the generation of alpha rhythms in the visual cortex, there are systems of surface-parallel intracortical connections responsible for the propagation of alpha rhythms over the cortex. These oscillations appear to be generated in small patches of cortex that behave as epicenters, from which they propagate at relatively slow velocities (approximately 0.3 cm/sec). This type of spatial propagation has been confirmed, in general terms, by experimental and model studies. A comprehensive study of alpha rhythms in the visual cortex of the cat showed characteristics corresponding closely to those of alpha in man and dog. It was found that this rhythmic activity was localized to a limited part of the primary visual cortex area 18 and at the border between areas 17 and 18. In this context, additional insight into the sources of alpha rhythms in man has been obtained using MEGs integrated with anatomical information obtained from MRI. Different sources of alpha rhythms, the so-called "alphons," were found concentrated mainly in the region around the calcarine fissure, with most sources located within 2 cm of the midline. A typical distribution of sources of alpha rhythmic activity over the human cortex was recently obtained using whole-head MEG and analyzed using the MUSIC algorithm as shown in Fig. 2.

In addition to the alpha rhythms of the visual cortex, rhythmic activities with about the same frequency range (in man, 8–13 Hz, in cat; 12–15 Hz) have been shown to occur in other cortical areas, namely in the somatosensory cortex (SI areas 1–3). These activities are known as "rolandic mu rhythms" or "wicket rhythms," named after the appearance of the records on the scalp in man, and they have a typical reactivity since they appear when the subject is at rest and they are blocked by movement. The mu rhythm is particularly pronounced in the hand area of the somatosensory cortex and it reacts typically to the movement of closing the fists. In the cat, there is no significant coherence between the mu rhythm of the SI cortex and the alpha rhythm of the visual cortex, which supports the general idea that these two types of rhythms are independent. Furthermore, mu rhythms of the SI area also differ from the alpha rhythms of the visual cortex recorded in the same animal in that the former have systematically higher frequencies than the latter, the difference being about 2 Hz. Mu rhythms were also recorded in thalamic nuclei, namely in the ventroposterior lateral nucleus. The mu rhythm has also been identified in MEG recordings over the rolandic sulcus, particularly over the somatomotor hand area. The reactivity of the EEG/MEG mu rhythm to movement and other behavioral conditions has been analyzed in detail in man using advanced computer analysis. In addition, another spontaneous MEG activity, the so-called tau rhythm, was detected over the auditory cortex. This rhythmic activity was reduced by sound stimuli. This MEG tau rhythm, first described by the group of Riitta Hari in Helsinki, is apparently similar to an EEG rhythm that was found using epidural electrodes over the midtemporal region by Ernst Niedermeyer in Baltimore.

C. EEG Activities of the Limbic Cortex

Two main types of rhythmic EEG activities can be recorded from limbic cortical areas characterized by different dominant rhythmic components, one in the theta and one in the beta/gamma frequency range. The former was first described by Green and Arduini in 1954, and in several species it may cover the frequency range between 4 and 12 Hz. It is common practice to call this activity theta rhythm since in most species it is dominant between 4 and 7.5 Hz; however, since in rodents it can extend to 12 Hz, it is preferentially called rhythmic slow activity (RSA). The brain areas in which RSA is most apparent are the hippocampus and parahippocampal gyri, although it also occurs in other parts of the limbic system. It has been questioned whether RSA also occurs in humans. However, RSA was incidentally recorded in the human hippocampus and was clearly demonstrated in the hippocampus of freely moving epileptic patients using spectral analysis. The relative difficulty in recording RSA in the human hippocampus may be related to the decrease in amplitude and regularity of RSA encountered in higher primates. Therefore, it can be concluded that the human hippocampus is no exception among mammals with respect to the occurrence of RSA. Using MEG imaging in normal human subjects, Claudia Tesche showed that the activity centered on the anterior hippocampus consisted of spectral components lower than 12 Hz that included task-dependent peaks.

It is generally accepted that hippocampal RSA depends on intact septo-hippocampal circuits. The experimental evidence is based on the fact that lesions of the septal area result in the disappearance of RSA from the hippocampus and other limbic cortical areas. Furthermore, it was shown that subpopulations of medial septal/diagonal band neurons, particularly those lying within the dorsal limb of the diagonal band and in the ventral part of the medial septal nucleus, discharge in phase with hippocampal RSA. This population of septal neurons is capable of sustaining burst firing within the RSA frequency range even when disconnected from the hippocampus. These experimental findings have led to the general idea that in the septal area some neuronal networks can work as pacemakers of RSA. However, it must be emphasized that the hippocampal neurons do not act as simple passive followers of the septal neurons. The neuronal networks of the hippocampus and of other cortical limbic areas also contribute to the characteristics of the local RSA. Indeed, even hippocampal slices kept *in vitro* are able to generate RSA-like rhythmic field potentials on the application of the cholinergic agonist carbachol in a large concentration. Theta frequency oscillations were also recorded in hippocampal neurons, maintained in *in vitro* slices, induced by depolarization by current injection of long duration. This cholinergic activation is mediated by muscarinic receptors since it is blocked by atropine, and RSA elicited in hippocampal slices involves recurrent excitatory circuits of the CA3 region, mediated by glutamatergic (non-NMDA) synapses. It should be emphasized that this form of *in vitro* RSA mimics the so-called atropine-sensitive RSA of behaving rats that appears during motionless behavior and REM sleep. However, the atropine-insensitive RSA that appears during motor activity certainly involves other processes and depends on other neuromodulating systems.

In addition to the rhythmic activity in the theta frequency range, one can also record from the paleo- and archicortex other EEG activities within the frequency range from 30 to 50 Hz (i.e., beta or gamma activities). An interesting feature of these rhythmic activities of the basal forebrain is that they have a relatively large value of coherence over a wide range of brain areas involved in olfaction. This coherent domain of beta activity reflects the fact that there is a rostrocaudal spread of this activity along the olfactory bulb, prepyriform, entorhinal cortices.

The cellular origin of the beta activity of the olfactory areas (paleocortex) has been revealed by many comprehensive investigations in which both single and multiple neuronal activity or LFPs were recorded, and their relationships were analyzed using signal analysis techniques by Walter Freeman. A conclusion of Freeman's studies is that the interactions at the neuronal population level are mediated by synaptic somadendritic mechanisms, involving electrotonic spread of activity and the transmission of action potentials, that have nonlinear dynamical behavior. It is also assumed that the oscillations result primarily from synaptic interactions among interconnected populations of neurons and not from intrinsic neuronal oscillations since the paleocortex isolated from extrinsic connections remains silent.

It is noteworthy that computer simulation studies of Walter Freeman and collaborators showed that the typical complex nonlinear (possibly chaotic) dynamics of the olfactory cortical areas appear to depend on the presence of interactions between the olfactory bulb, the anterior olfactory nucleus, and the prepyriform cortex, which are interconnected by short and long pathways with the corresponding time delays. This implies that the dynamical behavior of neuronal networks should not be assumed to be determined only by local properties but also to depend on the interactions between networks at different locations, through reentrant circuits, such that new emerging properties arise from these functional assemblies of corticocortical and subcorticocortical systems.

D. Beta/Gamma Activity of the Neocortex

The identification and characterization of high-frequency rhythms in the neocortex has been concentrated mainly in two neocortical areas—the visual cortex and the somatomotor cortex. Here, some of the properties of these beta/gamma rhythmic activities for these two areas are discussed.

Commonly, the EEG or LFP of the visual cortex is associated with the alpha rhythm, with typical reactivity with closing and opening of the eyes as described previously. However, other types of rhythmic activities can be present in the same cortical areas, namely within the beta frequency range. In the dog, it was shown that the EEG spectral density was characterized by peaks within the beta/gamma frequency range while the animal was looking attentively at a visual stimulus. These findings in the awake animal are in line with the demonstration in the bulbospinal transected preparation that brain stem electrical stimulation causes not only desynchronization of alpha spindles but also the appearance of fast rhythms in the cortical EEG. Recently, Walter Freeman and Bob van Dijk found in the visual cortex of a rhesus monkey that fast EEG rhythms (spectral peak of 30 ± 3.7 Hz) occurred during a conditioned task to a visual stimulus. A possibly related finding is the discovery by the group of Charles Gray and Wolf Singer and by Eckhorn and collaborators of oscillations within the beta/gamma frequency range (most commonly between 30 and 60 Hz) in the firing of individual neurons of the visual cortex in response to moving light bars. Using auto- and cross-correlation analyses, it was demonstrated that neurons tended to fire in synchrony, in an oscillatory mode, within cortical patches that could extend up to distances of about 7 mm. The oscillations in neuronal firing rate were correlated with those of the LFPs. The cortical oscillations are modulated by the activation of the mesencephalic reticular formation (MRF), but the stimulation of the MRF alone does not change the pattern of firing of the cortical neurons. However, MRF stimulation increases the amplitude and coherence of both the LFP and the multiunit responses when applied jointly with a visual stimulus.

In the somatomotor cortex, beta/gamma oscillations of both neuronal firing and LFPs were described in the awake cat by the group of Rougeul-Buser, particularly when the animal was in a state of enhanced vigilance while watching an unreachable mouse. Also, in monkey during a state of enhanced attention, fast oscillations were found in the somatomotor cortex. Oscillations of 25–35 Hz occurred in the sensorimotor cortex of awake behaving monkeys both in LFPs and in single- /multi-unit recordings. They were particularly apparent during the performance of motor tasks that required fine finger movements and focused attention. These oscillations were coherent over cortical patches extending at least up to 14 mm that included the cortical representation of the arm. Synchronous oscillations were also found straddling the central sulcus, so they may reflect the integration of sensory and motor processes. The LFP reversed polarity at about 800 μm under the cortical surface, indicating that the source of the LFP is in the superficial cortical layers. It is noteworthy that at least some of the cortical beta/gamma rhythmic activities appear to depend on projecting dopaminergic fibers arising in the ventral tegmental area, but it is not clear to what extent the beta rhythms of the somatomotor cortex are related to thalamic or other subcortical activities.

It is relevant to correlate the characteristics of EEG beta/gamma activities found in experimental animals with those recorded from the scalp in man. Beta/gamma activity was reported by DeFrance and Sheer to occur over the parieto-temporo-occipital cortex in man, particularly in relation to the performance of motor tasks.

With respect to the origin of beta/gamma rhythmic activity, several experimental facts have led to the interpretation that these rhythmic activities are primarily generated in the cortex: (i) the fact that oscillations in the beta/gamma frequency range were easily recorded from different cortical sites but not from simultaneously obtained recordings from thalamic electrodes; (ii) the observation that in the visual cortex there are neurons that show oscillatory firing rates with a phase difference of about one-fourth of a cycle, indicating that a local recurrent feedback circuit can be responsible for the oscillations; and (iii) the finding of intrinsic oscillations in cortical neurons from layer IV of the frontal cortex of guinea pig *in vitro*. Nevertheless, it is possible that thalamic neuronal networks also contribute to the cortical beta/gamma rhythmic activity since about 40-Hz oscillatory behavior has been observed by Mircea Steriade and collaborators in neurons of the intralaminar centrolateral nucleus that projects widely to the cerebral cortex. The question cannot be stated as a simple alternative between a cortical versus a thalamic rhythmic process, both considered as exclusive mechanisms. As discussed in relation to other rhythmic activities of the mammalian brain, both network and membrane intrinsic properties cooperate in shaping the behavior of the population, including its rhythmic properties and its capability of synchronizing the neuronal elements.

VI. EVENT-RELATED PHENOMENA: EEG DESYNCHRONIZATION AND SYNCHRONIZATION

The electrical activity of the brain is ever changing, depending on both exogenous and endogenous factors. The spatiotemporal patterns of EEG/MEG activity reflect changes in brain functional states. These patterns are apparent as a sequence of maps of scalp activity that change at relatively short time intervals, on the order of seconds or even fractions of seconds. Dietrich Lehmann identified these series of maps as reflecting brain "microstates" and proposed that different modes of mentation are associated with different brain EEG microstates.

A classic phenomenon is the EEG/MEG activity that occurs in response to sensory events, the so-called sensory evoked potentials (EPs). In addition, another class of EEG phenomena of the same kind should be distinguished that consists of those changes of the ongoing EEG activity that precede motor acts, such as the readiness potential, or "bereitschafspotential" of Kornhuber and Deecke, and the premotor potentials. In order to detect EPs or, in more general terms, event-related potentials (ERPs), computer-averaging techniques are commonly used. The basic model underlying this approach is that the evoked activity is time and phase locked to a given event, or stimulus, while the ongoing EEG activity behaves as additive noise. Here, I do not consider this kind of phenomena in detail since this forms a specialized EEG field. Nevertheless, it should be noted that the discovery of evoked activity related to cognitive events has resulted in important contributions to neurocognitive research. One example is the contingent negative variation (CNV), first described by Grey Walter in 1964. The CNV is a slow potential shift with negative polarity at the cortical surface that precedes an expected stimulus and that is related to motivation and attention. Another example is a component of EPs that peaks at approximately 300 msec, with surface positivity, after infrequent but task-relevant stimuli that was discovered by Sutton, Zubin, and John in 1965. This component is called the P300, and it depends more on the meaning of the stimulus and the context of the task than on the physical properties of the stimulus. Still another EP phenomenon with relevant cognitive connotations is the so-called processing negativity described by Näätänen that is a large surface negative wave that can begin as early as 60 msec and can last for 500 msec. It is a sign of selective attention. Neurocognitive studies using ERPs and, recently, event-related magnetic fields have been successfully carried out. Such investigations have benefited much from the approach developed by Alan Gevins and collaborators, the so-called EP covariance methodology, that has provided interesting results concerning the cortical processes involved in working memory and in planning of movement. In these studies, the recording of EPs at different brain sites during the sequential processing of cognitive tasks allowed researchers to follow sequential and/or parallel activation of different cortical areas as cognitive tasks evolved. This approach has been particularly successful in studies of brain processes underlying language functions, such as the seminal investigation of Riitta Salmelin and collaborators in Helsinki. Using a whole-head MEG and event-related magnetic fields, they were able to trace the progression of brain activity related to picture naming from Wernicke's area to the parietal-temporal

and frontal areas of the cortex. Subsequent MEG studies of the same group in collaboration with that of Pim Levelt of Nijmegen revealed a more refined pattern of the dynamics of cortical activation associated with the successive stages of a psychological model of spoken word generation. These neurocognitive processes were approached using the novel methodology of combining fMRI and MEG in order to obtain high-resolution imaging, both in space and in time, of cortical activity during semantic processing of visually presented words. These studies confirmed that in general there is a wave of activity that spreads from the occipital cortex to parietal, temporal, and frontal areas within 185 msec during picture naming. Furthermore, they indicated that the effects of word repetition are widespread and occur only after the initial activation of the cortical network. This provides evidence for the involvement of feedback mechanisms in repetition priming (Fig. 5).

Since the focus of this article is the ongoing EEG/MEG activity, I consider in more detail a class of EEG/MEG phenomena that are time locked to an event but

Neuron
62

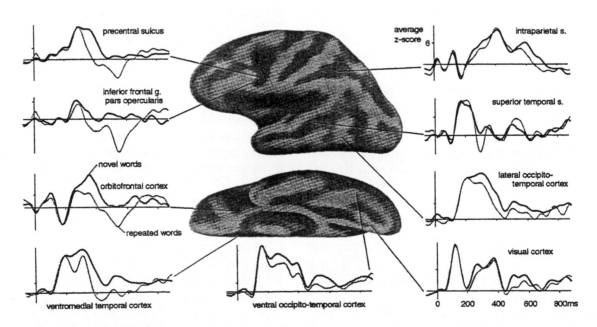

Figure 5 Estimated time courses of MEG signals corresponding to different cortical areas involved in processing of novel and repeated words. The MEG sources were estimated using noise normalization and were fMRI biased toward hemodynamically active cortical areas. The results represent averages across four subjects. Black lines show responses to novel words, and gray lines indicate the responses to repeated words. Waveforms are derived from single cortical locations (each representing 0.5 cm^2). Vertically, the z scores are shown: a score of 6 corresponds to a significance level of $p < 10^{-8}$ (reproduced with permission from Dale *et al.*, 2000).

not phase locked. These phenomena cannot be extracted by simple averaging but may be detected by spectral analysis. An event-related phenomenon may consist of either a decrease or an increase in synchrony of the underlying neuronal populations. The former is called event-related desynchronization (ERD), and the latter is called event-related synchronization (ERS) (Fig. 6). Gert Pfurtscheller and collaborators extensively studied these phenomena. When referring to ERD or ERS, one should specify the corresponding frequency band since, for example, there may be ERD of the alpha band and ERS of the beta band at the same time. The term ERD is only meaningful if the EEG activity during the baseline condition shows a clear spectral peak at the frequency band of interest, indicating the existence of a specific rhythmic activity. Complementarily, the term ERS has meaning only if the event results in the emergence of a rhythmic component, and therewith of a spectral peak that was not detectable under baseline conditions. In general, ERD/ERS reflect changes in the activity of neuronal networks that take place under the influence of specific and/or modulating inputs, which alter the parameters controlling the oscillatory behavior of the neuronal networks.

Even within the alpha frequency band, ERD is not a unitary phenomenon since we have to distinguish at least two patterns of alpha ERD: Lower alpha (7–10 Hz) desynchronization is found in response to almost any kind of task and appears to depend mainly on task complexity. Thus, it is unspecific and tends to be topographically widespread over the scalp. Upper alpha (10–12 Hz) desynchronization has a more restricted topographic distribution, particularly over the parieto-occipital areas, and it is most often elicited by events related to the processing of sensorisemantic information, as shown by the investigations of Wolfgang Klimesch. In general, many psychophysiological variables that cause ERD of rhythms within the alpha frequency range are related to perceptual and memory tasks, on the one hand, and voluntary motor actions, on the other hand. Voluntary movements can result in

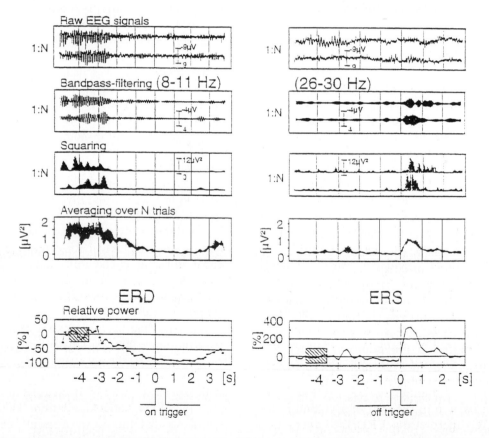

Figure 6 Principle of ERD (left) and ERS (right) EEG processing. A decrease of power within a given band (8–11 Hz) indicates ERD and an increase of band power (26–30 Hz) indicates ERS. Note that ERD precedes the trigger, a finger movement, and that ERS follows the trigger (i.e., it occurs at the cessation of the movement) (adapted with permission from Pfurtscheler and Lopes da Silva, 1999).

an ERD of the upper alpha (also called mu rhythm) and lower beta bands localized close to the sensorimotor areas. This desynchronization starts about 2 sec prior to movement onset, over the contralateral rolandic region in the case of a unilateral movement, and becomes bilaterally symmetrical immediately before movement execution. It is interesting to note that the ERDs for the different frequency bands have specific topographical distributions, indicating that different cortical populations are involved. For instance, in relation to a hand movement, the 10- to 11-Hz mu ERD and the 20- to 24-Hz beta ERD display different maxima over the scalp, although both activities are localized around the central sulcus. The mu rhythm ERD has maximal magnitude more posteriorly than the beta activity, indicating that it is generated mainly in the postrolandic somatosensory cortex, whereas the low beta activity is preferentially generated in the prerolandic motor area. In addition, after a voluntary movement the central region exhibits a localized beta ERS that becomes evident in the first second after cessation of the movement, at a time when the rolandic mu rhythm still presents a desynchronized pattern. The exact frequency of this rebound beta ERS can vary considerably with subject and type of movement. This beta ERS is observed not only after a real movement as shown in Fig. 6 but also after an imagined movement. Furthermore, ERS in the gamma frequency band (approximately around 36–40 Hz) can also be found over the central egions during the execution of a movement, in contrast with the beta ERS that has its maximum after the termination of the movement. A prerequisite for detecting this gamma ERS is that alpha ERD takes place at the same time.

A particular feature of ERD/ERS phenomena that we have recently analyzed is that under some conditions one can find a localized ERD at the same time as ERS in a neighboring region. This antagonistic ERD/ERS phenomenon can occur between two different modalities—for example, ERD of the alpha over the occipital region elicited by visual stimulation accompanied by ERS of the mu rhythm of the central somatosensory region—but it can also occur within the same modality. For example, a voluntary hand movement can result in an ERD over the cortical area representing the hand and simultaneously an ERS over the cortical area representing the leg/foot (Fig. 7). The opposite can be seen in the case of a voluntary foot movement. We interpret this ERD/ERS antagonistic phenomenon as indicating that at the level of the thalamic reticular nucleus, cross talk between the neuronal networks processing different inputs takes place. This may occur as follows: The specific movement would engage a focal attentional process that results in a desynchronization of a module of thalamocortical networks called the target module. This attentional signal is most likely mediated by the activation of modulating cholinergic inputs. These cholinergic inputs hyperpolarize the inhibitory neurons of the reticular neurons and depolarize the thalamocortical relay neurons of a given module. Consequently, the thalamocortical feedback loop responsible for the rhythmic activity becomes open, which is reflected in the ERD that is recorded over the corresponding cortical projection areas. At the same time, the neurons of the reticular nucleus that are adjacent to those of the target module become disinhibited. This results in an increase in the gain of the feedback loops to which the latter belong, thus resulting in an increase in the magnitude of the corresponding rhythmic activity that is reflected at the cortex by ERD. In this way, the analysis of ERD/ERS phenomena has led to the formulation of a hypothesis concerning the neurophysiological processes underlying the psychological phenomenon of focal attention/surround inhibition.

In short, ERD can be interpreted as an electrophysiolgical correlate of activated cortical areas involved in the processing of sensory, motor, or cognitive information. The mirror image of alpha ERD, of course, is alpha ERS (i.e., a pronounced rhythmic activity within the alpha frequency range), indicating that the corresponding neuronal networks are in a state of reduced activity. Thus, these rhythmic activities are sometimes called "idling rhythms," although one should be cautious about the literal interpretation of this term since the underlying neuronal populations are not really "idle"— they are always active but may display different dynamical properties. An important point is that ERD and ERS cannot be considered as global properties of the brain. Indeed, ERD and ERS phenomena can be found to coexist in neighboring areas and may affect specific EEG/MEG frequency components differently.

Understanding the significance of ERS of the beta frequency range that typically occurs after a movement has been aided by the observation that at the time that this form of ERS occurs the excitability of the corticospinal pathways decreases, as revealed by transcranial magnetic stimulation. This supports the hypothesis that the postmovement beta ERS corresponds to a deactivated state of the motor cortex. In contrast, the ERS in the gamma frequency band appears to reflect a state of active information

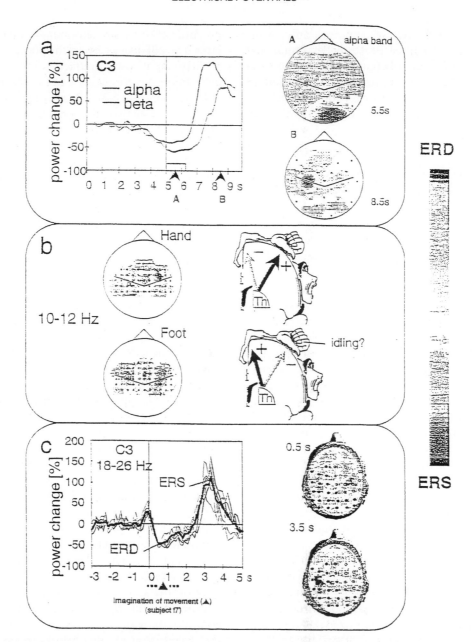

Figure 7 Event-related desynchronization (ERD) and event-related synchronization (ERS) in relation to movement. (a) Average ($n = 9$) of ERD curves calculated in the alpha and beta bands for a right-hand movement task; recording from C3 (left). The maps were calculated for a 125-msec interval during movement (A) and after movement offset in the recovery period (B). (b) Maps displaying ERD and ERS for an interval of 125 msec during voluntary movement of the hand and movement of the foot. The motor homunculus model is shown on the right-hand side to give an indication of the localization of the hand and the foot cortical areas. (c) (Left) Superimposed ERD curves and beta ERS rebound from eight sessions with right-hand motor imagery in one subject within the frequency band 18–26 Hz and for electrode C3. The average is superimposed. (Right) ERD maps displaying simultaneously occurring ERD (contralateral) and ERS (ipsilateral) during imagery and ERS (contralateral) after motor imagery. Color code: dark areas indicate power decrease (ERD) and light areas power increase (ERS) (reproduced with permission from Pfurtscheller and Lopes da Silva, 1999).

processing. Indeed, recordings by Bressler and collaborators from the monkey motor cortex during the performance of a visual-guided motor task showed increased neuronal activity at relatively high frequen-

cies that corresponds in time to the gamma ERS found in human. Furthermore, these gamma band activities recorded from the striate and motor cortex were correlated when an appropriate motor response was made but were uncorrelated when no response occurred. Similarly, the group of Pfurtscheller found that there was an increase in coherence between the EEG recorded from the sensorimotor and supplementary motor areas over one hemisphere, within the gamma range, during the performance of contralateral finger movements.

VII. WHAT ARE THE ROLES OF OSCILLATIONS IN THE PROCESSING OF NEURAL INFORMATION?

This question is sometimes answered in a negative way with the implication that brain oscillations are irrelevant for the functioning of the brain and should be considered simple epiphenomena. This point of view, however, is superficial since is does not take into account what is happening at the neuronal level during EEG oscillations. In order to answer the question, it is necessary to identify the specific neuronal processes underlying such oscillations. Only in this way we may reach an understanding of the functional implications of an EEG oscillation. In other words, we have to analyze the state of a neuronal population that displays an oscillatory mode in terms of the membrane potentials of the neurons that belong to the population. Of course, during an oscillation the membrane potentials of the constituting neurons vary in synchrony. Since the membrane potential controls the transfer of information of a neuron, we must analyze what happens to the membrane potential of the main neuronal population (i.e., the collective membrane potential) during specific oscillatory modes. Two essentially opposite states of the collective membrane potential may occur during an oscillatory state: The membrane potential of the main population changes in either a hyperpolarized or a depolarized direction with respect to the resting membrane potential.

The former case occurs during a sleep spindle or during a burst of alpha or mu waves since in these circumstances the mean membrane potential of the thalamocortical neurons is in a hyperpolarized state. The main neuronal population displays phased inhibitory potentials with only a few occasional action potentials. Consequently, the functional unit formed by this population is in an inhibitory mode and the transfer of information is blocked. In other words, a gate is closed for the transfer of information. Thus, the oscillatory mode of activity characterized by a dominant alpha frequency represents a "closed gate" functional state. In cases in which the mean membrane

potential of the main neuronal population is hyperpolarized at still deeper levels, the population will present oscillations at lower frequency in the delta or ultra-delta frequency range, as it occurs during deep sleep.

In the opposite case, the mean membrane potential of the main neuronal population is displaced in a depolarized direction and it shows oscillations phased with the occurrence of action potentials, sometimes in the form of bursts. The implication is that the probability that series of action potentials of different sets of neurons are time locked increases. This can be the basic mechanism ensuring that neuronal firing becomes synchronized (i.e., that binding occurs). This form of oscillation is usually manifest at relatively high EEG frequencies in the beta/gamma band. Note that this does not imply that oscillations at about the same frequency will have the same functional connotation at the neuronal level. This can be illustrated with two examples that show that different types of beta oscillations may correspond to different functional states of corticospinal pathways. In one case, the beta burst that occurs over the central areas of the scalp at the end of a hand movement corresponds to a state of decreased excitability of the corticospinal pathways. In contrast, the MEG beta activity that occurs over the motor cortex during isometric contractions of the muscles of extremity is directly related to the EMG of the corresponding muscles. A common denominator of both cases, however, is that during the oscillatory mode the main neuronal population displays coherent activity. We may hypothesize that this coherent activity serves a goal in binding the neurons within the underlying population so that they may form a functional unit. The ultimate behavioral result corresponding to the EEG oscillatory mode will depend not only on the state of the membrane potentials of the neurons within the population but also on their connectivity with other networks. The complexity of the circuits that are involved in this process makes it difficult to assign a well-defined functional state to a given EEG/MEG oscillatory mode without precise knowledge of the related processes at the level of neurons and of interconnections between subsystems.

Nevertheless, two main functional connotations of brain oscillations can be put forward: (i) binding or linking of single neurons within a population such that they can form a functional unit of information processing, and (ii) gating the flow of information through given circuits. In addition, we should also consider the possibility that oscillatory modes of activity may contribute to other aspects of brain functions. One aspect is that neuronal networks in general have frequency-dependent properties (e.g., they may show resonance behavior or frequency selectivity). This implies that the transfer of information between two neuronal networks coupled by way of anatomical pathways is likely to depend on the frequency of the sets of action potentials that are transferred between both. This means that oscillatory modes of activity can have another function, namely that of matching, which is the transfer of information between networks from distinct but related areas such that this transfer may be facilitated or optimized.

In this context, it has been demonstrated that in the hippocampus during the theta rhythmic mode of activity, the transmission of impulses through the synaptic path from the CA3 to the CA1 region is reduced. During the theta mode of activity, impulses arising in the entorhinal cortex may pass the two first synapses of the trisynaptic pathway (i.e., to the dentate gyrus and CA3 area) but cannot reach the CA1/subiculum areas. As a consequence, they will be rerouted and will be lead from the CA3 area to target structures of the forebrain, such as the septal area, instead of back to the entorhinal cortex through the subiculum.

Another functional implication of brain oscillatory modes of activity derives from the observation that the strength of synaptic transfer can change, either in the sense of potentiation or depression, depending on frequency of stimulation. This has been evidenced mainly in the case of the theta rhythm of the limbic cortex, particularly of the hippocampus, since it was shown that electrical stimulation at the theta frequency can induce long-term potentiation, whereas stimulation at much lower frequencies may lead to long-term depression. This implies that brain oscillatory activities may be associated with modulating processes of synaptic transmission and plasticity, even promoting the latter in specific synaptic systems.

One general principle of the functional organization of the brain is that it must keep track of different flows of information in the appropriate circuits while it establishes dynamical associations between several sets of processes through multiple reentrant pathways. This means that multiple neuronal networks, at both the cortical and the subcortical levels, are simultaneously active (i.e., that most cognitive processes involve the parallel activity of multiple cortical areas). In this way, different rhythmic activities may be present simultaneously in distinct brain areas or systems.

Another general principle is that processing of information takes place in populations of neurons organized in networks or assemblies of neurons and not just in single neurons. In this respect, evidence obtained recently from studies in which recordings of multiple neurons and LFPs in the visual cortex were obtained simultaneously is strongly indicative that coherent oscillations in a population of neurons could be the basic mechanism to ensure feature binding in the visual system. To underscore this finding, the concept of the linking or association field has been introduced, which is the equivalent—at the level of a neuronal population—of the classic receptive field of the single neuron. The linking field represents the area in visual space in which a stimulus can induce synchronized oscillations in assemblies of cortical neurons. In general, synchronized oscillations occur in different cortical populations if they have similar, or overlapping, receptive field properties and if the appropriate stimulus is present. Therefore, stimulus-induced synchronized oscillations in a given neuronal network may be the basic unit from which attentive percepts that require iterative processing between different neuronal groups are formed.

A third principle of organization, mentioned previously, is that the functional assemblies are interconnected by multiple reentrant connections. The experimental finding that the rhythmic firing of most neurons in an assembly tend to oscillate with zero-degree phase shift results from this property of multiple-level feedback and feedforward.

In summary, note that the change in the activity of a neuronal population from a random mode of activity to an oscillatory mode yields two important consequences for the functioning of the corresponding systems. First, it changes the value of the mean membrane potential in a relatively large group of neurons simultaneously: thus, it sets a bias on the activity of a neuronal population. Accordingly, the transfer function of the population can change in a dynamic way. It appears that the occurrence of synchronized oscillatory activities provides an efficient way to switch the behavior (i.e., to cause a qualitative bifurcation within an assembly of neurons) between different modes of information processing. In this way, neuronal groups with a similar dynamical functional state (linking fields) can be formed. Second, the oscillatory activity may have a frequency-specific role. This role is evidenced by two types of phenomena: (i) matching between interconnected neuronal networks in order to facilitate the transfer of information and (ii) modulation of synaptic plasticity. It is likely that this optimal transfer of information takes place bidirectionally between any two populations of neurons, ensuring what Gearld Edelman called the reentry process. In this way, large groups of neurons can interact optimally. We may speculate that these processes of facilitating the transfer of information between populations of neurons distributed over different brain areas, such that they can form functional units (although with distinct patterns of local activity), could constitute the physiological basis of consciousness. Under specific conditions consciousness would be impaired, as occurs when these brain areas are recruited into a generalized oscillatory mode, such as the 3-Hz oscillations typical of an epileptic absence seizure.

Finally, the fact that neuronal networks tend to oscillate in a synchronized way, depending on local circuit properties and intrinsic membrane mechanisms, is gradually receiving more attention from physiologists and theoreticians. This is important since it is becoming apparent that the functional units of the brain, by means of which information is processed and transmitted, are dynamical assemblies of neurons. It is indeed necessary to determine how such functional networks are formed in order to be able to understand how the brain subserves cognitive functions. To reach these goals, it is clear that new techniques are necessary that combine the analysis of elementary physiological properties of neurons, *in vitro* and/or *in vivo*, with the study of groups of neurons working as dynamical systems in the intact brain.

VIII. CONCLUSIONS

Knowledge of the electrical and magnetic fields generated by local neuronal networks is of interest to neuroscientists because these signals can give relevant information about the mode of activity of neuronal populations. This is particularly relevant to understanding high-order brain functions, such as perception, action programming, and memory trace formation, because it is becoming increasingly clear that these functions are subserved by dynamical assemblies of neurons. In this respect, knowledge of the properties of the individual neurons is not sufficient. It is necessary to understand how populations of neurons interact and undergo self-organization processes to form dynamical assemblies. The latter constitute the functional substrate of complex brain functions. These neuronal assemblies generate patterns of dendritic currents and action potentials, but these patterns are usually difficult to evaluate experi-

mentally due to the multitude of parameters and the complexity of the structures. Nevertheless, the concerted action of these assemblies can also be revealed in the local field potentials that may be recorded at the distance of the generators. However, extracting information from local field potentials about the functional state of a local neuronal network poses many nontrivial problems that have to be solved by combining anatomical/physiological with biophysical/mathematical concepts and tools. Indeed, given a certain local field potential, it is not possible to precisely reconstruct the behavior of the underlying neuronal elements since this inverse problem does not have a unique solution. Therefore, it is necessary to assume specific models of the neuronal elements and their interactions in dynamical assemblies in order to make sense of the local field potentials. This implies that it is necessary to construct models that incorporate knowledge about cellular/membrane properties with that of the local circuits, their spatial organization, and how they are modulated by different mechanisms.

I have presented many arguments and suggestions in line with the concept that the synchronized activity of populations of neurons in general, and the occurrence of rhythmic oscillatory behavior of different kinds in particular, is not an epiphenomenon of the functional organization of neuronal networks; rather, brain oscillatory activities can play essential functional roles within the brain.

See Also the Following Articles

ACTION POTENTIAL • CIRCADIAN RHYTHMS • ELECTROENCEPHALOGRAPHY (EEG) • EVENT-RELATED ELECTROMAGNETIC RESPONSES • GABA • ION CHANNELS • LIMBIC SYSTEM • NEOCORTEX • NEURAL NETWORKS • SLEEP DISORDERS • THALAMUS AND THALAMIC DAMAGE

Suggested Reading

Basar, E., and Bullock, T. H. (Eds.) (1992). *Induced Rhythms in the Brain.* Birkhäuser, Boston.

Dale, A. M., Liu, A. K., Fischl, B. R., Buckner, R. L., Belliveau, J. W., Lewine, J. D., and Halgren, E. (2000). Dynamic statistical parametric mapping: Combining fMRI and MEG for high-resolution imaging of cortical activity. *Neuron* **26,** 55–67.

Gray, C. M. (1999). The temporal correlation hypothesis of visual integration: Still alive and well. *Neuron* **24,** 31–47.

Hari, R. (1993). Magnetoencephalography as a tool of clinical neurophysiology. In *Electroencephalography. Basic Principles, Clinical Applications, and Related Fields* (E. Niedermeyer and

F. H. Lopes da Silva, Eds.), pp. 1035–1061. Williams & Wilkins, Baltimore.

Lamme, V. A., Supèr, H., and Spekreijse, H. (1998). Feedforward, horizontal, and feedback processing in the visual cortex. *Curr. Opin. Neurobiol.* **8**(4), 529–535.

Lehnertz, K., Arnhold, J., Grassberger, P., and Elger, C. E. *Chaos in Brain?* World Scientific, London.

Lopes da Silva, F. H. (1991). Neural mechanisms underlying brain waves: From neural membrane to networks. *Electroencephalogr. Clin. Neurophysiol.* **79**, 81–93.

Niedermeyer, E., and Lopes da Silva, F. H. (Eds.) (1999). *Electroencephalography. Basic Principles, Clinical Applications, and Related Fields*, 4th ed. Williams & Wilkins, Baltimore.

Nunez, P. L. (1995). *Neocortical Dynamics and Human EEG Rhythms.* Oxford Univ. Press, New York.

Pfurtscheller, G., and Lopes da Silva, F. H. (1999). Event-related EEG/MEG synchronization and desynchronoization: Basic principles. *Clin. Neurophysiol.* **110**, 1842–1857.

Regan, D. (1989). *Human Brain Electrophysiology.* Elsevier, New York.

Singer, W. (1989). Neuronal synchrony: A versatile code for the definition of relations? *Neuron* **24**, 49–65.

Steriade, M. (1999). Coherent oscillations and short-term plasticity in corticothalamic networks. *Trends Neurosci.* **22**, 337–345.

Steriade, M., Jones, E. G., and Llinás, R. R. (1990). Thalamic Oscillations and Signaling. Wiley–Interscience, New York.

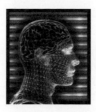

Electroencephalography (EEG)

PAUL L. NUNEZ

Tulane University

GLOSSARY

cerebral cortex The outer layer of mammalian brains; in humans, approximately 2–5 mm thick with a surface area of approximately 1500–3000 cm^2.

coherence A squared correlation coefficient measuring the phase consistency between two signals, expressed as a function of signal frequency.

conductivity (ohm^{-1} mm^{-1}) The property of a material (e.g., living tissue) that determines the ease with which charges move through the medium to produce current.

current density (μA/mm^2) The flux of positive plus negative charge passing through a cross-sectional area.

electric potential (μV) The negative gradient of the local electric field vector.

electrocorticogram Electric potential recorded directly from the brain surface.

electroencephalography Electric potential generated by brain tissue, recorded from locations outside of nerve cells, either from scalp or from inside the cranium.

event related potential Brain electric potential produced by a combination of sensory stimulus and cognitive task.

evoked potential Brain electric potential produced as the direct result of a sensory stimulus.

Ohm's law for a volume conductor Vector current density equals the product of conductivity and vector electric field. Ohm's law simplifies to the usual scalar expression, voltage change = current × resistance, for current flow confined to one spatial direction, for example, in electric circuit wires.

The first recordings of electrical activity [electroencephalography (EEG)] from the human scalp were obtained in the mid-1920s. EEG provides functional, as opposed to structural, brain information and has important applications in medicine and cognitive science. The field of EEG encompasses evoked and event-related potentials and spontaneous EEG. This article focuses on spontaneous EEG recorded from human scalp.

I. WINDOW ON THE MIND

Human electroencephalography (EEG) provides a convenient but often opaque "window on the mind," allowing observations of electrical processes near the brain surface. The outer brain layer is the cerebral cortex, believed to be largely responsible for our individual thoughts, emotions, and behavior. Cortical processes involve electrical signals that change over times in the 0.01-sec range. EEG is the only widely available technology with sufficient temporal resolution to follow these quick dynamic changes. On the other hand, EEG spatial resolution is poor relative to that of modern brain structural imaging methods—computed tomography, positron emission tomography, and magnetic resonance imaging (MRI). Each scalp electrode records electrical activity at large scales, measuring electric currents (or potentials) generated in cortical tissue containing approximately 30–500 million neurons.

Electrodes may be placed inside the skull to study nonhuman mammals or human epilepsy patients. Such intracranial recordings provide measures of cortical dynamics at several small scales, with the specific scale dependent on electrode size. Intracranial EEG is often uncorrelated or only weakly correlated with cognition and behavior. Human "mind measures" are more easily obtained at the large scale of scalp recordings. The technical and ethical limitations of human intracranial recording force emphasis on scalp recordings. Luckily, these large-scale estimates provide important measures of brain dysfunction for clinical work and cognition or behavior for basic scientific studies.

EEG monitors the state of consciousness of patients in clinical work or experimental subjects in basic research. Oscillations of scalp voltage provide a very limited but important part of the story of brain functioning. For example, states of deep sleep are associated with slower EEG oscillations of larger amplitude. More sophisticated signal analyses allow for identification of distinct sleep stages, depth of anesthesia, epileptic seizures, and connections to more detailed cognitive events. A summary of clinical and research EEG is provided in Fig. 1. The arrows indicate common relations between subfields. Numbers in the boxes indicate the following:

1. Physiologists record EEG from inside skulls of animals using electrodes with diameters ranging from approximately 0.001 to 1 mm. Observed dynamic behavior generally depends on measurement scale, determined by electrode size for intracranial recordings. In contrast, scalp-recorded EEG dynamics is exclusively large scale and mostly independent of electrode size.
2. Human spontaneous EEG occurs in the absence of specific sensory stimuli but may easily be altered by such stimuli.
3. Averaged evoked potentials (EPs) are associated with specific sensory stimuli, such as repeated light flashes, auditory tones, finger pressure, or mild electric shocks. They are typically recorded by time averaging to remove effects of spontaneous EEG.
4. Event-related potentials (ERPs) are recorded in the same way as EPs but occur at longer latencies from the stimuli and are associated more with endogenous brain states.
5. Because of ethical considerations, EEG recorded in brain depth or on the brain surface [electrocorticogram (ECoG)] of humans is limited to

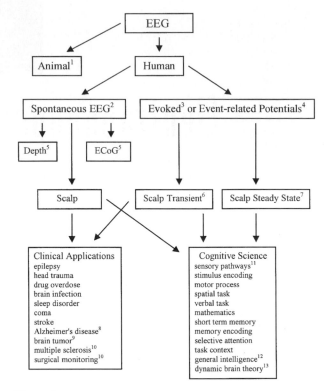

Figure 1 Common relationships between EEG subfields. Clinical applications are mostly related to neurological diseases. EEG research is carried out by neurologists, cognitive neuroscientists, physicists, and engineers who have a special interest in EEG.

patients, most of whom are candidates for epilepsy surgery.
6. With transient EPs or ERPs the stimuli consist of repeated short pulses. The number of pulses required to produce an average EP may range from approximately 10 to several thousand, depending on the application. The scalp response to each pulse is averaged over the individual pulses. The EP or ERP in any experiment consist of a waveform containing a series of characteristic component waveforms, typically occurring less than 0.5 sec after presentation of each stimulus. The amplitude, latency from the stimulus, or covariance (in the case of multiple electrode sites) of each component may be studied, in connection with a cognitive task (ERP) or with no task (EP).
7. Steady-state EPs use a continuous sinusoidally modulated stimulus (e.g., a flickering light) typically superimposed in front of a TV monitor showing the cognitive task. The brain response in a narrow frequency band containing the stimulus

frequency is measured. Magnitude, phase, and coherence (in the case of multiple electrode sites) may be related to different parts of the cognitive task.

8. Alzheimer's disease and other dementia typically cause substantial slowing of normal alpha rhythms. Traditional EEG has been of little use in dementia because EEG changes are often only evident late in the illness when other clinical signs are obvious. However, recent efforts to apply EEG to early detection of Alzheimer's disease have shown promise.

9. Cortical tumors that involve the white matter layer (just below neocortex) cause substantial low-frequency (delta) activity over the hemisphere with the tumor. Application of EEG to tumor diagnosis has been mostly replaced by MRI, which reveals structural abnormalities in tissue.

10. Most clinical work uses spontaneous EEG; however, multiple sclerosis and surgical monitoring are exceptions, often involving EPs.

11. Studies of sensory pathways involve early components of EPs (less than approximately 50 msec) since the transmission times for signals traveling between sense organ and brain are short compared to the duration of multiple feedback associated with cognition.

12. The study of general intelligence, often associated with IQ tests, is controversial. However, many studies have reported substantial correlation between scores on written tests and different quantitative EEG measures.

13. Mathematical models of large-scale brain function are used to explain or predict observed properties of EEG in terms of basic physiology and anatomy. Although such models represent vast oversimplifications of genuine brain function, they contribute to a general conceptual framework and may guide the design of new experiments to test this framework.

II. RECORDING METHODS

A. EEG Machines

Human EEG is recorded using electrodes with diameters typically in the 0.4- to 1-cm range, held in place on the scalp with special pastes, caps, or nets as illustrated in Fig. 2. EEG recording procedures are

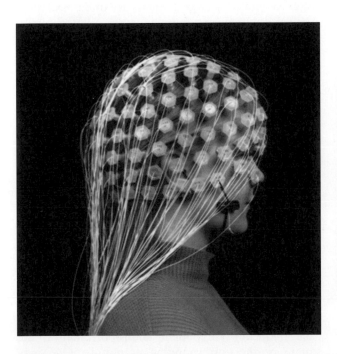
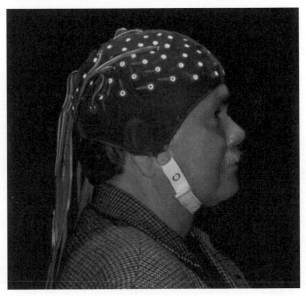

Figure 2 Two kinds of EEG scalp electrode placements are shown in which electrodes are held in place by tension in a supporting structure. (Left) A geodesic net with 128 electrodes making scalp contact with a sponge material (courtesy Electrical Geodesics, Inc.). (Right) An electrode cap containing 131 metal electrodes (courtesy Electro-Cap International, Inc., and the Brain Sciences Institute, Melbourne, Australia). Alternate methods use special pastes to attach electrodes.

noninvasive, safe, and painless. Experimental subjects used in research laboratories are often the same students or senior scientists conducting the research. Special gels are applied between electrodes and scalp to improve electrical contact. Wires from scalp electrodes connect to special EEG machines containing amplifiers to boost raw scalp signals, which are typically in the 5- to 200-μV range or approximately 100 times smaller than EKG (heart) signals. With older EEG machines, analog signals are displayed by rotating ink pens writing on chart paper that moves horizontally across machine surfaces. Modern machines typically replace such paper tracing with computer displays (*digital EEG*) and provide software packages to analyze unprocessed data.

B. Electrode Placement

In standard clinical practice, 19 recording electrodes are placed uniformly over the scalp (the *International 10–20 System*). In addition, one or two reference electrodes (often placed on ear lobes) and a ground electrode (often placed on the nose to provide amplifiers with reference voltages) are required. Potential differences between electrode pairs are recorded with EEG machines containing amplifiers, filters, and other hardware. In *referential recordings*, potentials between each recording electrode and a fixed reference are measured over time. The distinction between "recording" and "reference" electrodes is mostly artificial since both electrode categories involve potential differences between body sites, allowing closed current loops through tissue and EEG machine. *Bipolar recordings* measure potential differences between adjacent scalp electrodes. When such bipolar electrodes are placed close together (e.g., 1 or 2 cm), potential differences are estimates of tangential electric fields (or current densities) in the scalp between the electrodes. Electrode placements and the different ways of combining electrode pairs to measure potential differences on the head constitute the *electrode montage*.

Many research and some clinical laboratories use more than 21 electrodes to obtain more detailed information about brain sources. However, more electrodes may add very little useful information unless supplemented by sophisticated computer algorithms to reduce raw EEG data to a manageable form. Often, 48–131 recording electrodes are used in research; laboratories may soon use as many as 256 channels. The resulting multichannel data are sub-

mitted to computer algorithms that estimate potentials on the brain surface by accounting for distortions caused by intervening tissue and the physical separation of electrodes from brain. The combined use of high electrode density and computer algorithms providing such "inward continuation estimates" to the brain surface is called *high-resolution EEG*. Another approach using sophisticated computer methods is *dipole localization*. This method can estimate the location of source regions in the brain depths in a few specialized applications in which EEG is generated mainly in only one or two isolated source regions. However, in most applications, the sources are distributed over large regions of cerebral cortex and possibly deeper regions as well.

C. Artifact

Potentials recorded from the scalp are generated by brain sources, environmental and hardware system noise, and biological artifacts. Biological artifacts often contaminate EEG records and generally pose a more serious problem than environmental or system noise. Common artifact sources include whole body movement, heart, muscle, eyes, and tongue. EEG records containing large artifacts are often discarded. Artifact removal by computer is typically successful only for the largest artifacts. Such automated artifact editing is severely limited because the frequency bands of biological artifacts substantially overlap the important EEG bands, making distinctions between artifact and brain signal difficult.

III. TIME DEPENDENCE

A. Oscillatory Waveforms

Voltage traces of EEG signals recorded from each electrode pair oscillate with mixtures of component waveforms. Each component may be defined in terms of three parameters: its amplitude (A_{nm}), frequency (f_{nm}), and phase (ϕ_{nm}). The subscript n denotes the frequency component and the subscript m indicates the electrode pair. The electrical power associated with each frequency component is proportional to the square of the corresponding amplitude. One may express any physical waveform as a sum of components with different frequencies, amplitudes, and phases called a Fourier series. Fourier series are analogous to expressions of music or other sounds as compositions of tones or of white light composed of many colors. The EEG voltage $V_m(t)$ recorded from any electrode pair m may be expressed generally as a sum over frequency components:

$$V_m(t) = \sum_{n=1}^{N} A_{nm} \sin(2\pi f_{nm}t - \phi_{nm}) \qquad (1)$$

Waveform frequencies f_{nm} are expressed in terms of the number of cycles per second (or Hz). EEG frequency ranges are categorized as *delta* (1–4 Hz), *theta* (4–8 Hz), *alpha* (8–13 Hz), and *beta* (> 13 Hz). Very high frequencies (typically 30–40 Hz) are referred to as *gamma* activity. These distinctive labels correspond approximately to frequency ranges (or bands) that often dominate particular human brain states. For example, delta activity with frequencies lower than about 1 or 2 Hz provides the largest EEG amplitudes (or power) during deep sleep and in many coma and anesthesia states. Alpha, often mixed with low-amplitude delta, theta, and beta, is typically predominant in awake–resting states. It also occurs in *alpha coma* and is superimposed on delta activity during some sleep stages. Distinct rhythms can also occur in the same frequency range. Disparate rhythms may be associated with behavioral or cognitive state, brain location, or by other criteria. Thus, the plural terminology (alpha rhythms, beta rhythms, etc.) appropriately describes the wide variety of EEG phenomena.

B. Alpha Rhythms

Alpha rhythms provide an appropriate starting point for clinical EEG exams. The following are some initial clinical questions. Does the patient show an alpha rhythm, especially over posterior scalp? Are its spatial–temporal characteristics appropriate for the patient's age? How does it react to eyes opening, hyperventilation, drowsiness, etc.? For example, pathology is often associated with pronounced differences in EEG recorded over opposite hemispheres or with low alpha frequencies. A resting alpha frequency lower than about 8 Hz in adults is considered abnormal in all but the very old.

Alpha rhythms may be recorded in approximately 95% of healthy adults with closed eyes. The normal waking alpha rhythm usually has larger amplitudes over posterior regions, but it is typically recorded over widespread scalp regions. Posterior alpha amplitude in most normal adults is in the range 15–50 μV; alpha

amplitudes recorded from frontal electrodes are lower. A posterior rhythm of approximately 4 Hz develops in babies in the first few months of age. Its amplitude increases with eye closure and is believed to be a precursor of mature alpha rhythms. Maturation of the alpha rhythms is characterized by increased frequency and reduced amplitude between ages of about 3 and 10.

Normal resting alpha rhythms may be substantially reduced in amplitude by eye opening, drowsiness, and, in some subjects, moderate to difficult mental tasks. Alpha rhythms, like most EEG phenomena, typically exhibit an inverse relationship between amplitude and frequency. For example, hyperventilation and some drugs (e.g., alcohol) may cause reductions of alpha frequencies together with increased amplitudes. Other drugs (e.g., barbiturates) are associated with increased amplitude of low-amplitude beta activity superimposed on scalp alpha rhythms. The physiological bases for the inverse relation between amplitude and frequency and most other properties of EEG are largely unknown, although physiologically based dynamic theories have provided several tentative explanations.

C. Spectral (or Fourier) Analysis

The modern methods of time series analysis are often used to simplify complicated waveforms such as EEG. Many industrial applications involve such methods as electric circuits, signal processing (television, radar, astronomy, etc.), and voice recognition. Most time series analyses are based on spectral (or Fourier) methods. Computers extract the amplitudes A_{nm} and phases ϕ_{nm} associated with each data channel (m) and frequency (n) from the often complicated EEG, represented by Eq. (1). The computer "unwraps" the waveform $V_m(t)$ to reveal its individual components. Such spectral analysis is analogous to the physical process performed naturally by atmospheric water vapor to separate light into its component colors. Each color is composed of electromagnetic waves within a narrow frequency band, forming rainbows.

D. Alpha Spectra

Figure 3 shows a 4-sec period of alpha rhythm recorded from four scalp locations. The subject is a healthy waking adult, relaxed with eyes closed. Amplitude spectra recorded from left frontal (top left), right frontal (top right), left posterior (bottom left),

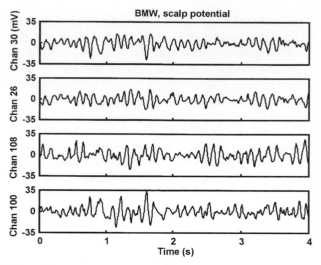

Figure 3 Alpha rhythm recorded from a healthy relaxed subject (age 25) with closed eyes using an electrode on the neck as reference. Four seconds of data are shown from four scalp locations (left frontal channel 30, right frontal channel 26, left posterior channel 108, and right posterior channel 100). The amplitude is given in microvolts. This EEG was recorded at the Brain Sciences Institute in Melbourne, Australia, using the electrode cap shown in Fig. 2 (right).

and right posterior (bottom right) scalp based on 5 min of EEG are shown in Fig. 4. The amplitude spectra show mixtures of frequencies that depend partly on scalp location; however, alpha rhythm is dominant at

all locations in this typical example. This subject has two frequency peaks near 10 Hz, a relatively common finding. These two alpha oscillations are partly distinct phenomena as revealed by their separate distributions over the scalp and their distinct behaviors during mental calculations.

E. Alpha, Theta, Cognitive Tasks, and Working Memory

Two prominent features of human scalp EEG show especially robust correlation with mental effort. First, alpha band amplitude normally tends to decrease with increases in mental effort. Second, frontal theta band amplitude tends to increase as tasks require more focused attention. In addition to amplitude changes, tasks combining memory and calculations are associated with reductions in long-range coherence in narrow (1 or 2 Hz) alpha bands, whereas narrowband theta coherence increases. Large alpha coherence reductions at large scalp distances (e.g, > 10 cm) can occur with no appreciable reduction in alpha amplitude and simultaneously with increases in short-range (< 5 cm) alpha coherence.

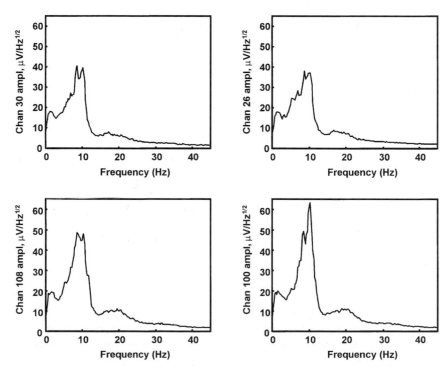

Figure 4 Amplitude spectra for the same alpha rhythms shown in Fig. 3 but based on the full 5-min record to obtain accurate spectra. Frequency resolution is 0.25 Hz. The double peak in the alpha band represents oscillations near 8.5 and 10.0 Hz.

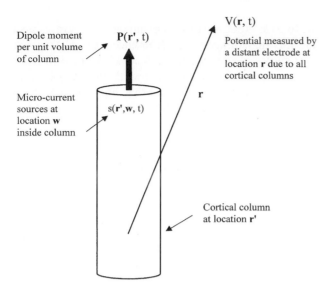

Figure 5 A single column of cerebral cortex with height equal to cortical thickness (2–4 mm) and diameter in the approximate range 0.03–1 mm (the mesoscopic scale). The volume microcurrent sources $s(\mathbf{r}', \mathbf{w}, t)$ ($\mu A/mm^3$) are generated by synaptic and action potentials at cell membrane surface elements, located by the vector $\mathbf{w}$ inside the column. A part of the column (e.g., the center) is located at $\mathbf{r}'$. The microcurrent sources integrated over the volume of the column produce a dipole moment per unit volume of the column $\mathbf{P}(\mathbf{r}', t)$, given by Eq. (2) and expressed in $\mu A/mm^2$. In Eq. (3), the electric potential $V(\mathbf{r}, t)$ at any tissue location $\mathbf{r}$ external to columns (including scalp) is due to the summed (cortical volume or surface integral) contributions from all column sources $\mathbf{P}(\mathbf{r}', t)$.

A common but oversimplified view of alpha rhythms is one of brain idling. However, upper and lower alpha band amplitudes may change independently, depending on scalp location and task. Some tasks cause lower alpha band amplitude to decrease while upper alpha band amplitude increases. Alpha amplitude reductions may be local cortical phenomena occurring in task-relevant brain areas, whereas task-irrelevant regions may be unchanged or even produce larger alpha amplitudes. Another (possibly complementary) hypothesis is that increases in higher frequency alpha amplitudes reflect a specific memory processing function and not simple idling.

Generally, intracerebral electrodes record a variety of alpha rhythms. Some intracerebral alpha rhythms are blocked by opening the eyes and some are not. Some respond in some way to mental activity and some do not. The alpha band rhythms recorded on the scalp represent spatial averages of many alpha components. For an alpha rhythm of a particular type to be observed on the scalp, it must be synchronized (roughly in phase) over a large cortical area.

F. The Rhythmic Zoo

Human EEG exhibits many waveforms, especially in the experience of clinical electroencephalographers (neurologists with specialized training). Some EEGs have known clinical significance and some do not. Any complicated waveform can be described as a mixture of oscillations with different frequencies and amplitudes, as indicated by Eq. (1). However, more picturesque descriptions are often preferred by electroencephalographers to characterized the "zoo" of EEG waveforms. Such labels include *paradoxical alpha, spike and wave, delta focus, sharp transient, sleep spindle, and nonspecific disrhythmia.*

Cortical EEG (ECoG) typically consists of complex waveforms composed of rhythms with different frequencies, locations, and spatial extent. This normal ECoG differentation between cortical areas is eliminated by anesthesia, suggesting a transition from more locally to more globally dominated brain dynamics. Highly localized cortical rhythms are not recorded on the scalp. Cortical beta rhythms are often strongly attenuated between cortex and scalp because they are more localized than some of the alpha band activity. EEG during sleep, coma, and anesthesia typically exhibits large scalp amplitudes, implying widely distributed cortical source activity.

IV. TOPOGRAPHY

A. Dynamic Measures that Depend on Spatial Location

EEG recorded from a single electrode pair is fully characterized by its time dependence, as in Eq. (1). In spatially extended systems, however, dynamic behavior generally depends on both time and spatial location, the usual independent variables of dynamical systems. Thus, multichannel recordings potentially introduce many new measures of brain dynamic behavior. Amplitude, phase, and frequency may vary with scalp or cortical spatial location, for example.

B. Spatial Distribution of Alpha Rhythms

Alpha rhythms have been recorded from nearly the entire upper cortical surface (ECoG), including frontal and prefrontal areas. High-resolution EEG scalp recordings also show widespread distribution of alpha rhythms over nearly the entire scalp in healthy, relaxed subjects. EEG clinical populations differ, typically involving patients who are older, have neurological problems, and may be anxious during recording. These factors all tend to work against production of robust, widespread alpha rhythms. Second, the clinical definition of alpha is based on raw waveforms rather than spectra. Often, alpha is identified simply by counting the number of zero crossings of recorded waveforms. This can sometimes provide a misleading picture because raw EEG composed of broad frequency bands can appear very "non-alpha" to visual inspection, even though its amplitude spectrum shows substantial contribution from the alpha band. Such alpha rhythms may consist of mixtures of both localized and widely distributed activity.

Larger amplitude frontal alpha often occurs as subjects become more relaxed, for example, by employing relaxation or meditation techniques. Alpha rhythms of unusually large amplitude or exhibiting frontal dominance may be associated with mental retardation and some types of epilepsy. Large amplitude and dominant frontal alpha rhythm may also be recorded in some coma and anesthesia states. In summary, frontal alpha rhythms of moderate amplitude are common in healthy relaxed subjects with closed eyes, but very large frontal alpha is associated with disease or anesthesia. The physiological relationships between these disparate alpha phenomena are unknown, but they appear to share some underlying physiological mechanisms since their frequencies and widespread distributions are similar.

C. Coherence

Other dynamic measures involve a combination of location and time measures. For example, the (normalized) covariance of two signals is a correlation coefficient expressed as a function of time delay for characteristic waveforms recorded at the two locations. Covariance is used in ERP studies of cognition. A measure similar to covariance is the coherence of two signals, which is also a correlation coefficient (squared). It measures the phase consistency between pairs of signals in each frequency band. Scalp potential (with respect to a reference) recorded at many scalp locations, for example, over 1-min record may be represented by Eq. (1). Consider any two locations with time-dependent voltages $V_i(t)$ and $V_j(t)$. The methods of Fourier analysis may be used to determine the phases ϕ_{ni}^p and ϕ_{nj}^p associated with each 1-sec period or *epoch* (indicated by superscript p) of the full 60-sec record. The frequency component is indicated by subscript n and

the two electrode locations are indicated by subscripts i and j. If the voltage phase difference $(\phi_{ni}^p - \phi_{nj}^p)$ is fixed over successive epochs p (*phase locked*), the estimated EEG coherence between scalp locations i and j is equal to 1 at frequency n. On the other hand, if the phase difference varies randomly over epochs, estimated coherence will be small at this frequency.

An EEG record involving J recording electrodes will generally provide $J(J-1)/2$ coherence estimates for each frequency band. For example, with $J = 64$ electrodes and 1-sec epochs, coherence estimates may be obtained for all electrode pairs (2016) for each integer frequency between 1 and 15 Hz. The generally very complicated coherence picture may be called the *coherence structure of EEG*. This dynamic structure provides information about local versus global dynamic behavior. It provides one important measure of functional interactions between oscillating brain subsystems. EEG coherence is a different (but closely related) measure than EEG "synchrony," which refers to sources oscillating approximately in phase so that their individual contributions to EEG add by superposition. Thus, *desynchronization* is often associated with amplitude reduction. Sources that are *synchronous* (small phase differences) over substantial times will also tend to be coherent. However, the converse need not be true; coherent sources may remain approximately 180° out of phase so their individual contributions to EEG tend to cancel.

V. SOURCES OF SCALP POTENTIALS

The *generators* of scalp potentials are best described as microcurrent sources at cell membranes. Relationships between such very small-scale sources and macroscopic potentials at the scalp are made easier by employing an intermediate (*mesoscopic*) descriptive scale. This approach makes use of the columnar structure of neocortex, believed to contain the dominant sources of spontaneous scalp potentials. For macroscopic measurements, the "source strength" of a volume of tissue is defined by its electric dipole moment per unit volume:

$$\mathbf{P}(\mathbf{r}', t) = \frac{1}{W} \int \int_W \int \mathbf{w} s(\mathbf{r}', \mathbf{w}, t) dW(\mathbf{w}) \qquad (2)$$

Here, the three integral signs indicate integration over a small, local volume W of tissue, where $dW(\mathbf{w})$ is the tissue volume element. $s(\mathbf{r}', \mathbf{w}, t)$ is the local volume source current ($\mu A/mm^3$) near membrane surfaces inside a tissue volume with vector location $\mathbf{r}'$. $\mathbf{w}$ is the vector location of sources within $dW(\mathbf{w})$ as indicated in Fig. 5. The current dipole moment per unit volume $\mathbf{P}(\mathbf{r}', t)$ in a conductive medium is fully analogous to charge polarization in a dielectric (insulator). Macroscopic tissue volumes satisfy the condition of electroneutrality at EEG frequencies. That is, current consists of movement of positive and negative ions in opposite directions, but the total charge in any mesoscopic tissue volume is essentially zero. Cortical morphology is characterized by its columnar structure with pyramidal cell axons aligned normal to the local cortical surface. Because of this layered structure, the volume elements $dW(\mathbf{w})$ may be viewed as cortical columns with height ≈ 2–5 mm, as shown in Fig. 5. For purposes of describing scalp potentials, the choice of basic cortical column diameter is somewhat arbitrary. Anything between the cortical *minicolumn* (≈ 0.03 mm) and *macrocolumn* scales (≈ 1 mm) may be used to describe scalp potentials.

The microsources $s(\mathbf{r}', \mathbf{w}, t)$ are generally mixed positive and negative due to local inhibitory and excitatory synapses, respectively. In addition to these active sources, the $s(\mathbf{r}', \mathbf{w}, t)$ include passive membrane (return) current required for current conservation. Dipole moment per unit volume $\mathbf{P}(\mathbf{r}', t)$ has units of current density ($\mu A/m^2$). For the idealized case of sources of one sign confined to a superficial cortical layer and sources of opposite sign confined to a deep layer, $\mathbf{P}(\mathbf{r}', t)$ is approximately the diffuse current density across the column. This corresponds to superficial inhibitory synapses and deep excitatory synapses, for example. However, more generally, column source strength $\mathbf{P}(\mathbf{r}', t)$ is reduced as excitatory and inhibitory synapses overlap along column axes.

Increased membrane capacity tends to confine the microsources $s(\mathbf{r}', \mathbf{w}, t)$ within each column to produce smaller effective pole separations—that is, smaller strengths $\mathbf{P}(\mathbf{r}', t)$. However, capacitive effects at macroscopic scales are negligible in normal EEG frequency bands. Also, tissue conductivity is only very weakly dependent on frequency. As a result of these two properties, a single dipole source implanted in the brain generates a time dependence of scalp potential that is identical (except for amplitude attenuation) to that of the source. Amplitude attenuation is independent of source frequency in the EEG range if the sources are equally distributed in location. The selective attenuation of different EEG frequency bands occurs as an indirect result of distinct spatial distributions of the sources.

Human neocortical sources may be viewed as forming a large *dipole sheet* (or *layer*) of perhaps 1500–3000 cm^2 over which the function $\mathbf{P}(\mathbf{r}', t)$ varies continuously with cortical location $\mathbf{r}'$, measured in and out of cortical folds. In limiting cases, this dipole layer might consist of only a few discrete regions where $\mathbf{P}(\mathbf{r}', t)$ is large, consisting of localized or *focal sources*. However, more generally, $\mathbf{P}(\mathbf{r}', t)$ is distributed over the entire folded surface. The question of whether $\mathbf{P}(\mathbf{r}', t)$ is distributed or localized in particular brain states is often controversial. The averaging of EPs over trials substantially alters the nature of this issue. Such time averaging strongly biases EPs toward (trial-to-trial) time stationary sources (e.g., sources confined to primary sensory cortex).

VI. VOLUME CONDUCTION OF HEAD CURRENTS

Scalp potential may be expressed as a volume integral of dipole moment per unit volume over the entire brain provided $\mathbf{P}(\mathbf{r}', t)$ is defined generally rather than in columnar terms. For the important case of dominant cortical sources, scalp potential may be approximated by the following integral of dipole moment over the cortical volume Θ:

$$V(\mathbf{r}, t) = \int \int_{\Theta} \int \mathbf{G}(\mathbf{r}, \mathbf{r}') \cdot \mathbf{P}(\mathbf{r}', t) d\Theta(\mathbf{r}') \qquad (3)$$

If the volume element $d\Theta(\mathbf{r}')$ is defined in terms of cortical columns, the volume integral may be reduced to an integral over the folded cortical surface. Equation (3) indicates that the time dependence of scalp potential is the weighted sum (or integral) of all dipole time variations in the brain, although deep dipole volumes typically make negligible contributions. The weighting function is called the vector Green's function, $\mathbf{G}(\mathbf{r}, \mathbf{r}')$. It contains all geometric and conductive information about the head volume conductor. For the idealized case of sources in an infinite medium of scalar conductivity, σ, the Green's function is

$$\mathbf{G}(\mathbf{r}, \mathbf{r}') - \frac{\mathbf{r} - \mathbf{r}'}{4\pi\sigma /\mathbf{r} - \mathbf{r}'/} \qquad (4)$$

The vector $\mathbf{G}(\mathbf{r}, \mathbf{r}')$ is directed from each column (located at $\mathbf{r}'$) to scalp location $\mathbf{r}$, as shown in Fig. 5. The numerator contains the vector difference between locations $\mathbf{r}$ and $\mathbf{r}'$. The denominator contains the (scalar) magnitude of this same difference. The dot product of the two vectors in Eq. (3) indicates that only the dipole component along this direction contributes to scalp potential. In genuine heads, $\mathbf{G}(\mathbf{r}, \mathbf{r}')$ is much more complicated. The most common head models consist of three or four concentric spherical shells, representing brain, cerebrospinal fluid, skull, and scalp tissue with different electrical conductivities σ. More complicated numerical methods may also be used to estimate $\mathbf{G}(\mathbf{r}, \mathbf{r}')$, sometime employing MRI to determine tissue boundaries. The accuracy of both analytic and numerical methods is limited by incomplete knowledge of tissue conductivities. MRI has also been suggested as a future means of estimating tissue conductivities.

Despite these limitations preventing highly accurate estimates of the function $\mathbf{G}(\mathbf{r}, \mathbf{r}')$, a variety of studies using concentric spheres or numerical methods have provided reasonable quantitative agreement with experiment. The cells generating scalp EEG are believed to have the following properties: First, in the case of potentials recorded without averaging, cells generating EEG are mostly close to the scalp surface. Potentials fall off with distance from source regions as demonstrated by Eq. (4). In genuine heads, tissue inhomogeneity (location-dependent properties) and anisotropy (direction-dependent properties) complicate this issue. For example, the low-conductivity skull tends to spread currents (and potentials) in directions tangent to its surface. Brain ventricles, the subskull cerebrospinal fluid layer, and skull holes (or local reductions in resisitance per unit area) may provide current shunting. Generally, however, sources closest to electrodes are expected to make the largest contributions to scalp potentials.

Second, the large *pyramidal cells* in cerebral cortex are aligned in parallel, perpendicular to local surface. This geometric arrangement encourages large extracranial electric fields due to linear superposition of contributions by individual current sources. Columnar sources $\mathbf{P}(\mathbf{r}', t)$ aligned in parallel and synchronously active make the largest contribution to the scalp potential integral in Eq. (3). For example, a 1-cm^2 crown of cortical gyrus contains about 110,000 minicolumns, approximately aligned. Over this small region, the angle between $\mathbf{P}(\mathbf{r}', t)$ and $\mathbf{G}(\mathbf{r}, \mathbf{r}')$ in Eq. (3) exhibits relatively small changes. By "synchronous" sources, it is meant that the time dependence of $\mathbf{P}(\mathbf{r}', t)$ is approximately consistent (phase locked) over the area in question. In this case, Eq. (3) implies that individual synchronous column sources add by linear superposition. In contrast, scalp potentials due to asynchronous sources are due only to statistical fluctuations—that is, imperfect cancellation of positive and negative contributions to the integral in Eq. (3). Scalp potential may be estimated as approximately proportional to the number of synchronous columns plus the square root of the number of asynchronous

columns. For example, suppose 1% ($s_1 \approx 10^3$) of the gyrial minicolumns produce synchronous sources $\mathbf{P}(\mathbf{r}', t)$ and the other 99% of minicolumns ($s_2 \approx 10^5$) produce sources with random time variations. The 1% synchronous minicolumn sources are expected to contribute approximately $s_1 / \sqrt{s_2}$ or about three times as much to scalp potential measurements as the 99% random minicolumn sources.

Third, the observed ratio of brain surface (dura) potential magnitude to scalp potential magnitude for widespread cortical activity such as alpha rhythm is approximately in the 2–6 range. In contrast, this attenuation factor for very localized cortical epileptic spikes can be 100 or more. A general clinical observation is that a spike area of at least 6 cm^2 of cortical surface must be synchronously active in order to be identified on the scalp. Such area contains about 700,000 minicolumns or 70 million neurons forming a dipole layer. These experimental observations are correctly predicted by Eq. (3).

Finally, for dipole layers partly in fissures and sulci, larger areas are required to produce measurable scalp potentials. First, the maximum scalp potential due to a cortical dipole oriented tangent to the scalp surface is estimated to be about one-third to one-fifth of the maximum scalp potential due to a dipole of the same strength and depth but orientated normal to the surface. Second, tangential dipoles tend to be located more in fissures and (deeper) sulci and may also tend to cancel due to opposing directions on opposite sides of the fissures and sulci. Third, and most important, synchronous dipole layers of sources with normal orientation covering multiple adjacent gyri can form, leading to large scalp potentials due to the product $\mathbf{P}(\mathbf{r}', t) \cdot \mathbf{G}(\mathbf{r}, \mathbf{r}')$ having constant sign over the integral in Eq. (3).

VII. DYNAMIC BEHAVIOR OF SOURCES

EEG waveforms recorded on the scalp are due to a linear superposition of contributions from billions of microcurrent sources or, expressed another way, by thousands to millions of columnar sources $\mathbf{P}(\mathbf{r}', t)$ located in cerebral cortex, as indicted by Eq. (3). However, the underlying physiological bases for the dynamic behavior of the sources are mostly unknown. The 10-Hz range oscillations of alpha rhythm, the 1-Hz range oscillations of deep sleep, and other waveforms in the EEG zoo must be based on some sort of characteristic time delays produced at smaller scales. Such delays can evidently be developed in *neural networks* that cover a wide range of spatial scales.

Locally generated activity in small networks and more globally generated activity involving spatially extensive networks up to the global scale of the entire cerebral cortex may be reasonably assumed. The local network category includes so-called *thalamic pacemakers* that could possibly impose oscillations in specific frequency ranges on cortex (*local resonances*). Other possible mechanisms occur at intermediate scales between local and global. These involve feedback between cortex and thalamus or between specific cortical locations. Preferred frequencies generated at intermediate scales may be termed *regional resonances*. At the global scale, the generation of resonant frequencies (*global resonances*) due to *standing waves of synaptic action* has been proposed.

Delays in local networks are believed due mainly to *rise and decay times of postsynaptic potentials*. In contrast, global delays occur as a result of *propagation of action potentials* along axons connecting distant cortical regions (*corticocortical fibers*). Delays in regional networks may involve both local and global mechanisms. A working conjecture is that local, regional, and global resonant phenomena all potentially contribute to source dynamics. However, the relative contributions of networks with different sizes may be quite different in different brain states. The transition from awake to anesthesia states is an example of a local to global change. The ECoG changes from rhythms depending strongly on location to rhythms that look similar over widespread cortical locations. Another example is desynchronization (amplitude reduction) of alpha rhythms that occurs with eye opening and certain mental tasks.

Several mathematical theories have been developed since the early 1970s to explain the physiological bases for source dynamics—that is, the underlying reasons for specific time-dependent behaviors of the source function $P(r',t)$. Distinct theories may compete, complement each other, or both. Some common EEG properties for which plausible quantitative explanations have emerged naturally from mathematical theories include the following observed relations: frequency ranges, amplitude versus frequency, spatial versus temporal frequency, maturation of alpha rhythm, alpha frequency–brain size correlation, frequency versus corticocortical propagation speed, frequency versus scalp propagation speed, frequency dependence on neurotransmitter action, and mechanisms for cross-scale interactions between hierarchical networks. Because the brain is so complex, such theories must involve many approximations to genuine physiology and anatomy. As a result, verification or falsification of specific theories for the physiological bases for EEG is difficult. However, such mathematical theories can profoundly influence our general conceptual framework of brain processes and suggest new studies to test these ideas.

See Also the Following Articles

CEREBRAL CORTEX • ELECTRICAL POTENTIALS • EVENT-RELATED ELECTROMAGNETIC RESPONSES • IMAGING: BRAIN MAPPING METHODS • MAGNETIC RESONANCE IMAGING (MRI) • NEOCORTEX

Suggested Reading

Braitenberg, V., and Schuz, A. (1991). *Anatomy of the Cortex. Statistics and Geometry.* Springer-Verlag, New York.

Ebersole, J. S. (1997). Defining epileptogenic foci: Past, present, future. *J. Clin. Neurophysiol.* **14**, 470–483.

Gevins, A. S., Le, J., Martin, N., Brickett, P., Desmond, J., and Reutter, B. (1994). High resolution EEG: 124-channel recording, spatial enhancement, and MRI integration methods. *Electroencephalogr. Clin. Neurophysiol.* **90**, 337–358.

Gevins, A. S., Smith, M. E., McEvoy, L., and Yu, D. (1997). High-resolution mapping of cortical activation related to working memory: Effects of task difficulty, type of processing, and practice. *Cerebral Cortex* **7**, 374–385.

Klimesch, W. (1996) Memory processes, brain oscillations and EEG synchronization. *Int. J. Psychophysiol.* **24**, 61–100.

Malmuvino, J., and Plonsey, R. (1995). *Bioelectromagetism.* Oxford Univ. Press, New York.

Niedermeyer, E., and Lopes da Silva, F. H. (Eds.) (1999). *Electroencephalography. Basic Principals, Clinical Applications, and Related Fields,* 4th ed. Williams & Wilkins, London.

Nunez, P. L. (1981). *Electric Fields of the Brain: The Neurophysics of EEG.* Oxford Univ. Press, New York.

Nunez, P. L. (1995). *Neocortical Dynamics and Human EEG Rhythms.* Oxford Univ. Press, New York.

Nunez, P. L., Srinivasan, R., Westdorp, A. F., Wijesinghe, R. S., Tucker, D. M., Silberstein, R. B., and Cadusch, P. J. (1997). EEG coherency I: Statistics, reference electrode, volume conduction, Laplacians, cortical imaging, and interpretation at multiple scales. *Electroencephalogr. Clin. Neurophysiol.* **103**, 516–527.

Nunez, P. L., Wingeier, B. M., and Silberstein, R. B. (2001). Spatial–temporal structures of human alpha rhythms: Theory, microcurrent sources, multiscale measurements, and global binding of local networks. *Human Brain Mapping* **13**, 125–164.

Nuwer, M. (1997). Assessment of digital EEG, quantitative EEG, and EEG brain mapping: Report of the American Academy of Neurology and the American Clinical Neurophysiology Society. *Neurology* **49**, 277–292.

Sato, S. (1990). *Advances in Neurology, Vol. 54, Magnetoencephalography.* Raven Press, New York.

Scott, A. C. (1995). *Stairway to the Mind.* Springer-Verlag, New York.

Srinivasan, R., Nunez, P. L., and Silberstein, R. B. (1998). Spatial filtering and neocortical dynamics: Estimates of EEG coherence. *IEEE Trans. Biomed. Eng.* **45**, 814–825.

Uhl, C. (Ed.) (1999). *Analysis of Neurophysiological Brain Functioning.* Springer-Verlag, Berlin.

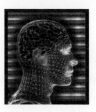

Emotion

RALPH ADOLPHS and ANDREA S. HEBERLEIN

University of Iowa College of Medicine

I. Introduction

II. Animals

III. Humans

IV. Development and Evolution of Emotion

V. The Future

GLOSSARY

amygdala (from Greek *amygdala* = "almond"). A collection of nuclei located deep in the medial temporal lobe bilaterally. Extensively connected with cerebral cortex, it projects also to hypothalamus and brain stem nuclei.

basic emotions A limited set (usually six) of emotions thought to be primary; exhibited and recognized cross-culturally and observed early in human development. The standard list of basic emotions is anger, fear, sadness, happiness, disgust, and surprise.

emotional reaction The physiological components of an emotion, including but not limited to changes in heart rate, blood pressure, and piloerection.

feeling The subjective experience of emotion.

orbitofrontal cortex (used interchangeably here with ventromedial frontal cortex). The area of cerebral cortex on the ventral and medial side of the frontal lobes. This area is heavily connected to the amygdala.

periaqueductal gray matter Several columns of cells in the midbrain, surrounding the aqueduct.

social emotions A set of emotions thought to exist only in social species, in which emotional states are elicited by specific social situations and require some awareness of other individuals. Social emotions include embarrassment, pride, and guilt.

valence The pleasant or unpleasant aspect of an emotional feeling.

ventral striatum Components of the basal ganglia, including the nucleus accumbens septi and ventral parts of the caudate nucleus. These structures receive input from areas including amygdala and

orbitofrontal cortex and project to the ventral globus pallidus (which projects via other structures back to amygdala and orbitofrontal cortex).

Emotions are internal states of higher organisms that serve to regulate in a flexible manner an organism's interaction with its environment, especially its social environment. Emotions can be divided into three functionally distinct but interacting sets of processes: (i) the evaluation of a stimulus or event with respect to its value to the organism, (ii) the subsequent triggering of an emotional reaction and behavior, and (iii) the representation of (i) and (ii) in the organism's brain, which constitutes emotional feeling. On the one hand, emotions are continuous with more basic motivational behaviors, such as responses to reward and punishment; on the other hand, emotions are continuous with complex social behavior. The former serve to regulate an organism's interaction and homeostasis with its physical environment, whereas the latter serves an analogous role in regard to the social environment. Studies in animals have focused on the first of the two previously mentioned aspects of emotion and have investigated the neural systems whereby behavior is guided by the reinforcing properties of stimuli. Structures such as the amygdala, orbitofrontal cortex, and ventral striatum have been shown to play critical roles in this regard. In humans, these same structures have been shown to also participate in more complex aspects of social behavior; additionally, there are structures in the right hemisphere that may play a special role in the social aspects of emotion. Emotions influence nearly all aspects of cognition, including attention, memory, and reasoning.

Encyclopedia of the Human Brain
Volume 2

181

Copyright 2002, Elsevier Science (USA).
All rights reserved.

I. INTRODUCTION

In order to interact flexibly with a changing environment, complex organisms have evolved brains that construct an internal model of the world. Two necessary components of such a model are (i) a representation of the internal environment (i.e., a self-model) and (ii) representations of the external environment, including the other individuals constituting the social environment. An organism must continuously map self and external environment as the two interact in time. Emotion refers to a variety of different aspects of nervous system function that relate representations of the external environment to the value and significance these have for the organism. Such a value mapping encompasses several interrelated steps: evaluation of the external event or situation with which an organism is confronted, changes in brain and body of the organism in response to the situation, behavior of the organism, and a mapping of all the changes occurring in the organism that can generate a feeling of the emotion.

A. Historical Overview

William James, writing in the middle of the 19th century, made the somewhat counterintuitive claim that the subjective experience, or feeling, of emotion is caused by and follows the bodily changes of emotion. Thus, for example, one sees an angry animal approaching quickly, and one's gut tenses, one's heartbeat rises, and one's hair stands on end, all *before* one feels afraid. In fact, James argued, we depend on these physiological changes *in order* to have a feeling of an emotion.

Charles Darwin focused on emotional expressions and described similarities between human emotional expressions, such as smiles and frowns, and nonhuman animal reactions to positive and negative situations. These similarities supported his claim that human emotional expressions were innate and had evolved from once-adaptive muscle movements. Darwin also emphasized the social communicative function of emotional expressions—for example, between mother and infant or between fighting conspecifics.

These historical viewpoints have counterparts in our commonsense, or folk-psychological, concepts of emotion: Important components of emotion include observable expressions of emotion and perceptions of our own feelings, both of which follow the perception and evaluation of an emotionally salient stimulus. These components are also important in most modern theories of emotion, which share the view that emotions are adaptations sculpted by evolution, and that emotions in humans are on a continuum with emotions in animals.

B. The Functional Structure of Emotion

Emotion can be broadly viewed as a relation between an organism and its environment, pertaining both to the evaluation of external stimuli and to the organism's dispositional and actual action on the environment in response to such evaluation. To analyze this view in more detail, we can identify three components of emotion: (i) recognition/evaluation/appraisal of emotionally salient stimuli; (ii) response/reaction/expression of the emotion (including endocrine, autonomic, and motor changes); and (iii) feeling (the conscious experience of emotion). These components, and some of the neural structures that participate in them, are schematized in Fig. 1.

However, it is important to keep in mind that emotion is a broadly integrative function for which recognition (appraisal), experience (feeling), and response (expression) typically all overlap and influence one another. Several lines of evidence point to a correlation between the experience and expression of emotion, at least in many circumstances. For example, production of emotional facial expressions and other somatovisceral responses directly causes changes in emotional experience, brain activity, and autonomic state. Additionally, viewing emotional expressions on others' faces can cause systematic changes in one's own facial expression and emotional experience.

C. Basic Emotions and Facial Expression

It is widely thought that a small number of emotions are basic or primary. Data suggest that there are six basic emotional expressions: happiness, surprise, fear, anger, disgust, and sadness. However, these categories are without clearly demarcated boundaries and show some overlap (e.g., facial expressions can be members of more than one category). The conceptual structure of emotions may thus bear some similarity to the conceptual structure of colors. As with primary colors, there are basic emotions, and, like colors, an emotion can be a blend of other emotions. Basic emotions correspond closely to the emotions signaled from human facial expressions. The basic emotional expressions are recognized easily by normal subjects and are recognized consistently across very different cultures, as shown in the work of the psychologist Paul Ekman.

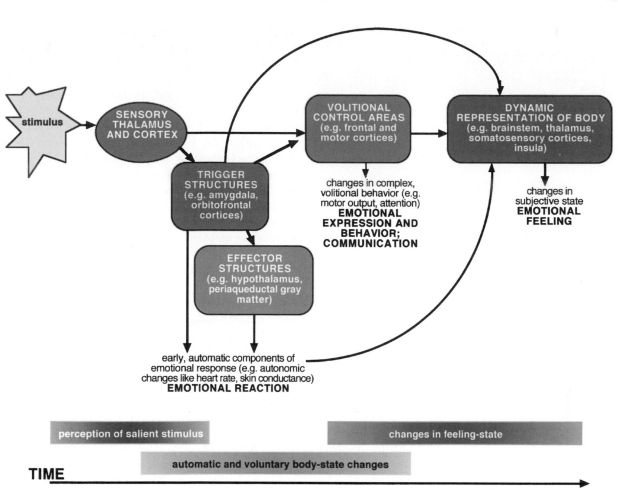

Figure 1 Time line relating the different components of emotion. A stimulus is perceived via a sensory organ, in most cases relayed through the thalamus to sensory cortex. The amygdala and other trigger structures receive projections from thalamus and from sensory cortex at many different levels. These trigger structures then project both to effector structures, such as hypothalamus, that effect changes in autonomic and endocrine activity and to volitional control areas, which are responsible for motor behavior and higher order cognition. All of these areas also project to areas which represent the body state and contribute to the subjective experience, or feeling, of emotion.

Although basic emotions may rely on largely innate factors, they do not appear immediately in infancy. Rather, like the development of language, emotions mature in a complex interplay between an infant's inborn urge to seek out and to learn certain things and the particular environment in which this learning takes place. Considerable learning important to emotion takes place between an infant and its mother. Some emotions that are present very early on, such as disgust, can be elaborated and applied metaphorically to a very large number of situations in the adult. For instance, all infants make a stereotyped face of disgust (as will most mammals) when they have ingested an unpalatable food. In adulthood, both the lexical term "disgust" and the facial expression are applied more broadly, for example to include responses to other

people whom one finds distasteful. Although the circumstances in which an emotional expression may be elicited can be complex and can depend on the culture, a basic core set of emotional reactions are likely shared across different cultures.

Each of the basic emotions is distinct at the level of concept, experience, and expression, but psychological studies have also examined the possibility that there might be factors shared by these emotions. There is evidence from both cognitive psychology and psychophysiology that valence (pleasantness/unpleasantness) and arousal are two orthogonal factors that may capture the entire spectrum of basic emotions. Data from normal subjects show that emotions, as depicted both in facial expressions and in verbal labels, can be represented on a two-dimensional grid with valence

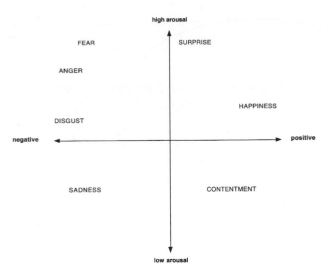

Figure 2 Valence and arousal emotion coordinates. Basic emotions can be placed on this two-dimensional grid.

and arousal as orthogonal axes (Fig. 2). Although such a representation makes sense intuitively, one need not conclude that emotions are analyzed completely in terms of their valence and arousal. A more pragmatic view might treat valence and arousal as two attributes of emotions that are useful for investigation but that may not exhaust all there is to know about emotion.

In addition to the previously mentioned ways of conceptualizing emotions, there are also the terms in our language by which we describe emotions. Certainly, these are much more numerous than just terms for basic emotions, and these include many combinations between emotions and varying shades of intensity of an emotion. Furthermore, we include so-called social emotions, such as guilt, embarrassment, and shame,

which may be found only in very social animals and which may be distinct from basic emotions. Table I provides a summary of some of the different schemes used to classify different emotions. It remains an open question how these different schemes are related to one another. Currently, there is no clear classification scheme that stands out as uniquely suited for scientific investigation: In all likelihood, we will have to use different schemes for different purposes, and we will have to be able to translate research findings from one scheme to provide answers to questions posed under a different scheme. This issue becomes especially pressing when we are using data obtained from studies in nonhuman animals, which often investigate emotion at the level of reward and punishment, to provide insights into emotion at the psychological level in humans. Here, we provide an overview of research findings from both animals and humans that considers some of these issues.

II. ANIMALS

A. Historical Research Findings in Animals

Early studies of the neural substrates of emotion-related behavior in nonhuman animals used both lesion and stimulation methods. In the 1920s, Philip Bard and Walter Cannon observed behaviors in decorticate cats that appeared similar to extreme anger or rage. Brain transections produced increased autonomic activity and behaviors including tail lashing, limb jerking, biting, and clawing. They termed this *sham rage* because they thought it occurred without

Table I
Some Schemes Used to Classify Emotions

Classification schemes	Theory/function
Reward/punishment, approach/withdrawal, and positive/negative valence and high/low arousal	All emotions are reducible to and/or based on basic and opposing principles
Basic emotions: happiness, sadness, anger, fear, disgust, and surprise (sometimes others)	Evolved for adaptive value relative to commonly encountered situations
Basic/primary emotions: desire, anger, fear, sadness, sexual lust, joy, and maternal acceptance/nurturance	Come from subcortical brain mechanisms; evolved for adaptive value; there are several categories of emotions involving progressively greater levels of higher cognitive involvement
Social emotions: guilt, embarrassment/shame, and pride (possibly flirtation)	Occur in addition to basic emotions; elicited only in social situations
All the emotions we have words for in our language	Probably many more distinctions made in language than there are separable brain systems subserving emotions

conscious emotional experience and because it was elicited by very mild stimuli, such as light touches. Further research showed that when the lateral hypothalamus was included in the transected region, sham rage was not observed. More focal lesions of the lateral hypothalamus were found to result in placidity and lesions of medial hypothalamus to result in irritability. This observation correlated with the results of stimulation experiments performed at approximately the same time by Walter Hess. Hess implanted electrodes into different areas of the hypothalamus and observed different constellations of behaviors depending on electrode placement. Stimulation of the lateral hypothalamus in cats resulted in increased blood pressure, arching of the back, and other autonomic and somatic responses associated with anger. These results led to a concept of the hypothalamus as an organizer and integrator of the autonomic and behavioral components of emotional responses.

A second key neuroanatomical finding in animals was that by Klüver and Bucy in 1937, who showed that large bilateral lesions of the temporal lobe, including amygdala, produced a syndrome in monkeys such that the animals appeared unable to recognize the emotional significance of stimuli. For instance, the monkeys would be unusually tame, and would approach and handle stimuli, such as snakes, of which normal monkeys are afraid.

On the basis of these animal findings, as well as on the basis of findings in humans, early theorists proposed several neural structures as important components of a system that processes emotion. One of the most influential of these, put forth by Paul MacLean in the 1940s and 1950s, was the notion of a so-called "limbic system" encompassing amygdala, septal nuclei, and orbitofrontal and cingulate cortices. This system was interposed between, and mediated between, neocortical systems concerned with perceiving, recognizing, and thinking, on the one hand, and brain stem and hypothalamic structures concerned with emotional reaction and homeostasis, on the other hand.

Although the concept of a specific limbic system is debated, the idea is useful to distinguish some of the functional components of emotion, as we have done previously. A key insight is the need for specific structures that can link sensory processing (e.g., the perception of a stimulus) to autonomic, endocrine, and somatomotor effector structures in hypothalamus, periaqueductal gray, and other midbrain and brain stem nuclei. In the next section, we discuss various structures that play a role in either linking sensory processing to emotional behavior or effecting the body state changes of emotion.

B. Brain Structures Studied in Emotional Behavior in Animals

1. Amygdala

The amygdala is a collection of nuclei deep in the anterior temporal lobe which receives highly processed sensory information and which has extensive, reciprocal connections with a large number of other brain structures whose function can be modulated by emotion. Specifically, the amygdala has massive connections, both directly and via the thalamus, with the orbitofrontal cortices, which are known to play a key role in planning and decision making. The amygdala connects with hippocampus, basal ganglia, and basal forebrain—all structures that participate in various aspects of memory and attention. In addition, the amygdala projects to structures such as the hypothalamus that are involved in controlling homeostasis and visceral and neuroendocrine output. Consequently, the amygdala is situated so as to link information about external stimuli conveyed by sensory cortices, on the one hand, with modulation of decision-making, memory, and attention as well as somatic, visceral, and endocrine processes, on the other hand.

Although the work of Klüver and Bucy implicated the amygdala in mediating behaviors triggered by the emotional and social relevance of stimuli, by far the majority of studies of the amygdala in animals have investigated emotion not at the level of social behavior but at the level of responses to reward and punishment. These studies have demonstrated the amygdala's role in one type of associative memory—the association between a stimulus and the survival-related value that the stimulus has for the organism. The amygdala is essential to link initially innocuous stimuli with emotional responses on the basis of the apparent causal contingencies between the stimulus and a reinforcer. Although such a mechanism is in principle consistent with the amygdala's broad role in real-life social and emotional behaviors, it has been best studied in the laboratory as "fear conditioning." Fear conditioning uses the innate response to danger, which is similar in many mammals and includes freezing, increase in blood pressure and heart rate, and release of stress hormones. This response is elicited in fear conditioning by a noxious stimulus such as an electric shock to the foot. If this shock is preceded by an innocuous stimulus such as a bell, the bell comes to be associated with the shock, and eventually the subject will exhibit the fear response to the bell. Joseph LeDoux and colleagues used this paradigm to study the neural substrates of conditioned fear responses in rats. By using anatomical tracing techniques to determine candidate structures and then lesioning these to observe changes in conditioning behavior, LeDoux determined that two nuclei in the amygdala are vital for associating an auditory stimulus with a fear response. The lateral nucleus receives projections from the auditory thalamus and cortex, and the central nucleus coordinates the response in various effector systems (freezing, increase in blood pressure, etc.).

The amygdala's role in associating sensory stimuli with emotional behaviors is also supported by findings at the single cell level. Neurons within the amygdala modulate their responses on the basis of the rewarding or punishing contingencies of a stimulus, as shown in the work of Edmund Rolls and others. Likewise, the responses of neurons in primate amygdala are modulated by socially relevant visual stimuli, such as faces and videos of complex social interactions. Again, it is important to realize that the amygdala is but one component of a distributed neural system that links stimuli with emotional response. There are several other structures, all intimately connected with the amygdala, that subserve similar roles (Fig. 1).

2. Orbitofrontal Cortex

Lesions of the orbitofrontal cortex (discussed in more detail later in regard to humans) produce impairments very similar to those seen following amygdala damage. As in the amygdala, single-neuron responses in the orbitofrontal cortex are modulated by the emotional significance of stimuli, such as their rewarding and punishing contingencies, although the role of the orbitofrontal cortex may be more general and less stimulus bound than that of the amygdala. Amygdala and orbitofrontal cortex are bidirectionally connected, and lesion studies have shown that disconnecting the two structures results in impairments similar to those following lesions of either structure, providing further support that they function as components of a densely connected network.

3. Ventral Striatum

Structures such as the nucleus accumbens also receive input from the amygdala and appear to be especially important for processing rewarding stimuli and for engaging the behaviors that cause an organism to seek stimuli that predict reward. Amygdala, ventral striatum, and orbitofrontal cortex all participate jointly in guiding an organism's expectation of reward on the basis of prior experience. Recent elegant single-unit studies by Wolfram Schultz and colleagues dissect some of the specific component processes. An important neurochemical system subserves the functional connectivity between ventral striatum and frontal cortex: the neurotransmitter dopamine. This system and the specific neurotransmitters involved are currently being intensively investigated as models of drug addiction.

4. Other Trigger Structures

There are several other structures that link stimulus perception to emotional response. Work by Michael Davis and colleagues has highlighted nuclei situated very close to the amygdala, such as the bed nucleus of the stria terminalis, and emphasized their role in anxiety. Other structures in the vicinity, such as nuclei in the septum, are also important and may mediate their effects through the neurotransmitter acetylcholine.

There are a collection of nuclei in the brain stem that can modulate brain function in a global fashion by virtue of very diverse projections. The locus ceruleus, a very small set of nuclei, provides the brain with its sole source of noradrenergic innervation. Similarly, the Raphe nuclei provide a broad innervation of serotonergic terminals. These neuromodulatory nuclei, together with the dopaminergic and cholinergic nuclei mentioned previously, are thus in a position to alter information processing globally in the brain. It is important to emphasize that these changes in the brain's information processing mode are just as important as the somatic components of an emotional reaction —and just as noticeable when we feel the emotion.

5. Effector Structures

The structures involved in emotional reaction and behavior include essentially all those that control motor, autonomic, and endocrine output. Some of these structures have further internal organization that permits them to trigger a coordinated set of responses. For instance, motor structures in the basal ganglia control some of the somatic components of emotional response (facial expressions in humans), and distinct regions in the hypothalamus trigger concerted emotional reactions of fear or aggression, as mentioned previously. Another important structure is the periaqueductal gray matter (PAG), which consists of multiple columns of cells surrounding the aqueduct in the midbrain. Stimulation of these areas has long been known to produce panic-like behavioral and autonomic changes in nonhuman animals as well as reports of panic-like feelings in humans. Moreover, different columns within the PAG appear to be important for different components of emotional response. In a recent functional imaging study, structures in brain stem and hypothalamus were active when human subjects were experiencing emotions, further supporting the roles of brain stem and hypothalamic structures in the coordination of emotional reaction and behavior.

III. HUMANS

Not surprisingly, the neural structures that are important for emotional behavior in nonhuman animals are also important for emotional behavior in humans (Fig. 3). Again, these can be divided into (i) structures important for homeostatic regulation and emotional reaction, such as the hypothalamus and PAG, and (ii) structures for linking perceptual representation to regulation and reaction, such as the amygdala and orbitofrontal cortex. We will discuss the role of frontal

and parietal regions in representing the organism's own changes in body state, focusing on right frontoparietal cortex as well as other somatosensory structures such as the insula. It is again important to remember, however, that all these structures are heavily interconnected, and that most play at least some role in multiple components of emotion. Next we discuss those structures for which the most data are available from humans: the amygdala, the orbitofrontal cortex, and right somatosensory-related cortices.

A. The Human Amygdala

Data on the amygdala in humans have come primarily from lesion studies and from functional imaging studies [e.g., positron emission tomography (PET) or functional magnetic resonance imaging] that image brain activity in neurologically normal individuals. These studies have provided evidence that the amygdala responds to emotionally salient stimuli in the visual, auditory, olfactory, and gustatory modalities. Lesion studies involve patients who have had amygdala damage because of encephalitis (such as Herpes simplex encephalitis) or other rare diseases or who have had neurosurgical resection of the amygdala on one side of the brain to ameliorate epilepsy.

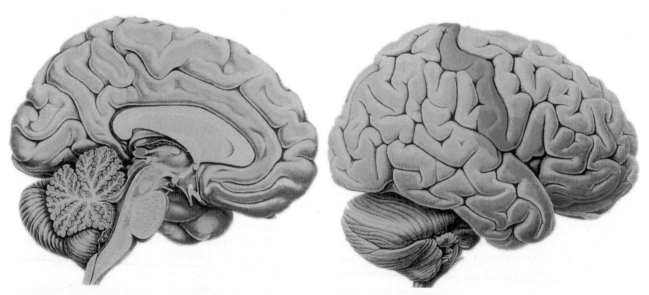

Figure 3   Some of the human brain areas important for emotion. (Left) Medial view of left hemisphere showing orbitofrontal cortex and, deep within the temporal lobe, amygdala, as well as hypothalamus and periaqueductal gray. (Right) Lateral view of the right hemisphere showing orbitofrontal cortex and, buried in temporal cortex, amygdala and also somatosensory cortex and, buried under overlying cortex, insula. As shown schematically in Fig. 1, amygdala and orbitofrontal cortex receive perceptual information and project to effector structures including, principally, hypothalamus and periaqueductal gray. These latter structures effect automatic changes in body state, including blood pressure and heart rate etc. The representation of body state (feeling) depends critically on somatosensory areas, including somatosensory cortex and insula. (See color insert in Volume 1).

As in animals, the human amygdala appears to be important for fear conditioning—for associating conditioned sensory stimuli with an aversive unconditioned stimulus. A variety of neuropsychological tasks have been used in humans to investigate in more detail both the recognition of emotion from stimuli (such as the recognition of emotions from viewing facial expressions of other people) and the experience of emotion triggered by emotional stimuli or emotional memories. Studies of the amygdala's role in emotion recognition have primarily used photographs of emotional facial expression (such as those developed by Paul Ekman). One subject with selective bilateral amygdala damage has been studied extensively with regard to her recognition of emotion in these photographs of facial expressions. This subject, SM046, has been shown in several different tasks to be specifically and severely impaired in regard to faces of fear. When rating the intensity of emotions in facial expressions, SM046 consistently failed to rate the emotions surprise, fear, and anger as very intense. She was particularly impaired in rating the intensity of fear, on several occasions failing to recognize any fear whatsoever in prototypical facial expressions of fear.

SM046's spontaneous naming of the emotions shown in faces in a labeling experiment using identical stimuli was impaired relative to normal controls: She virtually never used the label "fear," typically mislabeling such faces as surprised, angry, or disgusted. Thus, subject SM046's impairment in recognizing emotional facial expressions is disproportionately severe with respect to fear. However, she also has lesser impairments in recognition of highly arousing emotions that are similar to fear, such as anger. This is consistent with a more general impairment in recognition of negative emotions observed in other subjects with bilateral amygdala damage, and it leads to the question of how specific the amygdala's role is in recognition of certain emotions. Interestingly, SM046 is also impaired in her ratings of the degree of arousal present in facial expressions of emotion. When asked to place photographs of emotional facial expressions on a grid with valence (positive/negative) and arousal (low/high) as orthogonal axes, SM046 was normal in her valence ratings but abnormal in the level of arousal that she assigned to negative facial expressions. Thus, it is not the case that bilateral amygdala damage impairs all knowledge regarding fear; rather, it impairs the knowledge that fear is highly arousing.

A likely interpretation of the previous results from SM046, in conjunction with results from other subjects with bilateral amygdala damage, is that the amygdala is part of a more general neural system for recognizing highly arousing, unpleasant emotions—in other words, emotions that signal potential harm to the organism—and rapidly triggering physiological states related to these stimuli. Such physiological states involve both specific sets of behavioral responses and the modulation of cognitive processes, including those involved in knowledge retrieval necessary for normal performance on the previously mentioned tasks. In animals, the amygdala may trigger predominantly behavioral reactions; in humans, it may trigger both behavior and conscious knowledge that the stimulus predicts something "bad." How it is that conceptual knowledge about the arousal component of emotions comes to depend on the amygdala, in addition to emotional arousal itself depending on the amygdala, is a key issue for future research.

Functional imaging studies in normal individuals have corroborated the lesion studies implicating the amygdala in recognition of signals of unpleasant and arousing emotions. Visual, auditory, olfactory, and gustatory stimuli all appear to engage the amygdala when signaling unpleasant and arousing emotions. These studies have examined the encoding and recognition of emotional stimuli, as well as emotional experience and emotional response, but it has been exceedingly difficult to disentangle all these different components. Although there is now clear evidence of amygdala activation during encoding of emotional material, it is less clear whether the amygdala is also activated during retrieval. Two findings suggest that the amygdala's role may be specific to linking external sensory stimuli to emotion and not for triggering emotional responses that are internally driven. First, subjects with bilateral amygdala lesions can volitionally make facial expressions of fear. Second, when normal subjects induced a subjective experience of fear in themselves while undergoing a PET scan, no activation of the amygdala was observed.

Further insight has come from studies that used stimuli that could not be consciously perceived. Amygdala activation was observed when subjects viewed facial expressions of fear that were presented so briefly they could not be consciously recognized, showing that the amygdala plays a role in nonconscious processing of emotional stimuli. In summary, an important function of the amygdala may be to trigger responses and to allocate processing resources to stimuli that may be of special importance or threat to the organism, and ecological considerations as well as the data summarized here all appear to argue for such a role especially in regard to rapid responses that need not involve conscious awareness.

B. Orbitofrontal Cortex

The importance of the frontal lobes in social and emotional behavior was demonstrated in the mid-1800s by the famous case of Phineas Gage. Gage, a railroad construction foreman, was injured in an accident in which a metal tamping rod shot under his cheekbone and through his brain, exiting through the top of his head. Whereas Gage had been a diligent, reliable, polite, and socially adept person before his accident, he subsequently became uncaring, profane, and socially inappropriate in his conduct. Extensive study of modern-day patients with similar anatomical profiles (i.e., bilateral damage to the ventromedial frontal lobes), has shed more light on this fascinating historical case. These patients show a severely impaired ability to function in society, even with normal IQ, language, perception, and memory. The work of Antonio Damasio and others has illuminated the importance of ventromedial frontal cortices (VMF; we use ventromedial frontal cortex and orbitofrontal cortex interchangeably here) in linking stimuli with their emotional and social significance. This function bears some resemblance to that of the amygdala outlined previously but with two important differences. First, it is clear that the ventromedial frontal cortices play an equally important role in processing stimuli with either rewarding or aversive contingencies, whereas the amygdala's role, at least in humans, is clearest for aversive contingencies. Second, reward-related representations in VMF cortex are less stimulus driven than in the amygdala and thus can play a role in more flexible computations regarding punishing or rewarding contingencies.

Antonio Damasio and colleagues tested VMF-lesioned patients on several types of tasks involving the relation of body states of emotion to behavioral responses. When patients with bilateral VMF damage were shown slides of emotionally significant stimuli such as mutilation or nudity, they did not show a change in skin conductance (indicative of autonomic activation). Control groups showed larger skin conductance responses to emotionally significant stimuli, compared to neutral stimuli, suggesting that VMF patients are defective in their ability to trigger somatic responses to stimuli with emotional meaning. In a gambling task in which subjects must develop hunches about certain decks of cards in order to win money, VMF-lesioned patients made poor card choices and also acquired neither subjective feeling regarding their choices nor any anticipatory autonomic changes before making these poor choices. All these findings support the idea that the VMF cortices are a critical component of the neural systems by which we acquire, represent, and retrieve the values of our actions, and they emphasize the close link between emotion and other aspects of cognitive function, such as reasoning and decision making. Damasio presented a specific neuroanatomical theory of how emotions play a critical role in reasoning and decision making—the *somatic marker hypothesis*. According to this hypothesis, our deliberation of choices and planning of the future depend critically on how we feel about the different possibilities with which we are faced. The construction of some of the components of an emotional state and the feeling that this engenders serve to tag response options with value and serve to bias behavior toward those choices associated with positive emotions. This set of processes may operate either under considerable volitional guidance, and as such may be accessible to conscious awareness, or it may play out in a more automatic and covert fashion.

Both the amygdala and the orbitofrontal cortex function as components of a neural system that can trigger emotional responses. The structure of such a physiological emotional response may also participate in attempts to reconstruct what it would feel like to be in a certain dispositional (emotional or social) state and hence to simulate the internal state of another person. In the case of the amygdala, the evidence thus far points toward such a role specifically in regard to states associated with threat and danger; in the case of the orbitofrontal cortex, this role may be somewhat more general.

C. The Right Hemisphere

One generally defined neural area whose importance in emotional behavior and perception has been explored in primates much more than in other animals is the right hemisphere. Both clinical and experimental studies have suggested that the right hemisphere is preferentially involved in processing emotion in humans and other primates. Lesions in right temporal and parietal cortices have been shown to impair emotional experience, arousal, and imagery. It has been proposed that the right hemisphere contains systems specialized for computing affect from nonverbal information; these may have evolved to subserve aspects of social cognition.

Recent lesion and functional imaging studies have corroborated the role of the right hemisphere in emotion recognition from facial expressions and from prosody. There is currently controversy regarding the extent to which the right hemisphere participates in emotion: Is it specialized to process all emotions (the *right hemisphere hypothesis*), or is it specialized only for processing emotions of negative valence while the left hemisphere is specialized for processing emotions of positive valence (the *valence hypothesis*)? It may well be that an answer to this question will depend on more precise specification of which components of emotion are under consideration.

Recognition of emotional facial expressions can be selectively impaired following damage to right temporoparietal areas, and both PET and neuronal recordings corroborate the importance of this region for processing facial expressions of emotion. For example, lesions restricted to right somatosensory cortex result in impaired recognition of emotion from visual presentation of face stimuli. These findings are consistent with a model that proposes that we internally simulate body states in order to recognize emotions.

In contrast to recognition of emotional stimuli, emotional experience appears to be lateralized in a pattern supporting the valence hypothesis, in which the left hemisphere is more involved in positive emotions and the right hemisphere is more involved in negative emotions. Richard Davidson posited an approach/withdrawal dimension, correlating increased right hemisphere activity with increases in withdrawal behaviors (including feelings such as fear or sadness, as well as depressive tendencies) and left hemisphere with increases in approach behaviors (including feelings such as happiness).

D. Neuropsychiatric Implications

Emotion is a topic of paramount importance to the diagnosis, treatment, and theoretical understanding of many neuropsychiatric disorders. The amygdala has received considerable attention in this regard and has been shown to be involved in disorders that feature fear and anxiety. Moreover, specific neurotransmitters, acting within the amygdala and surrounding structures, have been shown to contribute importantly to fear and anxiety. Anxiolytic drugs such as valium

bind to GABA-A receptor subtypes in the amygdala and alter the neuronal excitability. Corticotropin-releasing factor is an anxiogenic peptide that appears to act in the amygdala and adjacent nuclei. Several functional imaging studies have demonstrated that phobic and depressive symptoms rely on abnormal activity within the amygdala, together with abnormalities in other brain structures.

With regard to depression, the frontal lobes have also been investigated for their contribution to emotional dysfunction in psychiatric disorders. Evoked potential recordings and functional imaging studies have revealed their participation in depression, which may engage regions below the frontal end of the corpus callosum. Moreover, individual differences in affective style, independent of any overt pathology, may rely on hemispherically asymmetric processing within the frontal lobes.

IV. DEVELOPMENT AND EVOLUTION OF EMOTION

Both the developmental and the evolutionary aspects of emotion remain important issues for further research. A large body of findings, primarily from developmental psychology, has shown that the highly differentiated sets of emotions seen in adult humans develop over an extended time course that requires extensive interactions between an infant, its parents, and its cultural environment. The importance of many of the structures discussed previously in the development of emotional behavior is underscored by findings that damage to these structures relatively early in development causes more severe impairments than damage during adulthood. Although newborns do show some relatively undifferentiated emotional responses (such as general distress), and although they have an innate predisposition to respond to emotionally salient stimuli (such as the mother's face), the subsequent development of emotion depends both on the presence of critical neural structures and, crucially, on the child's environment. As with language, humans are predisposed to have a rich and complex set of emotional processes, but the precise details require maturation and learning in a socially rich environment.

Phylogenetically, human emotion depends on the more basic sets of emotions and motivational processes that we share in common with other animals. Clearly, the neural circuitry that subserves the processing of reward and punishment must be in place before more differentiated emotions can evolve. However, higher mammals, and especially highly social mammals such as primates, did evolve additional circuitry in order to permit them to respond in a more flexible and adaptive manner to environments that change rapidly in time. The most dynamic environment of all, of course, is the social environment, and keeping track of and responding rapidly and appropriately to numerous conspecifics requires a rich repertoire of emotional regulation.

The comparative and developmental investigations of emotion raise important questions about how emotion contributes to behavior and about how emotion contributes to other aspects of cognition. A point of fundamental importance is that more complex behavior, and more complex cognition, requires more complex and differentiated emotions.

V. THE FUTURE

Emotion is now a hot topic in cognitive science in general and in neuroscience in particular. Future directions can be classified under two general topics: (i) development of a theoretical framework for thinking about emotion and for generating hypotheses regarding its component processes and (ii) further empirical investigations using new methods and using new combinations of methods and species. Especially important will be studies that combine different techniques, such as functional imaging and lesion methods, and studies that combine the same paradigms in different species, such as infant humans and monkeys. Such a multifaceted approach to investigating emotion is in fact being pursued by many laboratories. Currently, neuroscientists, psychologists, and anthropologists are collaborating on several of these issues.

A very difficult, but very important, problem to address in the future is the relation between emotion and consciousness. Recent proposals, for instance, by Antonio Damasio and Jaak Panksepp, have stressed that a proper understanding of emotion may in fact provide the key to understanding one particular feature of conscious experience: the fact that consciousness is always experienced from the particular point of view of the subject. The subjectivity of conscious experience shares in common with the feeling of an emotion that it requires a neural instantiation of a subject; that is, both require a set of structures in the brain that map and represent the organism and its ongoing state changes as the organism interacts with its environment. This proposal is in line with findings that damage to right hemisphere structures involved in self-representation also impairs the ability to experience emotions. The further investigation of the neural basis of such a mechanism, and of its enormous elaboration in humans, may provide us with a better understanding not only of emotion but also of the nature of conscious experience and its role in human cognition.

See Also the Following Articles

ANGER • AGGRESSION • BEHAVIORAL NEUROGENETICS • COGNITIVE PSYCHOLOGY, OVERVIEW • CREATIVITY • EVOLUTION OF THE BRAIN • HUMOR AND LAUGHTER • INHIBITION • PSYCHONEUROENDOCRINOLOGY • SEXUAL BEHAVIOR

Suggested Reading

Adolphs, R. (2002). Recognizing emotion from facial expressions: psychological and neurological mechanisms. *Behav. Cogn. Neurosci. Rev.* **1,** 21–61.

Adolphs, R. (1999b). Social cognition and the human brain. *Trends Cognitive Sci.* **3,** 469–479.

Aggleton, J. P. (Ed.) (2000). *The Amygdala: A Functional Analysis.* Oxford Univ. Press, New York.

Damasio, A. R. (1994). *Descartes' Error: Emotion, Reason, and the Human Brain.* Grosset/Putnam, New York.

Davidson, R. J., and Irwin, W. (1999). The functional neuroanatomy of emotion and affective style. *Trends Cognitive Sci.* **3,** 11–22.

Davis, M. (1992). The role of the amygdala in fear and anxiety. *Annu. Rev. Neurosci.* **15,** 353–375.

LeDoux, J. (1996). *The Emotional Brain.* Simon & Schuster, New York.

Panksepp, J. (1998). *Affective Neuroscience: The Foundations of Human and Animal Emotions.* Oxford Univ. Press, New York.

Rolls, E. T. (1999). *The Brain and Emotion.* Oxford Univ. Press, New York.

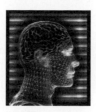

Endorphins and Their Receptors

CATHERINE ABBADIE and GAVRIL W. PASTERNAK

Memorial Sloan–Kettering Cancer Center

GLOSSARY

alternative splicing A way in which different portions of a gene are put together to yield more than a single protein.

analgesic A substance capable of relieving pain without interfering with other sensations.

endorphins Peptides naturally present in the brain with morphine-like actions. They function by activating a family of opioid receptors, which are also responsible for the effects of drugs such as morphine, methadone, and heroin.

opiates Compounds acting on the opioid receptors. Initially defined by their pharmacological similarity to morphine and other analgesic alkaloids present in opium, a product of the poppy plant.

respiratory depression A decrease in breathing.

The opiates, initially derived from opium obtained from the poppy plant, have opened new insights into many aspects of functioning of the brain. The opiates have been used since ancient times and represent one of the most important classes of medications currently in use. In ancient times, opium and extracts of opium were primarily used, although opium also was smoked. Morphine and codeine were isolated and purified from opium in the 1800s, providing physicians with a pure drug with a constant level of activity. Since then, thousands of analogs have been developed in an effort avoid side effects. The structures of these agents vary greatly: however, they share many pharmacological properties.

I. INTRODUCTION

The opiates have a wide range of actions. The opiates remain the most widely used drugs for the relief of moderate to severe pain (Fig. 1). Their actions on pain perception are unique. Rather than blocking the transmission of pain impulses into the central nervous system, like local anesthetics, or working on the sensitization of pain fibers, like the antiinflammatory drugs, opiates relieve the "suffering component" of pain. Patients often report that the pain is still there, but it just does not hurt anymore. This ability to relieve the pain without interfering with other aspects of sensation provides a major advantage. Furthermore, opiates do not display a "ceiling effect," implying that even very severe pain can be successfully relieved at sufficiently high drug doses. Unfortunately, side effects become increasingly troublesome as the dose is increased and the ability of the patient to tolerate these unwanted actions may interfere with the ability to administer adequate doses of the drug.

The actions of the opiates are not limited to pain. The additional actions most often encountered when treating patients are constipation, sedation, and respiratory depression. All these actions are mediated through opioid receptors and can be reversed by opioid antagonists, although evidence is mounting that they may be produced by different opioid receptor subtypes. Opiates influence gastrointestinal transit both centrally and peripherally. Although this action can be troublesome in pain management, it is valuable in the treatment of conditions associated with increased gastrointestinal motility, such as diarrhea.

Respiratory depression is another important opioid action. Opiates such as morphine depress respiratory

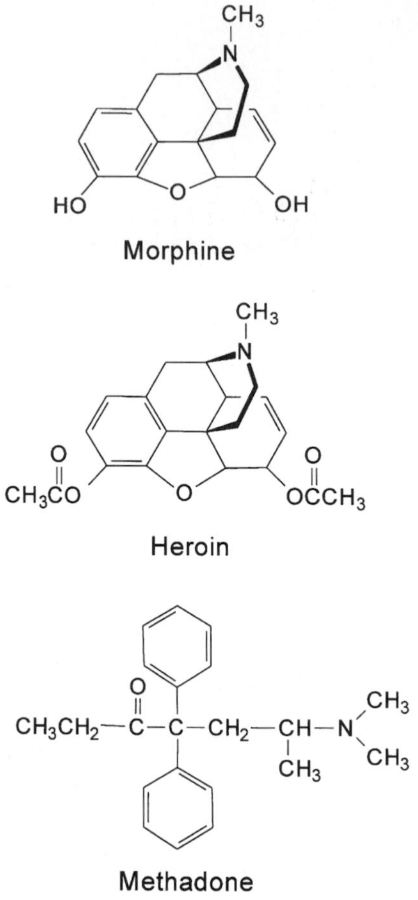

Figure 1 Structures of selected opiates.

the endorphins (Table I). The concept of peptide neurotransmitters has expanded dramatically, the endorphins are now only one family of many active endogenous peptides. This article discusses the four major groupings of opioid and opioid-like peptides and their receptors and also their physiological and pharmacological importance.

II. THE OPIOID AND RELATED PEPTIDES

Soon after the initial description of opioid binding sites using morphine-like radioligands, several laboratories identified endogenous peptides within the brain that bind to these opiate receptors (Table I). These peptides were then termed "endorphins," connoting their endogenous morphine-like character. Although their actions are likely to be very diverse, the only ones examined in detail involve analgesia and all the opioid peptides are active analgesics.

A. Enkephalins

The first peptides identified were the two enkephalins (Table I). These pentapeptides shared the same first four amino acids, differing only by a leucine or methionine at the fifth position. They are the endogenous ligand for the delta opioid receptor. The enkephalins are present throughout the brain and have been implicated in many actions. It is interesting that the enkephalins are present at high concentrations in the adrenal medulla, where they are colocalized with adrenalin. They also have been identified in other, nonneuronal tissues, including immune cells and the testis.

B. Dynorphins

Additional peptides with opioid-like actions were subsequently isolated. Dynorphin A is a heptadeca-peptide that contains the sequence of [Leu⁵]enkephalin at its amino terminus (Table I). Dynorphin A is the endogenous ligand for the kappa₁ receptor, although it retains high affinity for mu and delta receptors as well. Its actions were difficult to evaluate until highly selective, stable drugs were synthesized. These agents have established an important role for dynorphin A and its receptors in pain perception.

depression in a dose-dependent manner and at sufficiently high doses breathing stops. The potential of respiratory arrest is a concern with very high doses of the drugs in naive patients, but typically it is not an issue with patients chronically on the drugs due to the development of tolerance to the action.

Sedation is also a common effect of morphine and related drugs. Indeed, morphine was initially named for Morpheus, the god of sleep. Like other opioid actions, tolerance will develop to sedation, but it may develop more slowly and to a lesser degree than tolerance to the analgesic actions of the drug. Opioids have many other actions. Their effects on the endocrine system are extensive and recent studies have also implicated them in immune function.

Morphine and related opiates produce their actions by activating receptors in the brain, mimicking a family of peptides with similar actions that are naturally occurring within the nervous system, termed

Table I
Opioid and Related Peptides

[Leu⁵]enkephalin	**Tyr-Gly-Gly-Phe-Leu**
[Met⁵]enkephalin	**Tyr-Gly-Gly-Phe-Met**
Peptide E (amidorphin)	**Tyr-Gly-Gly-Phe-Met**-Lys-Lys-Met-Asp-Glu-Leu-Tyr-Pro-Leu-Glu-Val-Glu-Glu-Glu-Ala-Asn-Gly-Gly-Glu-Val-Leu
BAM 22	**Tyr-Gly-Gly-Phe-Met**-Lys-Lys-Met-Asp-Glu-Leu-Tyr-Pro-Leu-Glu-Val-Glu-Glu-Glu-Ala-Asn-Gly-Gly
BAM 20	**Tyr-Gly-Gly-Phe-Met**-Lys-Lys-Met-Asp-Glu-Leu-Tyr-Pro-Leu-Glu-Val-Glu-Glu-Glu-Ala-Asn
BAM 18	**Tyr-Gly-Gly-Phe-Met**-Lys-Lys-Met-Asp-Glu-Leu-Tyr-Pro-Leu-Glu-Val-Glu-Glu-Glu
BAM 12	**Tyr-Gly-Gly-Phe-Met**-Lys-Lys-Met-Asp-Glu-Leu-Tyr
Metorphamide	**Tyr-Gly-Gly-Phe-Met-Arg-Val**
Dynorphin A	**Tyr-Gly-Gly-Phe-Leu**-Arg-Arg-Ile-Arg–Pro-Lys–Leu-Lys-Trp-Asp-Asn-Gln
Dynorphin B	**Tyr-Gly-Gly-Phe-Leu**-Arg-Arg-Gln-Phe-Lys-Val-Val-Thr
α-Neoendorphin	**Tyr-Gly-Gly-Phe-Leu**-Arg-Lys-Tyr-Pro-Lys
β-Neoendorphin	**Tyr-Gly-Gly-Phe-Leu**-Arg-Lys-Tyr-Pro
β$_h$-Endorphin	**Tyr-Gly-Gly-Phe-Met**-Thr-Ser-Glu-Lys-Ser-Gln-Thr-Pro-Leu-Val-Thr-Leu-Phe-Lys-Asn-Ala-Ile-Ile-Lys-Asn-Ala-Tyr-Lys-Lys-Gly-Glu
Endomorphin-1	Tyr-Pro-Trp-Phe-NH$_2$
Endomorphin-2	Tyr-Pro-Phe-Phe-NH$_2$
Orphanin FQ/nociceptin	**Phe-Gly-Gly-Phe**-Thr-Gly-Ala-Arg-Lys-Ser-Ala-Arg-Lys-Leu-Ala-Asp-Glu
Orphanin FQ2	Phe-Ser-Glu-Phe-Met-Arg-Gln-Tyr-Leu-Val-Leu-Ser-Met-Gln-Ser-Ser-Gln
Nocistatin	Thr-Glu-Pro-Gly-Leu-Glu-Glu-Val-Gly-Glu-Ile-Glu-Gln-Lys-Gln-Leu-Gln

C. β-Endorphin

The third member of the endogenous opioid family is β-endorphin, a 31-amino acid peptide that is localized primarily in the pituitary and the cells of the arcuate nucleus within the brain. The initial amino terminus of β-endorphin is identical to that of [Met⁵]enkephalin, raising the question as to whether the enkephalins might simply be degradation products of longer peptides. However, this is not the case, as clearly demonstrated with the cloning of the peptide precursors.

The enkephalins and dynorphins are rapidly broken down by peptidases. Their extreme lability leads to very short durations of action, hampering early work on their pharmacology. However, substituting the glycine at the second position with a D-amino acid stabilizes the enkephalins and many stable derivatives have now been synthesized. The selectivity of these synthetic peptides for the opioid receptor classes can also be dramatically affected by their amino acid sequences. β-Endorphin, on the other hand, is more stable with a more prolonged duration of action. When steps are taken to minimize degradation, all three families of peptides share many actions, including the ability to produce analgesia. These actions are reversed by opioid-selective antagonists, confirming an opioid mechanism of action for the peptides.

D. Processing of Opioid Peptide Precursors

All these opioid peptides are generated by processing longer precursor proteins, which have been subsequently cloned. There are three distinct genes responsible for generating these peptides (Fig. 2).

1. Pre-Proenkephalin

The pre-proenkephalin gene contains four copies of Met-enkephalin and one copy each of Leu-enkephalin, the heptapeptide Met-enkephalin-Arg-Phe, and the octapeptide Met-Enkephalin-Arg-Gly-Leu (Fig. 2A). No dynorphin sequences are present within this precursor. However, the sequence of the gene predicts many additional putative peptides that also contain the sequence of met-enkephalin as the N terminus and thus might have opioid activity and be physiologically important. For example, peptide F contains [Met⁵]enkephalin sequences at both its N terminus and its C terminus. The carboxy-terminally amidated peptide

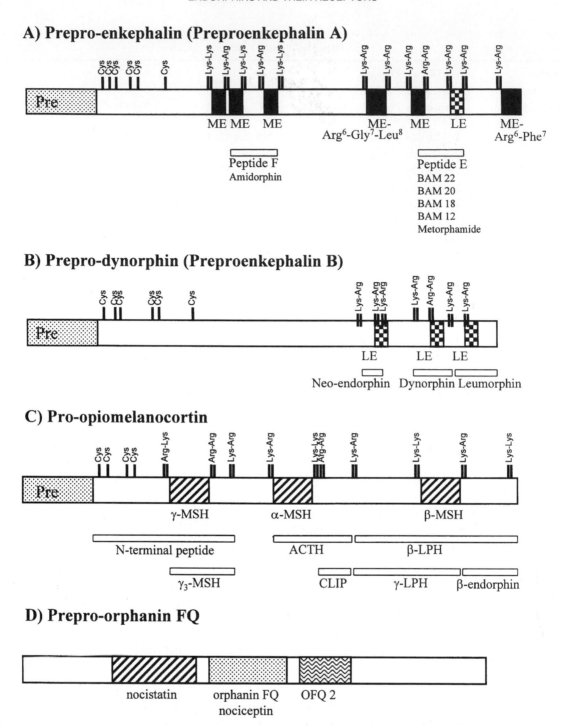

Figure 2 Structures of the precursors of the opioid peptides. Schematics of the precursor proteins for (A) the enkephalins, (B) the dynorphins, (C) β-endorphin, and (D) orphanin FQ/nociceptin.

comprising the first 26 amino acids of peptide F is named amidorphin. Peptide E has a [Met^5]enkephalin sequence at its N terminus and that of [Leu^5]enkephalin at its C terminus. Several peptides in which peptide

E has been truncated at the C terminus have also been isolated: BAM 22, BAM 20, BAM 18, BAM 12, as well as an amidated octapeptide corresponding to the first 8 amino acids of peptide E termed metorphamide or adrenorphin. The physiological significance of these additional peptides remains unclear. They may represent distinct neuropeptides with their own actions. However, the presence of dibasic amino acids following the enkephalin sequence in most of them raises the possibility that they might simply be further processed to the enkephalins. Although they were described many years ago, little work has been reported on these compounds for many years.

2. Pre-Prodynorphin

The pre-prodynorphin gene encodes a larger precursor that has many additional putative opioid peptides (Fig. 2B). The dynorphin precursor is quite distinct from the enkephalin precursor. It contains three [Leu^5]enkephalin sequences, each flanked by pairs of basic amino acids. If Lys–Arg pairs were the only processing signals, pre-prodynorphin would be cleaved into three larger opioid peptides: β-neoendorphin, dynorphin A, and leumorphine. However, several other peptides derived from pre-prodynorphin have been identified. Thus, the formation of dynorphin B results from the cleavage of leumorphin, whereas dynorphin A (1–8) is generated from dynorphin A. In addition, several larger peptides have been identified as putative processing products: a peptide containing dynorphin A at the N terminus and dynorphin B at the C-terminal end have been isolated. Dynorphin 24 contains dynorphin A with a C-terminal extension of Lys–Arg and the sequence of Leu–Enk. There is also evidence for a peptide comprising dynorphin A and leumorphin. In addition to dynorphin A (1–17), the truncated dynorphin A (1–8), and dynorphin B, this precursor also generates α-neoendorphin and β-neoendorphin. Again, the significance of these different peptides remains uncertain. Pharmacologically, they have opiate-like actions, but their physiologically relevance has not been proven.

3. Pre-Opiomelanocortin

β-Endorphin has the most interesting precursor peptide, pre-opiomelanocortin (Fig. 2C). Unlike the other opioid precursor peptides, the β-endorphin precursor makes many important, biologically active peptides that are not related to the opioid family. The precursor for β-endorphin also generates ACTH, an important stress hormone, α-melanocyte-stimulating hormone (MSH), and β-MSH. The association of β-endorphin with stress hormones is intriguing in view of the many associations between stress and a diminished percep-

tion of pain. In the pituitary, stimuli that release ACTH also release β-endorphin.

E. Endomorphins

For many years, the endogenous ligand for the mu opioid receptor was unknown. The recent identification of two tetrapeptides, endomorphin 1 and endomorphin 2, has resolved this issue. These peptides have a very interesting pharmacology and display the selectivity expected of a morphine-like, or mu, opioid peptide. It is assumed that the two peptides are also generated from a larger precursor, but this protein has not been identified. Although the evidence supporting the endomorphins is quite strong, the identification of its precursor is needed to fully establish its importance pharmacologically.

F. Orphanin FQ/Nociceptin

Recently, an opioid-related peptide has been identified termed orphanin FQ or nociceptin (OFQ/N). OFQ/N is the endogenous ligand for the fourth member of the opioid receptor gene family, ORL-1. Although it has some similarities to the traditional opioid peptides, it also has many significant differences. Like dynorphin A, OFQ/N is a heptadecapeptide (Table I) and its first four amino acids (Phe-Gly-Gly-Phe-) are similar to those of the traditional opioid peptides (Tyr-Gly-Gly-Phe-). However, OFQ/N has very poor affinity for the traditional opioid receptors, whereas the opioid peptides show no appreciable affinity for the ORL-1 receptor. Functionally, OFQ/N is also quite distinct from the opioid peptides. Although high doses of OFQ/N can elicit analgesia, low doses given supraspinally functionally reverse the opioid analgesia. The precursor for OFQ/N has been cloned, and it too contains additional putative neuropeptides, including nocistatin and OFQ2 (Fig. 2D).

III. OPIOID RECEPTORS

The opioid receptors were first demonstrated in 1973 with the binding of radiolabeled opiates to brain membranes. To date, three distinct families of opioid receptors have been identified that share many features. On the molecular level, they all are members of the G protein-coupled receptor family, which is a large family of receptors located within membranes. Members of this receptor family span the membrane seven times, providing both intracellular and extracellular domains (Fig. 3). The opioids and opioid peptides bind to the extracellular component of the receptor and activate G proteins inside the cell. The opioid receptors are almost exclusively coupled to inhibitory systems, primarily G_o and G_i. Each receptor is encoded by a separate gene, but there is high homology between them.

A. Mu Receptors

Morphine and most clinical drugs act though the mu opiate receptors, making these receptors particularly important. Morphine has many actions, including analgesia, respiratory depression, and constipation. Early studies raised the possibility that these actions may be mediated though different subtypes of mu opioid receptors based on results using highly selective opioid antagonists. Antagonists have been developed that selectively block morphine analgesia without influencing respiratory depression and the inhibition of gastrointestinal transit. Another antagonist has also been reported that can reverse the actions of heroin without interfering with those of morphine. Thus, there is extensive pharmacological evidence for multiple subtypes of mu receptors.

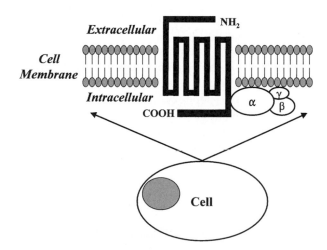

Figure 3 Structure of G protein receptors. G protein-coupled receptors span the cell membrane seven times, with the amino terminus located extracellularly and the carboxy terminus inside the cell. They are coupled to G proteins, which are composed of three subunits (α, β, and γ) and located on the inside surface of the cell. When the receptor is activated, it changes the G proteins, which then influence transduction systems.

Recently, a mu opioid receptor gene has been identified, *MOR-1* (Fig. 4). Additional cloning work has isolated seven different splice variants of this gene, implying the existence of at least seven different mu opioid receptor subtypes at the molecular level. Thus, the molecular biological approaches have uncovered far more mu receptor subtypes than even suggested from pharmacological studies. Correlating these variants with specific opioid actions is not simple. We know that a major disruption of the *MOR-1* gene eliminates all mu analgesia. However, more subtle disruptions of the gene leading to the elimination of only some *MOR-1* variants block the analgesic actions of some, but not all, mu analgesics. At this point, it appears that most mu analgesics will activate more than one mu receptor subtype. Thus, differences among the mu analgesics may reflect differences in their pattern of receptor activation.

B. Delta Receptors

Delta receptors were first found following the discovery of the enkephalins, their endogenous ligand. Early attempts to define the pharmacology of the delta receptors were limited by the lability of the enkephalins and their limited selectivity. The development of highly selective delta peptides, and recently organic compounds, has revealed important actions. Like mu receptors, activation of delta receptors produces analgesia but with far less respiratory depression and constipation. There is evidence for subtypes of delta receptors based on a series of antagonists, but functional splice variants have not been reported. The full functional significance of delta receptor systems is not entirely established.

C. Kappa₁ Receptors

Kappa receptors were first proposed from detailed pharmacological studies using a series of opiates long before the identification of its endogenous ligand, dynorphin A. Like the delta receptor, efforts to define kappa receptor pharmacology have been difficult due to the stability and selectivity of dynorphin A. The synthesis of highly selective ligands has helped to define the kappa₁ receptor, both biochemically and pharmacologically. Kappa₁ receptors can produce analgesia, but they do so through mechanisms different from those of the other receptor classes. However, kappa receptor ligands have also been associated with

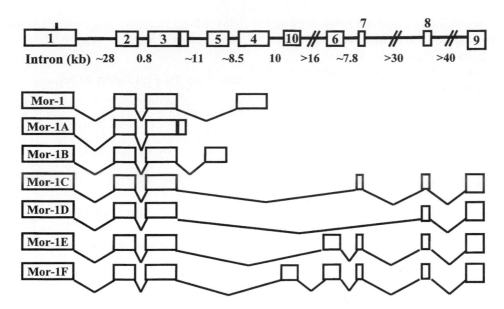

Figure 4 The murine *MOR-1* gene has been extensively studied. Ten different exons, the DNA sequences that end up in mRNA, are spliced together in different patterns to make seven different mu receptor variants. Although the human gene has not been explored as completely, there is little reason to believe that it differs significantly.

a variety of psychomimetic effects, making their clinical utility somewhat limited.

A kappa receptor with the appropriate pharmacological profile has been cloned, KOR-1. It has high homology with the other receptors and is localized within the brain. However, kappa$_1$ receptors also appear to be present in a variety of immune cells, as demonstrated by binding and molecular biological approaches.

Functionally, the ORL-1 receptor has some unusual actions. Depending on the dose and the site of administration, OFQ/N can be a potent antiopioid peptide, functionally reversing the actions of morphine and other opioid analgesics. However, at higher doses the peptide is analgesic. Antisense mapping studies have suggested that the kappa$_3$ receptor is related to the ORL-1 receptor, but they are not identical. Thus, the pharmacology of OFQ/N and its receptor is quite complex and many issues remain to be evaluated.

D. The Opioid Receptor-like Receptor

A fourth member of the opiate receptor family has been cloned that is highly selective for OFQ/N. As noted previously, OFQ/N has many similarities to the opioid peptides, but it has very poor affinity for the traditional opioid receptors. Similarly, the opioid peptides do not label the ORL-1 receptor. ORL-1 has an interesting pharmacology. Evidence from both binding and pharmacological studies has suggested multiple subtypes of receptors.

The relationship of ORL-1 to the opiate family is unusual. Although there is high homology at the molecular level, traditional opiates do not bind to this site, and its endogenous ligand, OFQ/N, has poor affinity for all the opiate sites as well. It is interesting, however, that OFQ/N is also a heptadecapeptide.

E. Kappa$_2$ and Kappa$_3$ Receptors

Several other kappa receptor classes have been proposed. U50,488H is a potent and highly selective kappa$_1$ receptor agonist. Binding studies revealed additional kappa receptor binding sites insensitive to U50,488H. The first site was termed kappa$_2$ to distinguish it from the U50,488H-sensitive kappa$_1$ site. The difficulty with defining this site pharmacologically resulted from the lack of highly selective ligands. Recently, it has been suggested that the kappa$_2$ receptor may actually represent a dimer consisting of a kappa$_1$ and a delta receptor. Together, the receptors display binding characteristics quite distinct from either kappa$_1$ or delta receptors alone and may correspond to the kappa$_2$ receptor originally observed in binding studies.

The kappa$_3$ receptor was originally proposed using naloxone benzoylhydrazone (NalBzoH), which is a potent analgesic. Its actions are not reversed by highly selective mu, delta or kappa$_1$ receptor antagonists, giving it a very unique selectivity profile. Recently, its actions have been associated with the ORL-1 receptor. Antisense mapping studies revealed that KOR-3, the cloned mouse homolog of the ORL-1 receptor, and the kappa$_3$ receptor are both encoded by the same gene but are not identical and may be splice variants of the *KOR-3/ORL-1* gene. The exact relationship between the kappa$_3$ receptor and the *KOR-3/ORL-1* gene has not been completely defined.

IV. CONCLUSION

The opioid system, composed of a family of receptors and their endogenous peptide ligands, is quite important within the central nervous system. It has many functions, some of which are readily demonstrated. However, the complexity of the system is quite extensive and a full understanding is not available. Many questions remain, including the role of the many unexplored opioid peptides postulated to be generated within the brain. Furthermore, splicing appears to play a major role in generating multiple subtypes of the various opiate receptor families. Although our knowledge of this system is growing, many unknowns remain.

See Also the Following Articles

CHEMICAL NEUROANATOMY • DOPAMINE • GABA • PAIN • PEPTIDES, HORMONES, AND THE BRAIN AND SPINAL CORD • PSYCHOACTIVE DRUGS • PSYCHONEUROENDOCRINOLOGY • RESPIRATION • STRESS: HORMONAL AND NEURAL ASPECTS

Suggested Reading

Evans, C. J., Hammond, D. L., and Frederickson, R. C. A. (1988). The opioid peptides. In *The Opiate Receptors* (G. W. Pasternak, Ed.), p. 23. Humana Press, Clifton, NJ.

Hughes, J., Smith, T. W., Kosterlitz, H. W., Fothergill, L. A., Morgan, B. A., and Morris, H. R. (1975). Identification of two related pentapeptides from the brain with potent opiate agonist activity. *Nature* **258**, 577.

Pan, Y. X., Xu, J., Bolan, E. A., Abbadie, C., Chang, A., Zuckerman, A., Rossi, G. C., and Pasternak, G. W. (1999). Identification and characterization of three new alternatively spliced mu opioid receptor isoforms. *Mol. Pharmacol.* **56**, 396.

Reisine, T., and Pasternak, G. W. (1996). Opioid analgesics and antagonists. In *Goodman & Gilman's: The Pharmacological Basis of Therapeutics* (J. G. Hardman and L. E. Limbird, Eds.). McGraw-Hill, New York.

Snyder, S. H. (1977). Opiate receptors and internal opiates. *Sci. Am.* **236**, 44.

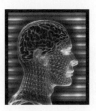

Epilepsy

BETTINA SCHMITZ

Humboldt University, Berlin

GLOSSARY

antiepileptic drugs (anticonvulsants) Drugs with different modes of action that prevent epileptic seizures.

epilepsy surgery A surgical treatment that includes the removal or disconnection of epileptogenic tissue and that aims at complete seizure control.

focal (partial) seizures Epileptic seizures with clinical or electro-encephalographic changes indicating initial activation of neurons limited to one part of one cerebral hemisphere.

generalized seizures Epileptic seizures in which the first clinical changes indicate involvement of both hemispheres.

hippocampal sclerosis Typical pathology in mesial temporal lobe epilepsy characterized by loss of neurons in the CA1 region and endfolium (CA3/4) but with relative sparing of the C2 region.

Epilepsy is a heterogeneous condition characterized by recurrent seizures. Because the epileptic seizure is a nonspecific neurological symptom, it is important to distinguish epilepsy from isolated seizures and acute symptomatic seizures provoked by acute systemic or cerebral disorders. Epilepsy is one of the most common

neurological disorders, with peak prevalence rates in early childhood and old age. Two international classification systems are used to differentiate seizure types and epileptic syndromes. The major distinction is between localization-related and generalized seizures. The former are most often symptomatic and caused by a circumscribed lesion, and the latter are typically idiopathic and associated with an inherited imbalance in excitatory and inhibitory mechanisms. There may be an association with learning disability or other neurological problems, particularly in symptomatic epilepsies. Idiopathic epilepsies are characterized by a specific age of onset, a good response to drug treatment, and a relatively benign course. The genes responsible for some rare syndromes have recently been identified; however, the suspected genetic background of the more common idiopathic epilepsies is complex and likely involves multiple susceptibility genes. The differential diagnosis of epilepsy includes a large spectrum of medical, neurological, and psychiatric disorders. The diagnosis of epilepsy is primarily based on history. Technical investigations include electroencephalography, functional and structural imaging techniques, and neuropsychological assessments. Treatment of epilepsies involves anticonvulsant drugs and behavioral recommendations and also surgery in suitable patients who are resistant to conservative strategies. Anticonvulsant drugs can be categorized into three groups according to their mode of action: GABAergic drugs, antiglutamatergic drugs, and membrane-stabilizing drugs that act through the modulation of the sodium channel. The choice of antiepiletic drugs depends on the type of epilepsy. The aim of drug treatment is complete seizure control without causing any clinical side effects.

Complications of active epilepsy are not only injuries but also psychiatric disorders such as depression. The social impact of epilepsy is more significant than with most other neurological disorders because of stigmatization and discrimination of seizure disorders. Professional training and employment are further limited by restrictions with respect to driver's licenses, working night shifts, and handling potentially dangerous machines.

I. CLASSIFICATION

How best to classify epileptic seizures and epileptic syndromes has occupied epileptologists for centuries. In the middle of the 19th century the epilepsy literature was dominated by psychiatrists who tried to systematize epilepsy based on their experiences with chronic patients in asylums. They spent more time on the psychopathological classification of psychiatric symptoms in epilepsy than on describing epileptic seizures. Specific psychiatric syndromes, especially short-lasting episodic psychoses and mood disorders, were regarded as being of equal diagnostic significance for epilepsy as convulsions.

With the introduction of electroencephalography (EEG) in the 1930s many episodic psychiatric states were identified as nonepileptic in origin. Epileptic seizures, however, showed very different ictal EEG patterns. Since then, epileptologists have concentrated on the electroclinical differentiation of epileptic seizures. Problems of terminology became obvious with increasing communication between international epileptologists in the middle of the 20th century. The first outlines of international classifications of epileptic seizures and epileptic syndromes were published in 1970. The proposed classifications by the Commission on Classification and Terminology of the International League against Epilepsy (ILAE) from 1981 and 1989 (Tables I and II) are based on agreements among international epileptologists and compromises between various viewpoints. They must not be regarded as definitive; a revision is currently being developed.

A. Classification of Seizures

Most authors in the 19th century simply differentiated seizures according to severity ("petit mal" and "grand mal"). Hughlings Jackson was the first to recognize the need for an anatomical description, physiological

delineation of disturbance of function, and pathological confirmation. In the 20th century clinical events could be linked to ictal electroencephalographic findings. More detailed analysis of seizures became possible with simultaneous EEG video monitoring and ictal neuropsychological testing. In the former, patients are monitored by video cameras and continuous EEG recordings for prolonged periods. The data can be simultaneously displayed on a split-screen television monitor (Fig. 1).

The International Classification of Epileptic Seizures (ICES) from 1981 is based on this improved monitoring capability, which has permitted more accurate recognition of seizure symptoms and their longitudinal evolution. The current classification of seizures is clinically weighted and gives no clear definitions in terms of seizure origin. The ICES does not reflect our most recent understanding of the localizing significance of specific seizure symptoms, which has grown significantly since 1981 due to increased data from intensive monitoring and epilepsy surgery. Some parts of the ICES are therefore outdated and in need of revision. Complex focal seizure types, for example, are not yet distinguished according to a probable origin in the frontal or the temporal lobe.

The principal feature of the ICES is the distinction between seizures that are generalized from the beginning and those that are partial or focal at onset and may or may not evolve to secondary generalized seizures (Table I). In generalized seizures there is initial involvement of both hemispheres, reflecting an epileptogenic generator in subcortical structures. Consciousness may be impaired and this impairment may be the initial manifestation. Motor manifestations are bilateral. The ictal EEG patterns are initially bilateral. Spikes, spike–wave complexes, and polyspike–wave complexes are all typical (Fig. 2).

Focal seizures are those in which the first clinical and EEG changes indicate initial activation of a system of neurons limited to a part of one cerebral hemisphere. The other important feature of the ICES is the separation between simple and complex partial seizures depending on whether there is preservation or impairment of consciousness.

B. Classification of Syndromes

"Epilepsy is the name for occasional sudden, excessive, rapid, and local discharges of the gray matter." This simple definition was formulated by Jackson in 1866

Table I
International Classification of Epileptic Seizures[a]

Clinical seizure type	Ictal EEG
Focal (partial, local) seizures	
A. Simple partial seizures	Local contralateral discharge starting over corresponding area of cortical representation (not always recorded on the scalp)
1. With motor symptoms	
a. Focal motor without march	
b. Focal motor with march (Jacksonian)	
c. Versive	
d. Postural	
e. Phonatory (vocalization or arrest of speech)	
2. With somatosensory or special sensory symptoms (simple hallucinations, e.g., tingling, light flashes, and buzzing)	
a. Somatosensory	
b. Visual	
c. Auditory	
d. Olfactory	
e. Gustatory	
f. Vertiginous	
3. With autonomic symptoms or signs (including epigastric sensation, pallor, sweating, flushing, piloerection, and pupillary dilatation)	
4. With psychic symptoms (disturbance of higher cortical function); these symptoms rarely occur without impairment of consciousness and are much more commonly experienced as complex partial seizures.	
a. Dysphasic	
b. Dysmnesic (e.g., déja vu)	
c. Cognitive (e.g., dreamy states and distortions of time sense)	
d. Affective (fear, anger, etc.)	
e. Illusions (e.g., macropsia)	
f. Structured hallucinations (e.g., music and scenes)	
B. Complex focal seizures (with impairment of consciousness; may sometimes begin with simple symptomatology)	Unilateral or frequently bilateral discharge; diffuse or focal in temporal or frontotemporal regions
1. Simple partial onset followed by impairment of consciousness	
a. With simple partial features (as in A, 1–4) followed by impaired consciousness	
b. With automatisms	
2. With impairment of consciousness at onset	
a. With impairment of consciousness only	
b. With automatisms	
C. Focal seizures evolving to secondarily generalized seizures (this may be generalized tonic–clonic, tonic, or clonic)	Above discharge becomes secondarily and rapidly generalized
1. Simple partial seizures (A) evolving to generalized seizures	
2. Complex partial seizures (B) evolving to generalized seizures	
3. Simple focal seizures evolving to complex focal seizures evolving to generalized seizures	

(continues)

Table I *(continued)*

Clinical seizure type	Ictal EEG
Generalized seizures	
A. Absence seizures	Usually regular and symmetrical 3-Hz but may be 2–4 Hz spike and slow-wave complexes and may have multiple spike and slow-wave complexes; abnormalities are bilateral
1. Absence seizures	
a. Impairment of consciousness only	
b. With mild clonic components	
c. With atonic components	
d. With tonic components	
e. With automatisms	
f. With autonomic components	

2. Atypical absence
    a. Changes in tone that are more pronounced than in A.1
    b. Onset and/or cessation that is not abrupt
	EEG more heterogeneous; may include irregular spike and slow-wave complexes, fast activity, or other paroxysmal activity; abnormalities are bilateral but often irregular and asymmetric

B. Myoclonic seizures, myoclonic jerks (single or multiple)	Polyspike and wave, or sometimes spike and wave or sharp and slow waves
C. Clonic seizures	Fast activity (10 c/sec or more) and slow waves; occasional spike and wave patterns
D. Tonic seizures	Low-voltage, fast activity or a fast rhythm of 9–10 c/sec or more, decreasing in frequency and increasing in amplitude
E. Tonic–clonic seizures	Rhythm at 10 or more c/sec decreasing in frequency and increasing in amplitude during tonic phase, interrupted by slow waves during the clonic phase
F. Atonic seizures	Polyspikes and wave or flattering or low–voltage fast activity

[a]From the Commission on Classification and Terminology of the International League against Epilepsy (1981).

long before the introduction of electroencephalography. It has not lost its justification today. Recurrent epileptic seizures are pathognomonic for all types of epilepsies. The clinical spectrum of epilepsy, however, is much more complex and an epileptic syndrome is characterized by a cluster of signs and syndromes customarily occurring together; these include such features as type of seizure, etiology, structural lesions, precipitating factors, family history, age of onset, severity, chronicity, diurnal and circadian cycling, and prognosis.

In contrast to a syndrome, a disease is characterized by a specific etiology and prognosis. Some recognized entities in the International Classification of Epilepsies and Epileptic Syndromes (ICEES) are diseases and others are syndromes, some of which may turn out to be diseases—a specific etiology may still be discovered.

The ICEES distinguishes generalized and localization-related (focal, local, and partial) epilepsies. Generalized epilepsies are syndromes characterized by generalized seizures in which there is involvement of both hemispheres from the beginning of the seizure. Seizures in localization-related epilepsies start in a circumscribed region of the brain. The other important classification criterion refers to etiology. The ICEES distinguishes idiopathic, symptomatic, and cryptogenic epilepsies. Idiopathic means that a disease is not preceded or occasioned by another. The major pathogenetic mechanism is genetic predisposition. Symptomatic epilepsies and syndromes are considered the consequence of a known or suspected disorder of the central nervous system. In cryptogenic disorders, a cause is suspected but remains obscure, often due to limited sensitivity of diagnostic techniques.

Table II
International Classification of Epilepsies and Epileptic Syndromes[a]

Localization-related (focal, local, and partial) epilepsies and syndromes

    Idiopathic (with age-related onset)

Currently, the following syndromes are established, but more may be identified in the future:

      Benign childhood epilepsy with centrotemporal spikes

      Childhood epilepsy with occipital paroxysms

      Primary reading epilepsy

    Symptomatic

      Chronic progressive epilepsia partialis continua of childhood (Kozhevnikov's syndrome)

      Syndromes characterized by seizures with specific modes of precipitation

      Temporal lobe epilepsy

        With amygdala–hippocampal seizures

        With lateral temporal seizures

      Frontal lobe epilepsy

        With supplementary motor seizures

        With cingulate seizures

        With seizures of the anterior frontopolar region

        With orbitofrontal seizures

        With dorsolateral seizures

        With opercular seizures

        With seizures of the motor cortex

      Parietal lobe epilepsies

      Occipital lobe epilepsies

Generalized epilepsies and syndromes

    Idiopathic, with age-related onset, listed in order of age

      Benign neonatal familial convulsions

      Benign neonatal convulsions

      Benign myoclonic epilepsy in infancy

      Childhood absence epilepsy (pyknolepsy)

      Juvenile absence epilepsy

      Juvenile myoclonic epilepsy (impulsive petit mal)

      Epilepsy with grand mal seizures (GTCS) on awakening

      Other generalized idiopathic epilepsies not defined previously

      Epilepsies precipitated by specific modes of activation

    Cryptogenic or symptomatic (in order of age)

      West syndrome (infantile spasms, Blitz–Nick–Salaam Krämpfe)

      Lennox–Gastaut syndrome

      Epilepsy with myoclonic–astatic seizures

      Epilepsy with myoclonic absences

    Symptomatic

      Nonspecific etiology

(continues)

(continued)

      Early myoclonic encephalopathy

      Early infantile epileptic encephalopathy with suppression burst

      Other symptomatic generalized epilepsies not defined previously

    Specific syndromes

      Epileptic seizures may complicate many disease states. Under this heading are included diseases in which seizures are a presenting or predominant feature.

Epilepsies and syndromes undetermined as to whether they are focal or generalized

    With both generalized and focal seizures

      Neonatal seizures

      Severe myoclonic epilepsy in infancy

      Epilepsy with continuous spike waves during slow-wave sleep

      Acquired epileptic aphasia (Landau–Kleffner syndrome)

      Other undetermined epilepsies not defined previously

    Without unequivocal generalized or focal features

[a]From the Commission on Classification and Terminology of the International League against Epilepsy (1989).

1. Localization-Related Epilepsies and Syndromes

Seizure symptomatology and ictal EEG findings are the most important criteria for anatomical classification of localization-related epilepsies. As mentioned, the 1981 version of the ICES, with its emphasis on the formal structure of seizures, is of limited help in the detailed localization of seizures required in the ICEES from 1989. The 1989 classification has been criticized because reliable localization often requires invasive EEG techniques. It is hoped that with more data from taxonomic studies, clinical symptoms or symptom clusters will be identified that eventually will allow classification on clinical grounds in most cases.

Temporal lobe epilepsies are classified as those with lateral temporal seizures with auditory hallucinations, language disorders (in the case of dominant hemisphere focus) or visual illusions, and those with amygdala–hippocampal (mesiobasal limbic or rhinencephalic) seizures. The latter are characterized by simple seizure symptoms, such as increasing epigastric discomfort, nausea, marked autonomic signs, and other symptoms including borborygmi, belching, pallor, fullness of the face, flushing of the face, arrest of respiration, pupillary dilatation, fear, panic, and

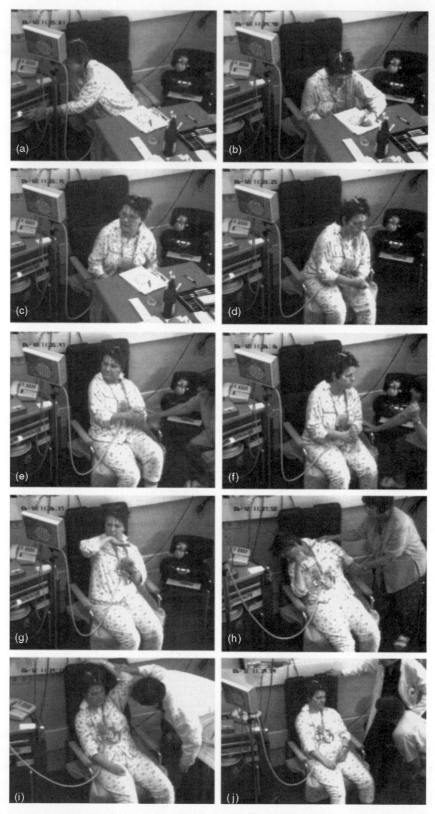

Figure 1 Video recording of a complex partial seizure with secondary generalization (frontal lobe epilepsy): (a) interictal normal behavior; (b) patient pushes alarm button; (c) patient describes aura of fear; (d) automatisms: hand rubbing; (e) alternating tapping of legs; (f) patient does not respond when asked to name a pair of glasses; (g) tonic elevation of right arm; (h) generalized myoclonic movements; (i) reorientation; (j) end of seizure, patient answers adequately.

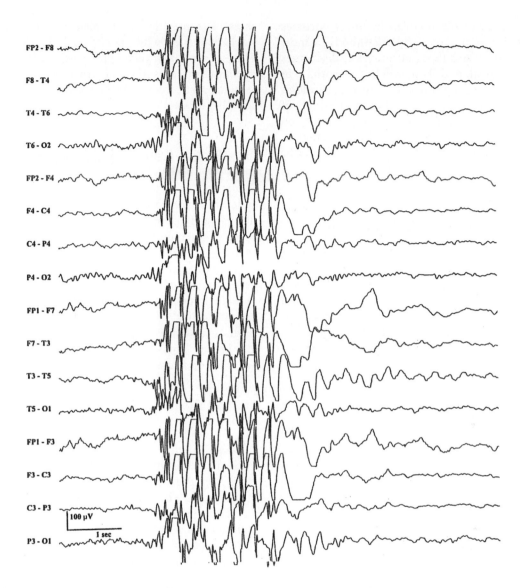

FP2 - F8

F8 - T4

T4 - T6

T6 - O2

FP2 - F4

F4 - C4

C4 - P4

P4 - O2

FP1 - F7

F7 - T3

T3 - T5

T5 - O1

FP1 - F3

F3 - C3

C3 - P3

100 µV

1 sec

P3 - O1

Figure 2   EEG in idiopathic generalized epilepsy (juvenile myoclonic epilepsy) with generalized polyspike–wave pattern.

olfactory hallucinations. Complex focal seizures often begin with a motor arrest, typically followed by oroalimentary automatisms. The duration is typically more than 1 min and consciousness recovers gradually.

Frontal lobe epilepsies are characterized by seizures of short duration, minimal or no postictal confusion, rapid secondary generalization, vocalization, prominent motor manifestations that are tonic or postural, complex gestural automatisms, and nocturnal clustering. Ictal scalp EEGs may show bilateral or multilobar discharges or are often normal. Accurate localization of frontal lobe epilepsies may therefore be difficult.

2. Generalized Epilepsies and Syndromes

Idiopathic generalized epilepsies are characterized by an age-related onset that reflects the ability of the brain to produce certain seizure types depending on cerebral maturation. In general, patients are asymptomatic between seizures. Radiological investigations are negative. Frequently, there is an overlap of idiopathic generalized epilepsies, especially of those manifesting in later childhood and adolescence. Response to antiepileptic drug treatment and psychosocial prognosis are good.

Symptomatic generalized epilepsies and syndromes usually start in infancy or early childhood. In most children several seizure types occur. EEG discharges are less rhythmical and less synchronous than in idiopathic generalized epilepsies. There are neurological, neuropsychological, and radiological signs of diffuse cerebral disease. The only difference between cryptogenic and symptomatic syndromes is that in cryptogenic syndromes the presumed cause cannot be identified.

3. Epilepsies and Syndromes Undetermined as to Whether They Are Focal or Generalized

There are two groups of patients who cannot be classified as focal or generalized. The first group consists of patients with both generalized and focal seizures (e.g., patients with both focal seizures and absence seizures). The second group comprises patients without unequivocal generalized or focal features (e.g., patients with nocturnal generalized tonic–clonic seizures).

4. Specific Syndromes

These are isolated seizures and situation-related syndromes, such as febrile seizures and seizures occurring only when there is an acute metabolic or toxic event due to factors such as alcohol, drugs, eclampsia, or hyperglycemia.

II. EPIDEMIOLOGY

A. Prevalence and Incidence

Epidemiological studies of epilepsy are often difficult to compare because of different study designs and definitions of epilepsy. Calculated incidence rates of epilepsy range between 20 and 70/100,000 per year. The incidence is age dependent, with a maximum in early childhood and lowest rates in early adulthood. Incidence rates rise again in older age groups, probably due to the higher prevalence of cerebrovascular disease. The overall risk for epilepsy is slightly higher in males than in females. The point prevalence of active epilepsy is of the order of 3–5/1000. The cumulative lifetime prevalence has been estimated to be 3.5%.

There is thus a 10-fold difference between the point prevalence and the lifetime prevalence, suggesting that the disease remains active in only a small proportion of cases. The prevalence of epilepsy is higher in third world countries, with rates of up to 37/1000 in Africa. This is probably related to a higher frequency of infectious diseases of the nervous system diseases such as neurocysticercosis and the higher risk of perinatal complications.

B. Relative Frequency of Epileptic Syndromes

Studies of the distribution of epileptic syndromes and epileptic seizures in the population have had conflicting results. In population-based studies, epilepsies with complex focal and focal seizures secondarily evolving to tonic–clonic seizures are most frequent, occurring in 69% of all patients. This is followed by primary generalized tonic–clonic seizures in 30% and absence or myoclonic seizures in less than 5%. In hospital-based studies, the numbers of subtle generalized seizures (absences and myoclonic seizures) are generally higher, almost certainly related to the increased accuracy and sensitivity of diagnosis.

C. Etiology

In most patients with epilepsy, the etiology remains unclear. According to an epidemiological survey in Rochester, New York, 65% of cases are idiopathic or cryptogenic. The most frequent cause of epilepsy is vascular disorder (10%), followed by congenital complications (8%), brain trauma (6%), tumor (4%), degenerative disorders (4%), and infectious diseases (3%). The etiology of epilepsy is largely dependent on the age of onset, with congenital disorders dominating in childhood epilepsies, trauma and tumors being most common in early adulthood, and cerebrovascular and degenerative disorders becoming more frequent with older age. Recent studies using advanced imaging techniques have revealed a high number of patients with subtle cortical dysgenesis or hippocampal sclerosis—patients who were formerly classified as cryptogenic.

III. PROGNOSIS

A. The Natural Course of Epilepsy

The natural course of untreated epilepsy is unknown. For obvious ethical reasons no one has ever conducted a controlled study, and there are no systematic data from the days before antiepileptic drugs were introduced. Nineteenth century epileptologists emphasized the poor prognosis in epilepsy, but their experience was limited to institutionalized patients. Gowers (1885) believed that seizures may beget more seizures: "The tendency of the disease is to self-perpetuation, each attack facilitates the occurrence of another, by increasing the instability of nerve elements." Gowers studied the recurrence of seizures in 160 cases. A second seizure followed the first within 1 month in one-third of patients and within 1 year in two-thirds.

B. Recurrence Risk after a First Seizure

In an unselected sample of the population, isolated seizures occur in 20–40% of people with one or more seizures. It is methodologically extremely difficult to investigate the recurrence risk after an initial epileptic seizure. Estimates in the literature range between 27 and 71%, depending on inclusion criteria, duration of follow-up, and whether or not patients are treated after a first seizure. The most important source of error has been the exclusion of patients with early recurrences of seizures before presentation. The longer the interval between first seizure and inclusion into the study, the lower the recurrence rate.

The recurrence risk within 24 months of a first seizure calculated from a meta-analysis of 14 studies was 42%, with a higher risk in the group of patients with symptomatic seizures and pathological EEG findings (65%) compared to those patients with idiopathic seizures and a normal EEG (24%).

C. Prognostic Studies

Recent prospective and population-based studies have challenged previous views that epilepsy is likely to be a chronic disease in as many as 80% of cases. In a population-based survey in Rochester, 20 years after the initial diagnosis of epilepsy 70% of patients were in 5 years of remission and 50% of patients had successfully withdrawn medication. In an English study, 15 years after diagnosis 81% of patients were seizure free for at least 1 year. In another study of 104 patients who were followed up after onset of treatment, 60% were in 1-year remission after a follow-up period of 24 months. By 8 years of follow-up, 92% had achieved a 1-year remission. It is recommended that antiepileptic drugs be withdrawn after a minimum

seizure-free period of 2 years or 5 years in severe cases. Relapses occur in 12–72% of patients after a 2-year remission and in 11–53% after a 3-year remission.

Approximately 5–10% of all patients with epilepsy eventually have intractable seizures despite optimal medication; most of these patients have complex partial seizures. Despite the overall favorable prognosis of epilepsy and the good response to treatment, the mortality rate of epilepsy is 2.3-fold higher than that in the general population, and it is 3.8-fold higher in the first years of the illness. The incidence of sudden unexpected death in epilepsy was estimated to be in the order of 1/525.

The prognosis of epilepsy largely depends on the syndromatic diagnosis. Idiopathic localization-related epilepsies such as Rolandic epilepsy have an excellent prognosis in all respects. Prognosis in terms of seizure remission, social adjustment, and life expectancy, on the other hand, is extremely poor in symptomatic generalized epilepsies such as West syndrome and in progressive myoclonic epilepsies.

Several studies have examined prognostic factors independent of the syndromatic diagnosis. Most studies have consistently shown that diffuse cerebral damage and neurological and cognitive deficits are associated with a poor outcome. There has been less agreement on the significance of other possible risk factors for poor prognosis, such as EEG features and positive family history of epilepsy. Whether early treatment and medical prevention of seizures improves the long-term prognosis as suggested by Gowers and indicated by experimental data from animal epilepsy models is not clear and subject to controversy. A recent Italian study showed that the treatment prognosis risk after a first seizure is not lower in patients treated with antiepiletic drugs (AEDs) compared to patients not treated after a first seizure.

IV. BASIC MECHANISMS

Epileptic syndromes are characterized by a tendency to paroxysmal regional or generalized hyperexcitability of the cerebral cortex. Because of the phenomenological diversity and the etiological heterogeneity of epilepsies, it is likely that there are multiple underlying cellular and molecular mechanisms.

The mechanisms responsible for the occurrence of seizures (ictogenesis) and the development of epilepsy (epileptogenesis) have been studied in animal models and by *in vitro* studies of surgical human brain tissue. The exact mechanisms remain to be clarified. They represent complex changes of normal brain function on multiple levels, involving anatomy, physiology, and pharmacology. There are categorical differences in the pathophysiology of idiopathic generalized and symptomatic focal seizures. The latter are caused by a regional cortical hyperexcitation due to local disturbances in neuronal connectivity. Synaptic reorganization may be caused by any acquired injury or congenital abnormalities, such as in the many subforms of cortical dysplasia. Some areas of the brain seem more susceptible than others, the most vulnerable being mesial temporal lobe structures. The pathophysiology of hippocampal sclerosis, the most common etiology of temporal lobe epilepsy, has been a topic of much controversy. It is most likely that the hippocampal structures are damaged by an early trauma, typically prolonged febrile seizures. The process of hippocampal sclerosis involves a synaptic reorganization with excitotoxic neuronal loss, loss of interneurons, and GABA deficit.

Epileptic neurons in an epileptogenic focus may produce bursts of action potentials that represent isolated spikes in the EEG as long as they remain locally restricted. Depending on the failure of local inhibitory mechanisms, these bursts may lead to ongoing and repetitive discharges. If larger neuronal networks are recruited in this hypersynchronous activity, this leads to an epileptic seizure that is either focal or secondary generalized depending on the extent of seizure spread. The local seizure threshold is regulated by influences on excitatory and inhibitory postsynaptic potentials. The membrane excitability is regulated by ion channels that are modulated by excitatory transmitters, particularly glutamate and aspartate, and the inhibitory transmitter GABA. These three levels are the major targets for antiepileptic drugs (Table III).

Primary generalized seizures are accompanied by a bilateral synchronous epileptic activity. Therefore, they cannot be explained by cortical dysfunction alone. They are caused by an imbalance of pathways between the thalamus and the cerebral cortex. These thalamocortical circuits are modulated by reticular nuclei. Excessive GABAergic inhibition and dysfunction of thalamic calcium channels also play a role in the pathogenesis, at least in the pathogenesis of absence seizures. These cortical–subcortical circuits are also responsible for circadian rhythms, which may explain the increased seizure risk after awakening and following sleep withdrawal in idiopathic generalized epilepsies. The appearance and disappearance of primary generalized seizures is strongly age dependent, a phenomenon that has been explained by disturbances in brain maturation processes.

V. GENETICS

Genetic factors play a major role in the etiology of idiopathic epilepsies. Progress in molecular genetics has revealed several susceptibility loci and causative gene mutations in many rare human epilepsies with monogenic inheritance, such as the progressive myoclonus epilepsies. Mutations in the gene encoding the α_4 subunit of the neuronal nicotinic acetylcholine receptor gene have been identified as predisposing to autosomal-dominant nocturnal frontal lobe epilepsy. Mutations of two genes encoding potassium channels cause benign neonatal familial convulsions. A gene encoding the β subunit of the voltage-gated sodium channel has been identified in a rare syndrome called generalized epilepsy with febrile seizures plus. These findings suggest that at least some epilepsies are related to ion channel dysfunction.

Table III
Mode of Action of Old and New Antiepileptic Drugs

	Sodium channel[a]	GABA[b]	Glutamate[c]	Calcium channel[d]
Old AED				
Benzodiazepines	+	+ +	0	0
Carbamazepine	+ +	±	±	?
Ethosuximide	0	0	0	+
Phenobarbitone	+	+	+	0
Phenytoin	+ +	±	±	0
Valproate	+ +	+	±	0
New AED				
Felbamate	+	+	+ +	?
Gabapentin	±	+	±	0
Lamotrigine	+ +	0	±	0
Levetirazetam	0	0	0	0
Oxcarbazepine	+ +	0	?	?
Tiagabine	?	+ +	?	?
Topiramate	+	+	+	?
Vigabatrin	0	+ +	?	?
Zonisamide	+	±	?	?

[a]Blockade of voltage-gated sodium channels.
[b]Potentiation of GABAergic mechanisms.
[c]Blockade of glutamatergic mechanisms.
[d]Blockade of thalamic calcium channels.

In the common idiopathic generalized epilepsies, positional cloning of susceptibility genes was less successful due to the underlying complex genetic disposition. Many chromosomal regions (on chromosomes 6 and 15) are thought to harbor susceptibility genes for generalized seizures associated with juvenile myoclonic epilepsy.

In the genetic counseling of patients with epilepsies with complex modes of inheritance, empirical risk estimates are used. The recurrence risk for the offspring of probands with idiopathic generalized epilepsies is on the order of 5–10%.

VI. DIAGNOSIS

A. Clinical Diagnosis and Differential Diagnosis

Epilepsy is a clinical diagnosis, defined by recurrent epileptic seizures. The most important tool for the accurate classification and optimal diagnosis is the clinical interview. This should cover seizure-related information, such as subjective and objective ictal symptomatology, precipitation and frequency of seizures, history of seizures in first-degree relatives, and also information relevant for etiology, such as complications during pregnancy and birth, early psychomotor development, and history of brain injuries and other disorders of the central nervous system. Other important information that should be obtained refers to doses, side effects, and efficacy of previous medical or nonmedical treatment; evidence of psychiatric complications in the past; and psychosocial parameters, including educational and professional status, social independence, and psychosexual history.

The neurological examination may reveal signs of localized or diffuse brain damage. One should also look for skin abnormalities and minor stigmata suggestive of genetic diseases and neurodevelopmental malformations. There may be signs of injuries due to epileptic seizures, such as scars from recurrent falls, burns, and tongue biting. Hirsutism, gingival hyperplasia or acne vulgaris are indicative of side effects of long-term antiepileptic medication.

The clinical interview and the neurological examination are often sufficient to distinguish between epilepsy and its wide spectrum of differential diagnoses (Table IV) in most cases. However, there is a substantial problem with pseudoseizures.

For the correct interpretation of functional and structural diagnostic techniques it is important to understand that in focal epilepsies different concepts of pathological cerebral regions have to be distinguished. The epileptogenic zone is defined as the region of the brain from which the patient's habitual seizures arise. Closely related but not necessarily anatomically identical are the irritative zone, defined as the region of cortex that generates interictal epileptiform discharges in the EEG; the pacemaker zone, defined as the region of cortex from which the clinical seizures originate; the epileptogenic lesion, defined as the structural lesion that is usually related to epilepsy; the ictal symptomatic zone, defined as the region of cortex that

Table IV
Differential Diagnosis of Epilepsy

Neurological disorders
  Transitory ischemic attacks
  Migraine
  Paroxysmal dysfunction in multiple sclerosis
  Transient global amnesia
  Movement disorders (hyperexplexia, tics, myoclonus, dystonia, paroxysmal choreoathetosis)
  Drop attacks due to impaired CSF dynamics
Sleep disorders
  Physiologic myoclonus
  Pavor nocturnus
  Somnambulism
  Enuresis
  Periodic movements in sleep
  Sleep talking
  Bruxism
  Nightmares
  Sleep apnea
  Narcolepsy (cataplexy, automatic behavior, sleep attacks, hallucinations)
  REM behavior disorder
Psychiatric disorders
  "Pseudoseizures"
  Panic attacks and anxiety disorders
  Hyperventilation syndrome
  Dissociative states, fugues
  Episodic dyscontrol, rage attacks
  Catatonia and depressive stupor
Medical disorders
  Cardiac arrhythmias
  Syncope (cardiac, orthostatic, reflex)
  Metabolic disorders (e.g., hypoglycemia)
  Hypertensive crisis
  Endocrine disorders (e.g., pheochromocytoma)

Table V
Localization of Pathological Zones in Focal Epilepsies[a]

Epileptogenic zone	Ictal EEG with special electrode placements
Irritative zone	Interictal EEG, MEG
Pacemaker zone	Ictal EEG with special electrode placements
Ictal symptomatic zone	Ictal EEG with special electrode placements
Epileptogenic lesion	CCT, MRI
Functional deficit zone	Functional imaging, neurological examination, neuropsychological testing, nonepileptiform interictal EEG abnormalities

[a]From Lüders and Awad (1991).

generates the ictal seizure symptomatology; and the functional deficit zone, defined as the region of cortex that in the interictal period is functioning abnormally. The diagnostic techniques applied in epilepsy are characterized by a selective specificity for these various pathological regions (Table V).

B. EEG

The interictal surface EEG is still the most important method in the diagnosis and assessment of all types of epilepsy. A routine EEG is recorded over 30 min during a relaxed condition, including photic stimulation procedures and 5 min of hyperventilation. Paroxysmal discharges strongly suggestive of epilepsy are spikes, spike waves, and sharp waves. These epileptiform patterns, however, are not specific for epilepsy. They may be observed in patients suffering from nonepileptic neurological diseases and even in a small proportion of normal subjects.

The sensitivity of the routine EEG is limited by restrictions of spatial and temporal sampling. About 50% of patients with epilepsy do not show paroxysmal epileptiform discharges on a single EEG recording. Their detection depends on the epileptic syndrome and the therapeutic status of the patient. In untreated childhood absence epilepsy the EEG almost always shows generalized spike–wave complexes either occurring spontaneously or provoked by hyperventilation. In mild cryptogenic focal epilepsies, on the other hand, the interictal EEG is often negative. The temporal sensitivity can be increased by repeating the EEG or by carrying out long-term recordings with mobile EEGs.

Paroxysmal discharges may also be identified by performing an EEG after sleep deprivation while the subject is asleep (Table VI).

Simultaneous video EEG recordings of seizures are useful for differentiating between different types of epileptic seizures and nonepileptic seizures. Ictal EEGs are also required for exact localization of the epileptogenic focus when epilepsy surgery is considered.

Surface EEGs record only a portion of the underlying brain activity. Discharges that are restricted to deep structures or to small cortical regions may not be detected. The spatial resolution of the EEG can be improved by special electrode placements, such as pharyngeal and sphenoidal electrodes.

Invasive EEG methods with chronic intracranial electrode placement are necessary for complex analysis in cases in which there are discordant or multifocal results of the ictal surface EEG and imaging techniques. These include foramen ovale electrodes positioned in the subdural space along the amygdala–hippocampal formation, epidural and subdural strip electrodes, and grids to study larger brain areas. Stereotactic depth electrodes provide excellent sensitivity for the detection of small areas of potentially epileptogenic tissue. The definition of exact location and boundaries of the epileptogenic region, however, is limited by the location and number of electrodes placed. Because of the limited coverage of implanted electrodes it may be difficult to distinguish whether a seizure discharge originates from a pacemaker zone or represents spread from a distant focus. Complications, the most severe being intracerebral hemorrhages, occur in 4% of patients.

Table VI
EEG Methods in the Diagnosis of Epilepsy

Interictal EEGs
  Routine surface EEG
  EEG after sleep withdrawal, during sleep
  Mobile long-term EEG
Ictal EEG
  Long-term video EEG
Special electrode placements (in increasing order of invasiveness)
  Nasopharyngeal electrodes
  Sphenoidal electrodes
  Foramen ovale electrodes
  Epidural electrodes (strips, grids)
  Subdural electrodes (strips, grids)
  Depth electrodes

C. Magnetoencephalography

Multichannel magnetoencephalography (MEG) is in some centers used in the presurgical assessment as a supplementary method to EEG. The electrical activity that can be measured by EEG produces a magnetic field perpendicular to the electric flow. This magnetic signal can be measured by MEG. In contrast to EEG, MEG is not influenced by intervening tissues, with the advantage of noninvasive localization of deep electric sources. Disadvantages are high costs and the susceptibility to movement artifacts, which makes it almost impossible to perform ictal studies.

D. Structural Imaging

Imaging studies should always be performed when a symptomatic etiology is suspected. Cranial computed tomography (CCT) is a quick, easy, and relatively cheap technique. The sensitivity can be improved by scanning in the axis of the temporal lobe (in cases of Temporal Lobe Epilepsy) and by using intravenous contrast enhancement. Except for a few pathologies such as calcifications, magnetic resonance imaging (MRI) is superior to CCT in terms of sensitivity and specificity in detecting epilepsy-related lesions such as malformations, gliosis, and tumors. With optimized MRI techniques, including T2-weighted images, inverse recovery sequences, and coronal images perpendicular to the hippocampus and thin sections, the sensitivity in depicting mesial temporal sclerosis reaches 90% (Fig. 3). Diagnosis of hippocampal pathology can be improved by quantitative MRI techniques such as T2 relaxometry and volumetric studies.

MR spectroscopy (MRS) is a noninvasive method for measuring chemicals in the body. MRS does not produce images but instead generates numerical values for chemicals. With phosphate spectroscopy it is possible to study energy metabolism in relation to seizure activity. Proton MRS is a technique that measures neuronal density, which has been found to be significantly decreased in the mesial temporal lobe of patients with mesial temporal sclerosis. MRS is a time-consuming procedure and therefore not routine.

E. Functional Imaging

Single photon emission computed tomography (SPECT) in epilepsy has mainly been confined to the

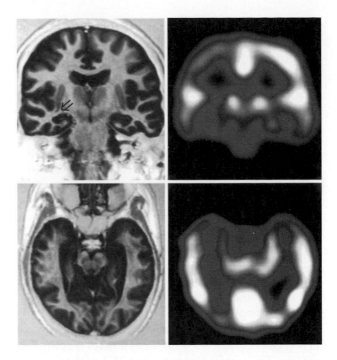

Figure 3 Imaging findings in temporal lobe epilepsy with hippocampal sclerosis. Left: MRI coronal (top) and horizontal (bottom), inversion recovery sequence. Hippocampal sclerosis (arrow). Right: Interictal HMPAO SPECT shows extensive ipsilateral hypoperfusion.

imaging of cerebral blood flow in focal epilepsy. The tracer most widely used is ^{99}Tc-HMPAO. Interictally, there is localized hypoperfusion in an area extending beyond the epileptogenic region. Initially, there was considerable skepticism about the clinical value of the technique because the early studies were of low resolution and the correlations with electroencephalographic findings were imprecise. The sensitivity of interictal focus detection of SPECT in the literature ranges from 40 to 80%. In recent years there have been major technical developments in instrumentation. Using brain-dedicated multiheaded camera systems, the sensitivity of SPECT is similar to that of [18F] fluorodeoxyglucose (FDG) positron emission tomography (PET).

^{99}Tc-HMPAO is distributed within a few minutes after injection in the brain, where it remains fixed for about 2 hr. If the radioisotope is injected during or shortly after an epileptic seizure, scanning can be carried out postictally without problems due to involuntary movements. Postictal and ictal SPECT is more sensitive than interictal SPECT and typically shows hyperperfusion ipsilateral to the epileptogenic

focus. Another ligand used for SPECT is ^{123}I-iomaze-nile, which is used to demonstrate benzodiazepine receptor binding, which is decreased in the epileptogenic region.

Compared to SPECT, PET is superior with respect to spatial and contrast resolution. PET, however, is expensive and requires an on-site medical cyclotron. Ictal studies are difficult with PET because of the short half-life of positron emitting radioisotopes. PET has mainly been used to study interictal blood flow with nitrogen-13-labeled ammonia and oxygen-15 and also glucose metabolism with FDG in focal epilepsy. Localized hypoperfusion and hypometabolism in the epileptogenic area as shown by PET are seen as a reliable confirmatory finding in the presurgical assessment of temporal lobe epilepsy. PET has also been used for imaging of benzodiazepine receptor binding and opiate receptor binding in epilepsy.

The major application of functional MRI in epilepsy is the noninvasive mapping of eloquent cortex in the presurgical evaluation of patients based on activation studies. The clear advantage over PET is the superior spatial resolution, which is on the order of 3 mm. The coregistration of a high-resolution MRI allows excellent localization of activated regions.

F. Neuropsychology

Identification of neuropsychological deficits is important for optimizing education, professional training, and rehabilitation in patients with epilepsy. Another aim of neuropsychological testing is to establish cognitive effects of antiepileptic drugs, seizure frequency, and "subclinical" EEG activity.

In the presurgical assessment neuropsychological evaluation is used to identify localizable deficits that can be related to the epileptogenic lesion. Crucial for lateralizing temporal lobe epilepsies is the function of verbal and nonverbal memory. Another neuropsychological task in the presurgical assessment is forecasting postsurgical cognitive outcome, which sometimes requires the intracarotid sodium amylobarbital procedure (Wada test).

G. Magnetic Cerebral Stimulation

Recently, magnetic cerebral stimulation has been used to lateralize the epileptogenic region in focal epilepsies. The technique of repetitive stimulation is also being evaluated for antiepileptic properties.

VII. TREATMENT

Once a diagnosis of epilepsy has been made and the decision to treat has been taken, many options are available. Pharmacological, surgical, and behavioral approaches may be taken. The majority of patients with epilepsy are treated with anticonvulsants. Recently, there has also been renewed interest in attempts at behavioral and nonpharmacological approaches to the management of seizures. A minority of patients with drug-resistant epilepsy may proceed to have surgery.

These strategies should not be viewed as being mutually exclusive. Hence, although in the following section, these treatments will be described separately, in practice they may be combined. Indeed, if surgery is pursued it is very likely that patients will receive antiepileptic medication both before and after the operation.

A. Antiepileptic Drugs

Ideally, patients should be managed on a single drug that leads to complete seizure freedom without causing any side effects. Approximately 75% of patients with epilepsy can be fully controlled on monotherapy (50% with initial monotherapy and 25% with second monotherapy), with the choice of agent determined by the epilepsy syndrome and seizure type (Table VII). Carbamazepine and valproate are the recommended substances for simple, complex partial, and secondary generalized tonic–clonic seizures. For most generalized seizures, sodium valproate is the most useful treatment. These drugs are generally thought of as the first-line treatments. Of the remaining patients not controlled on monotherapy, addition of another first-line drug will gain control in 15%. However, some patients will develop chronic seizures unrelieved by these treatments. In such circumstances, alternative monotherapies or adjunctive therapies will be considered. Many of the recently introduced anticonvulsants, often considered as second-line treatments, may be introduced, either alone or in combination with a first-line agent.

In Europe and the United States, nine novel anticonvulsants have been introduced in the past decade: vigabatrin, lamotrigine, felbamate, tiagabine, gabapentin, oxcarbazepine, topiramate, levetiracetam, and zonisamide. Because of serious side effects, two of these drugs are used only in a highly selected group of patients. Felbamate has caused fatal hepatotoxic and

Table VII
Selection of Antiepileptic Drugs According to the Epileptic Syndrome

Type of syndrome	First-line drugs	Second-line drugs
Focal epilepsies		
All seizure types	Carbamazepine	Lamotrigine
	Valproic acid	
		Gabapentin
		Topiramate
		Tiagabine
		Levetiracetam
		Oxcarbazepine
		Phenytoin
		Clobazam
		Primidone
		Acetazolamide
		Vigabatrin
		Felbamate
Generalized epilepsies		
Idiopathic		
Absences	Ethosuximide	Lamotrigine
	Valproic acid	
Myoclonic	Valproic acid	Lamotrigine
		Primidone
		Levetirazetam
Awakening grand mal	Valproic acid	Lamotrigine
		Primidone
		Topiramate
Symptomatic		
West syndrome	Vigabatrin	Clobazam
	ACTH	
	Valproate	
Lennox–Gastaut syndrome	Valproic acid	
		Lamotrigine
		Clobazam
		Topiramate
		Felbamate

hematotoxic adverse events, and vigabatrin leads to irreversible visual field constriction in 30% of patients.

An important feature in the clinical use of the first-line treatments is therapeutic drug monitoring (TDM). This should not be done as a routine procedure, but it may be useful in certain circumstances (e.g., to detect noncompliance and to explore changes in pharmaco-

kinetics). There are significant interindividual variations in the relationship between drug levels and clinical side effects. Therefore, the measurement of serum concentrations should not be used for the optimization of treatment (with few exceptions); decisions to alter dosages should be based on efficacy and tolerability of AEDs. For appropriate agents, indications for TDM may include drug initiation or dose change, investigation of the absence of or change in therapeutic response, investigation of suspected toxicity, and situations in which pharmacokinetics may change such as during pregnancy and related to renal or hepatic disease. Sampling should occur once steady state has been achieved, four to six half-lives after treatment has been modified or introduced. TDM is particularly important for phenytoin because its hepatic metabolism is saturable and therefore a small increase in dose can result in a disproportionate and unpredictable increase in serum concentration.

B. Behavioral Treatment

Pharmacological treatments of epilepsy are not uniformly successful. Even if good seizure control is obtained, many patients experience troublesome side effects of treatments that must often be continued for many years. The need to take medication on a long-term basis has obvious implications for women wishing to become pregnant. In addition, many individuals describe feelings of oppression and an increased fear of being labeled as ill because of their ongoing need for regular drug taking. Surgical treatment is only an option for a minority of patients and is also not without physical and psychological sequelae. That alternative treatment approaches should be sought is therefore not surprising.

It has been suggested that many patients with epilepsy have a mental mechanism that they use in an attempt to inhibit their seizures. In one study of 70 patients, 36% claimed that they could sometimes stop their seizures. A behavioral approach to the treatment of epilepsy is based on observations that epilepsy can be manipulated in a systematic way through environmental, psychological, and physical changes. The initial stage in this approach is a behavioral analysis of the ways in which environmental and behavioral factors interact with seizure occurrence.

It has been demonstrated that significant reductions in seizure frequency may be achieved by teaching patients a specific contingent relaxation technique that they must be able to employ rapidly when they identify a situation in which they are at high risk of having a seizure. In a subsequent study of three children with intractable seizures it was found that contingent relaxation alone did not significantly reduce seizures but that such a reduction was obtained following the addition of specific countermeasures aimed at changing the arousal level relevant to and contingent on early seizure cues—for instance, suddenly jerking the head to the right when it would habitually move to the left with a feeling of drowsiness at the onset of a seizure.

Some patients suffer from reflex seizures in that their seizures are precipitated by external stimuli. A proportion of people can identify specific environmental or affective triggers and may be able to develop specific strategies to abort or delay a seizure. These methods may involve motor or sensory activity or they may be purely mental. However, in one study it was found that 50% of patients who inhibited their seizures at times had to "pay the price in subsequent discomfort."

Primary seizure inhibition describes the direct inhibition of seizures by an act of will; for instance, a man whose seizures were precipitated by a feeling of unsteadiness dealt with this by keeping his gaze fixed on a point when walking down an incline. The nature of the successful act varies from person to person, and if this treatment approach is to be pursued then it must be tailored to each individual, based on an analysis of their seizures and of any actions they may already have noticed modify their seizures.

The term secondary inhibition is employed by Fenwick to describe behavioral techniques that are thought to act by changing cortical activity in the partially damaged group 2 neurons around the focus without deliberately intending to do so, thereby reducing the risk both of a partial seizure discharge and of a generalized seizure discharge that may otherwise follow recruitment of surrounding normal brain by group 2 neurons firing abnormally. An example of this is the act of maintaining alertness by a patient whose seizures appear in a state of drowsiness. Treatment in this case starts with trying to identify situations in which the subject reliably tends to have seizures or, alternatively, to be free of them.

In addition to these seizure-related approaches, more general psychological strategies have also been investigated. Several anecdotal reports have been published demonstrating benefit from reward programs that aim to reward seizure-free periods. Based on the observation that some patients with olfactory auras can prevent progression of the seizure by applying a sudden, usually unpleasant olfactory coun-

terstimulus, "aromatherapy" techniques have been studied in the control of epilepsy. Currently, it is not clear what the relative contributions of specific olfactory stimuli and the general relaxation that is a part of the treatment are to any clinical benefit that might be observed.

Specific biofeedback techniques have also been explored. Measurement of scalp electrical activity has demonstrated that there is an increase in surface-negative slow cortical potentials (SCPs) in the seconds before a seizure occurs. These SCPs represent the extent to which apical dendrites of cortical pyramidal cells are depolarized and hence indicate neuronal excitability. Studies using visual feedback of this effect have demonstrated that some patients are able to modulate cortical electrical activity with an associated decrease in seizure frequency. However, it appears that patients with epilepsy are less able than normal controls to regulate their cortical excitability. This impairment can be minimized by extending the amount of training received by those with epilepsy. In a study that gave 28 1-hr training sessions to 18 patients followed up for at least 1 year, 6 became seizure-free. However, not every patient who achieved reliable SCP control experienced a reduction in seizure frequency.

It has been noted that the teaching of any of these methods of self-control of seizures may increase morale not only by reducing seizures but also by providing patients with a sense of control over their epilepsy. An important aspect of many "nonmedical" treatments of epilepsy is that although still of very limited proven benefit, they aim to consider seizures in the wider setting of the patient's life. In mainstream clinical management it is sometimes easier to focus purely on seizure response to the latest change in anticonvulsant therapy.

C. Surgical Treatment

In all patients with persistent epilepsy unrelieved by AED treatment, it is appropriate to consider surgical intervention. The aim of epilepsy surgery is the removal of the epileptogenic brain tissue in order to achieve seizure control without causing additional iatrogenic deficits. Only in rare cases, such as those with diffuse pathology and catastrophic seizures, are palliative surgical procedures performed. Approximately one-third of patients with refractory epilepsy are suitable for epilepsy surgery. The prerequisites of surgery are frequent epileptic seizures and a minimum of 3–5 years of unsuccessful AED treatment including at least two first-line AEDs in monotherapy and combination. This is a minimal condition that only applies to patients who are ideal candidates for epilepsy surgery. These are patients with unilateral mesial temporal lobe epilepsy and hippocampal sclerosis, extratemporal epilepsies with localized structural lesions, and some types of catastrophic epilepsies in childhood. The poorer the individual prognosis of surgery, the longer the requested presurgical attempts to achieve seizure control with AEDs and complimentary nonsurgical treatments.

1. Presurgical Assessment

Treatment centers that engage in routine surgical management of epilepsy generally have a standardized assessment process for patients being considered for such treatment. Although the program may vary between centers, the general procedure is similar. A first hypothesis with respect to the suspected epileptogenic region is based on clinical history, neurological examination, and interictal EEG. These procedures focus particularly on searching for etiological factors, evidence of localizing signs and symptoms, and a witnessed description of the seizures. In addition, psychosocial information must be gathered relating to education, employment, social support, and past and present mental state findings. In a second step of presurgical assessment, all patients undergo more specific investigations. In general, these include several days of continuous video telemetry using surface electrodes. The aim of telemetry is to obtain multiple ictal recordings, which give more valuable localizing information than interictal records. Often, patients will reduce their AED prior to telemetry in order to facilitate the occurrence of seizures. Recent advances in structural and functional neuroimaging have made invasive EEG recording less necessary. MRI using optimized techniques has increased the sensitivity for the detection of subtle structural lesions not seen on CCT and standard MRI and is now used routinely. Functional imaging techniques using SPECT and PET are used to further delineate the epileptogenic region. If results from all investigations are concordant, patients will have surgery. If results are discordant, invasive EEG recordings using subdural grid electrodes or intracerebral depth electrodes may be applied in order to identify the critical epileptogenic region.

All patients being considered for epilepsy surgery should have a neuropsychological assessment. This is important both to detect focal brain dysfunction and to predict the results of surgery, especially temporal lobe surgery. The intelligence quotient may be measured using the Wechsler Adult Intelligence Scale. In some centers a score of less than 75 has been taken as evidence of diffuse neurological disorder and, hence, as a relative contraindication to surgery. It is important before proceeding to surgery to investigate the hemispheric localization of language and memory. This is generally performed using the Wada test. Sodium amylobarbitone is injected into one internal carotid artery, and while that hemisphere is briefly suppressed language and memory tests are performed. The procedure is then repeated for the other hemisphere.

2. Surgical Procedures

Many surgical procedures have been developed. Most patients who undergo surgery suffer from temporal lobe epilepsy. Most of these patients undergo one of two standard procedures: two-thirds anterior resection or amygdala hippocampectomy. In extratemporal epilepsies, lobectomies, lesionectomies, or individually "tailored" topectomies are performed. The latter techniques may involve preoperative stimulation in order to identify eloquent brain tissue that should be preserved from resection. A palliative method that can be applied in functionally crucial cortical regions is multiple subpial resections, which interrupt intracortical connections without destroying the neuronal columns that are necessary for normal cerebral function. Another palliative method that is performed mainly in patients with epileptic falls is anterior or total callosotomy.

3. Prognosis and Complications

The outcome of epilepsy surgery is classified according to four categories: class 1, no disabling seizures; class 2, almost seizure free; class 3, clinical improvement; and class 4, no significant improvement. According to a meta-analysis of 30 surgical series with a total of 1651 patients, seizure outcome is as follows: class 1, 59%; class 2, 14%; class 3, 15%; and class 4, 12%. In this study, predictors of a good surgical outcome were febrile seizures, complex partial seizures, low preoperative seizure frequency, lateralized interictal EEG findings, unilateral hippocampal pathology on MRI, and neuropathological diagnosis of hippocampal sclerosis. Predictors for a poor outcome were generalized seizures, diffuse pathology on MRI, normal histology of removed tissue, and early postoperative seizures.

Relative contraindications for temporal lobe resections are extensive or multiple lesions, bilateral hippocampal sclerosis or dual pathology within one temporal lobe, significant cognitive deficits, interictal psychosis, multiple seizure types, extratemporal foci in the interictal EEG, and normal MRI. The ideal patient has mesial temporal lobe epilepsy due to unilateral hippocampal sclerosis of the nondominant hemisphere. A negative MRI decreases the chances of surgery for seizure control and a focus in the dominant hemisphere increases the risk of postoperative neuropsychological deficits.

The nature of potential perioperative complications and postsurgical neurological, cognitive, and psychiatric sequelae depends in part on the site of surgery. Operative complications occur in less than 5% of patients. In two-thirds of patients who undergo temporal resection of the dominant hemisphere, verbal memory is impaired. Another possible complication of epilepsy surgery is psychiatric disorder. Only rarely does this manifest as *de novo* psychosis. Many patients, however, will go through a phase of depression and increased anxiety following surgery. Therefore, most surgery centers include a psychiatric assessment in the preoperative phase and also a psychiatric follow-up in order to avoid catastrophic reactions (including suicide) to either the failure of surgery or the success of surgery, which requires far-reaching psychosocial adjustment.

4. Vagal Nerve Stimulation

A different surgical approach is that of vagal nerve stimulation (VNS) using an implanted stimulator. This approach has the drawback that while the nerve is being stimulated, usually for 30 sec every 5–10 min, the voice changes. More intense stimulation may be associated with throat pain or coughing. Nevertheless, in one series of 130 patients, mean seizure frequency decreased by 30% after 3 months and by 50% after 1 year of therapy. Altogether, 60–70% of the patients showed some response, but seizure freedom has rarely been achieved. Therefore, VNS is only indicated in patients who are pharmacoresistant and who are not suitable for resective epilepsy surgery.

VIII. STATUS EPILEPTICUS

Status epilepticus (SE) is defined as a condition in which a patient has a prolonged seizure or has recurrent seizures without fully recovering in the interval. With respect to the most severe seizure type (primary or generalized tonic–clonic) a duration of 5 min is sufficient for diagnosis of status epilepticus. SE may occur in a person with chronic epilepsy (the most frequent cause being noncompliance) or in a person with an acute systemic or brain disease (such as hypoglycemia or stroke). The classification of SE follows the international classification of epileptic seizures. In clinical praxis, often only two major types are distinguished: convulsive and nonconvulsive status epilepticus. SE, particularly convulsive SE, is a life-threatening condition that requires emergency treatment. Prolonged seizure activity causes systemic complications and brain damage.

The incidence of SE is 50/100,000. In all studies the convulsive type is most common (80%). However, nonconvulsive SE is difficult to recognize and may therefore be underrepresented in epidemiological studies. Mortality of SE is on the order of 20%. Prognosis and response to treatment largely depend on the etiology of SE. SE occurring in the context of chronic epilepsy has a much better outcome than SE complicating acute processes (such as hopoxemia). SE should always be managed on an emergency ward. Traditionally, drug treatment of SE includes the immediate intravenous administration of a fast-acting benzodiazepine such as diazepam plus phenytoin. Alternatively, lorazepam may be used alone because its pharmacokinteics are such that the medium-term control is comparable to that of phenytoin. If SE persists, phenobarbitone is an alternative, with the next step being a general anesthesia using pentobarbital or propofol .

IX. PSYCHIATRIC AND SOCIAL ASPECTS OF EPILEPSY

A person with epilepsy, particularly if seizures are not immediately controlled, carries an increased risk of developing psychiatric complications. These may be related to the psychological burden of a disorder that is characterized by unpredictable loss of control and is often stigmatized in modern societies. Other risk factors are biological and include the consequences of recurrent epileptic cerebral dysfunction as well as the potentially negative psychotropic effects of AEDs. Psychoses in epilepsy can occur in direct relationship to seizure activity, most often triggered by a series of seizures. They may also occur when seizures are controlled—so-called "alternative psychoses" due to "forced normalization." More common than psychoses are depressive syndromes, and suicide accounts for about 10% of all deaths in persons with epilepsy. Other psychiatric disorders that are common in epilepsy are anxiety disorders and the coexistence of epileptic and nonepileptic pseudoseizures.

Epileptic seizures have a significant impact on the social life of a person with epilepsy. Depending on the type and frequency of seizures, patients are restricted in terms of their professional options as well as their leisure time activities. In all countries there are restrictions on driving. Patients and relatives often have false ideas about the nature and course of epilepsy and therefore need to be informed about individual dangers, restrictions, and liberties. Therefore, optimal treatment of epilepsy is a multidisciplinary and enduring task, in which not only the doctor but also the social worker and the psychologist play a significant role.

See Also the Following Articles

ANTERIOR CINGULATE CORTEX • BIOFEEDBACK • BRAIN DISEASE, ORGANIC • CEREBRAL CORTEX • GABA • MOOD DISORDERS • MOVEMENT REGULATION

Suggested Reading

Annegers, J. F., Hauser, W. A., and Elveback, L. R. (1979). Remission of seizures and relapse in patients with epilepsy. *Epilepsia* **20,** 729–737.

Berg, A. T., and Shinnar, S. (1991). The risk of seizure recurrence following a first unprovoked seizure: A quantitative review. *Neurology* **41,** 965–972.

Commission on Classification and Terminology of the International League against Epilepsy (1981). Proposal for revised clinical and electroencephalographic classification of epileptic seizures. *Epilepsia* **22,** 489–501.

Commission on Classification and Terminology of the International League against Epilepsy (1989). Proposal for revised classification of epilepsies and epileptic syndromes. *Epilepsia* **30,** 389–399.

Engel, J., and Pedley, T. A. (Eds.) (1997). *Epilepsy: A Comprehensive Textbook.* Lippincott–Raven, Philadelphia.

Fenwick, P. (1991). Evocation and inhibition of seizures: Behavioural treatment. *Adv. Neurol.* **55,** 163–183.

Lüders, H. O., and Awad, I. (1991). *Conceptual considerations.* In *Epilepsy Surgery* (H. Lüders, Ed.), pp. 51–62. Raven Press, New York.

Lüders, H. O., and Noachtar, S. (2001). *Atlas of Epileptic Seizures and Syndromes.* Saunders, Philadelphia.

Musicco, M., Beghi, E., Solari, A., and Viani, F. (1997). Treatment of first tonic–clonic seizure does not improve the prognosis of epilepsy. First Seizure Trial Group (FIRST Group). *Neurology* **49,** 991–998.

Schmitz, B., and Trimble, M. R. (2001). *Psychobiology of Epilepsy,* Cambridge Univ. Press, Cambridge, UK.

Shorvon, S. D. (1990). Epidemiology, classification, natural course and genetics of epilepsy. *Lancet* **336,** 93–96.

Shorvon, S. (1994). *Status Epilepticus.* Cambridge Univ. Press, Cambridge, UK.

Temkin, O. (1971). *The Falling Sickness.* Johns Hopkins Univ. Press, Baltimore, MD.

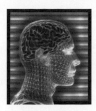

Event-Related Electromagnetic Responses

JOHN S. GEORGE

Los Alamos National Laboratory

GLOSSARY

electroencephalography (EEG) The noninvasive measurement of electrophysiological activity of the brain using electrodes attached to the scalp surface.

endogenous response An event-related response associated with voluntary movement, decision-making, or cognitive or other neural activity associated with internal processes of the experimental subject.

event-related potential (ERP) A spatiotemporal pattern in EEG data associated with a discernible event such as delivery of a stimulus or voluntary motion. The MEG analogs of these responses are sometimes called event-related fields.

event-related synchronization–event-related desynchronization (ERS–ERD) Neural population responses apparent as a resetting or reorganization of ongoing oscillatory activity.

evoked response An event-related response associated with sensory information processing of an external stimulus.

forward problem Computation of the physical consequences (e.g., an observable magnetic field or potential distribution at the head surface) associated with an assumed pattern of neural activation and a model of the properties of the head.

inverse problem Estimation of patterns of neural activation that can account for an observed pattern of experimental measures.

latency The timing of a response component or other feature relative to a defining event. Originally used to denote the period before any response was apparent (i.e., the latent phase of the response), in present usage often used to identify the peak of a response component.

magnetoencephalography (MEG) The magnetic analog of EEG, measuring magnetic fields associated with neural currents using ultrasensitive superconducting instrumentation.

response components Reproducible features in an event-related response. Typically identified on the basis of peaks and valleys in the response waveform in early work, components may be discriminated on the basis of response field topographies, consequences of stimulus properties, effects of behavioral modulations, or other criteria.

source localization Identification of the regions of neural activation that give rise to externally observable electromagnetic responses or other evidence of neural activation.

Event-related responses are spatial–temporal patterns of physiological responses associated with neural population activity, elicited by external stimuli or internal imperatives. Because these signals typically are much smaller than the ongoing activity, signal averaging, correlation, or related signal processing strategies are employed to recover the response.

I. INTRODUCTION

The function of neural systems, from the feeding and avoidance behaviors of the simplest multicellular organisms to the highest cognitive functions of the human brain, depends on dynamic spatial and temporal patterns of activation within linked networks of excitable cells. In the human brain, most purposeful function is mediated by correlated activity in substantial populations of neurons. The physical and physiological consequences of this activity can be detected with noninvasive measurement techniques, including electroencephalography (EEG) and magnetoencephalography (MEG). These techniques measure the integrated activity of thousands to hundreds of thousands of neurons. Many cells operating in synchrony are required to generate fields that can be detected centimeters away from the source. Fortunately, neural activation typically involves large clusters of neurons with similar response properties.

The information processing activities of individual neurons depend on a chain of biophysical processes: the integration of synaptic input (both excitatory and inhibitory) throughout the dendritic tree; electrical excitation mediated by the biophysical properties of ionic channel proteins in the cell membrane; transmission mediated by active and passive physical processes in the neuronal axon; and chemical or electrical relay of activation at the synapses on target cells. By linking together collections of excitable cells, networks can achieve complex behaviors beyond the capacity of individual cells.

MEG and EEG are not the only methods that can be employed with event-related and evoked response techniques. Essentially any technique that records a consistent transient response to neural activation can be used. Optical imaging methods employing sensitive video cameras have been used to record event-related responses from exposed brain tissue in experimental animals and in humans undergoing neurosurgery. With small animals such as rats or mice, it is possible to acquire images of reasonable quality though the skull. Most studies to date have exploited changes in blood flow and oxygenation associated with neural activation—the same processes that serve as the basis of fMRI. Studies have shown that it is possible to image fast intrinsic responses of neural tissue with high-performance video technology *in vivo*. Fast optical responses tightly coupled with the electrophysiological processes of neural activation were described at least 30 years ago, and the roots of such work go back much farther.

Other investigators have recorded optical evoked responses from human subjects using noninvasive methods, i.e., by injecting and recording light at the head surface to detect changes in the optical properties of tissue buried deep beneath the skull. Impedance tomography techniques have been used in a similar way to detect transient changes in tissue conductivity associated with neural activity. Even sensitive temperature measurement techniques, based on thermal emission of infrared photons, or, more recently, MRI-based methods have been used to record event-related responses associated with neural activation.

Event-related experimental paradigms have been demonstrated with functional MRI (fMRI), in spite of the facts that the earliest detectable hemodynamic responses require several hundred milliseconds and that the response peaks several seconds after neural electrophysiological activation. It is possible to use sophisticated selective averaging or correlation techniques to identify fMRI evoked responses that are highly overlapping due to rapid stimulation rates.

MRI has other important and unique roles in functional neuroimaging. MRI is used to identify and visualize the anatomical substrate of functional activation through coregistration with other imaging modalities. MRI can be used to define the computational geometries required to model the physics of techniques such as MEG and EEG, facilitating three-dimensional (3D) source localization on the basis of data that is surface-based and, thus, topographic. By defining the geometry of cortex, MRI provides useful constraints on ill-posed source localization procedures. Functional MRI provides an alternative measure of neural activation that can increase confidence in the results of comparative or integrated analysis based on multiple imaging modalities. Event-related fMRI techniques allow the same experimental paradigms to be used for NEM and fMRI experiments, a useful feature for most purposes and a prerequisite for simultaneous measurements, for example, combining EEG and fMRI.

We will consider a range of methods within this article, but the major focus will be on neural electromagnetic measurement (NEM) techniques (MEG and EEG) and noninvasive measurements of neural population responses. These methods have challenges and limitations for localizing the source of neural responses, but the excellent temporal resolution of these responses can be exploited by clever experimental paradigms to probe the dynamic interactions between multiple cortical regions. These interactions serve as the basis of information processing and control by the human brain.

II. PHYSIOLOGICAL AND PHYSICAL BASIS OF NEM RESPONSES

A. Single-Unit Electrophysiological Responses

Much of our understanding of neural function stems from electrophysiological studies of single neurons. By placing microelectrodes made of wire or drawn glass capillary tubing into or next to neurons, it is possible to record signals generated by one or a few cells. Because of the stereotypical shape and amplitude of action potentials (spikes) recorded from a given cell in a given recording configuration, it is often possible to sort a complex record into contributions from a small set of cells. The intensity of neuronal activation is typically assessed on the basis of firing rate; in sensory systems, the intensity of a stimulus is often encoded logarithmically in the firing rate within the sensory nerve. The response properties of neurons are often defined in terms of the *receptive field*, the region of sensory parameter space (e.g., location on the retina or stimulus properties of an auditory or visual stimulus) that can influence the firing rate of a particular neuron. A growing body of evidence shows that the temporal pattern of firing may also encode information. For example, in measurements across an ensemble of auditory nerve fibers in response to a pure tone stimulus below 1 kHz or so, spikes tend to occur in phase with the stimulus, i.e., a temporal code captures the temporal structure of the stimulus. In the visual system, phase-locked oscillatory activity in widely spaced cells appears to encode higher order features, such as coherent motion, beyond the spatial limits of the conventional receptive field.

B. Multiple Areas, Discrete Sources

Macroscopic electrophysiological techniques can resolve the course of neural population activation with sub-millisecond temporal resolution. This is adequate to detect the synchronous volley of action potentials that can result from electrical stimulation or sharp physiological activation and allows the characterization of oscillatory activity that can emerge within a network or by interactions between brain regions. In practice, most responses measured noninvasively do not disclose significant structure at time scales below a few milliseconds. A few specialized methods such as auditory brain stem evoked responses or electrical stimulation of the median nerve elicit a tightly correlated volley of action potentials that can be measured externally. However, most NEM evoked responses are a few milliseconds to tens of milliseconds wide and occur tens of milliseconds to hundreds of milliseconds after a stimulus event.

Dynamic responses of neural tissue involve a number of distinct processes. In response to upstream neural activity (or by endogenous processes in certain specialized sensor neurons, such as retinal photoreceptors or hair cells of the auditory system), the neuron generates an electrical response. This response is typically initiated by the flow of ionic currents though transmembrane protein channels in the plasma membranes of the neuronal dendritic tree. These currents produce a change in the standing potential across the membrane and produce potential gradients along the neuron. These potential gradients give rise to passive currents that flow along dendritic processes to rapidly equilibrate the membrane potential. Most neurons contain other channel proteins whose properties are voltage-sensitive; an excursion of the membrane potential from its typical resting value across some threshold produces a conformational change that opens an ion-specific conductance. This transient conductance change gives rise to an action potential or spike. Subsequent responses by other voltage-sensitive channels within the neuronal membrane shut down the action potential and allow recovery of the membrane potential to resting levels.

C. Propagation and Transmission

Unlike the passive conduction processes of the dendrites, action potentials are active processes that are essentially regenerated locally as the response moves across the cell body and along the axon. This allows the action potential to propagate for long distances without significant degradation of response amplitude. In some neurons the axons are sheathed with an insulating material called myelin. The sheath is interrupted periodically at nodes where membrane proteins responsible for excitation are concentrated. Excitation in myelinated axons appears to hop from node to node at rates considerably faster than transmission in uninsulated axons.

Because a patch of membrane is insensitive or refractory for a period after firing and given the stereotyped spatial pattern of dendritic integration, action potentials normally propagate in one direction from the cell body to the far reaches of the axon. Electrical simulation can elicit backward—antidromic—transmission, and there is evidence that similar processes may operate in the recovery of dendrites. Electrophysiological transmission in some specialized neural tissue is mediated by direct conductive interconnections (gap junctions), but most interneuron transmission is mediated by electrochemical transmission at specialized sites known as synapses. At the presynaptic terminal, the arrival of an action potential causes ionic changes (including an influx of calcium) that lead to the release of a chemical neurotransmitter into the synaptic cleft. The neurotransmitter molecules diffuse across the synapse to bind to receptor proteins at the postsynaptic terminal. These receptors in turn activate ionic channels, which alter the local ionic composition and/or membrane potential within the postsynaptic dendrite, leading to another cycle of integration, excitation, and transmission.

D. Neural Population Responses

These processes are the basis of information processing by neural networks. The patterns of connectivity between cells define which cells can influence which other cells and, thus, define the architecture of

information processing. Spikes signal the generation of a response by a single neuron and trigger the transmission of that information to the next cell in the chain. However, most neurons are interconnected in such a way that a spike in a single presynaptic neuron is not sufficient to elicit a response. Given the transient nature of postsynaptic responses, the efficacy of excitation within any particular neuron is critically dependent on the detailed temporal dynamics of activity within the population of neurons that converge on it.

Macroscopic electrophysiological responses depend on the activation of a significant population of neurons activating in concert. This is primarily a consequence of the distance separating the neuronal current generators and the electrodes or magnetic field detectors at the head surface. Electric and magnetic fields drop off

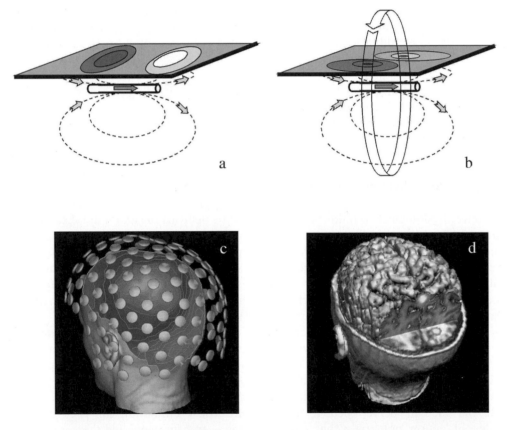

Figure 1 The physical basis of neural electromagnetic source localization. (a) Intracellular currents in tangential neural processes (parallel to the head surface) give rise to extracellular volume return currents. These currents interact with the head volume conductivity to set up a potential distribution, with surface extrema aligned with the current. (b) A detectable magnetic field is associated with the intracellular current. Extracellular currents tend to cancel in a spherical conducting volume. The extrema of the observed magnetic field distribution straddle and are orthogonal to the source current element. (c) An array of electrodes or SQUID-based magnetic field detectors are positioned on or over the surface of the head. Potential and field distributions consistent with one or more simple dipole-like sources are often observed. (d) Source localization based on a time-varying set of equivalent current dipoles. A simple source model is fit to the observed field distribution using nonlinear optimization techniques. In this figure, the uncertainty of source localization due to noise was estimated using Monte Carlo techniques, and a 3D histogram of dipole location was constructed.

rapidly with distance. EEG is further compromised by the insulating properties of the skull, which attenuate and diffuse the potential distributions that can be measured at the surface of the brain. Magnetic measurements are much less sensitive to the conductivity properties of the head, but the sensitivity of the method is reduced by the use of gradiometer sensors. Measurement of field gradients makes MEG less sensitive to interference from environmental influences, such as electric equipment, passing vehicles, or moving metal objects such as gurneys, at the expense of absolute sensitivity to neural responses.

E. Neural Electromagnetics

NEM responses are governed by the same physical processes that give rise to electric and magnetic fields in other systems. The vector currents set up by potential differences along cellular processes give rise to an electric field aligned with the current and an orthogonal magnetic field that encircles the current element. The sense (polarity) of the magnetic flux is predicted by the right-hand rule, which also predicts the direction of current flow induced in a coil penetrated by the flux. In a simple medium, charge is neither created nor destroyed; thus, all currents flow in closed loops. These relationships are summarized in Fig. 1.

Longitudinal, intracellular current flowing in the neuron during activation is matched by return current flowing through the extracellular space. These currents flow passively throughout the entire volume conductor, driven by the spatial potential gradient and limited by the resistance of the medium. In a spherical volume conductor, the magnetic contributions of these volume return currents integrate to zero, so that the measurement is dominated by the coherent currents flowing within neurons. The magnetic field is not strongly affected by the properties of biological tissue. EEG depends on the measurement of potential distributions set up by charge migration within the electric field and are critically dependent on the properties of the volume conductor. The potentials observed at the head surface arise from volume or capacitance currents that penetrate the highly resistive skull.

F. Spikes and Dendritic Responses

Although many investigators consider action potentials to be the most relevant observable consequence of neuronal activation, a number of factors limit their contribution to field and potential distributions measured at the head surface. The transmembrane currents that generate the action potential are radially symmetrical. The field cancellation associated with such distributions prevents their observation at a distance. The action potential itself is biphasic in both time and space: a depolarizing current flows along the axon, ahead of the region of excitation, and a repolarizing current flows in the opposite direction. This so-called quadrupolar current pattern is not readily detected in field measurements at a distance. Finally, the biphasic, temporally transient nature and stochastic timing of action potentials may limit their contribution to time-locked averages typically used in event-related or evoked response paradigms.

A number of lines of evidence suggest that electrophysiological responses observed at the head surface are dominated by postsynaptic dendritic currents. Such currents are typically gated by neurotransmitters, although they may have voltage-dependent characteristics. These channels often have a defined ionic specificity; some ions such as calcium may have powerful and specific effects on the response characteristics of the cell. Potentials set up by postsynaptic ion channels drive passive (i.e., ohmic) conduction along the dendrites.

G. Superposition and Integration

Electric and magnetic fields and the associated potential distributions obey the principle of superposition: the field distribution associated with a complex 3D pattern of currents is the integral over the contributions of all of the source currents flowing within the conducting volume. Within a small volume element (voxel), the distribution of cellular and volume currents can be modeled adequately by an equivalent point current with some orientation and magnitude, and the field of the entire volume can be computed as the sum over the contributions of all of the voxel currents.

Although the dendritic tree of a single neuron is often contained within a single voxel of an anatomical magnetic resonance image, each segment of current within the dendritic processes makes a contribution to the observed magnetic field and potential distributions. If the dendritic tree has a radially symmetrical geometry, the contributions may cancel and produce no effect observable at a distance. Cells of this configuration have been termed "closed field"

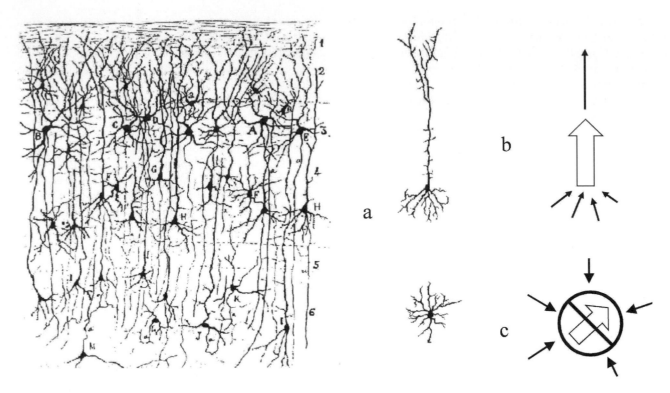

Figure 2 Vector summation of neuronal intracellular currents. (a) The regular array of cortical neurons is evident in this classic drawing of Golgi-stained neural tissue. (b) The partial symmetry of an open-field neuron (pyramidal cell) gives rise to a net intracellular current vector aligned normal to the cortical surface. (c) The radial symmetry of a closed-field interneuron produces current cancellation resulting in no net intracellular current vector.

neurons. Neurons with an asymmetric dendritic arborization have a net current vector and are termed "open field." These configurations are illustrated in Fig. 2. The neurons of neocortex have a net asymmetry that is normal (i.e., perpendicular) to the local cortical surface. Experimental validation of this prediction comes from experimental observations from linear arrays of microelectrodes penetrating the cortex. Such measurements find layered distributions of current sources and sinks across the thickness of cortex, whereas tangential potential differences are small within an extended area of activation. This basic prediction also is consistent with NEM measurements of responses from systematically arrayed sources in somatosensory or primary visual cortex.

III. THE METHODS

A. Measurement Technologies

Both MEG and EEG are passive technologies; they use sensitive instrumentation to detect the tiny electrical and magnetic perturbations associated with neural activity. Although some aspects of biological electricity can be measured directly even with primitive galvanometers, the practical application of EEG required the development of sensitive amplifiers. In particular, amplifiers with high input impedance [such as devices incorporating field effect transistors (FETs) on the front end] allow precise potential measurements without drawing significant current. This strategy has a number of advantages, including reduced sensitivity to high impedance electrodes or connections to the scalp.

EEG techniques traditionally employ a modest number of electrodes that are applied individually by hand. The most commonly used system (particularly for clinical practice) is the international 10–20 system —a montage of around 20 electrodes placed over the surface of the scalp with reference to anatomical landmarks. Electrodes are affixed to the scalp with conductive gel or other adhesives after preparation of the surface, typically by mild abrasion. This procedure produces lower contact resistance but is labor-intensive. Advances in source localization techniques, to some extent driven by MEG, have provided motivation to increase the density of potential sampling across the scalp surface. Over the past decade typical research systems have grown from 32 channels to 128 channels or more. The development of electrode arrays based on caps or mechanical tension structures (see Fig. 3) has made the application of such arrays considerably more practical, requiring minutes instead of the hours required to apply dense arrays using conventional techniques. Although it is not yet clear how many electrodes are required to capture the nuances of the scalp potential map, studies of the spatial Nyquist frequency for EEG suggest that useful new details are available using 128-channel electrode arrays and perhaps even larger arrays.

MEG is based on ultrasensitive magnetic field measurement technology, incorporating superconducting quantum interference devices (SQUIDs). The field sensors are typically superconducting pickup coils consisting of multiple loops configured for sensitivity to field gradients. Both SQUIDs and gradiometers can be constructed from high-temperature superconductors. In designs to date, the increase in noise associated with higher temperatures has proven unacceptable for brain measurements, although such systems are adequate for cardiac applications. From early in the history of MEG, it has been clear that sensor arrays of

256 channels or more would be required to adequately sample field distributions associated with superficial cortical sources. However, the first systems consisted of detector arrays of limited extent. Mapping studies involved multiple placements of the sensor array in the context of event-related or evoked response paradigms. Most current MEG and EEG systems still sacrifice spatial sampling in order to provide whole-head coverage with a practical and more affordable number of sensor channels.

MEG sensor arrays are housed in a dewar, essentially a double-walled, vacuum-insulated flask, designed to hold cryogenic fluids such as helium. The dewar limits the proximity of sensors to the head surface; most superconducting sensor arrays are separated from the outside world by 1 cm or more. With advanced designs and considerable care, this distance can be reduced to closer to 1 mm for some applications. The standoff distance produces a significant loss of sensitivity, but this is not the limiting factor for most human brain measurements. Sensor arrays must be constructed with a rigid housing designed to accommodate the majority of heads, and smaller heads will involve greater separations over at least portions of the sensor array. Even the most superficial areas of cortex are on the order of 1 cm below the head surface, and some subcortical structures of interest may be

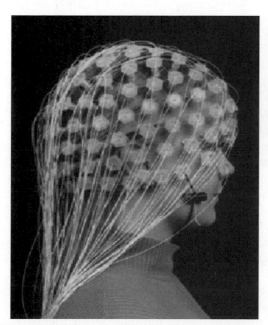 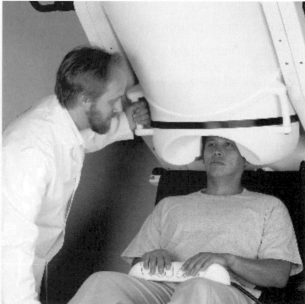

Figure 3 NEM measurement technologies. (Left) An EEG electrode array based on a mechanical tension structure (figure courtesy Electrical Geodesics, Inc.). (Right) A whole-head MEG system showing the helmet-shaped dewar that contains cryogenic fluids (figure courtesy of 4D Neuroimaging).

5–10 cm below the scalp. The fixed geometry of the MEG sensor array, the noncontact nature (and associated efficiency of subject preparation), and the relative insensitivity of MEG to head conductivity properties are all practical advantages of MEG for brain mapping applications. However, MEG sensor arrays providing full head coverage together with the magnetically shielded room used by most existing systems can cost as much as or more than a typical clinical MRI system with capabilities for functional neuroimaging.

B. Experimental Methodologies

Ongoing spontaneous activity can be recorded at the surface of the human head using MEG or EEG. Such activity typically is characterized by regions of relatively large amplitude oscillatory patterns that vary as a function of position on the head and state of the subject. Pathological responses such as certain forms of slow oscillation or the spikes and waves associated with epileptic activity often can be clearly resolved in the ongoing EEG record. The signals associated with responses to individual stimuli or other punctate cognitive or control processes typically are much smaller and require specialized experimental paradigms and signal processing techniques to pull the signals out of the noise.

1. Stimulus Evoked Responses

Brief presentations of sensory stimuli elicit a sequence of responses in the chain of specialized cortical and subcortical areas that process sensory information. In the primate visual system, over three dozen areas have been identified that are involved in the processing of visual information. Other sensory modalities such as auditory and somatosensory systems involve smaller numbers of areas and less cortical real estate but still employ distributed processing strategies.

In order to enhance the consistent aspects of the sensory response while suppressing the contribution of other physiological processes or environmental noise, most investigators employ averaging of temporal sequences time-locked to the stimulus. In this sort of *evoked response* paradigm, individual stimuli are typically presented in isolation. Different examples of a class of stimuli are often presented in a random sequence. The interstimulus interval typically is varied within some limits to minimize habituation and thwart the generation of temporal expectations by the subject;

such effects can influence the amplitude and timing of certain components of the response. The time course of the electrophysiological response to a single stimulus ranges from tens of milliseconds to a few hundred. Thus, by presenting stimuli at intervals of 500 msec or more, it is possible to examine the entire time course of the response with little or no overlap from preceding or subsequent responses. Figure 4 illustrates an example of some of the techniques used for visualizing a somatosensory evoked response.

2. Steady-State Paradigms

An alternative approach for evoked response paradigms is to present stimuli at high rates, accepting the response overlap. Instead of discrete stimulus presentations, such paradigms often impose rapid changes on an ongoing stimulus, such as amplitude modulation of a continuous tone or contrast reversal of a patterned video display. Because the response does not return to baseline between stimuli (i.e., residual activation is maintained between trials), this class of techniques is referred to as *steady-state* methods. However, when using typical AC-coupled recording methods, the response must be modulated in order to be detectable. The time-locked response is typically isolated using Fourier transform techniques. The amplitude at the stimulation frequency is taken as a measure of the evoked response, whereas the phase is taken as a measure of the temporal delay (or latency) of the response.

The primary advantage of this strategy is speed; steady-state methods provide an efficient way of collecting and analyzing topographic data produced by MEG or EEG. However, such methods also have disadvantages. Fast stimulus presentations produce a measure of sensory overload, often leading to habituation or reduced levels of attention to stimuli. Steady-state methods may also introduce phase ambiguities. For example, visual evoked responses show evidence of an initial activation in layer 4 of the primary cortical visual area, V1, followed by activation in other layers and eventually by feedback activation in V1 from higher visual areas. At high stimulation rates the temporal relationship between various phases of the V1 cortical response may be obscured. Further, the subsequent activation of other visual processing areas may produce field or potential topographies that overlap with the responses of earlier areas. The loss of timing information removes an important tool for the identification of sources and for studies of the dynamics of information processing.

Experimental studies employing MEG have demonstrated a clever application of high-frequency stimulation techniques. By modulating the stimulus at frequencies that may be too high to consciously perceive, it is possible to frequency-tag the downstream response. Such methods can be used to tag the hemifield of stimulation in a wide-field visual stimulus or to identify the stimulated ear in a dichotic listening paradigm. Residual modulation at the tag frequency can be used to identify the origin of a response even after the arrival of the signal at a higher sensory processing area with convergent bilateral inputs.

By presenting fast pseudo-random sequences of individual stimuli, it is possible to achieve much of the efficiency of steady-state techniques while avoiding several of the problems. For example, a video display can be divided into elements that are turned on and off in an apparently random sequence, such as an m-sequence. The temporal activation sequences are designed to be orthogonal, i.e., each element has its own unique activation sequence. This allows correlation techniques to be used to extract the spatial and temporal patterns of response to each element of the display. This method can be very efficient because many stimulus elements can be presented simultaneously. However, this leads to stimuli that are decidedly nonphysiological and may be a bit disconcerting. At present, the method appears to be more useful for rapid mapping of the systematic parametric organization of primary sensory areas (i.e., retinotopic, tonotopic, or somatotopic projections) than as a tool for probing higher cognitive processes.

Sensory evoked response paradigms provide a powerful and robust tool for probing the functional architecture and dynamics of the neural systems devoted to the processing of sensory information. However, this is only one of several classes of functional activity within the human brain.

3. Motor Control

The control of voluntary movement is another critical capability of higher organisms. Although the coordination and fine-tuning of movement appear to be distributed through several brain centers, the initiation of movement is a function of the motor cortex, located adjacent to primary somatosensory areas in humans. Some investigators have used cued trials to study motor function, hoping that the temporal jitter in the reaction time does not wash out the targeted motor response. This strategy also produces a time-locked response to the sensory cue, which can interfere with

the analysis of the motor response. An alternative strategy is to use self-paced tasks and to time-lock averaging to the motor response. For simplicity, the response can be a button press or similar action that is readily converted into an electronic timing signal. A bit more sophisticated strategy is to base experimental timing on a measured physiological response. For example, it is possible to record an electromyogram signaling the activation of specific muscle groups by using the same basic technology as EEG. These are large, robust responses that can be detected in a continuous recording, often using simple threshold techniques. This sort of activity, which may not be evoked directly by external stimulation but is associated with externally observable consequences, is referred to as an *event-related response*. In addition to motor processes or simple behavioral trials such as reaction time detection tasks, event-related experimental designs are often used to probe high order cognitive processing activity. In some cases, the "event" is only apparent as an internal state, e.g., conjunction of a particular stimulus with a specific behavioral or cognitive task.

4. Cognitive Processes

The general strategy for event-related cognitive studies is to employ a set of tasks designed to isolate and contrast the processes of interest. Measures derived from MEG or EEG are used as an index of activation and, thus, of the underlying cognitive processes. Such studies often employ well-balanced control trials, which account for sensory or motor components of a response while manipulating the relevance or difficulty of the cognitive component. Such strategies have been used to isolate and probe various aspects of selective attention. For example, many designs used for attention studies employ a cue stimulus presented before the probe trial to direct attention to one region of the visual field or another. The subject might be instructed to respond to a particular type of stimulus only when presented at the attended site. Thus, in the same experiment, a given physical stimulus might serve as the response target, an inappropriate stimulus at the attended site, or an irrelevant stimulus that can be ignored.

Other designs tap the endogenous cognitive skills of the subject. For example, a list of real words might be presented visually along with interspersed pseudo-words (i.e., pronouncible constructs that look like words but have no meaning) or nonwords. The nature of the observed response varies as a function of the

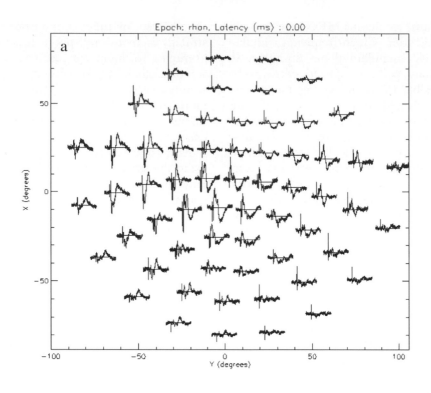

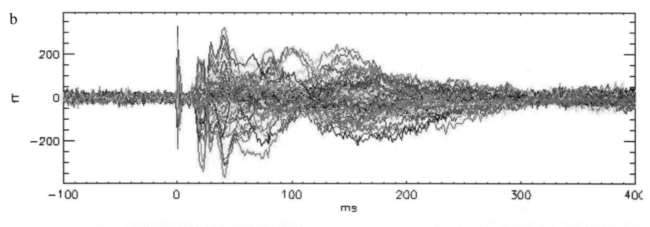

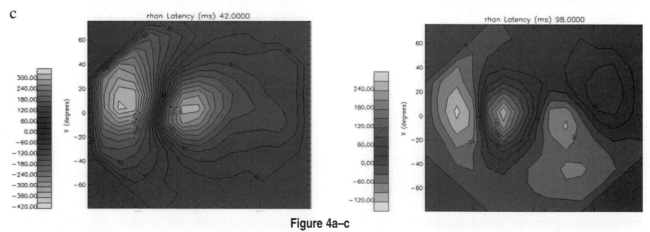

Figure 4a–c

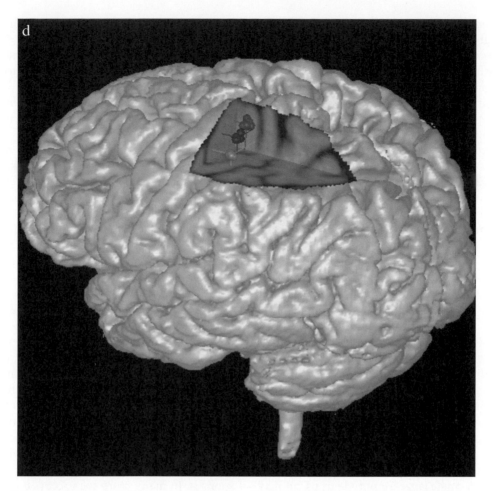

Figure 4 Several views of somatosensory evoked response recorded with MEG. (a) A depiction of the evoked response waveforms recorded over the surface of the head. Waveforms are positioned according to the polar projection of the corresponding sensor locations. (b) An envelope or "butterfly" plot of the stacked waveforms reveals the balanced polarity of MEG responses, allowing appreciation of temporal relationships between waveform features. (c) Contour plots of the field maps observed at two latencies of the evoked response. Field maps are plotted in polar coordinates. The left panel suggests a simple activation pattern early in the response. The right panel suggests the presence of an additional source in the contralateral hemisphere. (d) Equivalent current dipole sources estimated from early latencies localize to the posterior bank of the central sulcus.

lexical class of stimulus. A spoken sentence might be presented in which the final word either completes a reasonable semantic construct or renders the sentence nonsensical. Such paradigms can tap the mechanisms by which we comprehend language.

C. Signal Processing

Event-related and evoked responses in MEG and EEG are typically quite small compared to ongoing neural activity or other physiological activity or environmental noise. Effective signal processing strategies are essential for isolating the desired signals from other observed signals not of interest.

Temporal filtering is a ubiquitous initial step in the signal processing chain. Virtually all MEG and EEG systems employ some sort of analog filtering on the front end to reduce the signal bandwidth to avoid aliasing in digitization, if for no other reason. Many conventional EEG systems provide an extensive set of analog filtering capabilities, including high-pass and low-pass filters as well as notch filters (often tuned to the 50- or 60-Hz frequency of the power grid), to eliminate major sources of environmental interference. If the frequency content of the targeted signal is known or can be determined empirically, reduction of the bandwidth of the measurement reduces noise and can increase the efficiency of signal acquisition. However, as high-density sensor systems and digital acquisition and processing become more standard, instruments are increasingly designed with fixed analog front ends. Signal processing is increasingly performed by digital signal processing subsystems, general purpose computers embedded in the data system, or workstations used by investigators for subsequent analysis.

Digital filtering is cheaper and in many respects technically superior to the use of analog filters. Methods based on the fast Fourier transform (FFT) greatly simplify the algorithms required to implement digital temporal filters. Related techniques are used for the frequency domain analysis of the major rhythms characteristic of spontaneous EEG or MEG recording or for the extraction of steady-state responses at the stimulation frequency. Short time base analyses based on wavelets or special FFT algorithms may be used to identify periods of transient synchronization (or desynchronization) that are associated with (but not time-locked to) external stimuli or perceptual states. Such analyses are often based on trial by trial analysis of continuously acquired data. The averaging techniques used for most event-related response work would attenuate or eliminate such responses because they are not time-locked to the stimulus and may vary in time and phase from one response to another.

Eye blinks or other movements of facial muscles can produce strong signals in MEG or EEG. The startup of an electric motor or power-hungry instrument in the vicinity (or sharing a power circuit) can also introduce large artifacts. A single large-amplitude transient may leave significant residue in an averaged event-related response even after many trials. For this reason, *artifact rejection* is another common step applied in the analysis of MEG and EEG data. The digital data stream is monitored for values that exceed some criterion threshold. If the threshold is exceeded, the offending channels or, more commonly, the entire trial is excluded from further analysis. For some clinical applications, artifact rejection is typically accomplished by visual inspection. In epilepsy, the pathophysiological responses of interest may exceed the size of signals considered artifacts under other circumstances, and inspection by a trained clinician may be the most efficient and effective way to identify both artifacts and epileptiform activity. However, as data streams become more dense and algorithms become more sophisticated, there is increasing reliance on software that can categorize events in the experimental record on the basis of temporal waveforms, spatial topographies, or both. Such systems are often used to preprocess an extensive record, bringing interesting or suspicious events to the attention of the reviewer.

Time-locked selective averaging is the mainstay of most existing work with event-related or evoked responses. As a first step, epochs in the data are identified and characterized according to the nature of the stimulus, the response, or the task and its performance. Averaging can even be undertaken relative to a reproducible endogenous transient, such as an epileptiform spike. Segments of the waveform data across all channels are selected relative to the timing event, and within each channel the corresponding time points in the segment are averaged. In general, averages are segregated according to the particulars of the trial, e.g., the identity of the stimulus or the accuracy of task performance, although in many cases averages are collapsed across conditions that are considered irrelevant for a particular experimental question. Many studies report "grand averages" constructed by averaging responses across many subjects in order to increase the power of statistical inference, although this practice probably precludes reliable source localization.

The construction of *difference waves*, by subtracting a control condition from a particular response, is another time-honored method for the analysis of event-related response data. For example, such methods clearly disclose the increase in response amplitude associated with selective attention to a particular location in the visual field and isolate responses associated with certain endogenous cognitive responses. In many cases such records are reduced to a single response waveform, for example, by averaging (or summing power) across all channels or a selected subset. However, an increasing number of investigators construct difference topographies by subtracting control responses from the corresponding signal channels. These distributions are often analyzed in the same way as the underlying event-related signals, for example, subjected to source localization procedures.

Such analyses should be approached with caution. The methods will work, in principle, if the only differences between conditions are due to the strength of the underlying sources or the appearance of a new source under particular experimental conditions. Unlike PET and fMRI, which in effect produce an estimate of the distribution of source activity, EEG and MEG produce topographic maps with a complex relationship to source activity, driven by the physical properties of the measurement instrument and the system under study. Minor changes in the location or extent of activation (especially in cortical regions of high curvature) can produce big changes in the observed field topography and, thus, significant changes in computed difference fields.

Single-pass analytical methodologies are increasingly applied to the analysis of event-related response data. Frequency decomposition techniques (described previously) have been used to explore the putative role of transient phase-locking of oscillatory activity in certain perceptual processes. Correlation techniques can be applied to continuous evoked response data to identify consistent features in a manner analogous to signal averaging. Spatial filtering techniques compute a linear transform (based on a computed or assumed source model) that can be applied to the data to estimate the activation time course of the source. Several investigators suggest that techniques in this class (such as minimum variance beam-forming) are most useful if applied to single trial data rather than averaged responses. Some new methods such as independent component analysis (ICA), synthetic aperture magnetometry, or magnetic field tomography by the nature of the algorithm are most effectively applied to the analysis of single trial data.

IV. RESPONSE DYNAMICS

The principal strengths of neural electromagnetic methods stem from their capacity to define the dynamics of neural population activity. Even a single electrode pasted to the scalp may disclose a complex temporal waveform consisting of a series of peaks and valleys. In some cases, a peak in a waveform at a particular latency is observed across a large subset of the channels in a whole-head sensor array, even though the amplitude or the polarity of the peak changes. This pattern is characteristic of a single anatomical source or a set of sources acting in synchrony. In some cases, a close examination of the waveform montage collected from a sensor array discloses that what appears as a single peak in one waveform can be resolved as multiple overlapping temporal peaks observed at other locations. In such cases, the topographic map of the evoked response typically has apparent features that appear to shift systematically over the course of the response. A simple-minded analysis may suggest that the source is a single focus of activity moving through the brain volume. A more sophisticated source model may allow the same response to be decomposed into two or more component sources with stable NEM topographies and distinct but overlapping time courses.

In the absence of effective source localization techniques, there was a tendency in early work to focus on the peaks in the waveform as the unitary building blocks—the components from which complex event-related responses were built. Components were given names on the basis of the polarity and latency of the waveform peaks: e.g., the N100 (a negative-going response component peaking around 100 msec poststimulus) or the P300 (or P3, a positive peak in the response waveform around 300 msec poststimulus). As the characterization of response components proceeded, descriptions of the component scalp topography were sometimes added to aid identification and discrimination of named components. For endogenous cognitive response components, identifying criteria often included the nature of experimental manipulations required to elicit or enhance a particular peak in the waveform. Whereas such information is critical for investigators attempting to reproduce or extend a particular observation, it complicates the business of component quantification.

In an effort to address this concern, some investigators turned to blind decomposition techniques such as *principal components analysis* (PCA). PCA is a linear technique based on eigen analysis and singular value decomposition. The method attempts to find a set of basis functions—in this case, field or potential topographies—that can be used to reconstruct the original experimental data. In order to make the decomposition unique, principal components are constrained to be mutually orthogonal. Each principal component has an associated weighting vector that quantifies the representation in the data of each component as a function of time. In some well-behaved cases, principal components correspond to response components identified by other criteria. However, in general, the requirement for orthogonality precludes the proper identification of more than a few components. An alternative decomposition strategy has been developed that appears to hold an alternative decomposition strategy that appears to hold significant promise for functional neuroimaging applications. Independent component analysis identifies a basis set in which components are statistically independent though not necessarily orthogonal. Initial results with the algorithm are promising, although it will certainly be possible to find pathological cases that cause the algorithm to fail. It is not yet clear how effectively the algorithm will identify proper components in routine applications to event-related response data.

In a few cases, the idea that components reflect the successive activation of links in a processing chain appears basically correct. For example, in the *auditory brain stem evoked response* (ABER), the peaks in the waveform are associated with specific structures in the early auditory pathways, and the waveform morphology can be used to assess the integrity of the relay and processing circuitry. Similarly, the earliest components of somatosensory responses evoked by electrical stimulation appear to be associated with specific anatomical loci. In contrast, for visual evoked responses the situation is considerably more complex. Although some investigators have reported an early, relatively small EEG component (N70) that was identified as the initial activation of cortical V1, most analyses have focused on the more robust P100 component. A variety of source analysis techniques indicate that this component is a complex consisting of temporally overlapping responses from several distinct though nearby visual areas. Although there is an element of sequential processing in the early visual system as activation spreads through the information processing tree, there is also considerable parallel processing. There are also forward and feedback links that skip over portions of the schematic processing hierarchy and delays within areas that can further complicate the simple orderly picture of temporal response dynamics.

V. SOURCE LOCALIZATION

The existence of detectable magnetic fields and electric potential distributions at the head surface is a consequence of the physics of electromagnetism. Given an adequate description of the source currents and the conductivity properties of the medium, it is possible to compute the anticipated field topographies. Calculations to solve this so-called *forward problem* can employ models of greater or lesser detail, depending on the complexity of the system and the required degree of accuracy. Computation of the forward problem for more complex source distributions—extended regions of activation or multiple active sources—is more time-consuming, but not significantly more difficult. The principle of superposition tells us that the contributions for multiple source currents will sum linearly.

In principle, it may be feasible to invert the process—to compute the currents that give rise to an observed field or potential distribution at the head surface. Unfortunately, this *inverse problem* is not well-behaved. In general, many different current distributions can produce the same set of surface measure-

ments. To appreciate the problem intuitively, consider a homogeneous spherical volume that is conductive. It is possible to account for any given potential or magnetic field distribution measured at or above the surface, with a suitable collection of currents limited to the surface of the sphere. However, we can define another spherical shell 1 cm below the surface and derive another current distribution to account for the same set of observations. Given this fundamental ambiguity, how can we hope to reconstruct the proper set of current sources buried deep in the brain from the data available at the head surface?

The general strategy is to build a model of the sources that might produce the observed responses. The source model defines the structure of the solution. Model parameters define the details. In some cases, source models are very restrictive, so that a single, best-fitting set of model parameters can be found. In such cases, the accuracy of the solution depends on the applicability of the source model. As the complexity of the source model increases, generally the number of parameters also increases. This allows more complex source distributions to be modeled, but tends to increase the ambiguity of the reconstruction problem. By defining the criteria that we prefer in an acceptable solution it is generally possible to find a solution, but again, the accuracy of the solution depends on the validity of the assumptions.

A. Model-Based Approaches

Thus, source localization depends on the use of nested computational models that describe the distribution of neural currents and that predict the observable consequences of those currents. These models are based on implicit or explicit knowledge and assumptions about the nature of the system. The first 50 years of work with EEG involved little quantitative effort to localize the sources of observed topographies in the surface potential data. The development of MEG and the recognition that many observed field distributions could be explained by a simple forward model led to advances in procedures that have subsequently been applied to EEG data.

B. Forward Modeling

For electrical or magnetic measurements at a distance significantly larger than the extent of the source, the spatial fine structure of the field distribution is not detected, and the dominant contribution is the dipole associated with longitudinal intracellular currents. In MEG, the effects of ohmic currents through the head volume are minimal, and a reasonable analytical solution can be derived by treating the head as a homogeneous conducting sphere. The radius of the sphere is chosen to approximate the inner surface of the skull, based on individual anatomical images or external measures of head shape coupled with a knowledge of average anatomy. Unlike MEG, EEG signal topographies are strongly influenced by the conductivity properties of the head. Even simple models of elemental EEG signals must take into account the presence of multiple tissue layers of differing conductivity. Dipole response topographies for EEG can be computed in a volume model consisting of multiple spherical shells, with layers corresponding to brain, cerebral–spinal fluid, skull, and scalp, using a truncated series of Legendre polynomials. Many researchers in the field have argued that this class of model is more than adequate for source localization, given the uncertainties associated with the inverse problem. However, as inverse procedures have improved, a number of studies have underscored the value of more sophisticated forward models for source localization accuracy. Some of these approaches are summarized in Fig. 5.

A significant improvement in the accuracy of the forward calculation can be achieved by *boundary element* calculations incorporating the geometry of the major tissue classes within the head. Surface meshes are constructed to approximate conductivity boundaries. Because the conductivity of the skull is significantly lower than that of other tissues in the head, it is particularly important to capture the geometry of the skull near sensors. Most calculations of this sort are limited to simple topologies, e.g., nested compartments without intersections or penetrations. Conductivity values are typically taken from the literature and correspond to measurements originally made in cadaver tissue. Because there is no basis for further subdivision, conductivity is taken as homogeneous within a compartment. Although the boundary element method employs simple geometries, the calculations are relatively time-consuming, because the solution matrix typically contains terms for the interactions between every pair of nodes in the mesh. Numerical studies have demonstrated that it is possible to achieve accuracy approaching that of the boundary element methods at much lower computational cost by approximating the skull boundary with local spheres selected for each sensor.

3D methods provide an alternative strategy for high-resolution forward calculations. In *finite difference* (FD) or *finite element* (FE) forward calculations, the head volume is divided into a collection of volume elements that form the computational mesh. Potentials are computed at nodes, typically associated with boundaries or vertices of the volume elements. These calculations assume a current source that generates the potential and account for the conductivity properties of the volume elements that strongly influence the spread of potential. FE methods typically employ an irregular mesh composed of tetrahedral elements. This allows the mesh to closely match conductivity boundaries within the medium that may give rise to sharp gradients in the potential distribution, providing greater accuracy with a smaller number of volume elements. However, most present methods for mesh generation and refinement require considerable human intervention. FD methods typically employ a regular (e.g., rectangular) mesh. Segmentation or voxel classification schemes can be applied to regular volumetric data such as MRI to produce a data volume that can be used for calculations without constructing specialized meshes.

3D methods are most useful if we have access to external information that can be used to define the geometry or electrical properties of the conductive medium. MRI provides the most accessible and flexible measure of tissue properties, although X-ray CT provides a better definition of the geometry and microstructure of the skull. New and evolving MRI techniques will eventually provide even more useful information for forward modeling. *Current density MRI* operates by applying external currents at the head surface and measuring the perturbation of the image by local volume currents. This allows an estimation of head conductivity on a voxel by voxel basis. *Diffusion tensor MRI* measures the magnitude and characterizes the direction of diffusion of water within tissue. Structures such as white matter tracts give rise to anisotropic physical properties that can be described by a tensor, e.g., the apparent diffusion coefficient of water and the measured conductivity are much higher along a fiber tract than transverse to it. MRI can be used to estimate the anisotropic conductivity of such tissue. FE and FD methods can accommodate anistropic conductivity (though again the FD application is simpler). By passing currents through pairs of surface electrodes and estimating the induced potentials at other electrodes in the array, electrical impedance tomography (EIT) allows an estimation of the bulk properties of major tissue

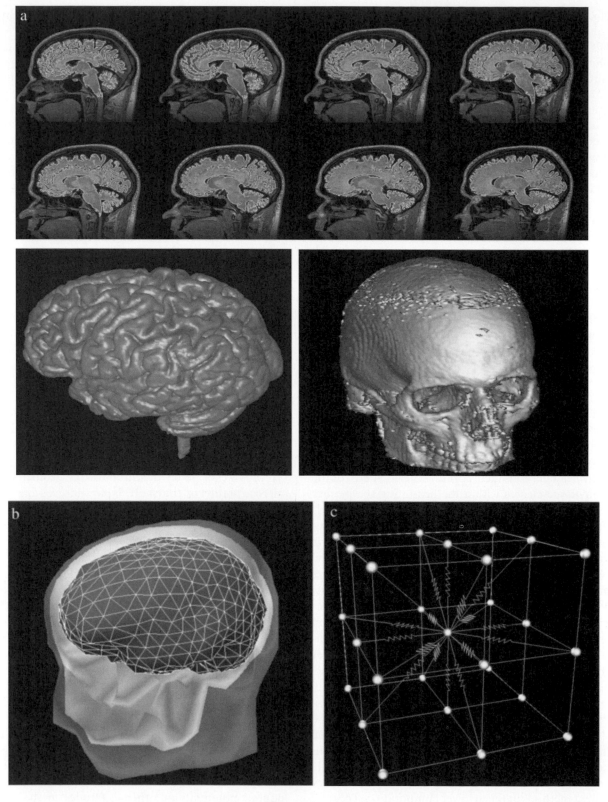

Figure 5a–c

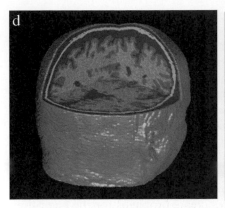
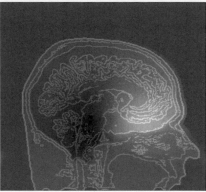
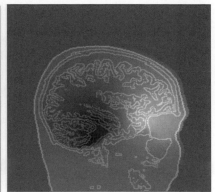

Figure 5 NEM forward modeling in realistic geometries. (a) Computational tools for interactive and semiautomatic segmentation of cortical anatomy allow extraction of computational geometries. Upper panel: Region-growing algorithms with adaptive criteria perform segmentation of white matter and identification of gray matter by dilation. Lower left: 3D rendering of the cortical surface identified by an automatic algorithm. Lower right: Rendering of the skull segmented by region-growing techniques from 3D MRI data. (b) Boundary element mesh based on simplified skull and scalp geometry derived from MRI volume imagery. (c) The regular computational mesh employed for finite difference computations in anisotropic media. The nodes for potential computation are at the corners of the spatial volume elements. (d) Finite difference calculation of potential distribution, using a detailed computational geometry derived from MRI. The current source is located within the temporal lobe, with a posterior to anterior orientation. The slices from the computed potential distribution show evidence of current leakage through the skull penetrations of the optic nerve.

classes within the head and even a measure of 3D reconstruction. Tomographic reconstruction of head conductivity requires 3D computational techniques and is greatly facilitated by accurate geometrical information drawn from MRI.

C. Source Model Estimation

Source localization from EEG and MEG began with educated inspection of surface field topographies. In EEG, a radially oriented current will produce a potential extremum over the source. In MEG, a radial current source produces little externally detectable magnetic field, but the tangential component of a neural source produces a field distribution with extrema that straddle the source. The distance separating the field extrema allows an estimation of the source depth, given assumptions regarding the nature of the current source. In both EEG and MEG, many observed response topographies can be explained by an *equivalent current dipole* (ECD) source, i.e., an isolated point current with a given location, orientation, and amplitude. Theory suggests that such a model provides a reasonable estimate of the field or potential distributions due to a small cluster of oriented neurons measured at a distance. Even extended patches of activated cortex often produce a

dipole-like distribution, although the estimated location and strength of the ECD will contain systematic errors. An extended patch of parallel current elements produces an ECD estimate that is deeper and stronger than the center of mass and integral current estimated from the actual source distribution.

Because field topographies are typically diffuse, source estimation by eye is a rather inexact process. Some investigators have employed image processing techniques to allow for easier detection of features in the field topography. For example, computation of the spatial derivative (the Laplacean) of the observed magnetic field or potential topography tends to place maxima over the current sources. Indeed, one form of MEG sensor—a first-order planar gradiometer— effectively implements this transform in the detector coil configuration.

Although *inspection of response topographies* is a useful starting point for finding NEM sources, model-based parameter estimation procedures provide a more objective strategy that allows quantitative assessment of the goodness of fit. Nonlinear optimization procedures such as simplex or gradient descent allow the estimation of a dipole source; current orientation and strength are linear parameters that can be optimized separately. If a single focal current source is active in a simple medium, such procedures can localize it very precisely. However, at any given instant in time, many sources may contribute to a given response topography. Because of superposition, a combination of several sources may give rise to a distribution that is adequately modeled by a single source at an entirely different location. Knowledge of the number and nature of active sources can reduce the ambiguity of the source localization problem. Spatio-temporal source localization techniques attempt to find a minimal set of sources, each with an associated time course, that explains the observed distribution across a defined interval within an event-related response. If the sources are activated asynchrously, this strategy can be very effective for decomposing and localizing the contributions of individual sources.

Nonlinear optimization methods can be used to find locations for a collection of simple current sources that might explain changing field topographies observed across time. Because the time course is an estimate of the source current amplitude as a function of time, linear methods can be used to optimize the estimates between iterative nonlinear optimization steps. This general strategy has been the most widely used approach for NEM source localization for over a decade, but modifications, extensions, or alternatives to the method can provide enhanced performance. A common problem with nonlinear methods is that they require a starting estimate of model parameters. This may be provided by an informed analyst or by a stochastic process. If the starting estimate is close enough, an optimization procedure that follows the error gradient can find the best-fitting model. If the starting estimates are far off and the error surface is complex (often the case with multiple-source models), the procedure may fall into a local minimum that is not globally optimal. A conscientious analysis can combat this problem by running the optimization procedure with multiple sets of starting parameters. *Multistart* procedures automate this process, employing a numerical algorithm to generate random starting parameter estimates. Such methods often find a consistent set of best-fitting source models that are globally optimal. Other methods such as *simulated annealing* or *genetic algorithms* employ alternative strategies to address the problem of local minima within the model parameter error space. Examples of these approaches are illustrated in Fig. 6.

The multiple signal classification (MUSIC) algorithm operates within the same framework (i.e., a multiple-dipole spatiotemporal model) but employs a more systematic strategy for finding sources. The array of measured potential or field values at any given instant in time is treated as a multidimensional vector in the space of possible measurements. Similarly, the topography associated with any given dipole is another vector in the same space. The algorithm operates by systematically stepping through a set of possible sources (e.g., a grid of locations within the brain) and evaluates the match between the source field vector and the collection of signal vectors across time. The sources that most closely match the observed signals across time are considered the most likely. The method is very effective and can be exhaustive, avoiding problems of local minima seen with nonlinear optimization techniques. Multiple sources with highly correlated time courses create problems for the algorithm, but enhanced methods such as recursively applied (RAP) MUSIC address this and other concerns.

A second general strategy is to use *linear inverse techniques* to solve a large and general source model. The reconstruction space is defined by a regular grid, a collection of voxels, or vertices from a computational mesh. One to three current elements are associated with each possible source location. The reconstruction procedure employs the Moore–Penrose pseudo-inverse to assign a current value to each model element. This procedure, based on singular value decomposition, estimates a source distribution with minimum power over the collection of driving currents. A number of variants on this *minimum norm* procedure have been described, mostly based on different strategies for weighting the lead field basis matrix in order to select a solution with desired properties. Anatomical constraints based on cortical geometry can improve accuracy and efficiency. However, even with substantial reductions in the source space based on anatomy, the inverse is a highly underdetermined problem. There are many more source model parameters to estimate than the number of independent measures available from MEG or EEG.

The major problem with minimum norm procedures is that there is no guarantee that the solution of minimum Euclidean norm (i.e., the sum of squared currents) will be representative of the true solution. Because of the strong dependence of measured magnetic field on distance from the source, the basic minimum norm procedure tends to produce diffuse, superficial current reconstructions, even when the reconstruction space is constrained to the cortical surface. Currents closer to the sensor array can account for more power in the field map with less current and therefore are favored by the method. However, more current elements are required to account for the shape of a field distribution that may actually arise from a more focal but deeper source.

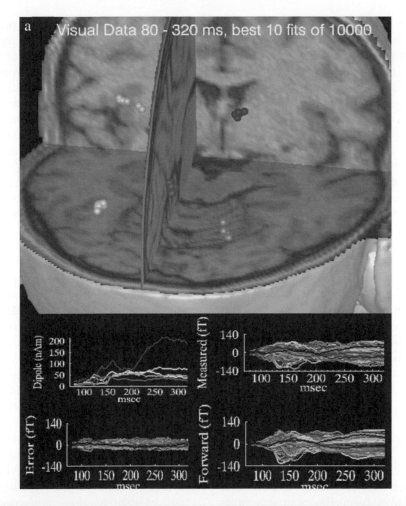

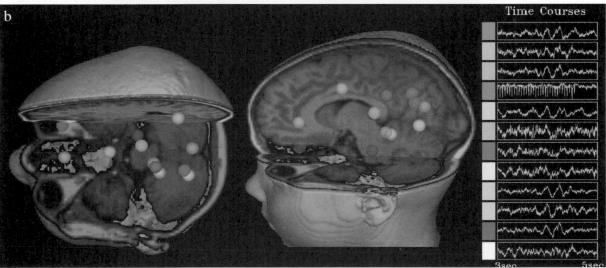

Figure 6 Source localization by multiple dipole spatiotemporal estimation procedures. (a) Dipole source locations and time courses estimated from visual evoked response data. This analysis used a multistart algorithm; the best 10 solutions from 10,000 generated are tightly clustered, suggesting that the algorithm has found a global best fit. (b) Dipole locations and time courses associated with an epileptic response from a photosensitive child. Dipole locations were estimated with a genetic algorithm. Note that the magnetic response of the eye contains evidence of the strobe flashes that triggered the response.

In order to combat this tendency, it is possible to scale the field distributions (or, alternatively, the strength of the unit currents) in order to normalize the field power associated with each elemental source. Pseudo-inverse procedures based on a normalized basis matrix offer some improvement in the fidelity of reconstructions. Explicit or implicit basis matrix weighting procedures have proven to be a useful general strategy for modifying the properties of reconstruction algorithms. The FOCUSS algorithm employs an iterative reweighting procedure to derive sparse reconstructions based on focal activated patches. The LORETA algorithm uses an alternative weighting scheme to find current reconstructions that are maximally smooth.

Given the fundamental ambiguity of the inverse problem and the complex error surface associated with the parameter space, there is no guarantee that the proper form of source model (e.g., the number of active sources) can be determined or that a single global minimum will be found. The estimated parameter values critically depend on model assumptions and may vary widely as a function of small amounts of noise in the data.

D. Bayesian Methods

Bayesian analysis techniques provide a formal method for integration of prior knowledge drawn from other imaging methods. In pure form, Bayesian techniques estimate a posterior probability distribution (a form of solution) based on the experimental data and prior knowledge expressed in the form of a probability distribution. In additional to providing a flexible mechanism for multimodality integration, these techniques allow rigorous assessment of the consequences of prior knowledge or assumptions about the nature of the preferred solution. Several investigators have explored traditional Bayesian methods, seeking a single "best" solution that satisfies some criterion, such as maximum likelihood, maximum *a posteriori* (MAP), or maximum entropy solution. However, any given single solution is effectively guaranteed to be inaccurate, at least in its details.

A technique for Bayesian inference has been developed that addresses this concern by explicitly sampling the posterior probability distribution. The strategy is essentially to conduct a series of numerical experiments and determine which solutions best account for the data. To make the method efficient, a Markov chain Monte Carlo (MCMC) technique is employed.

After the algorithm identifies regions of the source model parameter space that account for the data by a stochastic process, the algorithm effectively concentrates its sampling in that region. Thus, in the end, samples are distributed according to the posterior probability distribution—a probability distribution of solutions upon which subsequent inferences are based. The Bayesian inference method does not employ optimization procedures and does not produce an estimate of the best-fitting solution. Instead, it attempts to build a probability map of activation. This distribution provides a means of identifying and estimating probable current sources from surface measurements while explicitly emphasizing multiple solutions that can account for any set of surface EEG–MEG measurements.

This method for Bayesian inference uses a general neural activation model that can incorporate prior information on neural currents, including location, orientation, strength, and spatial smoothness. Instead of equivalent current dipoles, the method uses an extended parametric model to define sources. An active region is assumed to consist of a set of voxels identified as part of cortex and located within a sphere centered on cortex or a patch generated by a series of dilation operations about some point on cortex. In a typical analysis, 10,000 samples are drawn from the posterior distribution using the MCMC algorithm. Despite the variability among the samples, several sources common to (nearly) all are often apparent. Features such as these are associated with a high degree of probability. By keeping track of the number of times each voxel is involved in an active source over the set of samples, it is possible to build a probability map for neural activation and to quantify confidence intervals. In addition to information about the locations of probable sources, the Bayesian inference approach also estimates probabilistic information about the number and size of active regions. Figure 7 illustrates several aspects of this approach to Bayesian inference.

VI. MULTIMODALITY TECHNIQUES

A growing body of evidence suggests that there is a good if imperfect correspondence between neural electrical activation and the fMRI BOLD response and that convergent information can be used to improve the reliability of macroscopic electrophysiological techniques. Because of the ambiguity associated with the neural electromagnetic inverse problem, a number of investigators have pursued the strategy of using fMRI to define the locations of activation while using MEG or EEG to estimate time courses. Although this approach may have considerable value, it also has its pitfalls. In general, there is no guarantee that activation seen in one modality will be apparent in the other. The relationship between the precise areas of increased bloodflow and electrophysiological activation is not certain. If we assume that anatomical MRI constrains the location and orientations of possible source currents and that fMRI provides an estimate of the identity and relative strengths of active voxels, it is possible to compute the field topography associated with an extended source of arbitrary shape and size. Alternatively, fMRI can be employed as a method to *seed* dipole source estimates, which are optimized subsequently by using standard nonlinear procedures. This strategy provides a measure of flexibility to account for mismatches between assumptions and source model.

Other investigators have employed a form of weighted minimum norm to combine fMRI and NEM data. The inverse solution is constrained to lie within the cortical surface, and source current orientation may be constrained to lie normal to the local surface. By weighting the reconstruction according to the spatial pattern of apparent activation disclosed by fMRI, it is possible to guide the minimum norm reconstruction to preferentially place current in those regions. Because Bayesian methods explicitly employ prior knowledge to help solve the inverse problem, they provide a natural and formal method to integrate multiple forms of image data. The simplest strategy is to use fMRI data as a prior. This method can profitably employ strategies for the analysis of fMRI data that quantify the probability of activation in any particular voxel on the basis of fMRI data. Bayesian methods will also benefit from the efforts to develop probabilistic databases of functional organization. Figure 8 illustrates two approaches employed for the integration of MEG and fMRI data.

VII. TYPES OF EVENT-RELATED POTENTIALS

Model-based source localization, computational decomposition of complex responses, and quantitative estimates of the activation time courses of identified brain regions are all relatively new tools for the analysis of event-related neural electromagnetic data. However, 50 years of macroscopic electrophysiologi-

cal study of neurological, psychological, cognitive, and behavioral processes of the human brain have produced a rich legacy of experimental observations and interpretation. Many of these results are based on the analysis of features in the response waveform, often averaged across many sensor locations and sometimes across many individual subjects. A comprehensive summary of such results is well beyond the scope of this article. Excellent review articles and even entire volumes have been devoted to small corners of the field. We will briefly review some of the major classes of event-related responses that have been identified and characterized.

A. Evoked Responses

Evoked responses are elicited by sensory stimulation and are usually recovered by signal averaging time-locked to stimulus delivery. Response waveforms consist of a stereotypical series of peaks and valleys observed between 2 and 250 msec poststimulus. Such features reflect the sequential and parallel activation of multiple specialized processing waystations within the targeted sensory pathway, although individual response components may represent simultaneous activity in several distinct areas. The responses are a product of the network architecture and the dynamics of participating neurons and are reasonably robust. Sensory evoked activity can often be recorded even under anesthesia.

Evoked responses have been used to probe the architecture and the information processing activities of sensory systems. Such work has provided evidence for specialized processing modules, corresponding to the discrete areas identified through invasive physiology, and has disclosed systematic projection of the sensory parameter space onto cortex. Other studies have provided evidence for early modulation of sensory responses by selective attention and demonstrated dynamic plastic changes in the functional organization of cortex, based on patterns of sensory coactivation or neglect.

1. Somatosensory Evoked Responses

The somatosensory system can be activated through tactile stimulation of almost any body surface. Particularly robust responses can be elicited by electrical stimulation, for example, of the median nerve of the forearm. The earliest responses to somatosensory stimulation are observed from 9 to 15 msec poststimulus and represent responses generated in the spinal cord and brain stem. Initial responses in primary somatosensory cortex are observed around 20 msec poststimulus. An evolving complex of responses typically lasts over 150 msec. Source modeling studies identify at least 5–6 discrete regions of activation. Studies of the organization of the primary somatosensory area (S1) disclose a systematic projection of the body surface onto cortex adjacent to the central sulcus,

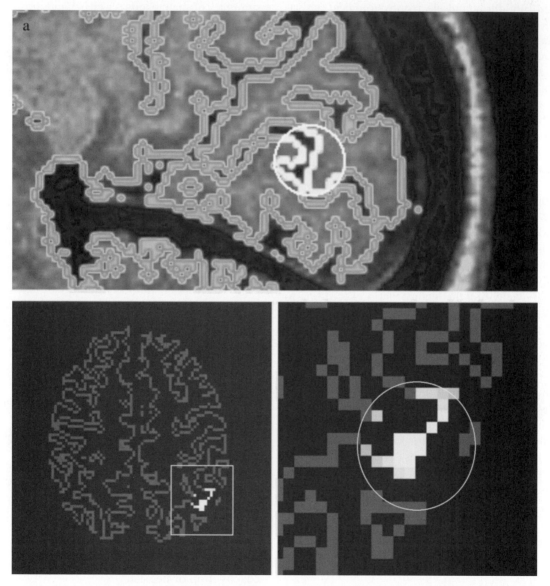

Figure 7 Analysis of MEG evoked responses by Bayesian inference. (a) Extended parametric source models used for Bayesian inference. Upper panel: A source defined by the intersection of cortex with a sphere centered on cortex. Note that adjacent sides of a sulcus or gyrus are often labeled together for extended sources. Lower panels: A source defined by a patch grown on the cortical surface. A location on cortex is seeded, and adjacent bands of voxels are labeled in a series of dilation operations. (b) A series of sample solutions from the posterior probability distribution. After 1000 iterations the MCMC algorithm found the same set of three sources in almost every sample, although additional extraneous sources also appear in some solutions. These data were simulated and thus known to contain three sources in the locations suggested by Bayesian inference. (c) Interactive visualization of spatial–temporal source probability maps coregistered with anatomical MRI for the same subject. The anatomical data set was used in the Bayesian inference procedure to constrain sources to lie in cortex. (d) Source probability maps estimated for visual evoked response data. Four views of a region found to contain activity at a 95% probability level. This example is for left visual field stimulation. For right field stimulation, the most probable source is lateralized to the calcarine fissure in the left hemisphere.

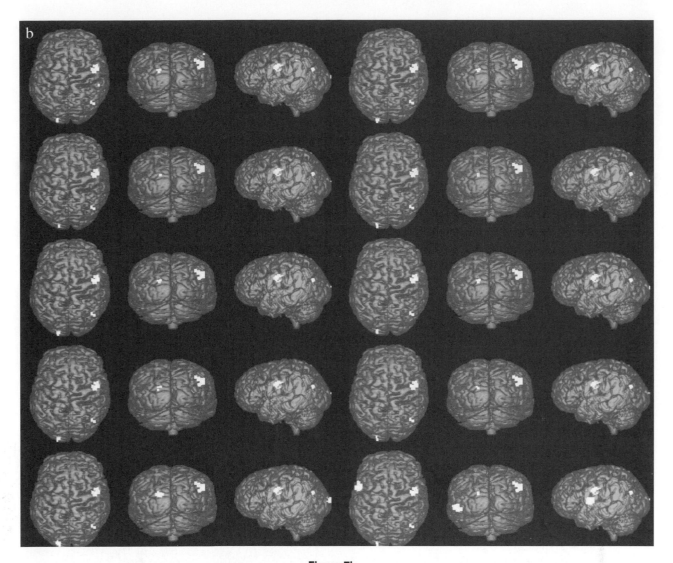

Figure 7b

generally consistent with the classic homunculus described by Penfield, based on intraoperative electrical stimulation.

2. Auditory Evoked Responses

Auditory evoked responses are typically elicited by clicks or tone bursts, which may be delivered to one or both ears. With appropriate electrode placement, it is possible to noninvasively measure electrical responses of the cochlea, including receptor potentials, and signals that reflect from neural encoding. From 1 to 12 msec poststimulus auditory brain stem responses can be measured. These responses consist of a series of mostly discrete waves labeled I–VII. Although the sources of these components are still a matter of some debate, there is general agreement that wave I is due to a compound action potential or graded dendritic potentials at the dictal (cochlear) end of the acoustic nerve. Waves III–V are generated in the brain stem. Waves V and VII are associated with higher brain stem structures—perhaps the medial geniculate body. Auditory brain stem responses are useful for hearing assessment in infants, uncooperative adults, and cases of functional deafness, as well as for evaluating brain stem function in suspected multiple sclerosis. The general temporal structure of auditory evoked responses is illustrated in Fig. 9.

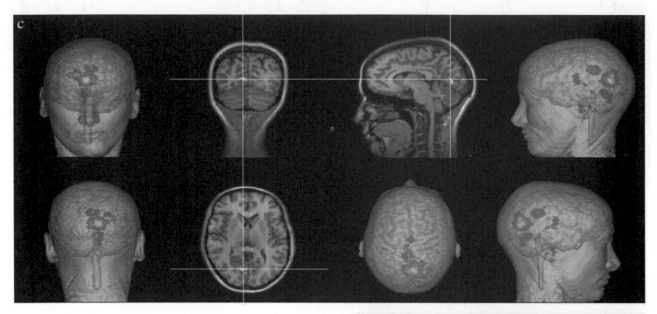

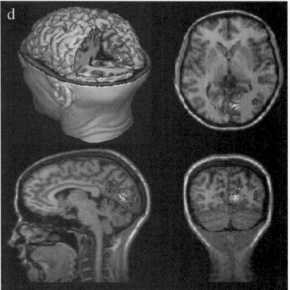

Figure 7c–d

Middle latency auditory evoked responses are typically observed from 12 to 50 msec poststimulus and are considered to represent subcortical activation.

Late auditory evoked responses (50 msec or more after the stimulus) are generally a product of neocortex. Such responses are best evoked by tone bursts and in EEG recordings show the highest amplitude over the vertex. MEG studies lave localized these responses to primary sensory areas along the Sylvian fissure and to nearby association areas. Such studies have also demonstrated clear tonotopic organization in primary cortical areas. With dipole localization techniques, very fine-grained discrimination of relative locations is possible. Auditory stimuli are often used for language studies, and in this role they may elicit an interesting array of endogenous responses that reflect the neural processing of language. However, at least one endogenous response appears purely acoustic: the mismatch negativity is observed when a repetitive auditory stimulus is briefly altered and may serve as an orienting response to cause a shift in the focus of attention.

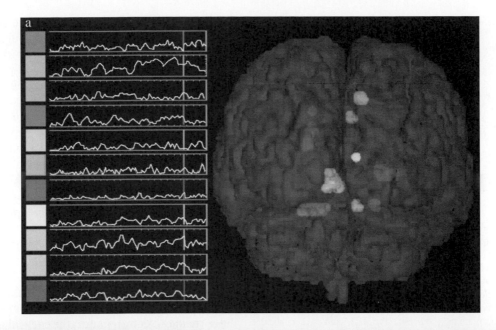

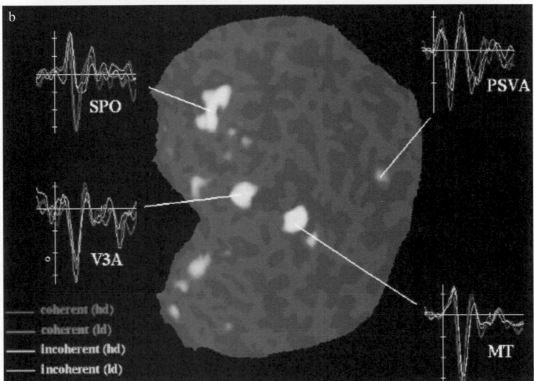

Figure 8   Integrated analysis of fMRI and MEG. (a) Time courses of fMRI equivalent sources estimated from MEG data. fMRI visual data were acquired using blocked steady-state stimulation, using the same video display from a previous MEG experiment. Currents were assumed to vary within the source according to the distribution of functional MRI activation. Currents were constrained to lie normal to cortex as indicated by anatomical MRI. Topographies were derived for each of the assumed sources and used as basis functions for a linear decomposition of the time-varying field maps. Estimated time courses for 11 areas are coded in color. (Figure courtesy of Dale *et al.*) (b) MEG time courses of fMRI sources using a weighted minimum norm procedure. Areas of activation from a visual fMRI experiment (involving visual motion) are shown on an unfolded cortex. A 0.9:0.1 weighted pseudo-inverse procedure was applied to field maps at each time point. Estimated time courses for activation in four identified visual areas are illustrated. Differences as a function of stimulus type are coded in color. (Figure courtesy of Dale *et al.*)

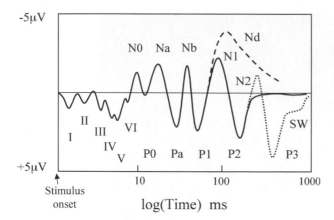

Figure 9 Component structure of the auditory event-related potential. The trace schematically represents the averaged evoked response of the auditory system to a brief stimulus such as a click or a tone. A logarithmic time scale allows visualization of the major response component peaks in a single trace. Components include auditory brain stem responses (I–VI), early positive (P) and negative (N) cortical components (Na, Nb, Pa, P1), and late cortical components (N1, P2). Other components that vary as a function of cognitive or attentive states are shown with dashed lines. (Figure courtesy of Hillyard and colleagues)

3. Visual Evoked Responses

In primates, the visual system is the largest and most distributed of the sensory modalities, consisting of over three dozen discrete areas and spanning at least one-third of the neocortical surface area. The system has been studied extensively with invasive electrophysiological techniques, as well as with MEG and EEG (and fMRI). The comparatively small signals and their dynamic complexity make this system a major challenge for sensory evoked response studies.

As in the auditory system, it is possible to measure the electrical response of the sensory organ—the eye. The electroretinogram (ERG) is typically measured using a contact lens electrode referred to a reference on the head surface. The response consists of receptor and neural components. Because the retina is a relatively accessible outpost of the brain, it has been the target of a number of studies of information processing by neural networks. In the future, optical techniques may allow noninvasive characterization of retinal network dynamics.

The visual evoked response observed with surface sensor arrays is dominated by primary cortical areas. The initial cortical activation in layer 4 of striate cortex probably occurs around 70–80 msec poststimulus, although this component is often small and difficult to detect. Other cortical responses are observed in striate

and nearby areas from 90 to 120 msec poststimulus, and evoked activity often lasts through 250 msec. Source localization studies have demonstrated the anticipated retinotopic organization of primary visual cortex as well as extrastriate areas. The visual field is systematically projected onto striate cortex, mostly buried in the fissure between the hemispheres along the calcarine fissure. The central field representation is found near the posterior pole of occipital cortex and may extend onto the posterior surface. The lower quadrants of the visual field are mapped onto the upper banks of the contralateral calcarine and interhemispheric fissure; the upper field projects to the lower banks, and the horizontal meridian projects to the depths of the calcarine in a scheme summarized by the cruciform model (due to its appearance in coronal section). Noninvasive studies have confirmed the outlines of this model, although individual departures appear common. Such studies also support the idea of the cortical projection factor: the cortical area devoted to a given size patch of the visual field systematically decreases from the center to the periphery of the visual field.

Noninvasive techniques so far have largely been used to confirm in humans results suggested by invasive studies in animals. Thus, a number of specialized areas have been identified in humans analogous to those identified in electrophysiological studies in nonhuman primates, including areas specialized for processing visual motion, color, texture, and even faces. The visual system appears to be organized into two major processing chains or streams. The dorsal stream, arrayed mainly across occipital cortex and the upper surface of the parietal lobe, operates in low contrast and is involved in processing visual motion. The system is probably involved in orientation and allocation of attention and may interact with motor control. The ventral stream flows along the base of the occipital and temporal cortices, and is involved in the processing of color, texture, and other detailed attributes of visual information. This system probably interacts with language processing centers. Some investigators have dubbed these streams the *what* and *where* systems.

B. Motor Control

The control of voluntary movement can also be studied with event-related response techniques. In a typical experiment, the subject is instructed to perform a series of self-paced voluntary movements, and the signal is averaged relative to the movement as registered by a button press or an electrical response recorded from muscle. The response appears as a slowly developing negative potential shift somatotopically arrayed along the central sulcus, starting approximately 1 sec before movement. This response is called *the readiness potential* and is taken as an index of motor preparation; the amplitude of the response is correlated with the complexity of the subsequent movement as well as the force and speed developed. The readiness potential preceding a lateralized response (such as a hand movement) is maximal over the contralateral hemisphere. Some investigators use signal subtraction techniques to remove the ipsilateral contribution to the signal. In addition to the readiness potential, other movement-related responses can be resolved, as well as somatosensory and proprioceptive feedback generated as a consequence of the movement.

C. Cognitive Event-Related Responses

The readiness potential is considered an *endogenous response* because no external (exogenous) stimulation is required to elicit it. Although motor cortex is certainly involved in responses that involve sensory processing, typical paradigms do not employ sensory cues because stimuli would elicit sensory evoked responses and trigger a set of cognitive processes that might complicate interpretation. Cognitive responses to assigned tasks involving search, discrimination, classification, or decision processes also have been studied extensively, often in the absence of any observable (behavioral) response.

1. CNV

Studies of the effects of classical conditioning led to the identification of the *contingent negative variation* (CNV), one of the first of the endogenous responses clearly linked to a cognitive process. In these experiments, an initial stimulus was delivered, followed by a delay and then a second stimulus. During the interval between the stimuli, a slowly growing negative potential was observed at the scalp. In many experiments the second stimulus was intended to cue a behavioral response, although a response is unnecessary and, as outlined above, would presumably elicit motor potentials that would complicate interpretation. Studies with variable intervals between the stimuli suggest that the CNV reflects at least two processes: an *orienting*

response (o-wave) associated with the initial (warning) stimulus and an *expectancy response* (e-wave) that develops in anticipation of the imperative stimulus.

2. P300

One of the most extensively studied cognitive event-related responses is the P300 (or P3) complex, sometimes referred to as the family of late positive responses. The form of this response is relatively independent of the sensory modality used to elicit it. The generic paradigm associated with the response is an oddball discrimination task: for example, two or more stimuli are presented in a random series so that one occurs infrequently. This oddball elicits a response that begins around 300 msec poststimulus and may last 100 msec or more. Since the initial reports, the response has been resolved into at least two components that are differentiated on the basis of scalp topography and sensitivity to paradigm manipulation. The P3A is larger in amplitude over the central and frontal electrode sites. The response may be an alerting response arising in frontal cortex; in any case it is the component most strongly associated with the oddball response. The P3B appears to reflect subsequent allocation of attentional resources and encoding of stimulus memory. Some authors have argued that the response reflects information transfer via the corpus callosum with subsequent activation of hippocampal and parietal processes.

3. Selective Attention

The processing of information from the environment can be effectively suppressed or significantly enhanced depending on the state of attention. Event-related responses have been used extensively to study the time course and anatomical basis of *selective attention* in the human brain. Such experiments are typically conducted with contingencies that are manipulated within or between blocks of stimuli, so that the same physical stimulus may be the target of a discrimination task, may share some features with the target, or may be irrelevant. Data are typically analyzed by taking differences between responses to the same stimuli that differ in assigned task. The so-called negative difference or processing negativity is constructed by subtracting the response to an unattended stimulus from the response to the same stimulus while attended. In focused auditory attention, this effect may be observed as early as 20 msec poststimulus and is most apparent around the latency of the N1; however, the time course does not reflect a simple scaling of the N1.

In visual evoked responses, tasks involving spatial selective attention, spatial cueing, or visual search produce enhanced P1 and N1 components, although controversy remains regarding whether the sources of the difference component are the same as for the underlying evoked response component. Visual selection on the basis of features such as shape, texture, or color elicits a difference signal termed the selection negativity and is observed from 150 to 250 msec poststimulus with a maximum over posterior electrodes. Taken together, these observations suggest that attention to location in the visual field is an early process, perhaps mediated by facilitation and/or suppression in prestriate relays such as the thalamus. Attention to other features or conjunction of features probably is mediated by specialized visual areas further along the processing chain.

4. ERN

In discrimination trials in which a fast choice is enforced by a reaction time task, an *error-related negativity* (ERN) is observed in trials in which the wrong response is performed. This response, predominantly observed over midline frontal areas, appears to reflect a process of rechecking that is initiated in parallel with the response. In many cases the ERN appears before the behavioral response; presumably when the response is optimized for speed, the motor system is committed before the decision–recheck cycle is complete.

5. Language-Related Responses

Event-related potential studies have been used to identify a number of responses associated with language processing. Word stimuli presented in spoken or written form elicit a response peaking around 280 msec (N280 or *lexical processing negativity*) typically characterized by a negative peak over left frontal regions of the scalp. This is considered to be a generic correlate of word processing, though in an experimental context the latency can be manipulated as a function of the frequency of the word. Another prominent response is elicited by semantic incongruity in written text or speech. The N400 is a right posterior scalp negativity the begins around 200 msec and peaks around 400 msec following the presentation of a word that violates semantic expectation. Because the response is associated with meaning and context, the N400 is considered an index of higher order language processing. A

number of response components have been associated with processing of the form and structure of language. The *syntactic positive shift* (P600) is a late positive response elicited by certain types of grammatical errors (such as subject–verb agreement), even though the meaning of such a sentence may be clear. Figure 10 illustrates an example of a language-related ERP.

6. ERS–ERD

Event-related or evoked responses are generally considered to reflect transient, discrete processes associated with responses to external stimuli or internal imperatives. The time courses of many event-related response components look suggestively like the postsynaptic potentials that are recorded directly from neural tissue, perhaps reinforced by population activation and broadened by timing jitter. However, in some cases the response of neural populations appears to reflect a reorganization of ongoing activity; either an increase in synchronized oscillatory activity (*event-related synchronization*) or a decrease (*event-related desynchronization*). Although most authors consider these to be distinct phenomena, others have argued that all event-related responses might reflect transient phase locking of spontaneous activity. For example, the waveforms associated with some auditory evoked responses look like a damped oscillation. Perhaps the most interesting responses of this class are transient oscillatory population responses that may reflect phase locking within a network. Such processes are not phase-locked with respect to the stimulus and appear to reflect detection or "binding" of features such as coherent motion or a shared contour that may extend well beyond the receptive field of any individual neuron.

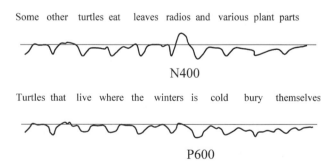

Figure 10 ERP effects elicited during language processing. Average ERP data from written sentences read one word at a time for comprehension. Upper trace: An N400 elicited by semantic violation. Lower trace: P600 elicited by grammatical violation. (Figure courtesy of Kutas and Dale.)

VIII. APPLICATIONS

A great deal of scientific effort has been devoted to the study of event-related neural responses: characterizing the spatial distribution and temporal structure of responses, probing the underlying physiology and biophysics, dissecting the consequences of cognitive and behavioral manipulations, and developing the analytical techniques and computational tools that allow more powerful inferences based on such measures. Event-related and evoked responses have recognized utility for a variety of applications in clinical and basic research.

A principal clinical application of evoked responses has been *for assessment of the patency of sensory information processing pathways.* Measurements of the ABR and early VEP have been used as objective diagnostics for the integrity and proper development of the auditory and visual pathways in infancy and childhood. The latency of the VEP has been used for the assessment of multiple sclerosis. Demyelination associated with this progressive degenerative disorder causes decreases in conduction velocity apparent as increases in the latency of cortical response components. Endogenous response components such as the P300 have been used as a generic probe of psychological and cognitive processes in disorders ranging from schizophrenia to Alzheimer's to alcoholism. In many cases the link between the diagnostic measure and the underlying pathology is tenuous, but statistical differences between normal and affected individuals can be observed.

The development of source localization techniques has led to applications for *presurgical mapping of eloquent cortex.* When neurosurgeons need to resect portions of brain tissue to remove a tumor or an epileptic focus, a principal requirement is that they spare the cortical tissue responsible for language and movement. Otherwise the pathology is often considered inoperable, even if life-threatening. The deleterious consequences for quality of life are considered too severe. MEG has been used to map the cortical regions responsible for these functions, in some cases even when the anatomical substrate has been distorted or displaced by the disease process. Such studies are typically undertaken as part of the process leading to a commitment to surgery; the conclusions are typically confirmed by conventional procedures during surgery. Because the questions are fundamentally issues of static functional architecture, fMRI is increasingly used for such purposes.

NEM techniques have clear advantages for *presurgical mapping of certain cortical pathology.* Disorders such as epilepsy are fundamentally disorders of dynamic neural function. Although the generator region is sometimes associated with an obvious lesion, sometimes the area appears normal on anatomical MRI. Typically, patterns of seizure and other epileptiform activity are first studied with EEG. MEG is used if available in an attempt to better localize the initial focus of the time-evolving response. In present practice, localization is usually confirmed by grids of electrodes placed over the surface of cortex or depth electrodes inserted in key locations. Many physicians believe that source localization based on noninvasive methods will eventually be accurate and reliable enough for surgical decisions.

Seizures can be triggered in some individuals, often children, by stroboscopic visual stimulation, providing a useful measure of experimental control. However, most epileptic seizures are not scheduled and may be relatively infrequent. Capture of an ictal event during an experimental session is, to some extent, a matter of chance. For practical reasons, many clinical researchers have studied interictal activity. Such studies suggest that interictal activity often arises at or near the locations that can trigger a seizure. Other researchers have noted a strong correlation between computed sources of slow waves with the margins of lesions that give rise to seizures. Slow waves are also associated with regions of closed head trauma. Abnormal low-frequency activity is sometimes seen in such cases even when the tissue appears normal in MRI and no significant cognitive or behavioral deficits can be detected.

NEM measures and event-related response methods have been used for other applications in *physiological and behavioral research.* EEG has been used extensively in human factors studies, for example, to assess the effects of workload, stress, and sustained effort on intellectual performance and attention. Although many of these studies have employed correlation or coherence analysis of ongoing EEG activity, others have employed sensory or cognitive probe tasks to assess neurological performance. Several investigators have explored the use of EEG to generate control signals for electromechanical systems. Prosthetic devices for amputees have been built with electronic control systems, although to date the most successful have employed control signals derived from remnant muscle. Proof of principle has been demonstrated for the use of EEG for the control of vehicles or mobility aids for patients with little or no voluntary control of muscle function.

Basic neuroscience and cognitive research have become major applications of event-related neural response techniques. The advent of neural electromagnetic source modeling techniques has allowed localization of specialized sensory processing areas and disclosed interesting aspects of functional organization within areas. Such methods have disclosed evidence for neural plasticity in the form of use-dependent changes in the strength and extent of activation associated with stimulation. The greatest value of electromagnetic techniques is likely to come in studies of the dynamics of neural information processing within and between areas. To date, such studies have been largely qualitative and observational. However, by coupling the physical models used for electromagnetic source localization with computational neural network models, it should be possible to predict integrated responses of complex networks from the interaction dynamics of populations of model neurons. Such methods will allow us to frame and answer questions about the role of dynamic, spatio-temporal processes in the encoding and processing of information by neural systems.

See Also the Following Articles

ELECTRICAL POTENTIALS • ELECTROENCEPHALO-GRAPHY (EEG) • INFORMATION PROCESSING • MAGNETIC RESONANCE IMAGING (MRI) • NEURAL NETWORKS • NEURON

Suggested Reading

Dale, A. M., and Sereno, M. I. (1993). Improved localization of cortical activity by combining MEG and EEG with MRI cortical surface reconstruction: a linear approach. *J. Cogn. Neurosci.* **5**(2), 162–176.

George, J. S., Aine, C. J., Mosher, J. C., Ranken, D. M., Schlitt, H. A., Wood, C. C., Lewine, J. D., Sanders, J. A., and Belliveau, J. W. (1995). Mapping function in the human brain with MEG, anatomical MRI, and functional MRI. *J. Clin. Neurophysiol.* **12**(5), 406–431.

Hamalainen, M. S., Hari, R., Ilmoniemi, R. J., Knuutila, J., and Lounasmaa, O. V. (1993). Magnetoencephalography—Theory, instrumentation and applications to noninvasive studies of the working human brain. *Rev. Mod. Phys.* **65**(2), 413–497.

Hillyard, S. A., Mangun, G. R., Woldorf, M. G., and Luck, S. J. (1995). Neural systems mediating selective attention. In *The Cognitive Neurosciences* (M. S. Gazzaniga, *et al.*, Eds.), pp. 665–681. MIT Press, Cambridge, MA.

Kutas, M., and Dale, A. (1997). Electrical and magnetic readings of neural function. In *Cognitive Neuroscience* (M. D. Rugg, Ed.), pp. 197–242. MIT Press, Cambridge, MA.

Naatenen, R. (1990). The role of attention in auditory information processing as revealed by event-related potentials and other brain measures of cognitive function. *Behav. Brain Sci.* **13**(2), 201–232.

Niedermeyer, E., and Lopes da Silva, F. (1999). *Electroencephalography: Basic Principles, Clinical Applications and Related Fields.* Williams and Wilkins, Baltimore, MD.

Regan, D. (1989). *Human Brain Electrophysiology: Evoked Potentials and Evoked Magnetic Fields in Science and Medicine.* Elsevier, New York.

Schmidt, D. M., George, J. S., and Wood, C. C. (1999). Bayesian inference applied to the electromagnetic inverse problem. *Human Brain Mapping* **7**, 195–212.

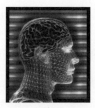

Evolution of the Brain

HARRY J. JERISON

University of California, Los Angeles

GLOSSARY

allometry Measured comparisons of two organs or organ-systems. In brain-body allometry, usually the regression of brain size on body size. Size is scaled logarithmically, and the allometric equation is usually a power function.

encephalization The degree to which actual brain size in a species is greater or less than that expected according to an allometric analysis. It is often measured as an "encephalization quotient" (EQ), which is the residual of the regression of log brain size on log body size.

neocortex A characteristically layered portion of the cerebral cortex unique to mammals, usually six-layered.

There are about 50,000 species of vertebrates, each unique in many traits but sharing "primitive" traits with close and distant relatives. The pattern of unique traits defines each species, and the suite of shared (older, more primitive) traits, depending on the size of the suite, helps define them as members of a higher taxon:

genus, family, etc. This is as true for neural traits as it is for other traits that differentiate animal species. All biologists accept the evolutionary dogma that the uniformities in traits across species are due either to common ancestry or to convergent evolution, and that the diversity of species should usually be explained by adaptations to specialized environmental niches.

I. GENERAL CONSIDERATIONS

This article emphasizes inferences from allometric analysis of brain/body relations and encephalization, the latter being a complex trait often attributable to convergent evolution. Although the diversity in organization of brains is at least as important, especially for understanding the phylogenetic trees, an adequate discussion of the evolution of diversified brain organization requires a more detailed review of comparative anatomy and physiology than is possible in a single article, and the conclusions, though important, are easily summarized for evolutionary neurobiology: Brain structure is appropriate to function, and specialized functions are appropriate to the environment (i.e., structure and function are adaptive). In short, the results are consistent with adaptation as a biological principle. Applied to the sizes (weight, volume, or surface area) of the subsystems in the brain, such as cortical projection areas and thalamic nuclei, this is the principle of proper mass.

Despite their simplicity, allometry and encephalization provide more unusual evolutionary insights. Allometry helps us understand the biological role of size; encephalization does the same for understanding neural information-processing capacity and its evolution. It will be enough to review the diversity of

---

This article is updated from one originally published in D. W. Zaidel, (Ed.), *Neuropsychology*. Academic Press, New York. (1994). For those with access to the Internet, an unusual collection of data is available for inspection and analysis at a site supported by the U.S. National Science Foundation, including photographs of brains and serial sections of brains in many living species of mammals. Fossil evidence is displayed at the same site and may be accessed at http://www.neurophys.wisc.edu/brain/paleoneurology.html.

organization by citing a few examples, the reports of which are extremely well documented.

The issues considered in this article are also relevant for the evolution of invertebrate nervous systems. The neuron, for example, probably appeared as a specialized cell early in metazoan evolution, more than 600 million years ago (Ma), and many of its features are identical in all instances in which it functions in a synaptic nervous system. This is evidently true for small networks of neurons as well as for isolated cells. Much of what is known about neural functions as single units and in small networks was learned from giant neurons of horseshoe crabs and from networks of cells in sea slugs and roundworms. The early appearance of the adaptation is deduced from a cladistic analysis of the time of divergence of species in which it is identifiable. It is most likely that the adaptation first appeared in a pre-Cambrian metazoan species that is the "common ancestor" of all the living species that share the adaptation. From an evolutionist's perspective, however, very complex behavior requiring integrated neural activity and involving more extensive neural circuitry that is common to vertebrates and invertebrates is as likely to be analogous ("homoplastic") rather than homologous. It may have evolved in independent evolutionary paths in the vertebrate and invertebrate groups in which it occurs.

A. Brain Structure and Function

Every vertebrate brain is hierarchically organized into forebrain, midbrain or mesencephalon, and hindbrain. The forebrain can be further divided into telencephalon and diencephalon, and hindbrain can be divided into rhombencephalon and myelencephalon. Brain tissue in all animals consists of neurons as information processing units and glia and other cells that are, in effect, supporting tissue. Neurons are often specialized with respect to neurotransmitters, shape, and size. Sizes, for example, range from the granule cells of the cerebellum (soma less than 10-μm diameter) to the giant Mauthner cells (soma about 100-μm diameter) that mediate startle responses in fish and in amphibian tadpoles. The full size of a nerve cell includes the arborization of axon and dendrites, which may account for 95% or more of the volume of a neuron and which varies enormously in pattern both within a brain and between species.

Underlying this diversity, there is surprising uniformity about principles of nerve action in the transmission of information, which makes it possible to use almost any neuron from any species as a model for neuronal action. There is, furthermore, a uniformity at the level of networks of cells in vertebrate brains, evident even in the neocortex in mammals, which encourages one to emphasize information-processing capacity for the brain as a whole as well as in its specialized component systems, such as those for color vision, binocular vision, sound localization, and olfaction.

B. Evolution

The facts of evolution are first, that it occurred and second, that it could occur because of the genotypic and phenotypic diversity both within species and between species. Charles Darwin's great contributions were to recognize the diversity and to explain it by the theory of natural selection. As currently understood, the theory is that given the variety of phenotypes in a species, some individuals will be more successful than others in surviving to produce offspring. Reproduction is the measure of success. The mean of the gene pool of the next generation shifts toward the mean of the successful phenotype. As the environment changes, the characteristics required to be successful change, and there is natural selection of individuals with those characteristics. This is a theory of the origin of species because there will eventually be enough change in the genotypic population to designate it as a new species.

There is so much support for the theory, in laboratory experiments and from field observations, that one might prefer a stronger word than "theory" to describe Darwin's integration. But there are disagreements among evolutionists, of course, which are sometimes taken incorrectly to be challenges to the credibility of the theory as a whole. The controversies are mainly about the relative importance of selection as opposed to random genetic drift, about the merits of various approaches to determining phylogenetic trees (cladistics), and about the rate of evolutionary change (gradualism versus punctuated equilibria). Despite their use and misuse in popular polemics, the controversies are on fairly technical questions and not on the fact of evolution.

II. THE EVIDENCE

A. Fossil Brains

The fossil record of the brain is from casts ("endocasts") that are molded by the cranial cavity of fossil skulls. Natural endocasts are made by the replacement of soft tissue in the skull by sand and other debris that eventually fossilizes. Artificial endocasts can be made by cleaning the cavity and filling it with a molding compound such as latex, from which plaster casts can be made. Errors in identifying "brain" areas in endocasts of birds and mammals are likely to be about the same as in brains when superficial markings rather than histological or physiological evidence are the basis for the identification. Endocasts of some fossil animals are so brainlike in appearance (Fig. 1) that they are often referred to as fossil brains.

Figure 1 presents lateral views of the endocast and brain from the same domestic cat, *Felis catus* (Figs. 1A and 1B), and a copy of a natural endocast from a fossil sabretooth (Fig. 1C). The sabretooth is *Hoplophoneus primaevus*, which lived in the South Dakota Badlands during the Oligocene epoch of the Tertiary Period, about 30 Ma. Although no more than a piece of rock, its endocast is unmistakably a picture of its brain as it was in life; it was clearly appropriate to name its parts as brain areas in Fig. 1D following the nomenclature for cat brains.

There are several lessons to be learned from Fig. 1. First, an endocast can provide an excellent picture of the whole brain. This is evident when comparing Fig. 1A with Fig. 1B: The endocast of the domestic cat provides an excellent picture of external features of its brain and correctly estimates its size. (The estimation from the endocast is as "correct" as that from the brain, which is probably slightly shrunken by fixation.) Second, the convolutional pattern in an endocast may be fairly constant in related species. Thus, despite their separation by 30 million years of felid evolution, the endocasts of the living cat and of the sabretooth (Figs. 1A and 1C) are clearly similar. This lesson is especially important because convolutions map the way a brain is organized, at least in a general way. A third lesson, therefore, is that the felid brain of 30 Ma was probably organized in a way similar to that of living felids. Finally, as counterpoint to the lesson of uniformity of organization, there is a lesson of diversity: Two gyri, the coronal and sigmoid gyral complexes, are differentiated in living domestic cats but are undifferentiated in the sabretooth. Increases such as these in the apparent complexity of the brain in felid evolution may be related to increases in information processing in the expanded areas in later species compared to earlier species.

The quality of an endocast as a model of the brain differs in different taxa. Endocasts from fish, amphibians, and reptiles (except in very small specimens) are poor models, useful mainly to estimate total brain size after suitable corrections, because the brain fills only a

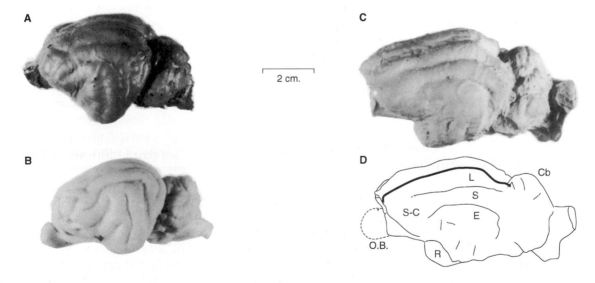

Figure 1 Brain and endocasts of felids. (A) Endocast of domestic cat (volume = 30 ml). (B) Brain of same cat (weight = 29.1 g). (C) Endocast of Oligocene sabretooth, *Hoplophoneus primaevus*, of 30 million years ago (volume = 50 ml; Specimen No. USNM 22538 at the United States National Museum, Smithsonian Institution). (D) Tracing of the endocast of Hoplophoneus with labels for several structures: Cb, cerebellum; E, ectosylvian gyrus; L, lateral gyrus; R, rhinal fissure; S, suprasylvian gyrus; S-C, sigmoid and coronal gyral complex (undifferentiated). Both endocasts are rotated about the anterior–posterior axis, exposing the longitudinal fissure (heavily inked in D). Olfactory bulbs (OB) are sketched in on the basis of more complete endocasts (e.g., AMNH 460 at the American Museum of Natural History). The unlabeled gyrus above the lateral gyrus is the lateral gyrus of the right hemisphere.

fraction of the cranial cavity. In mammals and birds, on the other hand, the brain actually helps shape the cranial cavity during development, and endocasts are usually excellent pictures of the outside of the brain. Olfactory bulbs, forebrain, and hindbrain are readily identifiable, as are most of the cortical gyri and sulci that are seen when a brain is first removed from the skull. Certain large-brained living mammals—namely, cetaceans, elephants, great apes, and humans—are exceptions to this rule, with little or no impression of their convolutions on their endocasts; even the boundary between cerebrum and cerebellum may be unclear.

Fossils provide other information for understanding brain evolution and for extrapolations to behavior. Body size, for example, estimated from postcranial skeletal data, is used to analyze encephalization of fossil vertebrates. Details of structure, such as the shape of teeth, forelimbs, and hindlimbs, can enable one to analyze feeding habits, gait, and other behavior. There is even fossil evidence on social behavior, for example, in dinosaurs, which has been reconstructed from the aggregation of fossils, their eggs, and their foot and tail prints. Perhaps most important for an analysis of brain evolution, there is a fossil record of sensory structures that is useful in reconstructing the information available to fossil animals. Olfactory bulbs, of course, are visible on the endocast, and their size is related to the evolution of the sense of smell. There are fossil middle ear bones and cochlea important for the analysis of the evolution of hearing; the orientation of the orbits of the eye provides evidence on the evolution of binocular vision, and the placement of the hyoid bones on fossil humans has been the basis for speculations on the evolution of the voice box and of articulated speech.

B. The Living Brain

Most of the evolutionary evidence on living brains is from anatomical and physiological studies of brain tracts and regions compared for unique and common features across species. There is growing interest in molecular evidence (e.g., on neurotransmitters), and one can anticipate increasing emphasis on that kind of information.

Braitenberg and Schüz have published a straightforward anatomical monograph, noteworthy for the quantitative analyses of the cerebral cortex of the mouse. Though not specifically concerned with evolutionary issues, they provided exemplars of data

necessary for an evolutionary analysis. The most striking facts are on the amount of information processing machinery in the mouse, with some suggestions on the human brain. There are about 40,000,000 neurons in the 0.5-g brain of a mouse; more astonishing, there are about 80,000,000,000 synapses in its neocortex. Taking into account the packing density of neurons and synapses, they reached the conclusion that a particular volume of cortex processes the same amount of information, whether it is in a mouse or a man. This is an outstanding uniformity for evolutionary analysis since it validates the use of brain size as a "statistic" to estimate the total information processing capacity of a brain.

Uniformity is balanced by diversity. All species differ in the details of the organization of the component systems of their brains. The raccoons and their relatives (family Procyonidae) provide an outstanding example reported by W.I. Welker. The fish-handling raccoon has a much enlarged forepaw projection area in its somatosensory neocortex, with separate representation in the brain for each of the pads on the forepaw. The coati mundi, kinkajou, and most other procyonids obtain this kind of information by nosing about, exploring their environment by touching things with the sensory skin around the nostrils. Their neocortical projections from that region are comparably expanded and their forepaw projection areas are much less extensive and not as differentiated as in the raccoon. The conclusion is inescapable that reorganization of the brain, like the differentiation of the behavior that it controls, occurred as part of the speciation of procyonids as they evolved, and that raccoons branched away from the main line by their specialized adaptations in their use of forepaws. Data like these can be used for formal cladistic analyses. The mammalian phylogeny constructed from brain features is essentially the same as that based on a more complete suite of traits.

I depend on the comparative quantitative data laboriously accumulated by Stephan and his colleagues on the volumes of many brain structures in "primitive" species represented by insectivores and their relatives and in "advanced" species (primates) for many of my analyses of allometry and encephalization. Theirs are the most complete data of this sort currently available. In their sample of 76 species, there were 26 from the order Insectivora (shrews, moles, and hedgehogs), 2 Macroscelididae (elephant shrews), 3 Scandentia (tree shrews), and 45 primates, of which 18 are from the suborder Prosimii (lemur-like species) and 27 from the suborder Anthropoidea (simian species, including humans). The brain structures are listed in Table I. These data are especially useful because of the large number of species that are in the sample and the good sample of brain structures on which measurements were taken.

III. QUALITATIVE ANALYSIS

There have been a number of outstanding evolutionary analyses of classic issues in neurobiology, and I describe three of these very briefly to suggest the topics and flavor: those by Ebbesson, by Karten, and by Killackey (complete citations for this discussion are in the chapter referred to in footnote on first page). Ebbesson provided a superb case history on the difficulties in interpreting and reasoning from available anatomical data on the brain. Ebbesson argued that connections are created by a process of "parcellation (segregation–isolation)" that occurs ontogenetically as well as phylogenetically, with originally diffuse and extravagantly proliferating neurons and connections eventually becoming reduced and segregated from one another during the course of development. Northcutt's commentary was noteworthy, pointing out not only the problems with the data used to support the position but also the semantic and philosophical difficulties: the need for rigorous specification of homologies and homoplasies in using comparative data for cladistic analysis.

Karten analyzed the origin of neocortex as a "uniquely" mammalian brain system, pointing out that neocortex is not functionally unique since its connections are comparable to those of the "neostriatum" in birds (and even in reptiles). The enlarged neostriatum in birds is homologous with mammalian neocortex. His microscopic analysis of these forebrain systems points to their comparability with respect to information processing, despite the very different ways that the brain is organized in these classes of vertebrates. This is in agreement with data that show birds and mammals to be comparable in "grade" of encephalization.

Killackey argued from ontogenetic data on the sequence of appearance of various neocortical regions, making the important point for evolutionists that the detailed organization of the neocortex is established to a significant extent by experience, and the evolution of its organization is therefore likely to be difficult to specify with standard genetic models.

Although informed by modern evolutionary theory, with the exception of Northcutt's commentary the discussion that I just reviewed was traditional in its evolutionary approach. The concern was to develop insight into the origin of neural systems and to the degree of specialization in different species. The analysis proceeded from data on morphology and development, and from educated intuition rather than from the rigorous application of cladistic methodology. All would agree that the nervous system parallels other systems in the body in reflecting adaptations to various environmental niches. Killackey and Ebbesson emphasized the lability of the fate of neural structures, and there is a consensus about the significant extent to which use determines fate for the circuitry of the brain—that brains can be normal only if they develop in a normal environment.

Comparative brain data have also been used for more formal analyses of relationships, either with the methods of modern cladistics or with other multivariate methods. The results of these analyses can be summarized in a few sentences. Performing a factor analysis on brain traits in fish helps to clarify issues on the classification of particular groups of fish. The most helpful traits were the size of the olfactory apparatus. The contribution, however, is primarily to taxonomic issues rather than to neurobiology. The cladistic analyses, using only data on brain traits in constructing a species-by-traits matrix, produce essentially the same phylogenetic tree as when a full suite of traits is used. The diversity of species as determined rigorously by a full suite of traits predicts the measured diversity as determined from brain traits. The similarity between *Hoplophoneus* and *F. catus* in Fig. 1 is the expected finding in any comparative analysis of mammalian brains and confirms the taxonomic conclusion that these are relatively closely related species despite their separation by 30 million years of evolution. The brain can serve as well as other organs of the body for evidence on phylogenetic relationships.

IV. QUANTITATIVE ANALYSIS: LIVING VERTEBRATES

Darwin's theory of natural selection emphasized evidence of selection as practiced by animal and plant breeders. The term natural selection implied that nature, like breeders, worked to select the "most fit" individuals relative to some criterion. In a breeder's case, the criterion might be plumpness, large size, docility, and so forth. Nature had other criteria, and animals well endowed on nature's criteria would be more likely to survive to produce more offspring than would less well-endowed animals. The unnatural docility of domestic animals suggested some deficit in their brains.

Darwin could explore the relationship by comparing brain size in wild and domesticated populations of animals known to be related to one another. In what was probably his only contribution to neurobiology, Darwin was the first to observe that the brain in domesticated rabbits was smaller than that in their wild cousins. This is evidently a general principle on the effect of domestication on brain size. It may even be true for human brain evolution if we think of ourselves as domesticated and our ancestors as savage or feral, although the available sample size is too small for a clear test. The earliest *Homo sapiens* were the neandertals, and they were slightly larger brained, on average, compared to their living conspecifics.

A. Uniformities in Structure in Living Brains: Allometry

Darwin's publications inspired several generations of comparative neuroanatomists to provide detailed pictures of the diversity of brains. The effort included studies of brain size and of brain-body relations, some of which stand up under appropriate analysis today. In this tradition, Brodmann tabulated data on brain surface area in mammals, and his results are included as 33 of the 50 data points in Fig. 2A. The validity of his

work is attested to by its consistency with data from more recent studies that used different methods of measurement. A single regression line fits the entire data set remarkably well. Both Fig. 2A and Fig. 2B are examples of uniformities of organization of the brain in mammals.

Analyses such as those in Fig. 2 are "allometric" in that they display the relationship between different morphological features, such as height and weight, as they can be measured in any animal. The relationships displayed in Fig. 2 transcend species and are so strong that they appear to reflect a fundamental feature of the body plan (*Bauplan*) of mammals. Evolutionists call shared ancestral features plesiomorphies, and although the term is not usually applied to functional relationships such as those shown in Fig. 2, the idea fits. The relationships should be thought of as representing a primitive feature in mammalian evolution.

Because of its unusually diverse sample of species, Fig. 2A provides important justification for using total brain size as a statistic that estimates the total neural information processing capacity of a brain, between species, in the mammals as a class. To understand this further, consider some candidates for the role of processing unit. A frequent candidate is the cortical column, and its cross sectional area appears to be relatively uniform across species. The neuron is another candidate, and the number of neurons under a given surface area of neocortex is more or less constant across species. Finally, the synapse is a candidate. Braitenberg and Schüz observed that the number of synapses per unit volume of cortical tissue is

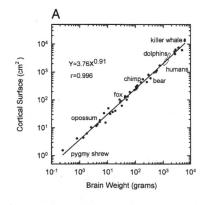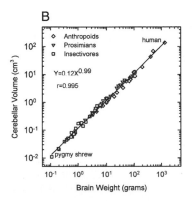

Figure 2 (A) Cortical surface area as a function of brain size in 50 species of mammals, including orders Monotremata, Marsupialia, Artiodactyla, Carnivora (including pinnipeds), Cetacea, Perissodactyla, Primates, and Xenarthra. Minimum convex polygons enclose individual human (*n* = 20) and dolphin (*Tursiops truncatus*: *n* = 13) data and indicate within-species variability. Some species are named to suggest the diversity of the sample. (B) Cerebellar volume as a function of brain size in 76 species of mammals (insectivores: 26 Insectivora, 2 Macroscelididae, and 3 Scandentia; primates: 18 Prosimii, 27 Anthropoidea (redrawn with permission from Jerison, 1991).

constant across species. There are qualifications to these generalizations, but they are reasonable first approximations. They reinforce the conclusion about the use of brain size as a statistic.

Figure 2B is another allometric analysis. It demonstrates the uniformity of cerebellar size in mammals—that, independent of species, if you know the size of the brain you can make a very good estimation of the size of the cerebellum. Although this analysis does not have the obvious theoretical significance of Fig. 2A, it demonstrates the fundamental orderliness of the construction of the brain. It validates the use of brain size as a statistic to estimate the size of other brain structures. To the extent that these other structures can be assigned special functional significance, one may be able to use quantitative data on brain size to assess the evolution of brain functions. This has been done by M.A. Hofman and by me for the analysis of the control of social behavior and of other neocortical functions. In general, anatomists emphasize the differences among the species that they examine, but I have been even more impressed by the uniformities. The example in Fig. 2B of the relationship between cerebellum and brain size is just one of these. Table I summarizes a multivariate analysis of an entire data set: 12 morphological measures in 76 species.

The most important fact in Table I is that just two factors were enough to account for all but 1.5% of the variance, and that 86% of the variance is explained by a single "size" factor. The size factor is a "general" factor in the sense that it is strongly represented in all the brain structures with the exception of the olfactory bulbs, and it is also represented in body weight. The loading of cerebellum on this factor (0.983, accounting for 97% of the variance in cerebellar volume) in conjunction with the even higher loading of total brain weight reflect the high correlation shown in Fig. 2B. All the measures with higher loadings would have produced bivariate graphs such as Fig. 2B. The mammalian brain hangs together well, and when one part is enlarged the rest of the brain tends to be correspondingly enlarged.

Perhaps the most surprising extension of this conclusion is the tentative discovery that even the size of prefrontal neocortex, the "executive organ" of the mammalian brain, appears to be determined by the size of the whole brain in mammals. The conclusion is tentative because it is based on evidence from only four primate species (marmoset, rhesus, orang, and human) and the laboratory rat, but there was an almost perfect correlation between neocortex volume and brain

Table I

Factor Loadings and Percentage Variance Explained by Two Principal Components (Factors) in Brain and Body in 76 Species of Mammals[a]

	Factor 1 (general brain size)	Factor 2 (olfactory bulbs)
Neocortex	0.991	0.059
Total brain weight	0.989	0.137
Diencephalon	0.987	0.144
Basal ganglia	0.987	0.133
Cerebellum	0.983	0.168
Mesencephalon	0.972	0.196
Medulla	0.966	0.224
Hippocampus	0.962	0.239
Schizocortex	0.954	0.274
Body weight	0.939	0.285
Piriform lobe	0.899	0.399
Olfactory bulbs	0.157	0.985
Percentage total variance	85.855	12.668

[a]Varimax rotation. Reproduced with permission from Jerison (1991).

volume in these five species (logarithmic measures; $r = 0.999$). Developmental and morphological evidence obtained by B.L. Finlay and her associates, essentially supporting the conclusions of the factor analysis, has resulted in much more extensive additional evidence for the fundamental uniformity of structure in the mammalian brain, that is, for the extent to which it "hangs together."

The second factor in Table I, accounting for 12.7% of the variance, is an olfactory bulb factor. It is represented primarily by the olfactory bulbs, with a modest representation in the parts of the brain that are classic "rhinencephalon" (piriform lobes, schizocortex, and hippocampus) and in body weight. Factor analyses are notoriously susceptible to artifacts of sampling, and I believe that the high fraction of variance accounted for by the olfactory bulb factor is such an artifact. Simian primates have much reduced olfactory bulbs, whereas insectivores are normal mammals in this regard. The distribution of olfactory bulb size in the sample on which the factor analysis was performed is, therefore, seriously bimodal. This inflates the measured variance of the size of the olfactory bulbs and enlarges its fraction of the total variance compared to what would be expected in a more representative sample of mammals. In any case, the important feature of the multivariate analysis is the almost uniformly heavy loadings of the other measures on the general size factor.

B. Diversity in Living Brains: Cladistics

Having emphasized uniformities so forcefully, I must warn against underestimating the importance of diversity. All brains are different, and there are major differences both within and between species. Differences in brains within species are often difficult to measure with conventional anatomical and physiological methods, but since the brain is the control system for behavior, behavioral differences are evidence of differences among brains. Differences among species, of course, are much more dramatic.

The qualitative differences among the procyonids described by Welker could be presented as quantitative differences as well by measuring the amount of tissue in, for example, forepaw and rhinarial projections to the neocortex of procyonids. Differences among orders of mammals or classes of vertebrates are even more striking, but they too have not been quantified, perhaps because they are so obvious. And even when differences are great, they may be surprisingly difficult to describe quantitatively. One recognizes in an instant that the human brain is an unusual primate brain, for example, but the analysis of the relative size of its major parts usually shows it to be a perfectly normal primate (or mammalian) brain. In Fig. 2 there is nothing other than gross size to distinguish the human data, which fell on or near the regression lines determined for all the mammals in each sample. Also, as mentioned earlier, even the size of the prefrontal neocortex, often assumed to be uniquely important in human performance, is exactly as large as expected for a mammalian brain the size of a human brain. The uniqueness of human behavior is related to the size of the entire neural control system, and the correct conclusion about prefrontal executive function is that its size is appropriate to the very large brain systems that it controls.

A rigorous, though not really quantitative, analysis of the diversity of organization of the brain has been in the application of cladistic methodology. As indicated earlier, the results of this kind of analysis with brain features are essentially the same as those when other morphological features are used in the traits-by-species matrix that provides primary data for the analysis.

A cladistic methodology was applied by P.S. Ulinski, who took as his goal the reconstruction of probable features of the internal anatomy of brains at nodal evolutionary points in the evolution of reptiles, birds, and mammals. He first used the results of cladistic classification to determine nodes at which branching occurred when an ancestral species split into two daughter species. Second, he examined the brains of living representatives of the daughter species (or higher taxa). Finally, he constructed a hypothetical ancestral brain as a kind of lowest common denominator of the brains of the daughter species. The approach can be applied only to nodes in which surviving species from both branches exist. For example, taking living turtles and crocodiles to represent surviving species from the node of the early reptilian branching that led to these species, the ancestral brain can be constructed as having only those features that turtles and crocodiles share. With this procedure Ulinski could suggest various details about the ancestral brain of birds, crocodiles, lizards, and turtles. (From a cladistic perspective birds may be thought of as specialized reptiles derived from dinosaurs.) The nodal point in the history of the mammals, unfortunately (for this approach), is late in a "reptilian" synapsid lineage, represented today only by mammals. The mammal–reptile transition brain could be reconstructed only if synapsids at a reptilian grade of brain evolution had survived; but none have. The reconstruction of the brain at the reptile–mammal transition is, therefore, impossible using his procedure.

It would be possible to temper this conclusion, which is based on qualitative internal features of the brain, by analyzing the superficial anatomy using data on fossil endocasts, although such data are sparse for synapsids. Where they exist, in therapsids, they suggest a size pattern comparable to that in living reptiles. The transition from mammal-like reptiles to mammals is documented in the endocasts, and at present it seems to be reflected primarily as both enlargement of the brain (encephalization) and a major reduction in body size.

In his analysis of mammalian brain evolution, particularly the diversity of organization of somatosensory neocortex, J.I. Johnson presents an impressive catalog of detail on differences but concludes that "a great many features are constant across all mammals, from platypus to monkey, rat, cat, and sheep." The major variations "include [amount of] multiplication of representations of certain body parts" and details of the representations. He also notes few general trends of organization but comments that the appearance of "association cortex" intercalated between somatosensory and visual neocortex is haphazard across species, and that its appearance seems "to have something to do with the use of limbs as information-gathering and manipulating organs." Johnson's conclusions are consistent with the notion that the pattern of organization of the brain in a species that differentiates it from other species follows no general principles in the mammals but is part of the specialization of each species. In cladistic analyses, Johnson and his associates found that the phylogenetic tree in mammals deduced from 15 brain traits was essentially the same as that deduced from other traits.

The quantification of diversity depends on the measurement of size. The evolution of brain size in mammals has led to the diversification that was already evident in the data of Fig. 2, with species having brains as small as 0.1 g (pygmy shrew) and as large as 8 kg (killer whale). These all evolved from a single species of mammal (according to the monophyly accepted today) that lived more than 200 Ma. I outline the history later, but we must first understand how the diversity of size is analyzed.

C. Allometry and Encephalization

Body size accounts for 80–90% of the variance in brain size between species, a relationship described by an allometric equation: the regression of the logarithms of brain size on body size. The distance of a species from the regression line is a measure of its encephalization. Because the scales are logarithmic, this distance, or residual, is an encephalization quotient—the ratio of actual brain size to expected brain size. Encephalization is a characteristic of a species; it is usually meaningless to discuss differences within a species in encephalization.

Allometry and encephalization do not have to be defined by regression equations and residuals, but most recent work on brain evolution involving brain body allometry uses this approach, which might be called "parametric" since it involves the estimation of the parameters of a normal probability distribution. Instead of the regression, the data can be described with minimum convex polygons enclosing the data points of the groups to be compared, but there are currently no quantitative methods to analyze the polygons.

Minimum convex polygons described the location of human and dolphin data in Fig. 2A, and the brain/body data for the same insectivores, prosimians, and anthropoids as in Fig. 2B are graphed in Fig. 3, with polygons drawn around each group to compare them

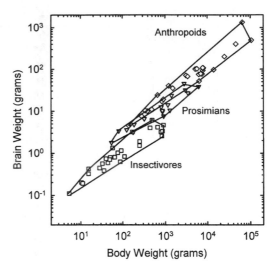

Figure 3 Convex polygons to differentiate insectivore, prosimian, and anthropoid data on brain weight and body weight (from a chapter for Zaidel; see footnote on first page).

with respect to encephalization. (Recall that Fig. 2B related the size of the cerebellum to the size of the whole brain; in Fig. 3 the relationship is of the whole brain to the size of the body.) It is not difficult to distinguish relative brain size among the groups since there is little overlap. All the polygons are oriented upward. There is slight overlap between the insectivores and prosimians and a bit more overlap between prosimians and anthropoids. From Fig. 3, one would describe the order of encephalization of these groups as follows: insectivores are least encephalized; prosimians are intermediate, and anthropoids are most encephalized. These data are also described by regression equations in Fig. 4.

The work by Stephan's group is especially relevant for evolutionary analysis because of the species they used. They worked with insectivores to represent a primitive grade of brain evolution and to provide an evolutionary perspective on the human brain. The issues are more complex, of course, but insectivores are reasonable models for the base group from which most placental species evolved. They resemble the earliest mammals both skeletally and in their endocasts. Although primates are currently a highly encephalized order of mammals, they are also a very ancient order, probably derived during the Late Cretaceous period from a species comparable to living insectivores or tree shrews. Comparisons between insectivores and primates are thus very appropriate for our topic.

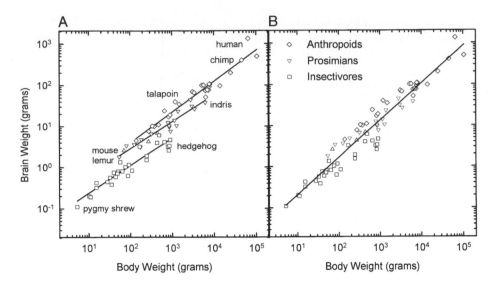

Figure 4   Regression analysis of the data shown in Fig. 3. Some species are named to indicate diversity of sample. (A) Separate regressions and correlation coefficients for the three groups: insectivores: $Y = 0.05\,X^{0.67}$, $r = 0.946$; prosimians: $Y = 0.14\,X^{0.66}$, $r = 0.960$; anthropoids: $Y = 0.13\,X^{0.75}$, $r = 0.972$. (B) Lumping the data for an overall regression for all 76 species: $Y = 0.05\,X^{0.91}$, $r = 0.966$. (redrawn with permission from Jerison, 1991).

D. A Bit of Theory

Issues in parametric quantification of encephalization as they apply to insectivores and primates are suggested in Fig. 4. The two graphs present the same data, fitted by straight lines in different ways. Fig. 4A shows the regression of log brain size on log body size computed separately for the three groups; Fig. 4B is a single regression for all 76 species. The three regression lines in Fig. 4A provide the same information as the polygons in Fig. 3. But if one is interested in curve fitting all the regression lines fit remarkably well ($r > 0.94$) despite their different slopes. These slopes on log–log axes are the exponents of the equations written as power functions, and the value of a "true exponent" has been the subject of considerable debate during the past decade. This is where a little theory may help.

The emerging consensus is that an exponent of 3/4 is the correct value. I have quarreled with this view, arguing in favor of a 2/3 exponent, which has theoretical significance for dimensional analysis of the brain's work in mapping information from the external environment. It is true that empirical analyses of large enough samples of species, or of properly sampled groups of species, lead to the 3/4 exponent when the fit is statistical, but I believe that the theoretical value of 2/3 is nevertheless correct. The point is that the 2/3 value is required by the dimensional problem in order to convert data about a surface

into data about a volume (a "mapping"). It reflects the fact that our information about the external world is spread across a surface consisting of sensory cells distributed throughout the body (skin, retina, organ of corti, olfactory epithelium, etc.) and that information is pumped up to neurons distributed through a kind of conceptual surface in a brain. I have assumed a fixed cortical thickness as representing that brain surface, and that the measure of brain volume in brainbody allometry is converted into a measure of that surface area. However, since the conversion is by a physical system that takes up space, one has to take into account the thickness of the map formed by the cortical "surface." To explain the difference between a 2/3 exponent required for the mapping and the 3/4 exponent found empirically, I have argued that this thickness as estimated by the thickness of neocortex is known to be greater in larger brains, varying approximately with the 1/9 power of body size. The value 3/4 is approximately the sum of 2/3 + 1/9. The theoretical value of 2/3, which is meaningful for the brain's mapping function, thus leads to an expected empirical value of 3/4.

E. Encephalization

The fact of encephalization is evident in the vertical displacement of the lines that are fitted to the three groups (Fig. 4A) or of the minimum convex polygons

(Fig. 3). Since the polygons do not require the dubious assumptions of statistical curve fitting, they may be preferred for describing encephalization. They are certainly preferred if they are adequate for answering questions about whether groups are equal or differ in encephalization.

The degree of encephalization in living vertebrates is summarized in Fig. 5. The polygons enclose all the available data on the indicated classes. The data were assembled from a variety of sources. The main inference from Fig. 5 is that one can characterize birds and mammals jointly as "higher" vertebrates, and reptiles, bony fish, and amphibians can be characterized as "lower" vertebrates. The polygons do an adequate job, although the addition of data on cartilaginous fish (sharks, rays, and skates), jawless fish (agnathans), and electric fish (bony fish: Mormyriformes) makes it difficult to distinguish the groups by inspection. The additions are of relatively few species. As mentioned previously, the present consensus recognizes about 50,000 vertebrate species. Of these, to the nearest thousand, about 25,000 are bony fish, 6000 are reptiles, 4000 are amphibians, 10,000 are birds, and 5000 are mammals. There are about 800 cartilaginous fish species and 70 agnathan species.

From the evidence presented earlier in Fig. 2A, it is appropriate to assume that the amount of encephalization measures the information processing capacity of a brain, adjusted for body size. It is therefore appropriate to consider the ecological requirements met by increments in processing capacity in different groups of species. Not much debate is required to see mammals and birds as higher vertebrates in this regard, given the normal complexity and plasticity of behavior observed in these groups. No reasonable speculations have been offered for the position of the cartilaginous fish as overlapping the higher and lower groups, but the place of electric fish reflects an unusually enlarged cerebellum in these species, related to processing information from their electric organs. It is unclear why that processing should require as great an investment in neural machinery. The position of jawless fish has been placed below the bony fish polygon, leading to speculations that there may have been a reduction in brain size related to the parasitic habits common in this group, particularly among lampreys. However, as evident from Fig. 5, agnathans, though relatively small-brained, fall more or less within the fish polygon, making such speculations unnecessary.

The approach signaled by Fig. 5 enables us to evaluate fossil endocasts with respect to encephalization, providing a direct evolutionary window to the patterns of change that led to the current diversity in brain size. I present such a nonparametric analysis as well as a parametric (regression) analysis of neocorticalization in the next section. In the analysis by convex polygons, I will be concerned with the evolution of birds and mammals from the reptiles and the utility of the method for some conclusions about dinosaur brains.

V. QUANTITATIVE ANALYSIS: FOSSILS

A. Vertebrate History

Vertebrates first appeared during the past 500 million years of the earth's 4.5 billion (4.5×10^9) year existence, and Table II provides a synopsis of their history. Here are some points to remember.

First, the world was very different in the distant past compared to the present. During the Paleozoic Era, there were times when there was only a single global continent (Pangea), but landmasses joined and separated with the passage of time. The global map was significantly different during the Mesozoic, with major masses (Gondwanaland and Laurasia) during the Paleozoic and Mesozoic Eras. There were warmer and more stable climates during the Mesozoic, and the continents were drifting toward their present loca-

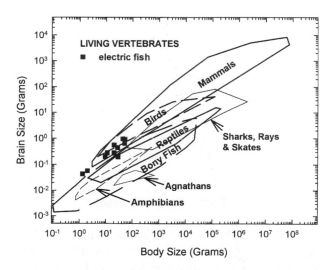

Figure 5 Brainbody relations in 2019 living vertebrate species enclosed in minimum convex polygons. The samples are 647 mammals, 180 birds, 1027 bony fish, 41 amphibians, 59 reptiles, 59 chondrichthyans (sharks, rays, and skates), and 6 agnathan fish (redrawn with permission from Jerison, Roth and Wulliman, 2001).

Table II

Synopsis of Vertebrate Evolution

Era	Period and epoch	Age (years $\times 10^6$)	Fauna (first appearance)
Cenozoic	Quaternary		
	Holocene	0.01–	No new megafauna
	Pleistocene	1.8–0.01	*Homo erectus, H. sapiens*
	Tertiary		
	Pliocene	5–1.8	Hominids: *Australopithecus, Homo habilis*
	Miocene	25–5	Hominoids (apes)
	Oligocene	35–25	"Progressive" brains
	Eocene	55–35	Progressive ungulates, Anthropoids
	Paleocene	65–55	Primates[a] and carnivores
Mesozoic	Cretaceous	140–65	Marsupials, Placentals
	Jurassic	210–140	Birds, mammal endocast
	Triassic	250–210	Mammals
Paleozoic	Permian	285–250	Primitive dinosaurs
	Carboniferous	360–290	Reptiles
	Devonian	410–360	Bony fish and amphibians
	Silurian	440–410	Jawed fish
	Ordovician	500–440	Jawless fish
	Cambrian	550	First chordates

[a] Primate teeth reported in late Cretaceous deposits. Paleocene primate identification is controversial. There is consensus recognizing early Eocene tarsier-like species, middle Eocene lemur-like species, and recently discovered late Eocene simian species.

tions. The Cenozoic was more variable in every way, with more diverse and sometimes chilling climates and periods of major mountain building. A burgeoning animal and plant life is evident in fossils from sediments laid down during all of these periods.

Second, there were several mass extinctions, with the greatest, at the end of the Permian Era, signaling the beginning of the Mesozoic. The most famous extinction, attributed to impact by a small asteroid, occurred at the end of the Mesozoic (the K–T, or Cretaceous–Tertiary boundary) 65 million years ago. Niches, emptied of their otherwise well-adapted organisms that could not survive the environmental catastrophe, could then be filled by suitably adapted birds, mammals, teleost fish, and snakes.

Third, although mammals were present during much of the 185 million years of the Mesozoic Era, all were small-bodied, none larger than living cats. They were probably nocturnal in their habits. Only during the Cenozoic did very large mammal species appear, and even today the average mammalian species is about cat size and nocturnal. Humans are giant vertebrates, physically larger and heavier than

90% or more of living species. Anthropoid primates are an unusual group of mammals; species of the suborder Anthropoidea (monkeys, apes, and humans) are diurnal and are well-adapted for color vision.

Finally, a major environmental event in human history may have been the Pliocene drying of the Mediterranean about 5 million years ago, which probably contributed to natural selection among chimpanzee-like primates for a species that became the earliest hominid. Extensive glaciation characterized the Pleistocene Epoch and may have driven the evolution of the human species to its present grade.

B. Fossil Brains Revisited

From the history of the brain in fish, amphibians, and reptiles as available from the fossil record, the most unusual inference is that these can all be treated as lower vertebrates in encephalization (Fig. 5). The exceptions are sharks and, perhaps, the ostrich-like dinosaurs (ornithomimids). Here is a list of a few more outstanding discoveries.

First, from the evidence of small (<15 cm long) Carboniferous (350 Ma) fossil fish, the diversity in living teleosts was probably foreshadowed by some of the earliest bony fish. They had optic lobes enlarged in ways comparable to those of living fish, such as trout, that feed at or near the surface of the water and rely on visual information.

Second, although sharks and other cartilaginous fish are often considered primitive, they are not primitive with respect to their brains. Many sharks are big-brained, overlapping the distributions of relative brain size of the lower vertebrates, on the one hand, and of birds and mammals, on the other hand. There is one uncrushed endocast known in a Paleozoic shark, the earliest evidence of encephalization beyond the grade of living bony fish. The species was comparable in both brain and body size to the living horned shark (*Heterodontus*).

Third, dinosaurs continue to be libeled with the walnut-size brain label despite evidence to the contrary. Their brains were within the expected size range for reptiles. The Tyrannosaurus 404-ml endocast implies a brain in the size range of those of living deer—small for an elephant-sized mammal but impressive for a reptile. The basic data are shown in Fig. 6.

Fourth, the major transition from water to land in the amphibians more than 350 Ma was accomplished without enlargement of the brain, and there has been no enlargement since if one compares present amphibians with their fossil ancestors. Of course, there was and is, considerable diversity in relative brain size within each of the classes of living lower vertebrates, just as there is in birds and mammals, and there has been significant reorganization of the brain across species of lower vertebrates, especially between classes but also within classes. By any standard, one must recognize the brain in living reptiles as more specialized than that of fish or amphibians.

Finally, of the major lateralization of function in the living human brain, and the recognized lateralization in the brains of many other living species, there is little or no evidence at a gross level. There is no good fossil evidence for such lateralization, although some has been claimed and evidence may be forthcoming. The problem is that asymmetries are difficult to establish, even in living brains, and are almost impossible to establish in fossils, which are often asymmetrically distorted and partially crushed.

These statements sum up the evidence on brain evolution in about three-fourths of the vertebrate species. There remains the story of about 10,000

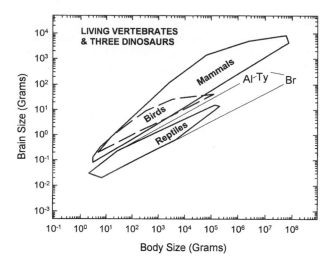

Figure 6 Data from Fig. 5 for mammals, birds, reptiles, and three dinosaurs (Al, *Allosaurus*; Ty, *Tyrannosaurus*; and Br, *Brachiosaurus*), showing extension of reptilian minimum convex polygon by adding dinosaur data.

species of birds and 5000 species of mammals, in which encephalization is a major feature. As background, and for a better sense of the potential and limitations of the method, I discuss the relevant data from Fig. 5, namely, those on reptiles, birds, and mammals. These are presented in Fig. 6, in which distracting information from the three classes of fish were removed and to which I have added data on three dinosaurs.

The three added species are the large well-known carnivorous dinosaurs, *Tyrannosaurus* and *Allosaurus*, and the largest of all dinosaurs in which there are reliable body size estimates, *Brachiosaurus*. To illustrate the method and its use, I will review the status of the "ostrich dinosaurs" from this perspective. One of these is a relatively small late Cretaceous carnivorous dinosaur, *Troodon*, which has been described as encephalized as large living birds and in the range of encephalization of living mammals. The analysis depends on estimating body size as well as brain size. There is a reliable estimate of *Troodon*'s body size as about 45 kg. Its brain size was first estimated by inspection and by perceived similarity to an ostrich's brain size of 40 g. However, with the help of a computer program recently developed and a quantitative analysis of its brain size, I now estimate its brain as about 20 ml in volume. This is somewhat smaller than the albatross's 27-ml brain as determined by the same computer analysis. If *Troodon* had a 20 ml brain in a 45 kg body, it would fit within the reptile polygon of Fig. 6. More analysis is needed, but it is evident that reports of the past 30 years of these large-brained dinosaurs need to be reevaluated. Other dinosaur data, such as those in Fig. 6, appear to be reasonably reliable, and provide an acceptable basis for evaluating dinosaur brain evolution. The ostrich that provided data for Fig. 6 weighed 133 kg and had a 42 g brain. It is the end-point of the avian polygon, which falls somewhat below the corresponding point on the polygon for living mammals. I have not entered data points for albatross at a body size of 12 kg, but it would fit comfortably within the avian polygon. *Troodon* fits within the reptilian polygon as extended in Fig. 6 to include a few dinosaurs. *Troodon* was indeed among the larger brained dinosaurs, but it probably did not reach either the mammalian or avian polygon.

The analysis with convex polygons is, in short, based on inclusion or exclusion of a particular species within the taxon described by a particular polygon. In Fig. 5, it was this approach that demonstrated the anomalous situation for living electric fish and cartilaginous fish and the "normal" position for agnathans. In Fig. 6, it indicates that dinosaurs were reptilian rather than avian in relative brain size.

C. Birds and Mammals

The history of the bird brain is not as well-known as that of mammals, and the present diversity in brains in birds does not appear to be as dramatic. However, the brain of *Archaeopteryx* was bird-like primarily because it filled the cranial cavity and was larger than that in comparable reptiles. There was no Wulst—that is, the dorsal enlargement of the forebrain in living birds that functions equivalently to primary visual cortex in mammals. The next significant evidence in the history of birds is from an Eocene whimbril-like bird, *Numenius gypsorum*, in which the brain is somewhat smaller than in comparable living birds of its body size but, most dramatically, its forebrain is clearly much smaller so that its optic lobes are more fully exposed than in living birds. Endocasts of later birds are indistinguishable from those of their living relatives.

In their early history, the mammals were small, probably nocturnal insectivorous creatures. Their adaptation for life in nocturnal niches could have been the major selection pressure to explain the "advance" to a mammalian grade of brain morphology and encephalization. The characteristic morphological feature of the brain of living mammals is the presence of neocortex, the six-layered neuronally rich outer covering of the forebrain. Its presence can often be established on an endocast because a major fissure, the rhinal fissure, is its ventral boundary.

The earliest mammalian brain is known from an Upper Jurassic endocast of *Triconodon mordax* and is about 150 million years old. The lateral surface of this endocast is not preserved well enough to indicate whether or not there was a rhinal fissure; thus, positive evidence regarding the presence of neocortex is not available. In encephalization, however, its brain was comparable to that of small–brained living species such as opossums and hedgehogs, in which neocortex is present. It is therefore likely that neocortex appeared at least 150 Ma. The best assumption from available information is that neocortex is, in fact, part of the suite of traits that characterized the mammals from the beginning of their evolution, at least 50 million years earlier.

Mammals in which the endocasts are sufficiently complete to show a rhinal fissure, if present, are about 75 Ma. They are from a unique assemblage of Late Cretaceous mammals from the Gobi desert, which includes early placentals. The most common mammals of the time, the multituberculates, were unrelated to any living species. Superficially, multituberculates probably looked like living rodents or insectivores. Their life span as an order was about 120 million years, between about 150 and 30 Ma, a very long span for a mammalian group. The specimen in which the endocast is best known, *Chulsanbaatar*, weighed no more than about 15 g, a small mammal even for the Mesozoic and smaller than most living species of mice. There is a suggestion of a rhinal fissure in its endocast, although there is disagreement about where it is located. Whether or not one can see a rhinal fissure, from its grade of encephalization it is very likely that neocortex was present in its brain.

D. Neocorticalization

Neocorticalization is a concept in comparative neuroanatomy, based on comparisons among living species. For example, it describes the fact that primates have relatively and absolutely more neocortex than insectivores. One makes the statement: Primates are more neocorticalized than insectivores. Of course, living insectivores did not evolve to change into living primates under natural selection. But there is an evolutionary translation of the statement: The ancestors of living insectivores were members of an order (or other taxon) of mammals that probably included at least one species from which primates evolved. This species has not been identified, but as evolutionists positing a relationship between insectivores and primates as "sister" groups, we have to assume that it existed. Neocorticalization is then understood as part of the differentiation of daughter species from parent species: One daughter species of a fossil insectivore, which had relatively more neocortex than the parent species, was the ancestral primate species. These statements are almost parodies of evolutionary analysis, but they approximate a correct analysis.

The concept of neocorticalization can also be used in another sense—as describing the history of a trait in successive populations of species. If we sample a broad range of species across geological time and determine that later species had relatively more neocortex than earlier species, we could state that neocorticalization had occurred, even though we would not be able to determine its phylogenetic history. Such a discovery would be enough to suggest that there was a selective advantage in an increase in neocortex. The analytic model to be applied might be an elaboration of simple models of phenotypic evolution within lineages. It would require theorizing about selective advantages above the species level—about broad evolutionary "landscapes" that are contexts for interaction among species.

Neocorticalization in this sense can be quantified as a feature of the history of the mammals. It is more or less evident from a simple inspection of endocasts, but the quantitative effect can only be demonstrated with the help of some statistical analysis. I present such an analysis in Fig. 7. For the analysis, I measured the planar projection of neocortex and olfactory bulbs in 59 species of living and fossil ungulates and carnivores. The sample included 38 Carnivora, 7 Creodonta, 4 Condylarthra, 5 species from extinct South American (neotropical) ungulate orders, 1 Eocene perissodactyl (*Hyrachyus*, an ancestral rhinoceros), and 4 progressive ungulates (artiodactyls). The complete sample consisted of 35 fossil species and 24 living species.

The results were analyzed as neocortical and olfactory bulb quotients, determined by partialling out the effect of body size much as in encephalization quotients. A quotient of 1.0 means that the size was as expected for a species at the centroid, 0.5 means it was half as big, and so on. As presented in Fig. 7, the results lead to four conclusions. There is first the fact of neocorticalization. Later species tended to have relatively more neocortex than did earlier species. This is the meaning of the significantly positive slope of the regression line of the neocortical quotient against geological time.

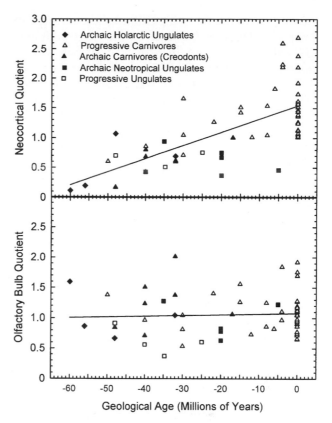

Figure 7 (Top) Change in relative neocortical surface area (neocortical quotient) as a function of geological age. "Progressive" change noted here (positive slope of regression line) indicates increased neocorticalization over time. Each point is a species. (Bottom) Absence of change in relative surface area of the olfactory bulbs as a function of geological age. (Redrawn with permission from Jerison, in Jones and Peters, 1990).

Second, species from archaic orders (Fig. 7, filled symbols) tended to have less neocortex than did species from progressive orders (Fig. 7, open symbols). Thus, 3 of the 4 archaic ungulate species, 5 of the 7 archaic carnivore (creodont) species, and 4 of the 5 Neotropical ungulate species (also archaic in that their orders are extinct) are below the regression line. Twelve of the 16 archaic species thus had less neocortex than would be predicted for their geological age by an unbiased regression analysis. For those who enjoy playing with statistics, a chi-square analysis contrasts this with an expected even split: $\chi^2 = 4$, $df = 1$, $p < 0.05$.

The third result in a comparison between progressive and archaic species limited to fossil Carnivora versus Creodonta. It is in two parts. First, the Carnivora points appear generally to be higher than those of the Creodonta. Second, the Carnivora points seem to show more "progress" over time than do those of the Creodonta. It is not possible to test the first part properly, because the species are from different geological times, and there is no obvious way to control the time variable. The second part, however, can be tested by simple regression analysis. The correlation between age and neocortical quotient for 15 Carnivora species was $r = 0.72$ ($p < 0.01$). For seven Creodonta it was $r = 0.42$ ($p > 0.05$). Only the Carnivora were demonstrably progressively neocorticalized.

The result is important for evolutionary analysis of the relations between true carnivores and creodonts. The argument is summed up by R. L. Carroll as follows: "Romer (1966) and Jerison (1973) stigmatized the creodonts as archaic and small brained, but Radinsky (1977) demonstrated that relative brain size increased as rapidly among creodonts as it did in the early members of the Carnivora, together with an increase in the extent of the neocortex." The quantitative analysis supports Romer's view as mentioned by Carroll. (My contribution in 1973 was mainly to quote Romer and to provide very limited quantitative data. The current confirmation of our older view is possible because of the additional data collected by Radinsky, which permitted a statistical test.)

The final conclusion is that unlike neocortex, the olfactory bulbs did not change in relative size with the passage of time. The correlation between the olfactory bulb quotient and geological time was $r = 0.1$, which is not significantly different from zero. This is an important point because it shows that this approach is fine enough to discriminate between the presence and absence of change. It also helps quash a myth about what is "primitive" and "progressive" in brain evolution.

Although careful students do not make the error, some neurobiologists assume that having large olfactory bulbs is a primitive mammalian trait and that the olfactory bulbs became relatively smaller as the mammals evolved. Fig. 7 corrects this error by showing that olfactory bulbs have been a stable feature of the brain in Tertiary carnivores and ungulates. The misconception is a bit of primate chauvinism, as it were. Primates (at least the anthropoids) are neocortical specialists, but they are deficient mammals in olfactory development. A reduced role for olfaction is part of the adaptive mosaic of the adaptive zone of simian primates and is not a broad feature of mammalian evolution. (It also complicated the factor analysis presented earlier.) Neocorticalization, on the other hand, appeared as a general trend in many mammalian groups and its relative absence in the

insectivores and many marsupials is correctly recognized as a primitive feature in these groups.

VI. CONCLUSIONS

First on neocorticalization. The fossil evidence indicates that there was neocorticalization in mammals and that it can be detected even in samples as small as 15 species of Carnivora. Evolution of the carnivores involved neocorticalization in another sense, in that the two great orders of Tertiary carnivores (Creodonta and Carnivora) differed in the extent of neocorticalization. This could have been a factor in the survival of true carnivores. In any event, the history of neocorticalization indicates that there was almost certainly some benefit derived from the expansion of neocortex. The fossil evidence therefore confirms conventional wisdom in neurobiology that it was a progressive thing for mammals to evolve neocortex and (perhaps within limits) more is better.

If the conclusions on neocortex are expected, those on the olfactory bulbs are not. These structures are surprisingly constant features in mammalian brains. There is no reason to have predicted that they would not evolve to large or small size relative to other parts of the brain, depending on the extent of olfactory specializations in particular species. But according to current evidence from fossil brains, the olfactory bulbs have been constant and relatively unchanging features that make a brain a mammal's brain. They are not unusually enlarged in any species; most mammals are olfactory specialists. Evolutionary changes in the olfactory bulbs occurred mainly in a negative way, by reduction. The reduced state of olfactory bulbs in humans and other primates (and their complete absence in some cetaceans) merely reflects the extremes of diversity that are possible as the brain evolved to control the activities of mammals in the variety of niches in which they function.

From these and related data it seems likely that encephalization in mammals was driven by neocorticalization. One mammalian trend was toward enlarged neocortex, and since neocortex is a fairly fixed fraction of total brain size the enlargement of the brain was presumably correlated with the increased size of neocortex. Because neocortical function is deeply involved with cognitive functions—knowledge of "reality," expanded neocortex would be associated with more elaborate cognition, a major suggestion about the evolution of mind.

It would be appropriate to look more closely at neocortical functions and assume that the evolutionary advantage conferred by these functions was the engine driving progressive brain evolution in mammals. However, it would be a mistake to make much of such an idea of progress. It is true that neocorticalized species are more prevalent now than in the distant past. It must also be true that some fitness is associated with this aspect of the brain's evolution. But there are many successful living species that are at a very ancient grade of mammalian neocorticalization. Hedgehogs in Europe and opossums in America are outstanding examples because they are very fit in the evolutionary sense. They may litter our highways because of their "stupidity" in refusing to yield the right of way to cars and trucks, but the litter is part of the evidence of their reproductive success. And they manage this at a grade of neocorticalization and encephalization that some mammalian species reached 150 Ma.

The analysis of neocorticalization suggests that comparable advances occurred in birds with the expansion of their forebrains. It is certainly true that the avian forebrain is much enlarged compared to that of reptiles, and the grade of encephalization in birds is probably related to forebrain enlargement. The optic lobes (midbrain, homologous to the superior colliculi in mammals) also seem much larger in birds than in reptiles, at least to an analysis by eye.

The final conclusion, however, must be that animals do not live by brains alone. The majority of living vertebrates get along with about as much brain as was present in their earliest ancestors. Adaptation to one's niche can be accomplished in many ways, and to adapt behaviorally by brain enlargement is expensive energetically. The brain is profligate in its use of energy, and almost any other solution to an adaptational problem is less costly. In those groups that adopted encephalization as an adaptive strategy, however, there was evidently a real gain in fitness. Encephalization appeared in many very distantly related species of birds and mammals. It is a general rather than specific adaptation for increased total information processing capacity. It is sometimes considered as the brain correlate of intelligence. If that is true, it must mean that there are many intelligences that evolved, since encephalization is an overall sum of enlargements of constituent regions within the brain. Because the different regional enlargements are correlated with different behavioral capacities, there would be different kinds of intelligences in different species.

See Also the Following Articles

BRAIN ANATOMY AND NETWORKS • BRAIN DEVELOPMENT • CIRCADIAN RHYTHMS • INTELLIGENCE • LANGUAGE ACQUISITION • LATERALITY • NEOCORTEX

Suggested Reading

Braitenberg, V., and Schüz, A. (1998). *Cortex: Statistics and Geometry of Neural Connectivity*, Second Ed., Springer Verlag, New York.

Butler, A. B., and Hodos, W. (1996). *Comparative Vertebrate Neuroanatomy*. Wiley–Liss, New York.

Carroll, R. L. (1988). *Vertebrate Paleontology and Evolution*. Freeman, New York. [References to Jerison, Romer, and Radinsky.]

Dawkins, R. (1987). *The Blind Wachmaker*. Norton, New York.

Deacon, T. W. (1997). *The Symbolic Species: The Co-evolution of Language and the Brain*. W.W. Norton, New York.

Falk, D., and Gibson, K. (Eds.) (2001). *Evolutionary Anatomy of the Primate Cerebral Cortex*. Cambridge University Press, Cambridge, UK. [Chapters by Finlay and by Jerison.]

Farlow, J. O., and Brett-Surman, M. K. (Eds.) (1997). *The Complete Dinosaur*. University of Indiana Press, Bloomington Indiana.

Harvey, P. H., and Pagel, M. D. (1991). *The Comparative Method in Evolutionary Biology*. Oxford Univ. Press, Oxford.

Jerison, H. J. (1991). *Brain Size and the Evolution of Mind*, 59th James Arthur Lecture on the Evolution of the Human Brain. American Museum of Natural History, New York.

Jones, E. G., and Peters, A. (Eds.) (1990). *Cerebral Cortex: Comparative Structure and Evolution of Cerebral Cortex (Parts I and II). Volumes 8A and 8B*. Plenum, New York. [Chapters by Jerison, Johnson, Ulinski, and Welker.]

Martin, R. D. (1990). *Primate Origins and Evolution: A Phylogentic Reconstruction*. Chapman & Hall, London.

Novacek, M. (1996). *Dinosaurs of the Flaming Cliffs*. Doubleday, New York.

Roth, G., and Wulliman, M. F. (Eds.) (2001). *Brain Evoluation and Cognition*. Wiley & Sons, New York. [Chapters by Hofman, Hodos, Jerison, and Schuez.]

Stephan, H., Baron, G., and Frahm, H. D. (1991). *Insectivora: With a Stereotaxic Atlas of the Hedgehog Brain, Comparative Brain Research in Mammals*, Vol. 1, Springer-Verlag, New York.

Taquet, P. (1992). Dinosaures et Mammifères du Désert de Gobi. Muséum National d'Histoire Naturelle, Paris.

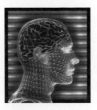

Eye Movements

CHARLES J. BRUCE and HARRIET R. FRIEDMAN

Yale University School of Medicine

I. Introduction

II. Why Move the Eyes?

III. How Do the Eyes Move? Phenomenology of Eye Movements

IV. Neural Circuits for Eye Movements

GLOSSARY

frontal eye field Motor cortex for eye movements. In man and monkey, the frontal eye field lies in premotor cortex, just rostral to the hand representation in motor cortex.

neural integrator Brain stem circuit that maintains the current position of the eye by integrating all eye velocity commands. Its tonically spiking output neurons (tonic neurons) are located in the nucleus prepositus hypoglossi, the interstitial nucleus of Cajal, and the medial vestibular nucleus.

nystagmus Any to-and-fro movement of the eyes. Nystagmus can be normal (e.g., continued optokinetic stimulation causes optokinetic nystagmus, such as watching a train go by) or pathological, both congenital and acquired. The waveform of pathological nystagmus often indicates the damaged structure (e.g., sawtooth nystagmus indicates vestibular system damage).

optokinetic reflex/nystagmus Smooth, relatively slow eye movements elicited by movement of the whole visual field. Prolonged optokinetic reflex becomes optokinetic nystagmus when the slow movement alternates with quick-phase movements in the opposite direction.

response field The spatial parameters for the sensory stimulation and/or motor behavior associated with the spiking (or maximal spiking) of a particular neuron.

saccade generator Circuitry in brain stem reticular formation that underlies all rapid eye movements. Its principal output cells are short-lead excitatory burst neurons (EBNs): Horizontal EBNs are in the caudal paramedian pontine reticular formation near the abducens nucleus, and vertical EBNs are in the midbrain near the oculomotor nucleus. Other key cell types are inhibitory burst neurons, long-lead excitatory burst neurons, and omnipause neurons.

saccades Short-duration, high-velocity (rapid) eye movements that quickly move the eyes to a new position; can include both voluntary saccades and the quick phase of vestibular or optokinetic nystagmus. Special saccade types include memory saccades, in which the eye movement is directed to the location of a remembered target not currently visible, and antisaccades, in which the movement is deliberately directed opposite to the target's location.

smooth pursuit Smooth, continuous eye movements used to track a moving target.

superior colliculus Midbrain visuomotor structure for triggering visually guided saccades.

vestibuloocular reflex Smooth, relatively slow eye movements elicited by the vestibular sense that serve to cancel movements of the visual stimulus on the retina (retinal slip) caused by head movements.

This article on the human brain's widely distributed circuitry for controlling the eyes stresses the functional significance of eye movements. It takes an evolutionary perspective by emphasizing the primacy of the image-stabilization system (vestibuloocular reflex, optokinetic reflex, and quick phases of nystagmus) and how the relatively new eye movements of primates (saccades, smooth pursuit, fixation, and vergence) serve the primate's high-resolution foveal vision by engaging the far older image-stabilization circuits. The anatomy and physiology of principal oculomotor structures are reviewed, with emphasis on the frontal eye field region of primate neocortex.

I. INTRODUCTION

Processing the visual sense is one of the most considerable endeavors of the human brain. One measure of the complexity of this function is that more than 30 distinct "visual" brain regions have been identified as contributing to the visual percept. Although eye movements are not required for visual function, they immensely improve the ability of primates to gather relevant, high-quality visual data for processing by this large expanse of neocortex. Thus, it is not surprising that a sizeable complement of cortical and subcortical circuits of the human brain is concerned with moving the eyes, nor that eye movements are often closely related to cognitive behavior.

This article is organized around three fundamental questions:

Why move the eyes? (What are the functions of eye movements?)
How do the eyes move? (What is the phenomenology and kinematics of eye movements?)
What moves the eyes? (Which neural structures and circuits effect eye movements?)

II. WHY MOVE THE EYES?

Eye movements serve vision in three principal ways (Table I): to stabilize images on the retina, especially against movements of the head and body (image-stabilization system); to image the important details of the visual world on the most sensitive part of the eye, the fovea (foveation system); and to align the retinal images in the two eyes in order to promote single vision and stereopsis (vergence-accommodation system). Eye contact and avoidance also have very important roles in interpersonal behavior.

A. The Image-Stabilization System

Ironically, one of the principal reasons for the eyes to move is to keep the direction of gaze stationary—that is, fixed in space. The underlying objective is to keep the visual image of the external world stationary on the retina despite movements of the head and body because even slight movements of this image across the retina (i.e., *retinal slip*) cause considerable visual blur. For this reason, seeing animals need image-stabilization strategies and reflexes, and for vertebrates this principally involves extraocular muscles that rotate the eyeball within its bony orbit so as to cancel

Table I
Principal Functions of Eye Movements

Image stabilization: Keep the visual image stationary on the retina

   Purpose: To prevent blurred vision caused by movements of the head and body

   Movements

      Vestibuloocular reflex in response to vestibular signals

      Optokinetic reflex in response to whole-field visual motion

      Quick phases of vestibuloocular and optokinetic nystagmus

Foveation: Capture and keep particular stimuli on the foveal part of retina

   Purpose: To facilitate fine, detailed viewing and visual analysis of important objects

   Movements

      Saccades to rapidly foveate new of different stimuli

      Smooth pursuit to track moving visual stimuli

      Fixation to maintain foveation of stationary visual stimuli

Binocular alignment: Foveate the same object/point in both retina

   Purpose: To facilitate single vision and steropsis in order to extract relative depth (3D) perception from fine disparities between the 2D images in the two eyes

   Movements

      Disjunctive eye movements, both convergent and divergent (other eye movements are conjugate/conjunctive, i.e., equal in the two eyes)

or minimize the retinal slip consequent to movements of the head. Furthermore, the anatomical and physiological substrates of image-stabilization eye movements are remarkably similar across vertebrate species, from primitive fish to modern apes.

Three distinctive types of eye movements are associated with image stabilization: the vestibuloocular reflex (VOR), the optokinetic reflex (OKR), and the extremely high-speed resetting movements called the "quick phase" (of nystagmus). The VOR is a very short latency reflex instigated by the vestibular system in response to body/head rotation. The OKR, on the other hand, is triggered by visual motion. In the laboratory, VOR and OKR can be separately studied; however, in the real world both are activated whenever the head moves, and they synergistically sum to compensate for most head movements and thereby minimize movement of the visual image on the retina. In contrast, the quick phase is an anticompensatory movement that very rapidly returns the eye to a more central position whenever it is taken to eccentric orbital positions by the vestibulooptokinetic reflexes.

These image-stabilization eye movements are reflexive and automatic. From an evolutionary perspective, they are the most basic, primary eye movements. Indeed, for most vertebrate species VOR, OKR, and the quick-phase movements of nystagmus are the only eye movements.

B. The Foveation System

As in most primates, the human retina has a tremendously specialized central zone, the fovea, where visual acuity is 1000 times better than vision just 10° eccentric. Hence, to "look at" something is effectively to foveate it. However, the fovea subtends only 1° of visual angle (equivalent to the full moon's subtend). Therefore, the second principal function of eye movements is to foveate important parts of the visual scene.

Foveation is accomplished by a triad of voluntary eye movements: saccades, fixation, and smooth pursuit. Of these, saccades are the most conspicuous because humans incessantly make saccades in order to maximize retrieval of high-quality visual information by foveal viewing. Although the saccadic movement is ballistic and stereotyped, saccades are voluntary with regard to the choice of whether or not to make a saccadic movement (when to look) and what saccadic vector to program (where to look). For example, reading is accomplished with a succession of voluntary saccades that march across each line (Fig. 1), and during each fixation (between saccades) the reader processes the foveated word(s) while simultaneously programming the next saccade.

Smooth-pursuit eye movements, the third member of the foveation triad, assists the viewing of objects moving in space by matching eye velocity to target velocity, up to 50–100°/sec. A record of smooth pursuit is shown in Fig. 2. Pursuit is sometimes confused with the OKR; however, they are very different movements, as described later, and pursuit often must override the combined vestibulooptokinetic reflexes (e.g., during combined head–eye tracking of a moving stimulus). Instead, pursuit is more equivalent to the continued fixation of a target that happens to be moving.

Whereas image stabilization is effected by a largely reflexive brain stem system, the more voluntary, cognitive foveation system and its constituent eye movements (saccades, fixation, and pursuit) involve many areas of neocortex, most notably the frontal eye field (FEF) region of the frontal lobe.

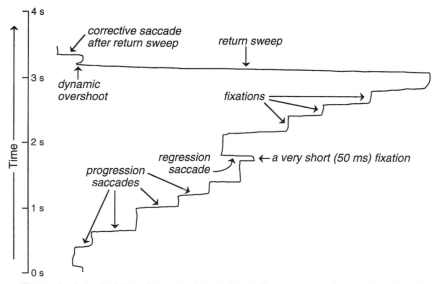

The main characteristics of eye movements in reading have been known since Javal.

Figure 1 Eye movements during reading. Eye movement records showing the pattern of saccades and fixations made while reading the sentence shown in the abscissa. Records were obtained using the infrared photoelectric scleral reflection technique (at 100 Hz). Time increases along the ordinate; therefore, to recreate the eye's movement the traces should be read from bottom to top. Notice that the sentence/line was read with 10 progressive (rightward) saccades and one regressive (leftward saccade), and the majority of the time spent reading the line is during the 11 fixations between the saccades (adapted from J. K. O'Regan, *Eye Movements and Their Role in Visual and Cognitive Processes* (E. Kowler, Ed.), copyright 1990, with permission from Elsevier Science).

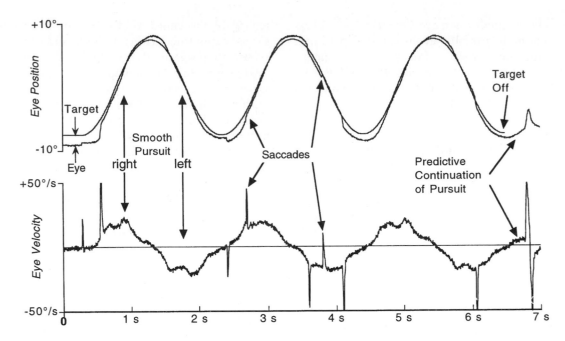

Figure 2 Smooth-pursuit eye movements. Horizontal eye position (top) and eye velocity (bottom) records of a monkey's smooth-pursuit tracking of a small spot with sinusoidal motion (amplitude ±7.5°, frequency 0.5 Hz). Tracking sinusoidal motion is equivalent to tracking the bob of a pendulum, a classic pursuit test. Maximum target velocity is 23.6°/sec, and maximum pursuit velocity was ~25°/sec. Saccades are easily identified by their spikes in the eye velocity traces. A total of seven saccades were made during the 6 sec of sinusoidal motion, starting with a large catch-up saccade shortly after the start of the target motion. At the end of the record smooth pursuit continued for part of a fourth cycle (predictive pursuit), even though the target was extinguished after three cycles (C. J. Bruce, unpublished data).

C. The Vergence-Accommodation System

As a consequence of frontally placed eyes (found in all primates and in predatory species of other vertebrate orders), the visual fields of the two eyes have considerable overlap. Stereoscopic depth can be extracted from the small differences in the these overlapping images, yielding detailed information about the three-dimensional (3D) structure of the visual world. However, good stereopsis requires that both eyes be directed at (i.e., foveate) the same object in visual space. Vergence (or disjunctive) eye movements provide such binocular alignment in response to changing fixation target distances, which necessitate that the two eyes point in different directions. In contrast, all of the aforementioned eye movement types are conjugate (or equivalently, conjunctive). Thus, the two eyes move as one during saccades, pursuit, VOR, etc. but not during vergence. The basic neural mechanisms of vergence and accommodation are in the brain stem, especially in midbrain regions immediately adjacent to the oculomotor nucleus (n. III). However, the vergence-accom-modation system is also dependent on neocortex, especially primary visual (striate) cortex and the frontal lobe cortex.

III. HOW DO THE EYES MOVE? PHENOMENOLOGY OF EYE MOVEMENTS

The oculomotor response can be reduced to seven basic types of eye movements (Table I) that achieve the three principal functions of image stabilization, foveation, and binocular alignment. Although these movements differ in many regards (e.g., whether they are fast or slow, voluntary or reflexive, as well as which of the three functions is served), the kinematics of eye movements are generic. All eye movements share a common final path represented by three cranial nerve nuclei and the six pairs of eye muscles that they control. This section describes the basic mechanics of eye movements and the muscles, nerves, and motor nuclei involved.

A. Eye Movements Are Three-Dimensional Rotations of the Eye in the Orbit

Eye movements can generally be regarded as rotations of the eye about the center of the eyeball. Like a ball in a socket, the eyeball spins inside its bony orbit in the skull. As shown in Fig. 3, any particular eye position can logically be obtained by a combination of rotations about the three axes through the center of rotation.

B. Each Axis of Rotation Is Controlled by a Pair of Opposing Muscles

Eye rotations are effected by six extraocular muscles that are organized as three opposed pairs. Each of these muscles has a major action: The medial and lateral rectus muscles effect horizontal eye movements, with the lateral rectus pulling the eye temporally (abduction) and the medial rectus pulling nasally (adduction). The primary actions of the superior and inferior rectus muscles are elevation and depression, respectively. The primary actions of the superior and inferior oblique muscles are torsional rotations of the

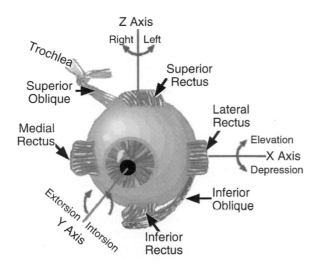

Figure 3 Axes of rotation and muscles of the eye. The eye rotates about three axes to effect horizontal, vertical, and torsional movements. These rotations are implemented via six extraocular muscles for each eye, as shown. Adduction and abduction about the z axis are accomplished by the lateral and medial rectus muscles. Raising and lowering the eyes (x axis rotations) are accomplished by the inferior and superior rectus muscles in association with the inferior and superior obliques. Likewise, torsional movements (y axis rotations) require the inferior and superior obliques together with the superior and inferior rectus muscles.

eye about the line of sight, with the superior oblique effecting intortion, and the inferior oblique effecting extorsion. However, the actions of the superior and inferior recti and the superior and inferior obliques are better regarded as "mixed" in that both pairs actually effect combined vertical and torsional eye movements. Vertical and torsional eye movements are further discussed later.

C. The Oculomotor Cranial Nerves and Their Brain Stem Nuclei

The six extraocular muscles are innervated by cranial nerves III (oculomotor), IV (trochlear), and VI (abducens). Nerve IV innervates the contralateral superior oblique, nerve VI the ipsilateral lateral rectus muscle, and nerve III the remaining four extraocular muscles as well as the eye lid. The neurons giving rise to these general somatic efferents are termed oculomotor neurons (OMNs). Their cell bodies are located in three eponymous nuclei that lie in pairs along the medial longitudinal fasciculus near the midline of the brain stem: the oculomotor, trochlear, and abducens nuclei, which are often grouped and simply termed the oculomotor nuclei.

D. Neural Activity in Oculomotor Neurons

In the early 1970s, several pioneering laboratories recorded the activity of single neurons in oculomotor nuclei while monitoring the eye movements of alert monkeys. They found that every OMN had the same characteristic firing pattern, organized about the eye's position and motion in the plane of its target extraocular muscle (Fig. 4). The clarity and constancy of the OMN responses galvanized sensorimotor neurophysiology, setting the stage for the analysis of circuits responsible for OMN responses and for tracing the antecedents of these activities further into the brain stem and then to the cerebral and cerebellar cortices.

1. Coding of Eye Position by Oculomotor Neurons

The relationship between the discharge rate of any OMN and the static position of the eye is a linear function of the eye's coordinate, θ, as measured along the pulling direction of the OMN's target muscle: $R_{OMN} = A \cdot (\theta - \theta_0)$, where R_{OMN} is spikes/sec, θ_0 is the

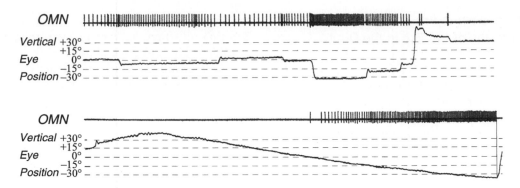

Figure 4 Discharge characteristics of a neuron in the oculomotor nucleus (OMN). The firing rate of this neuron increased in association with downward eye movement. The upper set of traces shows spontaneous saccadic eye movements with intervening periods of fixation. The lower set shows smooth pursuit brought about by moving an object in front of the monkey. In each part the top trace has the neuron's spikes during the eye movement; the **lower** trace (solid line) is the vertical eye position. The dashed lines represent degrees of deviation from straight-ahead gaze; upward deflection corresponds to elevation and downward deflection to depression of the eye (adapted with permission from P. H. Schiller, *Exp. Brain Res.* **10**, 347–362, 1970. copyright © 1970 by Springer-Verlag).

OMN's recruitment position, or threshold, and a typical value for factor A is 4 Hz/deg. Most θ_0 are more than 15° in the "off" direction (i.e., $\theta_0 \le 15°$), meaning that most motor units are active during central fixation. Two nonlinear constraints on R_{OMN} are necessary, however: $R_{OMN}=0$ for all $\theta \le \theta_0$, because neurons cannot have a negative rate, and $R_{OMN} \le 500$ because OMNs typically saturate at 500 Hz.

This linear relation reflects the passive physical properties of the eyeball in the orbit, namely the elastic forces that are constantly pulling the eye toward its central position with a force proportional to its eccentricity. Thus, larger deviations from the central position require proportionally larger muscular forces, which in turn require larger rates in the agonist muscle's OMNs. Larger eccentricities also require more relaxation in the antagonist muscle; however, the same equation, with the direction of θ reversed, provides for relaxation of the antagonist OMNs as well.

2. Coding of Eye Velocity by Oculomotor Neurons

For the eye to be rotated at any appreciable velocity, its extraocular innervation must also overcome the viscous drag of the orbit, which is approximately proportional to rotational velocity. Indeed, OMNs have significantly higher or lower spike rates when crossing a given eye position as a function of tracking direction and velocity. Thus, a velocity factor must be added to the OMN equation, yielding $R_{OMN}=A \cdot (\theta-\theta_0) + B \cdot (d\theta/dt)$. A typical value for velocity factor B is 1 Hz/deg/sec. The magnitude of this factor, like the threshold position (θ_0) and position factor (A), varies across the motor pool of each muscle; however, all OMNs require such a velocity term, as well as a position term, in their rate equation.

This basic equation holds for all OMNs during all types of eye movements. The velocity term has its most dramatic effect when the eyes move via saccades or quick phases (Fig. 4, top) because such rapid eye movements can approach 1000°/sec. Likewise, the nonlinear stipulation that $0 \le R_{OMN} \le 500$ is very important in relation to rapid eye movements; in fact, most OMNs are saturated at their maximal rate during large saccades in their on direction, and most are briefly silenced during saccades in their off direction.

3. Causality

The rate equation for OMNs is instructive, but it is causally backwards because the data are from recordings in alert monkeys making natural eye movements, not from direct experimental manipulation of eyeballs. Presumably, the brain arrives at a goal for θ and $d\theta/dt$ and then provides appropriate rates for all OMNs, including the few from which neurophysiologists record. Consequently, the extraocular muscles contract and the eye moves to position θ at velocity $d\theta/dt$. In other words, the causal equation is $\theta(t)=F(R_{OMN}(t-\tau))$, where τ is the ~5-msec delay from OMN spikes to actual eye movement. The substantive questions are (i) how an appropriate eye position and velocity are reckoned by a hierarchy of oculomotor structures distributed across the brain and then (ii) how the appropriate R_{OMN} for effecting that position and velocity are computed.

E. How the Eyes Are Coordinated and Constrained

The complexity of controlling 12 extraocular muscles is dramatically mitigated by several "laws" that reduce the degrees of freedom for controlling the eyes. These laws are implemented in the oculomotor anatomy near the output stage, and thus nearly all eye movements obey them.

1. Descartes–Sherrington's Law of Reciprocal Innervation

This law asserts that the six eye muscles of each eye act as three agonist/antagonist pairs (as discussed earlier), thus reducing the oculomotor system's degrees of freedom from 12 (the total number of extraocular muscles) to 6. Reciprocal innervation was implicit in the R_{OMN} equation because the agonist and antagonist muscles of each pair lie in the same plane with reversed sign.

2. Hering's Law of Motor Correspondence

Hering's law halves the oculomotor systems degrees of freedom from 6 to 3 because it asserts that the two eyes act in unison (conjugately) for all eye movements excepting vergence. Thus, the brain operates as if there is only one eye, a cyclopean retina. This motor correspondence is accomplished by yoking pairs of muscles in the two eyes. For example, the lateral rectus of the right eye and the medial rectus of the left eye comprise a yoked pair. They receive the same commands and both effect a rightward movement.

The brain stem circuits for both reciprocal innervation and motor correspondence in horizontal eye movements (medial and lateral rectus) are shown in Fig. 5 for rapid eye movements, such as saccades, and in Fig. 6 for smooth/slow eye movements, such as VOR. The yoking for horizontal movements is straightforward: Signals entering the right abducens nucleus not only innervate motor neurons of the right eye's lateral rectus but also innervate interneurons within the abducens nucleus. These interneurons relay this signal, via the medial longitudinal fasciculus, to the contralateral oculomotor nucleus, synapsing on OMNs of the left eye's medial rectus. For reciprocal

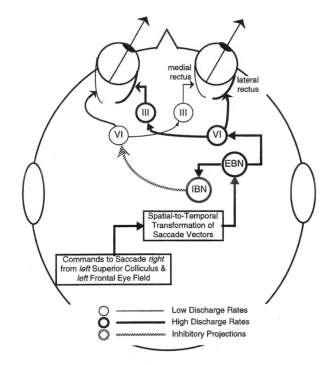

Figure 5   Neural circuit for a conjugate rightward eye movement. Making a conjugate eye movement, as in this figure, invokes activity in the diagrammed neural circuit that implements both Hering's law (motor correspondence) and Descartes–Sherrington's law (reciprocal innervation). For a rightward eye movement, the yoked agonist muscles contracted are the right lateral rectus and left medial rectus, and the antagonist muscles relaxed/inhibited are the left lateral rectus and right medial rectus. In the example shown, a signal to make a rightward saccade originates in the left hemisphere (cortex and colliculus) and is transmitted via the excitatory burst neurons (EBN) to the motoneurons of the right lateral rectus in n. VI (abducens). In order to also contract the yoked muscle in the left eye (the medial rectus), and thereby make the movement conjugate, a set of non-motor neurons in n. VI relay the movement signal to contralateral n. III (oculomotor). Reciprocal innervation (inhibition of the two antagonist muscles) is accomplished by inhibitory burst neurons (IBN) that project to the left n. VI and thereby both directly inhibit motoneurons of the left lateral rectus and indirectly diminish contraction in the right medial rectus via the n. VI to n. III projection. Similar circuits accomplish motor correspondence and reciprocal innervation for the other extraocular muscles in order to carry out conjugate vertical and torsional movements.

innervation, an inhibitory copy of the command signal is routed to the contralateral abducens, which relaxes the contralateral lateral rectus and, by the yoking circuit, relaxes the ipsilateral medial rectus as well.

For the remaining eight muscles, yoking is less obvious. Each superior oblique and the opposite inferior rectus constitute one yoked pair, and each inferior oblique and opposite superior rectus another.

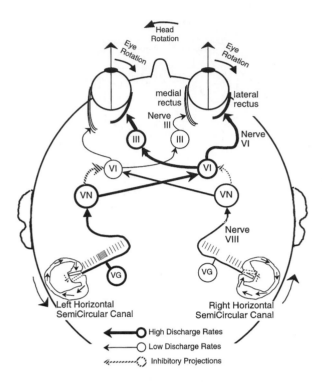

Figure 6 Neural circuit for the horizontal vestibuloocular reflex (VOR). The diagram depicts the rightward horizontal eye movements that compensate for leftward head rotation. The basic connectivity shown here serves all conjugate rightward eye movement (e.g., Fig. 5), regardless of the origin of the eye movement command signal. For the VOR, this signal originates in the semicircular canals and is communicated, via bipolar neurons in the vestibular ganglion (VG), to the vestibular nuclei (VN). The VN sends an excitatory projection to the contralateral oculomotor neurons in n. VI (abducens) and also sends an inhibitory projection to ipsilateral n. VI. The consequences of the increased activity from the left horizontal canal are reinforced by the decreased activity from the right horizontal canal, illustrating the push–pull operation of the canal pairs. An additional excitatory pathway (not illustrated) from the VN directly to the medial rectus motoneurons in ipsilateral n. III (oculomotor) gives the medial rectus its three-neuron VOR drive in addition to its four-neuron VOR drive via the contralateral n. VI.

These pairings reflect the true rotational axes of these muscles and their relation to the vestibular canals (Fig. 7).

3. Listing's and Donders' Laws and the Loss of Torsion

In primates torsional movements are severely constrained. For example, the human eye torts only a few degrees in response to a large sideways tilt (technically a "roll") of the head, whereas the rabbit eye torts up to

70°. The absence of significant torsional movement has an evolutionary advantage for stereoscopic vision.

Ocular torsion is classically summarized by the laws of Donders and Listing. Donders' law asserts that each eye direction (the combination of a particular azimuth and a particular elevation) has a unique torsion always associated with it, regardless of the sequence of eye movements used to achieve that particular azimuth/elevation. This has important implications. First, although it takes three coordinates to specify a general rotation, Donders' law means that the eye has only 2 degrees of freedom, and thus only two angles (azimuth and elevation) need be specified. This is analogous to navigation; longitude and latitude suffice, even though locations on the ocean surface have three coordinates in space. Second, whereas 3D rotations are not commutative, Donders' law stipulates that human eye movements effectively are commutative.

Listing's law asserts Donders' law and more because it specifies the particular torsion associated with any final eye direction, whereas Donders' law only ensured that this torsion is unique. To find the torsional position that the eye will always assume at a particular azimuth and elevation, Listing's law instructs to find the axis in the frontal plane through the center of the eye (Listing's plane) such that a single rotation about that axis takes the eye from the primary position to the particular azimuth and elevation in question. This single rotation will obtain the orientation that the eye will always have at that azimuth and elevation, no matter the sequence of eye movements actually used to get there. This means that the human eye has zero torsion following purely horizontal or purely vertical movements from the primary position (these are called "secondary" positions). However, for a typical oblique direction (a "tertiary" eye position) the eye appears to have undergone a torsional rotation because real-world vertical lines no longer fall along the vertical meridian of the retina when fixated. This is often called a "false torsion" because the eye did not have to make a true torsional movement about the line of sight but, rather, only a single rotation about an axis in Listing's plane, which is orthogonal to the torsional axis.

The role of the extraocular muscles in controlling ocular torsion is complex. The medial and lateral rectus have minimal torsional movements; however, as noted earlier, the four remaining muscles (inferior oblique, superior oblique, superior rectus, and inferior rectus) all have both vertical and torsional actions ("mixed" actions). Consequently, as Ewald Hering stated, elevation of gaze is effected "only by the cooperation of the superior rectus and the inferior

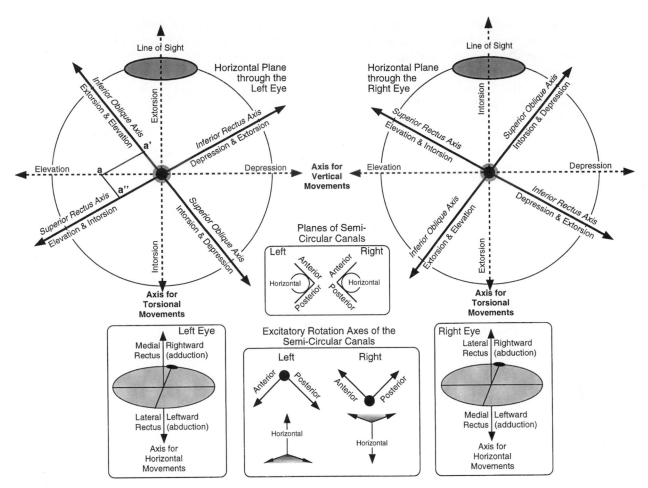

Figure 7   Rotational axes of the eye muscles and canals. (Top, left and right) The axis of rotation for all extraocular muscles, except for the medial and lateral rectus (bottom, left and right). For each muscle, the direction, or sign, of the eye rotation is given by the left-hand rule: Point the thumb along the arrow and the curve of the (slightly closed) fingers indicates the eye rotation. The rotation axes of the six semicircular canals (bottom middle) are perpendicular to the canal planes depicted above (upper middle) and show (by the left-hand rule) the eye rotation evoked by stimulation of individual canals. It is easy to see which muscle axis in each eye best aligns with each canal's axis; those muscles receive the three-neuron excitatory projection from that canal. Although in the primate, the eyes have migrated from the side of the head to the front, the canals are little changed, and the primate's extraocular muscles have maintained their rotation axes in correspondence with the canals axes. The figure also graphically depicts the rationale of yoking of the inferior oblique with the contralateral superior rectus and the superior oblique with the contralateral inferior rectus. The angular difference in both cases is far less than the difference between the left and right obliques axes or the left and right superior–inferior rectus axes. This figure was inspired by Fig. 51 in Hering (1942). His axis values, which were used here, have the axis of the superior–inferior rectus as being 29° off the axis for purely vertical movements and the axis of the superior–inferior obliques as being 38° off the torsional movement axis. The [a, a′, a″] parallelogram (top, left) is his geometrical construction of a pure elevation movement (with no torsion) from simultaneous contractions of the inferior oblique and superior rectus: Add the rotation axis vectors of these two muscles to obtain the axis for combined rotation.

oblique." Likewise, depression is effected by "cooperation of the inferior rectus with the superior oblique." This is analogous to lifting a barbell: If both arms lift with the same force, then the barbell will remain level, whereas if one arm exerts too much force then the barbell will tilt (tort) as it rises. Likewise, when the superior oblique and the inferior rectus are cocontracted, their downward forces are additive, but an extorsional force from increased tension in the superior oblique is canceled by an intorsional force from increased tension in the inferior oblique. Furthermore, the increased tension of the superior oblique and inferior rectus is always reciprocated by decreased tension of the inferior oblique and superior rectus, respectively. This results in a decrease in upward force, but with decreases in extorsion and intorsion canceling.

Thus, the eyes can move downward (or upward) with very little torsion, even though all four muscles involved have significant torsional actions.

Donders' and Listing's laws are not absolute or inherent in the passive properties of the eye. Large departures accompany convergence, head tilt, sleep, and certain neural pathologies. Torsional nystagmus, a clear violation of Donders' and Listing's laws, can be obtained with electrical stimulation of particular midbrain nuclei or individual canals and can also be a consequence of central disease.

IV. NEURAL CIRCUITS FOR EYE MOVEMENTS

A. Neural Circuitry of the Image-Stabilization System

The brain circuitry underlying image stabilization is organized around a vestibular apparatus in the temporal bone that can sense head rotations in any direction. The basic VOR is augmented by the OKR and several other specialized circuits, located in the brain stem and midline cerebellum, to become a very sophisticated system for minimizing retinal slip. These additional circuits are schematized in Fig. 8 and described next.

1. Circuit 1: The Three-Neuron Vestibuloocular Arc

How the brain fashions image-stabilization eye movements based on the vestibular sense has been extensively studied. Of prime importance is the vestibular sensory organ and the three-neuron arc composed of neurons in the vestibular ganglion, the vestibular nuclei, and the oculomotor nuclei.

On each side of the head within the labyrinth of the inner ear lie three semicircular canals filled with endolymph. Sensory receptor cells project hairs into a gelatinous mass, the cupula, that extends across the canal. When the head moves the bony canals move with it, but the endolymph lags behind, bending the cupula and the hairs embedded in it. Deforming the hairs hyperpolarizes their receptor cells for one direction of head rotation and depolarizes them for the opposite direction, and the resting discharge rate of bipolar neurons of the vestibular ganglion that innervate the receptor cells is modulated up or down by the receptor polarization (Fig. 6).

The central course of the bipolar cells' axons is the vestibular component of nerve VIII. They synapse in the vestibular nuclei, located in the medulla. Each canal projects to both the medial and the superior vestibular nucleus, and some vestibular afferents go directly to the cerebellum.

The three semicircular canals (horizontal, anterior, and posterior) lie in three different planes at approximately right angles to each other so that rotations of the head about any axis can be sensed. The planes of the three semicircular canals approximately correspond to the planes of action of the three pairs of extraocular muscles (Fig. 7), and the three-neuron pathway connects each canal to the extraocular muscles that move the eye in the canal's plane. This pathway was illustrated for the horizontal plane in Fig. 6. Horizontal head rotation excites the three-neuron pathway leading from the horizontal canal to the medial and lateral rectus, thus effecting an appropriate horizontal counterrotation of the eyes. Each canal also has a three-neuron inhibitory pathway to the corresponding antagonist muscles via inhibitory relay neurons in the vestibular nucleus. There are left and right sets of canals, and the symmetry of the VOR circuitry effectively uses the difference of the opposing signals from the left–right canal pair in each plane to increase the sensitivity of the VOR response, as shown in Fig. 6 for the horizontal canals.

The same principles hold for the anterior and posterior canals and the remaining four extraocular muscles, but in a less straightforward manner. The anterior and posterior canals lie in approximately vertical planes that are midway between the sagittal and coronal planes (Fig. 7). Thus, they do not correspond to the x–y–z axes of eye rotations described previously. Each anterior canal is paired with the contralateral posterior canal because they are in approximately the same plane and have the opposite responses to rotations in that plane. Also, each anterior–posterior pair controls a yoked pair of extraocular muscles that comes closest to its plane. For example, as can be deduced from Fig. 7, the excitatory three-neuron pathway of each anterior canal leads to the ipsilateral superior rectus muscle and the contralateral inferior oblique.

2. Circuit 2. Position Holding Mechanism (the "Neural Integrator")

The first problem for the basic three-neuron VOR circuit occurs when the head stops moving after a brief

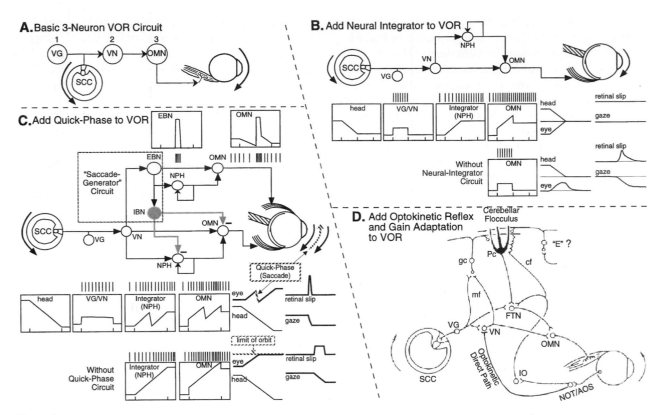

Figure 8 Neural circuits for image stabilization. (A) Basic three-neuron VOR circuit. Head rotations transduced by the semicircular canal (SCC) activate a three-neuron circuit that rotates the eye in the opposite direction. The circuit is as follows: neurons in the vestibular ganglion (VG) to neurons of the vestibular nuclei (VN) to oculomotor neurons (OMN) in one of the three oculomotor nuclei. (B) The VOR with the addition of a neural integrator. (Top) The neural integrator for horizontal eye movements is located in the n. prepositus hypoglossi (NPH) (and in the medial vestibular nucleus, which is not illustrated). Its integration function is symbolized by the recurrent connection of the NPH onto itself. (Middle) The plots show idealized spike rate functions for the components of this circuit, with idealized spikes above the plot boxes. With the neural integrator, retinal slip is minimal as gaze is held steady during and after the head movement. (Bottom) Without the integrator, the OMN does not cancel the elastic forces of the eye; thus, the eye slides back to the center of its orbit, both during and after the head movement, resulting in considerable retinal slip. (C) The quick-phase addition to the VOR. The quick-phase addition is symbolized by the inclusion of the saccade generator circuit with its excitatory (EBN) and inhibitory burst neurons (IBN) that enable the eye to be rapidly "reset" to the central position. Again, the plot boxes and spikes are hypothetical neural responses of the components of this circuit. (D) Addition of the optokinetic reflex (OKR) and a circuit for VOR gain adaptation. Visual motion signals from the nucleus of the optic tract (NOT) and the accessory optic system (AOS) go directly to the VN to add an OKR to the image-stabilization system. This OK signal is also sent to the inferior olivary nucleus (IO), and then to the cerebellar Purkinje cells (Pc) via their climbing fibers (cf). Likewise, the canal signal is relayed to the cerebellum's floccular Pc on mossy fibers (mf) that are axon collaterals of vestibular neurons via granule cells (gc) and their parallel T fibers. These inputs enable the flocculus to adaptively adjust VOR gain via its direct projections to the VN; the VN cells that receive this inhibitory projection are termed floccular target neurons (FTN). Pcs are also thought to receive a copy of the eye velocity signal, hence "E?" (adapted with permission from A. E. Luebke and D. A. Robinson, *Exp. Brain Res.* **98**, 379–390, 1994. Copyright © 1994 by Springer-Verlag).

turn. The canal signal quickly returns to baseline when the head stops moving because the cupula is no longer distended. However, if the innervation of the extraocular muscles also returns to its baseline level, then the elastic forces of the orbit would pull the eye back to the central position, thus negating the benefits of the VOR because vision would be blurred throughout this prolonged return.

Thus, for stable vision, the eye should not only stop rotating when the head stops turning but also must be held stationary at its current position and not slip back toward the central position. This is elegantly accomplished by the brain stem's neural integrator, a hypothesis of David Robinson, who reasoned that a command for eye position could be obtained by integrating eye velocity commands. Robinson's integrator now has a specific location, a neural signature (tonic activity coding static eye position), and distinctive neurological consequences of injury to it (e.g., gaze-evoked nystagmus).

The stabilization system, based on the VOR with the addition of the neural integrator, is shown in Fig. 8B, with the neural integrator represented by a local recurrent connection. Such a local recurrent connection was perhaps the earliest neural mechanism proposed for a short-term memory by Rafael Lorente de Nó and others. As the VOR "eye velocity signal" moves the eye, the integrator output grows, continually signaling where the eye should be held both during the VOR movement and after it. Thus, the neural integrator serves to exactly overcome the elastic force that accompanies increasingly eccentric eye rotations. Referring back to the equation $R_{OMN} = A \cdot (\theta - \theta_0) + B \cdot (d\theta/dt)$, the head velocity signal from the vestibular sensory nucleus is fed to the oculomotor nuclei as a command for eye velocity $(B \cdot (d\theta/dt))$ [where B is the synaptic strength] and the neural integrator obtains its eye position signal by integrating the eye velocity command, $d\theta/dt$, to obtain the $A \cdot (\theta - \theta_0)$ term for the OMN. This scheme is used for all types of eye movements: The command signal is formulated as a desired eye velocity (the velocity command hypothesis), and a common neural integrator integrates velocity commands of all types to continuously maintain the eye position signal.

3. Circuit 3. Quick Phases and Nystagmus

What if a large head rotation is made, or there are successive turns in the same direction? The eye can move only about 40–60° in any direction from its central position in the orbit. Thus, the VOR/neural integrator circuit will quickly drive the eye to the extreme of the orbit and the retinal image will begin to slip. Furthermore, in extreme orbital positions the eye's visual field is partially occluded.

Nature's solution is to periodically reset the eye back to the central position (usually slightly past it) during prolonged or large head rotations. Moving back to center results in considerable blur; however, the vertebrate solution is for the reset mechanism to recenter the eye as fast as possible in order to minimize the duration of the temporary blindness due to the high-velocity smearing of the retinal image. This requires near-maximal contraction of the agonist muscles coupled with complete relaxation of the antagonist muscles in order to produce eye movements approaching 1000°/sec and directed opposite the compensatory vestibuloocular movement.

The resets are obvious when prolonged rotation occurs, the resulting to-and-fro pattern of movement is called nystagmus (Fig. 9). In vestibular nystagmus, fast movements alternate with slow ones, yielding a characteristic sawtooth waveform. The slow phase is the compensatory reflex, and the rapid resets are called the quick phase. The quick-phase circuit is indicated by the addition of "burster" neurons in Fig. 8C. The excitatory burst neurons (EBNs), with their high spiking rate, project to the OMNs to realize the quick-phase movements. Actually, these EBNs are the output neurons of the "saccade generator" circuit, so labeled because it is appropriated by the foveation system to effect voluntary saccadic eye movements that are completely independent of the VOR. Moreover, the saccade generator is usually studied in the context of voluntary saccadic eye movements, in part because rotating subjects about different axes to achieve vestibular nystagmus can be a daunting experiment. Therefore, the saccade generator is further elaborated later in conjunction with voluntary saccades.

4. Circuit 4. The Optokinetic Reflex Complements the VOR

The VOR handles brief head movements very well, but it has trouble with prolonged rotation. This is because, with continued rotation of the head, the endolymph in the semicircular canals begins to catch up with the movement of the head, the cupula returns to its resting position, and hence the vestibular afferents return to their baseline rate, falsely indicating that the head is no longer rotating. Consequently, for continued rotation in the dark (or with the eyes closed) vestibular nystagmus will gradually slow down and completely stop after 30–60 sec. One solution to this problem of vestibular transducer adaptation is to let retinal slip help in driving this compensatory reflex. This is OKR, which is added to the basic VOR circuit in Fig. 8D. The principal sources of this retinal slip signal are two lesser known targets of the optic nerve: the nucleus of the optic tract (NOT) and the accessory optic system (AOS). Cells in these brain stem nuclei are tonically driven by the movement of large patterned visual stimuli, the best stimulus for eliciting OKR, with different neurons tuned to different directions of motion. In primates, the responses of these cells depends not only on their direct retinal inputs but also on pathways that involve neocortex, especially primary visual cortex and extrastriate motion areas. The direct and indirect projections of AOS/NOT to the vestibular nuclei complete the OKR circuit, which means that neurons in the vestibular nuclei also respond to visual (OK) stimuli. Moreover, despite

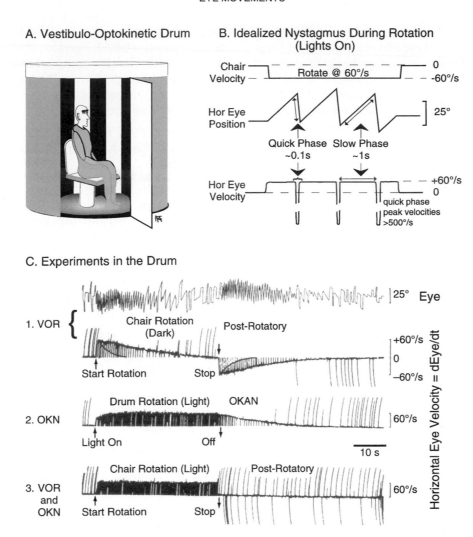

A. Vestibulo-Optokinetic Drum

B. Idealized Nystagmus During Rotation (Lights On)

C. Experiments in the Drum

Figure 9 The optokinetic reflex and nystagmus. (A) A depiction of a rotating chair and drum (with striped inner walls) used for testing the vestibuloocular (VOR) and optokinetic reflexes (OKRs), together and separately. Rotation of the drum (surround) alone, with illumination, elicits the OKR in a stationary subject. Rotation of the chair in the dark elicits the VOR. Rotation of the chair in the light activates both reflexes. (B) Idealized nystagmus during chair rotation with full illumination. (Top) The chair velocity plot indicates leftward rotation. (Middle) The horizontal (HOR) eye position record shows slow-phase movements, directed opposite the chair rotation, which compensate for the chair rotation, combined with quick-phase movements in the direction of rotation that periodically reset the eyes toward their central positions in the orbit. (Bottom) The "envelope" of the velocity trace also shows the rightward direction of slow-phase motion, which is quite distinct from the brief, high-velocity leftward-moving quick phase of the nystagmus. (C) Experimental nystagmus data (1) (Top trace) Horizontal eye movement record showing vestibuloocular nystagmus elicited by chair rotation in the dark. (Bottom trace) Eye velocity record from the same trial (see Fig. 9B). The velocity envelope shows that slow-phase rightward movements are elicited with a very short latency after rotation begins but taper off as rotation continues (adaptation). Note that the postrotatory response is in the opposite direction. The exponential dark lines, in both the adaptation and the postrotatory epochs plot the theoretical strength of the vestibular canal signal, which adapts much faster than the slow-phase velocity adapts. (2) Eye velocity during drum rotation in the light. Optokinetic nystagmus (OKN) refers to the combination of the slow-phase OKR response and the quick-phase resets. The OKN velocity envelope during rotation is similar to that of the VOR except that (i) there is no diminution in the response to ongoing rotation in the light and (ii) there is a more gradual rise time to the maximal slow-phase velocity. Also notice that the optokinetic after nystagmus (OKAN) is in the same direction as the OKN, whereas the postrotatory response was opposite the VOR. (3) Chair rotation in the light elicits both VOR and OKN responses. There is a quick rise in slow-phase velocity because of the VOR, no adaptation because of the OKN, and no postrotatory nystagmus because the OKAN cancels the postrotatory nystagmus from the canals (Fig. 9C adapted with permission from T. Raphan, V. Matsuo, and B. Cohen, *Exp. Brain Res.* **35,** 229, 1979. Copyright © 1979 by Springer-Verlag.

the addition of many refinements to the VOR, and the addition of new types of eye movements, the vestibular nuclei remain the principal gateway to the oculomotor nuclei.

Since the OKR is indefatigable, why not dispense with the VOR and base image-stabilization eye movements solely on the OKR? The reason is that the OKR is much slower to react than the VOR. OKR latency is 50–100 msec (reflecting the slow pace of visual processing), whereas VOR latency is ~10 msec. To demonstrate that OKR alone is poor, rotate the head left and right while reading. The text is legible because image stability is provided by the VOR. Now move the book left and right with the head still; the page will be blurred despite the OKR. This test hints at another reason the VOR is needed: Once a visual image is moving very fast across the retina, then it is blurred and hence is a poor stimulus for engaging the OKR in order to decrease its retinal slip and blur.

5. Circuit 5. Velocity Storage

VOR adaptation during prolonged rotation in the dark reflects the adaptation of the vestibular transducer in the semicircular canals. However, closer inspection of this phenomenon reveals that the vestibular apparatus adapts rapidly, with a time constant of ~6 sec, but the reflexive eye movement adapts with a much longer time constant (15–30 sec) (Fig. 9C.1). The reason is that a central neural process stores up the vestibular signal, thereby providing a more veridical representation of head motion than is provided by the raw VIIIth nerve signal.

This velocity-storage circuit stores optokinetic as well as the vestibular velocity (because they are merged in the vestibular nucleus). Indeed, the OKR does not stop immediately with the cessation of OK stimulation but continues, in the same direction, for several seconds after the lights go off (Fig. 9C.2). This continuation is called optokinetic afternystagmus (OKAN). Thus, the OKR is like charging a battery: It takes several seconds of stimulation for the OKR to reach its asymptote velocity (Fig. 9C.2) and to ensure robust OKAN after the optokinetic stimulation ceases.

This velocity storage underlies another aspect of the symbiosis between the VOR and the OKR regarding cessation of prolonged head rotations. If the VOR is adapted when rotation stops, the canal endolymph continues to move and produces a strong VOR in the opposite direction, called "postrotatory nystagmus" (Fig. 9C.1). It is accompanied by a loss of balance and vertigo and lasts several seconds. However, postrotatory nystagmus is best demonstrated by rotation in the dark so there can be no optokinetic stimulation. Indeed, there is usually no problem after rotation in the light (Fig. 9C.3) because OKAN serves to cancel postrotatory nystagmus.

6. Circuit 6. Gain Adjustment Mechanism for the VOR

Whereas the OKR is a closed-loop system in that the response cancels its own input signal, the VOR is an open-loop system because the counterrotation of the eye has no direct effect on the semicircular canal head-rotation signal. Also, because it is an open-loop system, the VOR reflex strength is critical. Ideally, VOR gain is exactly 1.0; however, it would seem too much for the genome to so completely specify the VOR circuitry so as to yield this ideal gain. Instead, an adaptation circuit continually adjusts VOR reflex strength so as to minimize the retinal image slippage that accompanies head movements. For example, wearing 2 × magnifying goggles for a few days will drastically increase VOR gain because 2 × goggles require that the VOR gain be 2.0 to cancel retinal slip when the head moves. In real life, less drastic but nevertheless critical adjustments of VOR strength need to be made—for example, when the head changes size during development, when people don spectacles (which more modestly magnify or minify the visual world), or whenever vestibular hair cells die or extraocular muscles weaken because of old age or other factors.

The crucial brain structure for VOR gain adaptation is the cerebellum, specifically the flocculonodular lobe that is interconnected with the vestibular nuclei that mediate the VOR (Fig. 8D). Monkeys without a cerebellum still have a robust VOR; however, VOR gain does not adapt in response to experimental goggles and other manipulations that induce adaptation in normal subjects. Other structures critical for VOR gain adaptation include the NOT and AOS, which provide an optokinetic signal not only directly to the vestibular nuclei but also to cerebellar cortex via the dorsal cap of the inferior olive. The overall goal of the gain-adjustment circuit (Fig. 8D) is to minimize the optokinetic signal that the cerebellum "sees"; the better the VOR works, the less the OKR is needed. Thus, the optokinetic signal serves two important purposes: It effects the OKR to assist the VOR and it provides the error signal for continually fine-tuning VOR gain.

B. Neural Circuitry of the Foveation System

The image-stabilization system (ISS) functions to ensure that the visual image as a whole is stationary on the retina. This suffices for many species, but with the evolution of the fovea came the need to deliberately shift the direction of gaze, independent of the ISS, in order to purposively foveate different stimuli. Because the foveal specialization covers only $\sim 1/10,000$ of the visual field, the eyes must be moved accurately. Furthermore, they must be moved intelligently to selected targets because systematic scanning of the whole visual field (like radar or television) would require hours and mostly be a waste of time. Therefore, the foveation system (FS) orchestrates eye movements that provide the fovea with an endless succession of the most important, informative, and pleasing visual stimuli.

As mentioned earlier, the primate FS uses three distinct eye movements: saccades, smooth pursuit, and fixation. These eye movements are voluntary in that they are controlled by, or made in the service of, the subject's choice to foveate a particular stimulus. In contrast, the ISS reflexively responds to the aggregate of vestibular and visual motion sensations and requires only a state of wakeful alertness.

Although choosing to foveate a particular stimulus is a voluntary action, doing so automatically activates the appropriate foveation subsystem(s). For example, after choosing to fixate a particular stationary target, (i) if the target moves quickly to a new location (e.g., a "step" motion), then a saccadic movement will be made in order to foveate it at its new location; (ii) if the target begins to smoothly move (e.g., "ramp" motion), then smooth-pursuit movements will match the target velocity and thereby both maintain foveation and reduce retinal blur; and (iii) if the target remains stationary, then fixation continues.

The cerebral cortex has a large role in these foveating eye movements. This seems obvious considering that occipital, temporal, and parietal neocortex are all heavily engaged in visual processing. Nor is involvement of the frontal lobe surprising, because the FS concerns voluntary movement. Although saccadic and smooth-pursuit eye movements are represented in separate cortical areas that have different subcortical projections, it is still likely that a common network of cortical areas mediates the target choice decisions for the FS as a whole.

Despite their functional differences, the FS and ISS engage the same basic brain stem neural circuits to effect eye movements. More precisely, the FS engages OMNs only indirectly via the ISS circuits: Voluntary saccadic eye movements exploit the quick-phase generating circuitry in the midbrain and pontine reticular formation and smooth-pursuit eye movements target the vestibular nuclei where the vestibulo-optokinetic velocity commands are assimilated. By engaging these established motor (as opposed to sensory) aspects of the ISS circuitry, foveating eye movements automatically achieve proper connectivity to the neural integrator in order to overcome elastic forces in the orbit and hold the eye steady wherever it has moved. Note that an important implication of this strategy is that the FS, like the ISS, ultimately formulates both its fast and slow eye movement objectives as eye velocity commands.

Usually the FS and the ISS work together; for example, while walking through a garden, saccades might foveate different flowers, with the VOR holding the image of each flower stationary on the retina despite movements of the head while walking. However, it is easy to pit the systems against each other, and in such situations the FS usually prevails. For example, given a small stationary spot in front of a background of moving stripes, one can elect to fixate the spot and thereby subdue the OKR ordinarily evoked by a large moving pattern. Conversely, given a moving spot on a stationary background of stripes, one can choose to pursue the spot smoothly across the stripes and the ensuing retinal slip of the pattern, caused by the pursuit eye movements, would be ignored. Finally, the FS can even suppress vestibular signals to move the eyes. For example, by looking at an object fixed relative to the head (e.g., the brim of a cap) and then rotating the head (like in Fig. 10), one can keep the brim fixated and thus keep the eye stationary in its orbit, despite the vestibular signals that indicate head rotation.

C. Neural Circuitry of Voluntary Saccades

The principal eye movement of the FS is the voluntary saccade. Humans average about two saccades/sec while awake, and thus most of the day is spent in brief fixations of different parts of the visual world, continually interrupted by saccades. This incessant visuomotor activity, the processing of foveal visual data during a fixation, as well as the planning and execution of the next saccade, occupies much of the human brain, as exemplified by the expansive zones of

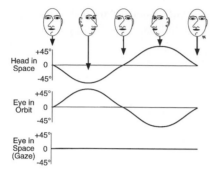

Figure 10 Retinal image stabilization during head rotation. As the head rotates about its vertical axis, the eyes reflexively rotate in the opposite direction to stabilize gaze, the direction of the eye in space. The two sinusoidal plots show the angular direction of the head in space (top) and the eye in its orbit (middle). The flat summation of these changes (bottom) signifies a steady gaze despite movements of the head.

cerebral activation revealed by functional magnetic resources imaging during simple and complex visuomotor tasks.

A few behavioral facts about saccades must be presented before considering their neural circuitry. First, saccades are open loop (i.e., ballistic and preprogrammed). As Gerald Westheimer stated, "once initiated, saccadic movements complete their predetermined course and cannot be modified or countermanded." In fact, 50–100 msec prior to its start, the saccade generally cannot be canceled or redirected on the basis of new sensory information. Second, saccades have long reaction times. Saccadic latency, the time from the appearance of an unpredictable visual target to the start of the movement, is 100–400 msec (200 msec being typical). Third, saccades have a long refractory period. It is usually difficult to initiate a second saccade for 100–200 ms after the previous saccadic movement ends. Fourth, saccades are highly stereotyped movements. Thus, the saccadic waveform and its parameters (duration, velocity, etc.) are almost completely determined by the dimensions of the movement vector being programmed. Finally, although saccades to foveate a stimulus can seem reflexive, and have been termed the visual grasp reflex, one can make accurate and advantageous predictive saccades that anticipate where a stimulus will appear. Thus, saccades can be guided by our experience, memories, guesses, purposes, and strategies as well as by overt visual stimulation.

1. The Saccade Generator

The first four properties mentioned previously reflect the fact that all saccades are ultimately "generated" or programmed in a very rigid, mechanistic fashion by a specialized circuit in the brain stem. This final common pathway for all rapid eye movements, called the saccade generator, is a network of several distinctive types of neurons embedded within the reticular formation near the oculomotor nuclei. This network originally evolved to generate the quick-phase movements of vestibulooptokinetic nystagmus. Thus, voluntary saccades of primates are accomplished by the relatively new FS triggering this ISS circuitry. If the saccade generator is damaged, then all rapid eye movements, both reflexive and voluntary, are disabled.

To accomplish a saccadic eye movement, the OMNs of the agonist muscle(s) need a special waveform of innervation: a pulse followed by a step. The pulse is a brief period of spiking at a very high rate, which is used to move the eye very quickly to its new location. The step is the new level of tonic discharge needed to hold the eye at its new location in the orbit. This pulse–step innervation is inherent in the OMN equation given earlier, and is illustrated in Fig. 11. Not shown is the fact that the pulse briefly but completely silences most OMNs of the antagonist muscles via inhibitory interneurons termed inhibitory burst neurons. This brief silence is also inherent in the basic OMN equation reviewed previously.

The pulse is provided by the principal output neuron of the saccade generator—the excitatory burst neuron (EBN). EBNs discharge with a high-frequency burst of spikes in conjunction with all saccadic eye movements and are silent between saccades. Their bursts begin ~12 msec before the eye starts to move (they have also been called short-lead bursters) and end just before the eye completes the saccade. Horizontal EBNs are located in the caudal portion of the paramedian pontine reticular formation, conveniently near the abducens nucleus. Their spike counts during each burst determine the horizontal displacement of the saccade (in the ipsilateral direction). Vertical EBNs are located in the rostral interstitial nucleus of the medial longitudinal fasciculus, with separate sets of neurons for the upward and downward components. Other EBNs here also represent torsional saccadic eye movements.

The tonic "step" change in the OMN innervation is provided by the neural integrator that adds the pulse (EBN spikes) to its current value and then maintains that new value. Thus, when each saccade is made, the

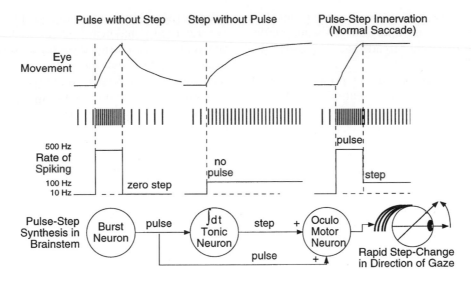

Figure 11   Pulse-step innervation of oculomotor neurons. A schematic showing eye position (top) and spike rates of burst and tonic neurons (middle) for real and hypothetical conditions producing abnormal and normal saccades. (Left) Given pulse activity but no tonic activity (step) to defend the new eye position, the eye slides back to its starting position (e.g., gaze-evoked nystagmus). (Middle) In the hypothetical case of a damaged pulse generator, the tonic/step activity alone causes very slow eye movements that "glide" exponentially to a target. (Bottom) Circuit diagram for pulse–step innervation of oculomotor neurons and the generation of saccades. The excitatory burst neurons are activated by signals from higher levels (e.g., the superior colliculus and frontal eye field). The activity of tonic neurons reflects ongoing integration of all eye velocity commands by neural integrator circuits in the pons and midbrain. Oculomotor neurons sum these phasic and tonic inputs to produce a high-velocity saccade and then to hold this new eye position.

neural integrator quickly "steps" from its old pre-saccadic level of activity to a new postsaccadic level. In contrast, the response of the neural integrator to a low-velocity long-duration signal from the VOR command is a "ramp" change in output rate. This short-term memory mechanism has been successfully modeled with recurrent neural networks and thus is schematized as a single recurrent feedback connection (Fig. 8C).

Several cell types antecedent to the EBNs have been identified. One of the most remarkable types is the omnipause neuron (OPN). The tonic activity of these inhibitory (glycine) neurons has the critical job of keeping all EBNs totally silent during the intervals between saccades. If EBNs had even a low spontaneous rate when not bursting, then the neural integrator would generate random "walks" between saccades instead of providing steady fixations. Only when OPNs temporarily stop spiking (which they briefly do in conjunction with all saccades, regardless of saccade size or direction) are EBNs given an opportunity to discharge. In fact, electrical stimulation at the OPN locus (nucleus raphe interpositus along the midline of the pons) during a saccadic eye movement will immediately brake the eye and (prematurely) end

the saccade, and continuous stimulation there prevents all rapid eye movements, but not slow eye movements, such as the VOR or smooth pursuit. Detailed consideration of OPNs and the other cell types that complete the saccade generator circuit are beyond the scope of this article.

2. Visually Guided Saccades and the Superior Colliculus

How can the brain stem's saccade generator be activated to produce useful saccades in the absence of head movements and VO/OK stimulation? The exemplar structure for this function is the superior colliculus (SC), which forms the roof of the midbrain. The SC is the mammalian version of the optic tectum, which is the vertebrate brain's prototype sensorimotor structure. The SC receives a strong projection directly from the retina as well as afferents from most other senses (auditory, somatosensory, etc.), and its efferents to the brain stem and spinal cord serve to orient the head and body toward localized sensory inputs. In the primate, and other mammals with a foveation system, a major role of the SC is to move visual stimuli appearing in the visual periphery into the foveal region of the retina by triggering a saccadic eye movement of the appropriate size and direction. This automatic, visually guided foveating saccade has been called the visual grasp reflex.

The functional anatomy of the primate SC that affords such visually guided foveation is forthright (Fig. 12): Neurons in the superficial layer of the primate SC constitute a topographic map of the contralateral visual hemifield (Fig. 12B; interestingly, this is only true of primates—for all other vertebrates each SC represents the entire contralateral eye). Neurons in the deeper, intermediate layer of the primate SC provide a topographic map of all contralaterally directed saccade vectors. These sensory and

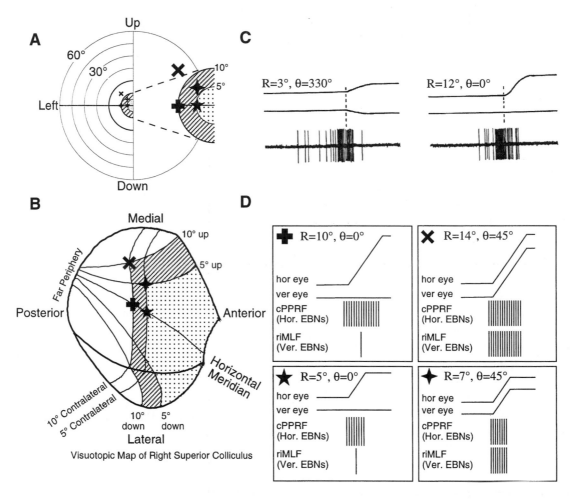

Figure 12 Spatial-to-temporal transformation of saccade vectors. Depiction of the necessity of a spatial-to-temporal transformation as saccade commands are relayed from the superior colliculus (SC) to the saccade generator, but the figure does not show how it is accomplished. (A) Spatial representation of four hypothetical visual stimuli. The stimuli are within the central-most 10° of the diagram and the dashed lines lead to enlargement of this region. (B) A visuotopic map of the SC showing the idealized representations of the visual stimuli depicted in A on the surface of the SC. Note that more than half the SC is used to map the central 10° (adapted with permission from M. Cynader and N. Berman, *J. Neurophysiol.* **35**, 187, 1972). (C) Saccade-related burst cells in the deeper SC layers code saccadic eye movements via their location in its spatial map of the contralateral visual hemifield. The top two traces are horizontal and vertical eye coordinates, and the bottom traces are spikes. These cells burst most robustly prior to a saccade matching their preferred vector (reprinted from D. L. Sparks, *Brain Res.* **156**, 1, copyright 1978, with permission from Elsevier Science). (D) Hypothetical response of the excitatory burst neurons (EBNs), the output stage of the saccade generator, to the visual stimuli shown in A and B. Top traces are eye position, and lower traces are the bursts of horizontal (Hor) EBNs [in the caudal paramedian pontine reticular formation (PPRF)] and vertical (Ver) EBNs [in the rostral interstitial nucleus of the medial longitudinal fasciculus (riMLF)]. Saccade dimensions are a quasilinear function of the number of spikes in the bursts. Since EBNs usually burst at near-maximal rates, their spike count is largely a function of burst duration, just as saccade size is largely a function of saccade duration. In contrast, the burst duration of the saccade-related bursters in the SC is independent of saccade size or duration.

motor maps are in perfect register for making foveating saccades. For example, if recording from a superficial layer neuron located near the center of the left SC, the visual response field center would be 10° right of the fixation point (cross in Fig. 12B). If the microelectrode were then advanced into the underlying intermediate layer, it would record a "saccade-related burst neuron" that responds optimally (i.e., has the most spikes in its burst) immediately prior to 10° rightward saccades (Fig. 12C), exactly the saccade needed to foveate visual stimuli appearing in the superficial (layer) neuron's visual response field (RF). Moreover, electrical stimulation there would yield a 10° rightward saccade as well.

3. Transformation from Spatial Code to Temporal Code

Saccades are clearly "spatially" coded in the SC in that the saccade vector is determined by which part of collicular "space" has active saccade-related bursters. In contrast, the output cells of the saccade generator, the EBNs, use a "temporal" code for saccade metrics: Saccade size is coded by the spike counts in their bursts (Fig. 12D) and not by which (or where) EBNs are spiking most. Exactly how this spatial-to-temporal transformation is carried out is unclear. Moreover, the cortical eye field signals need the same spatial-to-temporal transformation, and neither the cortex nor the colliculus projects directly to the EBNs. Another class of saccade generator neurons, the long-lead burst neurons (LLBNs), seem to be an intermediate stage in this transformation. LLBNs do receive direct projections from the SC and FEF. Moreover, individual LLBNs often prefer saccades with specific oblique directions and amplitudes, like SC and FEF neurons but unlike EBNs.

D. Cortical Eye Fields and Saccades

1. Cortical Pathways for Visually Guided Saccades

In primates, the cerebral cortex is a very important part of the saccadic circuitry. Although the SC seems to be the premier structure for visually guided saccades, it is not a critical component of saccade generation because the effects of SC lesions are largely transient, whereas the saccade structures downstream are vital. Thus, lesions of the saccade generator structures in the pontine and midbrain reticular formation permanently eliminate all rapid eye movements, including visually guided saccades, whereas SC lesions do not eliminate visually guided saccades at all. Following an acute period of visual neglect, there are few lasting oculomotor deficits following SC lesions in monkeys and man, with the most consistent lasting deficit being a modest increase in latency of visually guided saccades.

Visually guided saccades survive SC lesions because the primate also has an elaborate neocortical network for visually guided saccades. The connectivity diagram of Fig. 13 summarizes these cortical pathways and helps explain most effects of experimental lesions. For example, the sparing of visually guided saccades following SC lesions is mediated by FEF projections to the brain stem saccade generator; however, the SC normally provides a shorter path via its direct retinal projections, which explains the increase in saccade latency after SC damage. FEF lesions alone also spare visually guided saccades; however, FEF lesions combined with SC lesions eliminate most visually guided saccades. Thus, the SC and FEF provide parallel pathways for visual stimuli to activate the brain stem saccade generator for the purpose of accurate, foveating saccades. It is also the case that visually guided saccades are spared following lesions of primary visual cortex (V1) even though conscious awareness of the visual world is lost. However, combined V1 and SC lesions eliminate visually guided saccades most likely because, as Fig. 13 indicates, V1 removal eliminates most visual inputs to FEF and, hence, renders FEF incapable of triggering visually guided saccades.

2. Frontal Eye Field Anatomy and Physiology

David Ferrier discovered (~1875) that electrical stimulation in the frontal lobe of macaque monkeys deviated the eyes toward the contralateral side, and it was soon confirmed that many primate species, including man, have such an FEF. These electrically elicited eye movements are indistinguishable from naturally occurring saccadic eye movements, and each site in FEF yields saccades of a characteristic direction and amplitude, with the set of all possible contralaterally directed saccades represented in each hemisphere's FEF. The macaque FEF lies primarily in the anterior bank of the arcuate sulcus; the human FEF lies in the precentral sulcus, behind the middle frontal gyrus and in front of the hand representation in the precentral gyrus (Fig. 14).

FEF is not the only cortex specialized for eye movements. There is also the parietal eye field (PEF),

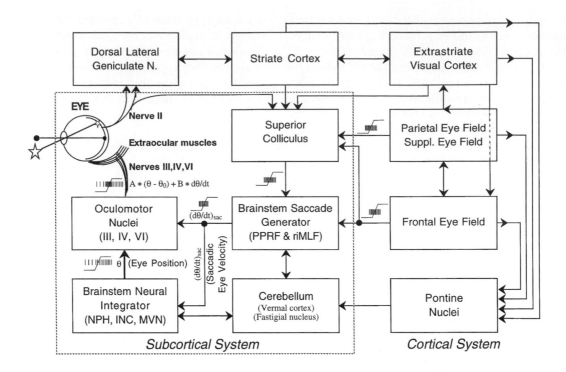

Figure 13 Pathways for visually guided saccades. Anatomical connections between cortical and subcortical structures involved in the control and generation of saccadic eye movements. The frontal eye field (FEF) receives visual information via pathways originating in the striate cortex, as does the parietal eye field (PEF) and the supplementary eye field (SEF). Notice that all these cortical areas project to the superior colliculus (SC), with FEF, PEF, and SEF all projecting primarily to its intermediate layers. In contrast, the superficial layers of SC receive direct visual projections from the retina and indirect visual projections from the striate and extrastriate cortices. The brain stem saccade generator is in the paramedian pontine reticular formation (PPRF) and in the rostral interstitial nucleus of the medial longitudinal fasciculus (riMLF). The brain stem neural integrator is in the medial vestibular nucleus (MVN), the adjacent nucleus prepositus hypoglossi (NPH), and the interstitial nucleus of Cajal (INC). Additional structures and pathways involved in saccades, such as the thalamus and basal ganglia, are omitted for simplicity.

located in the lateral bank of the intraparietal sulcus in the macaque, and the supplementary eye field (SEF), located in the frontal lobe near the midline. FEF, SEF, and PEF are reciprocally interconnected with each other; however, FEF seems to be the principal cortical eye field. FEF has the lowest thresholds for electrically elicited saccades, oculomotor behavior after FEF lesions is generally more impaired than after lesions of the other eye fields, and FEF is indispensable for visually guided saccades if the SC is damaged.

3. Effects of FEF Lesions

Gordon Holmes found that patients with frontal lesions had difficulty moving their eyes in response to verbal commands, even though they could follow visual objects and understood the verbal commands. In a 1938 lecture, he concluded that "the frontal centers make possible the turning of gaze in any desired direction and the exploration of space, but they also keep under control, or inhibit, reflexes that are not appropriate." In 1985, Daniel Guitton and colleagues used the antisaccade paradigm to demonstrate that "frontal lobe lesions in man cause difficulties in suppressing reflexive glances and in generating goal-directed saccades." In other words, their subjects could not launch saccades in the direction opposite the visual target (antisaccades), even though they understood that to be the task. Instead, they made inappropriate saccades toward the visual targets (prosaccades), exactly what they were instructed not to do. Similarly, subjects with FEF lesions have difficulty making memory saccades and in making predictive saccades to square-wave target motion. Thus, lesion studies show that FEF is important for "purposive" saccades, particularly when there is no visual target present to trigger the visual grasp reflex.

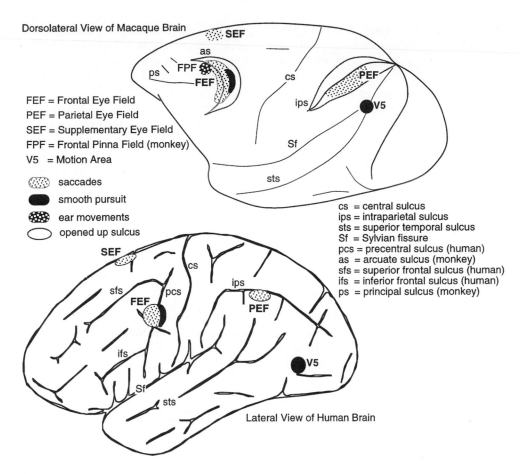

Dorsolateral View of Macaque Brain

FEF = Frontal Eye Field
PEF = Parietal Eye Field
SEF = Supplementary Eye Field
FPF = Frontal Pinna Field (monkey)
V5 = Motion Area

saccades
smooth pursuit
ear movements
opened up sulcus

cs = central sulcus
ips = intraparietal sulcus
sts = superior temporal sulcus
Sf = Sylvian fissure
pcs = precentral sulcus (human)
as = arcuate sulcus (monkey)
sfs = superior frontal sulcus (human)
ifs = inferior frontal sulcus (human)
ps = principal sulcus (monkey)

Lateral View of Human Brain

Figure 14 Cortex for eye movements in man and monkey. Cortical regions important for saccade and smooth-pursuit eye movements are highlighted on lateral views of a monkey brain (top) and human brain (bottom). In both monkey and man, FEF is in front of premotor cortex for the hand and neck and mostly lies within the sulcus marking the anterior limit of the precentral gyrus. In both species, the smooth-pursuit region of FEF is just posterior to the saccadic region of FEF. A dorsolateral view is used for the monkey brain in order to minimize distortion of the frontal lobe sulci.

4. FEF Bursts Precede All Types of Purposive Saccades

During the past three decades, single-neuron recordings in trained macaque monkeys have resulted in a detailed picture of FEF activity during all manner of voluntary oculomotor behavior. Presaccadic bursts are the signature activity of FEF and are manifest in more than 30% of FEF neurons. These bursts begin prior to saccade initiation, usually end sharply just after the saccade is completed, and are always tuned for particular saccade vectors, similar to saccade related bursters in the SC and vectorial LLBNs in the pons. Presaccadic bursts seem to constitute the FEF command to the saccade generator (both directly and through the SC), providing both an impetus to saccade and a saccade vector specification. Indeed, electrical stimulation through a recording microelectrode in FEF elicits natural-looking saccades that closely match the vector for the optimal presaccadic burst of nearby cells. Moreover, FEF-elicited saccades are very insistent and are still elicited with low currents even when subjects are intently fixating a stationary light.

a. Visually Guided Saccades FEF neurons have robust presaccadic bursts in conjunction with visually guided saccades. The average response of 51 FEF cells recorded in a single monkey during a "stable-target" type of saccade task is shown in Fig. 15A. This task was chosen to separate any phasic visual response to the appearance of the peripheral target from the presaccadic burst. This provides a baseline for assessing presaccadic bursts made without an overt target.

b. Memory Saccades Presaccadic bursts of FEF neurons in conjunction with saccades made to remembered targets are generally equivalent to bursts associated with visually guided saccades on the stable-target task. In this paradigm, as shown for a representative visuomovement neuron in Fig. 15B, a peripheral cue appears only briefly, and the saccade is made some time later and hence must be guided by a short-term memory of the cue.

c. Antisaccades FEF neurons also have robust presaccadic bursts in conjunction with antisaccades, as shown in Fig. 15C for another representative visuomovement neuron. The cell discharged preceding antisaccades into its visuomovement RF, even though the visual cue had been on the opposite side and thus not at all in the cell's RF.

d. Other Purposive Saccades FEF cells have also been demonstrated to reliably burst for some other types of purposive saccades (e.g., saccades made to the locations of sounds). It is interesting to speculate that FEF lesions might disrupt socially motivated saccades and that FEF cells would burst in conjunction with such saccades, but this has not been tested.

e. Spontaneous Saccades In contrast with most purposive saccades, FEF bursts are usually weaker in conjunction with spontaneous saccades made in the dark, presumably because such saccades are usually not purposive.

5. FEF Activities and Circuits

Just as the basic VOR reflex has a set of associated assisting circuits, a diverse set of functional activities and cortical circuits underlie FEF's programming of purposive saccades in the monkey. These serve to facilitate the generation of appropriate presaccadic bursts in diverse situations and paradigms.

a. Visual Activity More than half the neurons in FEF are visually responsive. Typically, they have large RFs centered in the contralateral hemifield and respond to the appearance of any stimulus within their RF, without much selectivity for color or form. Moreover, FEF visual responses do not require overt attention to the stimulus or the RF location or that the stimulus has functional significance to the monkey.

b. Alignment of Visual and Presaccadic Movement Fields Visuomovement FEF cells have both visual and presaccadic burst activities, and their visual RF generally corresponds with the optimal saccade vector for their burst (i.e., movement field) and also to the electrically elicited saccadic eye movement vector obtained at the cell's location. Thus, the FEF default is a foveating saccade. However, the presaccadic burst is independent of the location and/or the presence of RF stimulation as shown by the memory saccade and antisaccade tasks (Fig. 15B,C). Moreover, a minority of FEF cells are discordant with nonmatching, or even nonoverlapping, visual and movement fields.

c. Tonic Visual Activity The strongest aggregate visual response in FEF is to the initial appearance of visual targets, and many visual cells only respond to this appearance. However, other visual cells tonically respond as long as the target remains in their RF. Notice in Fig. 15A that the composite spike rate was elevated throughout the wait period (between the phasic visual response and the eventual presaccadic burst). Thus, FEF visual activity can guide saccades to old, "stable" visual targets as well as newly appearing targets.

d. Mnemonic Activity Usually tonic visual FEF activity is maintained even after the visual cue is extinguished, and this activity could provide a short-term memory of the visual cue location in the memory saccade test. Many individual FEF cells have robust mnemonic responses (Fig. 15B). However, when many FEF cells are averaged, the mnemonic signal is only a modest elevation of the overall spike rate, especially when compared to the size of the presaccadic burst. Tonic neural activity has a high metabolic cost; therefore, it is economical for overall tonic visual and tonic mnemonic activity to be minimal—just robust enough to inform spatially appropriate saccades whenever the go signal finally arrives.

e. Postsaccadic Activity Coding Executed Saccades (Efferent Copy) Postsaccadic activity in the FEF was first described by Emilio Bizzi, and ~25% of FEF neurons are excited after particular saccadic eye movements. This postsaccadic activity seems to be an efferent copy of saccades actually executed because it reliably follows every saccade made into the cell's postsaccadic movement field, even spontaneous saccades made in the dark or rapid phases of nystagmus. A timely efferent copy of saccadic displacements, as coded by postsaccadic activity in FEF, is critical for several of the following circuits. Interestingly, many FEF cells with presaccadic (visual, movement, or

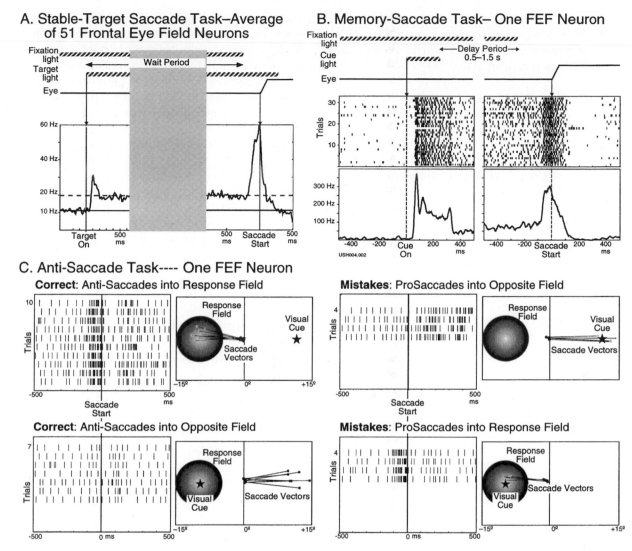

A. Stable-Target Saccade Task–Average of 51 Frontal Eye Field Neurons

B. Memory-Saccade Task– One FEF Neuron

C. Anti-Saccade Task---- One FEF Neuron

Correct: Anti-Saccades into Response Field

Mistakes: ProSaccades into Opposite Field

Correct: Anti-Saccades into Opposite Field

Mistakes: ProSaccades into Response Field

Figure 15 Frontal eye field activity for purposive saccades. (A) Aggregate activity of 51 FEF neurons recorded from one monkey during the stable-target type of visually guided saccade task. (Top) Task events: Shortly after the monkey fixates a central light, a peripheral target appears in the neuron's response field (RF). This target remains on for the remainder of the trial, but no saccade is permitted until the fixation light is extinguished at the end of the wait period. Thus, the target is a stable presence at the time of the saccade. (Bottom) The histogram aligned on the target appearance (left) shows the aggregate visual response. The histogram aligned on the saccade start (right) shows the large aggregate burst that starts just prior to the saccade. Thus, FEF activity manifests both visual (phasic and tonic) and movement activities (H. R. Friedman and C. J. Bruce, unpublished data). (B) Activity of a visuomovement FEF neuron from a second monkey tested on memory–saccade task. (Top) Task events: Shortly after the monkey fixates a central light, a peripheral cue briefly appears. Then, after a delay period, the fixation light is extinguished and the monkey must saccade to the location where the peripheral cue had been shown earlier. Thus, unlike in A, there is no visual target present at the time of the saccade. (Bottom) Rasters (by trial) and histograms of spike activity aligned on cue onset (left) show the burst of activity elicited by the visual stimulus and aligned on saccade onset (right) show the large burst of activity preceding the saccades. Note that the visual response has three components: a phasic high-rate burst to the initial appearance of the visual stimulus (with a latency of ∼ 50 msec), a robust tonic visual discharge while the cue remained on, and then, starting ∼ 50 msec after the cue was extinguished, a medium-level tonic mnemonic response that was maintained above the cell's baseline level of activity throughout the delay interval (M. S. Kraus, H. R. Friedman, and C. J. Bruce, unpublished data). (C) Activity of a visuomovement FEF neuron, from a third monkey, tested on an antisaccade task (memory version). As in B, the monkey must remember the position of a brief visual cue across a delay interval. However, unlike in B, the correct response (once the fixation light goes off) is a saccade to the location opposite to where the cue was shown. The visual RF of this cell was on the left when tested with conventional "prosaccade" tasks and its presaccadic bursts were maximal for leftward saccades. (Top, left) The cell discharged preceding leftward antisaccades, even though the visual cue had been in the right side and thus not in its RF. (Bottom, left) The neuron was silent before rightward antisaccades even though the visual cue had been in its RF. Interestingly, its bursts were completely predictive of erroneous prosaccades mistakenly made on some trials (right). (H. R. Friedman and C. J. Bruce, unpublished data).

both) activity also have postsaccadic activity for saccades directed opposite their presaccadic RF. This provides a mechanism for readily returning to the previous fixation (i.e., glances).

f. Suppression of Presaccadic Activities by Saccade Execution A striking aspect of FEF presaccadic activity of all types (e.g., anticipatory, visual, mnemonic, and movement) is that it quickly ceases upon the execution of a saccade into the RF. Notice in Fig. 15 that saccade execution actively suppresses both tonic visual (Fig. 15A) and mnemonic (Fig. 15B) activity as well as the presaccadic bursts.

This suppression could come from the postsaccadic coding of prior saccades (efferent copy) previously described. Such suppression is very important because visual or mnemonic activity coding a peripheral cue location becomes invalid once the monkey foveates the peripheral location. Without prompt suppression, persistent activity could lead to multiple triggering of the same saccade, much like the "staircase" of saccades evoked by continued electrical stimulation in FEF.

g. Fixation Status Signals (Tonic Foveation and Eye Position Activity) Some FEF cells provide tonic signals concerning the current fixation target rather than pertaining to possible saccade targets. One class is excited by fixation (foveal) stimulation; their activity could play a role in suppressing other saccade cells in FEF and elsewhere in the interest of maintaining fixation. Another class has the inverse activity, being suppressed by foveal stimulation and active thereafter, and thus signaling the extinction of the current fixation light. A small minority of cells tonically respond as a linear function of absolute eye position (e.g., elevation); they could be receiving an efferent copy from the common neural integrator, and some have foveal responses that are modulated by the current eye position.

h. Other Saccade-Related Activities and Responses Many FEF cells show anticipatory activity for predictable saccadic situations. This activity could decrease saccade latency by biasing FEF in favor of the predicted saccade dimensions. Sometimes, anticipatory activity is purely guessing. For example, in the "gap" paradigm, wherein the signal to saccade (e.g., fixation light off) precedes the peripheral target appearance by 100–200 msec, FEF neurons with presaccadic motor bursts will first discharge at an intermediate level in response to the fixation light extinction and then drastically accelerate or suppress

their rate after the peripheral target comes in the neuron's RF or opposite it. Saccade latencies in the gap paradigm are typically shorter than in conventional saccade tasks and are termed express saccades.

Cells in and near the medial FEF have responses to sound. Their auditory RFs are partially remapped from a craniocentric to a retinocentric framework, which should facilitate FEF bursts known to precede aurally guided saccades. Moreover, there is a pinna movement region adjacent to the medial FEF of the monkey (Fig. 14).

Finally, saccades to moving targets are usually directed at a predicted target location, based on both retinal position and velocity. Visual and movement RFs of FEF neurons evidence this predictive process, indicating that target motion information is being utilized.

E. Neural Circuitry of Smooth Pursuit

1. Tracking with Pursuit and Saccades

Smooth-pursuit eye movements support scrutiny of objects moving in space by matching eye velocity to target velocity in order to both reduce retinal blur of the moving object and facilitate its continued foveation. Smooth pursuit occurs when the FS selects a moving target or when a previously selected stationary target starts to move. However, target selection for pursuit also activates the saccadic system; hence, moving targets are usually tracked with a combination of smooth pursuit and saccades, with these two eye movement systems operating independently but synergistically to track the same chosen target (Fig. 2). Their synergy reflects control by separate parameters of the target's trajectory. The principal impetus for smooth pursuit is target velocity (i.e., retinal slip), and the pursuit system continuously endeavors to eliminate retinal slip by matching eye velocity to target velocity. In contrast, the principal concern of the saccade system is target position (i.e., retinal error), and saccades are intermittently generated to eliminate retinal error by foveating the target.

However, this division of labor is not absolute. Smooth pursuit is modestly affected by positional errors: Ongoing pursuit accelerates in response to small retinal positional errors, and it is even possible to initiate smooth pursuit with an afterimage placed near the fovea (although eccentric afterimages are usually tracked with a succession of saccades). The pursuit system also responds to the rate of change in retinal slip (i.e., acceleration). Thus, pursuit is a function of the zero-, first-, and second-order derivatives of the target's retinal image.

Conversely, the saccadic system attends to target velocity as well as location. Saccadic latency is shorter for targets moving centrifugally (away from the fixation point) and longer for targets moving centripetally. Moreover, saccades are usually directed to a predicted target location based on its position and velocity as acquired 100–200 msec before the saccadic movement starts.

Pursuit velocity ranges up to ~100°/sec; however, pursuit gain (defined, like VO and OK gain, as eye velocity/target velocity) is generally poor for target velocities above 25°/sec. When the pursuit gain is low, the eye will persistently fall behind the target and frequent, large "catch-up" saccades will be made; however, if gain is high (~1.0), then only a few, small saccades may be needed.

Interestingly, low smooth-pursuit gain is the principal symptom of the eye tracking dysfunction (ETD) of schizophrenia. Subsequent research has shown a cluster of oculomotor impairments that covary across the schizophrenic patient population and are often also present in first-degree relatives of schizophrenic patients. On the basis of the ETD and other cognitive aspects of schizophrenia, it has been hypothesized that schizophrenia reflects diminished frontal lobe function in general, and that the ETD specifically reflects impaired function in both the saccadic and the smooth-pursuit regions of the FEF.

2. Smooth Pursuit versus Optokinetic Following

Smooth pursuit can be confused with the OKR because both provide smooth, nonsaccadic ocular following in response to visual motion. However, the OKR is an automatic response to motion of large parts of the visual world (e.g., watching a train go by), whereas pursuit is the voluntary tracking of a discrete moving object (e.g., a bird flying across the sky).

In typical situations, smooth pursuit is in direct opposition to the OKR (and often to the VOR as well), and we choose to maintain foveation of the pursued target stimulus and reduce its retinal slip at the expense of increasing retinal blur of the rest of the visual field. For example, pursuit will need to override the OKR whenever tracking a target moving across a patterned background because as soon as pursuit starts the background necessarily becomes a stimulus for OKR in the opposite direction. Similarly, during combined head–eye tracking of a moving stimulus, the combined vestibulooptokinetic reflex must be overcome.

3. The Neural Pathway for Pursuit

The major pathways of the smooth-pursuit system are shown in Fig. 16. On the sensory and decision-making side, smooth pursuit is very much a neocortical behavior. It begins with the high-quality visual map in V1 that sends visual motion information into area V5 and other immediate extrastriate areas. Motion information is relayed to several other areas in the parietal and temporal lobe and to the smooth-pursuit zone of FEF. These cortical areas relay their visual motion signals and commands to oculomotor parts of the cerebellum, principally by way of their projections to the dorsolateral and medial pontine nuclei.

On the efferent side of the pursuit pathway, smooth movements are created by engaging the brain stem substrate for the slow-phase, compensatory part of VOR, much as visually guided saccades are made by engaging the mechanism that generates the quick phases of vestibuloocular nystagmus. Specifically, pursuit uses the VOR adaptation circuit that was shown in Fig. 8D. The key neurons are the Purkinje

Figure 17 Ac[...]
FEF, was activ[...]
all three cycles [...]
of sinusoidal tr[...]
three spikes on [...]
Sinusoidal (1.0 [...]
following a sma[...]
cycle, especially[...]
Friedman, and [...]

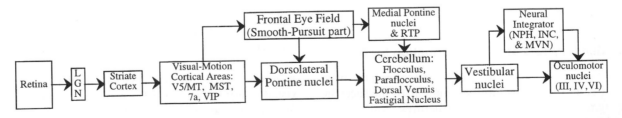

Figure 16 Pathways for smooth-pursuit eye movements. The flow-chart shows that the smooth-pursuit part of the frontal eye field receives visual motion information from extrastriate motion areas, e.g., from the middle temporal area (MT, V5) and the medial superior temporal area (MST) and from parietal regions such as 7a and the ventral intraparietal area (VIP). INC, interstitial nucleus of Cajal; LGN, lateral geniculate nucleus; MVN, medial vestibular nucleus; NPH, nucleus prepositus hypoglossi; RTP, nucleus reticularis tegmenti pontis.

cells
lus
smo
vest
extr
ect,
fron
thes
nucl
smo
rily
purs
mov
supp
the v
as by
head

4. E
Smo

Neoc
ticati
profc
ted p
prod
respo
Discr
pursu
(purs

FE
defici
conce
defici
durin
veloci
the d
lesion
deficit
ment
types
but ar

5. Se

Neurc
studie
systen
retina
closer
more
rons i

G. Neural Circuitry of the Vergence-Accommodation System

The primate has frontally placed eyes with highly overlapping visual fields (i.e., a large binocular field). The two retinal images are combined (fused) in the cyclopean retina (effectively located in V1). Fusion, however, requires that both eyes look in approximately the same direction so that visual objects fall on corresponding points of the two retinae. Consequently, most eye movements are conjugate because both eyes move in synchrony during nystagmus, saccades, and pursuit in order to maintain fused vision and obtain stereopsis, the extraction of relative depth from slight differences in the images of the two eyes. As discussed earlier, conjugate movement is accomplished by equal innervation of yoked muscle pairs in the two eyes (Hering's law).

However, when the distance of the fixation object varies, adjustments are needed that involve converging or diverging the relative horizontal directions of the two eyes. Cells in a region immediately lateral to the oculomotor nucleus are active during such disjunctive eye movements. These cells bilaterally innervate the nearby OMNs of the medial rectus and thus add a convergence command to the conjugate eye movement signal that medial rectus OMNs receive from interneurons in the abducens nucleus.

The two principal cues for vergence movements are retinal disparity, which occurs when a fixation target is not on the fovea of both eyes, and retinal blur, which occurs when a target is not in focus (as well as when it has retinal slip). Because vergence is tightly linked to accommodation, either cue evokes both responses. The "near triad" is a popular term for the response to viewing a near object: (i) The lens is compressed to bring the object into focus (accommodation), (ii) the eyes converge to image the object on the fovea of both eyes, and (iii) the pupils constrict to increase the depth of field. As noted earlier, cranial nerve III also has the efferents (from the Edinger–Westphal nucleus) that effect the lens accommodation and pupillary reflex components of the triad.

Although the complete circuitry of vergence is not known, it is clear that cortical visual areas, especially V1, are critical for processing disparity and blur. Paul Gamlin finds that a small region of frontal cortex, located just anterior to the saccadic FEF in the monkey, has cells that respond specifically during vergence movements and electrical stimulation there can elicit vergence eye movements. Moreover, cells throughout FEF can be sensitive to the depth location (or binocular disparity) of visual targets as well as to their azimuth and elevation. This depth information may be critical in allowing changes in vergence to be made simultaneously with saccades to targets differing in depth as well as in visual direction. Vergence movements are generally very slow and can last nearly a second. This slowness reflects in part the difficult task of processing vergence cues; however, saccadic vergence is accomplished much faster than pure vergence movements. Vergence changes can also accompany smooth pursuit in depth, and vergence could even be considered as part of the FS rather than as a separate, third oculomotor system or function.

See Also the Following Articles

COLOR PROCESSING AND COLOR PROCESSING DISORDERS • EVOLUTION OF THE BRAIN • NEUROIMAGING • SPATIAL VISION • SUPERIOR COLLICULUS • VISION: BRAIN MECHANISMS • VISUAL SYSTEM DEVELOPMENT AND NEURAL ACTIVITY

Acknowledgments

We gratefully acknowledge the critical comments of Gregory B. Stanton and Micheal S. Kraus.

Suggested Reading

Becker, W. (1991). *Saccades*. In *Vision and Visual Dysfunction* (R. H. S. Carpenter, Ed.), Vol. 8, pp. 95–137. CRC Press, Boca Raton, FL.

Bruce, C. J. (1990). *Integration of sensory and motor signals for saccadic eye movements in the primate frontal eye fields*. In *Signal and Sense, Local and Global Order in Perceptual Maps* (G. M. Edelman, W. E. Gall, and W. M. Cowan, Eds.), pp. 261–314. Wiley–Liss, New York.

Carpenter, R. H. S. (1988). *Movements of the Eyes*. Pion, London.

Emery, N. J. (2000). The eyes have it: The neuroethology, function and evolution of social gaze. *Neurosci. Biobehav. Rev.* **24,** 581–604.

Goldberg, M. E. (2000). *The control of gaze*. In *Principles of Neural Science* (E. R. Kandel, J. H. Schwartz, and T. M. Jessell, Eds.), pp. 782–800. McGraw-Hill, New York.

Henn, V. (1992). Pathophysiology of rapid eye movements in the horizontal, vertical and torsional directions. *Baillieres Clin. Neurol.* **1,** 373–391.

Hering, E. (1942). *Spatial Sense and Movements of the Eye*. American Academy of Optometry, Baltimore, MD.

Holzman, P. S. (2000). Eye movements and the search for the essence of schizophrenia. *Brain Res. Rev.* **31,** 350–356.

Kowler, E. (1990). *The role of visual and cognitive processes in the control of eye movement*. In *Reviews of Oculomotor Research 4. Eye Movements and Their Role in Visual and Cognition* (E. Kowler, Ed.), pp. 1–70. Elsevier, New York.

Leigh, R. J., and Zee, D. S. (1999). *The Neurology of Eye Movements.* Oxford Univ. Press, New York.

Rayner, K. (1998). Eye movements in reading and information processing: 20 years of research. *Psychol. Bull.* **124,** 372–422.

Robinson, D. A. (1987). The windfalls of technology in the oculomotor system. *Proctor lecture. Invest. Ophthalmol. Vis. Sci.* **28,** 1912–1924.

Schall, J. D., and Thompson, K. G. (1999). Neural selection and control of visually guided eye movements. *Annu. Rev. Neurosci.* **22,** 241–259.

Vilis, T. (1997). Physiology of three-dimensional eye movements: saccades and vergence. In *Three-Dimensional Kinematics of Eye, Head, and Limb Movements* (M. Fetter, T. Haslwanter, H. Misslisch, and D. Tweed, Eds.), pp. 57–72. Harwood Academic Publishing, Amsterdam. (See also http://www.med.uwo.ca/neuroscience/vilis/courses.htm)

Wurtz, R. H. (1996). Vision for the control of movement. The Friedenwald Lecture. *Invest. Ophthalmol. Vis. Sci.* **37,** 2130–2145.

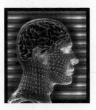

Forebrain

LUIS PUELLES* and JOHN RUBENSTEIN†

*University of Murcia, Spain and † University of California, San Francisco

GLOSSARY

prosencephalon Refers to the anteriormost major subdivision of the neural tube that gives rise to the forebrain. Consists of several major parts. The caudal part is the caudal diencephalon. The rostral part is the secondary prosencephalon; this region consists of the telencephalic and optic vesicles, and the rostral diencephalon.

prosomere Prosencephalic (forebrain) segment or neuromere. A transverse subdivision of the forebrain containing all the primary longitudinal subdivisions.

rostral diencephalon Unevaginated part of secondary prosencephalon, divided into hypothalamus proper (basal plate and floor plate) and prethalamus (alar plate).

telencephalon Large evaginated dorsal subdivision of the forebrain that contains primarily the cerebral cortex (pallium) and basal ganglia (subpallium).

The forebrain is the rostralmost portion of the central nervous system (CNS). It is an extremely complex assembly of structurally and functionally diverse structures that regulate most aspects of cognition, homeostasis, and behavior. In this brief overview, we describe the major components of the forebrain using a developmental viewpoint. Although the adult forebrain seems hopelessly complicated to most neuroa-

natomy students, a rudimentary understanding of its development provides a framework that simplifies its comprehension. Thus, we describe forebrain organization from a neuroembryological perspective. Most of the information that we will describe is valid for tetrapods (mammals, birds, reptiles, and amphibians). Available evidence supports the idea that the fundamental organization of the human forebrain differs little from that of less complex vertebrates. Most apparent differences are due to more extensive growth and larger morphogenetic deformation in the human brain of structures already found in other vertebrate brains. These differential aspects will be noted whenever this is appropriate.

I. EARLY DEVELOPMENT

The forebrain is derived from the anteriormost transverse domain of the neural plate that is generated during gastrulation (Fig. 1). Tissues adjacent to and within the neural plate produce molecules that regulate regional specification and morphogenesis of the CNS. Prospective subdivisions of the brain are specified through several mechanisms. Anteroposterior patterning generates transverse subdivisions: forebrain, midbrain, hindbrain, and spinal cord (Fig. 1A). Dorsoventral patterning generates longitudinally aligned domains, called floor plate, basal plate, alar plate, and roof plate (Fig. 1B). Within the forebrain, neuromeric theories postulate that there are further transverse subdivisions, which will be discussed later. Finally, regionally distinct molecular properties of the neuroepithelium and local signals from adjacent

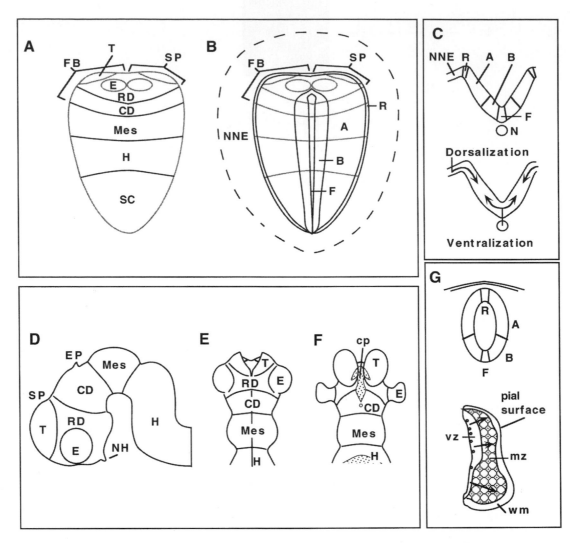

Figure 1 Early development of the forebrain. (A) Schema of transverse domains specified at the neural plate stage; the transverse boundaries are represented by black lines. Note that telencephalic and eye vesicles are separate outgrowths. (B) Schema of longitudinal domains at the same stage (boundaries in black; transverse and other limits in gray). (C) Schema of cross section through the neural plate showing the longitudinal domains and the relative position of the main tissues that regulate dorsoventral patterning, the notochord and the nonneural ectoderm. These exert ventralization and dorsalization effects, respectively, which are symbolized below. (D) Side view of the closed neural tube. The forebrain appears rostral to the mesencephalon and is composed of the caudal diencephalon, rostral diencephalon, eye vesicle, and telencephalon; the latter is shown as it starts to evaginate. (E) Dorsal view of the same stage as in D showing unfinished anterior closure of the neural tube and the bulging eye vesicles. (F). At a later stage, a dorsal view illustrates the stalks of the eye vesicles, the bilateral telencephalic vesicles, and the choroidal plexus primordium at the forebrain roof (cp; stippled area). (G) Schema of the closed neural tube in cross section and its longitudinal domains. Development of its wall is schematized below; a proliferating ventricular zone, a differentiating mantle zone, and a subpial layer of white matter (growing axons) can be distinguished.

tissues regulate the outgrowth of vesicles from the forebrain, such as the bilateral eye and telencephalic vesicles (secondarily also the olfactory bulbs), the neurohypophysis, and the epiphysis (pineal gland) (Figs. 1D–1F).

Dorsoventral patterning is regulated by nonneural tissues flanking the neural plate [the dorsalizing nonneural ectoderm (NNE) in Figs. 1B and C] and below the neural plate midline (the ventralizing notochord and prechordal mesendoderm) (N; Fig. 1C). Anteroposterior patterning is less fully understood, but it involves tissues underlying the neural plate, tissues at the anterior and posterior limits of the neural plate, as well as a later-appearing patterning

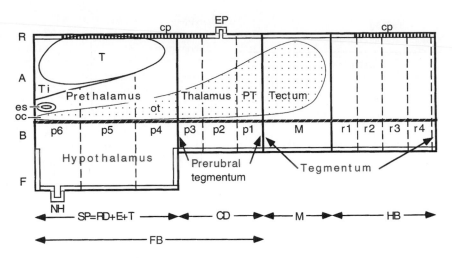

Figure 2 Topological schema of transverse and longitudinal subdivisions of the vertebrate forebrain (FB), midbrain (MB), and rostral hindbrain (HB). The longitudinal zones are indicated at the far left (R, roof plate; A, alar plate; B, basal plate; F, floor plate); the alar/basal boundary is represented by the thick black line with oblique white stripes. The transverse boundaries are vertical lines; black lines separate the main brain vesicles (identified underneath) and dashed lines separate the neuromeric subdivisions (prosomeres p1–p6), which are identified under the alar/basal boundary line. Various other specific names for different alar or basal territories are indicated. The choroidal plexi (cp) are marked by vertical stripes at the top. Note the position of the evaginated telencephalic vesicle (T) and the unevaginated telencephalon impar (Ti). The optic tract (ot) is schematized as a longitudinal domain extending from the optic chiasm (oc) to the optic tectum. See Table I for other abbreviations.

center at the midbrain–hindbrain junction. These stepwise processes generate a two-dimensionally regionalized specification map of prospective forebrain subdivisions (Fig. 2) Table I.

During the patterning stage, morphogenetic processes start to generate the shape of the forebrain. Neurulation folds the neural plate into the neural tube (Figs. 1C and G) and rapid cell divisions expand its surface area. The position-specific production of neurons and glia increases the thickness of the neural tube along the ventriculopial axis, which is the third dimension of the brain (Fig. 1G, arrows). Note that the internal, fluid-filled cavity of the neural tube and adult brain is called ventricular space, which is lined by the pseudostratified neuroepithelium; the outside of the neural tube contacts through a basement membrane the surrounding mesenchyme, which matures into a thin meningeal sheet called the "pia." Thus, the term "pial" means superficial, whereas "ventricular" means internal; most cell divisions occur in the "ventricular zone" (vz) of the neuroepithelium (Fig. 1G). Cell-type specification and differentiation processes generate postmitotic cells that migrate away from their site of origin in the vz toward the pial surface, under which they form the mantle zone (mz; Fig. 1G). Here, nuclei and laminar structures are gradually assembled. Many neurons and some glia cells only undergo radial

migrations to the mz (Fig. 1G, arrows), thus maintaining a fixed position relative to their site of origin. This is probably essential for the generation of topographic connectivity maps between different brain regions. On the other hand, some neurons and oligodendrocytes undergo tangential migrations away from their primary sites of entrance in the mantle layer, frequently into specific target loci. Tangential migrations enable certain cell types that can only be formed in specific neural tube areas to become functionally integrated in local circuitry elsewhere.

II. PRINCIPAL COMPONENTS

In this section, we describe the major components of the forebrain in the context of their developmental origins and following the framework of the prosomeric model of Puelles and Rubenstein (Fig. 2). Although this model is still changing as new data accrue (in fact, we introduce some changes here), we suggest that it provides a useful conceptual format to integrate developmental mechanisms with the complex morphology of the forebrain. It is important to note that other morphological models of the forebrain have been postulated, including neuromeric and nonneuromeric

Table I
Anatomical Abbreviations

(continued)

Abbreviation	Definition
A	Alar plate
Ac	Accoustic cortex
ac	Anterior commissure
Ac1-2	Primary and secondary accoustic cortical areas
ACC	Accumbens nucleus
AEP	Anterior entopeduncular area
AH	Anterior hypothalamus
AM	Amygdala (subpallial part)
B	Basal plate
BL	Basolateral amygdala
BM	Basomedial amygdala
BST	Bed nucleus of the stria terminalis
CAU	Caudate nucleus
cc	Corpus callosum
CD	Caudal diencephalon
Ce	Central amygdala
CLdl	Claustrum, dorsolateral part
CLvm	Claustrum, ventromedial part
cp	Choroid plexus tissue
DP	Dorsal pallium
DT	Dorsal thalamus
E	Eye vesicle
EMT	Eminentia thalami
EP	Epiphysis
es	Eye stalk
ET	Epithalamus
F	Floorplate
FB	Forebrain
FP	Frontal pole of telencephalon
GP	Globus pallidus
H	Hindbrain
hc	Habenular commissure
hic	Hippocampal commissure
iml	Internal medullary lamina
INS	Insular cortex
L	Lateral amygdala
LOT	Lateral olfactory tract
Lp	Lateral pallium
Mes	Midbrain
M	Motor cortex
M1–M3	Primary and secondary motor cortical areas
MAM	Mammillary region

Abbreviation	Definition
Me	Medial amygdala
MP	Medial pallium
mz	Mantle zone
N	Notochord
NH	Neurohypophysis
NNE	Non-neural ectoderm
OB	Olfactory bulb
oc	Optic chiasm
OP	Occipital pole of telencephalon
OT	Olfactory tuberculum
ot	Optic tract
p1–p6	Prosomeres 1–6
p1c	Floor commissure of p1
p3c	Floor commissure of p3
Pal	Pallium
pc	Posterior commissure
PEP	Posterior entopeduncular nucleus
PIR	Piriform (olfactory) cortex
POA	Anterior (telencephalic) preoptic area
poc	Postoptic (supraoptic) commissure
POP	Posterior (prethalamic) preoptic area
PT	Pretectum
PUT	Putamen nucleus
PV–SO	Paraventricular-supraoptic nucleus
R	Roof plate
r1–r4	Rhombomeres 1–4
RD	Rostral diencephalon
RM	Retromammillary area
rt	Retroflex tract
S	Somatosensory cortex
S1–S3	Primary and secondary somatosensory cortical areas
SC	Spinal cord
SCH	Suprachiasmatic nucleus
Se	Septum
SIA	Subincertal area
sm	Stria medullaris
SP	Secondary prosencephalon
Sp	Subpallium
ST	Striatum
T	Telencephalon
Ti	Telencephalon impar
TM	Tuberomammillary region
TP	Temporal pole of telencephalon

(continues)   *(continues)*

Table I *(continued)*

Abbreviation	Definition
TU	Tuberal region
V	Visual cortex
V1–V4	Primary and secondary visual cortical areas
VP	Ventral pallium
VPA	Ventral pallidum
VST	Ventral striatum
VT	Ventral thalamus
vz	Ventricular zone
wm	White matter
zl	Zona limitans

ones of Herrick and Kuhlenbeck. The primary prosencephalon, or early forebrain vesicle, soon divides into two principal transverse subdivisions: caudally, the caudal diencephalon, and rostrally, the secondary prosencephalon (sum of rostral diencephalon and telencephalon; Figs. 1D–1F, 2). In our description, the conventional hypothalamus is constituted exclusively by parts of the rostral diencephalon and is independent from the caudal diencephalon.

The caudal diencephalon abuts caudally the midbrain; it has three transverse subdivisions, postulated to be prosencephalic neuromeres (prosomeres p1–p3) (Figs. 2 and 3). These contain the pretectal (p1), dorsal thalamic/epithalamic (p2), and ventral thalamic (p3) regions. Each prosomere has alar (dorsal) and basal (ventral) components; the aforementioned three large regions are the respective alar components of p1–p3 (Fig. 3). The basal components jointly form the prerubral tegmentum.

The transverse organization of the secondary prosencephalon (SP) is more hypothetical, but it has been postulated to contain three prosomeres as well (p4–p6), which are readily distinguishable in the rostral diencephalon, though it is not clear how they relate to the overlying telencephalon (Fig. 2). The telencephalon is a dorsal evaginated region within the SP (T in Figs. 1D–1F), and lies strictly dorsal to the rostral diencephalon. The latter also appears divided into alar and basal plates, like its caudal counterpart. The alar plate extends from the telencephalon down to approximately the ventral limit of the optic tract. Thus, the optic stalk and the optic tract lie in a longitudinal alar plate domain that traverses the rostral diencephalon, thalamus, pretectum, and midbrain (Fig. 2). The

alar rostral diencephalon consists of three prosomeric subregions labeled caudal (p4), intermediate (p5), and rostral (p6) prethalamic areas (Fig. 4). The optic vesicles evaginate out of the rostral area at early neurulation stages (Figs. 1A–1F). Part of the prethalamus, particularly the rostral part, has been attributed to the hypothalamus, but it is convenient to restrict the term "hypothalamus" to the basal part of the rostral diencephalon. This includes mammillary/subthalamic (p4), tuberomammillary (p5), and tuberal hypophyseal regions (p6) (Fig. 4). In this way, the rostral diencephalon divides into optic vesicles and prethalamus (alar plate) and hypothalamus (basal and floor plates).

III. THE CAUDAL DIENCEPHALON

The pretectum (alar p1) is the caudalmost forebrain region. It is characterized by the posterior commissure, whose fibers cross the pretectal dorsal midline and then course transversally through the alar plate, just in front of the diencephalomesencephalic limit, before spreading longitudinally in the basal plate (pc in Fig. 3). The function of the posterior commissure is unclear. This region contains various pretectal nuclei involved in visual processing, including the centers for the pupillary and optokinetic eye reflexes. The subcommissural organ is a dorsal midline specialization that secretes glycoprotein (Reissner's fiber) into the ventricular fluid. The basal plate has dopamine-containing neurons that form part of the substantia nigra in addition to diverse reticular cell populations involved in motor circuits, like the parvocellular nucleus ruber (origin of the rubroolivary tract) and the interstitial nucleus of Cajal. The latter is a rostral source of descending preoculomotor axons in the medial longitudinal fasciculus, a tract that coordinates eye movements.

Anterior of the pretectum lies the dorsal thalamus and epithalamus complex (alar p2). Its dorsal midline includes the epiphysis (pineal gland), the habenular commissure, and choroid plexus rostrally. The epithalamus (ET or habenula) is the most dorsal nuclear complex; these neurons relate to the longitudinal stria medullaris tract (sm), which crosses the dorsal midline in the habenular commissure (hc in Fig. 3). The habenular nuclei produce the retroflex tract (habenulointerpeduncular tract). This compact transverse fascicle is a landmark that remains just anterior to the p1/p2 boundary throughout its dorsoventral extent; near the diencephalic floor it bends caudally (retroflects), continuing longitudinally across p1 and

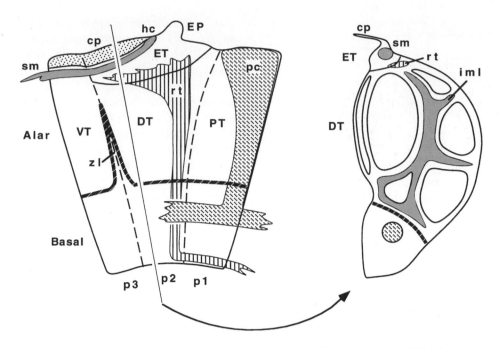

Figure 3   Schema of subdivisions of the caudal diencephalon and relevant anatomical landmarks in lateral view (rostral to the left; alar/basal limit as in Fig. 2): The pretectum (PT) in alar p1 contains the posterior commissure (pc); the dorsal thalamus (DT) and epithalamus (ET) in alar p2 contain to the retroflex tract (rt). The zona limitans (zl) separates dorsal and ventral thalami (VT) and seems to contain an expansion of the basal plate (according to gene expression data). The stria medullaris tract (sm) courses longitudinally near the roof choroidal plexus (cp). (Right) A schematic cross section through the dorsal thalamus, whose section level is indicated in the schema on the left, shows various nuclear groups (each of them is further subdivided into several nuclei), separated by the axon-rich internal medullary lamina (iml). See Table I for other abbreviations.

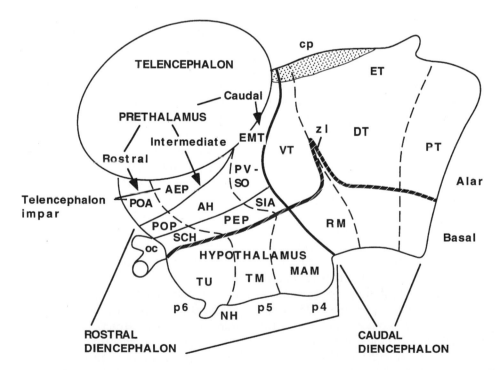

Figure 4   This schema highlights subdivisions in the rostral diencephalon in the context of the overlying telencephalon and caudal diencephalon. We call "hypothalamus" the basal part of the rostral diencephalon and "prethalamus" the alar part. These are both divided into three prosomeres (p4–p6) and various smaller areas. See Table I for abbreviations.

the midbrain into the interpeduncular nuclear complex in the isthmic floor plate (rt in Fig. 3).

The dorsal thalamus (DT) lies ventral to the epithalamus and consists of an elaborate complex of nuclei that generally project to the telencephalon (targeting both subcortical and cortical structures) (Fig. 3 and arrow 11 in Fig. 5A). These nuclei serve as relay centers for numerous telencephalopetal pathways with diverse functional implications. The telencephalic cortex sends topographically ordered projections to the respective thalamic relay centers. The main subdivisions of the DT contain groups of related nuclei. The *intralaminar* nuclei lie within the fiber-rich internal medullary lamina, which separates the other nuclear groups (iml in Fig. 3). These intralaminar nuclei form a separate projecting system with a modulatory role over the cortex and basal ganglia (embodying the final stage of the ascending activating system for mental arousal). The *sensory* nuclei process somatosensory and viscerosensory information (ventrobasal complex), visual input (dorsal lateral geniculate nucleus), and auditory input (medial geniculate nucleus), which are then relayed by these nuclei to the primary sensory areas of the isocortex via axons in the internal capsule (telencephalic peduncle; arrow 11 in Fig. 5A). Other thalamic nuclei are part of the *motor control* system (ventral anterior and ventrolateral nuclei); these process inputs from the globus pallidus and the cerebellar dentate nucleus and send efferents to the motor and premotor cerebral cortex. The anterior and periventricular thalamic nuclei are the *limbic* part of the thalamus, receiving hypothalamic (mammillary and other) projections and projecting to the limbic cingulate cortex, hippocampus, septum, and amygdala. Another important group of dorsal thalamic nuclei is conceived as the *associative* group (lateral dorsal, lateral posterior, pulvinar, and medial nuclei). These nuclei receive their major inputs from parts of the secondary sensorimotor, limbic, and associative cortex and project again into higher order cortical areas of the frontal, parietal, and temporal lobes. The associative nuclei are particularly developed and become secondarily subdivided and specialized in man.

The basal plate of p2 is poorly understood; it resembles that of p1 in that it contains a part of the dopaminergic neurons of the substantia nigra and of the median ventral tegmental area, in addition to some reticular populations participating in preoculomotor functions (i.e., the rostral interstitial nucleus).

The transition from p2 to p3 is characterized by several major changes in molecular and developmental properties. The p2/p3 limit appears as a fiber-rich gap between dorsal and ventral thalami; it is known as the zona limitans intrathalamica, or external medullary lamina (zl in Figs. 3 and 4).

Alar p3 is also known as the ventral thalamus for historical reasons, even though it is anterior to the dorsal thalamus (VT in Figs. 2 and 3; compare resulting position in bent forebrain, as in Fig. 1D). The choroid plexus of p2 extends through p3 and p4 into the telencephalon (cp; dotted roof domain in Figs. 1F, and 3 and 4; striped roof in Fig. 2). A choroid plexus is a neuroepithelial specialization where blood plasma is filtered into the brain ventricles as cerebral spinal fluid, which circulates and then flows out from holes in the hindbrain roof. Alar p3 consists of the ventral lateral geniculate nucleus (a superficial reflex visual center), the reticular thalamic nucleus (traversed by the thalamocortical fiber bundles), and a periventricular zona incerta. The latter two nuclei contain many inhibitory neurons, whose projections spread widely ipsi- and contralaterally in the alar and basal plates of the caudal and rostral diencephalon, perhaps reaching the midbrain. Inhibition exerted by the reticular nucleus on the dorsal thalamus organizes rhythmic electrical activity characteristic of sleep.

The basal plate of p3 consists of the so-called posterior hypothalamic area and the retromammillary area, which is frequently named the "supramammillary area." The latter is characterized by some dopaminergic neurons and other reticular cell populations.

IV. THE ROSTRAL DIENCEPHALON

As outlined previously, we use the term rostral diencephalon to refer to the extratelencephalic part of the secondary prosencephalon. We hypothesize that it is divided in basal and alar plates across three prosomeres (p4–p6), with its alar plate forming the prethalamus and its basal/floor plates representing the hypothalamus, as originally defined for human embryos by His in 1890 (Figs. 2 and 4). Although the diencephalic prosomeres p1–p3 represent the part of the extratelencephalic forebrain machinery that regulates information processing (and subsequent motor output) of signals coming in from the external world, the rostral diencephalic prosomeres p4–p6 attend mainly to the inner world of viscera, neurohumoral functions, and internal homeostasis. They also provide ascending (motivating) input into the limbic parts of

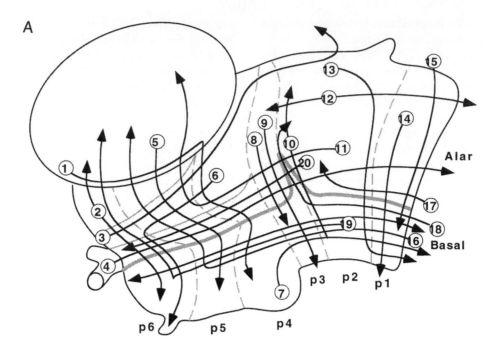

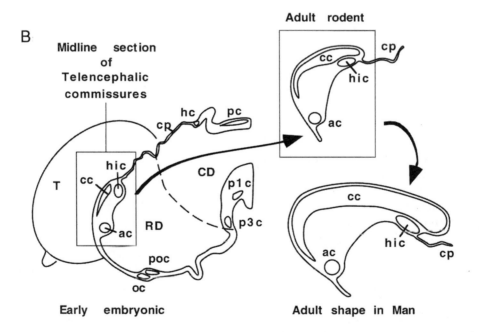

Figure 5 Schema of connectivity in the rostral and caudal diencephalon. (A) In general, tracts can be mapped within the prosomeric model as aligned with the transverse or longitudinal dimensions of the forebrain components. There are thus basically transverse tracts or tract portions and longitudinal tracts or tract portions. Individual tracts may change direction at specific decision points. This schema does not describe all the tracts present in the forebrain. It only exemplifies the previous general principle by illustrating 20 assorted tracts: 1, Fornix (hippocampomammillary) tract; 2, septohypothalamic tract; 3, stria medullaris (into habenular commissure); 4, optic tract; 5, amygdalohypothalamic tract; 6, supraoptohypophyseal tract; 7, mammillotegmental tract; 8, incertotegmental tract; 9, commissural ventral thalamic tract; 10, mammillothalamic tract; 11, thalamotelencephalic tract; 12, longitudinal alar interconnections; 13, retroflex tract; 14, commissural anterior pretectal tract; 15, posterior commissure; 16, nigrostriatal tract; 17, medial lemniscus; 18, superior cerebellar peduncle; 19, medial forebrain bundle; 20, intergeniculate–suprachiasmatic tract. (B) The various commissures present in the forebrain are illustrated in a median sagittal section. Emphasis is placed in the area where the telencephalic commissures develop, showing in the two schemas on the right the progressive relative increase in size of the corpus callosum over developmental time and from adult rodent to adult man. See Table I for abbreviations.

the telencephalon through the medial forebrain bundle, whereas the caudal diencephalon is connected to the telencephalon via the lateral forebrain bundle (internal capsule). The prethalamus and hypothalamus accordingly are a collection of neural centers that are involved in regulation of homeostasis, reproduction, the autonomic nervous system, and emotional states.

The caudal part of the hypothalamus (p4) includes the mammillary region, the subthalamic nucleus, the lateral hypothalamic area, and part of the posterior hypothalamus (MAM in Fig. 4). The prethalamic (alar) region of p4 reaches dorsally the forebrain roof (choroidal plexus) via the eminentia thalami at the caudal end of the telencephalic stalk (EMT in Fig. 4); this area possibly extends into the telencephalon through the medial amygdala. The p4 alar plate probably includes among its derivatives the subincertal area, the paraventricular and supraoptic nuclei (SIA and PV–SO in Fig. 4), and the perireticular nucleus (not shown), with the latter lying just in front of the ventral thalamic reticular nucleus. The eminentia thalami received its name due to its protrusion at the back of the interventricular foramen (tight passage interconnecting the prethalamic ventricular space with that of the telencephalic vesicle, or lateral ventricle) and the idea that it belongs to the thalamus. Its neuronal derivatives participate in the bed nuclei of the stria terminalis (posterior, or medial, parts) and the stria medullaris. This domain is characteristically traversed superficially by the telencephalic peduncle as it exits the telencephalon, incorporating as well the thalamotelencephalic projections. The fornix tract —hippocampal fibers passing from the caudal aspect of the commissural septum to the mammillary region —follows the dorsoventral dimension of p4 at an intermediate depth (arrow 1 in Fig. 5A).

The intermediate hypothalamus (p5) is represented by the tuberomammillary region, which also contains the premammillary nuclei and the dorsomedial hypothalamic nucleus (TM in Fig. 4). The corresponding alar or prethalamic area extends through the posterior entopeduncular area, the conventional 'anterior hypothalamus,' and anterior entopeduncular area into the telencephalic stalk (PEP, AH, and AEP in Fig. 4).

The rostral hypothalamus (p6) starts ventrally with the neurohypophysis, median eminence, and arcuate nucleus (floor plate derivatives) and includes the basal plate tuberal area, with the ventromedial hypothalamic nucleus and the anterobasal nucleus (retrochiasmatic area) (NH and TU in Fig. 4). The rostral prethalamic alar plate continues through the supra-

chiasmatic and posterior/anterior preoptic regions into the telencephalic stalk (SCH, POP and POA in Fig. 4).

The mammillary area is a complex of nuclei with a variety of inputs, including the fornix fibers from the hippocampus, as a part of the limbic circuit of Papez. These nuclei send their major outputs through the basal plate of p3, p2, and p1 to the brain stem tegmental nuclei (mammillotegmental tract), with a collateral projection to the anterior dorsal thalamus, via the mammillothalamic tract (arrows 7 and 10 in Fig. 5A); these are also part of the Papez limbic circuit, which returns from there to cingulate and hippocampal cortex.

The tuberal/infundibular region and pituitary stalk are traversed by neuroendocrine fibers carrying vasopressin and oxytocin from magnocellular secretory cells in the overlying alar plate (supraoptic and paraventricular nuclei) to the neurohypophysis (arrow 6 in Fig. 5A); the neurohypophysis liberates these substances into the bloodstream. The median eminence contains a profusion of nerve terminals that secrete the proteins that regulate the release of various hormones from the anterior pituitary (corticotropin, thyrotropin, gonadotrophin, and growth hormone) into the hypophyseal portal capillaries. These regulator proteins arise from discrete groups of parvocellular neurosecretory neurons in the anterior hypothalamus and preoptic area. Other modulation of the pituitary occurs directly via axon terminals of dopamine neurons in the arcuate nucleus. The anterobasal nucleus bridges the retrochiasmatic midline area as a bed nucleus of the postoptic (supraoptic) commissures (poc in Fig. 5B) and is the rostralmost component of the basal plate.

The prethalamus can be subdivided into two superposed longitudinal tiers across prosomeres p4–p6. The lower tier coincides with the subpial course of the optic tract and the optic chiasm (Figs. 2 and 5A). It contains the suprachiasmatic nucleus (p6; involved in the control of circadian rhythms in homeostatic functions), the posterior entopeduncular area (including the migrated posterior entopeduncular nucleus; p5) and the subincertal area (p4). Little is known about the functions of the more caudal area. The upper tier is the so-called optoeminential domain, which lies just under the telencephalic stalk and telencephalon impar (unevaginated parts continuous with telencephalic structures, such as the telencephalic preoptic and median septal areas; Ti in Fig. 2). The optoeminential domain starts rostrally (p6), with a prethalamic preoptic area found around the optic stalk recess (POP in Fig. 4). It includes the anterior hypothalamic area (p5), dorsal to the PEP, and the supraoptic and paraventricular nuclei, together with the derivatives of the eminentia thalami (p4; posterior bed nucleus striae terminalis and bed nucleus striae medullaris). At the boundary with the telencephalic stalk, this domain is traversed longitudinally by the stria medullaris, which continues caudalwards into the diencephalic roof (epithalamus) (arrow 3 in Fig. 5A). The overlying telencephalic stalk domain (telencephalon impar) consists of cell groups found at the peduncular transition into the evaginated telencephalic vesicles. From caudal to rostral, these contribute to the amygdala, the extrapyramidal system [entopeduncular nucleus (or internal segment of globus pallidus in highly evolved mammals), substantia innominata, and basal nucleus of Meynert], the anterior preoptic area/diagonal band formation, and the telencephalic preoptic area.

V. BASIC CIRCUITRY IN THE EXTRATELENCEPHALIC FOREBRAIN

The whole lateral wall of the rostral and caudal diencephalon is traversed by numerous transverse, longitudinal, and commissural fibers that interconnect the diverse prosomeric centers into interactive circuitry (Figs. 5A and 5B). These interconnecting fiber systems often reach the midbrain alar and basal plates (and extend from there into the rest of the brain stem), and they converge rostrally at the postoptic (so-called supraoptic) commissure or diverge into the telencephalic stalk. The commissures allow the left and right halves of the brain to interact for coordination of both analytical (alar) and motor/neurovegetative/neurohumoral (basal) functions.

Another pervasive fiber system, the optic tract, is subpial and is found largely in the alar plate (there is also an accessory basal optic tract targeting specific terminal centers in the basal and alar parts of p1). The main optic tract courses longitudinally from the optic chiasm, where half of its fibers decussate (in man), through the prethalamus, thalamus, and pretectum and up to the midbrain roof (tectum)—the superior colliculus. Along its way, the optic tract gives out collaterals or terminal fibers to prethalamic areas (such as the suprachiasmatic nucleus) and to thalamic (ventral and lateral geniculate nuclei, intergeniculate leaflet, and pulvinar nucleus) and various pretectal centers receiving topographically ordered (retinotopic) projections (anterior pretectal nucleus and nucleus

of the optic tract) or nonordered retinal projections (olivary pretectal nucleus). The retinorecipient posterior pretectal nucleus lies in the midbrain.

There are also many characteristic transverse fiber tracts normally coursing close to a given interprosomeric boundary (Fig. 5A), although other systems of transverse fibers course sheet-like throughout a given portion of the wall. Most of these fibers change course (i.e., become longitudinal) at a given decision point, generally coinciding with entrance into the basal plate; a few proceed into commissures across the roof or floor plate (mainly in p1 and p3; Fig. 5B).

Given the specialization of alar centers in analytic signal decoding/locating and associated relay functions, and the specialization of the basal centers in motor patterns, longitudinal alar or basal fibers crossing diverse neuromeres tend to integrate separately such functions (bilaterally, due to the commissures). Conversely, fiber tracts coursing transversally convey the diverse segmentally analyzed (and longitudinally cross-correlated) alar outputs into the responding basal plate net of reticular and motor neurons. Much of our subconscious brain activity and reflex behavior depend on this subtle multimodal neuronal machinery for its precise situation- and aim-dependent adaptations. Note that this system, which is able to respond in a large extent to external and/or internal multimodal stimuli autonomously, is also controlled by the telencephalon for a higher degree of contextual integration, or volitional control, as indicated by separate descending telencephalic projections to many alar and basal plate centers.

VI. THE TELENCEPHALON: BASIC PARTS AND MORPHOGENESIS

The telencephalic hemispheres evaginate bilaterally from the dorsalmost alar plate of the secondary prosencephalon (Fig. 1). This process includes within each vesicle a portion of the roof plate choroidal tissue, which later builds the choroidal plexi of the lateral ventricles (Figs. 1 and 2F). Rostrally, a thick median wall portion is the site where the telencephalic commissures develop (fibers interconnecting both vesicles; there are three major commissural pathways in mammals—anterior commissure, hippocampal commissure, and corpus callosum; Fig. 5B).

There are two principal subdivisions of the telencephalic vesicle: the roof, or pallium, and the basis, or subpallium (Fig. 6A). The subpallium consists

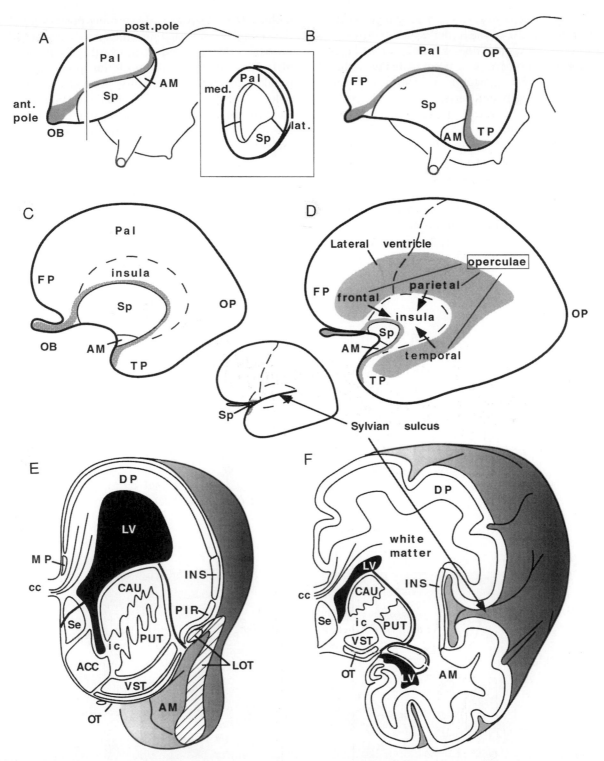

Figure 6 Morphological development of the telencephalon. (A–D) These drawings show lateral views of the left telencephalon at four developmental stages (see text). The inset in A shows a cross section and internal division into pallium (Pal) and subpallium (Sp). The olfactory tract is shaded in gray and helps to visualize the enormous growth of the pallium relative to the subpallium. (E) This drawing represents a section through the frontal part of the telencephalon, seen from the front; it shows in perspective the more caudal parts and the position of the temporal lobe. Within the section, the thick black lines mark the palliosubpallial boundary. Many subdivisions are indicated, as well as the lateral olfactory tract (LOT). (F) Similar to the drawing in E, representing a later stage in which further cortical expansions have introduced gyrification, internment of the insular cortex in the Sylvian sulcus (arrows) under the opercular overgrowths (compare with D and inset), and entrance of the temporal lobe (including its ventricular cavity) into the section plane (compare full shape in D). See Table I for abbreviations.

primarily of nuclei, the so-called basal ganglia (Figs. 7 and 8; note that use of the term "basal" here, or with regard to the amygdala, does not mean an embryological origin in the neural tube basal plate but, rather, a rough topographic indication of intratelencephalic position; all telencephalic parts are alar). The pallium contains primarily cortical structures but also some pallial nuclei (Fig. 8).

The area occupied by the basal ganglia in the hemisphere differentiates early and then its growth slows, whereas the overlying pallium is capable of prolonged surface growth. The increasing disproportion between these two parts leads to a characteristic morphogenetic deformation that in highly evolved mammals consists of a progressive incurvation and relative diminution in size of the subpallium, forced by anteroposterior and mediolateral expansion of the pallium (Fig. 6). The early forming posterior pole of the vesicle is converted into the temporal pole, which protrudes laterally and rostralwards (TP in Figs. 6B–6E). New anterior and posterior poles appear in parallel, forming the definitive frontal and occipital poles of the hemisphere (FP and OP in Figs. 6A–6E). An outgrowth at the early forming anterior pole forms the olfactory bulb, which gradually becomes displaced under the new frontal pole or orbitofrontal cortex (OB in Figs. 6A–6D). The lateral olfactory tract projecting from the olfactory bulb to the primitive posterior pole (gray in Fig. 6A) is transiently visible at the surface along the whole telencephalon, always just lateral to the palliosubpallial boundary (gray in Figs. 6C and 6D).

Internally, the subpallium forms an intraventricular bulge that affects the shape of the lateral ventricle

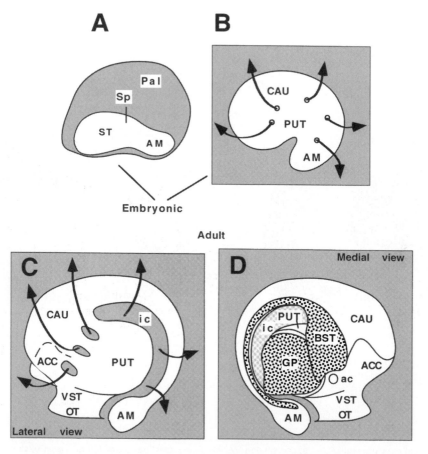

Figure 7 Development and subdivisions of the basal ganglia. (A). The common mass of subpallial formations is shown under the pallium. Its caudal part contains prospective subpallial amygdala (AM) and its rostral part the striatum (and pallidum, internally). (B). Early passage of fibers from the internal capsule (arrows) starts to divide the subpallial nuclei. (C, D). At the final stage, external (C) and internal (D) views show the different main portions that are distinguished. The stippled formations in D represent the pallidal components. See Table I for abbreviations.

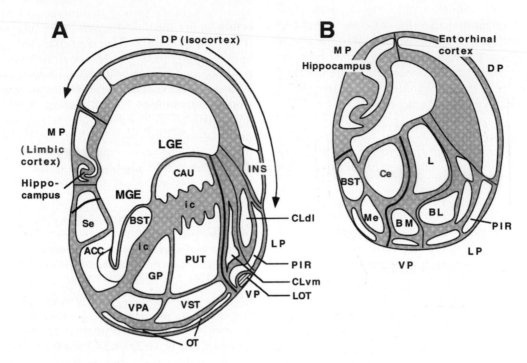

Figure 8 Pallial and subpallial subdivisions shown in schematic cross sections through the middle sector of an undeformed telencephalon (A) and through the amygdaloid complex at the temporal pole (B). The thick black line represents the palliosubpallial boundary. Note the pallium is subdivided into ventral, lateral, dorsal, and medial portions. See Table I for abbreviations.

(Sp in Figs. 6A, 6E and 6F, 7, and 8). The basal ganglia are traversed by the radiating fibers of the internal capsule (bidirectional thalamocortical axons) and become secondarily subdivided into several portions (Figs. 6E and 6F, 7B–D, 8A, and 8B). Pallial overgrowth also occurs mediolaterally, both in the main frontooccipital body of the hemisphere and in the temporal horn. This leads to the formation of the Sylvian (lateral) fissure and the progressive internment under the frontoparietal and temporal operculae of the piriform (olfactory) and insular cortexes (these are the earliest formed cortical parts, covering laterally the basal ganglia) (Figs. 6D–6F).

Additional adjustments of the pallial surface to more localized bouts of final surface growth lead to the partial or total burial of the oldest formed cortex (anchored by its more advanced connections) in the depth of other fissures (hippocampal, collateral, internal parietooccipital, and calcarine) and constant or variable sulci (central, frontal, parietal, temporal, cingulate, and rhinal). The intervening gyri protrude superficially in interlocked shapes, adapting to available space in the cranium (Fig. 6F). The main sulcal formations serve to separate the frontal, parietal, occipital, temporal, insular, and cingulate/entorhinal

lobes; the latter includes the hippocampus. The relative amount of gyrification increases in evolutionarily more advanced mammals. The increase in cortical surface that is found in complex mammals is thought to occur without fundamental changes in the radial organization of the cortex, which is divided into columnar modules of constant dimensions and cell density across mammals. Thus, one evolutionary trend tends to increase the number of cortical columnar modules (presumably improving the analytical capacity of the animal). At the interhemispheric surface, gyrencephalic animals also show a correlatively larger corpus callosum, the main interhemispheric commissure (Fig. 5B).

VII. TELENCEPHALIC COMPONENTS

A. The Pallium

Recently, the pallial cover of the telencephalic vesicle has been shown to be divided molecularly and structurally into four pallial territories, that are common to all vertebrates: the medial, dorsal, lateral, and ventral pallial domains (Fig. 8). The medial and dorsal pallial parts mature structurally into purely cortical centers. The medial pallium primarily forms the hippocampal cortex (allocortex; three-layered), although parts of the surrounding transitional cingulate/entorhinal cortex (mesocortex; four- or five-layered) may have the same origin. This functionally connected complex is subsumed under the term "limbic lobe" and is important in the evaluation of experiences, motivation of behavior, emotions and memory.

The dorsal pallium forms the isocortex (six- or seven-layered; predominant in relative surface extent). This domain specializes into separate sensory or motor cortical areas. Primary sensory cortex processes relatively simple sensory data; secondary cortex generates more complex perceptual constructs of the external world and the body. Associational cortical areas are

where higher mental functions are believed to occur (Figs. 9B and 9C). The ancestral dorsal pallium appears as a variably sized island surrounded by the rostrally and caudally interconnected medial and lateral pallia; the reduced sensory/motor and associative representations partly overlap (Fig. 9A). The dorsal pallium is the portion that expands more in mammalian evolution so that the isocortex represents the largest and most variably subdivided cortical domain in mammalian species (Figs. 9B and 9C). Major axonal outputs of the isocortex (apart from the massive layer II/III corticocortical projections, both within the same hemisphere and projecting into the contralateral hemisphere using the corpus callosum) are the corticoclaustral, corticostriatal, corticothalamic, corticopretectal–collicular, corticoreticular, corticopontine, corticonuclear, and corticospinal fiber pathways. They jointly constitute a potent means for

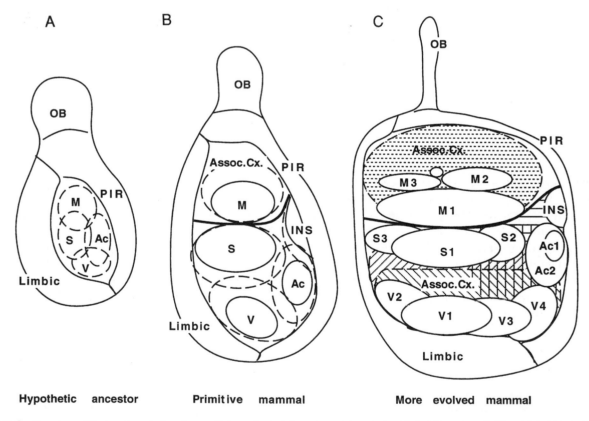

Figure 9 Drawings of flattened cortical surface, with hypothetical three stages of cortical evolution in mammals. The progressive expansion and diversification of specialized and associative fields within the isocortex is put in the context of its invariant topology, both externally [with respect to the surrounding limbic and piriform (PIR) cortexes] and internally (with respect to each area's topological relationship to the other isocortical areas). Dashed lines indicate imprecise boundaries. The thick black lines in B and C indicate the boundary between frontal lobe (action planning and motor functions) and the parietal, occipital, and temporal lobes (sensorial analysis and abstraction). The different patterns of lines in C symbolize associative multimodal intermixing of analysis properties. In man, the number of identified visual areas is approximately 20, and similar numbers may exist for the other specialized regions; this indicates the relative complexity of the functions performed in these domains. See Table I for abbreviations.

descending modulation of subjacent alar and basal centers, and they arise primarily from layer V pyramidal neurons (except those to claustrum and thalamus, which arise from layer VI neurons). The acquisition of direct cortical innervation of motoneurons seems to be a relatively recent evolutionary addition since it is absent in nonmammals.

The lateral and ventral pallial domains both give rise to portions of the olfactory cortex. In addition, each develops underlying pallial nuclei, which have been classified tentatively according to their molecular profiles (Figs. 8A and 8B). The lateral pallial nuclear formation consists rostrally of the dorsolateral claustrum and caudally of the endopiriform nucleus and basolateral parts of the amygdala (plus associated cortical amygdala domains). The ventral pallial nuclear formation is represented rostrally by the ventromedial claustrum and caudally by the lateral and basomedial parts of the amygdala (and associated cortical parts). Little is known of the functions of the claustrum, although the dorsolateral part has a bidirectional topographically ordered projection with the whole isocortex. The ventromedial claustrum may receive multimodal thalamic connections. The pallial nuclei of the amygdala are known to integrate multiple inputs from the isocortex, apparently integrating recognition of contextual Gestalts (characteristic sense data configurations) with entrainment of appropriate instinctive or learned (associated) behavior through motivational (limbic) and direct descending efferents onto extratelencephalic circuitry. It should be noted that the amygdala was long held to be only a part of the basal ganglia, but it has recently emerged as a heterogeneous complex of interactive pallial and subpallial elements (Fig. 8C). The same can be said for the telencephalic septum, found at the interhemispheric or medial wall, which also shows pallial and subpallial portions, although in this case the pallial part (the dorsalmost part of the septum) is much smaller than its subpallial constituents.

B. The Subpallium

The subpallium may be divided for descriptive purposes into a middle sector and two transitional domains at its rostral and caudal ends. The wall of the middle sector bulges into the ventricular cavity early in development, forming two ridges called the medial and lateral ganglionic eminences (MGE and LGE); these transient structures are perforated by the

major tract interconnecting the diencephalon with the telencephalon, the internal capsule (ic; arrows in Figs. 7B and 7C; Fig. 8A).

The mantle layer under the MGE matures earliest and gives rise to the globus pallidus (GP) or pallidum (there are dorsal and ventral pallidal formations; the dorsal pallidum divides into internal and external segments in hominids; in other mammals, the internal pallidal segment is called entopeduncular nucleus; Fig. 8A). The internal capsule fibers separate the GP from the periventricular pallidal derivative, which forms a curved complex called the bed nucleus of the stria terminalis (BST in Figs. 7D, 8A and 8B). The stria terminalis is a tract interconnecting the amygdala with the anterior commissure and surrounding areas (Fig. 7D). Together with the LGE, the MGE also produces numerous cohorts of neurons that migrate tangentially to invade the striatum and the whole cortical pallium (they largely become incorporated as cortical inhibitory interneurons).

The mantle developing under the LGE is the striatum [laterally there are dorsal and ventral striatum parts and a rostromedial part, the accumbens nucleus (ACC); Figs. 6E, 7C–7D, and 8A]. In man, the internal capsule partially divides the dorsal striatum into a peripheral portion called putamen and a periventricular portion called caudate nucleus (Fig. 8A). An obsolete anatomical conception artificially joined the putamen to the medially adjacent dorsal pallidum under the concept of "lenticular nucleus"; this term nevertheless still appears in clinical usage and in some tracts projecting out of the pallidum (lenticular tract and ansa lenticularis).

The respective dorsal and ventral parts of the striatum and pallidum are separated (arbitrarily) by the plane in which rostral and caudal components of the anterior commissure collect and course toward the midline commissural plate. At the subpial (ventral) surface of the subpallium, various superficially migrated cell populations form the laminated olfactory tuberculum. Toward the telencephalic stalk, this ventral area is contiguous with the substantia innominata, which contains both dispersed and dense groups of cholinergic neurons, such as the basal nucleus of Meynert. These constitute the main source of cholinergic input to the overlying cortex.

The striatopallidal complex is integrated into a circuit that modulates the motor output of the motor and premotor cortex. The cortex projects excitatory axons to specific areas of the striatum complex (characteristic afferents: accumbens and ventral striatum, limbic; caudate, associative; and putamen, sensorimotor). The striatum projects separately to the external and internal parts of the pallidum, where its effect is inhibitory, phasically breaking a tonic inhibitory activity of the pallidum over its targets. The external pallidal part interacts bidirectionally with the subthalamic nucleus, whose fibers counteract striatal inhibition in the pallidum. The internal part of the globus pallidus projects its tonic inhibition on the motor dorsal thalamic nuclei, which connect with the motor and premotor cortex. Phasic striatal inhibition of the pallidal tone thus decreases inhibition on thalamocortical neurons and thereby facilitates movement. Thus, motor plans are filtered through the basal ganglia to modulate the outputs of the motor cortex. It is thought that this circuit is important for regulating the dimensions of movements (e.g., tracing small or larger versions of one's signature) and for improving fluidity in opposite or alternating motions. There is an important ascending activation of striatal activity by nigrostriatal dopaminergic axons, in parallel with an important dopaminergic innervation of the premotor cortex. This input decreases in Parkinson's disease due to degeneration of the dopaminergic neurons in the substantia nigra and ventral tegmental area (partly in midbrain and partly in the basal/floor plate of diencephalon). These patients have hypokinesia (difficulty initiating movements), rigidity, and inexpressive faces. On the other hand, lesion of the subthalamic nucleus (p4 basal plate) diminishes the tonic inhibitory output of the pallidum, which leads to hyperactivity symptoms (involuntary movements are released, e.g., tics, hemibalismus, and choreoathetosis).

The amygdala is caudal to the striatum and pallidum. This massive nuclear formation, formed at the primitive caudal telencephalic pole and brought to the tip of the temporal lobe during morphogenesis (Figs. 6 and 7), can be divided into pallial and subpallial parts according to the expression of genetic markers and other characteristics (Fig. 8B). The numerous amygdaloid subnuclei traditionally have been grouped into central, medial, basal, lateral, and cortical groups (Fig. 8B). The pallial amygdaloid components have considerably increased in size in highly evolved mammals. The subpallial part of the amygdala is represented by the central amygdaloid nucleus, which shares some striatal characteristics, and the medial amygdaloid (plus amygdaloid BST) nuclei, which share some pallidal characteristics.

A recent variant conception of the subpallial amygdala adds the so-called "extended amygdala," which includes all the intratelencephalic supracapsular and subcapsular BST formation (relations to internal capsule) and other specific cell groups related to the anterior commissure. The extended amygdala, however, would belong to the middle and perhaps also the rostral subpallial sectors since it converges on the anterior commissure. According to our embryological formulation, the extended amygdala largely corresponds to pallidal areas surrounding the globus pallidus (Fig. 7D).

Finally, the rostral subpallial sector is constituted largely by the septum, found in front of or partially mixed with the telencephalic commissures in the medial hemispheric wall (See in Figs. 6E, 6F, and 8A). This nuclear complex can again be divided by use of genetic markers and other characteristics into subpallial and pallial portions (the pallial one being very small). The subpallial portion subdivides into an upper, striatum-like part and a ventral, pallidum-like part. Traditionally, the septum has been divided into "medial" and "lateral" septal nuclei, which embryologically correspond to superficial and periventricular strata, respectively. It is unfortunate that the term "lateral" was associated with a periventricular formation since this is somewhat counterintuitive (most other lateral structures in the brain are superficial, i.e., subpial).

See Also the Following Articles

EVOLUTION OF THE BRAIN • HINDBRAIN • HYPOTHALAMUS • NEOCORTEX • NEUROANATOMY

Suggested Reading

Ahlheid, G. F., de Olmos, J. S., and Beltramino, C. A. (1995). *Amygdala and extended amygdala.* In *Rat Nervous System* (G. Paxinos, Ed.), 2nd ed., pp. 495–578. Academic Press, San Diego.

Anderson, S. A., Eisenstat, D., Shi, L., and Rubenstein, J. L. R. (1997). Interneuron migration from basal forebrain: Dependence on Dlx genes. *Science* **278**, 474–476.

Medina, L., and Reiner, A. (2000). Do birds possess homologues of mammalian primary visual, somatosensory and motor cortices? *Trends Neurosci.* **23**, 1–12.

Puelles, L. A. (1995). Segmental morphological paradigm for understanding vertebrate forebrains. *Brain Behav. Evol.* **46**, 319–337.

Puelles, L., and Medina, L. (1994). Development of neurons expressing tyrosine hydroxylase and dopamine in the chicken brain: A comparative segmental analysis. In *Phylogeny and Development of Catecholamine Systems in the CNS of Vertebrates* (W. J. A. J. Smeets and A. Reines, Eds.), pp. 381–404. Cambridge Univ. Press, Cambridge, UK.

Puelles, L., and Rubenstein, J. L. R. (1993). Expression patterns of homeobox and other putative regulatory genes in the embryonic mouse forebrain suggest a neuromeric organization. *Trends Neuro. Sci.* **16**, 472–479.

Puelles, L., and Verney, C. (1998). Early neuromeric distribution of tyrosine hydroxylase-immunoreactive neurons in human embryos. *J. Comp. Neurol.* **394,** 283–308.

Puelles, L., Kuwana, E., Bulfone, A., Shimamura, K., Keleher, J., Smiga, S., Puelles, E., and Rubenstein, J. L. R. (2000). Pallial and subpallial derivatives in the embryonic chick and mouse telencephalon, traced by the expression of the Dlx-2, Emx-1, Nkx-2.1, Pax-6 and Tbr-1 genes. *J. Comp. Neurol.* **424,** 409–438.

Rakic, P. (1995). A small step for the cell, A giant leap for mankind: A hypothesis of neocortical expansion during evolution. *Trends Neurosci.* **18,** 383–388.

Rubenstein, J. L. R., and Beachy, P. A. (1998). Patterning of the embryonic forebrain. *Curr. Opin. Neurobiol.* **8,** 18–26.

Rubenstein, J. L. R., Shimamura, K., Martinez, S., and Puelles, L. (1998). Regionalization of the prosencephalic neural plate. *Annu. Rev. Neurosci.* **21,** 445–478.

Shimamura, K., Hartigan, D. J., Martinez, S., Puelles, L., and Rubenstein, J. L. R. (1995). Longitudinal organization of the anterior neural plate and neural tube. *Development* **121,** 3923–3933.

Smith-Fernandez, A., Pieau, C., Repérant, J., Boncinelli, E., and Wassef, M. (1998). Expression of the *Emx-1* and *Dlx-1* homeobox genes define three molecularly distinct domains in the telencephalon of mouse, chick, turtle and frog embryos: Implications for the evolution of telencephalic subdivisions in amniotes. *Development* **125,** 2099–2111.

Swanson, L. W., and Petrovich, G. D. (1998) What is the amygdala? *Trends Neurosci.* **21,** 323–330.

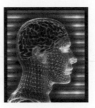

Frontal Lobe

LADA A. KEMENOFF, BRUCE L. MILLER, and JOEL H. KRAMER

University of California, San Francisco

GLOSSARY

dysarthria Disturbance of speech articulation or impairment of the speech mechanism, including muscle weakness. It is manifested by slurred pronunciation.

dysprosody Loss of the normal rhythm, melody, and articulation of speech.

gliosis Glial cells migrate to and proliferate in areas of neural tissue where damage has occurred.

hemiplegia Paralysis of one side of the body.

hypophonia An abnormally weak voice resulting from uncoordination of speech muscles, including weakness of muscles of respiration.

paraphasia The production of unintended syllables, words, or phrases during speech.

regional cerebral blood flow (rCBF) Amount of blood flow in a region of the cortex is positively correlated to the metabolic activity of that region. Imaging of the rCBF by scintigraphy with inhaled xenon-133 can be combined with psychological testing during the measurement of blood flow, allowing assessment of the effects of cognitive activation procedures on blood flow in specific regions of the cortex.

Commonly described as the anatomic seat of human self-awareness, the frontal lobes are the most evolutionarily advanced components of the human brain. Scientific advancements during the past decade have considerably improved our understanding of the frontal lobes and their complex role in cognition, personality, and neurological disease. This article presents a contemporary perspective on frontal lobe neuroanatomy; neuropsychological functions; and frontal lobe disorders.

I. NEUROANATOMY OF THE FRONTAL LOBE

The frontal lobes comprise the most anterior portion of the cerebral hemispheres. They are demarcated posteriorly by the central sulcus, laterally by the Sylvian fissure, and medially by the cingulate sulcus. The frontal lobes are anatomically and functionally heterogeneous, and the lateral surface of the frontal lobes can be divided into three major functional sectors: primary motor, premotor, and prefrontal cortex.

A. Primary Motor Cortex

The most posterior region of the frontal lobe, the precentral gyrus, represents the brain's primary motor area. This region forms a narrow strip of tissue along the lateral surface of the frontal lobe and continues down around the medial bank of the cortical apex. Primary motor cortex gives rise to the corticobulbar and corticospinal tracts and is responsible for the mediation of movement.

B. Premotor Cortex

Positioned immediately anterior to the primary motor region, the premotor cortex is composed of several functional areas. The lateral premotor area appears to be involved in the integration of motor skills and learned action sequences. The supplementary motor area on the medial surface in the superior frontal gyrus appears to mediate the initiation and programming of body movements. Broca's area is situated in the inferior, posterior frontal gyrus and is responsible for controlling voluntary speech.

C. Prefrontal Cortex

The prefrontal cortex is composed of the anterior portion of the frontal lobes. This region has robust connections with limbic and subcortical areas. In 1993, Jefferey Cummings described three frontal–subcortical circuits that mediate cognitive, motivational, and emotional processes: the dorsolateral prefrontal circuit, the orbitofrontal circuit, and the anterior cingulate circuit.

The dorsolateral prefrontal circuit includes the lateral convexity of the frontal lobe, dorsolateral caudate, portions of the globus pallidus and substantia nigra, and ventral anterior and dorsomedial thalamic nuclei. The dorsolateral circuit subserves executive functioning abilities, including response inhibition, fluency, working memory, and retrieval from long-term memory.

Jefferey Cummings also proposed an orbitofrontal circuit composed of two parallel subcircuits: the lateral and medial orbitofrontal circuits. The lateral orbitofrontal circuit projects from orbitofrontal cortex to ventral portions of the caudate; the medial circuit projects to the ventral striatum. Both circuits then project to medial portions of the globus pallidus, midbrain structures, and ventrolateral and dorsomedial thalamus. The orbitofrontal circuit mediates the modulation of social behavior; lesions can produce personality changes, including indifference to others, irritability, tactlessness, and impulsive behavior.

The anterior cingulate circuit projects from the anterior cingulate cortex and incorporates the ventromedial caudate, ventral putamen, and nucleus accumbens. This circuit is thought to mediate motivation; lesions are associated with apathy and disinterest.

II. NEUROPSYCHOLOGICAL FUNCTIONS OF THE FRONTAL LOBE

A. Executive Functioning

Damage to the dorsolateral prefrontal cortex has been associated with compromised performance on neuropsychological measures sensitive to executive func-

tioning. According to Muriel Deutsch Lezak, the term "executive functions" can be defined as the capacities that enable a person to engage in purposive, independent, and self-serving behavior. These functions include the ability to plan, to disengage from the immediate environment, to show flexibility of thinking, to fluently generate concepts, and to inhibit responses to overlearned patterns of behavior. Many researchers contend that executive functioning abilities remain among the most highly developed of human frontal lobe accomplishments.

B. Mental Flexibility

Mental flexibility requires the capacity to shift a course of thought or action according to rapidly changing situational demands. The Wisconsin Card Sorting Test (WCST) is a popular neuropsychological measure used to assess concept formation, abstract reasoning, and the ability to shift cognitive strategies in response to changing environmental contingencies. The subject is presented with four stimulus cards depicting figures of varying forms, colors, and numbers of figures (one red triangle, two green stars, three yellow crosses, and four blue circles). The task is to match each consecutive card from a deck of similar stimulus cards with one of the four key cards. In response to each matching, the subject is told only whether his or her choice was correct or incorrect. After the subject makes a specified number of correct matches, without warning the sorting strategy is changed. The subject is therefore required to use the examiner's feedback to develop a new sorting strategy.

Patients with frontal lobe damage have been found to perform more poorly on the WCST task than patients with nonfrontal damage. The required shifting response is particularly challenging for these patients because it entails the use of mental flexibility and reasoning skills. Frontal lobe patients commonly make perseverative errors by continuing to sort by a certain principle (e.g., by color) long after that sorting principle has been changed (e.g., to form). In some cases, patients appear almost oblivious to feedback and continue to make erroneous perseverations, despite their ability to verbalize the correct sorting strategy. Recent work by Kyle Boone suggests that perseverations on the WCST are more strongly associated with right frontal damage than left frontal damage.

The California Card Sorting Test is another useful measure of concept formation, shifting, and reasoning.

This unique card-sorting task was designed to isolate and measure specific components of problem-solving ability. The subject is asked to sort six cards spontaneously into two groups of three cards each, according to as many different rules as possible, and to report the rule after each sort. In another condition, subjects are required to report the rules for correct sorts performed by the examiner. This test examines several executive components, including the ability to generate and initiate different sorts, the ability to verbalize the principles of accurate sorts, and the ability to inhibit perseverative sorts. In 1992, Dean Dellis and colleagues found that patients with focal frontal lobe lesions and patients with Korsakoff's syndrome were impaired on eight of nine components of the task. Based on these results, the authors suggested that a wide array of deficits in abstract thinking, cognitive flexibility, and use of knowledge to regulate behavior contribute to the problem-solving impairment of patients with frontal lobe dysfunction.

C. Response Inhibition

Another important aspect of executive functioning is the ability to inhibit responses to established patterns of behavior. The Stroop Test is considered a measure of a person's ability to inhibit a habitual response in favor of an unusual one. During the interference condition of the Stroop, subjects are presented with a list of colored words (blue, green, red, etc.) printed in nonmatching colored ink. For example, the word *blue* may be printed in red ink, and the word *green* may be printed in blue ink. The subject's task is to name the ink color in which the words are printed as quickly as possible. This challenge involves suppressing the strong inclination to read the color name. Many patients with frontal lobe damage are unable to inhibit reading the words and thus show impairment on this task.

D. Verbal Fluency

Frontal lobe impairment can also produce deficits in a person's ability to rapidly generate words. The Controlled Oral Word Association Test (COWAT), also known as the "FAS," is a commonly used neuropsychological measure of verbal fluency. The COWAT consists of three word conditions. The subjects' task is to produce as many words as he can that begin with the given letter (F, A, or S) within a 1-min time period.

Subjects are also instructed to exclude proper nouns, numbers, and the same word with a different suffix.

The COWAT and other measures of verbal fluency have proven to be sensitive indicators of frontal lobe dysfunction. In 1989, Jerry Janowsky, Arthur Shimamura, and Larry Squire found that patients with circumscribed left or bilateral frontal lobe lesions produced significantly fewer words than did control subjects. Other researchers found that left frontal lesions resulted in lower word production than right frontal ones. Similarly, regional cerebral blood flow findings have shown left-sided frontal activation during the performance of verbal fluency tasks.

Frontal lobe damage can also impair performance on visual or design fluency tasks. Design fluency tests were developed as visual analogs to verbal fluency measures such as the FAS. The subjects' task is to generate as many unique designs as they can within a given time period. Although the left prefrontal region appears to be specialized in using verbal material, Christina Elfgren and Jarl Risberg reported bilateral frontal lobe activation during the performance of visual generation tasks.

E. Planning

Patients with frontal lobe dysfunction have been reported to demonstrate impairments in the ability to plan. A wide spectrum of neuropsychological measures have been designed to assess numerous aspects of planning behavior. The Porteus Maze Test is a maze tracing task commonly used to assess planning and foresight. The subject's task is to trace the maze without entering any blind alleys. Performance level is usually measured on the basis of completion time and the test age level of the most difficult task the subject is able to successfully complete. In 1991, Harvey Levin and colleagues reported that patients with frontal lesions solved the Porteus mazes more slowly than severely injured nonfrontal head trauma patients and control subjects.

A number of tower puzzles have been designed to gauge more abstract forms of planning ability. Some of the most popular are the Tower of London, Tower of Hanoi, Tower of Toronto, and Tower of California. In all these tasks, the subject sees a set of pegs on which a number of beads or disks are placed in an initial starting position. The subject is instructed to move the disks to the appropriate pegs in order to reach a predetermined goal state. Two common test rules include only moving one disk at a time and never placing a larger disk on top of a smaller disk.

In 1991, Tim Shallice and Paul Burgess found that patients with predominantly left anterior lesions performed more poorly on the Tower of London test than patients with posterior lesions and normal controls. Guila Glosser and Harold Goodglass reported similar results using the Tower of Hanoi: Patients with anterior lesions performed worse than the patients with posterior lesions.

Planning ability can also be measured by an individual's ability to prepare and execute target behaviors required for simulated real-life situations and events. In 1998, Eliane Miotto and Robin Morris developed the Virtual Planning Test with the intention of investigating the planning and organizational abilities of patients with frontal lobe neurosurgical lesions. The simulated planning tasks involved preparations for a fictional "trip" abroad or planning events that related to the subject's immediate environment. The frontal lobe patients were found to be impaired on this task and showed a tendency to select inappropriate activities associated with their immediate environment.

F. Memory

The frontal lobes play an important role in adequate memory functioning. Conventional research suggests that frontal lobe lesions do not produce a primary deficit in memory per se, but that they interfere with critical memory processes. Although encoding deficiencies can be observed in frontal lobe patients, they usually occur secondarily to executive functioning impairments. Thus, relatively speaking, frontal lobe damage does not significantly impair the ability to memorize material but does interfere with the ability to organize, attend to, and spontaneously retrieve information.

G. Retrieval

On measures of recent verbal memory, patients with frontal lobe impairment often demonstrate a pattern of poor recollection or retrieval of information in the context of relatively preserved recognition memory. In 1994, Donald Stuss and colleagues examined the memory abilities of patients with prefrontal, temporal, and diencephalic lesions. Patients with medial temporal and diencephalic lesions performed most poorly and did not improve with cueing. Patients with lateral

temporal and prefrontal pathology scored worse in the free recall condition than the controls, but they improved with cueing. In addition, their recognition memory performance was relatively better than their free recall performance.

In 1995, Felicia Gershberg and Arthur Shimamura found similar results in their examination of free recall strategies in a group of patients with unilateral frontal lobe lesions. An example of a typical memory strategy is the rehearsal of associations between words presented in a list learning task. This kind of organizational ability is thought to require considerable executive control. As such, one would expect diminished use of such strategies on the part of patients with frontal lobe impairment. Consistent with their hypothesis, Gershberg and Shimamura found that the frontal lobe patients demonstrated impaired free recall ability and reduced use of subjective organization strategies. The frontal patients also benefited from strategy instruction (e.g., category cues) at either study or test, suggesting that both encoding and retrieval processes may be impaired by frontal lobe damage. Based on these findings, the authors suggested that retrieval impairments by patients with frontal lobe lesions might be partly due to deficits in the use of organizational strategies.

Impaired encoding and retrieval functions in prefrontal syndromes can also be related to deficits in working memory. Allan Baddeley uses the term "working memory" to describe the "scratch pad" of the human memory system—the place where information can be held and manipulated while new information is being processed. Researchers suggest that the prefrontal cortex plays a critical role in these complex working memory abilities. In support of this view, several functional imaging studies have reported activation of the dorsolateral prefrontal cortex during both auditory and visual mental working tasks.

H. Temporal Sequencing

Frontal lobe patients have also demonstrated deficiencies in their ability to integrate temporally separated events. Temporal sequencing can be tested by assessing an individual's ability to recall or recognize the temporal order of recently presented lists of words, abstract designs, or pictures. Patients with prefrontal cortex damage have been shown to demonstrate impairment in recalling the temporal order of such items but have no item recognition problems for the same list of words, designs, or pictures. In 1994,

Raymond Kesner, Ramona Hopkins, and Bonnie Fineman conducted a study in which a group of prefrontal cortex-damaged patients were tested for item and order recognition memory for spatial location, word, abstract picture, and hand position information. Compared to controls, frontal patients showed severe deficits on all order recognition tests. However, relative to controls, the frontal patients showed no deficits in their ability to recognize these same items with the exception of a deficit for hand position. With regard to laterality, order recognition memory deficits for spatial location occurred for right and bilateral but not left prefrontal cortex-damaged patients. Both right and left prefrontal cortex subjects showed order recognition memory deficits for words, abstract pictures, and hand position.

I. Source Memory

In addition to deficits in sequencing temporal information, patients with frontal lobe dysfunction have been reported to show deficits in identifying the source of their knowledge. Thus, an individual with source amnesia may be able to remember a fact but will forget where and when that fact was learned.

In a 1989 study, Jerry Janowsky and colleagues found that patients with frontal lobe lesions exhibited impaired source memory for facts acquired in a recent test session, even though their memory for the facts was normal. During the first phase of the experiment, subjects were asked to learn some general information facts (not known prior to the study session). After a 6 to 8 day retention interval, subjects were asked to answer some additional questions. Some questions were the previously nonrecalled items from the initial study phase, some were new items from the same level of difficulty, and others were easy questions that had not been presented previously. When subjects correctly answered a question, they were asked to recollect where and when the information had been learned. Compared to their age-matched controls, the frontal lobe group made significantly more errors by attributing learned information to an incorrect source. Results of this study suggest that the frontal lobes play an important role in one's ability to associate information in memory to the context in which it was acquired.

J. Autobiographical Memory

The active process of recollecting information from one's earlier life requires the use of executive abilities such as attention, flexible searching, and organization. Given the dysexective syndrome characteristic of frontal lobe patients, it is not surprising that individuals with prefrontal cortex damage occasionally exhibit impaired autobiographical memory. Assessments of autobiographical memory usually involve a lengthy series of questions covering the major periods of a typical life span (childhood, adolescence, and adulthood). Subjects are asked to describe specific events in great detail, including the dates and the importance of the events, and to indicate the names of friends and family members who may have participated in the events. For example, a subject may be asked to remember the date of his or her wedding or to provide the name of the preschool that he or she attended. The subject's family members later corroborate all reported information.

In a 1993 study, Sergio Della Salla and fellow researchers examined autobiographical memory retrieval in a group of patients with frontal lobe lesions. The battery of tests administered included an autobiographical memory enquiry and a series of executive functioning measures. Six of 16 frontal lobe patients were impaired on the autobiographical memory measure. Moreover, poor autobiographical retrieval correlated significantly with impaired performance on the executive functioning measures. Thus, impaired ability to retrieve information from autobiographical memory may have been related to the frontal lobe patient's inefficient organizational and searching ability.

K. Language

Frontal lobe lesions can result in a variety of language disturbances, including loss of grammar (aggramatism) and the production of unintended syllables, words, or phrases during speech (paraphasic errors). The following sections highlight some of the most extensively researched frontal lobe language disorders.

L. Broca's Aphasia

Broca's aphasia is one of the most commonly known syndromes of frontal language disorder. The core features of this syndrome include nonfluent, effortful speech production, semantic and phonemic paraphasias, articulatory errors, agrammatism, and relatively preserved comprehension. Widely accepted definitions of Broca's aphasia also include poor repetition, reading, and writing ability.

The lesion in classical Broca's aphasia involves the left posterior, inferior frontal gyrus. With the advent of sophisticated neuroimaging techniques, researchers have discovered that circumscribed damage to Broca's area does not necessarily result in the complete syndrome of Broca's aphasia. Moreover, some individuals with Broca's aphasia do not have lesions in Broca's area. Therefore, it seems that the underlying pathology in Broca's aphasia can be relatively extensive and varied. Regions including the inferior central Rolandic area, the insula, subcortical regions, and the anterior parietal regions have also been implicated in this language syndrome.

M. Pure Motor Aphasia

Verbal apraxia or pure motor aphasia refers to the articulatory and prosodic disturbance of language output in the absence of the agrammatic component. The underlying lesion is said to involve the left lower motor cortex and posterior operculum. Recently, Nina Dronkers emphasized the relationship between articulatory deficits and damage to the precentral gyrus of the insula.

This clinical syndrome is characterized by impaired articulation, slow and effortful speech, segmentation, phonemic paraphasias, dysprosody, and occasional hypophonia. The outcome for pure motor aphasia ranges from full recovery to a status of normal language with persistent dysarthria and/or dysprosody.

N. Transcortical Motor Aphasia

Transcortical motor aphasia (TCMA) involves lesions of the left frontal lobe–supplementary motor area (SMA), just anterior and superior to Broca's area. During acute phases, patients may initially present as mute but later develop a clinical profile characterized by normal repetition and comprehension, with limited, slow, and perseverative spontaneous speech.

Some researchers hypothesize that the SMA represents the "starting mechanism" or center for initiation of speech. Others suggest that damage to the SMA results in a lack of a plan or program to carry out voluntary speech. In their 1984 study, Morris Freedman and colleagues studied 15 patients with TCMA or near variants of the syndrome. Consistent with TCMA literature, these researchers concluded that small lesions to SMA cause a pure disorder of speech initiation. Furthermore, damage to fibers from SMA to premotor cortex may disconnect the limbic starter mechanism of speech from the cortical regions that control the motoric aspect of speech.

O. Frontal–Subcortical Aphasias

Language deficits can also result from lesions to frontal–subcortical brain regions. Lesions of the putamen and internal capsule will produce a nonfluent language disorder that at times resembles Broca's aphasia. In 1982, Margaret Naeser and her colleagues examined nine cases of subcortical aphasia with capsular/putaminal (C/P) lesions documented by computed tomographic scans. Patients with C/P lesion sites with anterior-superior white matter lesion extension had good comprehension, grammatical but slow dysarthric speech, and lasting right hemiplegia.

III. NEUROPSYCHIATRY OF THE FRONTAL LOBE

A. Personality

One of the most well-known early cases of behavioral change following frontal lobe damage is that of Phineas P. Gage. On September 13, 1848, this young man became a victim of a bizarre accident in which a tamping iron rod caused severe damage to his frontal lobes. Prior to sustaining this injury, Phineas was described as a reserved, intelligent, and responsible individual. Following the mishap, he transformed into an irreverent, irresponsible, and careless human being. This famous case and many modern counterparts that followed sparked considerable interest in the wide spectrum of personality changes seen in frontal lobe pathology.

The diminished capacity to modulate emotional behavior has frequently been associated with damage to the frontal lobes. In the context of traumatic brain injury, the changes customarily involve either an exaggeration or muting of emotions. In some cases, previously outgoing and sociable individuals become apathetic, emotionally flat, disengaged, and withdrawn. On the opposite end of the spectrum, patients can demonstrate uncharacteristically aggressive, impulsive, disinhibited, and socially inappropriate behavior. The apathetic syndrome has been localized to damage to the convexity and medial aspects of the frontal lobes, whereas the aggressive and disinhibited syndrome has been attributed to the orbitofrontal regions.

A disturbance in self-awareness represents another common feature associated with frontal lobe damage. Deficient awareness may be reflected by the inability to appreciate performance errors on neuropsychological testing or to recognize the impact of one's impairments on others. Patients with compromised frontal lobe functioning have also been reported to demonstrate a failure to appreciate social and interpersonal norms. In an attempt to explain these deficits, some authors have suggested that frontal lobe pathology may actually impair an individual's personal consciousness or sense of self. Endel Tulving and colleagues used the term "autonoetic awareness" (awareness of oneself as a continuous entity across time) to describe this phenomenon. According to Donald T. Stuss, in this context disturbed self-awareness is "not lack of knowledge but impaired judgment of the objective facts in relation to one's own life."

IV. DISEASES OF THE FRONTAL LOBE

A. Frontotemporal Dementia

Frontotemporal lobar degeneration (FTLD) is a common cause of early onset dementia. There are three clinical syndromes that occur in FTLD: frontotemporal dementia (FTD), progressive nonfluent aphasia, and semantic dementia. The following sections are limited to a discussion of the core behavioral, neuropsychological, and pathological features of FTD.

1. Behavioral Features of FTD

The early stage of FTD is characterized by marked changes in personality and behavior. Patients typically become disinhibited, apathetic, and irritable. Gross disinhibition often leads to impulsivity, increased aggressiveness, and antisocial behavior. Antisocial acts can range from inappropriate comments to various forms of criminal behavior. In a 1997 study, Bruce Miller and colleagues compared the presence of antisocial conduct in FTD versus Alzheimer's dementia (AD) patients. Almost 50% of the FTD patients were involved in behaviors such as stealing, physical assault, public urination or masturbation, and unethical job conduct. In contrast, only one of the AD patients manifested these types of behaviors.

According to the FTD consensus criteria proposed by David Neary and colleagues in 1998, declines in social graces and decorum are commonly manifested in tactlessness and a loss of interpersonal etiquette and social awareness. For example, FTD patients often demonstrate increased talking, inappropriate laughter, singing, and invasion of personal space. Improper hygiene, grooming, and other aspects of personal awareness are also observed. These deficits in social and personal awareness are further complicated by the FTD patients' lack of insight into their behavioral disturbance and its impact on others.

FTD patients often lack empathy and are typically described as emotionally indifferent and apathetic. Some patients become self-absorbed and exhibit less concern about the welfare of friends and family members. Other characteristic affective symptoms in FTD include depression, anxiety, and psychotic features. Patients with FTD can also demonstrate hyperorality and dietary changes. Hyperorality may manifest in overeating, bingeing, and excessive consumption of liquids and/or alcohol. Some patients develop a strong preference for sweets and may also place inanimate objects in their mouths.

FTD patients progressively develop changes in speech production and structure. During the early phases of the disease patients may demonstrate excessive talking, frequent use of stereotyped phrases, and echolalia. Later stages may be characterized by mutism.

2. Neuropsychological Features of FTD

According to the 1998 consensus criteria proposed by David Neary and colleagues, the neuropsychological profile for FTD is characterized by significant impairments on frontal lobe measures in the context of relatively preserved memory, language, and visuospatial skills. Frontal lobe measures are tests designed to assess executive functioning abilities, such as planning, mental flexibility, verbal fluency, abstraction, and the ability to inhibit responses to overlearned patterns of behavior. Popular standardized neuropsychological measures of executive functioning include the WCST, Stroop Test, and Trail Making Test.

A number of studies have examined the patterns of executive functioning deficits found in FTD. In a 1996 investigation, Nancy Pachana and colleagues documented the neuropsychological changes that distinguish FTD patients from AD patients. They found that AD patients exhibited relatively greater impairment on memory than executive tasks, whereas the FTD group showed the opposite pattern.

FTD patients may perform poorly on measures of recent memory, language, and visuospatial tasks. However, these deficits are thought to occur secondarily to executive dysfuntion, such as inattention, inefficient organizational strategies, and poor self-monitoring. For example, on measures of recent verbal memory, FTD patients tend to have difficulty spontaneously recalling information (free recall), whereas their ability to recognize these same items is relatively preserved.

3. Pathological Features of FTD

According to the pathological criteria proposed by Arne Brun and colleagues in 1994, FTD results from bilateral and for the most part symmetrical distribution of pathology in the frontal and anterior temporal lobes. Upon inspection, mild atrophy of these brain regions is commonly observed. At the microscopic level, a degenerative process is noted in the frontal or frontotemproal cortex, characterized by microvaculation (spongiosis), neuronal loss, and gliosis. The presence of argyrophillic, ubiquitin positive inclusion bodies (Pick bodies) and swollen, achromatic neurons (Pick cells) can also be observed. The clinical syndrome of FTD can be seen with and without the presence of Pick bodies and Pick cells.

B. Traumatic Brain Injury

Brain damage following traumatic brain injury, particularly closed head injury (CHI), frequently involves the orbital and polar aspects of the frontal lobes. Commonly observed behavioral features of CHI following frontal lobe damage include posttraumatic amnesia, attentional deficits, and changes in personality. Posttraumatic amnesia (PTA) is thought to result from a disconnection or damage of the basal forebrain and orbitofrontal cortex. PTA usually occurs during the period of acute recovery following a severe head injury. Patients typically experience confusion and disorientation, and tend to confabulate, and have difficulty learning and remembering information. The duration of PTA usually depends on the severity and the outcome of the brain injury.

Attentional deficits are a relatively common behavioral consequence of severe head injury. Distractibility, problems with concentration, inability to focus, and an overall slowing are commonly reported complaints. Attention is considered a complex cognitive process composed of a number of components, including phasic alertness, selective attention, and sustained attention. Several studies of CHI patients suggest that individual attentional components can be selectively impaired following frontal lobe damage. For example, investigators have linked the midfrontal regions to deficits in sustained attention. Others attribute impairments in selective attention to damaged frontal–thalamic and subcortical structures.

Traumatic brain injuries that damage the frontal and temporal lobes can also result in profound changes in personality and social adjustment. Victims of traffic and other common head injury accidents frequently exhibit reduced drive, decreased awareness, blunted affect, and a lack of initiative. This apathetic syndrome is attributed to damage of the medial frontal lobes. Closed head injuries can also produce what is described as a euphoric syndrome, characterized by impulsivity, sexual disinhibition, socially inappropriate behavior, and aggressiveness. The orbitofrontal regions have been implicated in this class of personality deficits.

See Also the Following Articles

APHASIA • EVOLUTION OF THE BRAIN • LANGUAGE, NEURAL BASIS OF • MEMORY NEUROBIOLOGY • MODELING BRAIN INJURY/TRAUMA • MOTOR CORTEX • NEUROANATOMY • PHINEAS GAGE • SPEECH • TIME PASSAGE

Suggested Reading

Benton, A. L. (1968). Differential behavioral effects in frontal lobe disease. *Neuropsychologia* **6**(1), 53–60.

Brun, A., Englund, B., Gustafson, L., Passant, U., Mann, D. M. A., and Snowden, J. S. (1994). Clinical and neuropathological criteria for frontotemporal dementia. *J. Neurol. Neurosurg. Psychiatr.* **57**, 416–418.

Damasio, A. R., and Anderson, S. W. (1993). *The frontal lobes.* In *Clinical neuropsychology* (E. Kenneth, M. Heilman, E. E. Valenstein, *et al.*, Eds.), 3rd ed., pp. 409–460. Oxford University Press, New York.

Damasio, H., Grabowski, T., Frank, R., Galaburda, A. M., and Damasio, A. R. (1994). The return of Phineas Gage: Clues about the brain from the skull of a famous patient. *Science* **264**, 1102–1105.

Levin, H. S., Goldstein, F. C., Williams, D. H., and Eisenberg, H. M. (1991). *The contribution of frontal lobe lesions to the neurobehavioral outcome of closed head injury.* In *Frontal Lobe Function and Dysfunction* (E. Harvey, S. Levin, E. Howard, M. Eisenberg, *et al.*, Eds.), pp. 318–338. Oxford University Press, New York.

Levine, B., Black, S. E., Cabeza, R., Sinden, M., McIntosh, A. R., Toth, J. P., Tulving, E., and Stuss, D. T. (1998). Episodic memory and the self in a case of isolated retrograde amnesia. *Brain* **121**(10), 1951–1973.

Lezak, M. D. (1995). *Neuropsychological Assessment*, 3rd ed. Oxford University Press, New York.

Miller, B. L., and Cummings, J. L. (1999). *The Human Frontal Lobes: Functions and Disorders*. Guilford, New York.

Miller, B. L., Cummings, J. L., Villanueva-Meyer, J., Boone, K., Mehriinger, C. M., Lesser, I. M., and Mena, I. (1991). Frontal lobe degeneration: Clinical, neuropsychological and SPECT characteristics. *Neurology* **42,** 1374–1382.

Miller, B. L., Chang, L., Mena, I., Boone, K. B., and Lesser, I. (1993). Progressive right frontotemporal degeneration: Clinical, neuropsychological and SPECT characteristics. *Dementia* **4,** 204–213.

Neary, D., Snowden, J. S., Gustafson, L., Passant, U., Stuss, D., Black, S., Freedman, M., Kertesz, A., Robert, P. H., Albert, M., Boone, K., Miller, B. L., Cummings, J., and Benson, D. F. (1998). Frontotemporal lobar degeneration: A consensus on clinical diagnostic criteria. *Neurology* **51**(6), 1546–1554.

Perecman, E., and the Institute for Research in Behavioral Neuroscience (1987). *The Frontal Lobes Revisited*. IRBN Press, New York.

Prigatano, G. P., and Schacter, D. L. (Eds.) (1991). *Awareness of Deficit after Brain Injury: Clinical and Theoretical Issues*. Royal Chem. Soc., London.

Stuss, D. T., and Benson, D. F. (1984). Neuropsychological studies of the frontal lobes. *Psychol. Bull.* **95**(1), 3–28.

Stuss, D. T., and Benson, D. F. (1986). *The Frontal Lobes*. Raven Press, New York.

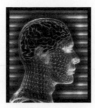

Functional Magnetic Resonance Imaging (fMRI)

ROBERT L. SAVOY

MGH/MIT/HST Athinoula A. Martinos Center

GLOSSARY

block design Experimental design for functional neuroimaging in which an attempt is made to put the subject's brain in a steady state of activity by using the same type of task for an extended period of time (typically 20–60 sec) and then comparing the brain activation during that block with other blocks that use a different task.

blood oxygen level dependent (BOLD) Refers to a general method of magnetic resonance imaging (MRI) for detecting changes in the nuclear magnetic resonance (NMR) signal that are caused by the varying concentration of deoxyhemoglobin, locally, in the blood near a part of the brain.

event-related design Experimental design for functional neuroimaging in which individual, brief (typically 1–2 sec in duration) stimuli of different types are presented in random order, and where the evoked responses for many such trials of a given type are averaged together to detect a measureable response.

flow via alternating inversion recovery (FAIR) Refers to a specific method of MRI for detecting changes in the NMR signal that are caused by the varying flow, locally, of blood in arteries near a part of the brain.

functional magnetic resonance imaging (fMRI) The use of MRI to detect changes in blood flow and blood oxygenation associated with local changes in neuronal activity in the brain.

gradient magnets Part of the technology of MRI used for supplying strong, operator-controlled linear gradients of magnetic field to enable the generation and detection of the NMR signal associated with a specific point in three-dimensional space.

hemodynamics Changes in the properties (volume, flow rate, and chemical composition) of blood over time.

magnetic resonance imaging (MRI) The use of a variety of operator-controlled electromagnetic fields to generate a NMR signal that can be associated with a particular point in space.

nuclear magnetic resonance (NMR) The physical phenomenon of absorption and reemission of electromagnetic energy associated with the quantum mechanical spin and magnetic field of the nuclei of some atoms.

principle component analysis (PCA) The re-representation of multidimensional data into a collection of components (sometimes called eigenimages and eigenvectors) via an algorithm that accounts for the most variance by the first principal component, the second most by the second component, etc.

retinotopy The regular spatial arrangement of the receptive fields of cortical neurons in many parts of the visual cortex that follows, in a systematic way, the two-dimensional spatial arrangement of the retina.

talairach coordinates The most widely used convention for orienting and scaling human brains to facilitate the averaging and/or comparing of data across multiple subjects.

Functional magnetic resonance imaging (fMRI) refers to the use of the technology of magnetic resonance imaging (MRI) to detect the localized changes in blood flow and blood oxygenation that occur in the brain in response to neural activity. This article presents the basics of fMRI-based research, including the physical and biophysical bases of the signals, the current developments in experimental design and data analysis, and other practical considerations attendant to the technique, and also provides an overview of the broad range of scientific and clinical questions to which fMRI is being applied.

I. INTRODUCTION

It has long been known that there is some degree of localization of function in the human brain, as indicated by the effects of traumatic head injury. Work in the middle of the 20th century, notably the direct cortical stimulation of patients during neurosurgery, suggested that the degree and specificity of such localization of function was far greater than had earlier been imagined. One problem with the data based on lesions and direct stimulation was that the work depended on the study of what were, by definition, damaged brains. During the second half of the 20th century, a collection of relatively noninvasive tools for assessing and localizing human brain function in healthy volunteers led to an explosion of research in what is often termed "brain mapping." The tool that has been developing the most rapidly, and the tool that currently supplies the best volumetric (three-dimensional) picture of activity in the human brain, is fMRI.

Functional MRI uses the physical phenomenon of nuclear magnetic resonance (NMR) and the associated technology of MRI to detect spatially localized changes in hemodynamics that have been triggered by local neural activity. It has been known for more than 100 years that neural activity causes changes in blood flow and blood oxygenation in the brain, and that these changes are local to the area of neural activation. Techniques using radioactive tracers were developed in the mid-20th century to detect metabolic activity correlated with neural activation and to detect blood volume changes correlated with neural activation. In the early 1990s the technique of MRI was successfully adapted to measuring some of these effects noninvasively in humans. The development of fMRI led to a dramatic increase in neuroscience research in human functional brain mapping across the spectrum of psychological functions—from sensation, perception, and attention to cognition, language, and emotion—in both normal and patient populations.

Functional MRI makes the future of functional brain imaging particularly exciting for at least three reasons. First, fMRI does not involve ionizing radiation, and therefore it can be used repeatedly on a single subject and even on child volunteers. This permits longitudinal studies and it permits improvement in signal-to-noise ratios if the task being used elicits the same general response when repeated multiple times. Second, technical improvements in fMRI (due to more powerful magnets, more sophisticated imaging hardware, and the development of new methods of experimental design and data analysis) promise to yield improvements in spatial and temporal resolution for the technique. Third, there is a growing effort to integrate the findings based on fMRI with those from other techniques for assessing human brain function, such as electroencephalography (EEG) and magnetoencephalography (MEG), which inherently have much greater temporal resolution. It is likely that major advances in functional brain imaging will be made in the near future, but the associated technologies are complicated. In particular, to understand the technique of fMRI, one must consider a collection of interrelated issues, from physics and physiology to the practicalities of experimental design, data analysis, safety, and costs.

II. PHYSICS AND PHYSIOLOGY

MRI operates by creating and detecting a signal generated by the physical phenomenon of NMR. Although an in-depth explanation of the physics of NMR and the technology of MRI is beyond the scope of this article, a basic understanding of how a MR scanner operates is useful in discussing fMRI in its applications to psychology and medicine. The following discussion is based on a description of the "classical electrodynamics" picture of NMR and MRI. A more rigorous and complete treatment of NMR would require quantum mechanics, but MRI is best understood in terms of classical electrodynamics.

A. The NMR Signal

To begin an MRI session, the subject is placed horizontally into the bore of a high-field magnet. In a typical clinical MRI system this magnet has a field strength of 1.5 T. A small fraction of the hydrogen nuclei (single protons) of the water molecules in the body of the subject become aligned with the field of this magnet. (Many other atoms and nuclei with magnetic moments are also aligned, but for the purposes of this article and almost all fMRI applications, it is the hydrogen nuclei of water molecules that are the source of the signal.) The hydrogen nuclei are oriented in a random collection of directions, relative to the main magnetic field, but there is a small statistical preference to have the longitudinal component of their orientations (i.e., the component in the direction of the main magnet) to be aligned with the main field. To the extent that a proton is not perfectly aligned with the main magnet, it will precess (spin) around the orientation of the main magnet. However, because the orientation of each proton is random (except for the component along the direction of the main field), and because it is only the randomly oriented transverse components (i.e., the components perpendicular to the main field) that generate a signal, the collection of spinning protons do not yield a net, detectable magnetic field.

Application of a radio frequency (RF) pulse of magnetic energy, presented at the frequency of the precession (i.e., the resonant frequency), causes all the hydrogen nuclei to change orientation (nutate). By controlling the power and duration of the RF pulse, the nuclei can be rotated to any desired angle relative to the main magnetic field. Typically, the parameters of the device are set so that the protons are rotated 90°. When the protons continue to precess in this new orientation, the net magnetic field that was originally induced in the body by the main magnet, and that was previously aligned with the main magnet, is now oriented 90° away and thus generates a detectable, changing magnetic field as it spins (precesses). A coil of wire around the subject will have a current generated within because of the changing magnetic field (Faraday's law). This current is the raw signal detected in a MRI scanner (Fig. 1).

B. Relaxation

The signal thus generated decays exponentially over time due to a number of processes. If the raw, exponential decay of the signal is measured (without doing anything else to create images), the process takes about 100 msec and the exponential time constant associated with that decay is conventionally called "T2*" (read "tee-two-star"). This decay in the measured signal is driven by a number of different physical processes.

First, the protons slowly (on the time scale of seconds for most brain tissue) realign with the main magnet. This is called longitudinal relaxation, and the time constant associated with this exponential process is called T1. Second, the signal generated by the collection of precessing protons is weakened by the

fact that each individual proton experiences a slightly different *local* magnetic field due to interactions with nearby water molecules and other biological tissues and thus precesses at a slightly different frequency from its neighbors. With time (typically on a scale of tenths of seconds for most brain tissue) these protons get out of phase so that their respective magnetic fields are no longer lined up and therefore do not generate a detectable, macroscopic signal in the surrounding coil of wire. This is sometimes called the spin–spin component of transverse relaxation because it is based on the interaction of the spins (which imply magnetic fields) of nearby nuclei. If the magnetic field were perfectly uniform, then the net decay rate of the signal would be given by the exponential decay rate T2, which is driven by the combination of spin–spin transverse relaxation and the T1 longitudinal component. In the brain tissue of interest, T2 is almost entirely determined by the spin–spin relaxation.

In reality, there are other sources of magnetic field nonuniformity. Imperfections in the main magnet, variable magnetic susceptibility of the differing parts of the human body that has been inserted into the magnet, and changes in blood chemistry caused by externally injected "contrast agents" all contribute to nonuniformities in the magnetic field experienced by the precessing protons. Most important for fMRI, some chemicals that occur naturally in the body also distort the magnetic field. Deoxyhemoglobin is such a molecule, and as its local concentration is varied, the amount of distortion also varies. The rate of exponential decay of the NMR signal is influenced by all of these factors (Fig. 1).

C. Creating an Image

The preceding description yields a single number: T2*, the decay rate of the net NMR signal. This signal is conventionally called the free induction decay (FID) of the NMR signal because it is elicited when nothing else is done to the protons—that is, if the system were left free to decay at its own rate. However, this signal represents the net effect of inducing an NMR signal from the *entire volume of tissue* being subjected to the main magnet and the orientation-flipping RF pulse. To create an *image* in which different NMR signals are measured for different points in the three-dimensional volume, nonuniform magnetic fields are applied intentionally. The basic idea is to use linear magnetic field gradients, applied at various times and in various orientations, to distinguish the NMR signals arising

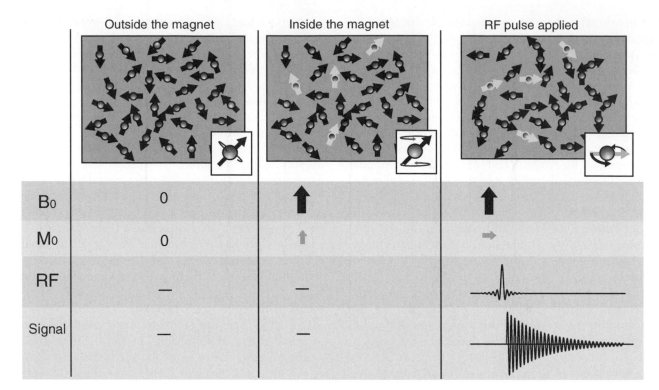

Figure 1 The basics of the NMR signal. The discussion of Section II.A is represented here in a simplified, cartoon form, with the story proceeding from left to right. Protons can be thought of conceptually as positively charged spheres that are always spinning, and this spin about an axis gives the proton an inherent orientation as well as a net magnetic moment along the axis of the spin. Before entering the magnet, the protons (with their magnetic field and spin direction indicated by arrows) are randomly oriented. There is no main field surrounding the body ($B_0=0$) and there is no induced field within the body ($M_0=0$). The body is placed in the main magnet ($B_0 \gg 0$). All the protons immediately start processing in a direction around B_0, but because the orientation and phases are random there is no net signal. After a few seconds, a small fraction of the protons change orientation to line up with B_0, which results in the creation of a net magnetic field in the body ($M_0>0$) oriented in the same direction as B_0. The individual protons are still precessing, now with a common net orientation, but the components of that rotation perpendicular to B_0 are still random so there is no detectable signal. A radio frequency (RF) pulse is applied for a brief period of time, causing all the protons to change their orientation by 90° so that the net induced magnetic field M_0 is now perpendicular to B_0. Now the individual precessing protons are aligned in such a way that the common component of orientation (M_0) goes around B_0 in a perpendicular direction and generates a macroscopically detectable current—the signal. The strength of that signal decreases exponentially with time for a variety of reasons described in Section II.B.

from different points in the three-dimensional volume. (The application of these nonuniform magnetic fields causes the raw NMR signal to decay even more rapidly than the FID, but the signal can still be measured, and various procedures can be used to create "echos" that enable the recovery of more information.)

The technology of MRI is based on the flexible (but complicated) application of multiple RF pulses and multiple gradients, synchronized precisely (and typically described in a pulse sequence diagram). The pulse sequence diagram indicates how a given slice of the brain is selected for imaging, how individual volume elements (voxels) are detected within each slice, and how the resulting signals are preferentially selected to obtain information about arterial blood flow or about the concentration of deoxyhemoglobin in venous

blood flow. Some imaging pulse sequences use multiple RF-pulses in the generation of NMR signals that will yield a single plane of imaging data. Some imaging pulse sequences [such as echo-planar imaging (EPI)] generate data for an entire plane from a single RF pulse. EPI is rapid (with an entire plane collected in less than 50 msec), but it is associated with more expensive hardware and various limitations in spatial resolution or susceptibility to imaging artifacts and distortions.

D. Contrast in an Image

As with any imaging modality, the key variable in producing a meaningful image is contrast. The signal measured at one point in space or time must be higher or lower than the signal at another point, and the variation in signal intensity across the image should systematically follow some variable of interest. In the endeavor of brain mapping, the ultimate variable of interest is neural activity. In order to measure local brain activity with MRI, one must exploit a chain of indirect linkages from neural activity (a constellation of electrical and chemical events) to changes in brain physiology and metabolism and finally to changes in the magnetic properties of substances within the brain.

Anything that causes a change in the NMR signal from a given voxel relative to other voxels at the same time is a source of *contrast* in the image. The density of protons in a given voxel (due to chemical composition) is one such source of contrast, though not an important one in fMRI. More commonly, it is the variation in rates of relaxation from voxel to voxel that generates contrast in the image.

In the earliest fMRI studies, exogenous contrasts (chemicals injected into the bloodstream of the subject) were used to obtain contrast. These blood-borne chemicals locally distorted the magnetic field, thus allowing increased blood perfusion to be detected. Subsequent studies demonstrated that endogenous contrast agents (i.e., naturally occurring molecules in the body, such as the concentration of deoxyhemoglobin in the blood) could also yield sufficient contrast between different states of neural activity. The use of endogenous contrast agents obviated the need for injecting foreign molecules into the bodies of normal (healthy) subjects, and this is one of the key reasons that fMRI has become so popular as a technique for assessing human brain function. In the short history of fMRI, a wide variety of techniques that produce various contrasts have been developed for detecting changes in brain physiology.

E. Neural Activation MRI

When neurons are active in the brain, there is an increase in blood flow and blood volume local to that region of activity. MRI can be used to detect the change in blood flow directly. The idea is that when fresh blood flows into the slice of the brain that is being imaged, it will have a different "spin history" (i.e., it will not have recently been hit by an orientation-flipping RF-pulse) and will thus have a greater degree of alignment with the main magnet. When another RF pulse is applied, the fresh blood will have a greater concentration of aligned protons to flip and will thus yield a greater NMR signal. The imaging of this signal

happens on a timescale that is rapid with respect to the blood flow, so the change is detected. This phenomenon is the basis for one kind of imaging in fMRI. It is largely sensitive to changes in arterial blood flow (where flow is the fastest).

There is a second, and more commonly used, process that yields an fMRI signal. The neural activity that elicited the local increase in blood flow and blood volume surprisingly does not elicit a correspondingly great increase in oxygen utilization. That is, although the neural activity leads to a small increase in oxygen utilization, it is dwarfed by the increase in blood flow. Thus, there is an increase in oxygenated hemoglobin in the venous portion of the circulatory system near the site of neural activity (as well as downstream from that site). The combination of increased oxygenated hemoglobin and increased blood flow results in a *decrease* in the instantaneous concentration of deoxygenated hemoglobin on the venous side of the capillaries. Deoxygenated hemoglobin (unlike oxygenated hemoglobin) is a strongly paramagnetic biological molecule, and it distorts the magnetic field locally. Thus, a *decrease* in the local concentration of deoxyhemoglobin leads to a *more* uniform magnetic field locally and to a longer time period during which the orientations of precessing protons stay in phase. Thus, the NMR signal in a region of decreased deoxyhemoglobin concentration *increases* relative to its normal (neuronally resting) state. This phenomenon is called the blood oxygen level dependent (BOLD) effect. It is the major source of contrast in most fMRI experiments.

F. Other Technical Issues in MRI

Operationally, fMRI differs from conventional MRI in two basic respects. First, it is tailored to be sensitive to contrasts in blood flow and/or oxygenation that reflect neural activity. Second, it is typically conducted with special hardware that permits the very rapid variation of the magnetic field gradients that are needed to create images. This permits much more rapid acquisition of whole-brain volumes than is conventionally done in MRI. This rapid data collection is crucial in most modern fMRI-based experiments.

Functional MRI is made practical and powerful by virtue of special pulse sequences (such as echo planar and spiral scanning) and hardware that permit the encoding of a brain slice while using a single RF pulse, allowing the entire brain to be imaged in a few seconds. A wide variety of different pulse sequences are used in fMRI, and this remains an area of continuous innovation. Moreover, the versatility of MRI for neuroscience extends beyond fMRI, and MR can also be used to assay various aspects of brain chemistry through a technique known as magnetic resonance spectroscopy (MRS). Because some variants of MRS can measure the presence of brain metabolites at temporal resolutions on the order of minutes and spatial resolutions similar to those of BOLD fMRI, MRS is in many ways conceptually related to fMRI.

G. Summary

A strong, spatially uniform magnetic field aligns a small but significant fraction of the hydrogen nuclei of water molecules in the brain. A carefully controlled sequence of gradient fields and RF pulses is used to generate NMR signals that can be reconstructed to form a three-dimensional image in which contrast is dependent, in part, on the blood flow and/or oxygenation changes caused by neural activity. Thus, MRI can be used noninvasively to detect changes in local neural activity in the human brain.

III. EXPERIMENTAL DESIGN

Designing experiments for fMRI-based studies presents unique opportunities and challenges. First, fMRI [like position emission tomography (PET) using O^{15}] depends on the indirect signals generated by hemodynamic changes (i.e., changes in blood flow and/or blood chemistry) rather than the more direct electrochemical changes associated with neural activity. Second, there are numerous technical challenges that follow from the particular physics of MRI when used for high-speed imaging of the human brain. Third, there are a number of practical considerations associated with both safety and the physical requirement for minimum movement of the subjects in fMRI studies that add to the challenges of fMRI experimental design. All these factors affect (and, in turn, are affected by) the current practical and future potential limits of spatial and temporal resolution associated with fMRI. Finally, as with any experimental approach to important questions concerning human psychology, the most fundamental and difficult problems arise in choosing tasks and stimuli that allow one to be convincing to one's self and to one's audience that the psychological question being asked is truly addressed by the experiment being performed. Can you convince your audience, for example, that when you

use fMRI to measure changes in brain activity during the color Stroop task you are actually studying some general attribute of inhibition and higher cognitive function?

A. Experimental Design and Hemodynamics

Functional MRI is dependent on hemodynamic changes rather than the electrical consequences of neural activity. The spatial and temporal characteristics of these hemodynamic effects must be taken into account when designing experiments and analyzing the data from these experiments. The spatial characteristics arise from the underlying vasculature; the temporal characteristics include a delay in the onset of detectable MR signal changes in response to neural activity and a dispersion of the resulting hemodynamic changes over a longer time than that of the initiating neural events.

With regard to the temporal aspects of the hemodynamics, fMRI experiments can be classified into two broad categories: block designs and event-related designs. In block designs, the experimental task is performed continuously in blocks of time, typically 20–60 sec in duration. The idea here is to ignore the details of the temporal characteristics by virtue of setting up a "steady state" of neuronal and hemodynamic change. The fact that there is a brief delay before the MR signal changes are detected is often unimportant when analyzing a long block of steady-state activity. This approach is conceptually simple; it is analogous to older PET experimental designs, and it is of great practical importance for fMRI because it is the optimal technique for *detecting* small changes in brain activity. The major weakness of block design is the requirement that all the stimuli or task characteristics remain unchanged for tens of seconds, precluding the use of many classic psychological paradigms (such as the "oddball" scheme).

The other major approach, event-related design, makes use of the details of the temporal response pattern in the hemodynamics as well as the largely linear response characteristics associated with multiple stimulus presentations. In event-related designs, the different stimuli are presented individually in a random order (rather than in blocks of similar or identical stimuli) and the hemodynamic response to each stimulus is measured. Event-related designs are further subdivided into spaced single-trial designs and rapid single-trial designs. In spaced single-trial designs, stimuli are presented with a long interstimulus interval

(ISI) relative to the hemodynamic response to a single stimulus. Specifically, an ISI of at least 10 sec, and more typically 12–20 sec, is used in an effort to allow the hemodynamic response to each stimulus to return to its resting state before the next stimulus is presented. This approach is conceptually simple but very inefficient in its use of imaging time, much of which is spent collecting data when the MR signal variation due to hemodynamcs is small or not detectable. (This is not only wasteful of expensive imaging time but also boring for the subject, who is only doing something approximately once every 15 sec.)

In contrast to *spaced* single-trial designs, *rapid* single-trial designs take advantage of the linearity and superposition properties of the hemodynamic responses to neural activity. To a first approximation, the hemodynamic changes associated with multiple stimulus presentations are additive and when presented at different times, are simple time shifts of each other. This permits the much more efficient design of experiments in which novel stimuli appear in quasi-random order and with variable ISIs (typically presenting a new stimulus every 1–3 sec). The associated data analysis is more difficult because the hemodynamic responses to the different stimuli overlap in time (and there are consequent weaknesses relative to block designs in terms of the detection of small effects) but the rapid single-trial designs are particularly powerful and useful when it is essential to have random order in the presentation of individual stimuli (i.e., in the situation in which a block design with long periods of the same type of stimulus would not permit the desired comparisons for neural activations). It is also more efficient in the use of imaging time and more engaging (less boring) for the subject.

One final approach to experimental design should be mentioned. All of the previously discussed techniques typically make use of averaging over multiple instances of a given trial type. In block design the trials all occur together, so the averaging is done as much by the hemodynamic and neural systems as by any data analysis software. In event-related designs the averaging over the effects of multiple stimulus presentations is done explicitly in software during data analysis. It is possible, however, to analyze spaced single-trial data on the basis of activation from a *single event* (rather than averaging over multiple instances of the same trial type). This technique has not been widely applied, primarily because the elicited signals to single stimulus events are generally weak. However, high-field MRI systems, and the selection of experimental paradigms that elicit strong, focal neural activity,

have been used to demonstrate the feasibility of single-event fMRI.

B. Spatial and Temporal Resolution in High-Speed MRI

The physiology of the circulatory system and the physics of the MRI devices constrain the spatial and temporal resolution of fMRI. Today, it is routine to obtain $1 \times 1 \times 1$-mm structural MR images and $5 \times 5 \times 5$-mm functional MR images. The temporal resolution of fMRI is on the order of 1–3 sec. Neither the spatial nor the temporal resolution numbers are indicative of absolute limits in terms of the physiology or the imaging hardware. Rather, they represent a snapshot in the development of ever-improving resolutions. Moreover, at any give stage of technical development in MRI, the various imaging parameters can be manipulated to emphasize one aspect of resolution in exchange for another.

When investigators approach experimental design in fMRI, they must recognize that the key physical variables—spatial resolution, temporal resolution, brain coverage, and signal-to-noise ratio—are quantities whose values can be manipulated by trading one off against the others. For example, extremely high spatial resolutions are possible, but the techniques needed to achieve them involve reduced temporal resolution, limited brain coverage, and/or decreased signal-to-noise ratio. Alternately, extremely rapid imaging can be performed, but at the cost of spatial resolution and/or brain coverage. Trade-offs will continue to exist even as the overall power of scanning technology improves.

As an indication of the numbers associated with these issues, and the manner in which they are changing, consider the issue of the rate at which individual images can be collected. The first whole-body high-speed (EPI) fMRI system could collect 20 images per second for about 1 min, and then it would overheat. At a slower operating rate of 10 EPI images per second (which was still very fast in 1992), there was no overheating, but the subject (in an fMRI experiment) had to wait a long time between scans for reconstruction of the images from the raw data. At an even slower rate of 5 EPI images per second, the scanner could operate continuously and reconstruct the images in real time, but the memory for buffering those images would fill after about 2000 images. In contrast, modern machines can operate at 20 images per second continuously.

Analogous improvement is ongoing in all of the mentioned domains. Higher field MRI (from 3 to 8 T) will improve spatial resolution and will yield the added signal that may improve the practicality of single-event fMRI designs and the possible use of the "initial dip" in oxygenation to improve temporal resolution. However, these high-field machines are not as widely available as 1.5 T machines, and they are considerably more expensive, difficult, and dangerous to use.

Currently, the message for experimental design is simply that these resolution limits must be taken into account. There is little point to designing a conventional experiment to detect changes in a structure that is much smaller than one's spatial resolution permits, nor in designing a study that requires the detection of temporal changes that are too rapid for one's current technology. At the same time, because these imaging parameters can be traded off, one should not dismiss difficult-sounding experiments too quickly.

C. Practicalities: Psychophysiological Laboratory in the Magnet, Safety, and Costs

The physical properties of MRI, as well as the financial costs, place a number of practical constraints on the design and execution of fMRI-based studies and thereby impact experimental design.

As indicated previously, the experiments take place in the bore of a large, powerful magnet. The presence of this large, static magnetic field precludes the participation of subjects who would be adversely affected by it. For example, subjects with pacemakers or other forms of implanted metalic devices that would be subjected to strong forces by the magnet are clearly ineligible. The fact that subjects must lie in a relatively confined space rules out volunteers who suffer from claustrophobia. The physical position and limitations of the subject's movement also constrain various experimental procedures that would be simple in an ordinary behavioral laboratory (Fig. 2).

In addition to the main, static magnetic field, there are strong varying electromagnetic fields from the gradient magnets (for generating images) and from the RF oscillator (for flipping the protons to obtain the NMR signal). Each of these fields has associated safety considerations. For the most part, this is a minor issue at 1.5 T. It can be more of an issue for some pulse sequences at higher fields. The manufacturers of MRI scanners are required to build in various safety measures to protect subjects (such as calculating the heating effects of the RF pulses for a person of a given

size and weight). Nonetheless, each imaging facility normally includes a screening form (and sometimes a metal detector) to prevent the inadvertent harming of subjects from a collection of (sometimes not so obvious) potential dangers.

In addition to these safety considerations, the physics of MRI has other practical consequences. All of the devices used to present stimulation (visual, auditory, etc.) and to obtain behavioral and physiological response measures (button pushes, breathing and heart rate, etc.) must be constructed in an MR-compatible manner. As fMRI has become a more widespread enterprise, various companies have made it a business to supply such equipment. However, custom design of devices for specialized experiments is still common.

The single most vexing problem in the practical application of fMRI is head movement. Although pulse sequences have been developed to collect an entire slice of brain data in less than 50 msec, and multiple slices (for entire brain coverage) can be collected in 2–3 sec, the amount of information in each such image is limited. That is, the amount of *functional contrast* in the images—the differences in the signals between two experimental states—is small. To make up for this, many images are collected over extended periods of time—at least minutes and sometimes hours. During these time periods it is important that the subject's head move as little as possible.

A variety of techniques are used to encourage subjects to keep their heads as motionless as possible, but none is perfect. For well-motivated healthy adult subjects, this is usually not an insurmountable problem. For children and older patient populations, it can be the main reason that data are discarded. Although there are data analytic procedures for transforming images of moving heads back to a fixed position, these procedures are limited. Indeed, because the moving head actually distorts the main magnetic field in different ways, no motion correction algorithms can fix the problem perfectly. There are many extra coils in an MRI scanner that are used to make the main magnetic field as uniform as possible, despite the irregularities introduced by the presence of a human head in the bore of the magnet. These "shimming" coils are supplied with electric current designed to minimize the magnetic field distortions introduced by the head at the beginning of a scanning session. However, they are not modified on the fly, during the session, so any subject head movement results in more than just a displacement of the image; it also causes distortions that are much more difficult to correct.

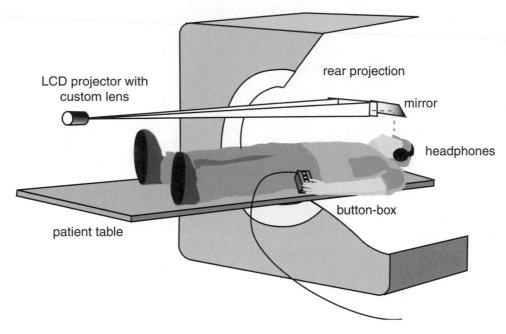

Figure 2   Subject in the magnet. Functional MRI is conducted in the environment of a MRI suite. There are many ways to present stimuli and obtain responses from the subject in such a suite, but all must be compatible with the difficult and hostile electromagnetic environment of MRI. In the example shown, visual stimuli are projected onto a rear-projection screen and are viewed by the subject via a mirror. Auditory stimuli can be presented via MR-compatible headphones or by the speaker systems typically included in MRI scanners. Finally, subject responses can be collected using an MR-compatible button box. A variety of commercial and custom approaches to the problems of presenting stimuli and recording responses in fMRI have been developed.

Finally, it should be noted that MRI time is not cheap. Charges for an hour of clinical imaging are in the hundreds of dollars. Therefore, when designing a study, the total number of imaging minutes is one of the parameters that must also be considered in the trade-offs.

D. Comparing Activation States

Fundamental to the understanding of fMRI as a tool for representing the localization of brain function is the idea that a single image, in isolation, conveys little if any useful information. Rather, it is the comparison of multiple images that are collected during different states of neural activity that supplies interpretable data. Note that this statement is *not* true for structural MR images. A single structural image conveys a great deal of useful information because data about *change* is not sought (except on a much longer timescale, as in developmental and longitudinal studies of brain structure). In contrast, functional imaging data are almost exclusively about *changes* in neuronal activity.

One might ask, Why isn't a single image, collected during rest, a useful definition of the "resting," "neutral," or "idling" state of the brain? In some ways, a single image might be interpretable this way. Indeed, some variants of PET can be used to yield a single snapshot of the metabolic state of the brain. However, the variation in local activity in the brain during "rest" is not very meaningful—the demonstration that one portion of the brain is more active during rest than another has limited value. On the other hand, the demonstration that a particular manipulation (of the stimulus or task requirements for the subject) causes a localized change in neuronal activity is far more useful.

The art of fMRI experimental design lies largely in the creation of tasks that accurately probe the cognitive function of interest. One natural way to design an experiment in functional neuroimaging is to create two tasks that are identical except for one minor difference. This is the basis of the classic subtraction method originally delineated by Donders and widely used in cognitive research. Such experimental designs are sometimes called "tight" task comparisons. The difference between experimental conditions in a tight task comparison is either in the *stimulus alone* (while keeping the response task of the subject fixed) or in the *response task alone* (while keeping the stimulus fixed).

Such an approach is particularly useful for testing specific hypotheses about the activation pattern in a single brain region.

However, there are practical and theoretical reasons for including experimental conditions that are more broadly different from the main conditions of interest. Frequently, this is accomplished via the use of a low-level control task, such as simple visual fixation or rest. This has sometimes been called a "loose" task comparison. It is particularly useful for seeing the simultaneous activation of many areas of the brain. The loose task comparison not only provides an internal check for the integrity of the data collected (because it typically includes robust activations of no direct experimental interest, but the absence of which could indicate a problem with the subject, the machine, or the data analysis) but also serves as an important point of reference for observed differences within the tight task comparison. For instance, a difference between two conditions in a tight task comparison could reflect either an increase in activity in one condition or a decrease in activity in the other. The addition of a loose task comparison provides a means of disambiguating such a situation by providing a baseline against which the two tight task conditions can be compared.

More generally, it is essential to have at least two conditions to be compared, but the power of fMRI-based experiments to test interesting theories is greatly enhanced by the presence of more conditions in the design. Sometimes these multiple conditions are qualitatively different (as indicated previously), but increasingly subtle experiments are being done that make use of quantitative (parametric) variation in the experimental conditions. In general, when attempting to model and understand the networks of the brain, all types of experimental sampling are needed.

Finally, the critical importance (and occasional irrelevance) of behavioral measures must be discussed. It might seem obvious that obtaining observable behavioral responses could only be a good thing in functional neuroimaging research. Certainly most investigators try to have an observable behavioral measure for their tasks when possible. (In "imagination" studies, such as imagining visual images or imagining performance of a motor task, it is sometimes impossible to have an observable *behavioral* response measure, but even in the context of something as "unobservable" as mental rotation, investigators have sometimes found ways to obtain associated reaction times and accuracy measures.) On the other hand, at least one prominent psychologist has argued against the necessity of behavioral response measures, suggesting that the imaging data are sufficient and that adding irrelevant behavioral tasks will only confuse the issue by eliciting neural activity unrelated to the particular cognitive task of interest. Also, several researchers have commented that, independent of anything else, it is good to have a behavioral task associated with the imaging study because it will help keep the subject awake in the scanner.

Each of these observations has merit, but there are more important uses for behavioral response measures in most studies, and for some studies they are critical. Specifically, a number of studies have made the analysis of the imaging data depend crucially on the observed *behavioral* responses. Examples from the study of memory and from the study of the effects of cocaine on brain activity are described in Section I.

E. Summary

Experimental design in fMRI-based experiments is challenging but rewarding. Practical limitations related to the safety and behavior of human subjects, technical limitations in MRI devices, underlying properties of the spatial arrangement of blood vessels, and the temporal characteristics of the coupling between neuronal activity and blood flow are all intertwined. In addition to these technical considerations there is the art of experimental design associated with any question in understanding human psychology. The application of the technology of fMRI to neuroscience entails a collection of trade-offs. Nonetheless, the current strengths of fMRI-based investigations include the best spatial and temporal resolutions for noninvasive, volumetric brain mapping, the most flexible experimental designs, and a constantly improving set of instrument-based limits to the technology's sensitivity and resolution.

IV. DATA ANALYSIS

A typical fMRI scanning session lasts 1–2 hr and results in the collection of hundreds of megabytes of data. The theory and practicalities associated with processing that data are complex and evolving. In contrast to functional neuroimaging associated with PET—in which the total amount of data is much smaller, the understanding and agreement about the sources and nature of noise in the data are well established, and there is a consequent widespread agreement about the basic issues in data analysis—the situation with fMRI data is much more complex. The sources of machine-related noise in the raw MR images are relatively well understood. However, the general consensus regarding noise in fMRI data is that the most important sources are physiologically based (in the subject) rather than machine based (from the scanner). There is less agreement about the details and the consequences of modeling these noise sources in terms of the practical consequences for data analysis.

Perhaps even more important, the present (and future) spatial and temporal resolution of fMRI data encourages modeling of brain systems at a level that may substantially exceed that of previous volumetric imaging systems. Some of these advances (e.g., the ability to obtain precise delineation of multiple visual areas in occipital cortex by virtue of their retinotopic regularities) require different kinds of data analysis and different kinds of visualization tools than made sense in the context of systems with poorer spatial resolution. Finally, the ability to image the same subject multiple times, and the associated potential for the collection of many kinds of functional data from that same subject, encourages novel approaches to data analysis.

Data analysis is a critical, time consuming, and sometimes controversial part of fMRI-based experimentation. Although the nature of many of the problems is well defined, the appropriate solutions are not. There is general agreement on how to handle some of the issues associated with data analysis (e.g., algorithms to detect head movement and correct for head movement) but there are no universally agreed on approaches to many other issues (e.g., the appropriate statistical tests to define the detection of neural activation, the best way to compare data across different subjects, and the best way to visualize and report the results of data analysis). There are a host of software tools for data analysis, each having its strengths and weaknesses. Because of the rapid development in all aspects of fMRI-based research, no *de facto* standard approach to data analysis has emerged. Figs. 3 and 4 indicate some of the procedures that are discussed in more detail in the following sections.

A. Preprocessing

Before the essential part of data analysis can begin, a number of preliminary steps are typically taken. Some spatial smoothing and temporal smoothing may be applied, but the first and most important step is the assessment of subject head movement during the imaging session.

The problem of subject motion is a pervasive one in fMRI and arises not only in constraining experimental design but also in the analysis of images of a brain that may have moved over the course of an experiment. The high-speed imaging techniques used in fMRI typically minimize the effects of movement in any one image. However, many images are collected in each run, which are typically 2–8 min long, and there are many runs in a typical 2-h session, representing more than 1000 brain volumes per session. Because the fMRI-based signal modulation is intrinsically small (typically 0.5–5%), data from all the images collected in these long runs are normally needed to gain statistical power. Thus, it is important that the images within a run and across runs are properly aligned. Head motion makes this process a challenge. In addition, even if the skull were perfectly immobile, the brain still moves. The pulsatile flow of arterial blood causes movement virtually everywhere in the brain, particularly in subcortical structures.

For all these reasons, the data analytic approach to motion detection and motion correction has been based on the brain images rather than on monitoring head movement externally. Efforts are made to *minimize* subject head movement, and it is not currently possible to correct for severe or rapid movement. All the current algorithms for correcting head movement assume rigid motion of the head. Although a single slice of brain imaging data is collected very rapidly compared to most head movement, the time needed to collect an entire brain volume—consisting of 20 or more slices—is much longer than many head movements. Such motion cannot be corrected with these algorithms. However, if the movement is not too great in amplitude and not too rapid, there are algorithms available in most fMRI data analysis packages that are adequate to detect the motion and to transform the data in an attempt to compensate for the effects of that motion.

A key feature of these algorithms is that they automatically reveal many kinds of movement, including stimulus-correlated movement. If a subject moves every time he or she is supposed to start a task, the movement could create MR signal artifacts that appear as a false activation signal. There is no good way to correct for such data, and these date must be detected and discarded.

Subject movement is generally regarded as the major problem for getting consistent data in fMRI-based experiments. Experienced, well-motivated subjects

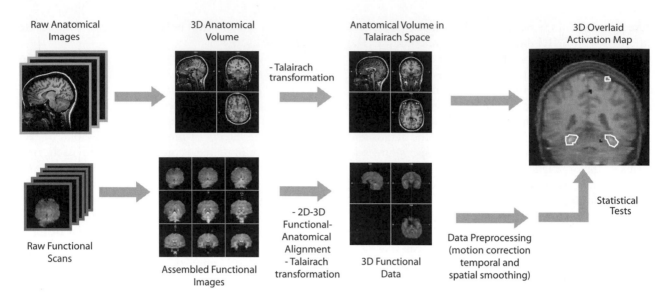

Figure 3 Highlights of an fMRI data processing stream. Data from fMRI-based experiments are analyzed in many steps. The number and order of these steps are still a topic of controversy, with variations across laboratories and software packages. This is a simplified representation of the generic steps. Both high-resolution structural MRI images, and lower resolution functional images pass through a variety of preprocessing steps. Early steps may transform the raw anatomical images from individual (two-dimensional) slices of the brain into volumetric (multislice, three-dimensional) arrays that are more suitable for the detection of head movement. At the same time, data are often transformed to a standard three-dimensional orientation and overallsize scale (Talairach coordinates). In addition to the essential step of *detecting* the presence of head motion in the data, several other (arguably optional) steps may be applied. Motion correction algorithms can help if head movement is not too much (although these algorithms are sometimes unnecessary or counterproductive if motion is little). There are both theoretical and practical reasons for smoothing the data in the spatial and/or temporal domains, although some investigators argue against performing these steps. Finally, statistical tests are performed contrasting the data collected during different experimental conditions. The resulting statistical maps are typically thresholded and overlaid on anatomical images, as indicated in Fig. 4. Further considerations are attendant to the comparisons across the brains of different subjects, as discussed in the text.

who use bite bars in the scanner can routinely be expected to yield data free of serious motion artifact. In contrast, in studies with clinical patients or other difficult subjects, as much as 20–30% of data may need to be discarded because of subject motion. There are methods for helping to minimize physical motion during data acquisition and to detect and possibly compensate for it after data acquistion, but none are fully satisfactory.

B. Basic Detection of Change

The first goal of any analysis of fMRI-based data is to determine whether the experimental manipulation has resulted in a measurable change in the MR signal and to specify where in the brain and when (in time) that change has occurred. In principle, any statistical method that can be applied to a time series can be used with fMRI data. In practice, the demands of the experimental paradigm, limitations of the tool, and the capabilities of distributed software packages constrain

the sorts of analyses that are typically performed. A few broad classes of common data analysis options are detailed here, although the presentation is not comprehensive. With the exception of principle component analysis (PCA) and other multivariate techniques, each of these tests is applied at the voxel level. When these statistics are computed for each voxel in the brain, and the resulting collection of statistics is presented in the form of an image in which color or intensity is used to represent the value of that statistic, the result is called a statistical map of brain activation.

High-speed imaging (e.g., EPI) is used to collect many images of the brain during each of the experimental conditions designed. The simplest (and, historically, the first) comparison was obtained by subtracting the average of all the images collected during one condition from the average of all the images collected during another condition. The resulting difference image clearly showed areas that were brighter, indicating greater MR signal during one condition than another.

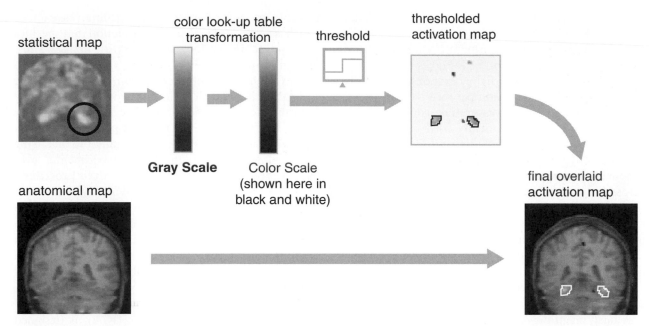

Figure 4 Production of a color–coded activation map. After preprocessing, comparisons of the values of the functional MR images collected during different experimental conditions are used to generate a statistical map. The underlying question is whether the collection of values from one condition is likely to have been generated by statistically different levels of brain activity, when compared with the collection of values obtained during a second condition. These statistics are computed on a voxel-by-voxel basis, resulting in a spatial map (left, top) in which gray-scale intensity indicates magnitude of the statistic. The midgray area represents little difference between the two experimental conditions in question; bright regions occur where the first condition elicited much stronger MR signals than the second condition; and darker regions occur where the first condition elicited much weaker MR signals than the second condition. Because of the need to collect many functional images in a short period of time, functional images typically have substantially less spatial resolution than structural (anatomical) images. (These differences are a consequence of the different pulse sequences that are used to collect functional versus structural MRI data.) In order to combine information from the statistical map with the higher resolution structural images, two transformations are applied to the statistical map. First, the gray-scale intensities used to represent the statistics are mapped into a color scale. Second, a threshold is applied so that statistical values that are within a user-defined range close to zero are mapped to transparency. This permits the combining of the two maps (thresholded pseudocolor map of statistics and high-resolution gray-scale map of anatomy) by overlaying the color map on top of the structural map. In this way, it is possible to get a better sense of the location of the changes in neural activity associated with the different experimental conditions.

This sort of comparison is the only one that, strictly speaking, is "subtraction," although the term is sometimes used informally during discussions of contrasts between conditions, even if those contrasts are based on some other statistic. Instead of subtracting (on a voxel by voxel basis) the averaged data from different conditions, the more general approach is to compute a statistic based on the collection of values at each specific spatial voxel, collected across the times of the many images. Such generic statistical computations on grouped images are more accurately described as "contrasts" or "comparisons" rather than subtractions.

C. Systematic Detection of Change

The most obvious and simple statistical test that can be used in fMRI data analysis is student's *t* test. This test assumes that each number in each group is independent, and that the underlying distribution of numbers is Gaussian (i.e., it is a parametric test). In fact, both of these assumptions are often violated in actual fMRI data. Nonetheless, parametric statistics like the *t* test are the most widely used measures of the difference between the groups of numbers collected in fMRI images across conditions. Other statistical tests are possible and sometimes used.

The most commonly used approach to the detection of systematic effects in fMRI data is the general linear model, which uses correlational analysis. Here, the fMRI data are compared with some kind of reference temporal function to determine where in the brain there are high correlations between the reference function and the MR data. The reference function is obtained from the experimental design. For example, because the brain's hemodynamic response follows a fairly consistent profile, a boxcar function defining the experimental paradigm is often convolved with an estimated hemodynamic response function to yield the reference function. The resulting reference function is smoother than a boxcar and better takes into account the shape of the hemodynamic response, generally resulting in better correlation between the MR signal time courses and the regressor time course. Several functions have been historically used to model the hemodynamic response, including a Poisson function and, recently, a gamma function. Often, a single canonical hemodynamic response function is used across the entire brain and across subjects, though there is evidence for variation in hemodynamic response shape across subjects and brain regions. Some software packages make provisions for this, allowing for independent modeling of the hemodynamic response function on a voxelwise basis.

There are a number of variations on this general scheme. For multiple experimental conditions, the previously mentioned scheme can be easily extended using multiple regression. In addition, it is also possible, though less common, to perform nonlinear regression on fMRI data, given some nonlinear prior model of expected brain response.

As with any statistical test, one must exercise some caution when using correlational analysis to ensure that incorrect inferences are not made due to violation of the assumptions inherent in the statistical test. In particular, the assumption of independence of consecutive samples is sometimes badly violated in fMRI data, inflating estimates of significance.

All of the preceding approaches make the assumption that the variations of interest in the data are those that occur in temporal synchrony with the experimental variations built in to the design. These tests cannot detect novel temporal variations triggered by the experiment but not part of the design. For instance, if a change was triggered at stimulus onset and stimulus offset, most standard data analytic packages, as they are typically employed, could not detect that response. In contrast, various multivariate approaches (such as PCA) seek regularities in the spatiotemporal structure of the fMRI data that are not specified beforehand. Such techniques typically detect the experimental variation that was designed by the experimenter as well as some physiological variations (such as those due to breathing or heartbeat). The challenge is to refine these tests so that it is easy to interpret the regularities that are detected.

Principal component analysis is not really a statistical test. Rather, it is a re-representation of the data that condenses as much of the variability in that data as possible into a small number of eigenimages, each of which is associated with an eigenfunction that specifies a temporal fluctuation for the entire image. Thus, instead of one temporal variation for each voxel in a brain volume, there are a small number of volumetric images, each of which varies as a single relative image according to some time course. The key virtue of PCA is that it has the power to pick out particular areas in the brain that exhibit a time course similar to that in the experimental design without the experimenter ever having specified that design to the analysis procedure. Similarly, it can detect temporal changes that are different from the ones built into the experiment. On the other hand, there is no obvious way to *know* which eigenimages and eigenfunctions actually correspond to an important or interpretable variation. PCA and related techniques have great theoretical appeal, but they have been rarely used in practical fMRI data analysis. A related multivariate technique, called independent component analysis (ICA), is designed to help with the interpretation of the data. Instead of projecting data into a lower dimensional space that accounts for the most variation (as PCA does), ICA finds a space in which the dimensions are as independent as possible, thus facilitating interpretation of the components.

D. Comparing Brains

Nearly all fMRI studies use multiple subjects and perform statistical analyses across data collected from multiple subjects. This practice introduces a number of practical problems that must be addressed.

A first, relatively simple step toward comparing activity across the brains of multiple subjects is to transform the representations of those brains so that they are similar in overall size and similarly oriented in space. To accomplish this, the brain images are rigidly rotated and linearly scaled into a common "box." The Talairach stereotactic coordinate system is the most widely used standard coordinate system box for comparing brains. In the full Talairach transformation, a rigid rotation and translation to a standardized orientation is followed by a piecewise linear scaling of the anterior, middle, and posterior portions of each hemisphere, independently. The standard orientation in three dimensions is determined by the line between two interhermispheric fiber bundles—the anterior commissure (AC) and the posterior commissure (PC)—and the plane between the two hemispheres. The anterior, middle, and posterior portions of each hemisphere are defined in terms of the AC–PC line: The portion of each hemisphere in front of the anterior commisure is the anterior, the portion of each hemisphere between the AC and PC points is the middle, and the portion behind the posterior commisure is the posterior.

In some software packages an abbreviated form of the Talairach transformation is performed in which the brain is scaled as a whole, without piecewise linear portions for each hemisphere. This has the advantage of being much faster and simpler to implement. Indeed, some packages compute this transformation automatically by comparing the given brain to a standard "average" brain that was generated by transforming the anatomical MR images of 305 brains to Talairach coordinates and averaging. This process eliminates the tedious and often tricky steps of finding the AC–PC line and other landmarks for each individual brain. Despite the fact that the individual anatomy of the AC–PC line is ignored and the transformation has fewer degrees of freedom than the full Talairach transformation, this automatic process yields data that are adequate for most purposes.

The more serious problems with either the simplified Talairach transformation or the full Talairach transformation are caused by the fact that real brains are not rigid transformations of one another. The simplified Talairach transformation, being strictly linear, cannot account for these differences. Even the full Talairach transformation, which is only piecewise linear with a small number of pieces, is clearly inadequate for dealing with these individual differences in brain anatomy. More powerful nonlinear approaches have therefore been developed.

There are a wide range of approaches to more general transformations of brains to facilitate data display and intersubject comparison. One approach is to permit complicated nonlinear warping procedures based on sulcal and gyral landmarks to guide computer-generated distortions of one brain into another (or to a standard). Another approach, which is also based on nonlinear transformations, is to try to match the perimeters of given brain slices between different brains. Perhaps the most widely used alternative to Talairach and these other nonlinear transformations is to "inflate" the brain as a means of removing all sulci and gyri. This inflation is often followed by cutting the inflated brain in a small number of places to permit "flattening."

The goal of inflating is to obtain a three-dimensional, smooth, nonconvoluted surface representation of cortex. The goal of flattening is to lay that surface representation on a flat plane. Given that a brain hemisphere (when inflated) looks like an ellipsoid, it is necessary to cut it in one or more places to allow it to be flattened. Qualitatively, this is similar to the need to cut a globe to get a flattened representation of the world. Quantitatively, however, for an inflated brain, the analogy is closer to a cylinder. When a globe is cut and flattened, it is necessary to create many cuts or else there will be some very large distortions. On the other hand, when a cylinder is cut, the resulting surface can be flattened with virtually no distortions. In these terms, the inflated cortex is more like a cylinder than a sphere, and the distortions are not terribly large.

Flattened representations are visually and logically very appealing. Unlike Talairach coordinates, however, they are not three dimensional and only apply to the cortical surface. Subcortical structures cannot be represented. (Talairach invented his system for subcortical structures, although it does not include the cerebellum.)

Given the good spatial resolution of fMRI and the ability to detect activations in individual subjects, some researchers eschew averaging across subjects. Their position seems to be that the right way to compare across subjects is to look at *each individual's functional map* (preferably in a flattened brain format to facilitate intersubject comparison). Elaborations on this approach can include warping within the flattened space and could therefore eventually include averaging in that space.

Recent developments in brain comparisons involve the use of more sophisticated algorithms to inflate the brain to a sphere but then warp the surface borders on that sphere (associated with major and almost universal sulcal/gyral landmarks) toward a common standard. This transformation permits a smoother and more effective comparison of activation sites across the brains of different subjects than do the Talairach transformations.

E. Comparing Groups

One of the most obvious and important classes of questions that are addressed with human functional brain imaging is the search for differences between groups. For example, can fMRI be used to detect the early onset of Alzheimer's disease? Does a remedial training program in reading cause changes in brain activity preferentially for one diagnostic classification of dyslexia versus another? Does a given drug treatment lead to greater area of functional brain activity? All these questions have as an essential component the attempt to make quantitative distinctions between different groups of subjects.

Functional MRI (and functional brain imaging more broadly) can be used to address at least two types of questions. One question might be thought of as the attempt to represent "typical" brain function and associated networks of activity. In that context, collecting increasingly more data about a single brain doing a single task might be useful because the error bars associated with any particular aspect of the brain activity might be expected to decrease with increased measurement. In statistics, this is called a fixed effects model. On the other hand, to determine whether there are differences in brain function and networks of activity between two putatively different *groups* of subjects, it is important to sample many of members of each group, even if the individual measurement of any one member of the group is noisy. In particular, knowing with extreme precision that two members of one group differ from two members of another group is only useful if the within-group variation (i.e., between brains) is as small as the within-brain variation (i.e., between multiple measurements of the same brain). If not, then the exceptional precision of the measurement of the small number of subjects is not useful. In statistics, this is the random effects model.

The practical implication of the fixed versus random effects model of variance for functional neuroimaging is that it is better to have measurements on many brains if the goal is to claim group differences. On the other hand, it may be better to have many measurements on a few brains if the goal is to delineate functional systems as precisely as possible.

V. RESEARCH APPLICATIONS

Human fMRI based on the endogenous contrast agent (deoxyhemoglobin) was first reported in 1991. In the ensuing 10 years the growth of fMRI-based research applications has been explosive. The easiest (and probably the most accurate) way to summarize the range of fMRI-based research applications is "all of psychology and neuroscience". In addition to widespread reports of results of fMRI-based research in general scientific and popular journals, there are two journals devoted exclusively to the technical developments and applications of human brain mapping, for which fMRI is a primary tool. Research applications range from the classical psychophysical questions of

sensation, perception, and attention to higher level processes of cognition, language, and emotion, in both normal and patient populations. Even domains ranging from psychotherapy to genetics are beginning to make use of fMRI-based experiments. The impact of fMRI on a few select areas of research is elaborated next.

A. Retinotopy/Multiple Cortical Visual Areas

The first application of fMRI-based research was in the domain of the early stages of visual processing. Indeed, the very first human fMRI study involved the demonstration that a region of the brain associated with early visual processing—occipital cortex in the calcarine fissure—yielded an NMR signal that varied as flashing lights were presented (or not) to a subject.

This demonstration was exciting, but the excitement was limited for several reasons. First, nothing "new" had been demonstrated about human visual cortex. Second, there were a host of technical concerns that, had they been correct, would have meant that the spatial resolution obtainable with fMRI would be seriously compromised. Finally, most of the following simple advances would not go beyond what we already know from (invasive) single cell recordings in nonhuman primates.

However, the development of fMRI in the ensuing years for the study of early visual processing addressed all these concerns and went far beyond them. First, retinopy was demonstrated for area V1 at a level of spatial resolution that exceeded any previously demonstrated with a noninvasive technique. Second, retinotopy was used to delineate multiple visual areas. Differences between the layout of human visual areas compared with those of other primate species were demonstrated, and new visual areas apparently unique to humans were claimed.

At the same time, some classic psychological effects, such as the motion aftereffect, were seen to be associated with detectable brain activity localized to specific parts of the cortex associated with visual motion processing.

The early dependence on the connection to known primate neurophysiology is being lessened. Several laboratories are now developing fMRI suites designed specifically to study nonhuman primates. The idea is to use the invasive technologies such as single cell recording, adapted for the MR environment, to obtain a deeper understanding of both the functional brain structures and the relationship between neural activity and hemodynamics using methods that would be unethical with human subjects.

B. Modulatory Effects of Attention

One early fMRI-based study demonstrated that the use of voluntary attention (deciding whether to attend to a subset of moving dots or to a subset of stationary dots in a field of moving and stationary dots) caused detectable changes in MR signals associated with a visual motion processing area in cortex (Fig. 5). This study did not have an overt behavioral measure to provide external evidence that subjects were actually performing their assigned tasks. However, the data were sufficiently clean and unambiguous that this study was published and gained considerable attention.

During the ensuing years the study was replicated and extended in a number of ways by different laboratories throughout the world. The initial basic demonstration of attentional modulation became the starting point for much more subtle experiments—experiments that were more tightly tied to behavioral measures. Importantly, both the qualitative and the quantitative measures of attentional modulation were replicated. For instance, the motion processing area was active whenever there was visual movement present, but that activity increased by about 50% when the subject was attending to the movement compared to when the subject was not attending to the movement. The studies that used analogous tasks as part of their design found quantitatively similar changes.

The basic paradigm was adapted to more complex stimulus situations in which subjects could attend to various different aspects of a complex scene. This permitted the testing of specific hypotheses about the allocation and connection of visual attention to different aspects of a stimulus. For example, it was demonstrated that when an object was attended because of one attribute (e.g., motion), there was increased processing of other attributes of that object (e.g., whether it was a familiar face or represented a familiar location) even though the other attributes were irrelevant to the attentional task. Thus, fMRI-based experiments were being applied to theoretical questions of long-standing interest in cognitive psychology.

C. Use of Behavioral Responses

The use of behavioral responses in fMRI-based studies began as a comforting demonstration that subjects were doing what the experimenter had asked them to do. However, behavioral measures can be much more useful. Two studies of memory, for example, made use of behavioral data collected after the MRI scanning session was over and the subject was out of the magnet to retroactively specify the data analytic process. One study of the effects of a drug used the subject's behaviorally reported mental state to obtain a temporal function that could be correlated with the brain imaging data.

The two memory studies each made use of the visual presentation of stimuli during the fMRI scanning session. In one case the stimuli were pictures; in the other case they were words. In both cases the subjects had an irrelevant task to perform related to these stimuli. After the scanning session was over, the subjects were given a memory task (without prior warning) to determine which of the test stimuli they recalled seeing. The key idea here was to group the imaging data according to whether the data were collected during the presentation of stimuli *that were subsequently remembered* versus the presentation of stimuli that were subsequently forgotten. The expectation (which was confirmed) was that various parts of the brain associated with long-term memory and encoding would have been more active on those trials in which the stimulus was subsequently recalled.

The drug study used behavioral measures more directly in analyzing the fMRI data. The study involved the challenging task of measuring fMRI changes during the administration of a psychoactive drug, cocaine. Subjects were regular cocaine users who had declined treatment but who had volunteered for a study. During the course of an imaging session they were given either a placebo or an injection of cocaine. (There were two imaging runs, so each subject received the cocaine on one run and the placebo on the other.) During the runs subjects regularly reported on their subjective state of "high," "low," "rush," and "craving"— terms that were known to be associated with cocaine experiences.

Note that there are unique technical challenges in this study. In addition to being a psychoactive drug, cocaine is also a cardiovascular stimulant. Therefore, before considering the possible effects of cocaine in its psychoactive and addicting role, it was necessary to demonstrate that such effects would not be masked by the circulatory effects of the drug. To accomplish this, the investigators used a standard stimulus (flashing light) to calibrate neuronally triggered hemodynamic responses. Also, they used two imaging pulse sequences: one that was sensitive to BOLD effects and

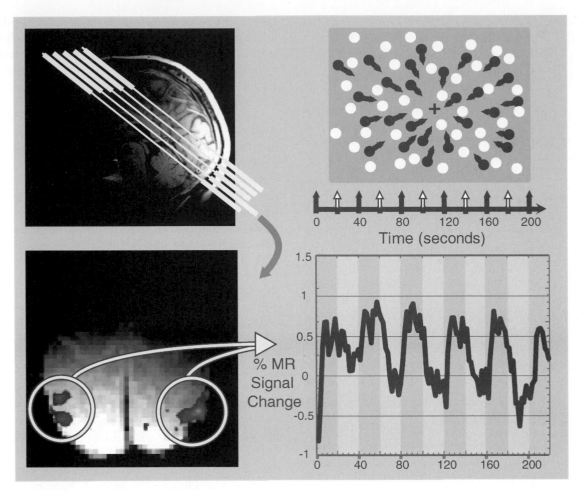

Figure 5 Voluntary attention modulates activity in human visual cortex. This collection of images summarizes an early fMRI-based experiment demonstrating the detection of neural modulation due to the exertion of voluntary attention. Subjects viewed a continuous movie consisting of a cross in the middle of the visual vield (on which they were instructed to fixate) and moving black dots and stationary white dots in the periphery. The cartoon at the upper right represents one frame of this movie, with arrows indicating the direction of motion. In the actual stimuli, of course, there were no arrows present—only moving, stationary dots and the fixation cross. The motion was always radial, toward the fixation point, to make it easy for the subjects to maintain fixation. Additional testing with an MR-compatible eyetracker revealed that subjects could maintain fixation. While looking at this movie for several minutes, subjects received verbal instructions to attend to one collection of colored dots or the other. These instructions alternated every 20 sec, as indicated in the figure by the black ("attend black") and white ("attend white") arrows on the timeline, below the visual stimulus. When the subjects heard "attend black," they would continue to fixate the central cross, but they were supposed to pay more attention to the black (moving) dots than the white (stationary) dots during that time. Similarly, when they heard "attend white," they were supposed to attend more to the white (stationary) dots. The imaging data were collected with a small coil of wire (about 13 cm in diameter) placed near the occipital cortex (the back of the head). This yielded a stronger signal in the brain regions of interest for the experiment, but it yielded weak signals from the rest of the brain, as indicated in the structural image shown at the upper left and the functional image shown in the lower left. Data for five slices, oriented parallel to the calcarine fissure (primary visual cortex), were collected (as indicated by the lines in the upper left). Data from one of those slices is shown in the lower left. As described for Fig. 4, a pseudocolor representation of the results of a statistical test comparing the MR data collected during one condition ("attend black") versus the other condition ("attend white") is displayed. There was a clear increase in activity on both the left and the right sides of this brain, in a region that corresponds anatomically to a known visual motion processing area of the cortex. Data from the voxels of the brain whose statistic exceeded the threshold used to specify the color map were averaged; the results are plotted as a function of time in the graph in the lower right. Data collected during the time that subjects were attending to moving stimuli (light background portions of the graph) were clearly higher in amplitude than the data collected during the time that subjects were attending to the stationary stimuli (dark background), *even though the visual stimulus was unchanged throughout the entire scanning period.* This experiment represents a simple, dramatic demonstration of the ability of fMRI to detect the neural consequences of changes in cognitive state (data and analysis courtesy of Kathleen O'Craven).

one that was sensitive to flow effects. This combination allowed them to demonstrate that cocaine influenced the flow-dependent MR signal changes but not the BOLD MR signal changes.

Thus, they could use the BOLD changes to study the effects of cocaine in its role as a psychoactive stimulant relatively independent of its role as a cardiovascular stimulant. Using the time course profile obtained from the behavioral ratings (specifically, the temporal modulation of craving and rush) they could find brain areas whose activity followed a similar profile, allowing them to conclude that those areas were implicated in the experience of these sensations.

D. Emotional Affect versus Cognitive Processing Load

A unique strength of functional brain imaging is the ability to test various intuitions and hypotheses about our mental activities by virtue of the quantitative nature of the MR signal changes. Sometimes the most salient aspect of a stimulus (such as its emotional valence) may be less cognitively engaging than the lack of that cue. Specifically, although the localization of function repeatedly found in studies of the low-level aspects of sensory processing appears to have analogs in other cognitive and emotional tasks, the tasks and stimuli that most effectively activate those areas may be counterintuitive. Higher contrast in visual stimuli generally evokes stronger modulation of early visual processing areas in the brain, but high contrast in an emotional domain does not always evoke the strongest variation in the brain areas associated with processing those stimuli. The data and experiment presented in Fig. 6 exemplify this idea.

Subjects were required to classify stimuli along an emotional scale as "neutral," "positive," or "negative." The stimuli were individual words (e.g., "calm," "delighted," and "insecure") intermixed with individual pictures of human faces (Fig. 6, top). There is ample evidence, both from the domain of human functional neuroimaging and from the literature of human brain lesions, that words and faces are exceptionally good stimuli for the activation of specific brain regions. Pictures of faces are good stimuli to activate the fusiform gyrus, especially on the right side. Single words, when associated with a semantic (rather than a purely perceptual) task, are effective stimuli for activating the inferior frontal region, almost always most strongly on the left side. One might reasonably expect that variation along the important dimension of emotional valence would modulate the strength of activation in these two areas. Given the demonstrated power of emotional stimuli to activate areas of the brain associated with general arousal, one might also predict that the most emotionally powerful stimuli (the positive and negative stimuli) would elicit greater neural activity than the neutral stimuli.

The stimuli were presented for 2 sec each, with 8 sec between the onset of each stimulus. This design, as one might deduce from Section II.A, is less than optimal because it does not take advantage of the power of rapid single trials, nor does it completely isolate the hemodynamic responses from the different stimulations. However, it was sufficient to address the preceding question, and it is useful in illustrating the way in which event-related fMRI data are often reported–via overlapping plots of the time course of the hemodynamic responses to the different stimulus types.

The stimuli were effective in eliciting emotional responses. Not surprisingly, the emotional faces (happy, in particular, and, to a lesser extent, sad) evoked stronger amygdala responses than neutral faces, with a weaker finding (but in the same relative order of strength) for words. Also not surprisingly, faces of any type elicited minimal response in left inferior frontal cortex and words of any type elicited minimal response in right fusiform cortex.

However, in the context of this categorization task, neutral stimuli (both faces and words) were far more effective activators of the regions known to be especially responsive to such stimuli (right fusiform and left inferior frontal, respectively) than were the emotionally powerful stimuli. The graphs in Fig. 6 show the time course of activity for each stimulus type in the relevant regions of the brain. The amplitude of the hemodynamic responses to the neutral stimuli was approximately twice as large as that to the positive stimuli, and it exceeded the response to the negative stimuli even more dramatically.

Interpretation of this result is not trivial. Behavioral measures of reaction time and accuracy for the words suggest one possible explanation. In the case of the word stimuli, the reaction times were longest, and percentage correct was lowest, for the neutral words. The fact that it was faster and easier to categorize positive and negative words could mean that the relevant brain area (left inferior frontal) was active for a shorter period of time during the emotional words, resulting in less time for the hemodynamic signal to grow. However, this kind of explanation cannot be the

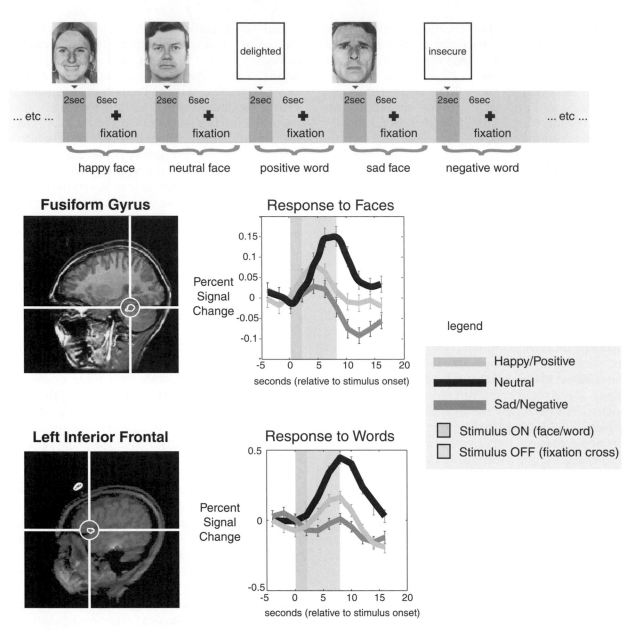

Figure 6 Strength of affect versus difficulty of processing. As described in Section II.A, detection of the hemodynamic responses to different types of events can reveal unintuitive effects. The stimuli and timing for this experiment are indicated in the top row. The stimuli were "positive," "negative," and "neutral" faces and words. One of these was presented for 2 sec every 8 sec in random order. Subjects were required to categorize each stimulus presentation as being positive, negative, or neutral. Two of the resulting activation foci are presented. A region of the brain known to respond strongly to face stimuli (the fusiform gyrus on the right side of the brain) and a region known to respond strongly to words (the inferior frontal region on the left side of the brain) were detected, and their locations are indicated by the crosshairs in the anatomical images shown on the left. The graphs on the right indicate the hemodynamic responses to the three classes of stimuli (positive, negative, and neutral). For words in the frontal region and for pictures of faces in the fusiform region, the most activity was elicited not by the most emotionally salient and affective stimuli but by the neutral stimuli. Apparently, categorizing happy or sad stimuli places a smaller processing load on these areas than categorizing a neutral stimulus (data and analysis courtesy of Patricia Deldin and David Cox).

whole story. In the case of face stimuli, it was the negative (rather than neutral) faces that had the longest reaction times and lowest percentage correct. Face stimuli were generally classified more quickly than words, but neutral faces may still evoke more processing because the observer tries harder to find positive or negative nuances (albeit quickly). However, these are speculations.

The point of recounting this study is to emphasize both the complexity of interpreting fMRI data and their potential nonintuitiveness. To an experimenter, it can naturally seem that positive and negative stimuli will, in one sense, evoke stronger responses than neutral stimuli. For some brain areas, this is no doubt true. However, the constraints of a classification task are different. In that context, the fact that neutral stimuli elicit more activity from their respective processing areas (for words and faces) can be plausibly interpreted as an indicator of greater processing effort.

VI. CLINICAL APPLICATIONS

The ability of fMRI to image brain activity *in vivo* makes it a promising tool for the diagnosis, interpretation, and treatment evaluation of clinical disorders involving brain function. A great deal of effort is currently being exerted to develop concrete clinical applications for fMRI as well as to use fMRI to better understand various psychiatric and neurological disorders. Until we better understand the wealth of data being generated from neurologically intact individuals, however, the use of fMRI-based data in actual clinical applications is likely to be limited.

The development of clinical applications of fMRI is of great importance to the fMRI community for many reasons. Functional MRI-based research has historically been closely tied to the medical community. Indeed, one reason why research using fMRI has been able to expand so rapidly and extensively is the availability of conventional MRI machines. MRI machines are very expensive, and any new, clinically relevant application would help subsidize costs of existing machines and the purchase of new machines (or the upgrading of existing machines) for fMRI use. Additionally, such demand encourages manufacturers to invest in the development of scanners that are more specifically designed with fMRI applications in mind. The widespread acceptance of the development costs for higher field (3 and 4 T) scanners by virtually all MRI manufacturers is almost certainly due to the potential promise of the neural-activation MRI and related imaging techniques, such as diffusion-weighted MRI and diffusion-tensor MRI (which are more relevant to the analysis of stroke and white matter anatomy, respectively).

There is at least one area of clinical importance in which fMRI is already playing an active role: presurgical planning. In situations in which a surgeon is going to be removing portions of a patient's brain, it is critical to know exactly where various motor and sensory functions are mapped in that individual's brain. Some information can be obtained during surgery via direct cortical stimulation or prior to the main surgery via a separate surgical procedure for the implantation of electrode arrays in the brain. Functional MRI, however, is a nonsurgical technique for obtaining similar information well before any surgical intervention starts. Furthermore, it is almost always the case that a structural MRI will be obtained prior to surgery, so it may be a relatively small incremental cost to obtain functional information during the same MRI session.

Many other areas of obvious *potential* clinical importance (in psychopharmacology, neurology, stroke treatment and recovery, drug addiction, and psychiatric disorders) are still largely in the stages of initial research. Although many studies have been performed, there are no specific clinical interventions that are driven by fMRI. A brief summary of some of the ideas in this area is presented in the following sections.

A. Preoperative Planning

One promising clinical application for fMRI is in preoperative planning and risk assessment. Since fMRI allows for the creation of maps of brain activity corresponding to the performance of a specific task, one natural use of fMRI is in identifying areas of the brain that are functionally important and therefore should be carefully avoided during neurosurgery. It should be emphasized that it is the creation of maps specific to the individual patient in question (rather than maps based on averages across many subjects) that is of use to the surgeon. Functional MRI is particularly well suited to the creation of such individualized maps.

Intractable focal epilepsy is sometimes treated by excising the epileptogenic focus surgically. In this context, "intractable" means "not successfully treated with drugs," and "focal" means that there is a single site that appears to be the source or trigger for the epileptic seizures.) The areas to be removed are often close to brain areas critical to language (so-called "eloquent" cortex), so surgeons must exercise extreme caution lest their patients acquire severe language impairments as a result of the operation. For most adults, language function is strongly lateralized, meaning that damage to one hemisphere (typically the left) has much greater consequences for language comprehension and production than damage to the other (typically the right) hemisphere. Approximately 95% of right-handed individuals are left lateralized for language, whereas left-handed individuals show a much more variable language lateralization (both in left versus right and in the degree of lateralization). Historically, the best procedure for assessing the side and degree of language lateralization in an individual patient has been the Wada test. In this procedure, amobarbitol is injected unilaterally into the left or right carotid artery, resulting in the anesthetization of the corresponding hemisphere of the brain. Both sides are tested in this way. If the subject is relatively unimpaired on language and memory tasks performed during the anesthetization of one hemisphere, then it is deemed safe to operate on that hemisphere. Functional MRI offers several advantages over the Wada test: It is completely noninvasive, and it provides a better estimate of areas important to language within each hemisphere. In the early days of attempting to use fMRI to assess language lateralization, the results were equivocal. Today, fMRI is a robust measure of language lateralization. On the other hand, fMRI has not been demonstrated to be as sensitive a measure of memory function as the Wada test, but progress is being made. At least one hospital in the United States has replace the Wada test with fMRI for presurgical planning, but use of this alternative is not widespread. Notwithstanding this slow start, it can be speculated that the first generally accepted clinical application of fMRI will be as a replacement for Wada test.

More detailed functional maps are being developed for presurgical planning and risk assessment relevant to other brain areas (besides eloquent cortex). For instance, during the surgical removal of tumors and other abnormalities near the central sulcus, one risk is the unnecessary removal of portions of primary motor cortex, resulting in serious impairments of motor control. Functional MRI has been used to map the boundaries of primary motor cortex in order to help weigh the risks and benefits of various treatment options. Obtaining an accurate, *individualized* functional map in this instance is particularly important because brain abnormalities in question often displace structures and make anatomical landmarks ambiguous as well as potentially disturbing the underlying functional maps of normal brain structures. Depending on the type of tumor, if fully resecting a tumor would endanger primary motor cortex, then partial resection might be in the patient's best interest. If, on the other hand, the entire tumor can be safely removed without endangering primary motor areas, then it is in the patient's best interest to remove the entire tumor.

B. Pharmacology

Pharmacology is another area in which fMRI has great potential. Although fMRI is poorly suited to identifying the binding sites of a drug (due to its inherent lack of sensitivity to chemicals in such relatively low concentrations), its good spatial resolution and moderate temporal resolution make it quite well suited to identifying which functional brain systems a drug influences. Studies of the action of clinically and socially significant drugs (such as addictive drugs) have revealed specific patterns and locations of activation via fMRI. Such studies (which include cocaine and nicotine and a growing list of psychoactive pharmaceuticals) are being conducted to learn more about how these drugs affect the brain. A better understanding of the anatomy and physiology of addiction may eventually lead to more effective treatments.

More generally, an important possible use of fMRI could be the determination, on an individual patient level, of whether or not a drug is affecting the appropriate brain systems and the quantification of the strength of that effect and thus potentially guide dosage. Since it is difficult to predict the dose–response effects of a drug on any given individual, fMRI could potentially speed the process of prescribing effective drugs in appropriate doses. Similarly, fMRI has the potential to aid drug development by quickly identifying the brain areas on which a drug acts, increasing knowledge about an existing drug, or helping to identify potential uses of a new drug. Finally, because fMRI has a temporal resolution that is rapid compared to most of the effects of psychoactive drugs, it is possible to use fMRI to follow the pharmacokinetic profile of such drugs.

C. Understanding Neurological and Psychiatric Disorders

In contrast to presurgical planning and some pharmacology, the application of fMRI-based studies to neurological and psychiatric disorders might better be characterized as occurring in the developmental rather than application stages. The primary thrust is in the area of refining diagnosis. The wealth of studies using neurologically intact subjects supplies a natural baseline for using fMRI to derive more sensitive and/or more specific diagnostic criteria. For every robust finding in the functional localization of tasks involving frontal cortex with healthy subjects, there will eventually be a comparison study involving patients with all manner of neuropsychiatric disorders, from Alzheimer's disease to psychosis, schizophrenia, and autism. Many such studies have been conducted already.

The strength of fMRI is in obtaining spatially localized maps of function, especially in the context of purely cognitive function. These may be of value in diagnosing a variety of disorders. On the other hand, a weakness of fMRI is its extreme lack of sensitivity for directly detecting the presence and concentration of specific drugs in the brain—the discussion so far has referred to the detection of huge numbers of hydrogen atoms in water molecules. In contrast, PET detects virtually every decay of a radioactive atom in a single molecule and is consequently an exquisitely sensitive measure for localizing the sites of activity for suitably labeled psychoactive drugs.

Functional MRI is an *imaging* modality—it generates pictures that have a great deal of spatial specificity. Magnetic resonance spectroscopy (MRS), in contrast, sometimes collects data from the whole head to detect the presence and concentration of some of the body's more plentiful chemicals (such as lactate). There is a trade-off between detecting weak signals (there are far more water molecules than lactate molecules in the body) and being able to make spatial maps. As the MRI devices are made more sensitive (via stronger main magnets, better coils, etc.), the "whole head" MRS data can be refined to yield greater spatial resolution. The clinical relevance of MRS will increase in the future, and some of that improvement will be associated with blood flow changes and hence to fMRI.

D. Dyslexia

A particularly active area of clinically relevant research using fMRI is the study of developmental dyslexia. What makes this effort especially promising is that reading is of such fundamental importance to society and education, but there is limited understanding of the development and actions of the relevant cognitive systems underlying reading, even in normal readers. Psychophysical studies of temporal processing, not only in the auditory domain but also in the context of motor activity and coordination and in the visual perception of motion, have all been implicated, by at

least some researchers, in the etiology of dyslexia. Coupling fMRI with behavioral studies in this context has especially rich appeal.

Again, as with some of the preceding potential clinical applications, the likelihood is not for a treatment based on fMRI, but, rather, an improved ability to differentially diagnose different types dyslexia and to monitor the effectiveness and modes of action of any behavioral or drug-based treatments. Dyslexia is a complex disorder, with an etiology that is likely to include low-level physiology, high-level cognitive structures, and other levels as yet undetermined. It is not clear whether fMRI-based research will be able to tap into all aspects of dyslexia, but initial work is encouraging. The discussion of clinical applications of fMRI closes with a simpler disorder than dyslexia, but one that couples directly with the particular strengths of hemodynamically based fMRI.

E. Migraine

A recent tour de force in fMRI-based experimentation brings together some of the most elegant work in a research application context (retinotopic mapping of visual cortex) and a long-standing phenomenon of clinical importance (migraine headaches). Migraines are an intense form of headache, often associated with visual auras (i.e., the perception of various strange visual patterns, typically around a circular arc or perimeter of some portion of the visual field, bilaterally) and an associated temporary blindness (a temporary scotoma) within that perimeter. The fact that these auras and scotomas appear to both eyes at the same portion of the visual field is very strong evidence that the underlying effect is being controlled at the cortical level, where these corresponding portions of the visual field share the same physical location in the brain. Moreover, migraines have long been understood to be associated with changes in dilation and constriction of the cerebral vasculature.

It is very difficult to study this phenomenon using fMRI both because it is relatively short-lived (sometimes 30–60 min and sometimes 2–4 hr) and because it is associated with aversion to loud noises and bright lights (on the part of the sufferer). Therefore, it is difficult to get migraine sufferers to volunteer for an fMRI study; even if they were willing, it would be rare that they got a migraine while they were near the scanner. One research group was fortunate enough to find a volunteer who predictably and regularly triggered his own migraine headache by dint of intense athletic activity (playing basketball). He was therefore available for repeated (schedulable) scanning immediately before and during the onset of his migraine attacks.

The investigators were experts in visual retinotopy and they designed a protocol that revealed, in exquisite detail, the neurological correlate of the patient's visual symptomotology. As the scotoma grew and as the aura changed in size (both of which phenomena could be reported subjectively by the patient), fMRI data revealed the location on the cortex and the functional variation in amplitude of response to a flickering checkerboard of visual stimulation. Combining this data with previously obtained retinotopic maps of the subjects visual cortex permitted a precise connection between measurable function and subjective loss. Although this study does not immediately suggest a treatment for migraine attacks, it certainly demonstrates a method for objectively assessing the effectiveness of candidate therapies.

VII. CLOSING

Given the strong technical components of fMRI, perhaps it is appropriate to close with a discussion of the ultimate spatial and temporal resolutions that might be obtainable in the near future. The temporal resolution of fMRI is not likely to be limited by the imaging tool but, rather, by the vagaries of the hemodynamic response. We are probably close to that limit already. Although there are aspects of temporal properties of hemodyamics that we can detect on the timescale of 100 msec, for most practical purposes the fMRI temporal resolution limit is likely to remain approximately 1 sec. Significant improvements in temporal resolution *associated* with fMRI are likely to result from integration with modalities such as EEG and MEG, whose intrinsic temporal resolution is the millisecond range.

Technological developments, especially in terms of higher field magnets and more sensitive and versatile imaging coils, will increase the effective spatial resolution of fMRI. Because higher field strength increases the signal-to-noise ratio, less averaging of signals across space is required, allowing for smaller voxels and thus greater spatial resolution. Although there are some safety issues that arise as field strength increases, there is no known reason why MRI cannot be done with humans at much higher field strength than the conventional 1.5 T. An increasing number of 3- and 4-T scanners are in routine use, and a handful of 7- and 8-T scanners for use on humans are either currently in use or are being built. Even without the higher field strengths, it would be possible to increase spatial resolution by using longer imaging times. However, the ultimate spatial resolution limits will not be determined by the MR scanner. Rather, they will be determined by hemodynamic limits, i.e., by the spatial resolution of the smallest vessels that show local changes with neural activity. Based on the available evidence, this limit is approximately the size of a cortical column—between 0.1 mm and 1 mm in linear dimension. If that spatial resolution could be achieved in routine fMRI-based experiments, it should represent a dramatic leap in the ability to develop and test far more interesting and explicit models of functioning neural systems in the human brain.

See Also the Following Articles

CEREBRAL CIRCULATION • DYSLEXIA • ELECTRO-ENCEPHALOGRAPHY (EEG) • EVENT-RELATED ELECTROMAGNETIC RESPONSES • HEADACHES • IMAGING: BRAIN MAPPING METHODS • MAGNETIC RESONANCE IMAGING (MRI) • PSYCHOPHYSIOLOGY • RECEPTIVE FIELD

Suggested Reading

Beauchamp, M. S., Cox, R. W., and DeYoe, E. A. (1997). Graded effects of spatial and featural attention on human area MT and associated motion processing areas. *J. Neurophysiol.* **77**(7), 516–520.

Breiter, H. C., Gollub, R. L., Weisskoff, R. M., Kennedy, D. N., Makris, N., Berke, J. D., Goodman, J. M., Kantor, H. L., Gastfriend, D. R., Riorden, J. P., Mathew, R. T., Rosen, B. R., and Hyman, S. E. (1997). Acute effects of cocaine on human brain activity and emotion. *Neuron* **19**(9), 591–611.

Brewer, J. B., Zhao, Z., Desond, J. E., Glover, G. H., and Gabrieli, J. D. E. (1998). Making memories: Brain activity that predicts how well visual experience will be remembered. *Science* **281**, 1185–1187.

Bushong, S. C. (1996). *Magnetic Resonance Imaging: Physical and Biological Principles*, 2nd ed. Mosby–Year Book, Boston.

Calvin, W. H., and Ojemann, G. A. (1995). *Conversations with Neil's Brain: The Neural Nature of Thought and Language*. Perseus, Reading, MA.

Gollub, R. L., Breiter, H. C., Kantor, H., Kennedy, D., Gastfriend, D., Mathew, R. T., Makris, N., Guimaraes, A., Riorden, J., Campbell, T., Foley, M., Hyman, S. E., Rosen, B., and Weisskoff, R. (1998). Cocaine decreases cortical cerebral blood flow but does not obscure regional activation in functional magnetic resonance imaging in human subjects. *J. Cereb. Blood Flow Meta.* **18**, 724–734.

Hadjikhani, N., Sanches del Rio, M., Wu, O., Schwartz, D., Bakker, D., Fischl, B., Kwong, K. K., Cutrer, M. F., Rosen, B. R., Tootell, R. B. H., Sorensen, A. G., and Moskowitz, M. A. (2001). Mechanisms of migraine aura revealed by functional MRI in human visual cortex. *Proc. Natl. Acad. Sci. USA* **98**(8), 4687–4692.

Moonen, C. T. W., and Bandettini, P. A. (Eds.) (1999). *Functional MRI.* Springer-Verlag, Berlin.

O'Craven, K. M., and Kanwisher, N. (2000). Mental imagery of faces and places activates corresponding stimulus-specific brain regions. *J. Cognitive Neurosci.* **12**(6), 1013–1023.

O'Craven, K. M., Downing, P. E., and Kanwisher, N. (1999). fMRI evidence for objects as the units of attentional selection. *Nature* **401**, 584–587.

O'Craven, K. M., Rosen, B. R., Kwong, K. K., Treisman, A., and Savoy, R. L. (1997). Voluntary attention modulates fMRI activity in human MT/MST. *Neuron* **18**, 591–598.

Savoy, R. L. (2001). History and future directions of human brain mapping and functional neuroimaging. *Acta Psychol.* **107**(1–3), 9–42.

Toga, A. T., and Mazziotta, J. C. (Eds.) (2000). *Brain Mapping: The Systems.* Academic Press, San Diego.

Tootell, R. B. H., Dale, A. M., Sereno, M. I., and Malach, R. (1996). New images from human visual cortex. *Trends Neurosci.* **19**(11), 481–489.

Wagner, A. D., Schacter, D. L., Rotte, M., Koutstaal, W., Maril, A., Dale, A. M., Rosen, B. R., and Buckner, R. J. (1998). Building memories: Remembering and forgetting of verbal experiences as predicted by brain activity. *Science* **281**, 1188–1191.

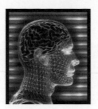

GABA

SOFIE R. KLEPPNER and ALLAN J. TOBIN

UCLA Brain Research Institute

I. Introduction

II. GABA Production and Degradation

III. GABA Response

IV. GABA Transport

V. GABA Function

VI. GABA and Development

VII. GABA and Disease

VIII. Summary

GLOSSARY

apoenzyme An enzyme without its obligate cofactor, which is therefore inactive.

carrier-mediated release Nonsynaptic release (usually of a neurotransmitter) by a plasma membrane transporter.

GABA γ-Aminobutyric acid; the major inhibitory neurotransmitter of the central nervous system; also found in extraneuronal tissues (e.g., the pancreas and reproductive tracts).

GABA receptor A protein that binds GABA and initiates downstream effects.

GABA-T GABA-transaminase; enzyme that degrades GABA.

GABA transporter A protein that moves GABA across either the plasma membrane or the vesicular membrane.

GAD Glutamic acid decarboxylase; enzyme that converts glutamate to GABA.

holoenzyme An enzyme bound to its obligate cofactor, which is therefore active.

inhibitory neurotransmitter A neurotransmitter that, when it activates its postsynaptic receptor, decreases the probability that the postsynaptic cell will fire.

phasic inhibition Short-term (milliseconds) decrease in excitability of a cell, usually synaptically mediated.

pyridoxal phosphate Vitamin B6; a cofactor required for GAD activity.

receptor agonist A substance that binds to a receptor and mimics or enhances the receptor response.

receptor antagonist A substance that binds to a receptor and blocks or decreases the receptor response.

tonic inhibition Long-lasting decrease in the overall excitability of a cell or cells, usually extrasynaptically mediated.

GABA (γ-aminobutyric acid; 4-aminobutyric acid) is an inhibitory amino acid neurotransmitter. Three separate groups published the first reports of GABA in the brain in 1950, although its function as a neurotransmitter was not recognized until later. Eugene Roberts, the author of one of the first reports, identified GABA in the course of chromatographic studies on the amino acid profiles of murine neuroblastomas. GABA from potatoes was used as a standard and comigrated with an unknown substance isolated from the tumors. Roberts rigorously pursued his studies of GABA synthesis and degradation in the brain and GABA is now recognized as the most prominent inhibitory neurotransmitter in the central nervous system (CNS).

I. INTRODUCTION

Approximately 30% of neurons in the brain produce GABA, and almost every neuron can respond to GABA. Some nonneural cells also make GABA, including the cells of the endocrine pancreas and the reproductive tracts. GABA in the pancreas presumably acts as a signaling molecule, in a similar manner to CNS signaling. GABA function in the reproductive tracts is unknown.

Encyclopedia of the Human Brain
Volume 2

The molecules associated with GABA synthesis, degradation, transport, and signaling include two synthesizing enzymes, one degrading enzyme, two transporting proteins, and two classes of receptors. These molecules, their functions, and their putative locations are listed in Table I and illustrated in Fig. 1.

GABA acts by binding to GABA receptors, which are located on both pre- and postsynaptic cells. Generally, GABA receptor binding hyperpolarizes the cell, producing an inhibitory effect. In some circumstances, however, GABA can exert excitatory effects by depolarizing the membrane. Excitatory GABA effects occur most notably during development but also in the rodent suprachiasmatic nucleus, where it may be related to circadian rhythms.

Table I
GABA-Related Proteins, Their Locations, and Their Functions[a]

Protein	Location	Function
GAD	Intracellular	Synthesizes GABA
GAD_{65}	Axon terminal	
GAD_{67}	Cytosol	
GABA-T	Mitochondria	Degrades GABA
GAT		Transports GABA across plasma membrane
GAT1	Neurons and glia	
GAT2	Glia and periphery	
GAT3	Glia and periphery	
GAT4	Brain and periphery	
vGAT	Synaptic vesicle membrane	Packages GABA into vesicle
$GABA_A$	Postsynaptic membrane	Ionotropic receptor (chloride channel)
α_{1-6}		
β_{1-4}		
γ_{1-3}		
δ		
ρ_{1-3}		
π		
ε		
$GABA_B$	Pre- and postsynaptic membrane	Metabotropic receptor (G protein linked)
R1		
R2		

[a]Abbreviations used: GAD, glutamic acid decarboxylase; GABA-T, GABA-transaminase; GAT, GABA transporter; vGAT, vesicular GABA transporter.

Beyond neurotransmission, GABA also acts as a signaling molecule during development, both in the CNS and elsewhere in the embryo. In the CNS, GABA can influence cell migration, neurite extension, differentiation, and synapse formation. GABA also plays an important role in the actions of steroid hormones in the brain. Outside the CNS, GABA is associated with developmental functions including palate formation.

GABA is found in organisms that lack synapses (e.g., bacteria and plants); therefore, it may have an important role outside of intracellular signaling. GABA can be degraded into succinate, which participates in the tricarboxylic acid cycle. Thus, GABA can provide energy for the cell, and this may be part of its role in nonsynaptic functions.

Alterations in GABA production, degradation, response, and transport have tremendous effects. Within the brain, changes in GABA signaling contribute to epilepsy, movement disorders (e.g., Huntington's disease and Parkinson's disease), anxiety, and panic disorder. Injury can influence the expression of glutamic acid decarboxylase, the enzyme that synthesizes GABA, suggesting that GABA may play a role in recovery. Outside of the brain, a lack of GABA in the embryo is associated with cleft palate, a craniofacial malformation. Autoimmunity to glutamic acid decarboxylase is associated with the death of pancreatic β cells and the development of insulin-dependent diabetes mellitus.

II. GABA PRODUCTION AND DEGRADATION

GABA is unique among neurotransmitters because it can be synthesized by either of two closely related enzymes. Almost all GABA derives from the decarboxylation of glutamate, catalyzed by glutamic acid decarboxylase [glutamate decarboxylase (GAD); L-glutamate 1-carboxylase, E.C. 4.1.1.15]. Pyridoxal phosphate [PLP; derived from pyridoxine (vitamin B_6)] is an obligate cofactor for GAD, as it is for many other decarboxylases. GABA can also be synthesized from ornithine via ornithine decarboxylase, although this is a minor route of synthesis. The GABA-synthesizing pathway is illustrated in Fig. 2.

A. GABA Synthesis

GAD consists almost entirely of homodimers of two distinct polypeptides—GAD_{65} (with M_r of 65,000)

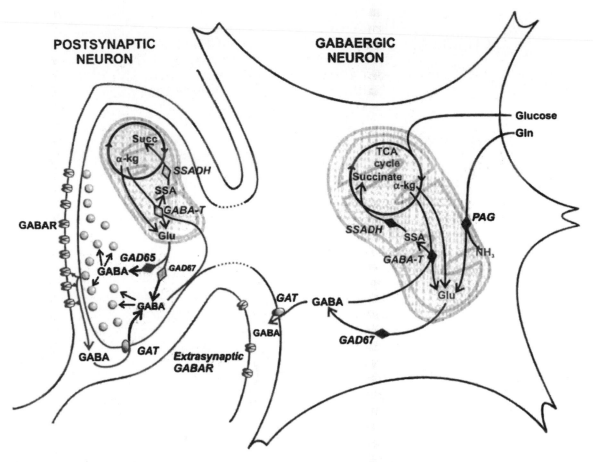

Figure 1 Schematic of GABA-related proteins and their locations within the cell. GAD_{65} or GAD_{67} synthesizes GABA from glutamate. GABA can be packaged into vesicles for release (vesicular GABA transporter not shown) at the synapse, where it binds to GABA receptors. GABA receptors are located on the presynaptic and postsynaptic neuron and can be found outside of the synapse. The plasma membrane GABA transporter (GAT) takes up unbound GABA from the synapse. GABA can also exit the cell via GAT. The GABA shunt is depicted within the mitochondria. Also shown are two sources of glutamate: α-Ketoglutarate can be converted to glutamate by GABA-T, and glutamine, provided by astrocytes, can be converted to glutamate by phosphate-activated glutaminase (PAG). GABAR, GABA receptor; GAD, glutamic acid decarboxylase; GABA-T, GABA-transaminase; α-kg, α-ketoglutarate; Succ, succinate; SSA, succinic semialdehyde; SSADH, succinic semialdehyde dehydrogenase; Gln, glutamine [from D. L. Martin and A. J. Tobin, Mechanisms controlling GABA synthesis and degradation in the brain. In *GABA in the Nervous System: The View at Fifty Years* (D. L. Martin and R. W. Olsen, Eds.). Lippincott, Williams & Wilkins, Philadelphia, 2000].

and GAD_{67} (with M_r of 67,000). The two GADs account for essentially all GAD activity in tissue extracts. Although other purified proteins reportedly have GAD activity, none is known to contribute substantially to GABA synthesis *in vivo*.

The two GAD polypeptides are the products of distinct genes and differ in sequence by about 35%. The two genes have identical exon–intron organizations, suggesting that they share a relatively recent common ancestor. The GAD_{65}s of humans, mice, and rats are 97% identical, as are the GAD_{67}s of humans, rats, and cats. Clearly, the two GADs have been under

strong selective pressure during the 150–200 million years since the beginning of mammalian radiation.

Almost every neuron that produces one form of GAD also produces the other, suggesting that the two genes share some transcriptional regulatory mechanisms. During the development of specific brain structures, GAD_{67} usually appears earlier than GAD_{65}. In the hippocampus and the spinal cord, however, GAD_{65} appears earlier in development than GAD_{67}. The ratio of GAD_{65} to GAD_{67} mRNA increases dramatically during synapse formation, both in the striatum and in the cerebellum.

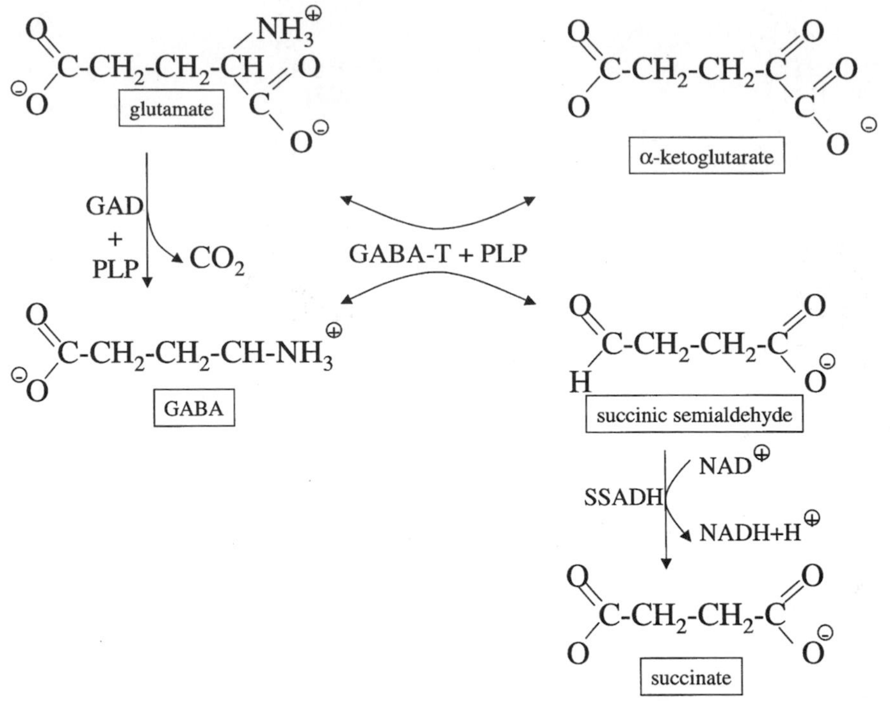

Figure 2   GABA is synthesized from the decarboxylation of glutamate. GABA is degraded to succinic semialdehyde and succinate by GABA-T and succinic semialdehyde dehydrogenase (SSADH). GABA-T can also convert α-ketoglutarate to glutamate, completing the first step of the GABA shunt.

The GAD_{67} gene produces two alternatively spliced transcripts during early development. The two embryonic forms of GAD are GAD_{25} and GAD_{44}, but only GAD_{44} is enzymatically active. GAD_{25} is not enzymatically active because it lacks the PLP binding site. As the embryo develops, the shorter transcripts are replaced by the mature GAD_{67}. GAD_{65} has no identified alternatively spliced transcripts.

GAD_{65} and GAD_{67} differ in their enzymatic characteristics. GAD_{67} exists mainly in the active, holoenzyme form (bound to PLP) and is less sensitive to small changes in neuronal GABA concentration than is GAD_{65}. Most GAD_{65} in the brain is in the apoenzyme form (inactive, not bound to PLP), and the GAD activity of brain extracts increases two- or threefold upon the addition of PLP. The loss of PLP from GAD is not a simple dissociation but a catalytic misstep that results in the formation of succinic semialdehyde and pyridoxamine phosphate (rather than GABA and PLP). This reaction is illustrated in Fig. 3. Pyridoxamine phosphate dissociates from GAD, generating an apoenzyme that lacks enzymatic activity until it again combines with PLP to reform $holoGAD_{65}$.

The interconversion of apoGAD and holoGAD is sensitive to ATP, phosphate (Pi), and GABA levels.

These influences may regulate GABA production in response to altered neuronal activity within GABA neurons. ATP favors the formation of apoGAD and inhibits the formation of holoGAD. Pi enhances the formation of holoGAD. GABA also favors apoGAD formation in the absence of PLP because the GABA-forming steps are readily reversible. Consequently, GAD_{65} is sensitive to small changes in neuronal GABA concentration. GAD has a K_m for glutamate of approximately 0.45 mM and a K_m for GABA of approximately 16 mM. Therefore, given similar concentrations of glutamate and GABA, glutamate is converted to GABA much faster than the reverse reaction.

GAD_{65} and GAD_{67} also differ in their subcellular locations. Both are present in cell bodies and axon terminals, but GAD_{65} is usually more concentrated in axon terminals, whereas GAD_{67} is more concentrated in cell bodies. GAD_{65} associates with vesicle membranes both in neurons and in pancreatic cells, and it is characterized by punctate immunostaining in mature neurons. GAD_{67} generally shows no such association with vesicles, and it is diffuse throughout the cell when examined by immunostaining.

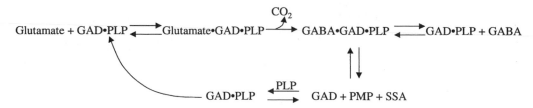

Figure 3 Interconversion of the GAD apoenzyme and holoenzyme. GAD can be converted from its active holoenzyme form, bound to pyridoxal phosphate (PLP), into its inactive apoenzyme form by a catalytic misstep that results in the formation of pyridoxal monophosphate (PMP) and succinic semialdehyde (SSA). GAD must reassociate with PLP to be active [adapted from Brain Glutamate Decarboxylase. In *Neurotransmitter enzymes* (Boulton, Baker, and Yu, Eds.) Humana Press, Clifton, NJ].

GAD_{65} undergoes at least two types of reversible posttranslational modifications—palmitoylation and phosphorylation. These modifications can anchor GAD_{65} to internal membranes, even in cells not specialized for exocytosis, but they are not required for membrane association. Palmitoylation and phosphorylation are limited to a distinct GAD_{65} polypeptide whose electrophoretic mobility is slightly less than that of GAD_{65}, but the structural basis for this difference in mobility is not well understood.

Although most GAD molecules are homodimers, GAD_{65} and GAD_{67} also form heterodimers. The association of some GAD_{67} with synaptic terminals and with the Golgi complex in genetically modified cells appears to depend on its association with membrane-targeted GAD_{65}. The presence of GAD_{67} in a restricted subset of synaptic boutons, observed in the mouse hippocampus, may reflect the distribution of GAD_{65}–GAD_{67} heterodimers.

B. GABA Degradation: The "GABA Shunt"

GABA-transaminase (GABA-T) is the main degradative enzyme for GABA, although steady state GABA levels are normally controlled by GAD. GABA is degraded to succinic semialdehyde (SSA) by GABA-T, a mitochondrial enzyme. Since SSA can be converted to succinate by succinic semialdehyde dehydrogenase (SSADH), GABA can serve as one step in a shunt that bypasses α-ketoglutarate dehydrogenase in the tricarboxylic acid (TCA) cycle. The GABA shunt begins with the conversion of α-ketoglutarate to glutamate by GABA-T, other transaminases, and glutamate dehydrogenase. Glutamate is then decarboxylated by GAD to form GABA, which is degraded to SSA by GABA-T. Finally, SSA is converted to succinate by SSADH. These reactions are summarized in Fig. 4. Normally, the conversion of α-ketoglutarate to succinate produces one NADH and one GTP. The GABA shunt therefore produces approximately 8% less total energy compared to the TCA cycle, although it provides 10–20% of the TCA cycle activity in most brain regions.

III. GABA RESPONSE

Responses to GABA depend on two classes of GABA receptor—$GABA_A$ receptors, which are located on the postsynaptic cell and produce fast (millisecond) responses, and $GABA_B$ receptors, which are found on both pre- and postsynaptic cells and produce slower (second) responses that depend on second messengers. A third class of GABA receptors, the $GABA_C$ receptors, is also ionotropic and is now generally considered to be a subset of $GABA_A$ receptors. The differences in GABA receptor structure, function, and location allow fine-tuning of GABA signaling and response.

A. $GABA_A$ Receptors

Most neurons express $GABA_A$ receptors. $GABA_A$ receptors are GABA-gated chloride channels located on the postsynaptic membrane. Upon binding GABA, the channel opens and chloride flows along its concentration gradient. The extracellular chloride concentration is usually higher than the intracellular concentration, so chloride usually flows into the cell. The inward chloride flux results in hyperpolarization of the postsynaptic membrane and a concomitant decrease in the probability of cell firing. In some cases, however, GABA evokes a depolarizing response, either because of high intracellular chloride concentrations resulting in an outward flow of chloride through the open channel or because of the flow of bicarbonate ions through the channel.

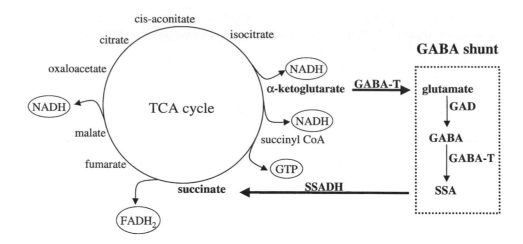

Figure 4   The GABA shunt. GABA can contribute to the TCA cycle via the GABA shunt, which converts α-ketoglutarate to succinate. The GABA shunt provides less energy than the complete TCA cycle because it bypasses the formation of one NADH and one GTP. Nonetheless, approximately 10–20% of TCA cycle activity in most brain regions is provided by the GABA shunt. SSA, succinic semialdehyde; SSADH, succinic semialdehyde dehydrogenase.

1. GABA$_A$ Receptor Topology

GABA$_A$ receptors are highly diverse. Each GABA$_A$ receptor consists of five transmembrane polypeptide subunits. At least 19 subunits exist, named $\alpha(1–6)$, $\beta(1–4)$, $\gamma(1–3)$, δ, ε, $\rho(1–3)$, and π. The recently identified subtype θ may be identical to β_4. Splice variants of several subunits exist as well. Receptor heterogeneity results from at least 20 different combinations of five subunits.

Each subunit consists of a long extracellular amino-terminal region, four transmembrane domains, and a large intracellular loop between the third and fourth transmembrane domains (Fig. 5A). This motif is shared by the channel superfamily that includes nicotinic acetylcholine receptors, glycine receptors, and serotonin 5-HT$_3$ receptors. Five subunits form a complex with a central pore (Fig. 5B). The amino-terminal domains of the α and β subunits are believed to be exclusively responsible for the GABA binding site. Receptor gating is almost certainly mediated by the M2 regions of all five subunits, which presumably line the pore, as is the case in related receptors.

2. GABA$_A$ Subunit Composition

The GABA$_A$ subunit genes are located on several chromosomes. For example, human α_1 is located on chromosome 5, α_2 on chromosome 4, and α_5 on chromosome 15. Many of the subunit genes occur in clusters. For instance, $\alpha_1/\alpha_6/\beta_2/\gamma_2$ are clustered on

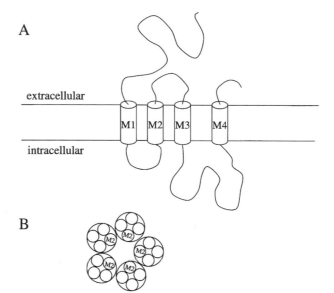

Figure 5   GABA$_A$ receptor subunit and complex topology. (A). Each GABA$_A$ subunit has four transmembrane domains (M1–M4). The amino terminus is extracellular and the carboxy terminus is intracellular. (B). Top view of five subunits that form the receptor complex with a central pore, which is likely lined by the M2 domains of each subunit [reprinted from Cherubini and Conti, *TINS* **24**(3), 155–162, 2001, with permission of Elsevier Science].

chromosome 5, whereas $\alpha_2/\alpha_4/\beta_1/\gamma_1$ are located on chromosome 4. The chromosomal arrangement of the subunit genes suggests that both gene and cluster duplication occurred during evolution.

Despite the number of potential subunit combinations, there are some common combinations, which are summarized in Table II. Both development and brain region regulate $GABA_A$ subunit composition and presumably each combination has unique properties based not only on each subunit but also on the assembly as a whole. The functional consequences of specific combinations are not well understood but can affect both receptor function and location.

The subunit composition affects receptor binding of GABA and other ligands, but it is also important in receptor targeting, assembly, and clustering. For instance, γ_2 knockout mice show reduced $GABA_A$ receptor clustering as well as reduced ligand binding. α_6 knockout mice also demonstrate decreased δ subunit expression, despite normal mRNA levels, indicating posttranscriptional control by the subunits.

3. Pharmacology of $GABA_A$ Receptors

The $GABA_A$ receptor is affected by a myriad of drugs, including those that both cause and prevent convulsions, those that relieve anxiety, and those that relax, sedate, and anesthetize. Receptor subunit composition is critical in determining drug action. The specific binding sites for many but not all compounds have been identified.

Benzodiazepines (BZs) constitute a class of drugs that act on the $GABA_A$ receptor with sedative, anxiolytic (antianxiety), muscle relaxant, and cognitive effects. BZs bind to the external surface of receptors with specific combinations of subunits: A combination of γ_2 with α_1, α_2, α_3, or α_5 and any β subunit confers BZ binding. Each α subunit may have its own BZ binding affinity. The BZ binding site is thought to be between the γ_2 and α subunits and is highly homologous to the GABA-binding site located between the α and β subunits. Recent work has shown that the α_1 subunit mediates the sedative but not the anxiolytic effect of BZs.

Anticonvulsant and anesthetic drugs can positively or negatively modulate the receptor response to GABA. For example, barbiturates can directly enhance the GABA response either by opening the chloride channel or by increasing the time for which it remains open after binding to GABA. Very high concentrations of barbiturates can block the channel entirely, however. Barbiturates bind within the $GABA_A$ receptor pore and can also act at other receptors, including glutamate and acetylcholine receptors. This

Table II

Common $GABA_A$ Receptor Subtype Combinations and Their Locations[a]

Subtype	Comments
$\alpha_1\beta_2\gamma_2$	Approx 50% of the total $GABA_A$ receptors; widespread; GABAergic interneurons
$\alpha_2\beta_3\gamma_2$	Approx 15–20% of total $GABA_A$ receptors; cortex, hippocampus, amygdala, septum, hypothalamus
$\alpha_3\beta_3\gamma_2$ ($\alpha_1\alpha_3\beta_3\gamma_2$)	Approx 15–20% of total $GABA_A$ receptors; cortex, amygdala, septum, raphe; monoaminergic, serotonergic neurons
$\alpha_4\beta_x\gamma_2$	<5% of total $GABA_A$ receptors in whole brain; cortex, hippocampus, thalamus, striatum
$\alpha_4\beta_x\delta$	<5% of total $GABA_A$ receptors in whole brain; cortex, hippocampus, thalamus, striatum
$\alpha_5\beta_3\gamma_2$	<5% of total $GABA_A$ receptors in whole brain; hippocampus (approx 20% of total $GABA_A$ receptors), cortex
$\alpha_6\beta_x\gamma_2$ ($\alpha_1\alpha_6\beta_x\gamma_2$)	<5% of total $GABA_A$ receptors in whole brain; cerebellar granule cells (30–40% of total $GABA_A$ receptors)
$\alpha_6\beta_x\delta$ ($\alpha_1\alpha_6\beta_x\delta$)	<5% of total $GABA_A$ receptors in whole brain; cerebellar granule cells (20–30% of total $GABA_A$ receptors); extrasynaptic
$\alpha_2\beta_1\gamma_1$	
$\alpha_2\beta_1\gamma_1\theta$	<10% of total $GABA_A$ receptors in whole brain; limbic regions, basal ganglia, tyrosine hydroxylase-positive neurons, Bergmann glia
γ_3-containing receptors	<5% of total $GABA_A$ receptors in whole brain; widespread, low abundance; little data available
ε-containing receptors	<5% of total $GABA_A$ receptors in whole brain; hippocampus, hypothalamus; little data available

[a]Adapted from P. J. Whiting, K. A. Wafford, and R. M. McKernan, Pharmacologic subtypes of $GABA_A$ receptors based on subunit composition. In *GABA in the Nervous System: The View at Fifty Years*. (D. L. Martin and R. W. Olsen, Eds.). Lippincott, Williams & Wilkins, Philadelphia (2000).

may reflect conservation of specific residues within the subunits. The anesthetic binding site is different from the GABA binding site, and it is probably located within the pore.

Alcohol acts on the GABA$_A$ receptor, although its route of action and potential binding site are unclear. In some cases, alcohol potentiates GABA function at the GABA$_A$ receptor, but this effect may depend on receptor subtypes or on an indirect action. Currently, there appear to be alcohol-sensitive and alcohol-insensitive GABA$_A$ receptors, but the basis for that sensitivity is unclear.

neurotransmitter and also decreases the action potential duration. Postsynaptic GABA$_B$ receptor activation causes inwardly rectifying K$^+$ channels to open, which increases K$^+$ conductance. Increased K$^+$ conductance causes an increase in extracellular K$^+$ and a concomitant hyperpolarization, rendering Na$^+$ channels inactive. Thus, the net result of GABA binding to GABA$_B$ receptors is a decrease in the probability of cell firing.

B. GABA$_B$ Receptors

GABA$_B$ receptors are located both pre- and postsynaptically and they appear to be largely extrasynaptic. GABA$_B$ receptors are G protein-coupled receptors that interact with a number of proteins on K$^+$ and Ca^{2+} channels as well as with adenylate cyclase. They belong to the class C metabotropic receptor family, which includes the metabotropic glutamate receptors. The GABA$_B$ receptor has only recently been cloned, and our understanding of this receptor is therefore more limited than that of the GABA$_A$ receptor.

GABA$_B$ activation is inhibitory both pre- and postsynaptically. Presynaptic GABA$_B$ receptor activation causes Ca^{2+} channels to close, which decreases Ca^{2+} conductance. Decreased Ca^{2+} conductance at the nerve terminal reduces exocytotic release of

1. Receptor Topology

GABA$_B$ receptors are unique within the metabotropic receptor family because they exist as heterodimers. Functional GABA$_B$ receptors require the GBR1 and GBR2 subunits in order to be expressed at the cell surface, to bind ligand, and to mediate action. Both GBR1 and GBR2 have seven transmembrane domains, with extracellular amino termini and intracellular carboxy termini (Fig. 6). The amino terminus of GBR1 provides a GABA binding site, whereas the intracellular loops and carboxy terminus participate in G protein binding. GBR2 does not appear to interact with GABA. GBR1 and GBR2 interact via the carboxy domain, and this interaction is necessary in order to direct GBR1 expression to the cell surface.

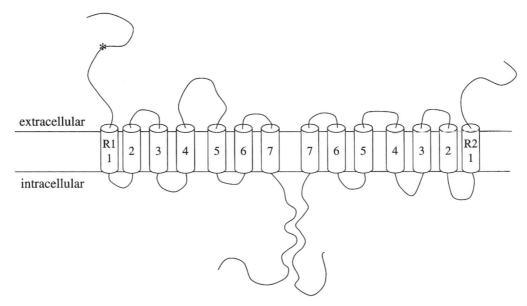

extracellular

intracellular

Figure 6 GABA$_B$ receptor subunit and complex topology. The GABA$_B$ receptor is composed of two similar subunits, each with seven transmembrane domains, extracellular amino termini, and intracellular carboxy termini. The putative GABA binding site, denoted by an asterisk, is on the amino terminus of GABA$_B$R1. The subunits interact via their carboxy domains.

2. Subunit Composition

There are at least four isoforms of GBR1, GBR1a–GBR1d, which range in size from approximately 100 to 130 kDa. The GBR1a isoform may be more prevalent at presynaptic sites, whereas the GBR1b isoform is predominantly found postsynaptically. GBR1 and GBR2 share 35% homology with each other but have little homology with other metabotropic receptors.

IV. GABA TRANSPORT

A. Plasma Membrane GABA Transporters

GABA is actively transported across the plasma membrane by GABA transporters (GATs). The four GATs identified so far (GAT1–3 and GAT4 or BGT-1) belong to the superfamily of Na^+- and Cl^--dependent transporters that include transporters for norepinephrine, serotonin, dopamine, and glycine but not for glutamate. The four GATs differ in pharmacology and in cell expression. For instance, GAT1 is inhibited by nipecotic acid and is predominantly found on neurons, although it is also expressed on some glia. GAT2 and GAT3 can transport both GABA and β-alanine. GAT3 is primarily a glial transporter, whereas GAT2 is found on neurons but its cell specificity remains unclear. BGT-1 was first identified in the kidney and transports GABA, betaine, and taurine.

GAT2 and GAT3 are also found in peripheral tissues, including the liver and kidney.

Na^+- and Cl^--dependent transporters rely on the ionic gradients across the membrane. GABA transport is an electrogenic process that cotransports approximately two Na^+ ions and one Cl^- ion with each GABA molecule. Since the ionic gradients normally favor inward transport, GABA usually is transported into the cell. Under conditions of high intracellular Na^+ or membrane depolarization, however, GABA can be released through the transporter.

1. Topology

The GATs are glycoproteins with a molecular weight of 70–80 kDa. The presumed topology predicts that both the amino and the carboxy termini are cytoplasmic and that there are 12 transmembrane domains. The GAT1 topology is illustrated in Fig. 7. There are three glycosylation sites between the third and fourth transmembrane domains. The fourth through sixth extracellular loops form a putative GABA-binding site.

2. Carrier-Mediated Release

The GABA transporters reverse to release cytosolic GABA when the Na^+ gradient across the membrane is perturbed and also when the membrane potential increases. Although these changes occur rapidly during an action potential, GAT-mediated GABA release (or carrier-mediated release) is probably not a

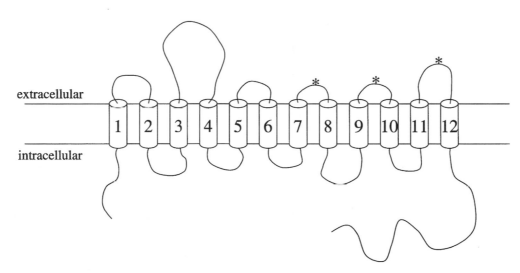

extracellular

intracellular

Figure 7 GAT has 12 transmembrane domains, and both the amino and carboxy termini are intracellular. The putative GABA binding site denoted by asterisks, is on the fourth through sixth extracellular domains.

major route of egress during cell firing because the changes in membrane potential are rapid and transient. However, several studies suggest that activation of the glutamate NMDA receptor causes intracellular Na^+ levels to increase sufficiently to produce GAT-mediated GABA release. Small perturbations in the extracellular K^+ concentrations, and concomitant membrane depolarization, can also cause carrier-mediated GABA release at levels sufficient to activate nearby $GABA_A$ receptors. Seizure activity and the accompanying changes in the extracellular ionic environment may therefore stimulate carrier-mediated GABA release.

B. Vesicular GABA Transporters

GABA is packaged into vesicles at the synapse by the vesicular GABA transporter (vGAT), which was recently cloned. Although vGAT transports GABA across a membrane, it bears no resemblance to the GATs. Both the amino and carboxy termini of vGAT are cytoplasmic, and there are 10 predicted transmembrane domains (Fig. 8).

vGAT, with a K_m for GABA in the millimolar range, depends on both pH and electrochemical gradients (ΔpH and $\Delta \Psi$) across the vesicular membrane to concentrate GABA into vesicles. These gradients are maintained by Mg^{2+}-activated ATPase, which belongs to the class of vacuolar ATPases. Vesicular transporters for other neurotransmitters have a different dependence on the same gradients. For instance, the vesicular dopamine transporter depends mostly on

ΔpH, whereas the vesicular glutamate transporter depends mostly on $\Delta \Psi$.

Glycine, an inhibitory neurotransmitter, can also be transported by vGAT. vGAT mRNA distribution in neurons coincides with other glycinergic and GABAergic markers. Immunohistochemical studies demonstrate vGAT in terminals and the neurotransmitter phenotype of the particular terminals can be GABA, glycine, or mixed.

V. GABA FUNCTION

The GADs differ in their PLP dependence, encoding gene, membrane association, and subcellular location, which suggests that the GADs may synthesize separate pools of GABA that serve different functions. Although GABA is a neurotransmitter, it also functions as a developmental molecule and can contribute to the tricarboxylic acid cycle to provide energy to the cell. Studies of GABA in transgenic mice deficient in one GAD support the hypothesis that GAD_{65}-synthesized GABA is predominantly packaged for neurotransmission, whereas GAD_{67}-synthesized GABA remains in the cytosol and is available for alternate functions.

A. Effects of GAD Deletions in Knockout Mice

Mice lacking GAD_{67} die shortly after birth, presumably as a result of cleft palate. Their brains contain only 7% of the GABA concentration of control brains and about 20% of the GAD activity. Morphological

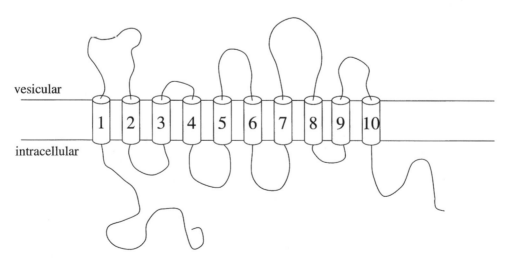

Figure 8   VGAT has 10 transmembrane domains, and both the amino and carboxy termini are intracellular (cytosolic).

analyses of their brains reveal no major abnormalities, but no detailed anatomical or electrophysiological studies of embryonic structures from GAD_{67} knockouts have been reported.

Mice lacking GAD_{65} appear to develop normally but are abnormally sensitive to seizures, particularly in a mouse line that is genetically susceptible to insulin-dependent diabetes mellitus. Perhaps significantly, these mice exhibit both humoral and cellular immune responses to both GAD_{65} and GAD_{67}.

Mice lacking GAD_{65} have a lowered capacity for depolarization-dependent GABA release *in vivo*. The GAD_{65} knockout mice also show impaired experience-dependent plasticity, as determined in monocular deprivation experiments. GAD_{65} may be selectively important in providing GABA to fill secretory vesicles and support exocytotic release of GABA. For example, GAD_{65} knockout mice cannot release normal amounts of GABA during and immediately after sustained stimulation of the retina or hippocampus. Moreover, in contrast to wild-type mice, these GAD_{65} knockout mice show no increase in the probability of GABA release after tetanic stimulation of the hippocampus. Although GAD_{67}-synthesized GABA can evidently be packaged into release vesicles under conditions of low demand, GAD_{67} alone seems to be unable to support the high-efficiency reloading of GABA vesicles required for normal function during conditions of high demand.

Mice lacking both forms of GAD die at birth, presumably from cleft palate. Although these mice have no detectable GABA, there do not appear to be any gross histological abnormalities in their brains. Therefore, GABA's role as a developmental molecule may be redundant, at least in some respects.

B. GABA as a Paracrine "Reset" Signal

GABA-producing cells increase GAD_{67} and GAD_{67} mRNA levels in response to injury, whereas GAD_{65} and its mRNA are usually unchanged. Injuries that produce increased GAD_{67} include chemical lesions of the substantia nigra and hippocampus, neuroleptic drugs, spinal cord transection, and acute stress. The increase in GAD_{67} can be observed as soon as 1 hr after insult, implicating immediate early genes in GAD_{67} regulation.

Most GAD_{67} is not associated with synapses, and GAD_{67} may be responsible for carrier-mediated GABA release. This direct release of cytoplasmic GABA occurs in cultured hippocampal neurons as well as in cells transfected with the GABA transporter and in a pancreatic cell line. Evidence from knockout mice suggests that GAD_{67}-synthesized GABA may not be effectively packaged into vesicles. Therefore, it either remains in the cytosol (where it is available for the GABA shunt) or crosses the plasma membrane via the GABA transporter.

Extrasynaptic GABA (either released via GAT or leaked from the synapse) could interact with extrasynaptic GABA receptors. Such diffuse GABA would cause inhibition diffuse with kinetics different from those at the synapse. Such inhibition would depend on the kinetics of GABA release, diffusion, reuptake, and degradation as well as on receptor composition.

Diffuse GABA could act in a paracrine manner on extrasynaptic $GABA_A$ receptors. Such receptors have been documented electrophysiologically in studies of GABA "spillover" in cerebellar synapses and microscopically by EM immunocytochemistry. The effect of such paracrine action would be to suppress neuronal firing in cells within damaged circuits. Sustained inhibition could allow the plastic remodeling of neural circuits, such as occurs during the retraining of the spinal cord. According to this view, paracrine GABA, synthesized primarily by GAD_{67}, could serve a "reset" function, giving the cells of damaged but plastic circuits the time to recover from challenge or injury. Observed parallel increases in GAD_{67} and extracellular GABA in the hippocampus of kainate-treated rats are consistent with this view. Therefore, GAD_{67} may contribute to a relatively slow mode of paracrine function, whereas GAD_{65} may be mainly responsible for the synthesis of GABA that participates in rapid point-to-point signaling.

C. How Much GABA Is Needed to Evoke a Response?

The cloning of $GABA_A$ and $GABA_B$ receptors has enabled researchers to study the properties of receptors of known covalent structure. In most of these *in vitro* studies, the K_D of the cloned receptors for GABA is in the micromolar range, but *in vivo* GABA often has an EC_{50} in the nanomolar or even subnanomolar range.

Within a synaptic cleft, the concentration of GABA is estimated to be in the millimolar range, enough to saturate postsynaptic $GABA_A$ (and $GABA_B$)

receptors. The occurrence of $GABA_A$ and $GABA_B$ receptors outside of synapses suggests that GABA may also act outside of synapses. The ability of cultured cells and partially purified receptors to bind GABA at nanomolar concentrations is consistent with a role for nonsynaptic GABA, particularly in response to injury, seizures, and other stresses.

D. Neurosteroids and GABA

GABA is involved in the actions of neurosteroids, which are steroid hormones that are synthesized in the brain and are particularly relevant to reproductive behavior and stress responses. Neurosteroids can enhance GABA release. For example, some GABAergic neurons are stimulated by testosterone, via androgen receptors, and may mediate the action or secretion of other hormones. GABA can affect lordosis, the steroid-modulated behavior exhibited by sexually receptive female rats. GABA facilitates or inhibits lordosis depending on the specific region of the brain that is stimulated.

Neurosteroids can directly bind to and activate $GABA_A$ receptors to produce sedative, anticonvulsant, and anxiolytic effects in animals. Neurosteroids can also influence $GABA_A$ subunit expression. Anesthetic effects from neurosteroids are modulated by a different site on the receptor than other types of anesthetics, but the binding site is probably also within the pore. The α, γ, and δ subunits affect neurosteroid response but not necessarily GABA binding.

E. GABA Affects Overall Excitability

GABA is synthesized in both projection neurons (e.g., neurons within the striatum that project to the substantia nigra and globus pallidus) and interneurons (e.g., the basket cells of the dentate gyrus). Projection neurons are thought to play a major role in initiating postsynaptic activity, whereas interneurons are thought to modulate postsynaptic activity. Interneurons within the hippocampus appear to also form large circuits that underlie the theta rhythms in the brain. These slow (4–9 Hz) rhythms are associated with learning and memory and may reflect an overall control of excitation that provides a more amenable environment for synaptic plasticity. Thus, GABA as a neurotransmitter not only provides straightforward

neuron-to-neuron signaling but also affects the overall excitability of large regions of the brain.

GABA can initiate two types of responses. Phasic responses occur when GABA binds to postsynaptic receptors. Phasic responses are characterized by fast postsynaptic changes. Tonic responses result from ongoing activation of GABA receptors outside of the synapse. This activation produces continuous inhibition of the postsynaptic cell, thereby controlling its overall excitability.

Tonic and phasic inhibition differ not only because of the receptor location but also in the receptor subunit composition. The extrasynaptic receptors that mediate tonic inhibition have a higher affinity for GABA than do the receptors responsible for phasic inhibition. Different affinities reflect the GABA levels to which the two sets of receptors are exposed. Extrasynaptic GABA levels are lower than those found within the synapse; therefore, extrasynaptic receptors must be sensitive enough to detect low levels, whereas synaptic receptors must not desensitize upon exposure to the high levels of GABA found within the synapse. The role of $GABA_B$ receptors, which are primarily extrasynaptic, has not been elucidated in these two types of inhibition.

VI. GABA AND DEVELOPMENT

GABA functions as more than a neurotransmitter. A growing body of evidence suggests that it also plays an important role in development. GABA appears in most CNS neurons at the beginning of neurogenesis (before synapse formation), as does the $GABA_A$ receptor. During this time, GABA is excitatory because a developmentally regulated chloride transporter maintains high intracellular chloride levels.

The pattern of GAD expression changes during development, again supporting a role for GABA at this time. In the spinal cord, the change from embryonic to mature GAD_{67} transcripts echoes the ventral to dorsal maturation of the cord. GAD immunoreactivity is diffuse early in development, suggesting that there is no vesicle-associated GAD present (which would be characterized by punctate staining) and therefore no synaptic GABA.

GAT-mediated GABA transport decreases from birth through adulthood, whereas vGAT-mediated transport increases from the time of synapse formation through adulthood. The differences in GABA trafficking may account for the developmental properties of

GABA because it does not necessarily act synaptically throughout development. GABA can stimulate both directed and random movement of young neurons, possibly through the GABA_B receptor. However, GABA may not be required during development since GAD knockouts have undetectable GABA but develop anatomically normal brains.

Outside of the CNS, compromised GABA signaling during development produces cleft palate, a craniofacial abnormality in which the roof of the mouth fails to close completely. Animal studies suggest that the barbiturate diazepam, which interacts with GABA_A receptors, can cause palatal defects. In addition, mice lacking GAD_{67} are born with cleft palate and die shortly after birth. The route by which GABA may be associated with cleft palate is not well understood.

VII. GABA AND DISEASE

Defects in GABA synthesis, release, and response have serious consequences. Since GABA is a ubiquitous neurotransmitter, it can be argued that it has a role (direct or indirect) in most neurological diseases. The direct loss of GABAergic neurons in the striatum, for instance, is a hallmark of Huntington's disease. Parkinson's disease, however, results from a loss of dopamine neurons in the substantia nigra. The lost neurons normally project to GABA neurons in the striatum, and those lost projections affect GABA signaling in Parkinson's disease.

A. Changes in GABA Signaling

Epilepsy describes a set of diseases characterized by hyperexcitability and synchronous firing of large groups of neurons. Although there are many different kinds of epilepsy, temporal lobe epilepsy (TLE) is the most common type in adults and is often difficult to resolve. TLE seizures usually begin in the hippocampus and spread to involve large parts of the brain. Genetic mutations, injury, or tumors can all result in TLE. TLE usually causes extensive changes within the hippocampus, including the death of subsets of neurons, neuritic sprouting, and sclerotic lesions. The hyperexcitability characteristic of TLE suggests that this disease compromises GABAergic inhibition.

GAD levels increase in parts of the TLE hippocampus, but GABA levels decrease. Since GAD increases

as a result of many types of injury, the changes observed in TLE may not serve to provide more GABA for signaling. Instead, the increase may reflect a general cellular response to injury, and the resultant GABA may be diverted to the GABA shunt to provide energy for the cell.

Hyperexcitability could reflect the loss of GABA neurons, but the neurons that die in TLE are mainly excitatory cells. Only a small subset of GABAergic neurons, which coexpress somatostatin, is lost. Several hypotheses address the compromised inhibitory capability of the TLE hippocampus. One possibility is that the excitatory inputs to some GABAergic neurons are lost, thus decreasing their inhibitory signaling. Another suggestion is that some GABAergic neurons lose their targets and redirect their outputs to many cells. The result is that one inhibitory cell now drives many excitatory cells, causing the synchronized firing that is a hallmark of TLE. A third hypothesis suggests that GABAergic neurons redirect their output to other GABAergic neurons, thus providing a net excitatory output relative to the normal state.

The multitude of changes within the TLE hippocampus may mean that one comprehensive treatment approach is impossible. Although GABA neurons are mainly intact, changes in connections may either increase or decrease net inhibition. GAD levels are increased, GABA receptors are increased in some cells but decreased in others, the GABA transporter is decreased only in some areas of the hippocampus, and overall GABA is decreased. Nonetheless, many of the drugs that are effective for treating TLE increase GABA action through potentiating GABA_A receptors (thus creating a more powerful response to endogenous GABA) or by interfering with GAT1 or GABA-T to increase available GABA.

B. Defects in GABA Receptors

Angelman syndrome is linked to deletions in human chromosome 15, specifically in the area that codes for the cluster of GABA_A receptor subunits $\alpha_5/\beta_3/\gamma_3$. Severe mental retardation, epilepsy, movement disorders, inappropriate laughter, and craniofacial abnormalities characterize this disorder. A similar syndrome, Prader–Willi syndrome, shows mild mental retardation, hypotonia, hyperphasia, and hypogonadism. The two syndromes are linked to the same gene; however, Angelman's is linked to the maternal gene, whereas Prader–Willi is linked to the paternal gene.

Epilepsy and craniofacial abnormalities are characteristic of other GABA-related disorders, highlighting GABA's role in both development and signaling, although the connection between gene deletions and symptoms is unclear.

C. Loss of GABA Neurons

Huntington's disease is an autosomal-dominant disease in which GABAergic projection neurons in the striatum are destroyed. Early symptoms include mood changes progressing to uncontrolled movements (chorea) and eventually to loss of movement and death. Disease progression can be correlated with the loss of three separate populations of GABAergic striatal neurons, although these are not the sole casualties. Cortical neuronal loss occurs later in the disease as well.

The gene for Huntington's disease codes for the huntingtin protein, which contains a long polyglutamine stretch. Normally, the number of glutamines in this protein is less than 40. Huntingtin mutations that include more than 40 glutamines are pathogenic. The number of glutamines is inversely related to the age of onset, and people with longer repeat lengths develop Huntington's disease at earlier ages. The function of the normal huntingtin protein is unknown, as is the reason for the susceptibility of GABAergic projection neurons.

The Huntington's disease gene is expressed throughout life, but disease symptoms normally begin in the fourth decade. This delay in symptom onset may reflect the ability of the brain to compensate for dysfunction for a period of time. Currently, there is no cure for Huntington's disease, and treatments are limited to palliative care.

D. Defects in GAD

Autoimmunity to GAD is a hallmark of two related conditions—insulin-dependent diabetes mellitus (IDDM, juvenile diabetes, or type 1 diabetes) and a rare neurological disorder called stiff-man syndrome (SMS).

1. Diabetes

IDDM is an autoimmune disease in which T cells mistakenly destroy pancreatic β cells, which are the sole producers of insulin. Several β cell proteins are targets of autoantibodies, including GAD_{65}, GAD_{67}, and insulin. These autoantibodies often arise several years before disease onset, possibly providing a window of opportunity for intervention.

The β cells of pancreatic islets contain high levels of GABA and GAD, comparable to those in neurons. GAD_{65} and GAD_{67} are both present in the pancreas of rats and mice, with GAD_{67} and its mRNA at higher levels than GAD_{65} and its mRNA. In humans, however, GAD_{65} greatly predominates and may also be present in pancreatic α cells. Species differences may reflect differences in gene regulation during the development of islet cell precursors. GABA from β cells is thought to act on $GABA_A$ receptors to inhibit glucagon release by α cells.

Autoantibodies to GAD, sometimes in combination with other autoantibodies, provide a highly specific and highly sensitive prediagnostic test for individuals at high risk for developing IDDM, sometimes many years before actual disease onset. GAD autoimmunity also provides a diagnostic marker that distinguishes between adult-onset non-insulin-dependent diabetes mellitus, which does not involve autoimmunity, and late-onset IDDM, which does. Whether it appears in children or adults, IDDM is an autoimmune disease, with GAD_{65} as the most common early target. Autoimmunity to GAD_{65} in IDDM could merely reflect the unmasking of a self-antigen after β cell destruction, but it may well have a causal role in the destruction of β cells.

2. Stiff-Man Syndrome

SMS is a rare neurological disease characterized by muscle rigidity that results from the simultaneous contraction of antagonistic muscle groups. As in the case of spasticity, GABA agonists can ameliorate symptoms.

About 60% of SMS patients have autoantibodies to GAD, but the causal role of GAD remains an open question since there is no apparent difference in the signs and symptoms of SMS patients with and without anti-GAD antibodies. Most SMS patients with GAD autoantibodies also have other autoimmune disorders (such as Hashimoto's thyroiditis and Grave's disease), whereas only a few percent of the GAD antibody-negative patients have any evidence of autoimmune disease. Despite years of attempts, the administration of GAD cannot provoke SMS in experimental animals, suggesting that GAD autoimmunity in SMS is probably not causal.

VIII. SUMMARY

In the 50 years since its identification as a neurotransmitter, GABA has emerged as a major force in normal CNS function, development, and disease. In addition to neurotransmission, GABA can provide energy through the GABA shunt and can mediate developmental events. Outside of the nervous system, GABA is involved with pancreatic glucagon release and is required for palate formation.

The variety of functions that GABA can perform may be governed in part by the different location and regulation of the two GABA-synthesizing enzymes. GAD_{65} appears to synthesize GABA largely for neurotransmission, whereas GAD_{67} synthesizes GABA that is available for the GABA shunt and also for release directly through GAT. The manner by which GABA leaves the cell may also be important in determining its function. GABA released via exocytosis is largely confined to the synapse, whereas that released through GAT is available to extrasynaptic receptors.

GABA receptors are an additional modulator of GABA function. Different subunit compositions impart different sensitivity, kinetics, and location. The $GABA_A$ receptor can confer inhibition or excitation, depending on the chloride gradient across the membrane. The $GABA_B$ receptor can exert both presynaptic and postsynaptic effects. The diversity of GABA actions is due in no small part to the great variation within the GABA receptor family.

GABA is the major inhibitory neurotransmitter and changes in GABA signaling have widespread effects. A role for GABA dysfunction can be argued even in diseases for which the primary pathology lies elsewhere. The molecules that synthesize, transport, respond to, and degrade GABA are all potential targets for therapy. Drugs that can selectively activate specific receptor subtypes or that can interfere with the kinetics of GABA transport and degradation will certainly be helpful in treating GABA-related diseases. Alternate approaches, including gene therapy, to control local GABA concentrations are also promising. Our understanding of the mechanisms of GABA regulation and signaling will therefore lead to new and effective therapies for a variety of diseases.

See Also the Following Articles

ALCOHOL DAMAGE TO THE BRAIN • DOPAMINE • ENDORPHINS AND THEIR RECEPTORS • EPILEPSY • NEURON • NEUROTRANSMITTERS • NOREPINEPHRINE • PEPTIDES, HORMONES, AND THE BRAIN AND SPINAL CORD

Suggested Reading

Barnard, E. A., Skolnick, P., Olsen, R. W., *et al.* (1998). International Union of Pharmacology. XV. Subtypes of gamma-aminobutyric acid A receptors: Classification on the basis of subunit structure and receptor function. *Pharmacol. Rev.* **50**(2), 291–313.

Blein, S., Hawrot, E., and Barlow, P. (2000). The metabotropic GABA receptor: Molecular insights and their functional consequences. *Cell Mol. Life Sci.* **57**(4), 635–650.

Martin, D. L., and Olsen, R. W. (Eds.) (2000). *GABA in the Nervous System: The View at Fifty Years.* Lippincott Williams & Wilkins, Philadelphia.

Jursky, F., Tamura, S., Tamura, A., *et al.* (1994). Structure, function and brain localization of neurotransmitter transporters. *J. Exp. Biol.* **196**, 283–295.

Kaufman, D. L., Clare-Salzler, M., Tian, J., *et al.* (1993). Spontaneous loss of T-cell tolerance to glutamic acid decarboxylase in murine insulin-dependent diabetes. *Nature* **366**(6450), 69–72.

Kaupmann, K., Huggel, K., Heid, J., *et al.* (1997). Expression cloning of GABA (B) receptors uncovers similarity to metabotropic glutamate receptors. *Nature* **386**(6622), 239–246.

Kaupmann, K., Malitschek, B., Schuler, V., *et al.* (1998). GABA (B)-receptor subtypes assemble into functional heteromeric complexes. *Nature* **396**(6712), 683–687.

Liu, Q. R., Lopez-Corcuera, B., Mandiyan, S., *et al.* (1993). Molecular characterization of four pharmacologically distinct gamma-aminobutyric acid transporters in mouse brain. *J. Biol. Chem.* **268**(3), 2106–2112.

Martin, D. L. (1986). Chapter 10. In *Neuromethods Series I: Neurotransmitter Enzymes* (A. A. Boulton, G. B. Baker, and P. H. Yu, Eds.). Humana Press, Clifton, NJ.

McIntire, S. L., Reimer, R. J., Schuske, K., *et al.* (1997). Identification and characterization of the vesicular GABA transporter. *Nature* **389**(6653), 870–876.

Mohler, H., Fritschy, J. M., Luscher, B., *et al.* (1996). The $GABA_A$ receptors. From subunits to diverse functions. *Ion Channels* **4**, 89–113.

Mohler, H., Benke, D., and Fritschy, J. M. (2001). GABA (B)-receptor isoforms molecular architecture and distribution. *Life Sci.* **68**(19–20), 2297–2300.

Olsen, R. W., DeLorey, T. M., Gordey, M., and Kang, M. H. (1999). GABA receptor function and epilepsy. *Adv. Neurol.* **79**, 499–510.

Smith, G. B., and Olsen, R. W. (1995). Functional domains of $GABA_A$ receptors. *TIPS* **16**(5), 162–168.

Soghomonian, J.-J., and Martin, D. L. (1998). Two isoforms of glutamate decarboxylase: Why? *TIPS* **19**, 505.

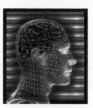

Glial Cell Types

CONRAD A. MESSAM, JEAN HOU, NAZILA JANABI, MARIA CHIARA MONACO,
MANETH GRAVELL, and EUGENE O. MAJOR

National Institute of Neurological Disorders and Stroke

I. Introduction

II. Astrocytes

III. Oligodendrocytes

IV. Microglial Cells

V. Ependymoglia Cells

VI. Conclusions

GLOSSARY

astrocyte The most abundant neuroglial cell type in the brain; named for its characteristic star-like shape due to processes extending radially from the cell body.

ependymoglial cells Glial cells that extend processes to the ventricular lumen in the brain and establish contact with the apical surface of neural tissue.

glial fibrillary acidic protein Type III intermediate filament protein used as a marker to identify mature cerebral astrocytes.

glial limitans Continuous layer at the surface of the cortex and cerebellum formed by the endfeet of radial glial cells.

gliosis Also called reactive astrocytosis; astrocytic response to injury or insult, marked histologically by the accumulation of glial fibers composed of glial fibrillary acidic protein.

microglia Resident macrophage of the brain; primary immune effector cell of the brain.

multipotential stem cells Cells derived from the neuroepithelium of the developing central nervous system that can give rise to different cell types.

myelin Specialized tissue high in lipid content that insulates the axons of neurons; produced in the brain by oligodendrocytes.

neuroglia The cells of the brain, excluding neurons; basic subtypes include astrocytes, oligodendrocytes, microglial, and ependymoglial cells.

oligodendrocyte Neuroglial cell type responsible for the production of myelin.

There are four major types of glial cells in the human brain—astrocytes, oligodendrocytes, microglia, and ependymal cells. This article will review the morphology and normal physiology of the various glial subtypes as well as their involvement in human brain disorders. Although glial cells comprise greater than 50% of the total population in the brain, historically they have been thought of solely as support cells for neurons. However, it has become apparent that the various glial cells perform critical functions during the development and normal functioning of the brain. Additionally, glial cells are central participants in almost all CNS disorders, taking part in both the protection or damage of brain tissue.

I. INTRODUCTION

More than a century and a half ago, Virchow (1846) introduced the word "neuroglia" to describe the tissue that fills the space between the nerve elements in the brain. Although simplistic when compared to our current concepts of neuroglia, the initial definition was correct. Almost four decades passed before the pioneering staining techniques developed by Golgi (1885) paved the way for others in the early 1900s to describe the morphology of the basic cell types that make up the neuroglia: astrocytes, oligodendrocytes, microglia, and ependymal cells.

With regard to establishing functions for neuroglia, His (1889) suggested that embryonic glial cells were responsible for guiding the migration of developing neurons to their final destination within the brain. In 1907, Lugaro proposed that adult astrocytes police the interstitial milieu and maintain it in a state compatible for neuronal function. He also postulated that astrocytes were the cells responsible for the chemical degradation and uptake of substances released by neurons, which allowed communication and excitation, thus establishing the basis for synaptic transmission of nerve impulses. The concept that glial cells and their processes insulate nerve fibers to enhance neural impulse transmission was proposed in 1909 by Ramón y Cajal. He further postulated that glial cells fill the spatial void created by pathologic neuronal death, setting the precedent for gliosis.

In the 1920s, del Rio Hortega, by use of an innovative and selective silver impregnation technique, was the first to give a detailed morphological description of oligodendrocytes. He also identified oligodendrocytes as the cells that produce the myelin sheath that enwraps the axons of central nervous system neurons. In 1932, by use of the same silver impregnation technique, Rio Hortega also gave the first morphological description of microglia. Unlike astrocytes and oligodendrocytes, microglia have markers normally associated with hematopoietic monocytes. The origin, lineage, and mode of differentiation of microglia are incompletely understood.

Beginning in the 1950s, electron microscopy yielded information about the ultrastructural characterization of the various organelles in glial cells. From these studies came the finding that fibrous and protoplasmic astrocytes contain gliofilaments, which were subsequently determined to be intermediate filaments containing glial fibrillary acidic protein (GFAP) and vimentin. Although not all astrocytes in the normal brain immunochemically stain positive for GFAP, especially those in the gray matter, GFAP immunoreactivity is a major characteristic used to identify astrocytes.

Later in the 20th century, the focus of neuroglial study shifted toward the understanding of various interactive processes that occur between different glial cell types and neurons. These interactions are required to establish, maintain, and regulate normal brain functions and to determine how they may contribute to pathology. In synaptic and nonsynaptic transmission of nerve impulses, neurons and glia were shown to communicate reciprocally. In nonsynaptic regions of the brain, neuron to glia and glia to glia signals were shown to be mediated by neurotransmitters. Prominent among other molecules that are involved in interactive signaling between glia and other cell types of the brain are growth factors, neurotrophic factors, hematopoietic factors, cytokines, and chemokines. In

the following sections, the morphology and functions of the subtypes of cells, which make up the "neuroglia," are described along with cellular activities associated with pathology or specific diseases.

II. ASTROCYTES

Astrocytes are generally divided into three subtypes, classified by morphology and anatomic location in the brain: radial, fibrous, and protoplasmic. All astrocytes express varying levels of GFAP, an intermediate filament that bundles together to form gliofilaments. The gliofilaments, 8–12 nm in diameter, are found mainly in the processes and less in the perinuclear region. Astrocytes can be visualized by Golgi impregnation; intracellular dye injection, which allows viewing of the entire cell body and processes; or immunocytochemical staining. Astrocytes are interconnected by gap junctions, which allow intercellular passage of ions and small molecules. The resulting cytoplasmic continuity suggests that astrocytes form a functional syncytium. Gap junctions are also observed between astrocytes and oligodendrocytes but not between astrocytes and neurons. Other characteristic features include the dense granules of glycogen in the cytoplasm and intramembrane "assemblies," observed by freeze fracture electron microscopy. These assemblies consist of 7-nm subunits bundled to form an array in the cell membrane, the function of which is not known. The endfeet of astrocyte processes terminate on the subpial glial limitans, blood vessels, nodes of Ranvier, and axons. Astrocytes are the most abundant cell type in the brain, comprising approximately 55% of the total population, and function in the maintenance of interstitial homeostasis and modulation of synaptic function. Astrocytes respond to almost any central nervous system (CNS) insult by activation and gliosis, which can limit edema, isolate damaged areas, and initiate an immune response.

A. Morphology and Subtypes

1. Radial Astrocytes

Radial astrocytes extend a single or group of long, thick, longitudinal processes that extend from the ventricle toward the surface of the brain. Radial astrocyte processes span the entire white matter and abut on the pia mater, the outermost surface of the brain. Because of their location in the ventricle and bipolar morphology, some of these cells are sometimes considered ependymal cells. There are three major subtypes of radial astrocytes. First, *Radial glial cells* are primarily observed during development. They extend processes from the ventricle throughout the neural tissue. The main function of these cells is to act as "cables" on which CNS progenitor cells can migrate to their final destination. Radial glial cells are transient since they are scarce in the adult brain. It is thought that some of these cells can later become other astrocyte subtypes. Second, *Bergman glial cells*, also called Golgi epithelial cells, are the radial astrocytes of the cerebellum. The cell bodies are located between the Purkinje neurons and send processes radially through the molecular layer of the cerebellar cortex. Endfeet of Bergman glia processes terminate at the surface of the cerebellum and form a continuous layer known as the glial limitans. Figure 1 demonstrates the immunohistochemical staining for GFAP on human fetal brain. Third, *tanycytes* are radial astrocytes found mainly in adult brain, the nuclei of which are located within or just below the ependymal, or innermost, lining of the ventricle. These cells extend processes radially through the white matter.

2. Fibrous Astrocytes

Fibrous astrocytes are located in the white matter of the brain, characterized by long, unbranched processes that radiate in all directions from the cell body but rarely reach the pia mater. Fibrous astrocytes can be found in the cortex and cerebellum, and they express high levels of GFAP in their processes. The endfeet of these processes terminate on blood vessels and synapses as well as on the cell bodies and processes of neurons.

3. Protoplasmic Astrocytes

Protoplasmic astrocytes are mainly found in the gray matter of the brain. These astrocytes possess numerous short, thin, ramified processes that radiate in all directions from the cell body. These processes express little GFAP and are better observed by Golgi

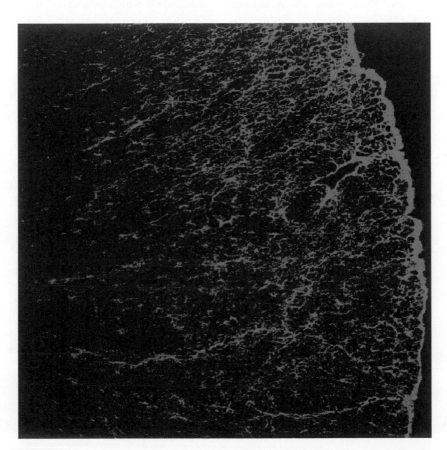

Figure 1 Immunohistochemical staining of adult human brain sections for GFAP. Note the radial morphology of the astrocyte tracts toward the outer surface of the brain. The area of intense GFAP staining at the periphery of the section is the glia limitans.

impregnation or dye injection. The endfeet terminate on blood vessels, synapses, and neuronal cell bodies, and the processes form the subpial glia limitans.

4. Astrocytes *in Vitro*

Astrocytes have varying morphologies in culture that may not fully reflect the range of morphologies found in the brain. *In vitro*, astrocytes can be separated from other neural cell types, thereby generating 95–99% astrocyte-enriched cultures. Figure 2 represents the immunofluorescent staining of cultured human astrocytes. In culture, most astrocytes derived from fetal brain appear fibroblast-like and immunostain with GFAP. These *in vitro* cultures maintain most of the functional properties of astrocytes *in vivo*. Cultured astrocytes are sometimes divided into two subtypes, type 1 and type 2, based on phenotypic characteristics as identified in rodent tissue cultures. Type 1 astrocytes stain with GFAP, whereas type 2 astrocytes costain for GFAP and A2B5, a sialoganglioside. The majority of astrocytes in culture are type 1. The type 2 astrocytes found in culture have not been observed in human brain tissue *in vivo* and may be an artifactual property of culturing.

B. Lineage and Development

Most of the information on development and lineage has been obtained from rodent brain developmental studies, with some confirmation using human fetal brain tissue. Astrocytes are derived from the neuroectodermal tissue of the neural crest. In the brain, the ventricular zone consists of a column of cells lining the ventricle that possesses the highly proliferative multipotential CNS stem cells. These stem cells give rise to progenitor cells of glial and neuronal lineage. Astrocytes are thought to originate from cells in the ventricular zone that migrate to the subventricular zone before traveling to the final destination in the brain. The process by which astrocytic progenitor cells migrate to specific brain regions is poorly understood. Radial glial cells, however, are recognized as the first glial subtype to appear in the brain. They express GFAP and nestin, an intermediate filament characteristic of immature cells. Radial and Bergman glia extend processes from the subventricular zone to the meninges at the outer surface of the brain and serve as the scaffold on which precursor cells migrate to their final location. The production and release of adhesion molecules and chemokines by astrocytes is also

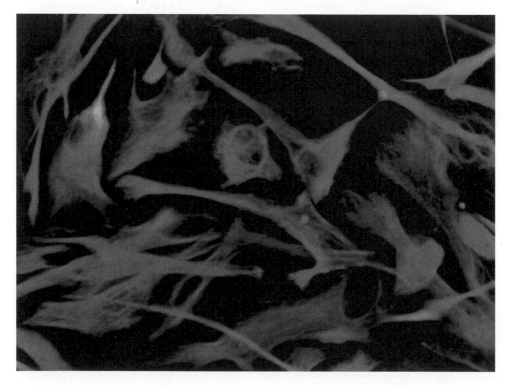

Figure 2 Immunofluorescent staining for GFAP in cultured human astrocytes. Note the filamentous ultrastructure of the cytoplasm. Magnification, × 200.

thought to contribute to the migratory process of progenitor cells during brain development. Additionally, astrocytes are known to produce a variety of trophic factors that assist in the maturation of other neural cells. Studies in rodent brain suggest that radial glia give rise to some astrocytes found in the gray and white matter. Little is known about the lineage progression of astrocyte progenitors and the factors responsible for directing the differentiation of the various astrocyte cell subtypes.

C. Normal Physiology and Function

1. Structural Functions

Astrocytes have several structural functions. They are necessary in conjunction with endothelial cells for the formation of the blood–brain barrier, an anatomic and metabolic barrier at the level of the capillary endothelial cells. The endfeet of astrocytes help to maintain a continuous layer between brain tissue and blood vessels, forming the perivascular glial membrane. The blood–brain barrier is the major obstacle preventing foreign compounds and toxins in the bloodstream from entering and damaging the brain. In effect, this barrier functionally and structurally sequesters the brain from the rest of the body. This protective barrier, however, also hinders the administration of drugs or other therapeutic compounds into the parenchyma of the brain. Another structural function of astrocytes is the formation of the glia limitans, a continuous lining of astrocyte processes, covered by a basal lamina, which is formed between the brain and the meninges. Again, the formation of the glia limitans by astrocytes helps to form the barrier to isolate the brain from other extraneural tissues. With their great abundance, astrocytes and their processes fill the extracellular space of the brain and insulate the various cell types from each other. This also occurs in brain injury, in which astrocytes hypertrophy and increase the size and number of processes at the site of injury to replace degenerated cells. The astrocytic response to CNS injury, termed gliosis, forms a scar that mechanically stabilizes the area of neuronal cell loss.

2. Maintaining Extracellular Homeostasis

Astrocytes contribute to the homeostasis of the extracellular fluid of the brain by helping to regulate pH and the extracellular concentration of K^+. There are several electrical properties characteristic of astrocytes that aid in maintaining K^+ homeostasis: electrical inexcitablity, higher membrane potential than neurons, precision in sensing and maintaining interstitial K^+ levels, and electrical linkage with neighboring astrocytes by gap junctions. The Na^+/K^+ pumps are highly concentrated on the endfeet of astrocyte processes in the vicinity of neurons. The pumps take up excess K^+ after neuronal depolarization, which can then be redistributed to more distal locations via gap junctions. The regulation of interstitial K^+ may limit excitation and be involved in fluid regulation. It is also hypothesized that astrocytes contribute to interstitial pH homeostasis. The Na^+/H^+ exchanger and the Cl^-/HCO_3^- exchangers regulate intracellular pH and may help to regulate extracellular pH as well. Astrocytes may also maintain homeostasis of the extracellular fluid by actively transporting material through the quasisyncytial network from capillary to brain tissue and vice versa.

3. Support and Interaction with Other Neural Cells

Astrocytes serve some essential functions for glutamatergic neurons and the glutamate synapse. The glutamate synapses involve the coordination between the presynaptic terminal of the axons, postsynaptic membrane, and surrounding astrocytes. The processes of astrocytes located around synapses possess high-affinity glutamate and GABA transporters that remove excess released neurotransmitters in order to limit neuronal excitation. Additionally, glutamate synthetase, found only in astrocytes, catalyzes the conversion of glutamate to glutamine, thereby providing neighboring neurons with the substrate for the production of glutamate. Therefore, glutamate synthetase also functions to detoxify neurotoxic levels of glutamate as well as ammonia. Glutamate dehydrogenase, another enzyme found in astrocytes, catalyzes the formation of glutamate from α-ketoglutarate and ammonia. Therefore, astrocytes are able to directly produce glutamate. Astrocytes may also modulate neuronal electrical activity through multiple interactions with neuronal cell bodies and nodes of Ranvier.

Astrocytes perform several functions that can modulate activity, survival, and development of other neural cells. During CNS development, radial glial cells form the highways from the subventricular zone to the parenchyma of the brain, on which the progenitor cells migrate to their final destination. The glycogen stores in radial glia are thought to provide energy for the migrating progenitor cells.

Additionally, astrocytes produce a variety of neuro-trophic factors, cytokines, and adhesion molecules that can contribute to neuronal maturation and survival in the normal brain. Table I provides a partial secretory profile of astrocytes during normal function and gliosis. In response to injury, astrocytes can release protective neurotrophic factors to promote neuronal survival or, in other cases, release factors that may exacerbate damage and contribute to neuronal death. Also, the termination of astrocytic endfeet upon the blood vessels facilitates the transport of nutrients from systemic circulation through gap junctions, thereby redistributing the nutrients to neural tissue.

Although there are several studies examining the cellular and biochemical properties of astrocytes,

Table I
Growth Factors, Cytokines, Chemokines, and Adhesion Molecules Produced by Astrocytes

Factor	Full name	Normal or gliosis[a]
FGF-1 (aFGF)	Acidic fibroblast growth factor	N
FGF-2 (bFGF)	Basic fibroblast growth factor	N
PDGF	Platelet-derived growth factor	N
NGF	Nerve growth factor	N
CNTF	Ciliary neurotrophic factor	N
TGF-α	Transforming growth factor-alpha	N
IGF-1	Insulin-like growth factor	N
GMF	Glia maturation factor	N
TNF-α	Tumor necrosis factor-alpha	R
LIF	Leukemia inhibitory factor	R
TGF-β	Transforming growth factor-beta	N/R
IL-1B	Interleukin-1 beta	N/R
IL-3	Interleukin-3	N/R
IL-6	Interleukin-6	N/R
G-CSF	Granulocyte colony-stimulating factor	N/R
M-CSF	Macrophage colony-stimulating factor	N/R
GM-CSF	Granulocyte and macrophage colony-stimulating factor	N/R
IP-10	Gamma-interferon inducible protein	N/R
MCP-1	Macrophage chemoattractant protein	N/R
IL-8	Interleukin-8	N/R
ICAM-1	Intracellular cell adhesion molecule-1	N/R
VCAM-1	Vascular cell adhesion molecule-1	N/R

[a]Abbreviations used: N, released by normal astrocytes; R, released by reactive astrocytes; N/R, released by both normal and reactive astrocytes.

relatively little is known about the molecular factors involved in astrocyte differentiation and normal function. Elucidating the molecular characteristics of astrocytes will be an area of active and intensive research for the future.

D. Contribution to Disease

1. Edema

Edema is one of the most common responses to brain injury resulting from astrocytic swelling. There are two types of edemas. The first is cerebral edema, which occurs after a disruption of the tight endothelial junctions of the brain vasculature. This causes fluid influx in the brain parenchyma, resulting in increased intracranial pressure. The second type of edema is cellular edema, which is astrocytic swelling after injury that may not result in a net influx of fluid into the interstitial space. Both types of edema may impair transporter function and the ability of astrocytes to maintain K^+ homeostasis. Acute abnormalities that cause edema include hemorrhage, trauma, and brain infarct. Subacute and chronic conditions such as status epilepticus, malignancy, Reye's syndrome, and encephalitis can also cause edema.

2. Gliosis

Gliosis, also called astrocytic gliosis or astrocytosis, is a common term that refers to the reactive astrocytic response to a brain injury or insult. Almost all brain lesions have a component of gliosis, even with different glial pathologies. Gliosis is a secondary event to CNS damage and may persist for weeks or months after brain injury. This condition occurs after infarct and is associated with infections and neoplasm as well as with demyelinating, toxic, and metabolic diseases. In gliosis, astrocytes hypertrophy, the nuclei become enlarged, and the chromatin becomes less dense while nucleoli become more prominent. There is an increased number of organelles and higher production of the intermediate filaments GFAP, nestin, and vimentin, which results in greater and more highly condensed glial processes and fibers. The increased glial processes replace injured CNS cells and form a gliotic scar. It is thought that the glial scar limits edema and prevents neuronal regeneration in the CNS by blocking regenerating axons from entering the damaged areas. With gliosis there is the release of cytokines, growth factors, and extracellular matrix proteins, which may be involved in immune response, neuroprotection, or possible further damage. The term "reactive gliosis" normally refers to massive hypertrophy of astrocytes; however, it is apparent that gliosis is inherently reactive.

3. Neoplasm

Astrocytomas are neoplastic cells largely derived from astrocytes. They are classified into four categories based on the level of malignancy, with grade I being the least malignant and grade IV being the most malignant. All astrocytomas express some level of GFAP, but less malignant tumors generally express higher levels. The more malignant tumors express higher levels of nestin than GFAP. *Grade I astrocytomas*, called pilocytic astrocytomas, are gray, firm, and often cystic, with tumor cells that have long, hair-like cellular processes. These tumors most often occur in children or young adults. The boundaries are clearly distinguishable from normal brain, and when amenable to surgical removal the prognosis is good with little chance of recurrence. *Grade II astrocytomas* are the low-grade astrocytomas, which occur most often in young adults. They are solid, gray homogeneous tumors, characterized by astrocytes with pleomorphic nuclei and dark, condensed chromatin. These tumors diffusely infiltrate the brain parenchyma, which allows only partial surgical removal. There is variable prognosis with these tumors, with average survival of 3–5 years. *Grade III astrocytomas*, called anaplastic astrocytomas, resemble grade II astrocytomas but have more pleomorphic nuclei and high mitotic activity. Even with surgical removal and radiation therapy, the prognosis is still variable, with average survival of 1–3 years. *Grade IV astrocytomas* are known as glioblastoma multiforme and are the most malignant and frequent brain tumors in adults. These tumors have exaggerated features of grade III tumors with additional coagulation necrosis, vascular proliferation, and occasional hemorrhage. These tumor cells have a very high mitotic rate and the poorest prognosis for survival (less than 1 year after diagnosis).

4. Astrocytes

a. Immune Involvement Astrocytes are immunocompetent cells that participate in local immunological reactions. At the site of CNS damage, these cells can phagocytose dead cells and act as an antigen presenting cell in the initial phase of the immune response.

Activated astrocytes express MHC II, which is involved in antigen presentation. Activation after CNS damage or pathogen infection results in the production of a variety of cytokines, interleukins, adhesion molecules, and chemokines. These released factors facilitate recruitment and activation of leukocytes and microglial cells to the area of insult and may contribute to disease development.

b. Involvement in Viral and Other Infectious Agents A variety of neurotropic viruses that cause neuropathogenesis in the human brain also infect astrocytes. Although in many cases infected astrocytes are not a primary target resulting in neuropathy, they contribute to viral latency and amplification of pathology through the release of cytokines. A good example is human immunodeficiency virus (HIV), the virus that causes acquired immunodeficiency syndrome (AIDS). HIV enters the brain and infects microglia and astrocytes, although astrocytic infection is nonproductive. It is hypothesized that astrocytes are a latent reservoir for HIV, complicating the task of complete virus eradication. Astroctyes, in conjunction with microglial cells, contribute to AIDS neuropathy by releasing cytotoxic factors that can amplify the immune response and further contribute to neuronal toxicity.

III. OLIGODENDROCYTES

Oligodendrocytes have a very clear functional definition. They are the cells in the CNS responsible for the production and maintenance of myelin, the insulating layer that surrounds the axons of neighboring neurons. As such, they are considered the most metabolically active cells in the brain. Due to an inherent resistance to early staining techniques, oligodendrocytes were the last cell type of the CNS to be discovered and characterized. Oligodendrocytes develop from the neuroepithelial cells of the neural tube in defined temporal and spatial patterns. In the gray matter of the adult human brain, oligodendrocytes are called satellite cells and function mainly in fluid and respiratory exchange, whereas oligodendrocytes found in the white matter are involved in the synthesis of myelin sheaths. In contrast to the functional diversity among astrocytes, oligodendrocytes appear to be a fairly homogenous population, with a unified purpose of myelinating axons. Structurally, however, oligodendrocytes exhibit a wide polymorphism, and classifying different variants has proven to be a difficult task.

A. Morphology and Subtypes

As a whole, oligodendrocytes are very refractive to stains. *In vivo*, the structure of the oligodendrocyte cell body is shrouded to some extent by the vast networks of myelin it produces as well as by its close association with neighboring axons. In fact, a cell may be identified as an oligodendrocyte based on its continuity with the outermost layer of the myelin sheath. The cells are morphologically diverse and can be classified into four subtypes. Type 1 oligodendrocytes have spherical or slightly polygonal cell bodies. They have several thin processes that emerge from the cell body in the direction of nerve fibers. This subtype can be found in the forebrain, cerebellum, and spinal cord, and these oligodendrocytes are usually arranged around blood vessels, neurons, and fiber tracts. Type 2 oligodendrocytes are polygonal or cuboid in shape, with fewer and thicker processes than those of the Type 1 subgroup. These cells are only found in the white matter and are closely associated with nerve fibers. Type 3 oligodendrocytes have even fewer processes directed toward nerve fibers and are found in the cerebral and cerebellar peduncles, medulla oblongata, and the spinal cord. Finally, type 4 oligodendrocytes are found near the entrance of nerve roots into the CNS and in association with large axons. These categories are arbitrary in nature because oligodendrocytes rarely fit perfectly into any one subgroup. Oligodendroglial cells may also be classified as interfascicular, perivascular, or perineuronal satellite cells, depending on their location.

Although the gross structure of oligodendrocytes varies widely, little difference in the fine structure has been observed in the CNS. The oligodendroglial cell body and the associated myelin membrane are enriched with sphyngoglycolipids such as galactosylceramide and its sulfated form, sulfatide. Immunocytochemical staining of the cell body *in vivo* may prove difficult because the vast network of myelin results in poor antibody penetration. Furthermore, the cell surface marker repertoire changes with different stages of differentiation. However, *in vitro*, isolated oligodendrocytes can be visualized by immunofluorescent staining, as shown in Fig. 3. Similarly, intracellular injection of dyes has revealed much about the ultrastructure of oligodendrocytes. The cytoplasm of the cells has well-developed Golgi apparati and abundant ribosomes, both free and bound to an extensive endoplasmic reticulum. This is to be expected since high-scale myelin protein synthesis and transport are the two main functions of this cell type. The greater density of the cytoplasm and nucleus, as well as the absence of glycogen granules or bundles of specific intermediate filaments, can distinguish oligodendrocytes from astrocytes. Oligodendrocytes do not contain intermediate filaments in the cytoplasm but, rather, actin microfilaments and a high content of microtubules, particularly in the processes. By electron microscopy, oligodendrocytes can be further subdivided into light, medium, and dark, distinguishable by decreasing size and increasing cytoplasmic density. It has been proposed that these structural differences are correlated to functional differences as well. For example, the light oligodendrocytes appear to be highly involved in the production of myelin, whereas the dark oligodendrocytes may be involved with myelin maintenance.

B. Lineage and Development

Most developmental studies of oligodendroglial lineage and development have been conducted in rodent models due to difficulty in culturing human oligodendrocytes. The maturation of oligodendrocyte precursors into mature oligodendrocytes is characterized by a distinct temporal expression of cell surface receptors and response to different growth factors. In mammals, oligodendrocytes originate from multipotential neural stem cells derived from the neuroepithelium of the developing CNS. In the adult brain, mature

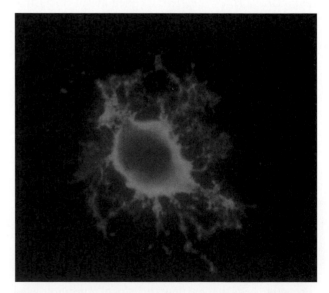

Figure 3   Immunofluorescent staining of a mammalian oligodendrocyte. Stained for Gal-C, a galactocerebroside expressed during the final stages of oligodendroglial development. Note the highly branched processes and intense staining of the cell membrane.

oligodendrocytes are distributed throughout the white and gray matter. In the developing CNS, however, induction of oligodendroglial precursors occurs in spatially restricted areas. Chemical factors released into localized areas of the extracellular environment can initiate changes in morphology and expression of growth factor receptor mRNA. In rodent studies, it is thought that the precursors are initially restricted to the ventral ventricular zone of the developing neural tube. The notochord and surrounding floor plate may release factors such as sonic hedgehog, which results in migration of the precursors dorsally and radially to populate the white matter. Furthermore, oligodendrocyte precursors located in the developing midbrain and forebrain may migrate into the thalamus and hypothalamus later in development, as well as to more dorsal regions of the cerebral cortex.

Induction of the oligodendrocyte progenitors from neuroepithelial stem cells in discrete locations must be followed by an active and large-scale migration throughout the CNS in order to myelinate all the white matter tracts. The cellular terrains or soluble factors utilized during this long-distance migration are unknown. The traveling precursors may interact with radial glial cells or may even utilize axons to guide them to their final destination. The oligodendrocyte precursors do possess a variety of integrin receptors, which may play important roles in migration and differentiation over various extracellular matrix components.

Extensive proliferation occurs in the white matter, and the expansion of the oligodendrocyte population is most likely regulated by a variety of growth factors. Once sufficient progenitor populations have been achieved, proliferation is downregulated and shifted toward differentiation. Again, maturation of the oligodendrocytes is highly influenced by growth factors and hormones. As the precursors mature, they will lose their motility and various cell surface receptors. Table II summarizes the proposed stages of oligodendroglial development and progressive changes in cell surface markers, morphology, and motility. Terminal differentiation of oligodendrocyte precursors and initiation of myelination requires dramatic and highly coordinated changes in the pattern of gene expression. The molecular mechanism by which oligodendrocyte-specific gene expression is regulated is most likely due to the combined action of multiple transcription factors. These include members of the homeodomain proteins in undifferentiated oligodendrocytes and zinc finger proteins in mature oligodendrocytes. Oligodendroglial survival factors secreted at the final destination induce the synthesis of myelin-specific mRNA, such as myelin basic protein (MBP) and proteolipid protein (PLP). MBP is actually a family of seven protein isoforms produced from a single gene by alternative splicing. Little is known about the precise structure of MBP in its native environment, although it is believed that the proteins are self-associating and may exist in an oligomeric form at the cell membrane.

Table II
Oligodendroglial Development[a]

Stage	Specific cell surface marker	Morphology	Motility
Preoligodendroglia, oligodendrocyte precursor (OP)	PDGFRα, O4 immunoreactivity		Highly motile
Immature oligodendrocyte	O1 immunoreactivity		Less motile
Mature oligodendroctye	CNP, PLP, MBP, MOG		None

[a]Abbreviations used: PDGFRα, platelet-derived growth factor receptor alpha; O4, antibody that recognizes cell surface constituents specific for oligodendrocyte precursors; O1, antibody against galactosylcerebroside; CNP, 2′,3′-cyclic nucleotide 3′-phosphotidase; PLP, proteolipid protein; MBP, myelin basic protein; MOG, myelin oligodendrocyte glycoprotein.

PLP is the most abundant protein in CNS myelin and also has alternative splice variants. With several transmembrane domains, functional studies have implicated a role of PLP as an ion channel.

C. Normal Physiology and Function

In the CNS, oligodendrocytes are responsible for the synthesis and maintenance of the myelin that surrounds the axons of neighboring neurons. The purpose of the myelin sheath is to allow saltatory propagation of nerve impulses along the length of the axon, resulting in a faster and more efficient neural impulse than in uninsulated nerve fibers. The exact cellular mechanisms responsible for the process of myelination are unclear. In humans, oligodendrocytes emerge several days or weeks before they actually start to synthesize myelin, and myelination takes place principally within the first year after birth. Recent studies have shown that initiation of myelination may be partially dependent on the activity of protein kinase C (PKC), a family of phospholipid-dependent enzymes ubiquitously present in the CNS. Not only do myelin-associated proteins appear to be excellent substrates for PKC-mediated phosphorylation but PKC activity also increases gradually after birth, coinciding with the temporal pattern of myelination in the human brain. Indeed, in cultures of human adult brain-derived oligodendrocytes, treatment with PKC agonists resulted in the increased synthesis of MBP as well as causing process extension, which are both myelogenic events.

Chemical or structural signals from neighboring axons are most likely the initiators of myelination by oligodendrocytes. An oligodendrocyte process extends from the soma and engulfs a segment of the axon, forming an inner and outer layer. As the cytoplasm is eliminated from the layers, the myelin condenses into compact myelin. The process will continue to encircle the axon, forming layers known as lamellae that abut one another and form a continuous spiral. Cross-linking of MBP oligomers on adjacent layers believed to condense the processes into thin, apposing sheets. Interestingly, the chemical composition of compact myelin is different from the chemical composition of the originating oligodendroglial cell membrane. Myelin has a much higher lipid content than the membrane of the cell body, despite the fact that compact myelin is continuous with the oligodendrocyte cell membrane. This is not surprising, however, since the insulating value of myelin is conferred in large part by its high

percentage of lipid constituents. The myelin sheath as a whole is discontinuous because each oligodendrocyte process furnishes the myelin for only one segment of the axon, leaving small areas of exposed axonal membrane called the nodes of Ranvier. The action potentials skip over the myelinated areas and are repropagated only at the nodes, greatly increasing the velocity at which impulses travel. Each oligodendrocyte is capable of myelinating up to 50 internodes at a significant distance. In fact, during periods of active myelogenesis, an oligodendrocyte is capable of producing up to three times its own weight in myelin a day.

Other than the obvious role in the CNS, oligodendrocytes have also been shown to be neurite inhibitors. They prevent abnormal axonal sprouting outside the already established nerve tracts, and they also lend structural integrity to the CNS. However, oligodendrocytes that prohibit axon growth can actually enhance axonal regeneration in instances of neural tissue damage, further contributing to the complexity in function and intercellular relationships of these cells. Satellite oligodendrocytes located in the gray matter may function in regulating ion concentrations and pH levels in the extracellular space by fluid and ion exchange. Further studies must be conducted on mechanisms responsible for the oligodendroglial ability to successfully remyelinate demyelinated regions resulting from traumatic injury or disease. Once elucidated, these cells may be critical for therapeutic purposes in treating demyelinating diseases of the CNS.

D. Contribution to Disease

Damage to oligodendrocytes can occur in a variety of ways, including microbial infections, injury, autoimmunity, genetic defects, inflammation, and exposure to toxins. Although great strides have been made in understanding the core features of many of these demyelinating actions, the molecular events leading to damage of oligodendrocytes and, in many cases, dysmyelation or demyelination are not totally understood.

1. Multiple Sclerosis

Multiple sclerosis (MS) is a major demyelinating disease with pathological features similar to those of the experimental animal model, experimental allergic encephalomyelitis (EAE). Blood vessels in the CNS of MS patients characteristically have inflamed perivascular cuffs containing T lymphocytes and monocytes recruited from peripheral circulation. Although much studied, the cause of oligodendrocyte death in MS is not clear. Some investigators have presented evidence that oligodendrocytes in acute and chronic demyelinated lesions undergo apoptotic death, whereas many others have found evidence of only necrotic cell death. Plaques of demyelination are present in the white matter, with chronic plaques devoid of both oligodendrocytes and myelin, as shown in Fig. 4. Reactive astrocytosis is also a prominent feature of MS lesions.

Many factors have been linked etiologically with MS. CD4$^+$ and CD8$^+$ lymphocytes have both been reported to lyse oligodendrocytes, with CD4$^+$ cells doing so by a non-MHC-restricted mechanism involving perforin release and CD8$^+$ by a MHC-restricted mechanism. Furthermore, $\gamma\delta$ T lymphocytes found in MS lesions may damage oligodendrocytes by a non-antigen-specific necrotic pathway. Activated macrophage/microglia also have the capacity to necrotically

kill oligodendrocytes. Although oligodendrocyte injury and death can be mediated by both antibody-dependent and antibody-independent complement pathways, as well as by exposure to nitric oxide, none of these factors can clearly be shown to be the sole cause of MS.

2. Human T Cell Lymphotropic Virus, Type 1

Human T cell lymphotropic virus type 1 (HTLV-1) is a retrovirus that causes human adult T cell leukemia. Frequently, however, it causes the demyelinating neurological disease tropical spastic paraparesis (TSP), so named because it was thought only to occur in tropical geographic areas of the world. However, it has been found multiracially, in many countries, and in a wide range of climates. Because TSP occurrence has also been documented in individuals residing in countries with temperate climates, the name TSP is considered a misnomer and it has been proposed that it be called HTLV-1-associated myelopathy (HAM).

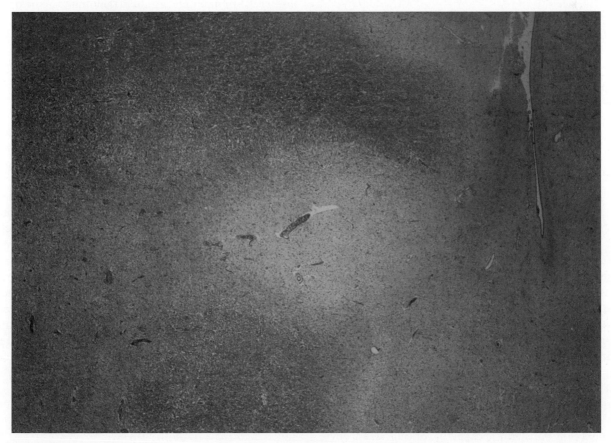

Figure 4 Demyelinated plaque occurring in the brain of a patient with multiple sclerosis. Tissue section staining with Luxol fast blue visualizes myelinated areas (dark) and regions devoid of myelin (light).

Symptoms associated with the chronic form of MS are similar to those of TSP/HAM, particularly in those patients exhibiting cerebellar signs. The occurrence of MS is rare in tropical regions, and the few patients from HLTV-l-endemic regions who were tested for HTLV-1 antibodies were negative. However, some individuals in temperate regions originally diagnosed as having MS in reality had TSP/HAM.

3. Progressive Multifocal Leukoencephalopathy

JC virus (JCV), a human polyomavirus closely related to BK virus and simian virus 40 (SV40), is the cause of the fatal demyelinating disease progressive multifocal leukoencephalopathy (PML), the only human disease known to be caused by infection with JCV. JCV infects 80% or more of the world's population, with initial infection occurring predominantly during childhood. The target of this ubiquitous virus is the myelin-producing oligodendrocyte. The virions can be detected in the nuclei of infected oligodendrocytes in a dense, crystalline arrangement called inclusion bodies. Prior to the AIDS pandemic, PML was a relatively rare disease affecting primarily immunosuppressed cancer patients with lymphoma or leukemia and transplant recipients receiving immunosuppressive therapy. It has been estimated that PML now occurs in about 5% of HIV-1-infected AIDS patients and is a major cause of death. Treatment of PML has been elusive. Some AIDS patients with PML receiving high-intensity antiretroviral therapy, including protease inhibitors, have shown clinical improvement, probably because the drug treatment regimen improved their general immunocompetence. Other AIDS patients with PML receiving high-intensity antiviral drug therapy showed no survival benefit from the treatment.

4. Other

Altered homeostasis of the neurotransmitter glutamate has also been postulated to cause excitotoxic death of oligodendrocytes. This depends on whether glutamate homeostasis is transiently or chronically altered. For example, exposure to short ischemic periods followed by transient increases in extracelluar glutamate may produce only limited damage to oligodendrocytes that can be repaired through the differentiation of oligodendrocyte precursors. Conversely, extended disturbances in glutamate signals may result in progressive oligodendrocyte cell death that exceeds the intrinsic capacity for oligodendrocyte repair, causing permanent damage to the oligodendrocyte population.

Toxic factors and genetic defects such as those seen in the leukodystrophies and Pelizaeus Merzbacher disease can also cause dysmyelination or demyelination. Exposure to free radical donors such as super-oxide (O_2^-) or nitric oxide (NO), to free radical generating systems such as catecholamines, heat shock, and irradiation, and to agents that increase intracellular calcium concentrations, such as calcium ionophores, kainite, and myelin basic protein, has also been shown to kill oligodendrocytes.

A small percentage of all gliomas, approximately 5%, are oligodendroglial in lineage. These relatively avascular oligodendrogliomas initially form in the white matter and grow into the gray matter as they progress. The tumors can be grouped into two categories: the low-grade, less aggressive oligodendrogliomas or the more aggressive, anaplastic oligodendrogliomas. As a rule, a tumor in the low-grade category tends to be a pure oligodendroglioma, whereas the anaplastic tumors are a mixture of astrocytomas and oligodendrogliomas, also known as oligoastrocytomas. Although oligodendrogliomas are seen mainly in adults, they can also occur infrequently in children. Treatment strategies for oligodendrogliomas include surgical removal, radiation therapy, and chemotherapy.

IV. MICROGLIAL CELLS

Microglia are the resident macrophages of the brain, comprising 10–20% of all glial cells. They have active functions similar to those of other tissue macrophages, including phagocytosis, antigen presentation, and the production of cytokines, eicosanoids, complement components, excitatory amino acids (glutamate), proteases, and oxidative radicals. The antigenic plasticity of certain microglial populations, the cross-reactivity of the antibodies for microglia and other tissue macrophages, and the lack of a fully microglia-specific antibody argue for a monocytic derivation of these cells. However, a direct lineage relationship between microglia and myelomonocytic will be debated until quantitative and qualitative differences in the expression of some cell surface proteins common to both cell types and in their functions can be evidenced.

A. Morphology and Subtypes

"Brain macrophage" is a general term that comprises several subtypes of cells based on morphology, localization, surface antigen markers, and function. Perivascular microglia, with an elongate shape, are located around blood vessels in adult tissue. They are thought to be regularly replenished by peripheral monocytes that infiltrate the CNS through the hemoencephalic or blood–brain barrier. The surface antigen profile is similar to that of circulating monocytes. *In vivo*, perivascular microglia are considered the most important antigen presenting cells, given their diversified, anatomical location. Intraparenchymal microglia, or resident microglia, are more numerous in gray matter than in white matter. They are maintained as a pool with a low turnover rate in normal adult brain. Parenchymal microglia can be subdivided into two populations. The first group includes ramified or resting microglial cells, which are highly branched cells with a small amount of perinuclear cytoplasm and a small, dense, and heterochromatic nucleus. The second population consists of ameboid microglial cells, which display migratory capacity and phagocytosis. These cells are particularly present during embryonic development and after CNS injury. In fact, ramified and retracted microglial processes can become ameboid-like, forming reactive microglia during brain injury. The best defined functions of microglial cells are related to microglial activation during pathological processes and include antigen presentation, cytotoxicity, neurovascularization, and phagocytosis. Some of these functions are also important for the normal physiology of the adult brain as well as the developing brain.

B. Lineage and Development

The origin of microglial cells has been debated since the initial silver staining by del Rio-Hortega. Although most macrophages are derived from monocytes, a subset can form locally by division of preexisting macrophages or from other progenitor cells. Here two contrasting theories are discussed in support of a mesenchymal or neuroectodermal origin of microglia.

During the development of the CNS, microglial cells are found after formation of blood vessels. During the vascularization of the CNS, the penetration of the endothelial cells is followed by focal degeneration of subadjacent glial endfeet, which attract monocytes from peripheral circulation. In fact, monocytes can infiltrate the CNS and have the potential to transform into macrophagic cells, giving rise to perivascular macrophages. However, there is not enough evidence that resident mature microglia in the parenchyma are

derived from monocytes. They are believed to belong to the mononuclear phagocyte system because they express Fc and CR3 receptors and are capable of phagocytosis. Furthermore, cytoplasmic enzymes expressed by microglial cells, such as lysozyme, nonspecific esterase, and peroxidase, are also found in cells of the mononuclear phagocyte system. Microglia can be identified in human fetuses as early as 13 weeks of gestation. An important accumulation of ameboid cells is observed in the ventricular zone (germinal matrix) of human fetuses at 13–24 weeks of gestation. Human fetuses less than 28 weeks of gestation also have a significant concentration of macrophages in the ventricular zone, perivascular sites, leptomeninges, and subependymal regions. However, there is no correlation between the density of the ramified microglia and areas where there has been a high incidence of cell death. Indisputably, hematopoietic macrophages are present and play an important role in the developing CNS. Nevertheless, as the system develops, the number of dying cells decreases, as does the number of hematopoietic macrophages. The development of ramified microglia seems to be an independent process because they appear later in development, proliferate to occupy the parenchyma, and develop close functional interactions with neurons and other glial cells.

In attempts to demonstrate that microglia can be replaced by hematopoietic monocytes, the use of bone marrow radiated chimeric animals suggests that monocytes–macrophages in leptomeninges, choroid plexus, and perivascular areas are indeed replaced by cells from the bone marrow. In contrast, parenchymal ramified microglia are not replaced by bone marrow-derived marked cells in a significant number. Thus, the majority of microglial cells come from locally present precursor cells, most likely of neuroectodermal origin. The theory of a neuroectodermal origin of microglia assumes that microglia originate from a common glial stem cell, the glioblast, in the ventricular zone and later in the subventricular zone of the developing neural tube. Thus, some of the precursor cells responsible for the turnover of macroglia might be responsible for the turnover of microglia. Another possibility is that the CNS is colonized by hematopoietic stem cells very early during development, and that stem cells become resident cells of the CNS. These cells are then responsible for the regular turnover of the intraparenchymal microglia in normal brain and increased numbers of microglia in pathologic conditions. To date, searches for hematopoietic stem cells in the CNS have been unsuccessful. Attempts to develop cultures of microglia initiated from the neuroepithelium of mouse embryos prior to vascularization and the appearance of monocytes–macrophages in the yolk sac strongly suggest that at least some microglial cells can originate from the neuroepithelium of the neural tube, as do other glia.

C. Normal Physiology and Function

The morphology and branching patterns of microglial cells display heterogeneity between different brain regions. Microglia in gray matter tend to be ramified, with processes extending in all directions. Cells in the white matter are bipolar and often align their cytoplasmic extensions in parallel, at right angles to nerve fiber bundles. Thus, the morphology of microglia adapts to the architecture of the brain region they populate, whereas their phenotype appears to be influenced by the chemical composition of the microenvironment. For example, MHC class II-positive and CD4-positive microglia are localized mostly in the white matter of normal brain. Regions lacking a blood–brain barrier show microglia and microglia-like cells with a different phenotype, suggesting that serum proteins influence the phenotype.

The microglial plasma membrane contains a large number of receptor and adhesion molecules as well as a wide variety of enzymatic activities (Table III). Therefore, a large number of antibodies can be used to stain microglial cells. Microglia in the human brain can be visualized using analogous antibodies against typical macrophage surface receptors. In addition to the expression of Fc and complement receptors, other cell adhesion molecules are expressed constitutively on resting microglia in normal brain. Belonging to the integrin superfamily of adhesion molecules, these include typical lymphocytic antigens, such as lymphocyte function antigen (LFA), CD4 antigen, and leukocyte common antigen. B lymphocyte antigens are also present on human microglia. Thus, the microglial surface membrane bears molecules associated with white blood cells. It is well documented that the normal brain contains MHC antigens and that the principal MHC-expressing cell type is the microglial cell. The constitutive expression of MHC antigens in the brain is not limited to microglial cells, however; it also includes endothelial cells and certain cell types located in the wall of cerebral blood vessels. MHC antigen expression is considerably increased in pathologic conditions or after systemic administration of cytokines, such as interferon-γ (IFN-γ). The

Table III
Phenotypic Characteristics and Secretory Activity of Microglial Cells[a]

	Antigen expression			Soluble mediator production
	Resting	Activated	Cell specificity	
Fc receptors	±	+	Macrophage	M-CSF
CD68	+	+	Macrophage	G-CSF
Lectin	+	+	Macrophage	TNF-α
CR3 complement receptor	+	+	Leukocytes	IL-1
MHC class I	±	+	Leukocytes	IL-6
MHC class II	−	+	Leukocytes	IL-10
CD4	±	+	T cells, monocytes	IL-12
LCA (CD45)	−	+	Leukocytes	TGF-β
ICAM-1 (CD54)	−	+	Leukocytes	Chemokines
VCAM-1 (CD106)	−	+	Leukocytes	NGF
LFA-1 (CD11a/CD18)	−	+	Leukocytes	NT-3
LFA3 (CD58)	+	+	Leukocytes	Prostaglandins
				Superoxide anions
				Matrix metalloproteinases

[a]Abbreviations used: ICAM, intercellular adhesion molecule; IL, interleukin; G-CSF and M-CSF, macrophage and granulocyte colony-stimulating factors; LCA, leukocyte common antigen; LFA, leukocyte function-associated antigen; MHC, major histocompatibility complex; NGF, nerve growth factor; NT-3, neurotrophin-3; TNF, tumor necrosis factor; TGF, transforming growth factor; VCAM, vascular cell adhesion molecule.

intermediate filament vimentin, which is evident in activated microglia and in brain macrophages, is absent from resting microglia. However, it can be upregulated rapidly in response to neuronal injury. Lectin histochemical staining of nervous tissue revealed that the B4 isolectin derived from *Griffonia simplicifolia* and the lectin from *Ricinus communis* resulted in the selective visualization of microglia. Both lectins have similar sugar-binding characteristics and recognize anomeric forms of galactose in the oligosaccharide side chains of nervous system glycoproteins in the microglial plasma membrane.

Perhaps the most well-known biological function of microglial cells is their role during the development of the CNS. Microglial cells remove dead cell fragments and eliminate transitory or aberrant axons. They can also play a more active role during cell degeneration by inducing the death of certain cells. Microglia support the development and normal function of neurons and glia by producing trophic factors as well as by participating in the growth and guidance of neurites within the developing CNS. They also promote the proliferation of astrocytes, increase myelinogenesis, and stimulate vascularization of the CNS. Many of these microglial effects are apparently mediated by active substances. Microglial cells in culture secrete a number of factors, such as nerve growth factor, neurotrophin-3, chemokines, macrophage and granulocyte colony-stimulating factors (M-CSF and G-CSF), interleukin-1 (IL-1), IL-6 and tumor necrosis factor α (TNF-α). In addition to acting on other populations of the nervous system, tissue culture studies have revealed microglial responsiveness to growth factors such as GM-CSF and CSF-1, which are potent inducers of microglial proliferation and function.

D. Contribution to Disease

Several arguments support a key role for microglia during immunopathologies. They are potentially phagocytic and have a pronounced microbicide and cytotoxic potential. Upon activation, microglia can rapidly upregulate the expression of several immunomolecules, such as MHC I and II, the CD4 antigen, and adhesion molecules. They are the most efficient and the most promptly inducible antigen presenting cells of the brain parenchyma, assuming an active immune surveillance in the CNS. Resting microglial cells stimulated with IFN-γ express MHC II products and display a capacity to present protein antigens in the molecular context of MHC II to CD4-positive T lymphocytes. In the context of MHC I expression, they can also become targets of cytotoxic CD8-positive T lymphocytes. Furthermore, microglia secrete as well as respond to several cytokines.

One of the characteristic features of microglia is the rapid activation in response to injury, inflammation, neurodegeneration, infection, and brain tumors. Microglial activation occurs after injury or changes in microenvironment, even before pathological changes or in the absence of obvious neuropathic changes, as part of an early CNS immune defense system. In terms of structural changes, many intermediate morphologies of activated microglia exist. Microglial hypertrophy begins with the formation of several stout processes, but they do not become phagocytic. If neuronal degeneration occurs in the brain parenchyma, activated microglia proliferate and transform into phagocytic cells. As the primary immune effector cells of the CNS, microglia respond to traumatic insult or the presence of pathogens by migrating to the site of injury, where they may proliferate. Activated microglia at the site of inflammation express increased levels of MHC antigens and become phagocytic. Like other tissue macrophages, microglia release inflammatory cytokines and mediators that amplify the inflammatory response by recruiting effector cells to the site of injury. In addition, microglia can release neurotoxins that may potentiate damage to CNS cells. The intense secretory activity of these cells is associated with diseases such as trauma, stroke, epilepsy, AIDS, and MS, in which the microglial response is prominent and deleterious to the brain tissue. The secretory activity of microglia has also been related to the neuronal destruction seen in Alzheimer's disease (AD).

1. Acquired Immunodeficiency Syndrome

HIV-1 causes an AIDS-associated psychomotor complex in a number of patients, who eventually develop either encephalitis or leukoencephalopathy. The main target cells of HIV-1 infection in the brain are microglia and macrophages, with a very limited infection of astrocytes and endothelial cells. Infected microglial cells can be detected by the presence of HIV antigens. The two pathological hallmarks of the HIV-1 infection of the CNS are multinucleated giant cells as a result of cell-to-cell fusion and microglial nodules (Fig. 5). Although microglial cells and macrophages seem to be the only cell types productively infected by HIV-1 within the brain, the replication rate of the virus remains relatively low in CNS tissue compared to other tissues. Thus, the neuropathological alterations in AIDS are more likely due to the neurotoxicity of certain viral products, toxic factors, and cytokines released by infected microglia and macrophages. Some of these putative toxic factors, such as viral proteins, are specific to HIV-1 infection of the CNS, whereas other potentially toxic factors are also involved in other diseases in which activation of microglia plays a key role in the pathological process. Among viral proteins, the viral surface glycoprotein gp120 can be released by infected microglia and macrophages. This protein induces excitoxicity in neurons via activation of glutamate receptors, it can inhibit myelin formation in oligodendrocytes, or it can alter Na^+/H^+ ion transport in astrocytes, leading to an increased secretion of glutamate and potassium. The infection of microglial cells and macrophages, and their subsequent activation, also results in the generation of a wide variety of secretory factors that are potentially neurotoxic, such as TNF-α, cytokines, chemokines, arachidonic acid metabolites, and nitric oxide. TNF-α released by infected microglia is particularly toxic to oligodendrocytes and can be an important factor in myelin damage. Arachidonic acid and its metabolites act mainly via potentiation of glutamate receptors on neurons, leading to an increase in intracellular calcium levels and neuronal death. They can also impair the transport of glutamate in astrocytes.

2. Multiple Sclerosis

Pathological studies of MS lesions suggest an important role of macrophages and microglia in MS demyelination. Active or recent plaques have areas of myelin degradation, infiltration by inflammatory cells, and collections of lipid-containing macrophages that may stain for myelin proteins such as myelin basic protein. In chronic plaques, macrophage-like cells remain lipid-laden but no longer express immunoreactive myelin proteins. Some of these macrophages represent phagocytic microglia and some may be of hematogenous origin. MS lesions are frequently localized in perivascular regions and contain not only demyelinated axons and microglia but also lymphocytes and plasma cells. The presence of MHC II molecules in macrophages and microglia in MS lesions indicates that microglia are activated and can exert phagocytosis and antigen presentation functions. They also express Fc receptors and have an increased number of chemotactic receptors, including C5a and IL8.

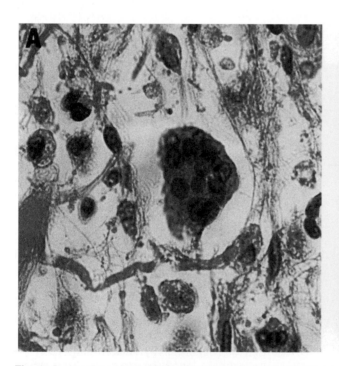
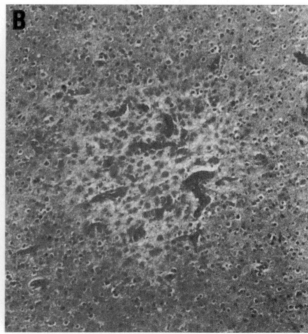

Figure 5 Neuropathological hallmarks of HIV infection. (A) Multinucleated giant cells are considered to be histological lesions directly attributed to HIV infection. (B) Microglial nodules, frequently observed in the brain of HIV-infected patients, are associated with opportunistic cerebral infections.

3. Alzheimer's Disease

Alzheimer's disease is a degenerative disorder characterized by memory loss eventually leading to dementia. Pathologically, AD is characterized by the presence of insoluble structures or depositions in cortical regions of the brain, namely β-amyloid (Aβ)-containing extracellular plaques and intraneuronal neurofibrillary tangles. The presence of large numbers of activated microglia and reactive astrocytes in brain tissue from AD patients has been interpreted as a secondary event. However, evidence suggests a significant role of these cells in the progression of the disease. Microglia cluster around Aβ-containing senile plaques with markedly enhanced MHC II protein expression on microglial cells associated with areas of degenerative pathology. Cytokines such as IL-1, IL-6, and TNF-α also have increased expression in microglia in the vicinity of senile plaques. These cytokines can potentially coordinate the majority of inflammatory changes found in AD brain tissue; however, a classic immune response as defined by the involvement of T cells or immunoglobulins does not appear to occur. The presence of microglia in the vicinity of amyloid plaques suggests a function in phagocytosis and plaque removal. Microglia can also uptake and degrade Aβ with a limited rate. In culture studies, synthetic Aβ not only recruits and activates microglia but also induces the secretion of cytotoxic products by these cells. Thus, rather than being protective, the activation of microglial cells may result in further neurotoxicity. Moreover, microglia can synthesize and secrete Aβ. Therefore, the stimulus of Aβ production may be Aβ.

V. EPENDYMOGLIA CELLS

The introduction of the term "ependyma" was meant to describe the cell layer lining the ventricles of the brain. However, a recent definition or classification of ependymoglial cells has been under debate. Some argue that certain members should be classified as astrocytes, whereas others argue that ependymoglial cells are distinct since they have many characteristics not shared by typical astrocytes. An ependymoglial cell is usually defined as a glial cell extending at least one of its processes to the ventricular space and having physical contact with the outer surface of neural tissue. Ependymoglia are made up of different members, including fetal radial glia, tanycytes, and Müller cells. Other cell types, such as Bergmann glia, have radial processes that extend to the ventricles of the brain.

However, since they do not actually establish contact with the apical surface of neural tissue, they are considered to be astrocytes and not ependymoglia.

A. Morphology and Subtypes

Structurally, ependymoglial cells are characterized by different types of processes that are determined by contact with various microenvironmental compartments. The type I process is a feature of every ependymoglia cell. The endfoot comes into contact with a fluid or space into which extend many microvilli. The apical pole contains abundant mitochondria, which indicates a high level of metabolic activity. Another characteristic of apical processes in some but not all ependymoglia is the presence of kinocilia, a simple cilia consisting of a ring of nine pairs of tubules. Type 1 processes are interconnected by various types of apicolateral junctions. In regions where no endothelial blood–barrier exists, ependymoglia cells form a cerebrospinal fluid (CSF) barrier by the expression of tight junctions. Ependymoglial type 2 processes are characterized by basal mesenchymal contact and a cytoskeleton with abundant intermediate filaments. These filaments consist primarily of vimentin when the endfoot is in contact with CSF, but they consist primarily of GFAP when in contact with a blood vessel. The basal processes extend to the basal lamina of the mesenchymal layer underlying the nervous epithelium, forming processes of type IIa. Processes extending to the basal lamina of blood vessels are termed type IIb. Type III processes are defined by contact with neurons. These processes are characterized by the formation of flat or lamellar sheaths that enclose the neuronal somata (type IIIa), synapses (IIIb), or axonal internodes (IIIc1) or by finger-like extensions that contact the nodal specializations of axons (IIIc2). These processes may act as stores of sodium or calcium ions and cannot be elaborated until neurons have completed their differentiation.

B. Lineage and Development

In the human brain, ependymoglial cells are thought to be derived from the developing neuroepithelium along a caudal-to-rostral gradient. Radial glial cells are the first subtype of neuroglia to appear during human fetal brain development. They stain intensely with GFAP and nestin early in development but lose immunoreactivity with time. It is thought that ependymoglia arise from a radial progenitor in a pathway that can also give rise to astrocytes. The radial progenitors differentiate into radial glial cells, which can then morphologically transform into the subtypes of ependymoglial cells mentioned earlier as well as into astrocytes.

C. Normal Physiology and Function

The function of ependymoglia cells is unclear. Physiological stimulation of brain compartments evokes specific reactions among ependymoglia. It has been reported that fetal ependymal cells play an important role during development of the nervous system by forming the cellular highway for the migration of progenitor cells. Furthermore, they arrest neurogenesis, facilitate motor neuron differentiation, and aid in transport of nutrients before development of capillary networks. Evidence of ependymal involvement in neuroendocrine function has also been reported as changes in ependymal cell morphology, coincident with changes in pituitary hormone secretion. In the adult brain, these cells provide only limited transport of ions, small molecules, and fluids between the brain and the CSF. The ependymal cells lining the ventricles act as a barrier for filtration of brain molecules and for the protection of the brain from potentially harmful substances in the CSF. From these examples, it is apparent that ependymoglia cells are continuously adapting to the changing needs of the neuronal tissue.

D. Contribution to Disease

Ependymomas and ependymoblastomas develop from the ependymal cells surrounding the ventricles and the central canal of the spinal cord. Intracranial ependymomas occur predominantly in children and tend to fill the ventricular lumen. The mean age at diagnosis of ependymoma and ependymoblastoma is 5 years. The incidence of these ependymal tumors in males and females is approximately equal. Clinical symptoms, although related to the location of the tumor, are usually due to blockage of CSF fluid flow, which may lead to a sudden increase in intracranial pressure. Ependymal tumors are sensitive to radiation.

Subependymomas are slow-growing, benign neoplasms originating from the subependymal glial matrix, consisting of a mixture of astrocytic, ependymal, and transitional cell clusters surrounded by their fibers. They generally project into the ventricular lumen. About one-fourth of the symptomatic intracranial tumors have mixed tumor cell populations and consist of a mixture of ependymomas and subependymomas. The prognosis in these cases is worse than that of a pure ependymoma. Another factor that affects the prognosis is the size of the neoplasm; symptomatic tumors tend to be large. Subependymoma is more common in men and has been reported in all decades of life, although no cases of subependymomas have been reported in children less than 2 years of age. The mean age for symptomatic tumors is 39 years, whereas that for asymptomatic lesions is 59 years. Microscopically, subependymomas consist of a nest of glial cells separated by glial fibers. Histologic studies have shown that some of the cells within these glomerate nests have attributes of ependymal cells and others of astrocytes; still others are transitional between the two.

VI. CONCLUSIONS

Neuroglial cells were described initially as specialized cells surrounding the neurons to provide structural support and insulation. In fact, neuroglial cells comprise a wide variety of phenotypes and functions. It is now known that complex intercellular communication exists not only between glial cells and neurons but also among the neuroglial members. This relationship becomes evident during pathological conditions of the brain. Selective damage of any one cell type can have severe ramifications on the functions of others as well as on the neuronal population. In the normal human brain, glial cells and neurons exist in a very delicate and highly coordinated balance. The diversity of neuroglial cells serves to contribute to the complexity of the human CNS.

See Also the Following Articles

ASTROCYTES • HOMEOSTATIC MECHANISMS • MICROGLIA • MULTIPLE SCLEROSIS

Suggested Reading

Adelman, G., and Smith, B. H. (Eds.) (1996). *Encyclopedia of Neuroscience,* Vols. 1 and 2. Elsevier, Amsterdam.

Beneviste, E. N. (1998). Cytokine actions in the central nervous system. *Cytokine Growth Factor Rev.* **9,** 259–275.

Bruni, J. E. (1998). Ependymal development, proliferation, and function: A review. *Microscopy Res. Techni.* **41,** 2–13.

Cuadros, M. A., and Navascues, J. (1998). The origin and differentiation of microglial cells during development. *Prog. Neurobiol.* **56,** 173–189.

Kettenmann, H., and Ransom, B. R. (Eds.) (1995). *Neuroglia.* Oxford Univ. Press, New York.

Kreutzberg, G. W. (1996). Microglia: A sensor for pathological events in the CNS. *Trends Neurosci.* **19,** 312–318.

Landis, D. M. D. (1994). The early reactions of non-neuronal cells to brain injury. *Annu. Rev. Neurosci.* **17,** 133–151.

Miller, R. H., Hayes, J. E., Dyer, K. L., and Sussman, C. R. (1999). Mechanisms of oligodendrocyte commitment in the vertebrate CNS. *Int. J. Dev. Neurosci.* **17**(8), 753–763.

Norenberg, M. D. (1994). Astrocyte responses to CNS injury. *J. Neuropathol. Exp. Neurol.* **53**(3), 213–220.

Stoll, G., and Jander, S. (1999). The role of microglia and macrophages in the pathophysiology of the CNS. *Prog. Neurobiol.* **58,** 233–247.

Wilkens, R. H., and Rengachary, S. S. (Eds.) (1996). *Neurosurgery,* Vol. 1. McGraw–Hill, New York.

Zhang, S. C., Ge, B., and Duncan, I. D. (2000). Tracing human oligodendroglial development in vitro. *J. Neurosci. Res.* **59,** 421–429.

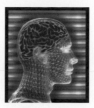

Hallucinations

JANE EPSTEIN, EMILY STERN, and DAVID SILBERSWEIG

Weill Medical College of Cornell University

GLOSSARY

delirium A state of altered attention, arousal, and thought, often caused by an acute medical condition.

delusion A false belief, not generally endorsed by the individual's culture, held despite contradictory evidence.

epilepsy A chronic disorder consisting of intermittent episodes of excessive neuronal electrical discharge (seizures).

ictal Relating to a seizure.

partial seizure An episode of excessive electrical discharge originating from a discrete region of cerebral cortex and remaining confined to one part of the cortex.

psychosis A condition in which unreal beliefs or experiences are believed to represent reality.

Hallucinations are involuntary sensory experiences perceived as emanating from the external environment, in the absence of stimulation of relevant sensory receptors. They were first defined in this manner in 1837 by Esquirol, who differentiated them from illusions, which are perceptual misinterpretations of existing external stimuli. Hallucinations can occur in a variety of contexts but are perhaps most striking and debilitating in the setting of schizophrenia, in which they are combined with a failure to realize that they do not represent reality. In this instance, they are generally experienced as real, emotionally significant, and related to concurrent delusions, and they represent a form of psychosis. Hallucinations can occur in any sensory modality or can involve multiple modalities, with auditory hallucinations most common in schizophrenia and other illnesses traditionally termed psychiatric and visual hallucinations most common in illnesses termed neurologic. This article presents a functional neuroanatomic approach to hallucinations, describing and analyzing them in terms of disorders of sensory input, midbrain/thalamus, and higher brain regions, including cortical sensory, limbic, and frontal regions. It also discusses other investigational approaches to hallucinations as well as treatment considerations. The focus is on visual and auditory hallucinations because they occur most frequently and have been most thoroughly investigated.

I. FUNCTIONAL NEUROANATOMIC APPROACH TO HALLUCINATIONS

The variety of forms, contents, and settings of hallucinations can be described and analyzed in a number of ways, each with its own strengths and weaknesses. Of these, a functional neuroanatomic approach, based on evolving data, is perhaps most heuristically satisfying. In order to present such an approach, we first review the functional neuroanatomy of normal sensory perception as set forth by Mesulam.

A. Functional Neuroanatomy of Normal Perception

External auditory, visual, tactile, gustatory, and olfactory stimuli are first detected by modality-specific receptors in the periphery. Information from most of these sensory receptors converges on modality-specific nuclei in the thalamus, where extraneous information is filtered out or "gated" and relevant information relayed to various parts of the cortex. At the cortex, the first regions to receive these inputs are the primary sensory areas: visual at the occipital pole and banks of the calcarine fissure, auditory at Heschl's gyrus on the posterior supratemporal plane, and somatosensory at the postcentral gyrus. These highly differentiated, or distinctly structured, regions carry out the most specialized processing within each modality, extracting basic features of sensory information. Output from these regions flows to adjacent unimodal association cortices, where modality-specific sensory elaboration occurs. Output from multiple unimodal association areas converges on heteromodal association cortices in temporoparietal and prefrontal regions, where unimodal percepts are linked with associated information to form multimodal constructs.

The path of information flow can be illustrated by considering the well-studied visual system. In this sensory modality, unimodal processing is mediated by regions stretching from the occiput anteriorly, with information flowing along two major pathways. The first, known as the ventral pathway, begins in association areas adjacent to primary visual cortex, where individual features of visual information, such as color and shape, are processed in separate subregions. As the information moves along the lower surface of the brain toward anterior temporal regions, these features are integrated and complex patterns are extracted, permitting discrimination of individual objects such as faces. Information from anterior temporal regions flows to heteromodal cortex, where highly processed visual percepts are integrated with input from other sensory modalities and with stored information about their characteristics, history, and emotional/motivational relevance, leading to object recognition. Integration is achieved via interconnections with limbic and paralimbic regions involved in mnemonic and emotional processing. The second, dorsal pathway leads from occipital unimodal association areas on the upper side of the brain to adjacent heteromodal regions in the posterior parietal cortex that mediate object localization. As information flows from more differentiated primary sensory areas to less differentiated heteromodal regions, specialized perception merges into complex cognition. Higher level cognitive processes are mediated by prefrontal heteromodal cortices involved in monitoring, categorizing, modifying, and integrating multiple streams of information processing to form

an overview of the current situation and generate a relevant plan of action. This serial, hierarchical flow of information occurs within a context of bidirectional feedback projections and concurrent parallel processing.

Although much remains to be learned about the nature and precise localization of the neural phenomena that give rise to hallucinations, the existing data, along with our knowledge of the pathways involved in normal perception, allow for the categorization and analysis of hallucinations based on their probable neuroanatomic substrates.

B. Disorders of Sensory Input Associated with Hallucinations

Hallucinations produced by disorders of the peripheral sensory system appear to result from ongoing cortical sensory processing in the setting of degraded or absent sensory input. Sometimes referred to as "release" phenomena, the use of the term in this context can be misleading because it has traditionally been used to connote neural activity released by the failure of higher level inhibitory centers rather than by disordered lower level input. The probable mechanism by which these hallucinations are generated is best understood by considering the interplay between peripheral and central processing in normal perception. Although the previous description of sensory processing emphasizes the flow of information from periphery to thalamus to cortex ("bottom-up" processing), the connections between thalamus and cortex are in fact bidirectional, as noted. This pattern of connectivity enables the cortex to play a role in selecting from among the massive array of inputs to the thalamus those most likely to be relevant in light of past and current experience. Thus, perceptions arise from an interplay between cortically generated expectations ("top-down" processing) and data (confirmatory or otherwise) from peripheral sensory receptors. In this setting, a dearth of peripheral input might give rise to perceptions dominated by expectations rather than current environmental conditions.

Hallucinations caused by disordered peripheral input are most frequently seen in the visual system. The term Charles Bonnet syndrome has been applied to such phenomena, but without a consistent definition. The hallucinations are most often vivid, colorful, and complex representations of people, animals, scenery, trees, buildings, or flowers that fill the entire visual field. They frequently appear smaller than normal, or Lilliputian, and may move. Hallucinations tend to have an abrupt onset, can last seconds to hours, and may disappear with movement or closure of the eyes. They can occur in the setting of acute blindness following altered blood flow or trauma to the eye, a phenomenon sometimes referred to as phantom vision, or during a gradual visual decline. In either case, they may fade as the visual disturbance continues. Notably, the individuals experiencing the hallucinations are aware that they do not represent reality and generally have no strong emotional association or reaction to them. Although primary abnormalities within the central nervous system may increase the risk of developing Charles Bonnet syndrome (a hypothesis supported by its greater prevalence in the elderly, who are at increased risk of subtle brain dysfunction), it can occur on the sole basis of peripheral visual system dysfunction. Indeed, its prevalence rate of 20% in people who develop blindness is similar to the 19% of normal individuals who experience visual hallucinations during sensory deprivation experiments—a clear example of hallucinations caused solely by disordered peripheral input.

Conditions such as stroke, that involve destruction of primary visual cortex or the cerebral pathways leading to it can also lead to complex visual hallucinations. Although the lesion in this instance is central, the phenomenology and mechanism are similar to those seen with peripheral lesions because primary visual cortex provides input to the unimodal association areas involved in the generation of complex hallucinations. The major phenomenologic difference derives from the organization of visual processing in primary cortex, where the right visual field is mediated by left occipital cortex and vice versa. When central lesions are limited to one hemisphere, hallucinations occur only in the affected contralateral visual field.

In the somatosensory system, a striking example of hallucinations caused by disordered sensory input occurs in the phantom limb syndrome, as described by Melzack. After amputation of a limb, approximately 95% of adults experience the limb as still present, able to move in space, and to feel pain or tingling. Over time, the perception weakens such that the proximal part of the limb no longer seems to exist, leaving the hand or foot hanging in midair, or the entire limb seems to "telescope" into the body, leaving the hand or foot directly connected to the stump. Phantom experiences have also been reported after the loss of eyes, teeth, external genitalia, and breasts. They are not dependent on sensory input from the residual scar and

can occur even in those with congenitally absent limbs, suggesting a central representation of the body that is at least partly innate.

In the auditory system, individuals with peripheral dysfunction can develop complex hallucinations, such as music (either instrumental or vocal) or voices, or simple hallucinations, such as ringing, buzzing, or isolated tones of various pitches. Although more common with bilateral dysfunction, hallucinations can accompany unilateral peripheral auditory disease, in which case they are experienced as emanating from the affected side.

C. Midbrain/Thalamic Disorders Associated with Hallucinations

Hallucinations similar to those produced by peripheral lesions can occur with lesions of the upper midbrain and adjacent thalamus. First described in 1922 by Lhermitte, who attributed them to a lesion in the midbrain peduncular region, they remain known as "peduncular" hallucinations. Like Charles Bonnet hallucinations, they are often vivid, complex visual hallucinations (although other sensory modalities may be involved), frequently of people or animals (sometimes Lilliputian) often engaged in animated activities. Unlike those produced by peripheral lesions, peduncular hallucinations are generally associated with disturbances in sleep and arousal and may at times be interpreted as real.

These disturbances in sleep and arousal provide clues to the mechanism by which hallucinations are generated by midbrain and thalamic lesions. Frequency-specific oscillations in thalamocortical circuits have been associated with the temporal binding of perception and with dreaming. As pointed out by Manford and Andermann, brain stem connections to the thalamus are important in switching thalamic relay nuclei out of waking relay mode, in which they faithfully transmit sensory inputs to the cortex, into sleeping mode, in which they do not. This is accomplished via neurotransmitters, notably acetylcholine and serotonin, whose cell bodies lie within the basal and brain stem reticular regions involved in modulation of arousal, selective attention, and cortical processing. Abnormalities of acetylcholine and serotonin transmission brought on by disease, medication, or drug use (including such hallucinogens as LSD) are frequently accompanied by hallucinations. Similarly, transitions between states of sleep and wakefulness are associated with hallucinations, usually in the setting of sleep disorders such as narcolepsy or insomnia. Hypnagogic hallucinations occur prior to falling asleep, whereas hypnopompic hallucinations occur upon awakening. Both are generally multimodal, vivid, and emotionally charged. Common examples are the feeling or experience of being about to fall into an abyss or attacked, of being caught in a fire, or of sensing a presence in the room. Hallucinations in the settings of delirium and sedative drug withdrawal are also associated with disturbances in sleep and arousal.

Abnormal thalamic activity was also present in a functional neuroimaging study, performed by our group with colleagues (as described below), of hallucinations in the setting of schizophrenia. This may relate to the modulatory and integrative roles of thalamocortical circuits in the generation of perceptual experience. A possible role for the thalamus in this setting is supported by a number of electrophysiologic, neuropathologic, structural, and functional imaging studies revealing sensory gating deficits and thalamic abnormalities in individuals with schizophrenia.

D. Disorders of Higher Brain Regions Associated with Hallucinations

Hallucinations are also associated with primary pathology at higher levels of the brain. Most prominent in this category are those that occur in migraine, epilepsy, and schizophrenia. Investigation of cerebral activity associated with hallucinations in these settings has been aided in recent years by the development of techniques such as electroencephalography (EEG), evoked potentials, single photon emission computed tomography (SPECT), positron emission tomography (PET), and functional magnetic resonance imaging (fMRI). Combined with data from other avenues of investigation, studies employing these tools have implicated a number of higher brain regions in the generation of hallucinations, corresponding to their form, content, and setting.

1. Cortical Sensory Activity Associated with Hallucinations

Regardless of the mechanism by which they are generated (primary peripheral, midbrain/thalamic, or higher brain disturbances), hallucinations appear to be associated with activity in cortical sensory regions corresponding to their modality and complexity. The

hallucinations described previously may be described as complex or formed. Noncomplex hallucinations are referred to interchangeably as simple, unformed, or crude. In the visual system, these are known as photopsias, and they occur frequently with migraines. In this setting, the most common forms are colorless glittering spots and black-and-white zigzag patterns known as fortification lines. They often occur unilaterally but may fill the entire visual field. Photopsias can also occur, briefly, at the onset of partial seizures and for the first few days following an infarction of the central visual system. In both settings they tend to be brightly colored and unilateral. In addition, disorders of visual input may give rise to photopsias. Simple hallucinations are believed to reflect activity in primary sensory or adjacent early unimodal association areas and to correspond in form to the area's functional specialization. For example, colored photopsias would be associated with activity in occipital subregions involved in color processing, as described previously.

Complex hallucinations are associated with activity in sensory association areas, with or without involvement of primary sensory cortex. As with simple hallucinations, their form and content correspond to the location of activity. We investigated neural activity associated with auditory/visual hallucinations in a 23-year-old man with schizophrenia. The subject underwent PET scanning while experiencing frequent hallucinations of colored, moving scenes containing disembodied, rolling heads that spoke to him in a derogatory fashion. Using techniques that allow for identification of activity simultaneous with hallucinatory events, we detected activations in occipital and temporal visual association cortex (higher order visual perception), temporal auditory–linguistic association cortex (speech perception), and temporoparietal and prefrontal heteromodal association cortex (intermodal processing) (Fig. 1). Activations were bilateral but more extensive on the left, perhaps reflecting the dominance of that hemisphere for language.

2. Limbic/Paralimbic Activity Associated with Hallucinations

The previously mentioned study included five other subjects, all of whom experienced frequent auditory/verbal hallucinations in the setting of schizophrenia. Although each had a somewhat different pattern of sensory cortical activation, perhaps reflecting differences in the form and content of their hallucinations, group analysis revealed a highly significant pattern of common activations in thalamic, limbic, and

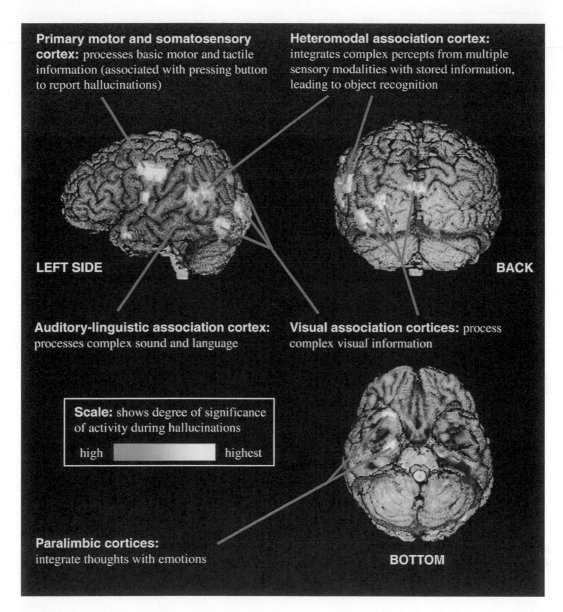

Primary motor and somatosensory cortex: processes basic motor and tactile information (associated with pressing button to report hallucinations)

Heteromodal association cortex: integrates complex percepts from multiple sensory modalities with stored information, leading to object recognition

LEFT SIDE

BACK

Auditory-linguistic association cortex: processes complex sound and language

Visual association cortices: process complex visual information

Scale: shows degree of significance of activity during hallucinations

high   highest

Paralimbic cortices: integrate thoughts with emotions

BOTTOM

Figure 1   Brain regions active in a schizophrenic patient experiencing auditory–visual hallucinations of disembodied, rolling heads speaking to him. The functional PET results are superimposed on the subject's own structural brain MRI scan. The bright areas pinpoint regions of heightened cortical activity associated with hallucinatory events [reproduced with permission from D. A. Silbersweig *et al.* (1995), A functional neuroanatomy of hallucinations in schizophrenia. *Nature* **378,** 176–179].

paralimbic regions that may be involved in the generation or modulation of hallucinations (Fig. 2). Limbic structures, the least differentiated, or least distinctly structured, older regions of the cortex, are involved in the linking of drives with experience and the processing of emotion. Paralimbic regions are intermediate in structure between, and interconnected with, limbic and heteromodal association areas and serve to integrate emotion and drive with highly processed sensory information. Because limbic and paralimbic structures are closely interconnected and functionally integrated, they are often referred to collectively as the limbic system.

In our study, activation in limbic regions involved hippocampi (extending to the adjacent amygdalae) and ventral striatum. The hippocampal formation, a convoluted structure within the medial temporal lobe, is involved in memory and the processing of contextual

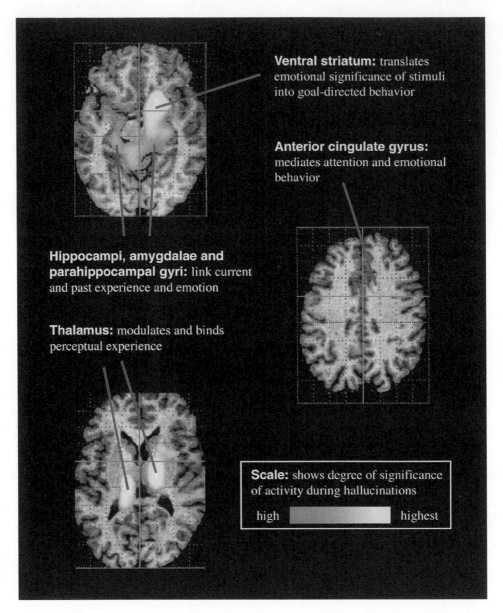

Figure 2   Common areas of brain activity in a group of schizophrenic patients experiencing auditory/verbal hallucinations. The functional PET results are superimposed on an anatomical MRI template. The bright areas pinpoint regions of heightened thalamic, limbic, and paralimbic activity associated with hallucinatory events [reproduced with permission from D. A. Silbersweig *et al.* (1995), A functional neuroanatomy of hallucinations in schizophrenia. *Nature* **378,** 176–179].

aspects of emotional evaluation. The amygdaloid complex, a collection of nuclei adjacent to and interconnected with the hippocampus, plays a central role in evaluating the emotional significance of internally and externally generated stimuli. Both of these structures send output to the ventral striatum, the limbic portion of the subcortical basal ganglia, where emotional significance is translated into goal-directed behavior. Activation in paralimbic regions involved

parahippocampal gyri, anterior cingulate, and orbito-frontal cortex. The parahippocampal gyrus, which lies on the medial surface of the temporal lobe, integrates sensory output from heteromodal and more complex unimodal association areas with limbically processed information. The anterior cingulate, the frontmost portion of a band running from medial frontal to parahippocampal regions, is involved in attention and social/emotional behaviors. The orbital frontal cortex is located in the medial ventral frontal lobes. Like the amygdala, it participates in the evaluation of emotional significance and sends output to the ventral striatum. In contrast to the amygdala, the orbital frontal region is able to modulate emotional responsivity and readjust behavioral responses to stimuli when their reinforcement value is changed or when a more complex assessment of the current context suggests the need for modification.

Just as abnormal activity in cortical sensory regions is correlated with the form and content of hallucinations, it is likely that aberrant activity in limbic/paralimbic regions gives rise to the marked emotional significance of hallucinations in the setting of schizophrenia. Further evidence of a role for limbic system dysfunction in the generation of schizophrenic symptoms is provided by postmortem, neuropsychological, and neuroimaging studies that reveal structural and functional abnormalities of limbic regions in individuals with schizophrenia, including hyperactivity of temporal regions (left greater than right) associated with psychosis. Activity of the limbic system is closely interconnected with that of dopamine, a neurotransmitter implicated in the generation of hallucinations and delusions in the settings of schizophrenia, medication toxicity, and drug abuse. Dopaminergic activity is regulated, in part, by input from limbic system structures and in turn appears to modulate the responsiveness of ventral striatal neurons to limbic inputs. Recent work suggests that glutamate, an excitatory neurotransmitter, may also play a role in both limbic dysregulation and schizophrenia. Hallucinations that occur in the context of severe emotional stress may also involve abnormal limbic activity.

Temporolimbic structures also play a role in the generation of hallucinations associated with epilepsy. In addition to photopsias, the onset of partial seizures can be accompanied by simple hallucinations in any modality, reflecting ictal discharges in primary sensory areas, or by complex hallucinations, reflecting discharges in limbic and sensory association areas. These often involve temporal regions including hippocampus and amygdala, which have the lowest seizure thresholds of all brain structures, as well as sensory association areas. Like the complex hallucinations seen in schizophrenia, these are often emotionally charged. Unlike those seen in schizophrenia, they are more often visual than auditory and are not usually believed by the person experiencing them to represent reality. Relatedly, electrical stimulation of temporal lobe regions, including the amygdala, can give rise to hallucinatory experiences. In addition to hallucina-

tions experienced during seizures, there is evidence that individuals who have suffered from epilepsy for more than 10 years may develop hallucinations between seizure episodes. These are more likely to resemble fully those seen in schizophrenia as they are often emotionally charged, are as likely to be auditory as visual, are accompanied by delusions, and are believed to represent reality. As in schizophrenia, they appear to be associated with temporal lobe abnormalities (left more often than right).

3. Frontal/Executive Activity Associated with Hallucinations

The lack of awareness that hallucinatory experience does not correspond to reality is a striking feature of schizophrenia. In addition to temporal lobe abnormalities, numerous studies have revealed frontal dysfunction and abnormal frontotemporal connectivity associated with schizophrenia. The frontal lobes, in concert with interconnected regions, mediate the higher, more complex aspects of cognition, such as judgment, insight, and self-monitoring. These are termed executive functions. Although relevant studies have produced mixed results, there is evidence that frontal dysfunction may contribute to the inability of individuals with schizophrenia to identify the internal origin of their hallucinatory experience and its relation to their illness. Temporal lobe epilepsy may also be accompanied by executive as well as other forms of cognitive dysfunction and by abnormalities of frontal activity.

II. OTHER INVESTIGATIONAL APPROACHES TO HALLUCINATIONS

The descriptive and analytic framework employed in this article represents one approach to hallucinations. Others tend to be complementary, rather than exclusive, with their boundaries increasingly blurred as convergence and integration occur. The resulting interdisciplinary synthesis has enhanced our understanding of hallucinations. At the cognitive level of analysis, numerous mechanisms have been posited to play a role in the generation of hallucinations, with support derived from psychologic, electrophysiologic, and animal studies. Several theories focus on abnormalities in the processing of input or its comparison with past experience. These can be seen to dovetail with the sensory input, midbrain/thalamic, sensory cortical, and limbic/paralimbic disturbances described previously. Others focus on cognitive abnormalities that may give rise to deficits in the ability to discriminate between external and self-generated events. These theories, in turn, are related to frontal/executive disturbances. At the neurochemical level, much work has been done on the relation between disturbances in neurotransmitter systems, such as dopamine, serotonin, and glutamate, and hallucinations. This is clearly relevant to the limbic and midbrain/thalamic disturbances noted previously. At the computational level, neural networks models have been used to investigate links between posited cognitive or physiologic abnormalities and hallucinations, with intriguing results. At the social/psychological level, investigations and clinical observations suggest that personal, social, and cultural factors play a role in the development and content of hallucinations—a role likely to be mediated by limbic and cortical brain regions involved in learning and complex cognition.

III. TREATMENT OF HALLUCINATIONS

For hallucinations in the setting of schizophrenia, medications that alter transmission of dopamine and related neurotransmitters, termed neuroleptics, are the mainstay of treatment. In other settings, the first step in the treatment of hallucinations is to address the condition that underlies their existence. When this is impossible or ineffective, neuroleptic medications may be tried. However, these tend to be less effective in settings that do not involve limbic, striatal, or dopaminergic pathology. Fortunately, hallucinations in the setting of sensory input disorders, where neuroleptics are least effective, are often less disturbing to those experiencing them, as described previously. Such hallucinations sometimes respond to carbamazepine, a medication often used for seizure prevention, mood stabilization, or control of pain originating in the nervous system. This is consistent with models of aberrant neural activity described previously.

When hallucinations are distressing and unresponsive to medication, psychological treatments may be helpful. Cognitive–behavioral approaches involve distracting activities or sensory input as well as behavioral and cognitive tasks. Supportive approaches involve helping patients understand their condition, solve problems, and adapt to reality. Psychological approaches tend to decrease distress associated with hallucinations and improve overall functioning rather than ameliorate hallucinations per se.

Future developments in the treatment of hallucinations are likely to be guided by the functional neuroanatomic approach. Recent investigations into the mechanism of action of antipsychotic medications have increasingly focused on the specific cerebral regions modulated by relevant neurotransmitters. In addition, a recent study examined the efficacy of transcranial magnetic stimulation (TMS), a novel technique for altering focal cortical activity through application of a magnetic pulse, in the treatment of persistent auditory hallucinations in schizophrenic patients. The results suggest that administration of TMS to the left temporoparietal regions noted (in the PET study discussed previously) to be active during auditory hallucinations can markedly decrease the severity of such events.

IV. FUTURE DIRECTIONS

The approach to hallucinations presented in this article represents an attempt to organize and synthesize current knowledge from a functional neuroanatomic perspective. It should be regarded as a framework on which further data from disciplines relevant to neuroscience can be laid. As new data emerge and interdisciplinary integration proceeds, our understanding of hallucinations will undoubtedly gain increased specificity and complexity and grow in new directions.

See Also the Following Articles

BODY PERCEPTION DISORDERS • DREAMING • EPILEPSY • LIMBIC SYSTEM • MIDBRAIN • PHANTOM LIMB PAIN • SCHIZOPHRENIA • SENSORY DEPRIVATION • STROKE • THALAMUS AND THALAMIC DAMAGE • VISUAL DISORDERS

Suggested Reading

Amador, X., and David, A. (Eds.) (1998). *Insight and Psychosis.* Oxford Univ. Press, New York.

Devinsky, O., and Luciano, D. (1991). Psychic phenomena in partial seizures. *Sem. Neurol.* **11**(2), 100–109.

Esquirol, J. (1837/1965). *Mental Maladies.* Hafner, New York.

Frith, C. (1998). The role of the prefrontal cortex in self-consciousness: The case of auditory hallucinations. In *The Prefrontal Cortex: Executive and Cognitive Functions* (A. Roberts, T. Robbins, *et al.*, Eds.), pp. 181–194. Oxford Univ. Press, New York.

Hoffman, R., Boutros, N., Berman, R., Roessler, E., Belger, A., Krystal, H., and Charney, D. (1999). Transcranial magnetic stimulation of left temporoparietal cortex in three patients reporting hallucinated "voices". *Biol. Psychiatr.* **46,** 130–132.

Krystal, J., Abi-Dargham, A., Laruelle, M., and Moghaddam, B. (1999). Pharmacologic models of psychoses. In *Neurobiology of Mental Illness* (D. Charney, E. Nestler, and B. Bunney, Eds.), pp. 214–224. Oxford Univ. Press, New York.

Lhermitte, J. (1922). Syndrome de la calotte pedonculaire. Les troubles psychosorielle dans les lesions du mesencephale. *Rev. Neurologique* **38,** 1359–1365.

Manford, M., and Andermann, F. (1998). Complex visual hallucinations: Clinical and neurobiological insights. *Brain* **121,** 1819–1840.

Melzack, R. (1990). Phantom limbs and the concept of a neuromatrix. *TINS* **13**(3), 88–92.

Mesulam, M.-M. (2000). Behavioral neuroanatomy: Large-scale networks, association cortex, frontal syndromes, the limbic system, and hemispheric specializations. In *Principles of Behavioral and Cognitive Neurology* (M.-M. Mesulam, Ed.), pp. 1–120. Oxford Univ. Press, New York.

Silbersweig, D., and Stern, E. (1996). Functional neuroimaging of hallucinations in schizophrenia: Toward an integration of bottom-up and top-down approaches. *Mol. Psychiatr.* **1,** 367–375.

Trimble, M., and Schmitz, B. (1998). The psychoses of epilepsy: A neurobiological perspective. In *Psychiatric Comorbidity in Epilepsy: Basic Mechanisms, Diagnosis, and Treatment* (H. McConnell, P. Snyder, *et al.*, Eds.), pp. 169–186. American Psychiatric Press, Washington, DC.

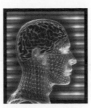

Hand Movements

J. RANDALL FLANAGAN* and ROLAND S. JOHANSSON[†]

*Queen's University, Canada and [†] Umeå University, Sweden

GLOSSARY

grasp stability control The control of grip forces such that they are adequate to prevent accidental slips but not so large as to cause unnecessary fatigue or damage to the object or hand.

haptic perception Perception through the hand based on tactile and somatosensory information.

internal models Neural circuits that mimic the behavior of the motor system and environment and capture the mapping between motor outputs and sensory inputs.

precision grip The grip formed when grasping an object with the distal tips of digits. Usually refers to grasping with the tips of the thumb and index finger on either side of an object.

sensorimotor control The use of both predicted and unexpected sensory information in the control of action.

The human hand and the brain are close partners in two important and closely interconnected functions: exploration of the physical world and reshaping of parts of this world through manipulation. The highly versatile functions of the human hand depend on both its anatomical structure and the neural machinery that supports the hand. This article focuses on the sensorimotor control of hand movements in object manipulation–a hallmark of skilled manual action. The article also examines relationships between the two main functions of the hand–object perception and object manipulation.

I. THE ACTING AND PERCEIVING HAND

Many of our cultural and technological achievements that mark us as human depend on skilled use of the hand. We use of our hands to gesture and communicate, make and use tools, write, paint, play music, and make love. Thus, the human hand is a powerful tool through which the human brain interacts with the world. We use our hands both to perceive the world within our reach (haptic perception) and to act on this world. These two functions of the hand, which are largely accomplished by touching and manipulating objects in our environment, are intimately related in terms of sensorimotor control. Haptic perception requires specific hand movements that are tailored to the kinds of information the perceiver wishes to extract. For example, to obtain information about the texture of an object, people rub their fingertips across the object's surface, and to obtain information about shape they trace the contour of the object with their fingertips. Conversely, in object manipulation sensory and perceptual information is critical for precise motor control of the hands. The fact that individuals with numbed digits have great difficulty handling small objects even with full vision illustrates the importance of somatosensory information from the fingertips.

To control both the exploratory and manipulatory functions of the hand, the brain must obtain accurate descriptions of various mechanical events that take place when objects are brought into contact with the hand. Mechanoreceptive (tactile) sensors in the glabrous skin of the volar aspect of the hand play an essential role in providing such information. The density of mechanoreceptors increases in the distal direction of the hand and is exquisitely high in the fingertips. As a perceptual organ, the hand has several advantages over the eyes. The hand can effectively "see around corners," allowing us to explore all sides of an object, and it can directly appreciate object properties such as weight, compliance, and slipperiness.

The numerous skeletal and muscular degrees of freedom of the hand, orchestrated by highly developed neural control systems, provide for tremendous dexterity that allows for both delicate exploration and versatile manipulation of objects. With approximately 30 dedicated muscles and approximately the same number of kinematic degrees of freedom, the hand can take on all variety of shapes and functions, serving as a hammer one moment and a powerful vice or a delicate pair of tweezers the next. The utility of hand movements is further enhanced by our ability to amplify the functions of the hand by using tools.

Different primates have very different hand movement capacities, with humans demonstrating the greatest dexterity. For example, true opposition between the thumb and index finger is only observed in humans, the great apes, and Old World monkeys. New World monkeys can manage pseudo-opposition, but prosimians are only capable of crude grasping. It seems improbable that the tremendous dexterity of the human hand can be explained solely by differences in anatomical factors given that the structural anatomy of the hands of different primates seems similar. This is not to say, however, that anatomical differences do not contribute. For example, the human thumb is much longer, relative to the index finger, than the chimpanzee thumb. This allows humans to grasp small objects precisely between the distal pads of the thumb. Similarly, the greater independence of finger movements in humans compared to monkeys arises, in part, from differences in the passive biomechanical connections among tendons. Humans have more individuated muscles and tendons with which to control the digits.

In addition to structural factors, a major contributor to differences in hand movement capacity among primates, and between primates and lower mammals, is the neural machinery underlying hand movement. Compared to lower mammals, primates have evolved extensive cerebral cortical systems for controlling the hand and the corticospinal pathways have taken on an increasingly dominant role in controlling movement.

Moreover, in primates the corticospinal tracts include direct connections between neurons in cortical motor areas and spinal motorneurons. Through these corticomotoneuronal connections, the cerebral cortex possesses monosynaptic control over motorneurons whose axons connect, in particular, with the hand muscles. In effect, these direct connections have moved the hand "closer" to the cerebral cortex. Furthermore, through cortical motor areas the corticospinal tracts provide rapid access to the hand from most other cortical areas and from subcortical structures, including the cerebellum and the basal ganglia, tightly involved in motor control.

The development of cortical systems for controlling the hand in primates parallels the evolution of the arm from a prop for balance and locomotion (in four-legged mammals) to a free and dexterous tool for sensing and acting on objects in the environment. The denser neuronal substrate for hand control provides more flexibility in the patterning of muscle activation and supports the ability to perform independent finger movements. Interestingly, across primates, there is a linkage between the number of corticomotoneuronal connections and manual dexterity in terms of performing tasks that require independent finger movements. Although there are many advantages in terms of control, the reliance on cortical control comes at a cost. Lesions to the motor cortex or corticospinal pathways due, for example, to cerebral vascular accident can be particularly devastating in humans.

The importance of the cortical involvement in fine fingertip control can be further appreciated by considering parallels between the ontogenetic development of central neural pathways and that of hand function. The efficacy of the corticomotoneuronal system can be probed using transcranial magnetic stimulation (TMS) of the brain. TMS applied over the hand area of the motor cortex activates muscles of the contralateral hand. During development the latency of this activation, and the stimulation strength required to elicit a response, decreases as the corticomotoneuronal connections are established. The conduction delays in these motor pathways, as well as in the somatosensory pathways conveying signals from the sensors of the hand, rapidly decrease during the first 2 years after birth and thereafter remain constant at adult values. Responses within the adult latency range appear during the age range in which young children demonstrate important improvements in their ability to grasp objects using the tips of the index finger and thumb. Similar parallels between hand function and corticomoto neurone (CM) system development have been demonstrated in monkeys using various electrophysiological and anatomical techniques.

II. SENSORIMOTOR CONTROL OF HAND MOVEMENTS IN OBJECT MANIPULATION

To understand and appreciate how the brain controls movements of the hand, it is best to study the natural behavior of the hand in everyday manipulatory tasks. During the past 20 years, the sensorimotor control of the hand in precision manipulation task has been investigated in great detail. In this section, we review what has been learned about the sensorimotor control of natural hand movements when grasping and manipulating objects with the fingertips.

The remarkable manipulative skills of the human hand are the result of neither rapid sensorimotor processes nor fast or powerful effector mechanisms. Rather, the secret lies in the way manual tasks are organized and controlled by the nervous system. Successful manipulation requires the selection of motor commands tailored to the manipulative intent, the task at hand, and the relevant physical properties of the manipulated object. For instance, most tasks require that we stabilize the object within our grasp as we move the object or use it as a tool. To prevent slips and accidental loss of the object we must apply adequately large forces normal to the grip surfaces (*grip forces*) in relation to destabilizing forces tangential to the grip surfaces (*load forces*) (Fig. 1). At the same time, excessive grip forces must be avoided because they cause unnecessary fatigue and may crush fragile objects or injure the hand. Hence, the term grasp stability entails prevention of accidental slips as well as excessive fingertip forces.

When grasping and manipulating objects, the forces needed to ensure grasp stability depend on the physical properties of the object. Object properties such as weight, slipperiness, shape, and weight distribution all impose constraints on the fingertip forces (including their magnitudes, directions, and points of application) required for stability. Thus, a basic question for understanding the control in manipulation is how do people adapt their fingertip forces to the constraints imposed by various object properties. Although visual information about object properties may be helpful in terms of force selection, ultimately people adapt to such constraints by using sensory information provided by digital mechanoreceptors. Individuals with impaired digital sensibility have great difficulty performing manipulation tasks even under visual gui-

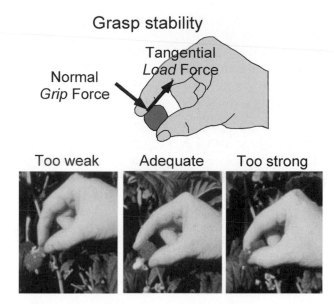

Figure 1 When manipulating objects grasped with a precision grip, we must carefully control the balance between grip force, normal to the contact surfaces, and load force tangential to the grasp surfaces. If grip force is too weak for a given load force, we risk having the object slip from our grasp. If grip force is too strong, we may crush the object or damage our hand and we waste energy.

dance. For instance, they often drop objects, may easily crush fragile objects, and have difficulties in dressing themselves because they cannot complete such apparently simple tasks as buttoning a shirt. Thus, it is clear that critical sensorimotor control processes required for manipulation are lost with impaired digital tactile sensibility.

The control of grip and load forces in object manipulation involves subtle interplay between two types of control: reactive control based on sensory feedback and predictive or feedforward control. These two control mechanisms are closely linked. On the one hand, reactive control mechanisms are invoked when errors arise between actual sensory feedback and the expected sensory feedback predicted from feedforward mechanisms. On the other hand, errors in sensory prediction are not only used for feedback control but also used to update feedforward mechanisms to reduce future prediction errors. In the following sections, we consider these two control processes in detail.

A. Feedback Control Based on Digital Sensors

One way to use digital sensors to adjust the force output would be to engage these sensors in feedback loops. However, such loops imply large time delays. These time delays arise from impulse conduction time in peripheral nerves, conduction and processing time in the central nervous system, and the inherent sluggishness of muscles. In humans, these factors sum to at least 100 msec for the generation of a significant force response. Consequently, closed-loop feedback is not effective for rapid movement involving frequencies above 1 Hz. In natural manipulation tasks, movement frequency components up to 5 Hz can be observed. Thus, feedback control alone cannot sup-

port control of grip force for grasp stability in these movements.

Despite these control limitations, feedback control is essential in certain types of manipulative tasks. For example, feedback control is required in reactive tasks in which we restrain "active" objects that generate unpredictable load forces tangential to the grip surfaces. Examples of tasks in which we must deal with active objects are holding a dog's leash, restraining a child by holding his or her arm, or operating power tools. Consider the situation depicted in Fig. 2A

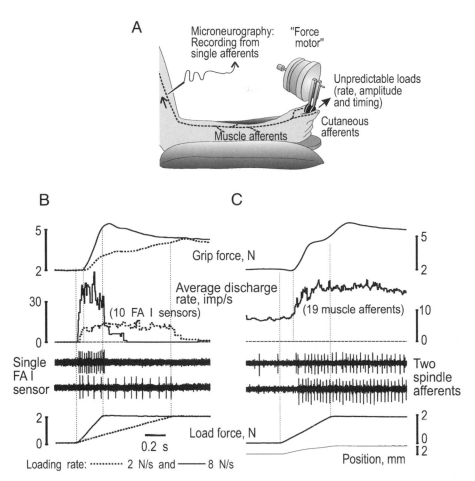

Figure 2 Peripheral afferent and reactive grip force responses to unpredictable loading of the precision grip by a pulling force. (A) The subject grasped the manipulandum with the tips of the thumb and index finger contacting parallel grip surfaces 25 mm apart. The force motor could deliver load forces pulled away from or pushed toward the hand. The grip and load forces, normal and tangential to the grip surfaces, respectively, and the position of the manipulandum were recorded. Afferent activity was recorded from the median nerve, with percutaneously inserted tungsten needle electrodes impaling the nerve about 10 cm proximal to the elbow. (B) Grip responses and average discharge rate of 10 FA I sensors to 2 N pulling loads delivered to the receptor-bearing digit at 2 N/sec (dashed lines) and 8 N/sec (solid lines). The two traces of single unit recordings are examples of responses in a single FA I sensor during load trials at 8 N/sec (upper trace) and 2 N/sec (lower trace). (C) Grip response and average discharge rate of 19 muscle afferents located in the long flexor muscles of the index, middle, or ring finger to 2.0 N pulling loads delivered at 4 N/sec. The single unit recordings are examples of responses in two different muscle spindle afferents. (B and C) The averages of forces and discharge rates are synchronized to the onset of the loading ramp; discharge rate represents average instantaneous frequency (adapted with permission from Macefield, V. G., Häger-Ross, C., and Johansson, R. S., *Exp. Brain Res.* **108**, 155–171, 1996; and Macefield, V. G., and Johansson, R. S., *Exp. Brain Res.* **108**, 172–184, 1996. Copyright © 1996 by Springer-Verlag).

in which an individual grasps an object attached to a force motor using a precision grip with the tips of the thumb and index finger on opposing vertical surfaces. The motor is used to generate increasing load forces (tangential to the grip surfaces) that are unpredictable in terms of onset time, amplitude, and direction (loading and unloading). To prevent the object from slipping, people automatically respond to increases in tangential load by increasing grip force normal to the grip surfaces in parallel with the load force changes (see load and grip force signals in Figs. 2B and 2C). When the load stops increasing, the grip force also stops increasing and may decrease slightly. Importantly, the changes in grip force lag behind the load force changes because they are reactively generated. A reactive grip response is initiated after a delay of approximately 100 msec but this varies with the load force rate. Because of this time lag, the object will slip from grasp unless the background grip force prior to a load increase is strong enough to meet the initial load increase. Indeed, following slips and trials with a high rate of load force increases, people learn to increase the initial background grip force as an adaptation to the expected range of loadings.

Figure 2A also shows signals, recorded using the technique of microneurography, from single nerve fibers of the median nerve that supply cutaneous, muscle, and joint sensors. Experiments with cutaneous anesthesia have demonstrated that reactive fingertip force responses are driven primarily by digital cutaneous inputs. Signals from fast adapting (FA I) cutaneous afferents seem most important, but slowly adapting cutaneous afferents may also contribute. As illustrated in Fig. 2B, the intensity of the cutaneous afferent responses is scaled by the rate of load force increase, and the afferent responses commence before the onset of the grip response. Furthermore, the size and duration of the grip force increase is scaled with the intensity and duration of the afferent response. This scaling is an attractive feature for feedback-based control.

Whereas cutaneous afferents contribute to the initiation and initial scaling of grip force responses, afferents from intrinsic and extrinsic hand muscles and interphalangeal joints do not respond to load increases early enough to allow them to contribute to the initiation of these grip responses. The muscle afferents respond reliably after the onset of the reactive grip force response and their discharge rates are related to changes in force output and, hence, to muscle activity (Fig. 2C). Thus, these muscle afferents are primarily concerned with events in the muscle itself rather than

functioning as exteroceptors sensing mechanical events at the fingertips.

B. Feedforward Control Processes

Almost everyone will recall having fallen victim to an older sibling, cousin, or friend who passed us an empty box while pretending it was very heavy. When we took the box, our arms flailed upwards. This trick demonstrates that when we interact with objects, we anticipate the forces required to complete the task. Although it may occasionally result in large movement errors, anticipatory or feedforward control is essential for skilled object manipulation. Feedback control is important when our predictions are erroneous or, as in reactive tasks, when predictions are unavailable. However, because of the long time delays, feedback control cannot support the swift and skilled coordination of fingertip forces observed in most manipulation tasks that involve ordinary "passive" objects. Instead, the brain relies on feedforward control mechanisms that take advantage of the stable and predictable physical properties of these objects. These mechanisms parametrically adapt force motor commands to the relevant physical properties of the target object.

Figure 3 illustrates parametric anticipatory adjustments of motor output to object weight, friction between the object and skin, and shape of the contact surface. The task is to lift a test object from a support surface, hold it in air for a couple of seconds, and then replace it. To accomplish this task, the vertical load force increases until liftoff occurs, stays constant during the hold phase, and then starts to decrease when the object contacts the support surface during replacement. When lifting objects of different weight (Fig. 3A), people scale the rate of increase of both grip force and load force to object weight such that lighter and heavier objects tend to be lifted in about the same amount of time. The scaling occurs prior to liftoff–before sensory information about object weight becomes available–and is therefore predictive. To deal with changes in friction, the motor system adjusts the balance between grip force and load force. As shown in Fig. 3B, when lifting equally weighted objects of varying slipperiness, people scale the rate of increase of grip force while keeping the rate of change of load force constant. Thus, the ratio of these force rates is a controlled parameter that is set to the current frictional conditions. A similar scaling of the grip-to-load force ratio is observed when object shape is varied. A larger

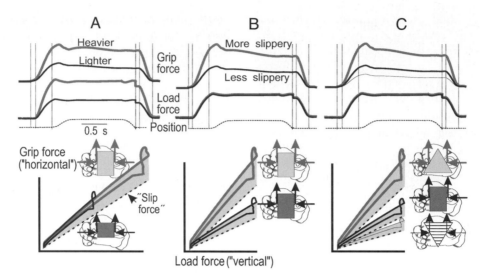

Figure 3 Feedforward adjustments of motor output to object weight (A), frictional conditions (B), and object shape (C) in a task in which a test object is lifted with a precision grip, held in air, and then replaced. The top graphs show horizontal grip force, vertical load force, and the vertical position of the object as a function of time for two superimposed trials. The bottom graphs show the relation between load force and grip force for the same trials. The dashed line indicates the minimum grip-to-load force ratio required to prevent slip. The gray area represents the safety margin against slip. After contact with the object (left most vertical line, top), grip force increases by a short period while the grip is established. A command is then released for simultaneous increases in grip and load force (second vertical line). This increase continues until the load force overcomes the force of gravity and the object lifts off (third vertical line). After replacement of the object and table contact occurs (fourth line), there is a short delay before the two forces decline in parallel (fifth line) until the object is released (sixth line) (adapted with permission from Johansson, R. S., and Westling, G., *Exp. Brain Res.* **56**, 550–564, 1984 by Springer-Verlag; Johansson, R. S., and Westling, G., *Exp. Brain Res.* **71**, 59–71, 1988. Copyright © 1988 by Springer-Verlag; and Jenmalm, P., and Johansson, R. S., *J. Neurosci.* **17**, 4486–4499, 1997 Copyright © 1997 by the Society for Neuroscience).

ratio is used when the grip surfaces are tapered upward compared to downward (Fig. 3C).

In each example shown in Fig. 3, grip force increases and decreases in phase with (and thus predicts) changes in vertical load force. This parallel coordination of grip force and load force ensures grasp stability. The grip force at any given load force is controlled such that it exceeds the corresponding minimum grip force, required to prevent slip, by a small safety margin (gray areas in the bottom of Fig. 3). This minimum grip force depends on the weight of the object, the friction between the object and skin, and the shape (e.g., angle) of the contact surfaces.

This parallel coordination of grip force and load force is a general feedforward control strategy and is not specific to any particular task or grip configuration. Parallel force coordination is observed when grasping with two or more digits of the same hand or both hands, when grasping with the palms of both hands, and even when gripping objects with the teeth. Moreover, it does not matter whether the object is moved by the arm or, for example, by the legs as when jumping with the object in hand. Importantly, the

parallel coordination of grip and anticipatory load force is not restricted to common inertial loads. People also adjust grip force in parallel with load force when pushing or pulling against immovable objects and when moving objects subjected to elastic and viscous loads. Figure 4 illustrates parallel coordination of grip and load forces under varying load conditions. People alternately pushed and pulled an object instrumented for force sensors and attached to a simple robot that could simulate various types of opposing loads acting tangential to the grasp surfaces (Fig. 4A). Figures 4B and 4C show kinematic and force records obtained under three different load conditions: an acceleration-dependent inertial load, a velocity-dependent viscous load, and an elastic load that largely depended on position but also contained viscous and inertial components. In all three cases, the grip force normal to the grasp surfaces changes in parallel with the magnitude of the load force tangential to the grasp surface. Importantly, the relationship between arm movement motor commands and the load experienced at the fingertips depends on the type of load being moved. Thus, to adjust grip force in parallel with load

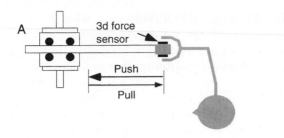

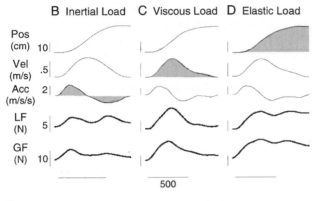

Figure 4 Kinematic and force records from one subject under the three load conditions. Shaded regions indicate the primary kinematic variable on which load depended. Under all three load conditions, grip force (GF) is adjusted in parallel with fluctuations in load force (LF), with the resultant load tangential to the grasp surface. The dashed vertical lines indicate movement onset (modified with permission from Flanagan, J. R., and Wing, A. M., *J. Neurosci.* **17**, 1519–1528, 1997. Copyright © 1997 by the Society for Neuroscience).

force under the different load conditions, people had to alter the mapping between the motor command driving arm movement and that driving the grip force.

In most everyday tasks, destabilizing loads acting on the grasp include not only linear load forces but also torques tangential to the grasped surfaces. Such torsional loads occur whenever we tilt an object around a grip axis that does not intersect the vertical line through the object's center of mass. In addition, torque loads arise in many natural manipulatory tasks due to changes in the orientation of the grip axis with respect to gravity. For example, this occurs when we hold a book flat by gripping it between the fingers beneath and the thumb above (vertical grip axis) and then rotate it by a pronation movement to put it in a bookshelf (horizontal grip axis). Because we rarely take a book such that the grip axis passes through its center of mass, a torque will develop in relation to the grasp. Importantly, the sensorimotor programs for object manipulation account for torsional loads by predicting the consequences of object rotation both

when we rotate objects around the grip axis and when we rotate the grip axis in the field of gravity. Rotational slips are prevented by automatic increases in grip force that parallel increases in tangential torque. The sensorimotor programs thus model the effect of the total load in terms of linear forces, tangential torques, and their combination.

C. Internal Models Underlying Predictive Force Control

As illustrated in Fig. 3A, with objects of different weight, people use different rates of force increase prior to liftoff. Since there is no sensory information available about object weight until liftoff, this behavior indicates that people predict the final force requirements. Likewise, with objects of different friction (Fig. 3B) and shape (Fig. 3C), the force output is tailored to the properties of the object from the start of the initial force attack, well before sensory information from the digits obtained after contact with the object could have exerted any influence. Thus, in all three cases, the motor controller operates in a feedforward fashion and uses motor command parameters determined by internal models that capture the physical properties of the object. Figure 4 further illustrates that such internal models also capture dynamic properties of objects. The question arises as to how such models are selected and updated for different objects and after changes in object properties.

1. Prediction Based on Object Shape

Figures 5A and 5B show three consecutive trials taken from a series of lifts in which the angle of the grasped surfaces was changed between trials in a pseudorandom order. The sequence is 30°, −30°, and −30° and thus includes a transition from an upward tapered object (30°) to a downward tapered object (−30°). In the trials preceding this sequence, a 30° object was lifted. First consider the trials in which vision of the objects is available (Fig. 5A). When the shape of the object is changed, the grip force is adjusted from the very start of the lift in anticipation of the lower grip force required to lift the object. In particular, grip force is now increased more slowly before sensory feedback from the digits could have influenced the motor output. The predictive adjustment in grip force observed in the first trial after the switch in object shape is very accurate. Indeed, no further adjustment is

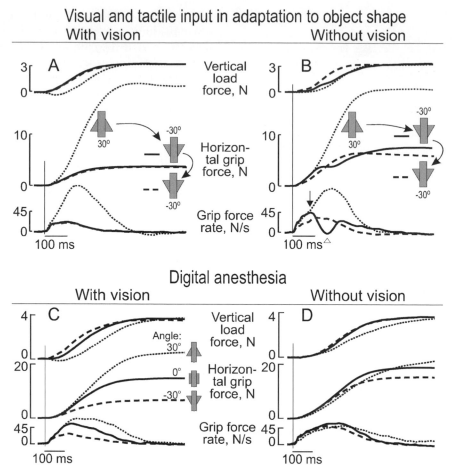

Visual and tactile input in adaptation to object shape

Figure 5 (A and B) Force adjustments to changes in surface angle during lift series in which surface angle was unpredictably varied between lift trials. Vertical load force, horizontal grip force, and grip force rate shown as a function of time for trials with (A) and without (B) vision and with normal digital sensibility. The dotted curves are from the last trial before the switch with the 30° object. The solid curves show the next trial with the −30° object. These curves illustrate adjustments to the smaller angle. The dashed lines show the following trial again with the −30° object. The downward arrow in B indicates the point in time when the new surface angle was expressed in terms of motor output. (C and D) Adaptation to surface shape during digital anesthesia with (C) and without (D) vision. Vertical load force, horizontal grip force, and grip force rate as a function of time for trials with 30° (dotted lines) 0° (solid lines and −30°, (dashed lines) surface angle (modified with permission from Jenmalm, P., and Johansson, R. S., *J. Neurosci.* **17**, 4486–4499, 1997. Copyright © 1997 by the Society of Neuroscience).

observed on the second trial after the change when information about shape has been obtained through tactile sensory signals. These results demonstrate that visual geometric cues can be used to efficiently specify the force coordination for object shape in a feedforward manner. These cues are used to parametrically adapt the finger force coordination to object shape in anticipation of the upcoming force requirements.

When vision of the object is not available, a very different pattern of force output is obtained. On the first trial after the switch to the −30° object, grip force develops initially according to the force requirements in the previous trial. This indicates that memory of the previous surface angle determines the default force

coordination in a feedforward manner. However, about 100 msec after the digits contacted the object, the grip force was modified and tuned appropriately for the actual surface angle (see first trial with the −30° in Fig. 5B). This amount of time is required to translate tactile information into motor commands, a process that likely involves supraspinal processing. By the second trial after the switch, the force output is appropriately adapted to the −30° surface angle from the onset of force application. Thus, an internal model related to object shape determines the force coordination in a feedforward fashion and tactile sensory information obtained at initial contact with the object mediates an updating of this model to changes in object shape. Furthermore, a single trial is enough to update the relevant internal model.

Sensors in the digits are thus used to update the force coordination for object shape when visual cues are unavailable or misleading. When digital sensibility is removed by local anesthesia, leaving neither visual nor somatosensory cues about shape, the adaptation in force output is severely impaired (Fig. 5D). Although grip force and load force still change in parallel, force output is no longer updated following contact. People adapt to the loss of both visual and tactile sensory cues about shape by applying strong grip forces regardless of surface angle. When vision is available during digital anesthesia, people are able to adapt their forces to object shape with only minor impairments (Fig. 5C). Thus, visual geometric cues can be used effectively for feedforward control even in the absence of somatosensory cues about shape.

The curvature of the grasp surfaces is another aspect of object shape. Surprisingly, the curvature of spherically curved symmetrical grasp surfaces has little effect on grip force requirements for grasp stability under linear force loads. However, it becomes acute in tasks involving torsional loads. The relationship between the grip force and tangential torque is parametrically scaled by surface curvature: For a given torque load, people increase grip force when curvature increases. As with linear force loads, this scaling of grip force is directly related to the minimum grip force required to prevent slip. Under torsional loads, people maintain a small but adequate safety margin against rotational slip. As with surface angle, visual information about surface curvature can be used for feedforward control of force. Likewise, people use cues provided by tactile afferents to adapt force once finger contact is established.

2. Prediction Based on Object Weight

When we manipulate familiar or common objects that we can identify either visually or haptically, we are extremely adept at selecting fingertip forces that are appropriately scaled to the weight of the object. That is, during the very first lift of a common object, before sensory information related to weight becomes available at liftoff, the force development is tailored to the weight of the object. This indicates that we can use visual and haptic cues to select internal models that we have acquired for familiar objects and can use these models to parametrically adjust our force output to object weight. For "families" of familiar objects that vary in size (e.g., screwdrivers, cups, soda cans, and

loafs of bread), we can exploit size–weight associations, in addition to object identity, to scale our force output in a feedforward fashion. However, as we have all experienced, our force output may sometimes be erroneous. Such situations can be created experimentally by unexpectedly changing the weight of a repeatedly lifted object without changing its visual appearance. In such cases, the lifting movement may be either jerky or slow. For example, if the object is lighter than expected from previous lifting trials, the load force and grip force drives will be too strong when the load force overcomes the force of gravity and liftoff takes place. Although somatosensory afferent events, evoked by the unexpectedly early liftoff, trigger an abrupt termination of the force drive, this occurs too late (due to control loop delays) to avoid an excessively high lift. Burst responses in FA II (Pacinian) afferents, which show an exquisite sensitivity to mechanical transients, most quickly and reliably signal the moment of liftoff. Conversely, if the object is heavier than expected, people will initially increase load force to a level that is not sufficient to produce liftoff and no sensory event will be evoked to confirm liftoff (Fig. 6A, solid curves). Importantly, this *absence* of a sensory event at the expected liftoff causes the release of a new set of motor commands. These generate a slow, discontinuous force increase until terminated by a neural event at the true liftoff (Fig. 6A, afferent response during the 800-g lift following the 400-g lift). Taken together, these observations indicate that control actions are taken as soon there is a mismatch between an expected sensory event and the actual sensory input. Thus, the absence of an expected sensory event may be as efficient as the occurrence of an unexpected sensory event in triggering compensatory motor commands. Moreover, this mismatch theory implies that somatosensory signals that represent the moment of liftoff are mandatory for the control of the force output whether or not the weight of the object is correctly anticipated. Finally, once an error occurs, the internal model of the object is updated to capture the new weight. In natural situations, this generally occurs in a single trial. As shown in Fig. 6A, in the trial after the switch trials when the weight of the object was unexpectedly increased from 400 to 800 g, the forces were correctly scaled for the greater weight (dashed curves).

3. Prediction Based on Friction

Whereas people use visual information about object size and shape to scale fingertip forces, there is no

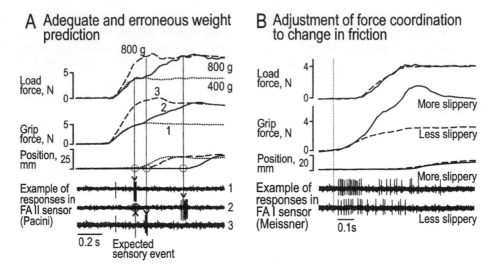

Figure 6 Single unit tactile afferent responses and adjustments in force to changes to object weight (A) and to the frictional condition between the object and the digits (B). Data are from single lift trials. (A) Three successive trials in which the subject lifted a 400-g object (dotted curves), an 800-g object (solid curves), and then the 800-g object again (dashed curves). The forces exerted in the first lift are adequately programmed because the subject had previously lifted the 400-g object. The forces are erroneously programmed in first lift of the 800-g object because they are tailored for the lighter 400-g object lifted in the previous trial. The vertical lines with arrowheads pointing downward indicate the moment of liftoff for each trial and they indicate the evoked sensory events exemplified by signals in a single FA II afferent. The absence of burst responses in FA II afferents at the expected point in time for the erroneously programmed 800-g trial is used to initiate a new control mode. This involves slow, discontinuous, and parallel increases in grip force and load force until terminated by sensory input signaling liftoff. (B) The influence of friction on force output and initial contact responses in a FA I unit. Two trials are superimposed, one with less slippery sandpaper (dashed lines) and a subsequent trial with more slippery silk (solid lines). The sandpaper trial was preceded by a trial with sandpaper and therefore the force coordination is initially set for the higher friction. The vertical line indicates initial touch (modified with permission from Johansson, R. S., and Westling, G., *Exp. Brain Res.* **66**, 141–154, 1987. Copyright © 1987 by Springer-Verlag; and from *Curr. Opin. Neurobiol.* Johansson, R. S., and Cole, K. J., **2**, 815–823, Copyright © 1992, with permission from Elsevier Science).

evidence that they use visual cues to control the balance of grip and load force for friction. However, tactile receptors in the fingertips are of crucial importance. The most important adjustment after a change in friction takes place shortly after the initial contact with the object and can be observed about 100 msec after contact (Fig. 6B). Prior to this force adjustment, there are burst responses in tactile afferents of different types but most reliably in the population of FA 1 (Meissner) afferents. The initial contact responses in subpopulations of excited FA I afferents are markedly influenced by the surface material as exemplified in Fig. 6B with a single afferent. The adjustment of force coordination to a change in frictional condition is based on the detection of a mismatch between the actual and an expected sensory event. This adjustment involves either an increase in the grip-to-load force ratio if the surface is more slippery than expected (as shown in Fig. 6B) or a decrease in the ratio of the surface if less slippery than expected. The adjustment also includes an updating of the internal model so as to capture the new frictional

conditions between the object and the skin for predictive control of the grip-to-load force ratio in further interactions with the object. However, sometimes these initial adjustments to frictional changes are inadequate and an accidental slip occurs at a later point, often at one digit only. Burst responses in dynamically sensitive tactile afferents to such slip events promptly trigger an automatic upgrading of the grip-to-load force ratio to a higher maintained level. This restores the grip force safety margin during subsequent manipulation by updating the internal model controlling the balance between grip and load force.

In summary, skilled manipulation involves two major types of control processes: *anticipatory parameter control* and *discrete event, sensory-driven control.* Anticipatory parameter control refers to the use of visual and somatosensory inputs, in conjunction with internal models, to tailor finger tip forces for the properties of the object to be manipulated prior to the execution of the motor commands. For familiar objects, visual and haptic information can be used to identify and select the appropriate internal model that is used to parametrically adapt motor commands, prior to their execution, in anticipation of the upcoming force requirements. People may also use geometric information (e.g., size and shape) for anticipatory control, relying on internal forward models capturing relationships between geometry and force requirements. There is ample evidence that the motor system makes use of internal models of limb mechanics, environmental objects, and task properties to adapt motor commands.

Discrete event, sensory-driven control refers to the use of somatosensory information to acquire, maintain, and update internal models related to object properties. This type of control is based on the comparison of actual somatosensory inflow and the predicted somatosensory inflow—an internal sensory signal referred to as corollary discharge. (The somatosensory input provided by tactile signals in the digital nerves is obviously critical in the control of skillful manipulation.) Thus, when we lift an object, we generate both efferent motor commands to accomplish the task and this internal sensory signal. Together, these are referred to as the sensorimotor program. Predicted sensory outcomes are produced by an internal forward model in conjunction with a copy of the motor command (referred to as an efference copy). Disturbances in task execution due to erroneous parameter specification of the sensorimotor program give rise to a mismatch between predicted and actual sensory input. For example, discrete somatosensory events may occur when not expected or may not occur when they are expected (Fig. 6A). Detection of such a mismatch triggers preprogrammed patterns of corrective responses along with an updating of the relevant internal models used to predict sensory events and estimate the motor commands required. This updating typically takes place within a single trial. With respect to friction and aspects of object shape, the updating primarily occurs during the initial contact with the object. In trials erroneously programmed for object weight and mass distribution, the updating takes place when the object starts to move (e.g., at liftoff in a lifting task).

III. ONTOGENETIC DEVELOPMENT OF SENSORIMOTOR CONTROL IN MANIPULATION

The ability to grasp using a precision grip involving the tips of the thumb and index finger first emerges in

humans at approximately 8–10 months of age. However, fully mature patterns of grasping, lifting, and holding objects are not observed until about 8 years of age. During this period, there is gradual improvement in grasping behavior as well as qualitative improvements in the capacity to produce independent finger movements. These changes parallel the gradual maturation of the ascending and descending neural pathways that link the hand with the cerebral cortex. These observations strongly suggest that the control of the skilled precision lifting and manipulation relies to a large extent on cerebral processes.

As noted previously, when adults lift objects, they increase grip force and load force in phase such that the two forces increase and decrease together. As a consequence, a linear relationship between these forces is observed (Figs. 3B, 3C, and 7B). The motor system adapts the slope of this relationship to factors such as the frictional conditions and the shape of the contact surfaces but robustly maintains this force synergy (Figs. 3B and 3C). However, before 18 months of age, children do not exhibit such parallel control of grip and load forces (Fig. 7). Instead, they tend to increase grip force in advance of the load force in a sequential fashion. The transition from sequential force coordination to the mature parallel coordination is not completed until several years later. Young children also produce comparably slow increases in fingertip force before liftoff and these increases are discontinuous, featuring multiple peaks in force rate (Fig. 7A). In contrast, adults smoothly increase grip force and load force with a single peak in force rate. The discontinuous or start-and-stop force increases observed in young children suggest that they employ a feedback control strategy rather than feedforward control. That is, they continue to increase force in small increments until liftoff occurs. It is not until they receive somatosensory information that liftoff has occurred that they stop these increases. This feedback strategy is similar to that observed when adults underestimate the weight of an object and then have to increase force again until liftoff occurs (Fig. 6B, solid lines). These observations suggest that young children may not have the cognitive resources for accurate feedforward control.

In addition, very young children appear to be relatively inefficient at integrating sensory information into sensorimotor programs. In precision lifting, people start to increase grip force and load force soon after the digits contact the object. Signals from tactile afferents related to object contact trigger the next phase of the lift. In very young children, there is a

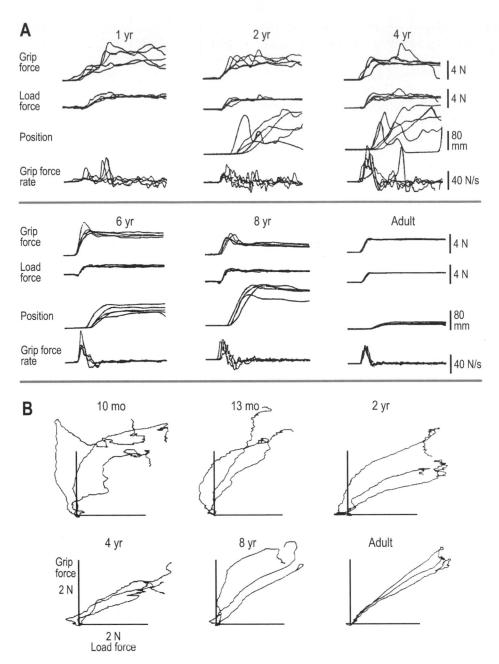

Figure 7 Ontogenetic development of the coordination of grip and load forces during precision lifting. (A) Grip force, load force, and grip force rate as a function of time during several consecutive trials (superimposed) for individual children of various ages and an adult. Note the large variability and excessive grip forces used by young children compared to the adults. (B) Relationship between grip force and load force during the initial parts of lifting trials by children of various ages and an adult. Note the nonparallel increase in grip and load forces for young children compared to adults. (A and B) Surface material and object's weight are constant (adapted with permission from Forssberg, H., Eliasson, A. C., Kinoshita, H., Johansson, R. S., and Westling, G., *Exp. Brain Res.* **85,** 451–457, 1991. Copyright © 1991 by Springer-Verlag).

relatively long delay between initial contact and the onset of increases in grip and load force. This long delay indicates immature control of hand closure and inefficient triggering of the motor commands by cutaneous afferents. The decrease in this delay during subsequent years parallels a maturation of cutaneous reflexes of the hand as assessed by electrophysiological methods.

During the latter part of the second year, children begin to use sensorimotor memory, obtained from previous lifts, for scaling forces in anticipation of object weight. However, adult-like lifting performance with precise control of the load force for smooth object acceleration does not appear until 6–8 years of age. At about 3 years of age, children start to use vision for weight estimation through size–weight associations for classes of related objects. Thus, additional cognitive development is apparently required before the necessary associative size–weight mapping can take place. Unlike adults, once children begin to use visual size cues, they are unable to suppress adequately their influence when the cues are misleading (i.e., in situations in which weight and size do not reliably covary). This observation is consistent with the view that vision has a particularly strong influence on motor coordination in children. Thus, the context-related selective suppression of visual cues appears to require even further cognitive development.

Young children display a limited capacity to adapt the ratio of grip force and load force to frictional conditions. These children use unnecessarily high grip forces in trials with high friction (or low slipperiness) and their behavior is reminiscent of that of adults with impaired digital sensibility. This increased grip force may be a strategy to compensate for immature tactile control of precision grip because overgripping will prevent slips when handling slippery objects. Nevertheless, even the youngest children (1–2 years) show some capacity to adjust grip force to friction if the frictional conditions are kept constant over several consecutive precision grip lifts. The need for repetitive lifts suggests a poor capacity to form sensorimotor memory related to friction and/or to use this memory to control force output. Older children require fewer lifts to update effectively their force coordination to new frictional conditions, and adults require only one lift.

IV. DISSOCIATIONS AND INTERACTIONS BETWEEN PERCEPTION AND ACTION

An important concept in neuroscience is the idea that sensory information is processed in multiple pathways for different uses. For example, in the visual system, there is strong evidence that neural systems that process visual information for use in guiding action are at least partly distinct from neural systems involved in processing visual information for perception and cognitive reasoning. Similarly, there is evidence that sensory information obtained from the hand can have differential effects on action and perception. Here, we discuss evidence for a dissociation between perception and action related to hand movement. However, first we discuss how manipulatory actions can influence perception.

A. Influences of Action on Weight Perception

Because haptic perception of objects generally involves manipulation, the question arises as to whether the perception of particular object properties is influenced by other object properties or by the way in which the object is handled. For example, does the perceived weight of an object depend on the angle of its contact surfaces or the friction between the object and the digits, both of which influence the grip force required to lift the object? Here, one question is whether the grip forces in lifting influence weight perception even though the grip forces are not directly involved in overcoming the force of gravity. For example, does the greater effort required to lift a slippery object give rise to the perception of it being heavier than a less slippery object of the same weight?

More than 150 years ago, Ernst Heinrich Weber observed that the ability to discriminate weight is better when the weights are actively lifted by the hand than when they are supported by a passive hand. This observation suggests that a sense of effort, associated with voluntary muscular exertion, contributes to the perception of weight. Although afferent signals contribute to weight perception, at least under some conditions there is ample evidence that effort, defined as the level of central or efferent drive, contributes to weight perception. The idea is that when we generate motor commands to lift an object, a copy of the commands (efference copy) generates an internal sensation (corollary discharge) that influences perceived weight. The centrally generated sensation is referred to as the sense of effort.

Figure 8A shows the results of an experiment in which people were asked to compare the weights of a reference object and a series of randomly presented test objects of varying weight both heavier and lighter than the weight of the reference. The test objects had the same size and shape as the reference object, and the objects were lifted using a precision grip with the tips of the index fingers on either side. In one condition, the reference object was covered in less slippery sandpaper and the test objects were covered in more slippery satin (Fig. 8, solid circles and solid curve), whereas in a second condition the reference object was covered in satin and the test objects were cover in sandpaper

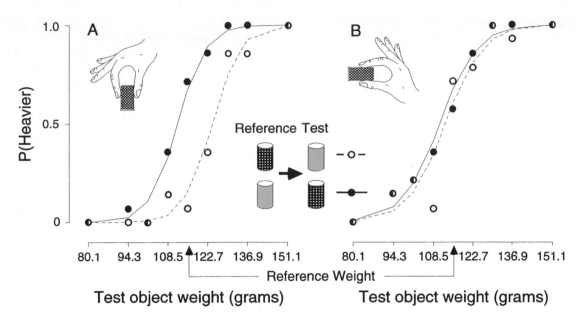

Figure 8 Probability ($n=14$) of responding that the test canister is lighter than the previously lifted reference canister as a function of the test canister weight. In different experiments, the canisters were lifted with either a vertical (A) or horizontal (B) precision grip. Open circles and dashed lines code the condition in which the test canister was covered in less slippery satin, and the closed circles and solid lines code the condition in which the test canister was covered in less slippery sandpaper. The triangles indicate the reference weight (modified with permission from Flanagan, J. R., Wing, A. M., Allison, S., and Spencely, A., *Perception Psychophys.* **57**, 282–290, 1995).

(Fig. 8, open circles and dashed curve). Figure 8A shows the probability of judging the test object to be heavier than the reference as a function of the weight of the test object. In both conditions, when the test object is much heavier (151.1 g) than the reference (115.6 g) the test object is always judged to be heavier. Conversely, when the test object is much lighter (80.1 g), it is never judged to be heavier. However, in between these extremes, the probability of judging the test object to be heavier is greater when the test object is covered in slippery satin. (Note that there is a general tendency to judge the second of two successively lifted weights, in this case the test object, to be heavier.) This indicates that when lifting with the fingertips on the sides of the object, a more slippery object is judged heavier than an equally weighted object that is less slippery. One interpretation of the results shown in Fig. 8A is that humans judge the more slippery object to be heavier because the grip force used in lifting is greater. When people hold the reference and test objects with a horizontal grip (Fig. 8B), in which surface slipperiness has little influence on the required grip force, there is no effect of surface slipperiness on weight perception.

The results shown in Fig. 8A suggest that people fail to fully distinguish between the effort related to grip force and that related to load force when judging weights lifted with a precision grip. However, this overflow effect may only pertain to muscle actions that are functionally related. Support for this view comes from the observation that the perceived heaviness of a given weight, lifted by one digit, increases if a concurrent weight is lifted by any other digit of the same hand. When the foot or other hand lifts the concurrent weight, the perceived heaviness is not affected.

Although differences in grip force influence weight perception when these differences are determined by frictional conditions, grip force does not appear to influence perceived heaviness when it is manipulated by changing surface shape. When people compare the weights of triangular blocks lifted either on the angled or flat side, there is no effect of angle of perceived weight. It may be that when the grip force requirements strongly match those prescribed by visual cues, people suppress the effort related to grip force differences in evaluating weight. Recall that visual cues related to surface angle can be used effectively for feedforward force control but that there is no evidence that visual information related to frictional condition can be exploited for anticipatory force control.

B. Independent Sensorimotor and Perceptual Predictions of Weight

As discussed previously, people use visual information about object size and shape to estimate parametrically the impending force requirements in manipulation. Thus, people will increase grip and load force more rapidly when lifting a large object than a similar looking small object. This feedforward strategy takes advantage of the link between size and weight that normally pertains to a class or family of similar objects; for example, big cups should weigh more than small ones. However, it fails when this link is altered. In such a case, people must rely on reactive control mechanisms to correct for their erroneous prediction and on feedback mechanisms to tune the internal models used for predictive control. Such a situation arises in the classic size–weight illusion in which people are asked to compare the weights of two equally weighted objects of similar form but unequal size. This illusion, first documented more than 100 years ago, refers to the fact that people reliably judge the smaller of the two objects to be heavier when lifted, even after many lifting trials.

A leading theory of the size–weight illusion is that the illusion arises from a mismatch between predicted and actual sensory feedback. The idea is that when we lift the smaller object, the actual sensory feedback about liftoff will not occur when predicted and the object will thus be judged heavier. Conversely, the larger object, which is lighter than expected, will be judged heavier.

The sensory mismatch seems entirely plausible when one considers lifting the two equally weighting objects the very first time. Here, visual size cues will be misleading and we would expect people to use too much force for the larger object and too little force for the smaller object. However, we also know that people acquire sensorimotor memory related to object weight over repeated lifts. The question arises whether people will continue to misjudge the force required when repeatedly lifting large and small objects of equal weight. Figure 9 reveals the answer. People were asked to repeatedly lift a small and a large cube (Fig. 9A) in alternation. Predictably, when the two objects are lifted for the first time, the forces required for the large object are overestimated and the forces required for the small object are underestimated (Fig. 9B, left). Compensatory, reflex-mediated adjustments in force are triggered in either case. When lifting the small object, the initial increase in grip force and load force is too small and liftoff does not occur when expected. As

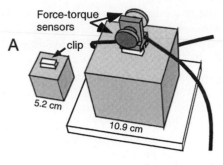

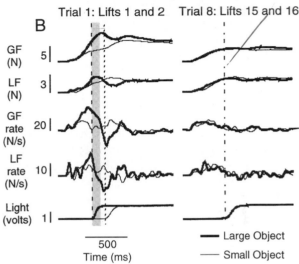

Figure 9 Independent sensorimotor and perceptual predictions of weight. (A) Drawing showing the relative sizes of two equally weighted cubes. Subjects lifted the cubes using a precision grip with the tips of the index finger and thumb on either side of a handle. The handle was attached by clips located on top and in the center of each object. The handle was instrumented with two sensors that measure the forces and torques applied by each digit. Plastic contact disks (3 cm in diameter) were mounted on each sensor and covered in medium-grain sandpaper. A light-sensitive diode embedded into the center of the lifting platform recorded liftoff. (B) Grip force (GF), load force (LF), grip and load force rates, and light-sensitive diode recorded in the first trial (lifts 1 and 2) and the eighth trial (lifts 15 and 16). The subjects lifted the large object (thick traces) and then the small object (thin traces) in each trial. In all trials, subjects grasped the object and increased grip and load force together until liftoff, signaled by the light diode, occurred. In the first trial, peak grip and load force rates were scaled to object size, whereas by the eighth trial the peak force rates were similar for the two objects and appropriately scaled to object weight. Although the subjects adapted their motor output to the true object weights, they still reported verbally that the small object was heavier (adapted with permission from Flanagan, J. R., and Beltzner, M. A., *Nature Neurosci.* **3,** 737–741, 2000).

a result, the forces increase again until liftoff is achieved. When lifting the large object, overshoots occur in the grip and load forces and liftoff occurs earlier than expected. The unexpected early liftoff triggers a decrease in force approximately 100 msec later. However, a very different pattern of force output is observed by the time the cubes are lifted for the eighth time (Fig. 9B, right). Now the force and force rate functions for the small and large cubes are very similar and liftoff occurs at about the same time for both cubes. In contrast to the initial lift trials, grip and load force neither overshoot nor undershoot their final levels, and no corrective adjustments in force are observed. These results illustrate that people adapted their force output, and thus their sensory predictions used for force control, to the actual object weights. Thus, sensorimotor memory about object weight, obtained from previous lifts and based on somatosensory information, comes to dominate visual size cues in terms of feedforward force control.

Although the motor system gradually adapts force output to the true, equal weights of the size–weight stimuli, the perceptual system that mediates awareness of object weight does not adapt. After lifting the two cubes 20 times each, people still reported that the small object was heavier. Moreover, the strength of the size–weight illusion—measured using magnitude estimation techniques—is equally strong. That people experience the size–weight illusion while accurately predicting the fingertip forces required for lifting clearly debunks the theory that the perceptual illusion is accounted for by a sensory mismatch. Instead, the results indicate that the illusion can be caused by high-level cognitive factors. Although the size–weight illusion occurs while there is no evidence of mismatch at the sensorimotor level, the mismatch theory may still operate at a purely perceptual level. For example, people may continue to make erroneous *perceptual* predictions about weight based specifically on visual size cues. A mismatch between these perceptual predictions and actual sensory feedback may give rise to the size-weight illusion. This implies separate comparison processes for perceptual and sensorimotor predictions.

The finding that people continue to experience the size–weight illusion even though they learn to make accurate sensorimotor predictions about object weight indicates that sensorimotor systems can operate independently of perceptual systems. This idea is supported by a growing body of research on visuomotor control showing that partly distinct neural pathways are used depending on whether the sensory information is used to control actions or make perceptual judgments.

See Also the Following Articles

LEFT-HANDEDNESS • MOTION PROCESSING • MOTOR CONTROL • MOTOR SKILL • NEUROFEEDBACK • OBJECT PERCEPTION • SPATIAL VISION • TACTILE PERCEPTION • VISUAL AND AUDITORY INTEGRATION

Suggested Reading

Flanagan, J. R., and Beltzner, M. A. (2000). Independence of perceptual and sensorimotor predictions in the size–weight illusion. *Nature Neurosci.* **3**, 737–741.

Johansson, R. S. (1998). Sensory input and control of grip. In *Sensory Guidance of Movement. Novartis Foundation Symposium, 218* (pp. 45–59). Wiley, Chichester, UK.

Jones, L. A. (1986). Perception of force and weight: Theory and research. *Psychol. Bull.* **100**, 29–42.

Lemon, R. N. (1993). The G. L. Brown Prize lecture. Cortical control of the primate hand. *Exp. Physiol.* **78**, 263–301.

MacKenzie, C. L., and Iberall, T. (1994). *The Grasping Hand.* North-Holland, Amsterdam.

Napier, J. R. (1980). *Hands.* Allen & Unwin, London.

Porter, R., and Lemon, R. N. (1993). *Corticospinal Function and Voluntary Movement.* Oxford Univ. Press, Oxford.

Wing, A. M., Haggard, P., and Flanagan, J. R. (Eds.) (1996). *Hand and Brain: Neurophysiology and Psychology of Hand Movement.* Academic Press, San Diego.

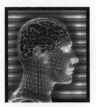

Headaches

SEYMOUR DIAMOND and GEORGE J. URBAN

Diamond Headache Clinic and Finch University of Health Sciences, Chicago, Illinois

GLOSSARY

aura A complex of focal neurological symptoms mostly in a visual form preceding some migraine attacks.

basilar Originating from the basilar artery at the base of the skull, supplying the brain stem.

biofeedback A behavioral treatment, relaxation technique that involves displaying, on monitors, some physiologic functions with the goal of attaining voluntary control over them.

hemiparesis Weakness of one side of the body.

hemiplegic Related to total paralysis of one side of the body.

ophthalmoplegia Weakness of one or more ocular nerves leading to double vision.

osmophobia Sensitivity to odors.

phonophobia An increased sensitivity to sound.

photophobia An increased sensitivity to light.

postdrome A set of symptoms occurring following remission of the headache.

prodrome A set of symptoms starting as early as 48 hr before the onset of a headache.

rebound headache A headache caused by or worsened by the withdrawal of analgesics, ergotamine, or caffeine.

status migrainosus Migraine attack lasting more than 72 hr.

Headache is defined by *Webster's* **as "a pain in the head"** and "a vexation or baffling situation or problem." Attempting to understand the source of headaches, and efforts at selecting appropriate treatment, is indeed a vexing problem. Headache is one of the oldest and the most common medical complaints, with references to it as early as 4000 BC. In the United States, the prevalence of headaches is about 70%. Headache has an enormous socioeconomic impact on society and personal lives. Headache can be a primary disorder or a symptom of another disease of benign or malignant origin, and it can occur at any age. The most simple classification divides headache types into three major categories; vascular (migraine and cluster), tension type, and traction and inflammatory (organic). Every major type of headache is defined, and the clinical picture, pathophysiology, and therapy are described.

I. VASCULAR HEADACHES

A. Migraine

By definition, migraine is an idiopathic, recurring headache disorder manifesting in attacks lasting 4–72 hr (untreated or unsuccessfully treated), usually unilateral location, of pulsating quality, and of moderate to severe intensity that may inhibit or prohibit daily activities. Pain is aggravated by routine physical activity and is associated with nausea and/or vomiting, photophobia, and phonophobia. History, physical, and neurological examinations do not suggest a secondary headache due to other disorders.

Migraine is an inherited neurological condition. A parental history can be obtained in 50–60% of patients with migraine. The form of inheritance has not been identified, although some genetic studies suggest an autosomal-dominant type in familial hemiplegic migraine. For the more frequent types of migraine, genetic influence is less clear.

Migraine has a marked impact on the economy and society. Surveys show that 8% of men and 14% of women miss all or part of a day of work or school in any given month. In the United States, the annual cost of lost productivity due to migraine has been estimated between $5.6 and $17.2 billion.

1. Clinical Features

Typically, there are five stages of a migraine attack: the prodrome, the aura, the headache, resolution, and the postdrome. The two major types of migraine are distinguished by the occurrence of an aura, a set of warning symptoms, that can precede the headache by 10–60 min. Migraine with aura was previously known as classical migraine, and migraine without aura was common migraine.

The aura is a complex set of focal neurological symptoms that precedes or accompanies an attack and may occur in almost 40% of patients, although not necessarily before each acute migraine headache. The frequency of aura may vary. The most common and most recognizable aura is visual occurring in more than 90% of patients with aura. There are three groups of visual aura: positive—fortification spectra or zigzag lines, flashing of lights and colors, stars, circles, and angles mostly appearing in both visual fields and migrating across the visual field at the rate of 3 mm per minute; negative—scotoma or blind spots, transient loss of vision, grayout, whiteout, heat waves, or the opaque glass-like experience; and metamorphopsia —illusion of distorted size, shape, and location of fixed object and Alice in Wonderland syndrome consisting of complex visual hallucinations. Other auras may consist of sensory phenomena (occurring in 30% of patients), such as numbness in the extremities and/or face, which may be fixed or may migrate. Motor disturbances (6%) and difficulty speaking or understanding language (18%) can also occur. The headache following the aura has rapid onset and graduation, is more lateralized, and has the same quality as the migraine without aura.

During the prodrome phase, patients with migraine with aura or migraine without aura may experience vague symptoms. These forerunners may precede the attack by up to 48 hr and gradually increase in intensity up to the headache onset. These signs are usually ambiguous and consist of mental, neurological, or generalized constitutional symptoms. Mental symptoms include euphoria, depression, restlessness, irritability, mental slowness, fatigue, drowsiness, and hyperactivity. Neurological symptoms may include hypersensitivity to light, sound, and smells. Constitutional symptoms may present with a feeling of cold, sluggishness, thirst, increased urination, fluid retention, decreased appetite or food craving, diarrhea or constipation, or equivocal symptoms of non-well-being.

The onset of headache is usually gradual. The pain is unilateral in 60% and on both sides in 40% of cases. The pain is localized most commonly in the temple, but it may radiate to the upper or posterior part of the head, including the neck and shoulders. Pain may travel from one part to the other or from one side to the other, or it may become generalized. Scalp tenderness may also develop in about two-thirds of patients. The headache usually last from 4 to 72 hr; in children, the headache may be briefer. The pain peaks and then subsides, but in some patients it may plateau for longer intervals. The pain varies in intensity, from annoying to debilitating, and is described as throbbing, pulsating, deep-seated pressure or aching and can be aggravated by routine physical activity such as walking or moving the head. During an attack, patients prefer to remain still in a dark and quiet room.

Accompanying symptoms are very common and are one of the criteria for migraine. The most common associated symptoms are gastrointestinal disturbances, including anorexia, nausea in more than 80%, vomiting in more than 50%, and diarrhea in 16%. Stomach motility is reduced as well as the absorption from the stomach including medications. Neurophysiological accompaniments include photophobia in 82%, phonophobia, blurred vision, osmophobia, lightheadedness in more than 70%, vertigo in one-third of patients; short-lasting numbness and weakness, and mood and mental changes. Visible distension of veins and arteries on the forehead and temples is not unusual. Fluid retention with edema and weight gain may occur in a weight-dependent part of the body, such as the feet, ankles, legs, face, and around the eyes. Increased urination may occurs during and after the headache.

Vomiting and sleeping may be the culmination of the migraine attack leading to the recovery phase. Following the headache, during the postdrome, patients may feel tired, irritable, exhausted, and washed out, may describe hangover-like symptoms, and may experience impaired concentration, muscle aching, and anorexia.

About one-third of migraineurs report severe disability with their attacks. It is estimated that in the United States approximately 30 million individuals experience severe migraine headache. Twenty-five percent of migraine sufferers experience four or more severe attacks per month, 35% experience one to three severe attacks per month, and the remaining migraine sufferers complain of one or less severe attacks per month.

2. Diagnostic Features

Initial onset of migraine usually occurs during adolescence or the early twenties, but it can start in childhood. In a classic study from Sweden, headaches of all types increase in a stepwise manner between ages 7 and 15. By age 15, 5% of all children have experienced a migraine, and another 15% complain of daily or almost daily tension-type headaches. In a follow-up completed 40 years later, in girls from age 11 years, there was a gradual increase in migraine headache. The original subgroup of 73 children with migraine reported being headache-free by age 25, with a more significant number of males reporting complete migraine remission. The data from an epidemiological study in Washington County, Maryland, revealed that 56% of boys and 74% of girls between the ages of 12 and 17 complained of a headache during the past month. Migraine prevalence (i.e., the proportion of the population with the disease) increases from 12 to 38 years of age in both females and males and is highest between ages 25 and 55 years. The lifetime prevalence of migraine ranges between 14 and 18%. However, many migraine sufferers remain undiagnosed. The highest incidence of new cases of migraine peaks between ages 12 and 17. In older patients, the prodromal aura symptoms may continue after the headaches disappear. Initial onset of migraine is rarely reported after age 50 years.

In children under the age of 14 years, no significant difference in migraine prevalence has been demonstrated. The female-to-male ratio is suggested to be between 2:1 and 3:1. This proportion peaks at about age 42, but thereafter it declines.

Migraine can start at any time of the day, and in many cases the headache will be present upon awakening. In some patients, the acute migraine attack will occur after a stressful episode or on weekends or vacations—the so-called "let down" headaches. Migraine patients may be hyperresponsive to various internal and external stimuli that, under certain conditions, can provoke a migraine attack. Environmental precipitants include weather changes (in 50% of migraineurs), high humidity, glare, bright light, fluorescent lighting, high altitude, cigarette smoke, and pungent odors. Nitrites, monosodium glutamate,

tyramine, aspartame, histamine, and other chemicals contained in certain foods or beverages are recognized migraine precipitants. Alcohol, chocolate, aged cheeses, pickled, cured and fermented products, caffeinated drinks, and nuts are frequently named offenders for susceptible migraine sufferers. Too much or lack of sleep as well as jet-lag, alternating shift work, and physical exertion can provoke migraine.

Emotional stress of positive or negative character, anxiety, anticipation, anger, fear, and worry are common precipitants. Menstruation or other hormonal changes, including hormonal treatment (oral contraceptives or hormone replacement therapy), play a major role in migraine in 60% of female migraineurs. Some medications, including nitroglycerine, blood pressure agents, antidepressants, and arthritis agents, as well as vitamins and herbal remedies in excess, can provoke an acute migraine attack.

3. Pathophysiology

The mechanism of the attack is still poorly understood. Three basic pathophysiological changes take place during the process of migraine: vascular, neurogenic, and neuropeptides abnormalities or dysfunction. It is unclear which process is primary and which is secondary. In the brain stem of migraine patients, there is evidence of a dysfunctional area of neurons, a so-called "central migraine generator," with abnormal reactivity to varying internal or external stimuli. This dysfunction is a result of genetic abnormalities and leads to a cascade of pathophysiological alterations producing the migraine attack. Initially, vasoconstriction occurs in the blood vessels of the brain, during the prodromal or aura stage. When a stimulus crosses a pain threshold, which differs in every individual and is determined by a complexity of physiological and emotional conditions, the migraine generator sends signals that lead to dilation of certain blood vessels in the brain. Migraine pain is thought to arise when intracranial blood vessels become dilated and as a consequence activate the terminals of trigeminal sensory nerves that surround them. Activation of those terminals leads to release of vasoactive neuropeptides, such as calcitonin gene-related peptide, substance P, bradykinin, prostaglandin, and other neurokinins. Vasoactive neuropeptides exacerbate blood vessel swelling and increase pain transmission back to the brain stem. From there, the signals are relayed to higher cortical centers, where the migraine pain is registered and other symptoms are produced, including nausea, vomiting, and photo- and phonophobia. Serotonin and serotonin receptors play a major role in this cascade and mediate many of these processes.

4. Therapy

Migraine therapy can be classified into four types: general measures, abortive therapy, pain relief measures, and prophylactic (preventive) therapy. Overall, the treatment consists of behavioral and pharmacological interventions and is individualized for each patient. General measures includes behavioral therapy, such as recognition and avoidance of migraine triggers, regulation of sleep and meal schedules, dietary modification, stress management, exercise, and biofeedback and other relaxation techniques.

The other three types of migraine treatment include pharmacological agents. Abortive medications used to stop the process of migraine in its development include the triptans, ergotamine preparations, and isometheptene. These drugs act on serotonin receptor sites, reducing activation of neuropeptides as well as constricting dilated intracranial blood vessels.

If abortive therapy is unsuccessful, the pain relief measures are indicated to reduce the symptoms of migraine, such as pain, nausea, vomiting, irritability, and anxiety. The agents used for symptomatic treatment include single or combined analgesics, antinauseants, nonsteroidal antiinflammatory agents (NSAIDs), sedatives, and tranquilizers.

Prophylactic treatment is instituted to reduce the frequency, duration, and intensity of migraine attacks. It may be considered if the patient is experiencing more than two migraine attacks per month or if the severity of the headache and its associated symptoms impact on the individual's ability to function. Beta blockers, methysergide, and divalproex sodium have been approved for the indication of migraine prophylactic therapy. Other medications that have been beneficial in migraine treatment include the calcium channel blockers, anticonvulsants, NSAIDs, and antidepressants.

5. Other Forms of Migraine

Migraine with prolonged aura, perviously termed complicated or hemiplegic migraine, is characterized by one or more aura symptoms lasting more than 60 min and less than 1 week. Any of the various forms of aura may occur. This type of migraine is relatively rare.

The headache usually starts within 1 hr of aura onset, becomes progressively more intense, and may linger for a prolonged period. Different forms of aura can be experienced at the same time. The intensity of the pain is usually less than that in the more common types of migraines. The aura persists into the headache stage and may continue after the pain subsides. The typical clinical features of the headache are the same with this complicated form of migraine.

The etiology or mechanism of migraine with prolonged aura and related symptoms is unclear. It has been assumed that a neurological deficit of longer duration is caused by prolonged vasoconstriction or limited spasm of a cerebral artery occurring as a part of the migraine syndrome. It appears that the constriction is probably secondary as the part of a complex cascade of migraine process. Computed tomography (CT) scan and magnetic resonance imaging performed during the attack of a migraine with prolonged aura show no abnormalities.

In patients with this form of migraine, risk factors such as smoking and estrogen use should be avoided. Hypertension and diabetes should be treated vigorously. Vasodilatory medications, such as calcium channel blockers mainly of a rapid onset of action (e.g., sublingual nifedipine) and sublingual nitroglycerine, have been shown to be effective in prompt alleviation of prolonged aura or neurological symptoms. Similar effects have been demonstrated with isoproterenol, administration of CO_2, and papaverine. These vasodilators are known to cause headache. However, interestingly, if they are used at the onset of an attack, the headache does not occur or is lessened. The use of ergotamine and triptans is controversial and generally not recommended due to the increased risk of complications such as stroke.

a. Hemiplegic Migraine Hemiplegic attacks usually start during childhood. The headache may occasionally precede the hemiparesis or be absent. The onset of hemiparesis may be abrupt, lasting for days, and may imitate a stroke. The headache is on same side as the weakness in about 20% of patients, on the other side in almost 50%, and can be generalized in 30%. Nausea and vomiting are unusual. Speech difficulty occurs in about 44% of patients in association with hemiparesis, and confusion can occur in one-third. The diminished sensitivity of the half of the body or extremities on one side accompanies the weakness. Visual aura and hemiparesis occur together in 88%. In most patients, the weakness continued for up to 1 hr, in 14% it lasted for up to 3 hr, in 12% from 3 to 24 hr, and in 16% of patients between 1 day and 1 week. The longer lasting episodes are associated with more profound weakness. A higher incidence of neurological symptoms accompanying the migraine attacks has been noticed in middle-aged patients. Hemiplegic migrainous attacks occur infrequently and irregularly. Typically, the patients experience complete recovery.

b. Ophthalmoplegic Migraine In this form of complicated migraine, repeated attacks of headache are associated with paresis of one or more of the ocular cranial nerves in the absence of demonstrable intracranial lesions. It is relatively rare, and its victims are usually children, affecting males six times more often than females. Adults may experience their first attack during the fourth and fifth decade. The most commonly affected nerve is the third cranial nerve (oculomotor), occasionally the fourth and sixth nerves are affected, and the ophthalmic division of the fifth cranial nerve may also be involved. The headache that precedes the ocular symptoms is of migrainous quality, usually localized behind or around the affected orbit with radiation to the same side of the head. The pain may last 1–4 days, and as it subsides other symptoms appear—the ptosis (droopy eyelid) on the same side, diplopia (double vision), and blurred vision. The ophthalmoplegia may persist for several weeks but usually completely resolves. After repeated attacks, some weakness of the ocular muscles may persist with permanently dilated pupil and deviated eye.

The isolated involvement of the cranial ocular nerves suggests that the anatomic localization of the lesion is the cavernous sinus. Research demonstrated narrowing in the internal carotid artery, probably due to edema of the wall. The swelling of the carotid wall is probably responsible for compression of the involved nerve or reduced blood flow to the nerve through the nourishing arteries.

These attacks are treated symptomatically with analgesics and antinauseants. Corticosteroids in large doses, instituted at the beginning of the attack of ophthalmoplegia, may reduce inflammation and edema and hasten the recovery. Ergotamine agents and triptans should not be used during the acute attacks as abortive drugs because it is unknown if the vasoconstricting effect of these medications would not further reduce the blood flow to the affected nerve. Prophylactic drugs are indicated if the attacks occur frequently. Neuroimaging is imperative to exclude an aneurysm or tumor.

c. Familial Hemiplegic Migraine This form of migraine with aura, which may be prolonged, includes some degree of hemiparesis and is characterized by the patient having at least one first-degree relative with identical attacks. The pattern of occurrence in family members suggests that familial hemiplegic migraine is an autosomal-dominant genetic disease. Researchers have found a locus on chromosome 19 in the majority of the investigated families.

d. Basilar Migraine This type of complicated migraine is also known as basilar artery migraine, Bickerstaff's migraine, and syncopal migraine. Its symptoms clearly originate from the brain stem or from both occipital lobes. To fulfill the criteria, two or more aura symptoms must be of the following types: visual symptoms in both the temporal and nasal fields of both eyes, difficulty articulating, vertigo, tinnitus, decreased hearing, double vision, ataxia (difficulty controlling bodily movements), numbness on both sides of body, weakness and numbness on both sides of the body, and decreased level of consciousness.

Originally considered to be mainly a migraine disorder of adolescent girls, it affects all age groups and both sexes. These attacks often occur with relationship to menstruation. The aura commonly lasts less than 1 hr. The neurological symptoms, of various duration, are consistent with dysfunction of the posterior part of brain supplied by the vertebrobasilar artery system. These symptoms usually precede the headache but may also begin during the actual headache. Typically, the numbness is bilateral, starting in the periphery of all four extremities, with slow and gradual radiating up the limbs. Confusion and disorientation are not uncommon. Syncopal episode occurs in 7% of the patients with this form of migraine. Various levels of decreased consciousness, including stupor and coma, can last for hours or days. The headache of basilar migraine is often bilateral and localized in the posterior part of the head, but it may radiate to the temporal and frontal areas. The pain is of a pulsatile quality and moderate in intensity. Associated nausea may become severe and progress to prolonged and intractable vomiting. Commonly, the attack ends with sleep. Typical attacks of basilar migraine infrequently occur in these patients, and more common forms of migraine occur in between the attacks. Basilar migraine is very rare after the fourth decade, and any episode in this circumstance should be considered nonmigraine in origin. Symptoms of basilar migraine are consistent with a disturbance in the vertebrobasilar artery supplying the territory of the brain stem and brain and are probably the result of ischemic changes.

6. Migraine Aura without Headaches

Another term for migraine equivalent is acephalic migraine, which is a migrainous aura unaccompanied by headache. It is quite common in individuals with migraine with aura to experience the aura with the headache absent. As patients age, the headache may lessen in frequency and eventually disappear, even if the aura continues. Recurring symptoms of aura for which no underlying organic cause has been found should be considered a possible manifestation of migraine aura without headache or a migraine equivalent. These symptoms may occur in a person with a strong family history of migraine or who has previously experienced attacks of migraine. Symptoms of aura without headache may occur in 20% of all migraineurs and in more than 40% of patients who have migraine with aura. Symptoms usually last about 20–30 min and only occasionally for longer periods. The most common symptoms are visual. They have a similar presentation as the typical aura. Patients with monocular visual defects should be evaluated to exclude the presence of ocular or other diseases. The recurrent abdominal pain and cyclic vomiting may also represent a migrainous phenomenon but only after organic disease has been excluded. The neurological episodic symptoms may represent this form of migraine and include numbness, weakness, vertigo, confusion, and amnesia lasting 1 hr or less. The sensory symptoms continue as long as a typical aura. These symptoms may slowly spread up one arm from the fingers to the body and descend the opposite arm. This march is slower than the abrupt onset of similar symptoms occurring with a typical transient ischemic attack. A neurogenic and vasoconstricting origin has been implicated.

Treatment is not necessary if symptoms of migraine aura without headache do not occur often and do not cause significant discomfort. With frequent attacks, the usual prophylactic agent such as the beta blockers, calcium channel blockers, and GABA-receptor agonist anticonvulsants (divalproex sodium, gabapentin, and topiramate) may be utilized. Sublingual nifedipine and sublingual nitroglycerine have been shown to be effective in prompt alleviation of prolonged aura. Isoproterenol, administration of CO_2, and papaverine have demonstrated similar efficacy.

a. Migraine with Acute Onset Aura In migraine with acute onset aura, the warning symptoms fully develop in less than 5 min. The subsequent headache has all the features of migraine. Transient ischemic attack and other intracranial lesions should be ruled out by appropriate investigation. The neurological symptoms develop within 5 min and last as a typical aura for 20–60 min. The presence of a typical headache phase is required to establish the diagnosis, and previous migraine attacks of another type or a strong family history of migraine support diagnosis. Extensive investigations are necessary to rule out a transient ischemic attack.

b. Childhood Periodic Syndromes These syndromes may be precursors to, or associated with, migraine. The syndromes are characterized by multiple, repeated brief attacks of neurological symptoms without headaches, or the headaches cannot be detected because of the young age. Abdominal migraine and cyclic vomiting are included in this group.

c. Benign Paroxysmal Vertigo of Childhood This disease is characterized by brief attacks of vertigo in otherwise healthy children. Neurological examination and electroencephalogram are normal. It has been found that in 13% of reported cases of benign paroxysmal vertigo of childhood, the individual subsequently developed migraine. Multiple, short-lasting, sporadic spells of disequilibrium are often associated with nystagmus, nausea, vomiting, and anxiety. In 14%, vertigo is accompanied by headache. The pathophysiology is unknown.

Treatment of an acute attack is symptomatic. Beta-blocking agents, as well as cyproheptadine, may reduce the frequency of attacks.

7. Complications of Migraine

a. Status Migrainosus Previously, this condition was called intractable migraine or persistent (pernicious) migraine. It is distinguished as a migraine attack with the headache phase lasting more than 72 hr despite treatment. A headache-free interval of less than 4 hr may occur. Any episode of migraine, in any form of migraine, may evolve into an intractable, daily, continuous headache attack, unresponsive to standard treatments. The headache may be unilateral or global, pulsatile or pressure-like, or may have characteristics of both migraine and tension-type headaches. The headache progressively intensifies to a debilitating pain, accompanied by the usual characteristics of migraine. Typically, the associated nausea and vomiting are severe, leading to osmophobia, dehydration, refusal to eat, and prostration. The photophobia, phonophobia, and headache exacerbated by any movement forces the patient to remain in a dark and quiet room, unable to function at even a basic level. Some patients will even wear dark sunglasses indoors because of excessive sensitivity to light. Dehydration and anorexia may cause electrolyte disturbances, further complicating their condition. Emotional despair and depression with suicidal ideation are generally present. Status migrainosus is considered "headache urgency" requiring immediate care, preferably in an inpatient setting for rehydration, pain control, and reversal of continuous headache.

Status migrainosus, is often iatrogenically induced due to overuse or inappropriate use of analgesics, ergotamine preparations, narcotics, caffeine, or triptans or due to inadequate treatment of migraine. In susceptible patients, high stress, anxiety, and poor sleeping and eating habits may lead to this condition. Rebound headaches, transformed migraine, mixed headache, and chronic daily headaches may ultimately cause intractable debilitating headache. Status migrainosus is thought to be due to a sterile inflammation of the intracranial blood vessels involved in migraine process. The vasodilatation and inappropriate release of vasoactive neuropeptides, some of which are very potent vasodilators, as well as other active peptides that mediate neurogenic inflammation are self-perpetuating processes leading to endless activation of the trigeminal neurovascular system and fueling the central migraine generator. The plausible mechanism responsible for the refractoriness of status migrainosus is that the constant activation and release of neuropeptides downregulates serotonergic receptors and depletes endorphins.

Patients with acute status migrainosus may require hospitalization, particularly if the condition was induced by dependency on medication, is accompanied by dehydration, or if the patient is depressed or has a prior experience of adverse reactions to medications (Table I). The offending medication causing rebound headache phenomenon must be withdrawn. The withdrawal is usually done in an abrupt manner, but all precautions to prevent seizures and/or other withdrawal reactions should be instituted. Treatment for patients with status migrainosus should be aggressive and includes rest; rehydration and electrolyte replacement; detoxification; round-the-clock parenteral analgesic therapy; symptomatic treatment of nausea, anxiety, insomnia, and withdrawal symptoms; concurrent initiation of prophylactic therapy; and behavioral treatment. Corticosteroids and NSAIDs are

Table I
Criteria for Admission to Inpatient Headache Unit

Prolonged, unrelenting headache with associated symptoms, such as vomiting, that if continued would pose a further threat to the patient welfare

Status migraine

Dependence on analgesics, caffeine, narcotics, barbiturate, and tranquilizers

Habituation to ergots, with rebound headache

Pain accompanied by serious adverse reactions from therapy

Pain occurring in the presence of significant medical disease

Chronic cluster unresponsive to therapy

Treatment requiring copharmacy with drugs that may cause a drug interaction and necessitating careful observation within a hospital environment

Patients with probable organic cause to their headache requiring appropriate consultations, diagnostic testing, and perhaps neurosurgical intervention

used to reduce the neurogenic inflammation. Phenothiazine-based neuroleptics are utilized to control nausea and vomiting, reduce pain perception, and induce sedation. A series of intravenous dihydroergotamine (DHE) administered every 8 hr for 3 days is very effective in interrupting the painful cycle. It cannot be used when the patient is rebounding from ergotamine preparation or when DHE is contraindicated. Pain control is achieved by scheduled administration of parenteral narcotics, neuroleptics, benzodiazepines, and ketorolac. "As needed" pain control is not recommended because of reinforcement of dependency on analgesics. Appropriate prophylactic therapy, education, psychotherapy, and biofeedback should be concomitantly instituted.

b. Migrainous Infarction Occasionally, a migraine attack with one or more migraine aura symptoms is not fully reversible within 7 days and/or is associated with an abnormal neuroimaging test, confirming ischemic brain infarction. To fulfill the criteria, cerebral infarction must occur during the course of a typical migraine attack and other causes of infarction must be ruled out. The prevalence of migrainous infarction is about 3.36 cases in 100,000 adult migraineurs. Some studies indicate that women are more in risk, particularly those who are smokers, on oral contraceptives, and experiencing migraine with regular and prolonged aura. Neurological symptoms may occur abruptly or more slowly, may present as aura preceding the headache, or may start during the headache phase. Various symptoms and the intensity are dependent on anatomical location of infarction. The stroke must be confirmed by neuroimaging, and other causes of stroke must be ruled out. Prolonged, decreased blood flow during the migraine attack may cause ischemia in a susceptible migraineur. Abnormal blood coagulation, platelet changes, and other unrecognized factors also have a causative role.

Treatment consists of reducing the known risk factors, such as smoking, high cholesterol, and oral contraceptives. Supportive and analgesic treatment is indicated, and ergotamine and triptan preparations are contraindicated. Corticosteroids may reduce concomitant neurogenic inflammation and swelling. Calcium channel blockers facilitate vasodilatation and increase of blood flow in affected areas. Aspirin has been found to reduce risk of further stroke. Rehabilitation should be initiated in early stages.

B. Cluster Headache

This form of vascular headache has been known as histaminic cephalalgia, Horton's headache, migrainous neuralgia, sphenopalatine neuralgia, petrosal neuralgia, red migraine, Raeder's syndrome, Sluder's syndrome, erythromelalgia, and Bing's erythroprosopalgia. The defining characteristic of cluster headaches is their occurrence in cycles (clusters) that occur and disappear spontaneously. There are two forms of cluster headache—episodic and chronic. The majority of patients with cluster headaches experience the episodic form, in which the headache cycles or series last for several weeks or months and then may disappear for years. For those unfortunate few with the chronic form, headache remission is briefer than 14 days, or the cycle of headaches is continuous, without any headache-free intervals.

1. Clinical Features

The head pain and the associated symptoms characterize the acute cluster attack. During a cluster series, the acute headaches usually occur several times per day. The acute episodes are characterized by their brief duration (compared to migraine), usually lasting 15–180 min.

The headache is very severe, localizing at the orbital or supraorbital regions, and the patient may have temporal pain. The pain is strictly unilateral without alternating sides during a series, with a slight predominance of right-sided headaches. The side shift may

occur between cycles. The most common localization of pain is around and behind the eye, temporal and frontal lobes, and upper and lower jaw. The pain begins abruptly without any warning or just with a slight "awareness" or mild pain. It peaks in intensity within a few minutes and may last from 5–10 min up to more than 3 hr, but in most cases the average duration is 30–60 min.

The intensity of pain is excruciating, almost unbearable; it is said to be probably the most severe type of head pain known. The pain is described as boring, burning, pulsating, squeezing, deep knife-like pain, stabbing, piercing, or as a combination. In most cases, the frequency of attacks ranges from less than one to three per 24 hours up to six to eight per 24 hours. Attacks may occur at any time but usually happen in clockwork regularity at the same time each day or night. There is a high preponderance of nocturnal attacks, with frequent headaches occurring 2 or 3 hr after retiring to sleep. During an attack, patients tend to be restless, unable to remain still; many pace the floor, constantly moving, rocking, and engaging in bizarre activities and behavior that sometime lead to self-mutilation and even suicide.

Typically, the pain is accompanied by various autonomic phenomena. The most common, in descending order, are lacrimation, redness of the conjunctiva, nasal congestion, nasal discharge, forehead and facial sweating, small pupil, droopy eyelid, and eyelid swelling on the same side of the pain. Nausea and photophobia may present in some patients.

The most common triggers during a series are alcohol, nitroglycerine, and hypoxia. During the cluster cycle, patients will voluntarily avoid alcohol consumption and will not note any headache provocation by alcohol during the remission intervals.

2. Diagnostic Features

Cluster headache is the least prevalent of the primary headache syndromes, with an occurrence of about 1:1000 persons. The migraine-to-cluster ratio ranges from 7:1 to more than 20:1. Cluster headache is predominantly a male headache disorder, with the male-to-female ratio ranging from 4.5:1 to 6.7:1. The mean age of onset is approximately 27–30 years, with the youngest 6–8 years old. The incidence of the disease as well as the episodes of cluster headaches decrease after the age of 60.

The mean duration of a cluster cycle is approximately 6–8 weeks, with only about 3% of patients having bouts of 1-week duration and 4% having cycles lasting more than 26 weeks. The frequency of periods is less than one per year in 13%, one per year in 40%, two per year in 30%, and three per year in 8%. Cycles of one or two per year occur in 60% of patients. There appears to be a cyclic periodicity to the "clusters," with two seasonal peaks in early spring and early autumn. Rhythmicity in daily occurrence has also been noted, with attacks usually occurring 24 hr apart and frequently presenting at the same time of the day or night. During remission periods attacks spontaneously cease. The most frequently reported remissions last 7–12 months in 48%, 1–6 months in 20%, and 2 or more years in the remaining 32%. During the remission period the cluster attack cannot be provoked.

In the chronic form, there are no cycles, and by definition remission does not occur, nor does it last longer than 14 days. Patients with chronic cluster headaches have a tendency to habituation problems because of the continuous nature of the headache. The chronic form has similar clinical features as the episodic type. Attacks of cluster headache recur for a period of time at least 50 weeks in 1 year. The age of onset seems to be higher, with a mean onset of 39 years. Male preponderance of the chronic forms is at least as significant as that in episodic cluster. The mean frequency of attacks and duration are slightly higher. Pain localization, quality, and associated symptoms are the same as those in the episodic form.

3. Pathophysiology

The mechanism of cluster headache is unclear and involves vascular changes and impaired autonomic neuronal activity as well as biochemical, hormonal, and chronobiological changes. The abnormal autonomic neuronal activity is most likely due to a primary disorder of the central regulation of autonomic functions controlled by the hypothalamus. Several vasoactive substances, including histamine, serotonin, and substance P, have been observed to be activated during the cluster attack. Hormonal level changes, including those of testosterone and melatonin, have also been noted. Circadian and circannual rhythmicity suggest the pathological involvement of the "biological clock" in hypothalamus. Furthermore, hypoxia and the role of the carotid body (the most sensitive chemoreceptor for hypoxia) have been discussed in regard to the pathomechanism of cluster attacks. It appears that the origin of cluster headache is in the hypothalamus, with abnormal activation of the autonomic nervous system causing vascular and biochemical changes.

4. Therapy

Treatment for both the episodic and the chronic forms is similar and consists of abortive and prophylactic therapy. Because of the brief nature of acute cluster attacks, medication used to stop the pain requires rapid onset of action (within 30 min). The most effective and safest method is self-administration of 100% oxygen, via facial mask, at high flow of 8–10 liters per minute for 10–15 min. Dramatic termination of an acute attack has been achieved within 10–15 min in 80% of patients. Other effective abortive therapies include parenteral and intranasal administration of sumatriptan or dihydroergotamine; sublingual ergotamine; and intranasal instillation of viscous lidocaine, a local anesthetic, to the affected nostril. Parenteral ketorolac, chlorpromazine, and narcotic analgesics may help control the pain.

The prophylactic treatment should be initiated at the very onset of a cluster cycle and continued at least 2–4 weeks after the last acute cluster episode. Corticosteroids may hasten the interruption of the cycle. Verapamil (a calcium channel blocker), lithium, methysergide, ergotamine, and divalproex sodium have been found to be effective in reducing and preventing acute cluster attacks during the episodic cycle or the chronic form. In some inpatient headache centers, intractable cluster headaches have been successfully treated with intravenous histamine desensitization treatment.

5. Chronic Paroxysmal Hemicrania

Chronic paroxysmal hemicrania (CPH) is a rare disorder. It has the same characteristics as cluster headache, including similar associated symptoms. These episodes are briefer, more frequent, occur mostly in females, and responsive to indomethacin.

The patient with CPH will characteristically complain of 10–20 brief, intense focal episodes of head pain, localized mostly in the temporal, ocular, frontal, and upper jaw area. The pain has the same quality as cluster headache pain, but of even shorter duration (an average of 10–20 min). CPH attacks are associated with autonomic symptoms and signs that are characteristic for cluster headache. In some patients, head movement or pressure on certain points in the neck can trigger attacks. About 70% of diagnosed patients are female and the mean age of onset is 34 years. The pathogenesis is unknown, but it is considered to be a cluster variant. One of the diagnostic criteria for CPH is absolute responsiveness to indomethacin, an

NSAID. Indomethacin selectively stops the attacks, usually within 2 days of treatment.

6. Cluster Headache Variant

These headache attacks are believed to be a form of cluster headache or CPH but do not meet their criteria. Cluster headache variant, originally described by Diamond and Medina, is a syndrome consisting of a triad of symptoms: atypical cluster headaches, multiple jabs, and background continuous headache. The atypical cluster headache is irregular in location, duration, and frequency, occurring several times a day. Multiple jabs are sharp, variable, painful episodes, lasting only a few seconds and occurring several times a day. Background headaches are chronic, continuous, often unilateral, sharply localized and of variable severity, and have vascular features—throbbing and exacerbated by physical exertion. The pathophysiology is unknown. The therapy consists of indomethacin or lithium.

II. TENSION-TYPE HEADACHE

Tension-type headache was previously known by several terms: muscle contraction headache, stress headache, ordinary headache, essential headache, psychogenic headache, or psychomyogenic headache. It is defined as recurrent episodes of headache lasting minutes to days. There are two primary forms—episodic and chronic. The pain is bilateral, with pressing or tightening (nonpulsating) quality of mild-to-moderate severity. The headache is not aggravated by routine physical activity. Photophobia or phonophobia may be present, and nausea may occur in the chronic form. The episodic type has been experienced by almost everyone, is usually relieved by over-the-counter analgesics, and does not require a physician's intervention. The chronic type is daily or almost daily, and the victim is prone to dependency problems with analgesics, tranquilizers, or sedatives.

A. Diagnostic Features

The prevalence in the general population ranges from 30 to 80%. The 1-year prevalence of episodic tension-type headaches is about 55% in men and 70% in women; in the chronic form the prevalence is only about 2–5%. The prevalence decreases with increasing age.

The pain is usually described as steady, nonpulsatile, band-like, vise-like, tightness, ache, soreness, and pressure in a hat-like distribution. Feelings of increased tension may be also felt in the occipital and cervical areas. Muscles of the scalp and neck may be tender to the touch, with palpable, sharply localized nodules. Combing or brushing the hair or wearing a hat may elicit soreness. Electromyographic recording from the scalp and cervical muscles may or may not register increased activity. In many individuals, the headache starts during the afternoon or evening but rarely impacts on the sufferer's daily activity.

The various psychological factors associated with chronic tension-type headaches include anxiety, fear, hostility, and, very frequently, depression. Typically, in the chronic form, the victim may complain of a sleep disturbance. In chronic tension-type headache due to anxiety, the patient may complain of insomnia (difficulty falling asleep). However, in patients with chronic tension-type headaches due to depression, early or frequent awakening may be prominent complaints. Physical exercise may alleviate the headache. Chronic tension-type headache is often associated with concomitant cervicogenic disease. Trigger and aggravating factors are usually identifiable and may include stress in marital, social, occupational, sexual, and interpersonal relationship; fatigue; overwork; insomnia; personality traits; and methods of handling stressful situations.

B. Pathophysiology

The mechanism of tension-type headache is poorly understood. In the episodic form, more peripheral mechanisms seem to be involved, including slightly increased electromyographic activity during resting conditions that are due to insufficient relaxation or reflex contraction. Slightly decreased electromyographic activity during maximal voluntary contraction may be due to impaired recruitment of muscle fibers at maximal activity. In the chronic form, it appears that sensory information is abnormally processed. Plausible mechanisms have been proposed, including sensitization of peripheral myofascial nociceptors and spinal and trigeminal neurons; decreased antinociceptive activation from supraspinal structures; and increased sensitivity of supraspinal pain perception. Furthermore, neurochemical processes involved in depression are also thought to be part of the pathophysiology of chronic tension-type headache. There is strong evidence that depression lowers tolerance to pain.

C. Therapy

The patient should avoid identifiable trigger factors. The episodic form responds well to simple analgesics, muscle relaxants, relaxation techniques, biofeedback, and exercise. Mild headaches of shorter duration are self-limited and in order to prevent analgesic dependency do not need to be treated. Patients with the chronic form need to be evaluated for depression and other psychological and psychiatric comorbid conditions. The daily use of analgesics is inappropriate because of the potential for dependency problems or a rebound phenomenon.

The antidepressant drugs provide the most effective treatment for this condition. Antidepressant prophylaxis should be used even if depression is not detected. Only a few antidepressants in the tricyclic category have been tested in placebo-controlled studies for chronic tension-type headaches. However, clinical experience suggests that other tricyclic and nontricyclic antidepressants, including the newer serotonergic types, are similarly effective. There is a minimal difference in their efficacy, but the adverse reactions can be significant. The choice of antidepressants is therefore made on the avoidance or use of certain side effects. For instance, tricyclic antidepressants such as amitriptyline or doxepin, which have sedative effects, can be used in the patient who has a sleep disturbance. The average dose of antidepressant for treatment of chronic tension-type headache is lower than that used for depression. Pain control is achieved with muscle relaxants, simple analgesics, and NSAIDs. Narcotic-type analgesics and tranquilizers, particularly the benzodiazepine types, are not recommended because of their high propensity of dependency, abuse, and addiction, particularly in a patient with coexisting chronic tension-type headache and depression. Psychotherapy, stress management, and cognitive therapy are essential parts of successful treatment.

III. TRACTION AND INFLAMMATORY HEADACHES (ORGANIC)

Headaches due to organic disease are rare, occurring in about 2% of headache patients. The term traction and inflammatory headaches refers to any headache resulting from inflammation, traction and displacement, and distortion of the pain sources of the head, such as the cranial vessels. Headaches associated with traction include hematomas, abscesses, aneurysms, brain tumor, and nonspecific brain edema from lumbar puncture. Examples of inflammatory headaches include eye infection, iritis, and glaucoma; ear diseases; and acute sinus infections.

A patient presenting with recent onset or change in character of headaches should alert the physicians to a possible organic cause. It is essential to rule out possible morbid causes of the headache. The danger signals for headaches that may suggest the presence of serious illness include

- Headaches that do not fit a recognizable pattern or a pattern that is easily identified
- Headaches occurring for the first time in childhood or after age 50
- Headaches occurring for the first time that rapidly increase in frequency and intensity
- The presence of neurological symptoms, such as dizziness, blurred vision, or memory loss
- A patient who feels sick or "not right" with his or her headaches
- Abnormal physical symptoms, for example, heart murmurs or kidney problems
- Any rigidity (stiffness) of the neck accompanying a headache may indicate an infection or inflammation of the spinal fluid

These signals are important for all headache sufferers—even those with a prolonged history of migraine headaches.

A. Mass Lesions

This category includes brain tumors, hematomas, brain abscesses, and expanding aneurysms. Headache is one of the cardinal signs of a mass lesion but may not present until the size is sufficiently large or the lesion expands to press on structures that will trigger a headache and associated neurological symptoms. Headache will occur if the lesion is expanding rapidly and is producing traction on one of the pain-sensitive structures of the head, especially if the ventricular system is compromised, with obstruction of absorption or flow of cerebrospinal fluid (CSF) and a resulting hydrocephalus.

The headache resulting from a brain mass is usually associated with neurological signs, including seizures (focal or general), progressive loss of neurological function, and mental symptoms. Headache onset is usually intermittent, with dull and aching pain. The frequency and duration will progressively increase, and the headache will sometimes be altered by changes in posture and tone. A rapid increase in intracranial pressure will usually manifest as a headache.

The headache associated with a brain tumor may facilitate locating the tumor. If the tumor is above the tentorium, the pain is frequently at the vertex or in the frontal regions. If the tumor is below the tentorium, the pain is occipital, and cervical muscle spasm may be present. Headache is almost always present continually with posterior fossa tumor. If the tumor is midline, the pain may be increased with cough or straining or sudden head movement. However, this exacerbation also occurs with migraine. If the tumor is hemispheric, the pain is usually felt on the same side of the head. If the tumor is chiasmal, at the sella, the pain may be referred to the vertex. Colloid cysts of the third ventricle can cause an acute increase in intracranial pressure when the patient assumes certain positions and the tumor blocks the flow of CSF. The pain is relieved when the patient moves the head back to a position in which the flow of CSF is unobstructed. The management of mass lesions requires neurosurgical intervention.

B. Post-Lumbar Puncture Headache

If a patient complains of headache following a lumbar puncture, it is probably related to a loss of CSF secondary to leakage through a dural defect. The headache is often exacerbated in the upright position and relieved with recumbency. The pain has been described as a dull ache that may become throbbing. The headache onset starts within hours to days after the procedure and may persist for 2 to 3 weeks. The symptoms usually subside spontaneously.

Prevention is the key and the use of smaller needles has been recommended to decrease the incidence of these headaches. Treatment of the post-lumbar puncture headache consists of bed rest in the horizontal position. A blood patch to stop the leak may be beneficial.

C. Headaches of Ocular Origin

Headache is rarely due to the eye, with the exception of obvious ocular pathology. Photophobia, associated with migraine, is rarely caused by diseases of the eye, eye muscles, or the optic nerves. Reading, eye strain, eye muscle imbalance, or refractive errors are rare causes of headache.

The pain of glaucoma is due to an increased intraocular pressure within the globe. The severity is more directly related to the rate of increase of the intraocular pressure rather than the absolute pressure. Glaucoma can be easily classified as: (i) open if the anterior angle filtration is patent, (ii) closed if the chamber is blocked, or (iii) combined if the chamber is patent and blocked. The type of glaucoma with the most severe pain is caused by acute closure of the angle in the anterior chamber. On exam, the orbit is "rock hard" and immediate ophthalmologic referral is necessary.

D. Sinus Headache

Sinus headache is an often cited complaint of many patients, although the acute headache due to actual sinusitis occurs less frequently than the rate quoted by the advertising media. Acute sinusitis presents with fever, pain triggered by pressure or direct percussion, and headache. Fever is the cardinal sign of this infective process. The pain associated with sinus diseases is a constant, dull ache. If the patient is suffering from acute sinusitis, the headache will typically increase in intensity as the day progresses. To confirm the diagnosis, sinus X-rays or sinus CT should be performed. Treatment consists of antimicrobial therapy and decongestants.

E. Facial Pain

The facial pain syndromes are a group of disorders that usually occur in paroxysms and are characterized by pain of severe intensity. The most common types are trigeminal and glossopharyngeal neuralgia. Trigeminal neuralgia, also known as tic douloureux, is usually seen in the elderly. The nature of the pain and its intensity may cause the patient to wince or twitch. The patient can identify trigger points, and avoidance of these trigger points is a diagnostic feature. The patient avoids these points by circumventing them during shaving, washing the face, or applying makeup. Glossopharyngeal neuralgia is similar to trigeminal neuralgia in its presentation. However, the site of pain is located in the ear, tonsils, or pharynx and is triggered by swallowing, yawning, or eating.

The prophylactic treatment for facial neuralgias consists of the anticonvulsants, and carbamazepine has produced a dramatic response. Its initial dose is 100–200 mg, two or three times daily. Most physicians would use gabapentin or baclofen after carbamazepine. Neurosurgical intervention is indicated for approximately 25–50% of patients who are refractory to therapy. Due to the chronic nature of the pain, habituating analgesics should be avoided.

F. Temporal Arteritis

Temporal arteritis is caused by an inflammatory process to the cranial arteries, and headache is the most common presenting complaint. It is also associated with night sweats, weight loss, aching of joints, low-grade fever, and jaw claudication. The headache pain is usually localized to the affected scalp vessels. Many patients will complain of pain on chewing. Temporal arteritis should be ruled out in any patient over the age of 50 who presents with an initial onset of headache and who was previously asymptomatic. The female-to-male ratio is 2:1. The area around the temporary artery is tender and the skin may appear red, depending on which artery is involved. Diagnosis is suggested by an elevated sedimentation rate by the Westergren method and confirmed by temporal artery biopsy.

It is essential that a diagnosis be established early and treatment started immediately because 50% or more of untreated cases result in irreversible blindness. Therapy with corticosteroids can be initiated while awaiting the results of the biopsy to avoid delays in treatment.

G. Headache with Vascular Disorders

Fortunately, headaches due to disorders of the cerebral vessels are rare. Because of the gravity of these disorders, these potentially life-threatening disorders should be quickly diagnosed and appropriate treatment started immediately.

1. Epidural Hematoma

Bleeding into the cranium may occur into the epidural, subdural, or subarachnoid space or directly into the parenchyma of the brain. Severe headaches are commonly manifested by these hemorrhages. However, the headache may not be a dominant feature or may be absent in some cases. An epidural hematoma is usually caused by a tear in the middle meningeal artery as it passes under the surface of the temporal bone. Because the dura is sensitive to stretching as it is being torn away from the bone, headache often occurs. Restlessness and combativeness also occur and progress to an altered consciousness. Neuroimaging will confirm the diagnosis. Prompt neurosurgical referral is essential.

2. Acute Subdural Hematoma

Subdural hematoma can be due to either an acute or a chronic event. In acute subdural hematoma, a brief lucid interval occurs between the head trauma and the patient becoming comatose, although the patient is usually comatose from the time of trauma. The bleed may be unilateral or bilateral and is often accompanied by lacerations of the scalp and contusions to the brain and parenchyma. A CT scan will confirm the diagnosis in up to 90% of cases, although angiography may be necessary. Neurosurgical intervention is required.

Chronic subdural hematoma is usually precipitated by minor head injury, which is often forgotten by the patient, and the trauma may have occurred several months previously. This form of hematoma occurs more commonly in the elderly and in patients receiving anticoagulant therapy. In addition to the headache, the patient may have decreased mentation, confusion, and drowsiness. The headache is considered secondary to the stretching of the tributary veins that drain the vessels of the cerebral hemispheres into the sagittal sinuses. Neuroimaging will establish the diagnosis, although angiography may be required. Treatment consists of surgical burr holes and evacuation of the clot.

3. Subarachnoid Hemorrhage

Most subarachnoid hemorrhages (SAHs) are caused by a ruptured berry aneurysm. The patient with SAH will describe the "worst headache of my life." Other causes of SAH include arteriovascular malformations, bleeding disorders, and miscellaneous or cryptogenic causes. A berry aneurysm results from a congenital weakness in the arterial wall, usually occurring in the vessels of the circle of Willis and at these vessels' bifurcations. Frequently, patients are drowsy, may vomit, and have meningeal signs on physical exam. If SAH is being considered, an unenhanced CT scan should be performed and immediate neurosurgical consultation should be provided. A four-vessel cerebral angiogram is usually the next stage of the workup and serves as a road map for surgical intervention.

4. Arteriovenous Malformations

Unless there is active bleeding, arteriovenuous malformations (AVMs) do not usually cause headaches. If there is bleeding, the AVM can mimic the symptoms of SAH. A slow leak from an AVM could possibly occur and irritate the meninges, thus causing headache.

5. Hypertensive Headache

Hypertensive headache is typically bilateral and often presents in the occipital region. Characteristically, the headache is worse upon awakening and gradually improves throughout the day. The diagnosis can only be confirmed with a diastolic blood pressure of 110 mmHg or higher.

See Also the Following Articles

BIOFEEDBACK • BRAIN DISEASE, ORGANIC • BRAIN LESIONS • DEPRESSION • FUNCTIONAL MAGNETIC RESONANCE IMAGING (fMRI) • MILD HEAD INJURY • PAIN • PAIN AND PSYCHOPATHOLOGY • STRESS

Suggested Reading

Dalessio, D. J., and Silberstein, S. D. (1993). *Wolff's Headache and Other Head Pain*, 6th ed. Oxford Univ. Press, New York.

Diamond, M. L., and Solomon, G. D. (1999). *Diamond and Dalessio's the Practicing Physician's Approach to Headache*, 6th ed. Saunders, Philadelphia.

Diamond, S. (1998). Headache. In *Conn's Current Therapy* (R. A. Rakel, Ed.). Saunders, Philadelphia.

International Headache Society (1988). Classification and diagnostic criteria for headache disorders, cranial neuralgias and facial pain. *Cephalalgia* **8** (Suppl. 7).

Sjaastad, O. (1992). *Cluster Headache Syndrome*. Saunders, Philadelphia.

Raskin, N. H. (1988). *Headache*, 2nd ed. Churchill Livingstone, New York.

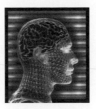

Hearing

JOHN F. BRUGGE

University of Wisconsin

MATTHEW A. HOWARD

University of Iowa

GLOSSARY

characteristic frequency The frequency of a tone (kilohertz) that excites an auditory neuron at the lowest threshold (decibel sound pressure level). Sometimes called the "best" frequency.

cytoarchitecture The structural organization of neuronal cell bodies in the brain as revealed by specific histological staining methods. The cerebral cortex in particular may be subdivided based on cytoarchitectural differences.

decibel (dB) The unit of sound intensity usually expressed as sound pressure level (SPL). Each 10-fold change in sound pressure is a 20-dB change in SPL.

Hertz (Hz) The unit of the frequency of a sound, defined as the number of cycles that a periodic signal undergoes each second. 1 kilohertz (kHz) = 1000 Hz.

Heschl's gyrus A gyrus (or in some cases multiple gyri) on the superior temporal plane that is the location of primary auditory cortex in the human.

response area The area within the threshold tuning curve.

superior temporal plane The dorsal surface of the superior temporal gyrus, buried in the Sylvian fissure, that contains much of auditory cortex in humans and in nonhuman primates.

threshold tuning curve A plot of an auditory neuron's sensitivity to sound frequency. Acoustic threshold (dB) is plotted as a function of stimulus frequency (kHz). The tip of the tuning curve is at the neuron's characteristic frequency.

tonotopy The orderly representation of stimulus frequency in the auditory system; often studied by mapping with a microelectrode the distribution of neurons' characteristic frequencies within an auditory structure.

transduction As related to hearing, it is the process by which sound energy is changed (transduced) into electrical energy (nerve impulses) within the inner ear.

Hearing engages a set of complex processes by which humans and other animals detect and discriminate sounds in the environment and determine the directions in space from which they arise. It also involves perceptual and cognitive processes that allow for sound source identification, for species-specific communication, and, in the apparently unique case of humans, for speech and language. Normal hearing is made possible through efficient sound transmission by the external and middle ears, transduction of sound energy into nerve impulses in the inner ear, transmission to the brain by the auditory nerve of information-bearing impulse trains, transformations of the transmitted information along the central auditory pathways, and integration of this information by widely distributed neuronal assemblies within and outside of the classical auditory pathways of the brain. Knowledge of the mechanisms underlying these processes in the human auditory pathways has been obtained from comparative anatomical, physiological, and behavioral studies in laboratory animals, from psychophysical experiments and noninvasive measurements of central auditory function in normal human subjects, and from intraoperative and chronic electrophysiological studies of auditory function in neurosurgical patients.

I. HUMAN HEARING

Human hearing operates over a wide range of frequency and intensity (Fig. 1), and within this range humans have a remarkable capacity to detect, discriminate, and locate sounds. A young listener hears sounds ranging in frequency from about 20 to 20,000 Hz, and over a considerable portion of this range a change in frequency as little as 0.15% is detectable. This same listener detects sounds that move the eardrum over a distance no greater than the diameter of a hydrogen atom, and yet hearing remains quite clear as sound pressure level is then raised by a factor of 106 or more. Within this dynamic range of 120 decibels (dB), a change in sound intensity of 1 or 2 dB is easily detected. Listeners also detect with uncanny accuracy the location of a sound in space and discriminate between two speakers located within a few degrees of each other on the horizontal plane.

Periodic envelope fluctuations, some highly complex, are common and important information-bearing features of natural sounds including speech. The even more complex process of speech communication, which in order to develop properly requires hearing ability, is normally acquired very early in life and shortly thereafter is carried out effortlessly even in environments filled with competing sounds.

II. TRANSMISSION OF SOUND BY THE EXTERNAL AND MIDDLE EARS

The functions of the external and middle ears are to capture sound energy and transmit it efficiently to the receptor organ of the inner ear. Figure 2A illustrates the structural relationships that underlie these functions.

The external ear consists of a highly convoluted protrusion, called the pinna (or auricle), and an ear canal (or external acoustic meatus). Together the pinna and ear canal amplify sound waves and guide them to the tympanic membrane (or eardrum).

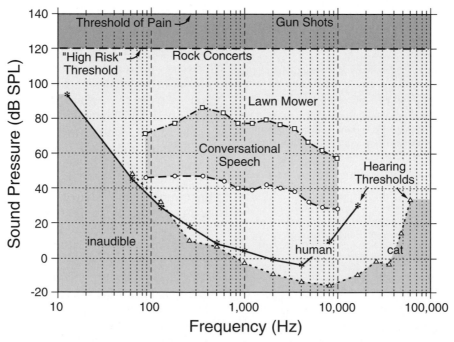

Figure 1 Hearing threshold and range of hearing for human listeners. Shown also are the ranges of frequency and sound pressure level of common environmental sounds, including human speech. The most intense sounds are capable of damaging the inner ear receptor organ. The hearing sensitivity of the cat, a laboratory animal commonly used in studies of the peripheral and central auditory systems, is illustrated as well (adapted with permission from Geisler, C. D, *From Sound to Synapse*. Oxford Univ. Press, New York, 1998).

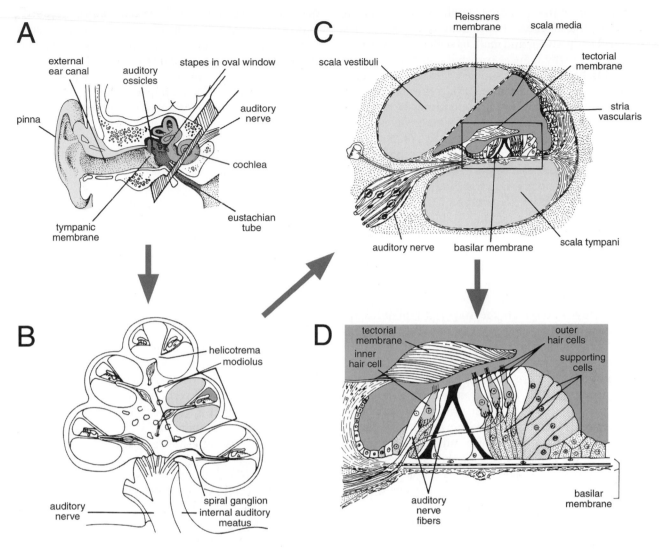

Figure 2 Structures of the external, middle, and inner ears [adapted with permission from Brugge, J. F., Auditory system. In *Encyclopedia of Neuroscience* (G. Adelman, Ed.). Birkhauser, Boston, 1987].

Amplification of sound ranges from 5 to 20 dB for frequencies within the speech range (about 1.5–7 kHz). This improvement in signal-to-noise ratio, which is due mainly to the resonant properties of the external ear canal, provides a way of enhancing speech intelligibility in the presence of many unwanted competing sounds. The pinna, on the other hand, acts as a directional amplifier for high frequencies. Spectrally transformed sound reaching the tympanic membrane provides cues for localizing the source of a sound in space, especially when the sound is on the midsagittal plane, where interaural time and intensity differences are small or nonexistent. Sounds originating from sources on either side of the midline reach the near ear

before reaching the far ear, thereby creating an interaural time difference (ITD). The head also acts as an acoustic barrier at high frequencies, creating an interaural intensity difference (IID). The magnitudes of the ITD and IID depend on the location of the sound on the horizontal plane, and neural circuits in the auditory central nervous system have evolved to detect them.

The middle ear cavity is located just behind the tympanic membrane. It is normally air-filled and in equilibrium with atmospheric pressure due to the periodic opening and closing of the Eustachian tube connecting the middle ear cavity with the nasopharynx. Three auditory ossicles (malleus, incus, and stapes) connect the tympanic membrane with the oval window of the inner ear. Reflex contraction of muscles attached to the stapes and malleus stiffens the ossicular chain and thereby reduces transmission of potentially damaging low-frequency sounds. The real need for a middle ear arises because the auditory receptor organ is an "underwater receiver" operating in the fluid environment of the inner ear. If sound waves in air were to strike this fluid boundary, 99.9% of the energy would be reflected. This interruption in the flow of sound to the inner ear would result in a conductive hearing loss, possibly as much as 30 dB. Thus, the role of the middle ear is to overcome this impedance mismatch between air and fluid and to transfer to the inner ear as efficiently as possible sound energy that impinges on the tympanic membrane.

The first, and most important, mechanism used to overcome impedance mismatch relies on the relatively large area of the tympanic membrane compared to the oval window into which the stapes footplate exerts pressure on the fluid of the inner ear. The force acting on the tympanic membrane is concentrated through the ossicles onto a small area of the oval window resulting in a pressure increase proportional to the ratio of the areas of the two membranes (approximately 20:1). Second, the lever arm of the malleus is longer than that of the incus with which it articulates, giving an additional mechanical advantage of about 1.3. Third, the conical shape of the tympanic membrane imposes additional force on the malleus. Sound energy transmitted to the inner ear is then transduced, through a cascade of mechanical and electrical events, to electrical nerve impulses in axons of the auditory nerve.

III. TRANSDUCTION OF SOUND BY THE INNER EAR

A. Structure of the Inner Ear

The inner ear, located in the temporal bone of the skull, is a complex structure serving both hearing and balance. Figures 2B–2D illustrate in detail the structures that make up that portion involved in hearing known as the cochlea (Fig. 2A). The cochlea is a coiled, tapered, and fluid-filled chamber divided along almost its entire length by a membranous partition. The two spaces thus formed, the scala vestibuli and scala tympani, are filled with a fluid called perilymph. The two scalae communicate with each other through an

opening at the top (apex) of the cochlea called the helicotrema. At the base of the cochlea each scala terminates at a membrane that faces the middle ear cavity. The scala vestibuli ends at the oval window into which the footplate of the stapes rocks when the ear drum moves; the scala tympani ends at the round window, a structure that provides a pressure relief for movement of the cochlear fluid. The partition that divides the cochlea lengthwise is a fluid-filled tube called the scala media or cochlear duct. Its fluid, endolymph, is chemically different from perilymph. The cochlear duct is bounded on three sides by a bed of capillaries and secretory cells (the stria vascularis), a layer of simple squamous epithelial cells (Reissner's membrane), and the basilar membrane, on which rests the receptor organ for hearing—the organ of Corti.

The organ of Corti contains the auditory receptor cells (hair cells) and a system of supporting cells that hold them in place. Hair cells are modified epithelial cells with hairs (stereocilia) protruding from their apical ends (Fig. 2D). Figure 3 is a drawing of a stereotypic ear hair cell. A kinocilium, which seems to play no active role in the transduction process, is seen throughout life in the vestibular epithelium but is no longer present in the adult cochlea. Within the organ of Corti two kinds of hair cell—inner (IHC) and outer (OHC)—are distinguishable by location, morphology, and connections with the auditory nerve. Approximately 3500 IHCs form a single linear array, from base to apex (Fig. 2D). About 12,000 OHCs are arranged in three or four rows, parallel to the IHCs (Fig. 2D). Approximately 100–150 stereocilia form a V or W pattern on each OHC, whereas approximately 40–50 stereocilia, arranged in a U shape, adorn each IHC. Displacement of stereocilia is the adequate stimulus for generating receptor currents in hair cells that eventually lead to action potentials in auditory nerve axons.

Spiral ganglion cells, located in the bony core of the cochlea, are the bipolar first-order neurons of the auditory pathway. Their distal processes make synaptic contact with the base of hair cells. The central axons, which in the human number approximately 35,000, form each auditory nerve bundle. The majority (~95%) of the central processes of spiral ganglion neurons originate at the base of IHCs. Thus, axons connected to IHCs transmit to the brain trains of nerve impulses that encode essentially all the acoustic information eventually perceived by a listener. The innervation is highly focused: Each auditory nerve is connected to one IHC, whereas each IHC is innervated

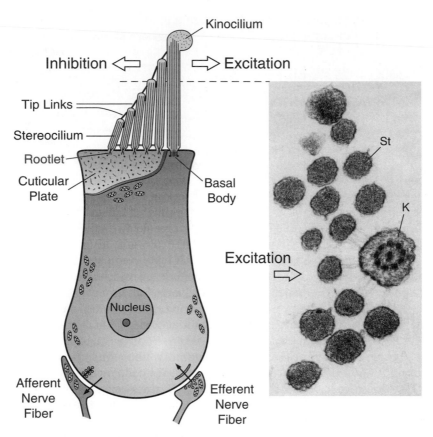

Figure 3 Stylized hair cell of the vertebrate inner ear (left). Deflection of stereocilia toward the kinocilium and basal body results in hair cell depolarization and excitation of auditory nerve fibers, whereas movement in the opposite direction leads to hyperpolarization and inhibition. Cross section of hair bundle is shown at the right (adapted with permission from Geisler, C.D, *From Sound to Synapse*. Oxford Univ. Press, New York, 1998).

by no more than approximately 10–20 spiral ganglion cells. The remaining 5% of axons of the auditory nerve are efferent fibers arising from cells in and around the superior olivary complex of the brain stem. Upon entering the organ of Corti they branch profusely, with each axon reaching many OHCs over considerable distance.

B. Mechanical Motion in the Inner Ear in Response to Sound

The basilar membrane is a resonant structure varying systematically in width and stiffness. It is wider (0.42–0.65 mm) and more flaccid at the cochlear apex than at the base (0.08–0.16 mm). When a sound wave is transmitted to the fluid of the inner ear, the basilar membrane is set in motion. Basilar membrane motion is best described as a traveling wave of deformation, which begins at the cochlear base and moves apically

toward a frequency-dependent place of maximal amplitude (Fig. 4). When very high-frequency sound waves reach the ear, only the region nearest the cochlear base vibrates. As the frequency of the sound is lowered, the place of maximal amplitude of vibration shifts toward the cochlear apex. Because of this resonance gradient, the basilar membrane is said to be "tonotopically" organized. Consequently, complex sound (e.g., speech) entering the inner ear is resolved into its component frequencies. This physical separation of sound energy into its spectral components, coupled with the focused innervation of the auditory nerve array, provides an orderly and spectrally segregated projection of the nerve into the auditory brain stem, thereby setting the stage for tonotopic organization along the entire central auditory pathway.

Normal cochlear vibration is not simply the result of passive mechanical resonance as once thought, but rather it involves active processes. Under certain conditions, OHCs are capable of changing shape,

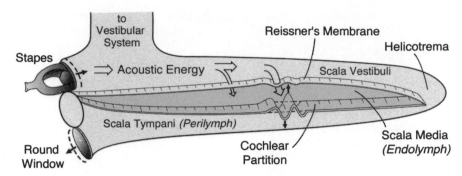

Figure 4 Stylized mammalian cochlea, shown uncoiled to illustrate the flow of energy and pattern of vibration of the cochlear partition in response to a midfrequency tone of modest intensity. The scalae vestibuli and tympani are assigned the same shading as in cochlear cross sections shown in Fig. 2. [Adapted with permission from Geisler, C.D. (1998). *From Sound to Synapse.* Oxford Univ. Press, New York].

which feeds energy back into the organ of Corti and alters the mechanical properties of the cochlear partition and possibly the transduction process. This active process may be controlled, in part, by feedback via olivocochlear axons originating in the auditory brain stem and profusely terminating at the base of OHCs. Apparently as the result of an active process, the organ of Corti acts not only to receive sound but also to generate it, as an otoacoustic emission (OAC) recorded by a microphone in the ear canal. There are several categories of OACs, reflecting perhaps more than one nonlinear active process in the cochlea. OACs are proving useful as an objective tool for diagnosing sensorineural hearing loss.

C. Transduction Process in Cochlear Hair Cells

Stereocilia of IHCs are in functional contact with an overlying auxiliary structure called the tectorial membrane. The base of the hair cell is in synaptic contact with the distal ends of auditory nerve axons. Sound waves that reach the inner ear set the basilar membrane, and hence the organ of Corti, into motion. This causes a shearing motion between the tectorial membrane and the tops of the hair cells that, in turn, displaces the stereocilia and triggers the flow of transducer currents. These changes in the receptor potential are mediated by the opening and closing of mechanically gated ion channels (transduction channels) at the tips of the stereocilia. This action leads to opening and closing of voltage-gated ion channels distributed over the basolateral surface of the cell body and then to the release of neurotransmitter at the afferent synapses at the base of the hair cell. The hair bundle is "polarized," which means that displacement of the stereocilia in the direction of the kinocilium (or

basal body) results in hair cell depolarization and an increase in firing of auditory nerve fibers, whereas displacement in the opposite direction leads to hyperpolarization and a decrease in firing (Fig. 3). Thus, the modulation of neurotransmitter release, and, as a consequence the pattern of action potentials in the auditory nerve, is linked tightly to the intensity, frequency, and temporal structure of sound waves entering the ear.

Inner ear structures are easily damaged by intense sound, drugs, viruses, and bacteria, and there are genetic causes of inner ear malformation. The resulting hearing loss is called sensorineural, and in such cases no treatment has been found to fully restore normal inner ear function. Some functional hearing may be restored, however, by electrically stimulating surviving spiral ganglion neurons through a cochlear prosthesis.

IV. TRANSMISSION OF SOUND INFORMATION BY THE AUDITORY NERVE

The term "code" as applied to the auditory system is simply a way in which information about a sound is represented in impulse activity of neurons. As in other regions of the central and peripheral nervous systems, the auditory system exhibits a variety of neural activities and, hence, a variety of candidate coding mechanisms. These include labeled lines (place), firing frequency (rate), temporal patterning, and ensemble firing. Each auditory nerve encodes the frequency, intensity, and temporal pattern of the sound reaching the ear. Coding for the direction of sound in space involves more complex processing in the central auditory pathway, where inputs from the two ears converge and where sound direction is computed from ITD and IID cues.

Auditory nerve fibers exhibit a frequency specificity that reflects the mechanical tuning properties of the basilar membrane and the highly focused innervation of IHCs. The discharge threshold of an auditory nerve fiber occurs around a particular frequency, referred to as the fiber's characteristic frequency (CF). Thus, a fiber's CF is directly related to the location along the basilar membrane innervated by that fiber. The fact that auditory nerve fibers and many central auditory neurons are frequency selective has been taken as evidence to support a place theory of hearing. The place theory is a labeled-line theory stating that the pitch of a tone (i.e., the psychological attribute associated with frequency) is determined by those fibers in the auditory nerve array (and, by extension, central auditory neurons) excited by that sound.

Not all sounds having pitch quality exhibit spectral energy at the pitch frequency; pitch is also perceived when a sound waveform is modulated in amplitude. Hence, frequency (or pitch) information may be transmitted from the ear to the brain in the temporal pattern of nerve impulses in auditory nerve fibers. Action potentials evoked by low-frequency tones (below about 4 kHz) or by temporally modulated sounds (below about 1000 Hz) occur at preferred times on a stimulus cycle, a phenomenon known as phase locking. Phase locking is the direct result of to-and-fro displacement of IHC stereocilia in response to low-frequency modulation of the basilar membrane. As a consequence of phase locking, nerve impulses tend to occur at integral multiples of the period of the stimulus time waveform, a behavior that is predicted by the volley theory of hearing. The volley theory states that the pitch of a sound is determined by the temporal rhythm of the discharges of an ensemble of auditory nerve fibers. High-fidelity transmission of temporal information from the cochlea to the brain serves at least two purposes. First, because much of human speech (especially vowel sounds) has its acoustic energy concentrated below about 4 kHz and contains amplitude-modulated components, phase locking serves to preserve temporal information found in human speech sound. Second, it serves to transmit temporal information to neural circuits of the brain stem capable of detecting ITD cues used by listeners for localizing the source of a sound in space. Neither the place theory nor the volley theory alone, however, fully account for a listener's ability to distinguish one tone from another, to encode the entire spectrum of speech, or to localize equally well both low- and high-frequency sounds. Hence, a duplex theory of hearing was postulated that states that temporal coding operates at low spectral frequency and that rate and place coding operate at high spectral frequency.

Sound intensity is likely encoded, in part, by the firing rate of auditory nerve fibers. As stimulus intensity is raised, the number of discharges steadily increases up to a plateau approximately 30–40 dB above threshold. Because a typical single auditory nerve fiber responds more or less linearly only over a 30- to 50-dB range of intensity, a second mechanism is needed to achieve the nearly 100 dB of dynamic range experienced by human listeners. This mechanism involves recruiting additional fibers with different discharge threshold into the active population.

Through the coding mechanisms outlined previously, the cochlear output faithfully reflects the time structure and intensity of speech and other naturally occurring sounds, with the spectrotemporal components of these coded messages distributed across the tonotopic array of primary afferent fibers. The representation of speech in the auditory periphery thus involves the full complement of temporal, rate, place, and ensemble encoding mechanisms operating in concert. Which mechanism dominates depends on the CF and spontaneous rate of the auditory nerve fiber and, in each instant in time, on the acoustic properties of the utterance and of the ambient environment.

Information transmitted in the auditory nerve array is received and transformed by neurons and neuronal circuits of the cochlear nuclei, and the resulting outputs are distributed over various pathways of central auditory system for further processing.

V. STRUCTURE AND FUNCTION OF THE CENTRAL AUDITORY PATHWAYS

The central auditory pathways have been studied extensively in many primate and nonprimate species using a wide range of anatomical and physiological methods. There are far fewer comparable studies in humans, but from them we may conclude that much of the neural circuitry and many of the neural mechanisms underlying mammalian hearing are, to the first approximation, shared by humans and nonhumans alike. Functional studies of the human central auditory system are discussed later. The top of Fig. 5 is a dorsal view of the human brain stem, midbrain, and thalamus showing the relative positions of the major nuclei in the ascending and descending mammalian auditory system. Auditory cortex on the temporal lobe is shown in cross section. The major connecting pathways are illustrated schematically below.

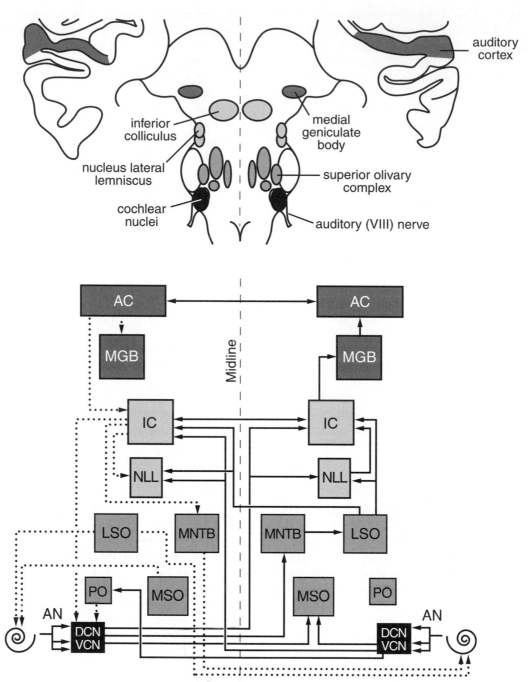

Figure 5 (Top) Dorsal view of the human brain stem, midbrain, thalamus, and cross section of the cortex showing the relative locations of the major nuclei in central auditory pathways. (Bottom) The major ascending (black lines and arrows) and descending (dotted lines and arrows) pathways connecting the major nuclei.

A. Cochlear Nuclear Complex: Initial Transformation of Sound Information Reaching the Brain

The cochlear nuclei, located bilaterally at the ponto-medullary junction, are the first synaptic stations in the central auditory pathway. The cochlear nuclei are obligatory relays, meaning that all information flowing from the cochlea must here encounter at least one synapse before being transmitted to higher auditory centers. In humans, as in all other mammals studied, two major cochlear nuclei are recognized: a dorsal cochlear nucleus (DCN) and a ventral cochlear nucleus (VCN). The latter is often subdivided into anterior and posterior divisions. Auditory nerve fibers penetrate this nuclear complex, bifurcate in an orderly (tonotopic) way, and terminate on neurons in both the DCN and the VCN. In addition to its major afferent supply from the inner ear, the cochlear nuclei receive input from a variety of other sources both intrinsic and extrinsic to the complex. Extrinsic sources include the other major brain stem nuclei. The role of these inputs in modulating the activity produced by primary afferent input from the ears is essentially unknown.

Cochlear nuclear neurons have been categorized based on their synaptic structure, cell morphology, pharmacology, connectivity, and acoustic response properties. Incoming spike trains that reach CN neurons are transformed by combinations of synaptic convergence and physiology, intrinsic membrane properties of target neurons, and feedback of excitation and inhibition via intrinsic or extrinsic circuitry. Cells of each category tend to extract particular features of sound that are transmitted by auditory nerve fibers, such as intensity, spectral composition, modulation amplitude and frequency, low-frequency time structure, and the timing of acoustic transients. Information received about human speech, for example, is thus distributed in such a way that one cell type preserves the temporal representation of vowels, whereas another cell type represents vowel information best in its rate of discharge. Similarly, other cell types extract formant transitions and still others transients (e.g., voice onset). Temporal information needed to detect ITD is preserved by still other cell types in the VCN having a highly specialized synaptic relationship (end bulb of Held) with auditory nerve fibers. Transformed information is sent to higher auditory centers for further processing over three pathways (stria).

Most axons leaving the VCN form a broad pathway that crosses the brain stem ventrally as the ventral stria or trapezoid body. A much smaller pathway, the intermediate acoustic stria, also leaves the VCN and joins the trapezoid body as it approaches the superior olivary complex, where many of its axons terminate. Axons of projecting neurons of the DCN form the dorsal acoustic stria, which reaches primarily the contralateral dorsal nucleus of the lateral lemniscus and the central nucleus of the inferior colliculus. At the level of the cochlear nuclei the input from the two ears has, for the most part, remained separated. One of the next levels of processing takes place in the superior olivary complex, where the inputs from the two ears converge and interact to encode sound direction.

B. Superior Olivary Complex: A Major Site for Integrating Input from the Two Ears

The superior olivary complex (SOC) comprises several interrelated nuclear groups located symmetrically on either side of the brain stem. There are three major SOC nuclei in most mammals studied: the lateral superior olivary nucleus (LSO), the medial superior olivary nucleus (MSO), and the medial nucleus of the trapezoid body (MNTB). In higher primates, including the human, the MNTB tends to be represented more by a collection of scattered neurons than by a coalesced structure. A number of periolivary nuclei (PO) are recognized as well. The major nuclei are the first stations in the auditory pathway that receive substantial bilateral input, and thus the SOC plays crucial roles in extracting and integrating information it receives from the two ears. Localizing the source of a sound in space is crucial to the survival of most animals, and to do so they rely on the fact that the positions of the ears on opposite sides of the head provide frequency-dependent ITD or IID. For human listeners, sound localization also plays an important role in identifying a talker in the presence of competing talkers (the so-called cocktail party effect). Sound localization in the horizontal plane is accomplished by engaging neural circuits in the SOC that compare these interaural time and intensity differences.

Principal neurons of the MSO have been shown in animal studies to receive direct input from particular cell types in the bilaterally placed ventral cochlear nuclei that preserve and transmit precise time information about a sound source in space. To a first approximation, these MSO neurons perform a cross-correlation on the spike trains arriving from the left and right ears. The projections from each ear form what may be considered a neural "delay line." As a result, phase-locked spikes transmitted over the two monaural channels arrive simultaneously at different MSO neurons depending on the interaural time delay and, hence, on the azimuthal (horizontal) location of a sound source. Next, the azimuthal location of a sound source is computed and is now represented at a "place" in the MSO.

In contrast, LSO neurons receive bilateral input from a different population of cochlear nuclear neurons. The ipsilateral input to the LSO is direct and excitatory, but the contralateral input involves an inhibitory interneuron in the MNTB. This arrangement renders LSO neurons particularly sensitive to IIDs. Hence, at this point in the central auditory system information concerning two of the major cues used by listeners in localizing the source of a sound in space has been extracted and to some extent segregated along two ascending pathways.

Periolivary nuclei in the human tend to encircle the MSO and LSO and are not easily distinguishable into subnuclei as they are in several other mammalian species. PO neurons in experimental animals have been shown to project profusely back to the cochlear nuclei as well as forward to midbrain auditory structures.

A bundle of axons arising in the SOC as well as passing axons form the CN is referred to as the lateral lemniscus. Two major cell groups embedded in this band of axons form the dorsal (DNLL) and lateral (VNLL) nuclei, respectively, of the lateral lemniscus. A third, intermediate (INLL) nuclear group has been identified in several animal species but not in humans. The VNLL receives its major input from the contralateral VCN via the trapezoid body and from the ipsilateral SOC. In contrast, the DNLL receives convergent input from a wide variety of sources, including the contralateral DCN and DNLL and ipsilateral SOC and VNLL. Ascending axons originating in the DNLL and VNLL contribute to the lateral lemniscus, which is now destined for the inferior colliculus.

Although the functions of the SOC and LL nuclei have not been studied directly in humans, synchronous firing of neurons in and around these auditory brain stem areas is believed to be the source of the wave IV–V complex in the sound-evoked averaged brain stem potential recorded from the scalp (Fig. 7).

C. Olivocochlear Efferent System: Central Modulation of Inner Ear Transduction

The cochlea, in addition to supplying afferent input to the brain stem, receives efferent projections that originate in the SOC. In animal studies it has been shown that two basic groups of brain stem neurons provide efferent innervation to the organ of Corti. Based on the general locations of their cell bodies in the SOC, they form the lateral (LOC) or medial (MOC) olivocochlear system. The LOC originates from AChE-positive neurons in and around the LSO and terminates primarily in the ipsilateral cochlea, at the base of inner hair cells. Small AChE-positive cells, believed to be LOC neurons, are found in this location

in the human brain stem. The MOC arises for the most part from neurons medial to the MSO and reaches the base of outer hair cells mainly in the contralateral inner ear. Collaterals of olivocochlear axons terminate in the cochlear nuclei. Both LOC and MOC neurons receive input from the ventral cochlear nucleus, with the MOC also receiving input from the inferior colliculus. Cochlear efferents are activated by sound and thereby provide reflex feedback to the cochlea. The consequence of this feedback is increased acoustic threshold due to reduced OHC amplification, which helps protect the cochlea from potentially damaging loud sounds and improves detectability of wanted sound in the presence of unwanted background masking noise. Sound induced reflex contraction of the middle ear muscles serves to complement the action of the olivocochlear system.

D. The Auditory Midbrain: Major Integrating Centers

The inferior and superior colliculi collectively form the roof of the midbrain. Both are major integrating centers, receiving converging input from a wide variety of sources representing the auditory, visual, and somatosensory systems.

Anatomically, the IC is subdivided into a central nucleus (ICC) and a surrounding cortex (divided into external and pericentral nuclei). The ICC forms an essential link in the mainline lemniscal auditory system and thus is critically involved in the transmission of auditory sensory information to the forebrain from lower auditory centers. The ICC also receives a rich supply of afferents from many other sources and directs its outputs to a variety of targets. This results in numerous feedback loops (Fig. 5) that involve essentially all major auditory areas of the forebrain, midbrain, and brain stem of the same side of the brain. In addition, several major axonal bundles (commissures) connect auditory areas of one side of the brain with their counterparts on the other. Hence, it is not surprising that essentially all information transmitted to the auditory forebrain is first transformed within the ICC. Transformations involve changes in the balance of excitation and inhibition exerted by converging afferent inputs—changes that are reflected in such fundamental attributes of coding as frequency tuning curves, timing of spike discharges, spontaneous background activity, sensitivity to modulations in frequency and intensity, binaural interactions, and spatial tuning. Remarkably, the diverse parallel input and output, and the transformations associated with them, are highly organized within the ICC tonotopic map, which is best described as being made up of frequency-specific layers or bands. Within each band are overlapping functional maps related to a wide array of response features and stimulus attributes such as amplitude modulation, pitch, intensity, threshold, onset latency, sharpness of frequency tuning, and binaural sensitivity. It is thought that these functional maps may provide the early substrates from which sound percepts are eventually derived. Information transformed by the ICC is carried to the auditory forebrain via the brachium of the IC.

The superior colliculus (SC) is a layered structure involved primarily in the control of movements of the eyes to an auditory or visual target. Thus, in the classical sense it is not a "sensory" structure. Auditory input carries information on the direction of a sound source to deep SC layers. Sound-source direction is represented by SC neurons having spatial receptive fields arrayed to form a map of auditory space. Visual input is received in the upper layers, and information on target direction is provided by its position on the SC visuotopic map. The auditory and visual maps are normally in alignment, presumably to coordinate visual and auditory directional information so that the eyes can move quickly and accurately to an object that appears in the visual and sound fields.

VI. FUNCTIONAL ORGANIZATION OF THE AUDITORY FOREBRAIN

The auditory forebrain consists of auditory thalamic relay nuclei and those cortical areas with which they have intimate reciprocal relationships. Together these forebrain areas carry out the highest levels of information processing in the auditory pathway.

A. Thalamus

The medial geniculate body (MGB) is a complex of nuclei that receive massive input from the IC and thus serve as major synaptic stations in the pathways for information reaching auditory areas of cerebral cortex. The MGB nuclei can be differentiated from one another on the basis of cytoarchitecture, chemoarchitecture, tonotopy, connectivity patterns, and acoustic response properties. Neighboring nuclei of the posterior complex and pulvinar also receive auditory input and project upon auditory cortex. The auditory

thalamus receives its input over pathways that originate in brain stem nuclei contributing to the lateral lemniscus as well as pathways that are nonlemniscal in origin. The cellular architecture of the human MGB is remarkably similar to that of OldWorld and New-World monkeys. Although the relative size and strength of each auditory cortical projection differ from one MGB subdivison to the next, each auditory cortical field receives highly convergent input from a subset of auditory thalamic nuclei and each auditory thalamic subdivision projects in a topographic way to a subset of auditory cortical fields. Thus, the auditory thalamocortical system, like auditory brain stem circuitry, exhibits widespread convergence and divergence. Tones evoke a characteristic pattern of cortical activation that reflects the thalamic projection to that active site. The earliest electrical response is thought to represent monosynaptic activation of neurons in cortical laminae 3 and 4, whereas later activity is considered polysynaptic activation through supragranular cortical layers. In addition to receiving massive ascending input from brain stem and midbrain auditory structures, the MGB also receives a substantial projection from those areas of cerebral cortex to which it projects. This reciprocal relationship provides opportunity for feedback control of ascending auditory input.

The ventral divison (MGBv) displays a high degree of tonotopy imposed by input from the similarly organized ICC. Nonauditory input to the ventral division is derived from the thalamic reticular and ventrolateral medullary nuclei. The MGBv projects heavily on the core areas of auditory cortex, including the primary field. Neurons in the MGBv preserve and convey to cortex with high fidelity the temporal and frequency-specific properties exhibited in the auditory brain stem. In the human, the dorsal division (MGBd) is larger and structurally more heterogeneous than the ventral division. It receives its auditory input from neurons primarily in the pericentral nucleus of the IC. Other afferents arise from the thalamic reticular nucleus, ventrolateral medullary nucleus, nucleus sagulum, superior colliculus, and brachium of the inferior colliculus. Neurons of the MGBd, in contrast to those of the MGBv, are poorly responsive to most sounds and are broadly tuned for frequency; hence, tonotopy is not a remarkable feature. The main targets of MGBd neurons are the belt areas of cortex. The medial, or magnocellular, division (MGBm) also exhibits diverse cellular architecture, and it receives input mainly from the external nucleus of the IC. Tonotopy is not a remarkable feature of this nucleus, again reflecting the organization of its main afferent source. Neighboring thalamic nuclei, including the posterior group and the pulvinar, receive auditory input and send projections to auditory cortical fields.

MGB neurons in all divisions appear to preserve ITD or IID information extracted at brain stem levels and widely disperse this information to auditory areas of cerebral cortex. Neurons within the MGB and auditory cortical fields respond best when the sound source is in the contralateral acoustic hemifield. There is no obvious anatomical specialization in MGB in humans for speech, nor is there evidence for bilateral asymmetry in the size of the MGB.

B. Auditory Cortex

1. Auditory Cortex Is Made up of Multiple Fields to Carry out Parallel and Serial Processing

In all mammals studied, auditory cortex is made up of multiple fields, which are distinguished from one another on both anatomical and functional grounds. The number of such fields varies among species studied from as few as 2 in rodents to as many as 15 in the rhesus monkey. The number, location, and organization of such fields in the human are not fully known. It would be highly desirable, however, to know the functional and structural counterparts of human and monkey auditory cortex. Although much less is known about the functional organization of temporal auditory cortex in the human than in the monkey, from available data there are some striking anatomical similarities between the two species. These data, together with modern imaging [functional magnetic resonance imaging (fMRI) and positron emission tomography (PET)] and direct [electrocorticography (ECoG)] and indirect [electroencephalography (EEG) and magnetoencephalography (MEG)] electrophysiological recording data in humans, enable us to tentatively apply to the human a model of functional organization of auditory cortex developed for the monkey. Figure 6C shows a schematic representation of monkey auditory cortex based on modern anatomical and physiological studies. Primary auditory cortex is combined with adjacent cortex to form a core area. Surrounding the core auditory cortex is an auditory belt area, and around that is a parabelt region. The belt and parabelt areas are often referred to as secondary or associational areas. Figures 6A and 6B show two views of the human brain showing the general locations and extent of what may be equivalent

core, belt, and parabelt areas in the human. There is general agreement about the location, extent, and tonotopic organization of the human primary auditory field (AI), on the mesial aspect of Heschl's gyrus (HG). There is less agreement about the organization of surrounding auditory. Whether this monkey model is adequate to describe the human auditory cortex is yet to be determined. Currently, however, it provides a tool for further exploration using modern recording and imaging technology.

We know from animal studies that auditory fields receive ascending input from the auditory thalamus, that they are richly interconnected on the same and opposite cerebral hemispheres, and that they provide afferent input to the MGB and IC as part of a massive parallel descending system of pathways that eventually reaches the lower auditory brain stem and the cochlea (Fig. 5). These auditory cortical areas are confined to temporal cortex and serve primarily a sensory function. This means that their neurons and neuronal circuits are sensitive mainly to changes in physical parameters of a suprathreshold acoustic signal reaching the ears, and thus they are designed to detect, discriminate, identify, and localize sound sources. Multiple auditory areas are thought to represent hierarchical processing levels. Some areas involved in higher order processing of acoustic stimuli, such as speech, lie outside of these "classic" auditory fields, on the frontal and parietal lobes.

2. Functional Organization of Primary Auditory Cortex: Maps of Stimulus Features

The primary auditory field (AI) has been identified anatomically and studied physiologically in a wide range of mammalian species, including humans. It is reciprocally and topographically tied to MGBv. Within AI, neurons are typically sharply tuned for frequency. Like other sensory cortices, AI exhibits a columnar representation of the peripheral sensory epithelium: Neurons occupying a vertical column tend to have the same or very similar CF. A tone just above threshold would activate a relatively small population of neurons in a cortical band having length, depth, and width (a cortical "sheet"). AI is thus said to be organized into isofrequency bands or sheets. The organization of the AI tonotopic map varies from one subject to the next, possibly suggesting that environmental factors may be involved in the formation and shaping of functional maps. It is now known that the AI tonotopic map exhibits plasticity because it undergoes dramatic change following a cochlear lesion. One can only

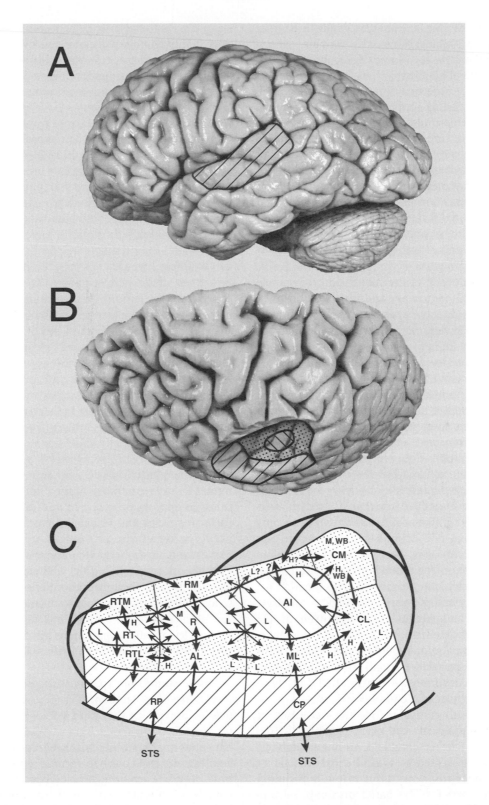

Figure 6 (A and B) Lateral and dorsal views, respectively, of the human brain showing the approximate extent and locations of known auditory fields on the lateral and superior surfaces of the superior temporal gyrus. (C) Diagram of the organization of auditory cortical fields on the same temporal lobe areas of the rhesus monkey (adapted with permission from Hackett, T. A., Stepniewski, I. and Kaas, J. H., *J. Comp. Neurol.* **394,** 475–495, 1998).

wonder if, for example, the improvement in hearing performance over time exhibited by subjects with a cochlear prosthesis may, to some degree, be attributed to auditory cortical plasticity.

In addition to a tonotopic representation within AI, studies of experimental animals have revealed spatial maps related to other functional properties associated with pure tones, ripple spectra noise, broadband transients, frequency sweeps, and binaural stimuli. The picture that emerges from this work is one of primary auditory cortex being made up of overlaid topographic representations of numerous independent stimulus features. To complicate matters even further, these representations, which are based on neuronal firing rate and spike timing, depend on stimulus intensity. Thus, individual stimulus features *per se* are probably not coded at the cortex simply by some fixed place within the primary auditory field. Instead, they may be coded by spatiotemporal activation patterns created by neuronal assemblies within cortex that change in dynamic ways to reflect the many and changing acoustic features that make up complex natural sounds, including speech.

Several auditory cortical maps represent fundamental acoustic features of a stimulus (e.g., spectrum and noise bandwidth), whereas others represent derived properties (e.g., binaural interactions) or perceptual qualities (e.g., pitch). The binaural organizational patterns distributed across AI are examples of computational maps representing the direction of a sound source in acoustic space. Because there is no extraction of spatial direction by the cochlea, such maps can only result from neural interactions taking place in the lower auditory brain stem, where spike trains arriving over the two monaural channels converge. Similarly, a cortical map of pitch may be laid out orthogonal to the tonotopic map. Pitch is the psychological attribute associate with fundamental frequency even in the absence of spectral energy at the pitch frequency. Hence, its representation on cortex would provide evidence for a higher order cortical representation of a percept rather than simply a sensation tied directly to the physical attributes of a complex stimulus.

AI cortical neurons may encode the frequency of temporal modulation of the sound envelope in the phase-locked activity of cortical neuronal assemblies. Indeed, the phase-locked thalamocortical input may provide the upper frequency limit of pitch encoding (approximatley 400–600 Hz) based on temporal mechanisms. Studies of cortical coding of species-specific vocalization and human speech in monkey have revealed no simple correlation between a single cortical neuron's response properties and a particular utterance. Thus, auditory cortical neurons may be specialized to respond more on the basis of the presence or absence of certain acoustic components embedded in a vocalization rather than on a unique vocalization per se. fMRI studies in humans have also revealed that activation of the core auditory area differed little from the surrounding cortex when speech and nonspeech sounds were presented to normal-listening subjects, again indicating that these fields are more involved in detecting the acoustic rather than linguistic parameters of speech. Indeed, the tonotopic constraints imposed on AI and the highly individualistic responses of its neurons to complex sounds suggest that specific mechanisms for identification of individual phonemes, for example, would not reside in this field and, moreover, that such specificity to speech or other species-specific communication sounds is more likely accomplished by ensembles of cortical neurons rather than by single cells. On the other hand, fields on the ventral aspect of the temporal lobe and on the temporal–parietal boundaries of the left cerebral hemisphere show greater activation to speech than to nonspeech sound.

3. Temporal Lobe Lesions Impair Acoustic Processing

Lesion behavioral studies, mainly in rat, cat, and monkey, have provided limited information on the function and organization of auditory cortex. Differences in species and in experimental paradigms have led to conflicting results across studies. One major impairment associated with auditory cortical lesions in cat and monkey, however, is localization of brief sounds in space. Lesioned animals exhibit an inability to localize sound in the acoustic hemifield opposite the side of the lesion. Additional consequences of auditory cortical lesions are impaired discrimination and retention of certain temporal patterns, including species-specific vocalizations.

Lesion studies in experimental animals usually aim to produce damage confined to a particular cortical field or portion of that field, often guided by electrophysiological mapping. This may be done repeatedly in a series of animals in which well-controlled behavior studies are carried out before and for varying period of time after the lesion is made. Far fewer systematic studies of human patients with auditory cortical lesions have been reported. Under ideal conditions a human subject communicates and cooperates well with the examiner in performing complex psychophysical tests. Specific deficits in auditory processing can then be quantified and correlated with anatomical data now obtainable from brain MRIs. Rarely, however, is this ideal achieved. For the most part, patients present with clinical symptoms resulting from large, spontaneously occurring lesions; hence, no two patients experience lesions of the same size and location. The damage is rarely, if ever, confined to a single cortical field. Patient–subjects are scattered geographically and thus examined by different investigators having different specific scientific interests using different experimental methods. Possible exceptions to this are studies of epilepsy patients undergoing temporal lobectomy. Even here, however, a unilateral temporal lobe resection varies in size from one patient to the next and usually does not extend into the core auditory cortex on the mesial aspect of HG. When a cortical lesion is made for clinical purposes, only rarely are preoperative baseline psychophysical data obtained. Even when this is done, however, attention is not always paid to the fact that following an acute brain lesion considerable recovery in function occurs over time. Futhermore, many cases may be overlooked because marked, clinically significant deficits in basic auditory functions are observed only in patients who have sustained bilateral temporal lobe damage. Hence, results of psychophysical testing in the chronic state may not provide a comprehensive picture of the functional significance of regions of auditory cortex affected by a lesion.

With these caveats, it is clear that apart from speech function, which strongly lateralizes to one (usually the left) hemisphere, basic auditory functions are subserved by both hemispheres. However, there does appear to be a degree of lateralization of musical processing to the right hemisphere. Bilateral lesions approximately confined to the core auditory areas are reported to result in transient auditory agnosia, which is a lack of awareness of auditory stimuli combined with abnormal pure tone thresholds in the absence of peripheral or brain stem damage (sometimes referred to as cortical deafness). With time, this condition may evolve into auditory agnosia for speech (pure word deafness), whereby patients regain near normal auditory acuity but remain impaired in their ability to interpret speech sounds. It is hypothesized that speech decoding requires more precise temporal analysis than is necessary for the detection and identification of most nonverbal sounds. This capacity to represent auditory stimuli with a high degree of temporal resolution is dependent on having intact core auditory cortex in at least one hemisphere. Conversely, the core regions can

be destroyed, but recognition of nonspeech sounds can remain intact, presumably mediated by surrounding auditory cortical fields that are functionally activated via parallel thalamic afferent inputs that do not synapse, or course through, the auditory core region. Anecdotal observations of localization ability in patients with temporal lobe lesions have suggested repeatedly that humans and nonhuman species suffer impairment in sound-localization ability. Recent and carefully controlled experiments indicate that such impairment is less marked than previously believed.

A small number of patients who have bilateral temporal lobe lesions that spare at least one core region while destroying portions of the middle and anterior regions of the superior temporal gyri (but not Wernicke's speech area) display a strikingly different pattern of auditory impairment than those with bilateral core lesions. Receptive speech function is preserved but there is a marked dysfunction of musical processing and of recognition of nonverbal auditory stimuli. It seems clear that lesions of auditory association cortex that spare core auditory regions are sufficient to impair melody discrimination and the perception of speech prosody. The existence of cases in which each one of these categories of nonverbal auditory processing is selectively impaired suggests that different subregions of auditory association cortex may serve a specialized role in representing different attributes of nonverbal auditory stimuli. It is not clear how these subregions, whose existence is implied by lesion study results, might correlate with cytoarchitectural or electrophysiologic findings in humans.

4. Functional Studies of the Human Central Auditory System

Studies of the neural mechanisms underlying hearing in humans have, with few exceptions, necessarily involved noninvasive and hence indirect methods of measurement of functional brain activity, including EEG, MEG, PET, and fMRI. These methods have proved to be most effective when used in complementary ways.

a. Electrophysiological Measures: EEG and MEG An electrode placed on the scalp records the summated electrical potentials generated by large groups of neurons in the brain. These neuronal assemblies at each station along the auditory pathway fire sychronously and in sequential order in response to a brief and abrupt acoustic stimulus. This orderly

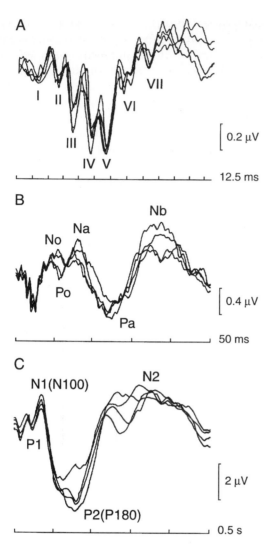

Figure 7 Auditory event-related potentials (ERPs) recorded from the scalp of a human subject in response to the presentation of brief sounds. The ERP is divided into three epochs: a short latency auditory brain stem response (ABR) (A), a middle latency response (MLR) (B), and a late, long-latency response (C) (adapted with permission from Picton, T.W., *et al.*, *EEG Clin Neurophysiol.* **36**, 179–190, 1974).

firing pattern is reflected in the sequence of peaks and valleys that make up the resulting evoked potential waveform, referred to as the event-related potential (ERP). The ERP typically is of very low amplitude and usually indistinguishable from the ongoing EEG. Thus, in practice, averaging the responses to hundreds or thousands of stimulus presentations is needed to reveal the ERP temporal waveform. The ERP is traditionally divided into three time epochs (Fig. 7). The seven waves arising during the first 10–15 msec

(Fig. 7A) after stimulus onset constitute the averaged brain stem response (ABR). Intraoperative recording from the human auditory nerve, cochlear nuclei, and inferior colliculi has provided the most compelling evidence that waves I and II are generated by the auditory nerve, wave III by the cochlear nuclei, and wave IV by the SOC. Wave V probably originates in or below the inferior colliculus, whereas waves VI and VII originate in the ICC or thalamocortical projection system. Thus, the temporal waveform of the ERP, its spatial distribution on the scalp, and its sensitivity to various acoustic parameters can provide information about the transmission and encoding properties of large neuronal assemblies at all levels of the central auditory pathway. The ABR is highly stable under a wide range of conditions, including various stages of consciousness, attention, sleep, wakefulness, and sedation. It is present at birth and mature by approximately 18 months. Today, it is used routinely to screen for hearing impairment in newborn babies. Overall, the ABR has proven to be a very useful noninvasive and objective way to test for hearing impairment and other disorders of the peripheral and central auditory pathways, especially in those subjects who are unwilling or unable to participate.

A cluster of three major wave peaks with onset latency beyond the ABR components (out to about 50–60 msec) are widely recorded over the frontal and temporal cortex and referred to as the middle latency response (MLR; Fig. 7B). The generation of the MLR may involve the interaction of many brain structures within and outside of the classic lemniscal auditory pathways. Lesions of auditory cortex in humans and animals disrupt MLR waveforms. MLR is influenced by the state of arousal of a subject, suggesting involvement of the reticular formation. The MLR is used clinically to assess hearing thresholds in the low-frequency range and to evaluate auditory pathway function in hearing individuals and in subjects who have cochlear implants.

When trains of brief stimuli are presented the MLR components become time locked to the individual stimuli at frequencies of approximately 40 Hz. This 40-Hz response to the appropriate stimulus is exhibited by other sensory systems as well, indicating that it represents a general mechanism for recognizing a sensory event. Spontaneous electrical oscillation in the human brain at frequencies of approximately 40 Hz and its resetting by a sensory stimulus have been postulated to reflect cortical mechanisms involved in temporal binding of sensory stimuli and perceptual scene segregation.

Finally, a series of peaks and valleys is recorded with latencies exceeding 50 msec (Fig. 7C). The amplitudes of the waves are higher but more variable than earlier ones, depending on the conscious state of the subject and the stimulus paradigm employed to evoke the waveform. This has led to the suggestion that the late components represent the convergence of input from a number of forebrain systems whose interactions are related to the attentive or cognitive state of the subject.

The currents that give rise to the electrical voltage recorded on the scalp also give rise to weak magnetic fields. These weak fields can be measured by an array of sensitive magnetometers (superconducting quantum interference devices) surrounding the head. The method is known as MEG, and the response to a sound is referred to as the auditory-evoked magnetic field (AEF) (Fig. 8). AEF data reveal many of the same

cortical processes as the ERP. Both methods yield similar waveforms with excellent response times capable of tracking with high fidelity neural events in time. In addition, the MEG offers relatively high spatial resolution, on the order of millimeters. Because of its differential sensitivity to currents flowing tangentially to the scalp, the MEG is particularly suited for noninvasive study of the cortex buried within fissures, including auditory cortex within the Sylvian fissure on the superior temporal plane. Because any electrical potential or magnetic signal may have more than one source in the brain (the so-called inverse problem), a source model is applied in which the orientation, strength, and location of the equivalent current dipoles are best accounted for on statistical grounds.

The ERP and AEF methods have been used effectively to study the neural activity associated with

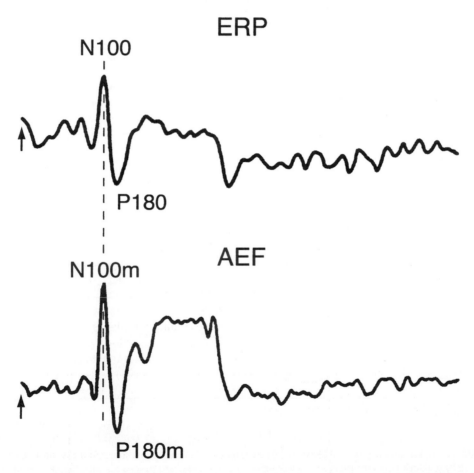

Figure 8 Electromagnetic waves generated by the cortex and recorded on or near the head in response to an acoustic stimulus. Event-related potential (ERP) represents electrical potentials recorded with an electrode in contact with the scalp. The auditory-evoked magnetic field (AEF) is the magnetic field recorded from a detector very near the head. The major component is a middle latency response because it occurs approximately 100 msec after stimulus onset (adapted with permission from Hari, R., *Adv. Audiol.* **6,** 222–282, 1990).

attentional and cognitive processes. Figure 9 (top) shows an example of the ERP obtained when a subject heard the same sound repeatedly and then when a rare, or odd-ball, stimulus was introduced at random times. The major changes associated with the waveform occurred relatively late, after about 200 msec. Similarly, the AES waveforms (Fig. 9, bottom) were obtained under conditions in which the subject was awake but reading and when the subject was attending to the stimulus. Like the ERP, the late components are the ones most affected by this difference in state of attention. These late components are thought to reflect the processing of auditory stimuli.

b. Functional Imaging: PET and fMRI   In recent years, the use of noninvasive functional imaging techniques—fMRI and PET—has provided a wealth of new information concerning the location and extent of regions of the human brain that are metabolically activated by acoustic stimulation. Both methods provide indirect evidence of neuronal activation based on the facts that when neurons become more active they require more oxygen and glucose and that this increased demand is met by a compensatory increase in regional cerebral blood flow. Using these indirect imaging methods, investigators have noted that broad regions of the supratemporal plane and lateral superior temporal gyrus are bilaterally activated by a wide

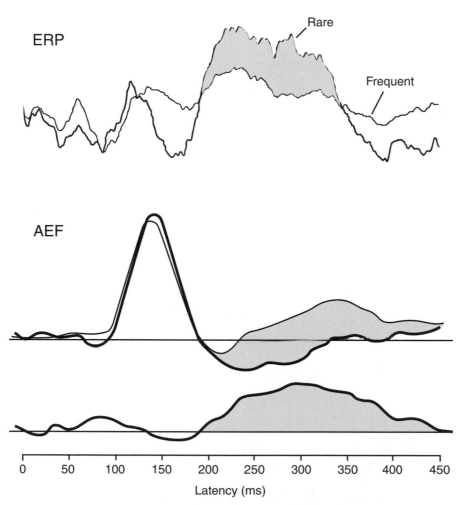

Figure 9   Sound-evoked event-related potential (ERP) and AEF are sensitive to unexpected changes in the sound and to shifts of the listener's attention. (Top) ERPs obtained when the same sound was repeated many times (frequent) and when that stream of repeated sound was interrupted occasionally by a different (rare) sound [adapted with permission from Kraus, N., and McGee, T., *The Mammalian Auditory Pathway*: Neuroanatomy (A. N. Popper and R. R. Fay Eds.). Springer-Verlag, New York, 1992]. (Bottom) The auditory-evoked magnetic field (AEF) obtained when listener attended (counting stimuli) or did not attend (reading) to the stimulus (adapted with permission from Hari, R., *Adv. Audiol.* **6,** 222–282, 1990). The main effect of both activities was seen in the late waves, beyond the 100-msec component.

range of acoustic stimuli, including speech sounds. Tones of different frequency induce localized changes in blood flow within subregions of HG, indicating a tonotopic organization, with higher frequency tones activating the more posterior–medial portion of HG. More complex tasks have been used in conjunction with fMRI to search for evidence of regional functional specialization within auditory cortex. Results from these investigations indicate that the right temporal lobe may play a more important role in the processing of musical stimuli (e.g., pitch and rhythmic temporal patterns) than the left. There have also been reports suggesting functional specialization of right-sided temporal (and parietal) lobe regions in processing information concerning the movement of sound sources. Both fMRI and PET methods have been used extensively to map patterns of cortical activation during speech sound processing.

Inherent limitations of these methods have prevented direct extrapolation of data obtained with these methods to results obtained in nonhuman primates using microelectrode recording techniques. In the future, however, the spatial resolution of fMRI may improve to the extent that the functional organization of human auditory cortex can be studied in far greater detail. Because activity-induced changes in blood flow patterns occur over a period of seconds, it is unlikely that fMRI techniques alone will be capable of delineating the fine temporal patterns of activity that characterize coding and processing of information at the level of auditory cortex.

c. Direct Recording (ECoG) and Stimulation of Auditory Structures in Human Direct electrical-stimulation mapping of the cortex during surgery to relieve medically intractable epilepsy or to remove a tumor is commonly carried out as a way of guiding the surgeon's decision on the location and extent of brain tissue to excise. When the primary auditory field on HG is stimulated, patients report hearing sounds, which are often referred to the ear contralateral to the stimulated cortex. Stimulation of the belt of cortex surrounding the primary field may result in the perception of more complex sounds, although it is now thought that some of this—especially the so-called experiential hallucinations—may be the result of spread of stimulus current to underlying limbic structures. In the caudal region of the superior temporal gyrus (Wernicke's area), and on the angular and supramarginal gyri electrical stimulation may result in the arrest of speech, which is similar to the results of stimulation of the classic Broca's area on the inferior frontal gyrus.

Direct recording from the human auditory cortex has also been carried out in neurosurgical patients both acutely in the operating room and chronically under more controlled experimental conditions. This recording is referred to as the ECoG to differentiate it from the scalp recorded EEG. Results from these experiments show acoustically evoked activity on the superior temporal plane and the lateral surface of the superior temporal gyrus. A field on HG is distinguished from a field on superior temporal cortex based on the HG tonotopic map and the properties of acoustically evoked potentials. Thus, cytoarchitectonic, electrophysiologic, and functional imaging data leave little doubt that the cortex on mesial HG is the primary auditory field of the human and the homolog of AI in nonhuman primates and other mammals. The cortex of the lateral surface of the superior temporal gyrus represents one or more separate auditory fields. Intraoperative electrophysiological studies show that single neurons in this cortex respond vigorously to complex sound, including speech—a finding similar to that in the rhesus monkey.

See Also the Following Articles

AUDITORY CORTEX • AUDITORY PERCEPTION • BRAIN STEM • FOREBRAIN • SENSORY DEPRIVATION • TEMPORAL LOBES • VISION: BRAIN MECHANISMS

Suggested Reading

Crocker, M. J. (Ed.) (1997). *Encylology of Acoustics.* Wiley, New York.

Ehret, G., and Romand, R. (1997). *The Central Auditory System.* Oxford Univ. Press, New York.

Geisler, C. D. (1998). *From Sound to Synapse. Physiology of the Mammalian Ear.* Oxford Univ. Press, New York.

Gilkey, R. II., and Anderson, T. R. (Eds.) (1997). *Binaural and Spatial Hearing in Real and Virtual Environments.* Erlbaum, Mahway, NJ.

Harrison, R. V., Kraus, N., Lütkenhöner, B., Rajan, R., and Schreiner, Ch. (Eds.) (1998). *Functional Organization and Plasticity of the Auditory Cortex. Audiology and Neuro-Otology,* **3,** 73–223. Karger, Basel.

Moore, J. K. (1987). The human auditory brain stem: A comparative view. *Hearing Res.* **29,** 1–32.

Moore, J. K. (1994). The human brainstem auditory pathway. In *Neurotology* (R. K. Jackier and D. E. Brachmann, Eds.), pp. 1–17. Mosby, St. Louis.

Nadol, J. B., Jr. (1988). Comparative anatomy of the cochlea and auditory nerve in mammals. *Hearing Res.* **34,** 253–266.

Peters, A., and Jones, E. G. (Eds.) (1985). *Cerebral Cortex: Association and Auditory Cortices*, Vol. 4. Plenum, New York.

Popper, A. N., and Fay, R. R. (Eds.) (1992). *The Mammalian Auditory Pathway: Neurophysiology*, Vol. 2. Springer-Verlag, New York.

Toga, A. W., and Mazziotta, J. C. (2000). *Brain Mapping, The Systems*. Academic Press, San Diego.

Webster, D. B., Popper, A. N., and Fay, R. R. (Eds.) (1992). *The Mammalian Auditory Pathway: Neuroanatomy*, Vol. 1. Springer-Verlag, New York.

Yost, W. A. (1994). *Fundamentals of Hearing. An Introduction*. Academic Press, New York.

Yost, W. A., Popper, A. N., and Fay, R. R. (Eds.) (1993). *Human Psychophysics*, Vol. 3. Springer-Verlag, New York.

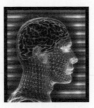

Heuristics

RALPH HERTWIG and PETER M. TODD

Max Planck Institute for Human Development, Berlin

GLOSSARY

algorithm A strategy for solving a problem that guarantees solution in a finite number of steps if the problem has at least one solution. An example of a very simple algorithm is that for obtaining temperature on the Fahrenheit scale when the value for the centigrade scale is known: Multiply the known value by 1.8 and add 32.

bounded rationality Principles underlying nonoptimizing adaptive behavior of real information processing systems working under conditions of limited time, information, and computational capacities. Among those principles specified by Herbert Simon is satisficing.

cognitive illusions or biases Systematic deviations of human judgments from rules of probability theory and logic. The occurrence of cognitive illusions is attributed to some judgment heuristics that are often useful but sometimes lead to predictable errors.

heuristic An approximate strategy or "rule of thumb" for problem solving and decision making that does not guarantee a correct solution but that typically yields a reasonable solution quickly or brings one closer to hand.

noncompensatory heuristic A heuristic is noncompensatory if, once it has used a piece of information to make a decision, no further information in any combination can undo or compensate for the effect of the original information. In contrast, a heuristic is compensatory if there is at least one piece of information that can be outweighed by other pieces of information. A compensatory strategy integrates at least some of the available information and makes trade-offs between the relevant pieces of information to form an overall evaluation of each of the available alternatives or options.

satisficing According to Herbert Simon, satisficing is using experience to construct an expectation (or aspiration level) of a reasonable solution to some problem and stopping the search for solutions as soon as one is found that meets the expectation.

unbounded rationality Decision-making strategies that have no regard for constraints of time, knowledge, or computational capacities. Modern mainstream economic theory is largely based on unbounded rationality models that portray economic agents as fully rational Bayesian maximizers of subjective utility.

Many decisions faced by people cannot be made in an optimal way because optimal solutions may take too much computation to find or may not even exist. Instead, real decision makers must often take shortcuts and use heuristics that yield reasonable solutions in a reasonable amount of time, even if they do not guarantee always reaching a good decision. These heuristics are thus an essential aspect of human intelligence, leading to adaptive behavior despite the challenging conditions of limited time, knowledge, and computational capacity under which people have to solve problems. Heuristics are most commonly studied in psychology, particularly within the domains of judgment and decision making, and in computer-based applications in artificial intelligence and operations research. This article focuses on research in psychology that has proposed heuristic models of how people search for information and make decisions and choices.

I. A SHORT HISTORY OF THE CONCEPT "HEURISTIC"

Recent research on decision heuristics descends from earlier schools of thought. For this reason, understanding current thought can be aided by first considering the history of the concept. In 1905, the 26-year-old Albert Einstein published his first fundamental paper in quantum physics, titled "On a Heuristic Point of View Concerning the Production and Transformation of Light." In that Nobel prize-winning paper, Einstein used the term heuristic to indicate that he considered the view he presented therein as incomplete, even false, but still useful. Einstein could not wholeheartedly accept the quantum view of light that he started to develop in this paper, but he believed that it was of great transitory use on the way to building a more correct theory. As used by Einstein, a heuristic (a term of Greek origin meaning "serving to find out or discover") is an approach to a problem that is necessarily incomplete given the knowledge available, and hence unavoidably false, but that is useful nonetheless for guiding thinking in appropriate directions.

A few decades later, Max Wertheimer (a close friend of Einstein's), Karl Duncker, and other Gestalt psychologists spoke of heuristic reasoning, but with a slightly different meaning from that of Einstein. Gestalt psychologists conceptualized thinking as an interaction between inner mental processes and external problem structure. In this view, heuristic methods such as "looking around" and "inspecting the problem" are first used to guide the search for appropriate information in the environment, which is then restructured or reformulated by inner processes.

Heuristic methods also play a prominent role in George Pólya's approach to mathematical problem solving. According to the Hungarian mathematician, effective problem solving consists of four main phases—understanding the problem, devising a plan, carrying out the plan, and looking back—all of which can incorporate heuristics. Devising a plan, for instance, can include heuristic methods such as "examine a simpler or special case of the problem to gain insight into the solution of the original problem," "work backward," or "identify a subgoal."

In the 1950s and 1960s, Herbert Simon and Allen Newell started to develop heuristics for searching for solutions to problems. They replaced the somewhat vague notion of heuristic reasoning of the Gestalt school and of Pólya's with much more precise computer-based models (e.g., in the General Problem Solver system) of human problem solving and reasoning largely based on the means–ends analysis heuristic. This heuristic found some way to reduce the distance between the current state and the goal state. With the advent of information processing theory in cognitive psychology, a heuristic came to mean a useful shortcut, an approximation, or a rule of thumb for guiding search through a space of possible solutions, such as a strategy that a chess master uses to explore the enormous number of possible moves at each point in a game.

Such general-purpose or "weak" methods as the means–ends analysis heuristic, however, proved insufficient to deal with problems other than artificial and well-defined mathematical problems or the games of chess and cryptoarithmetic that Newell and Simon investigated. As a consequence, research in artificial intelligence (AI) in the 1970s turned to collecting domain-specific rules of thumb from specialists in a particular field and incorporating these into expert systems. At approximately the same time, mathematicians working in operations research began dealing with new results from computational complexity theory indicating that efficient algorithmic solutions to many classes of challenging combinatorial problems (such at the traveling salesman problem) might not be found; as a consequence, they too turned to the search for problem-specific heuristics, although through invention rather than behavioral observation.

In psychology after 1970, researchers became increasingly interested in how people reason about unknown or uncertain aspects of real-world environments. The research program that spurred this interest was the heuristics-and-biases program initiated by Amos Tversky and Daniel Kahneman. This program's research strategy has been to measure human decision making against various normative standards taken from probability theory and statistics. Based on this strategy two major results about people's reasoning under uncertainty emerged: a collection of violations of the normative standards (that in analogy to perceptual illusions are often called "cognitive illusions" or "biases") and explanations of these illusions in terms of a small number of cognitive heuristics. According to Kahneman and Tversky, people rely on a limited number of heuristics—most prominently representativeness, availability, and anchoring and adjustment—that often yield reasonable judgments but sometimes lead to severe and systematic biases. Diverging from earlier usage, the term heuristics now gained a different connotation: fallible cognitive shortcuts that people often use when faced with uncertainty and that can lead to systematic biases and lapses of reasoning indicating human irrationality. This more negative view of heuristics—and of the people who use them as "cognitive misers" using little information or cognition to reach biased conclusions —has spread to many other fields, including law, economics, medical decision making, sociology, and political science.

Recently, however, a new appreciation is emerging that heuristics may be the only available approach to decision making in the many problems for which optimal logical solutions do not exist (as researchers in operations research realized). Moreover, even when exact solutions do exist, domain-specific decision heuristics may be more effective than domain-general logical approaches, which are often computationally infeasible (as AI found). This has led to research programs such as the study of ecological rationality by Gigerenzer, Todd, and colleagues. Their program focuses on precisely specified computational models of heuristics and how they are matched to the ecological structure of particular decision environments. It also explores the ways that learning and evolution can achieve this match in human behavior, something that has already been widely accepted for other animals in research on rules of thumb in behavioral ecology.

In the following sections, the focus is on research in psychology exploring heuristics proposed to model how people search for information and make decisions and choices. Researchers such as Payne, Bettman, and Johnson and Svenson have been concerned with psychological heuristics for preferences, but here we are mostly concerned with inference heuristics. Heuristics and shortcuts are also important in human perception and higher order reasoning processes (e.g., hypothesis testing), planning and problem solving, as well as in computer applications in these domains.

II. UNBOUNDED RATIONALITY VERSUS THE BOUNDED REALITY OF HUMAN DECISION MAKING

Both the heuristics-and-biases program and the recently emerging work on ecologically rational heuristics have been linked to Herbert Simon's notion of bounded rationality. This concept can be understood by contrasting it to the traditional decision-making approach embodied in unbounded rationality, illu-

strated by the following example. Imagine being faced with the decision of whether or not to marry. How can this decision be made in a rational way? Assume that you attempted to resolve this question by maximizing your subjective expected utility. To compute your personal expected utility for marrying, you would have to determine all the possible consequences that marriage could bring (e.g., children, companionship, and countless further consequences), attach quantitative probabilities to each of these consequences, estimate the subjective utility of each, multiply each utility by its associated probability, and finally add all these numbers. The same procedure would have to be repeated for the alternative "not marry." Finally, you would have to choose the alternative with the higher total expected utility.

Maximization of expected utility in this way is probably the best known realization of the prominent vision of unbounded rationality. Models of unbounded rationality have been criticized for having little or no regard for the constraints of time, knowledge, and computational capacities that real humans face. For instance, while you are deliberating about whether marrying is the right choice, considering each of the myriad conceivable consequences and assigning probabilities to each, any potential partner will probably have married someone else. To this criticism proponents of unbounded rationality generally concede that their models assume unrealistic mental abilities, but they nevertheless defend them by arguing that humans act as if they were unboundedly rational. In this interpretation, the models of unbounded rationality do not describe the process but merely the outcome of reasoning.

If the lofty ideals of human reasoning do not capture the processes of how real people make decisions in the real world, what then are those processes? In other words, what models take into account the challenging conditions under which people have to solve problems, including limited time, knowledge, and computational capacity? Herbert Simon proposed that these constraints force humans to use "approximate methods" (heuristics) to handle most tasks. These approximate methods form the basis of bounded rationality.

Simon's vision of bounded rationality has two interlocking components that act like a pair of scissors to shape human rational behavior. The two blades in this metaphor are the computational capabilities of the actor and the structure of task environments. First, the computational capability blade implies that models of human judgment and decision making should be built on what we actually know about the mind's limitations rather than on fictitious competencies assumed in models of unbounded rationality. There are two key limitations central to bounded rationality. First, contrary to models of unbounded rationality, humans cannot search for information for all of eternity. In computationally realistic models, search must be limited because real decision makers have only a finite amount of time, knowledge, attention, or money to apply to a particular decision. Limited search requires rules to specify what information to seek and in what order (i.e., an information search rule) and a way to decide when to stop looking for information (i.e., a stopping rule).

Another key limitation of the human mind is that the pieces of information uncovered by the search process are not likely to be processed in an overly complex way. In contrast, most traditional models of inference, from linear multiple regression models to Bayesian models to neural networks, try to find some optimal integration of all information available: Every bit of information is taken into account, weighted, and combined in some more or less computationally expensive way. Models of bounded rationality instead rely on processing steps that are computationally bounded. For instance, a bounded decision or inference can be based on only one or a few pieces of information, whatever the total amount of information found during search. The simple decision rule used to process this limited knowledge need not weigh or combine pieces of information, thus eliminating the need to convert different types of information into a single common currency (e.g., utilities). Note that decision rules and information search and stopping rules are connected. For instance, when a heuristic searches for only one (discriminating) cue, this largely constrains the possible decision rules to those that do not integrate information. On the other hand, if search extends to many cues, the decision rule will be less constrained. The cues may then be weighted and integrated, or only the best of them may determine the decision.

These two key limitations, limited information search and limited processing of information, can be instantiated into models of heuristics. The limitations help explain how heuristics achieve one of their most important advantages, namely, speed. In fact, for much decision making in the real world—the stock broker who decides within seconds to keep or sell a stock, or the captain of the firefighter squad who within a few moments must predict how a fire will progress and whether or not to pull out the squad— speed is often the crucial objective.

The second blade in Simon's scissors metaphor, operating in tandem with computational capability, is environmental structure. This blade is of crucial importance in shaping bounded rationality because it can explain when and why heuristics perform well, namely, if the structure of the heuristic is adapted to the structure of the environment (i.e., if the heuristic is ecologically, rather than logically, rational). Simon's classic example concerns foraging organisms that have a single need—food. An organism living in an environment in which little heaps of food are randomly distributed can survive with a simple heuristic: Run around randomly until a heap of food is found. For this, the organism needs some capacity for movement, but it does not need a capacity for inference or learning. For an organism in an environment in which food is distributed not randomly but in patches whose locations can be inferred from cues, more sophisticated strategies are possible. For instance, it could learn the association between cues and food and store this information in memory. The general point is that in order to understand which heuristic an organism employs, and when and why the heuristic works well, one needs to examing the structure of the information in the environment.

III. HEURISTICS FOR HUMAN JUDGMENT, CHOICE, AND SEARCH BEHAVIOR

The models of heuristics for human judgment, choice, and decision making that have been proposed in psychology since 1970 can be linked to two traditions of heuristics with earlier beginnings as described previously. These two traditions have employed different levels of description. First, following the line of the heuristic methods studied by the Gestalt psychologists, one class of heuristics consists of psychological principles that are verbally described. These models are only relatively loosely specified and usually do not explicate all the processes they involve (e.g., in terms of information search, stopping, and decision rules). Second, following from Simon and Newell's computer-based models of human decision making, another class of heuristics has been formulated as process models, with explicit specification of the processes involved. Because of this explication, the latter heuristics can be both mathematically analyzed and tested with the help of computer simulations. We consider each class of heuristics in turn.

A. Heuristics for the Judgment of Probability and Frequencies: Availability, Representativeness, and Anchoring and Adjustment

The heuristics most widely studied within psychology are those that people use to make judgments or estimates of probabilities and frequencies in situations of uncertainty (i.e., in situations in which people lack exact knowledge). Most prominent among these are the availability, representativeness, and anchoring and adjustment heuristics.

The availability heuristic leads one to assess the frequency of a class or the probability of an event by the number of instances or occurrences that can be brought to mind or by how easy it seems to call up those instances. For instance, which class of words is more common: seven-letter English words of the form "_ _ _ _ _ n _" or the form "_ _ _ _ i n g"? According to the availability heuristic, to estimate the frequency of occurrences people draw a sample of the events in question from memory. Specifically, for this case they retrieve words ending in –ing (e.g., "jumping") and retrieve words with "n" in the sixth position (e.g., "raisins") and then count the number of words retrieved in some period or assess the ease with which such words could be retrieved. They then answer that the more numerous or easier class of words is more common. Because people find it easier to think of words ending with –ing than to think of words with the letter "n" in the next-to-last position, they usually estimate the class "_ _ _ _ i n g" to be more common. This judgment, however, is wrong because all words ending with –ing also have "n" in the sixth position; in addition, there are seven-letter words with "n" the sixth position that do not end in –ing.

The availability heuristic has been suggested to underlie diverse judgment errors, ranging from the tendency to overestimate how many people die from some specific causes of death (e.g., tornado) and underestimate the death toll of others causes (e.g., diabetes) to why people's answers to life satisfaction questions ("How happy are you?") may be overly influenced by events that are especially memorable.

The representativeness heuristic has been proposed as a means to assess the probability that an object A belongs to a class B (e.g., that a person described as meek is a pilot) or that an event A is generated by a process B (e.g., that the sequence HTHTHT was generated by randomly throwing a fair coin). This heuristic produces probability judgments according to the extent that object A is representative of or similar to the class or process B (e.g., meekness is not representative of pilots, so a meek person is judged as having a low probability of being a pilot). This heuristic can lead to errors because similarity or representativeness judgments are not always influenced by factors that should affect judgments of probability, such as base rates. The representativeness heuristic has also been evoked to explain numerous judgment phenomena, including "hot hand" observations in basketball (the belief that a player is more likely to score again after he or she already scored successfully than after missing a shot) and the gambler's fallacy (the belief that a successful outcome is due after a run of bad luck).

Another heuristic, anchoring and adjustment, produces estimates of quantities by starting with a particular value (the anchor) and adjusting upward or downward from it. For instance, people asked to quickly estimate the product of either $8 \times 7 \times 6 \times 5 \times 4 \times 3 \times 2 \times 1$ or $1 \times 2 \times 3 \times 4 \times 5 \times 6 \times 7 \times 8$ give a higher value in the former case. According to the anchoring and adjustment heuristic, this happens because the first few numbers presented are multiplied together to create a higher or lower anchor, which is then adjusted upwards in both cases, yielding a higher final estimate for the first product.

Although it has been pointed out that availability, representativeness, and anchoring and adjustment are quite useful heuristics (because they often lead to good judgments without much time or mental effort), most of the large body of evidence amassed that is consistent with the use of these heuristics comes from studies showing where they break down and lead to cognitive illusions or biases (i.e., deviations from some normative standards). This heuristics-and-biases research program has caught the attention of numerous social scientists, including economists and legal scholars. There are good reasons for this attention, since systematic biases question the empirical validity of classic rational choice models (i.e., models of unbounded rationality) and may have important economic, legal, and other implications.

However, the exclusive focus on cognitive illusions has evoked the criticism that research in the heuristics-and-biases tradition equates the notion of bounded rationality with human irrationality and portrays the human mind in an overly negative light, with some researchers even arguing that cognitive illusions are the rule rather than the exception. It has also been criticized that, to date, the cognitive heuristics posited have not been precisely formalized such that one could either simulate or mathematically analyze their behavior, leaving them free to account for all kinds of experimental performance in a post hoc fashion. For instance, it is still an open question of how people assess similarity to make probability judgments with the representativeness heuristic or how many items (e.g., words ending with –ing) the availability heuristic retrieves before it affords a frequency estimate of a class of object (albeit theoretical progress has been made, for instance, by testing whether availability works in terms of ease of recall or number of items recalled). Moreover, the heuristics-and-biases program focuses on human computational capabilities (the first blade of Simon's scissors), largely ignoring the role of the environment by not specifying how such heuristics capitalize on information structure to make inferences. Finally, this program appears to consider heuristics as dispensable mechanisms (that would not be needed if people had the right tools of probability and logic to call on), in contrast to Simon's view of indispensable heuristics as the only available tools for solving many real-world problems.

Kahneman and Tversky have countered some of this critique by drawing a parallel between their heuristic principles and the qualitative principles of Gestalt psychology—the latter being still valuable despite not being precisely specified. Irrespective of the various criticisms, the heuristic and biases program has undoubtedly led to a tremendous amount of research into the idea that people rely on cognitive heuristics made up of simple psychological processes rather than on complex procedures to make inferences about an uncertain world. As a result, this insight has been firmly established as a central topic of psychology.

B. Fast and Frugal Choice Heuristics

More precisely specified models of heuristics have been studied by a another research program that emerged in psychology in the 1990s. This new program considers fast and frugal heuristics for making decisions as the way the human mind can take advantage of the structure of information in the environment to arrive at reasonable decisions. Thus, it focuses on how mental capabilities and structured environments together can lead to accurate and useful inferences rather than focusing on the cases in which heuristics may account for poor reasoning. Most of the fast and frugal heuristics that Gigerenzer, Todd, and colleagues have proposed model the way humans make choices rather than probability judgments (a few others deal with additional tasks, such as estimation and classification).

Many of the choices humans make involve an inference or prediction about which of two objects will score higher on a criterion: Which soccer team will win? Which of two cities has a higher crime rate or higher cost of living? Which of two applicants will do a better job? When making such choices, we may have different amounts of information available. In the most limited case, if the only information available is whether or not each option has been encountered before, the decision maker can do little better than rely on his or her own partial ignorance, for instance, choosing recognized options over unrecognized ones. This may not sound like much for a decision maker to go on, but there is often information implicit in the failure to recognize something, and this failure can be exploited.

This kind of "ignorance-based" decision making is embodied in the recognition heuristic. This heuristic states that, when choosing between two objects (according to some criterion), if one is recognized and the other is not, then select the former. For instance, if predicting whether Manchester United or Bayer Leverkusen will win the European Soccer Champions League, this heuristic would lead most of us to bet on Manchester United. Why? European soccer teams are often named after European cities (e.g., Arsenal London or AC Milano), and people who are ignorant of the quality of European soccer teams can still use city recognition as a cue for soccer team performance. Cities with successful soccer teams are likely to be large, and large cities are likely to be recognized; hence, Manchester, which is more than two times as large as Leverkusen, is also more likely to be recognized and thus chosen as the winner.

The recognition heuristic will yield good choices more often than would random choice in those decision environments in which exposure to different possibilities is positively correlated with their ranking along the decision criterion being used. Animals also behave as if they apply similar rules: Norway rats, for instance, prefer to eat things they recognize through past experience with other rats (e.g., items they have smelled on the breath of others) over novel items.

Employing the recognition heuristic can lead to a surprising phenomenon called the less-is-more effect. This is the analytical and empirical observation that an intermediate amount of (recognition) knowledge about a set of objects can yield the highest proportion of correct answers—knowing (i.e., recognizing) more than this will actually decrease the decision-making performance. A context in which this effect appears in the reasoning of people is judgments about demographics. When American students were asked to pick the larger of two cities, they scored a median 71% correct inferences when city pairs were randomly constructed from the 22 largest U.S. cities and 73% when city pairs were from the 22 largest cities in Germany. The result is counterintuitive when viewed from the premise that more knowledge is always better: The students knew a lifetime of facts about U.S. cities that could be useful for inferring population, but they knew little or nothing beyond mere recognition about the German cities—and they did not even recognize about half of them. The latter fact, however, allowed them to employ the recognition heuristic and to pick German cities that they recognized as larger than those they did not. This heuristic could not be applied for choosing between U.S. cities, however, because the students recognized all of them and thus had to rely on additional retrievable information.

In choosing one of two options, most of the time we have more information than just a vague memory of recognition to go on. The situation of American students comparing American cities is just one example. When multiple pieces of information (or "cues") are available for guiding decisions, how can a heuristic that limits search and processing of information proceed? A decision maker following the dictums of unbounded rationality would collect all the available information, weight it appropriately, and combine it optimally before making a choice. A more frugal approach is to use a stopping rule that terminates the search for information as soon as enough has been gathered to make a decision. One such approach is to rely on "one-reason decision making": Stop looking for cues as soon as one is found that differentiates between the two options being considered. This allows the decision maker to follow a simple loop, depicted in Fig. 1: (i) Select a cue dimension; (ii) search for the corresponding cue values of each alternative; (iii) if they differ, then stop and choose the alternative for which the cue indicates a greater value on the choice criterion; (iv) if they do not differ, then return to the beginning of this loop to search for another cue dimension.

This four-step loop specifies a stopping rule (stopping after a single cue is found that enables a choice between the two options) and a decision rule (deciding on the option to which the one cue points). Depending on how cue dimensions are searched for in the first step, (i.e., depending on what kind of specific information search rule the heuristic uses), different one-reason decision-making heuristics can be formed. The Take The Best heuristic searches for cues in the order of their ecological validity (i.e., their correlation with the decision criterion). Take The Last searches for cues in the order determined by their past success so that the cue that was used for the most recent previous decision is checked first during the next decision. Finally, the Minimalist heuristic selects cues in a random order.

For example, consider the task of inferring which of two cities in the United States has a higher homelessness rate. Assume that possible cues are "rent control," "temperature," "unemployment," and "public housing," each turned into a binary value (0 or 1) according to whether the actual value is below or above the median for U.S. cities. Rent control has the highest ecological validity, temperature has the second highest, and so on. The Minimalist heuristic only needs to know in which direction a cue "points." For instance, the heuristic needs to know only whether warmer or cooler weather indicates a city with a higher rate of homelessness (in the United States, warmer weather is indeed associated more often with higher homelessness rates than with lower rates). The strategy of Minimalist is to search for cues in random order,

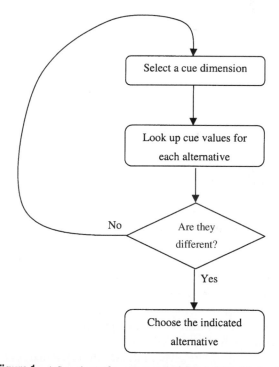

Figure 1   A flowchart of one-reason decision making. First, select a cue dimension and ascertain the corresponding cue values for each alternative; next, check whether the values for that cue discriminate between the alternatives. If so, then choose the indicated alternative; if not, select another cue dimension and repeat this process. Random choice can be used if no more cues are available.

stop cue search when a cue is found that discriminates between the two cities, and then choose the city that has the cue value 1 when the other city has cue value 0. For instance, when inferring whether New York or Los Angeles has a higher homelessness rate, the unemployment cue might be the first cue randomly selected, and the cue values are found to be 1 for both cities. Because this cue does not discriminate between the cities, search is continued, the public housing cue is randomly selected, and the cues values are 0 for New York and 1 for Los Angeles. Search is stopped at this discriminating cue and the inference is made that Los Angeles has a higher homelessness rate, as it indeed does.

The Take The Best heuristic is exactly like Minimalist except that it considers cues in order of their validity from highest to lowest. If the highest validity cue does not discriminate, the next best cue is tried, and so forth. Thus, Take The Best differs from Minimalist only in the information search rule, but it has the same stopping and decision rule. Take The Best (unlike the Minimalist, Take The Last, and recognition heuristics) is an instance of the class of lexicographic decision strategies. This term signifies that the cues are looked up in a fixed order of validity, and the first cue where choices differ is used alone to make the decision, like the alphabetic order used to arrange words in a dictionary. The Arabic number system is also lexicographic. To determine which of two numbers with equal digit length is larger, one has to start by examining the first (leftmost) digit: If this digit is larger in one of the numbers, the whole number is larger. If they are equal, one has to examine the second digit, and so on (a simple method that is not possible for Roman numbers). There is growing empirical evidence that people actually use lexicographic heuristics such as Take The Best, particularly when time is limited.

How well do these one-reason decision heuristics perform? Table I compares the performance of three fast and frugal heuristics (Minimalist, Take The Best, and Take The Last) to that of multiple regression and Dawes's and Franklin's rule. Unlike the heuristics, multiple regression is a computationally expensive linear strategy that calculates weights that reflect the covariances between predictors or cues. When the task is merely fitting the given data set, multiple regression is the most accurate strategy, by two percentage points, followed by Take The Best. However, when the task is to generalize from a training set to a test set, a simple heuristic such as Take The Best can outperform multiple regression (note that multiple regression has

Table I

Performance of Three Fast and Frugal Heuristics (Take The Best, Minimalist, and Take The Last) and Three Linear Strategies (Dawes's rule, Franklin's rule, and multiple regression) Averaged across 20 Empirical Data Sets[a]

Heuristic/strategy	Frugality	Accuracy	
		Fitting (% correct)	Generalization (% correct)
Take The Best	2.4	75	71
Minimalist	2.2	69	65
Take The Last	2.1	70	65
Franklin's rule	7.7	75	71
Dawes's rule	7.7	73	69
Multiple regression	7.7	77	68

[a]The average number of predictors available in the 20 data sets was 7.7. Frugality indicates the mean number of cues actually used by each strategy. Accuracy indicates the percentage of correct answers achieved by the heuristics and strategies when fitting data (i.e., fit a strategy to a given set of data) and when generalizing to new data (i.e., use a strategy to predict new data).

all the information Take The Best uses and more). The reason is that by being simple, the heuristics can avoid being too matched to any particular environment—that is, they can escape the curse of overfitting.

Overfitting refers to the problem of a model that is closely matched to one situation (set of data) failing to predict accurately in another similar situation (another set of data). This phenomenon can arise from assuming that every detail in a given environment is of great relevance. Consider forecasting of the U.S. presidential elections as an example. Beyond traditional variables such as incumbency and the state of the election-year economy, a plethora of additional variables have been suggested as predictors of recent U.S. presidential elections, including the voting behavior in Okanogan County (a rural stretch of north-central Washington), the rise or fall of women's hemlines, and the height of the candidates. General strategies such as multiple regression can in fact incorporate each of these and many more variables into the unlimited collection of free variables in their forecast models. As accurate as such parameter-laden forecast models may be for describing particular recent presidential elections, their accuracy in predicting other situations (e.g., earlier U.S. presidential elections or elections in other locations) may well be minimal. That is, these models can easily overfit the particular (training) data set and thereby fail to generalize to the new (testing) data set. In contrast, if a forecast model uses many fewer parameters, for instance, just incumbency and height of the candidates (which predicted the winner of every election since World War II, except in 1976 and 2000), it is likely to avoid overfitting and thereby generalize better to new situations.

Fast and frugal heuristics (like lexicographic strategies) are noncompensatory, meaning that once they have used a single cue to make a decision no further cues in any combination can undo or compensate for that one cue's effect. When the information in the decision environment is structured in a matching noncompensatory fashion (i.e., the importance or validity of cues decreases rapidly such that each weight of a cue is larger than the sum of all weights to come, e.g., one-half, one-fourth, one-eighth, and so on), the Take The Best heuristic can exploit that structure to make correct decisions as often as compensatory rules. Take The Best also performs comparatively well when information is scarce; that is, when there are many more objects than cues to distinguish them. Further research is needed to explore what environment structures can be exploited by different fast and frugal heuristics.

C. Heuristics for Multiple Alternative Choices

Not all choices in life are presented to us as convenient pairs of alternatives, of course. Often, we must choose between several alternatives, such as which restaurant to go to, which apartment to rent, or which stocks to buy. Table II lists various decision heuristics that have been proposed in the psychological literature for choosing one out of several alternatives, where each alternative is characterized by cue (or attribute) values and where the importance of a cue is specified by its weight (or validity). This collection is not exhaustive, and it only focuses on heuristics for inference rather than preference (albeit some could be applied to preferences as well). However, the heuristics represent a wide range of different information search, stopping, and decision rules. Among the heuristics for multiple alternative choice, lexicographic (LEX), lexicographic semiorder (LEX-Semi), and elimination by aspects (EBA) are noncompensatory, whereas the rest are compensatory heuristics, integrating (at least some of) the available information and making trade-offs

Table II
Description of Various Multiple Alternative Choice Heuristics[a]

Heuristic	Description
Franklin's rule or weighted additive rule	Calculates for each alternative the sum of the cue values multiplied by the corresponding cue weights (validities) and selects the alternative with the highest score.
Dawes's rule or additive rule	Calculates for each alternative the sum of the cue values (discretized to either 1 or −1) and selects the alternative with the highest score.
Good features	Selects the alternative with the highest number of good features: a good feature is a cue value that exceeds a specified cut-off.
Weighted pros	Selects the alternative with the highest sum of weighted "pros." A cue that has a higher value for one alternative than for the others is considered a pro for this alternative. The weight of each pro is defined by the validity of the particular cue.
LEX or lexicographic	Selects the alternative with the highest cue value on the cue with the highest validity. If more than one alternative has the same highest cue value, then for these alternatives the cue with the second highest validity is considered, and so on.
LEX-Semi or lexicographic semiorder	Works like LEX, with the additional assumption of a just-noticeable difference. Pairs of alternatives with less than a just-noticeable difference between the cue values are not discriminated.
EBA or elimination by aspects	Eliminates all alternatives that do not exceed a specified value on the first cue examined. If more than one alternative remains, another cue is selected. This procedure is repeated until only one alternative is left. Each cue is selected with a probability that is proportional to its weight.
LEX-Add or lexicographic additive combination	Represents a combination of two strategies. It first uses LEX-Semi to choose two alternatives as favorites and then evaluates them by Dawes's rule and selects the one with the highest sum.

[a]Defined in terms of alternatives (options), cues (information), and weights (importance of information).

between the relevant cues to form an overall evaluation of each alternative.

Weighing and summing of all available information has been used to define rational judgment at least since the Enlightenment: The concepts of expected value and utility, Benjamin Franklin's moral algebra, and Homo economicus all rely on these two fundamental processes. The heuristics for multiple alternative choices in Table II can be seen as various shortcuts of these two processes. Dawes's rule, for instance, questions the importance of precise weighting. In the 1970s and 1980s, Robyn Dawes and colleagues showed that tallying information (cues) in terms of simple unit weights, such as $+1$ and -1, typically led to the same predictive accuracy as the "optimal weights" in multiple regression (particularly when generalizing to new data). Thus, in situations in which the task is to predict what is not yet known (rather than to fit what is already known), weighting information does not seem to matter much, as long as one gets the sign right.

On the other hand, LEX (a generalization of Take The Best), LEX-Semi, and EBA do not require summing procedures. All three heuristics use a simple form of weighting by ordering the cues, but they do not sum the cues. Gigerenzer and colleagues collected counterintuitive evidence that this simple weighting without summing (as in the Take The Best heuristic) can be as accurate and in some circumstances (e.g., generalization) even more accurate than complex decision strategies such as multiple regression.

Among the choice heuristics listed in Table II, EBA, proposed by Amos Tversky, is the most widely known elimination model in psychology. In sequential elimination choice models, one alternative is chosen from a set of possibilities by repeatedly eliminating subsets of alternatives from further consideration until only a single choice remains. One of the motivating factors in developing EBA in particular as a descriptive model of choice was that there are often many relevant cues that may be used in choosing among complex alternatives. EBA deals with this challenge by probabilistically considering successive cues (which are chosen with a probability proportional to their importance), selecting one at a time, and eliminating all the alternatives that do not possess this current cue, until a single alternative remains as the final choice. Other elimination heuristics select cues in a different manner (e.g., deterministically or based on validity) or use them to process the alternatives in other ways (e.g., in terms of thresholds rather than presence or absence).

D. Heuristics for Sequential Search

The heuristics discussed so far for choosing one option from many operate with the assumption that all the possible options (e.g., cities to choose between) are presently available to the decision maker. In many real-world choice problems, though, an agent encounters options in a sequence spread out over time. The options typically appear in random order and are drawn from a distribution with parameters that are only partially known in advance. In this case, the search for possible options, rather than just for information about those already present, becomes central.

The traditional normative approach to such problems is to search until one finds an option below a precalculated reservation price that balances the expected benefit of further search against its cost; this requires full knowledge of the search costs and the distribution of available alternatives. Heuristics that simplify the reservation price calculation (by replacing an integral with a weighted sum) can come very close to normative performance (e.g., at selecting good prices during a shopping trip to several stores). Other heuristics require less knowledge, such as "Keep searching until the total search cost exceeds 7.5% of the best price found." Herbert Simon's bounded rationality principle of satisficing suggests setting an aspiration level equal to an alternative that is good enough for the decision maker's needs (rather than optimal) and searching until that aspiration is met. Exactly how the aspiration level can be set varies with the search setting (e.g., whether it is a one-sided search such as shopping or a two-sided mutual search such as finding a mate). Finally, another type of search heuristic that people use stops search after a particular pattern of alternatives is encountered rather than after some threshold is exceeded (despite the fact that pattern should not matter from a normative perspective). For instance, the "one-bounce" and "two-bounce" rules state that one should keep searching for a low price until prices go up for the last or two last alternatives, respectively.

E. Social Decision Heuristics

Decision-making mechanisms can exploit the structure of information in the environment to arrive at better outcomes. The most important aspects of an agent's environment are often created by the other agents with which it interacts. Two of the key problems social agents face are the questions of how to (fairly) divide up resources among one another and how to make cooperative decisions in situations in which the pursuit of self-interest by each agent would lead to a poor outcome for all. We consider each of these problems in turn.

The task of fairly dividing up resources is ubiquitous, ranging from distributing a cake among siblings to dividing an estate among heirs and splitting a fixed budget among a group of faculty members at an academic institution. Although there are a plethora of fair-division procedures, Brams and Taylor classified them according to a few dimensions, such as the number of players to which they are applicable ($n=2, 3, 4$, or more), the properties they satisfy (e.g., proportionality, envy-freeness, and efficiency), and whether or not the division has to be exact or only approximate. A simple but well-known decision heuristic that may be familiar to many parents is "one divides, the other chooses." Although this heuristic stipulates division of labor, it does not specify how the person who divides the resource (i.e., a cake) actually does it. If, however, the person who divides the cake understands the strategic interest of the other, the implied division rule is to divide up the resource such that one is indifferent between the two parts; the other person will then choose whatever he or she considers to be the larger piece. This way each person is assured of getting what he or she perceives to be at least half the resource, and neither party thinks that the other received a larger piece of cake. A fair-division procedure with these properties is said to be proportional and envy-free.

An example of a situation in which the pursuit of self-interest by each party leads to a poor outcome for all is that in which two industrialized regions of the world (e.g., the United States and the European Union) have established trade barriers to each other's exports. Because of the mutual advantages of free trade, both regions would be better off if these barriers were eliminated. However, if either region were to unilaterally give up the barriers, it would be faced with terms of trade that hurt its own economy. In fact, no matter what America does, the European Union (EU) is better off retaining its own trade barriers and vice versa. This strategic situation, in which the incentive to retain trade barriers for both regions produces a worse outcome than would have been possible had both decided to cooperate, is known as a prisoner's dilemma game. This game is just one among many situations that game theorists examine in order to analyze and model the strategic interactions of social agents.

If there is some likelihood that the players will encounter each other in the future, as in trade between the United States and the EU, the interaction become an iterated prisoner's dilemma game. There are a number of possible decision heuristics for this situation. A particularly simple but surprisingly successful decision heuristic is the tit-for-tat heuristic that Anatol Rapoport submitted to Axelrod's famous computer tournament. Given the possibility of cooperating with or defecting against the other player at each time step, tit-for-tat starts with a cooperative choice and thereafter does what the other player did on the previous move. In other words, tit-for-tat searches for a minimal amount of information (the counterpart's behavior in the last round) and cooperates if the last move was cooperative but defects if the last move was defective. Thus, akin to some of the heuristics described previously, tit-for-tat does not have to weigh and combine pieces of information in some more or less computationally expensive way. Many other successful heuristics, such as generous tit-for-tat and win–stay–lose–shift, have also been proposed for iterated prisoner's dilemma and other games.

IV. HOW TO MEASURE A HEURISTIC'S SUCCESS

The study of heuristics is a key approach to understanding how real minds make decisions for two main reasons. First, many of life's important problems, from choosing a mate to finding a job, cannot be solved in an optimal way because the space of possibilities that must be taken into account is often unlimited; hence, heuristic shortcuts are called for. Second, even when this space of possible solutions is limited and knowledge is complete, optimization may require unfeasible amounts of computation (as in trying to determine the best next move in chess) so that, again, heuristics will be an appropriate approach for the mind to take.

The fact that there are no optimal strategies for many real-world tasks, however, does not mean that there are no performance criteria. One set of criteria that is often used to evaluate judgments and decisions is their internal coherence, defined as accordance with the laws of probability theory and logic. For instance, if judgments are consistent (e.g., "I always think that event A is more likely than B") and transitive ("I think that A is more likely than B, B is more likely than C, and therefore that A is more likely than C"), this is taken as an indication that the underlying decision strategies are rational. If such criteria are violated, this is typically held to be a sign of irrationality on the part of the decision maker. The heuristics-and-biases research program has focused on such relatively abstract coherence criteria to indicate when a heuristic produces reasonable or unreasonable decisions.

Alternatively, the success of a heuristic can be measured by comparing its performance with the requirements of its environment, such as accuracy, frugality, and speed. Lexicographic strategies (e.g., Take The Best) are often evaluated via correspondence criteria relating to real-world decision performance (such as how often they correctly choose the larger object in a pair). Comparing heuristics' performance to the requirements of the external world rather than to internal consistency stems from the view that the primary function of heuristics is not to be coherent. Rather, their function is to make reasonable adaptive inferences about the real social and physical world given limited time and knowledge.

The two kinds of criteria, coherence and correspondence, can sometimes be at odds with each other. For instance, in social situations, including some competitive games and predator–prey interactions, it can be advantageous to exhibit inconsistent (and hence noncoherent) behavior in order to maximize adaptive unpredictability (and hence correspondence with real-world goals) and avoid capture or loss. As another example, the Minimalist heuristic violates the coherence criterion of transitivity but nevertheless makes fairly robust and accurate inferences in particular environments. Thus, intransitivity does not necessarily imply high levels of inaccuracy, nor does transitivity guarantee high levels of accuracy: Logic and adaptive behavior are logically distinct.

Finally, it is important to measure the performance of decision mechanisms in terms of how well they make decisions when applied to new data; that is, how they generalize to new situations rather than merely how closely they can be adjusted or fit to a static set of data. In this regard, simple heuristics will often do very well, being about as accurate as complex general strategies that work with many free parameters. The reason is that simple heuristics can avoid being too matched to any particular environment; that is, they can escape the curse of overfitting mentioned earlier. As a consequence, a computationally simple heuristic that uses only some of the available information can be more robust, making more accurate predictions for new data.

V. CONCLUSION

Simplicity in models has aesthetic appeal. The mechanisms are readily understood and communicated, and they are amenable to step-by-step scrutiny. Furthermore, Popper has argued that simpler models are more falsifiable. However, the idea that humans make many decisions using simple heuristic mechanisms is important not just because the resulting simple models are transparent and easily falsifiable. More important, simple heuristics may be the only approach available for real minds making decisions in the real, uncertain, time-pressured world.

See Also the Following Articles

ARTIFICIAL INTELLIGENCE • INFORMATION PROCESSING • INTELLIGENCE • LOGIC AND REASONING • NEURAL NETWORKS

Suggested Reading

Axelrod, R. (1984). *The Evolution of Cooperation*. Basic Books, New York.

Brams, S. J., and Taylor, A. D. (1996). *Fair Division: From Cake-Cutting to Dispute Resolution*. Cambridge Univ. Press, Cambridge, UK.

Dawes, R. M. (1979). The robust beauty of improper linear models in decision making. *Am. Psychologist* **34,** 571–582.

Gigerenzer, G., Todd, P. M., and the ABC Research Group (1999). *Simple Heuristics That Make Us Smart*. Oxford Univer. Press, New York.

Kahneman, D., Slovic, P., and Tversky, A. (Eds.) (1982). *Judgment under Uncertainty: Heuristics and Biases*. Cambridge Univer. Press, Cambridge, UK.

Newell, A., and Simon, H. A. (1972). *Human Problem Solving*. Prentice Hall, Englewood Cliffs, NJ.

Payne, J. W., Bettman, J. R., and Johnson, E. J. (1993). *The Adaptive Decision Maker*. Cambridge Univ. Press, New York.

Pólya, G. (1945). *How to Solve It: A New Aspect of Mathematical Method*. Princeton Univ. Press, Princeton, NJ.

Simon, H. A. (1955). A behavioral model of rational choice. *Q. J. Econ.* **69,** 99–118.

Simon, H. A. (1956). Rational choice and the structure of environments. *Psychol. Rev.* **63,** 129–138.

Simon, H. A. (1990). Invariants of human behavior. *Annu. Rev. Psychol.* **41,** 1–19.

Svenson, O. (1979). Process descriptions of decision making. *Organizational Behav. Hum. Performance* **23,** 86–112.

Tversky, A. (1972). Elimination by aspects: A theory of choice. *Psychol. Rev.* **79,** 281–299.

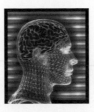

Hindbrain

JOEL C. GLOVER
University of Oslo

I. Anatomical and Functional Organization

II. Embryonic Development

III. Brief Considerations of Pathology

GLOSSARY

Hox genes Encode transcription factors bearing a DNA-binding portion called the homeodomain. Originally identified in *Drosophila* through the homoeotic effects of their mutation. In vertebrates their expression is strongly associated with the rhombomeric domains of the hindbrain.

Pax genes Encode transcription factors with a DNA-binding domain encoded by a sequence called the "paired box." Certain Pax genes are expressed in longitudinal domains within the hindbrain.

raphe Ventral seam of the brain stem, derived from the embryonic floor plate. Contains commissural axons and neuron populations termed the raphe nuclei.

reticular formation Central region of the brain stem extending from mesencephalon to medulla oblongata and containing relatively diffuse populations of neurons. Has a reticular appearance in histological sections stained to reveal nerve fibers. Regulates a wide variety of neural functions.

rhombencephalon Most caudal of the three primary brain vesicles; synonymous with the term "hindbrain." Assumes a form roughly approximating a rhombus during later development and eventually gives rise to the medulla oblongata, pons, and the greater portion of the cerebellar primordium.

rhombic lip Region of the hindbrain rimming the dorsolateral recess of the fourth ventricle.

rhombomeres Rhombencephalic segments, transiently visible as swellings or partitions during early stages of hindbrain development.

The hindbrain, or rhombencephalon, is an embryological term denoting the caudalmost of the three primary embryonic brain vesicles that form in the rostral neural

tube. It gives rise to the pons and medulla oblongata as well as the greater portion of the cerebellum. Here, we restrict our view of the hindbrain to that region encompassing the pontine and medullary divisions since the cerebellum is discussed in a separate article. The pons and medulla oblongata are complex anatomical structures that subserve a wide range of vital functions. This article provides a general description of the anatomical and functional organization of the pons and medulla and then discusses the embryonic development of the hindbrain, including mechanisms involved in patterning its anatomy and function. It concludes with some brief considerations of pathology.

I. ANATOMICAL AND FUNCTIONAL ORGANIZATION

A. General Features

The pons (metencephalon or "behind-brain") and medulla oblongata (myelencephalon or "medulla-brain") are the two most caudal divisions of the brain, lying between the mesencephalon and the spinal cord. Seen from the ventral surface (Fig. 1A), the boundaries between mesencephalon and pons (pontomesencephalic sulcus) and between pons and medulla oblongata (pontomedullary sulcus) are clearly demarcated by the massive population of transversely oriented pontocerebellar fibers. In contrast, there is a smooth transition from medulla oblongata to spinal cord the only indication being the pyramidal decussation. Most of the dorsal surface of the pons and medulla oblongata

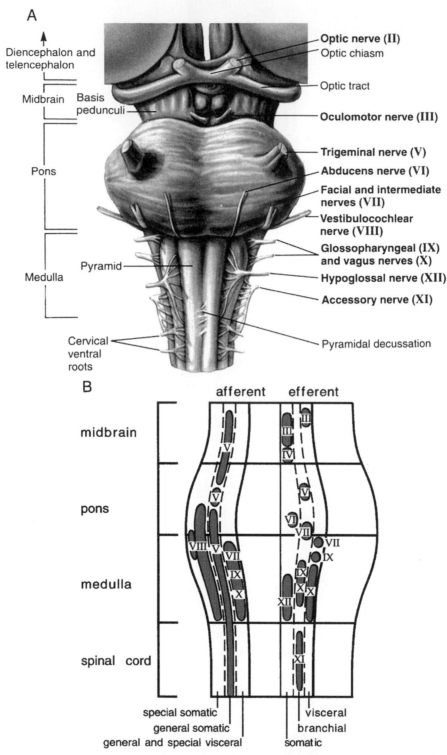

Figure 1 (A) Ventral view of the human brain stem showing the major structural features of the pons and medulla oblongata, including the cranial nerves (modified from Kandel *et al.*, 1992, *Principles of Neural Science*, 3rd ed., with permission of the McGraw-Hill Companies). (B) Organization of cranial nerve-associated nuclei into afferent (sensory) and efferent (motor) columns. The locations of nuclei relative to mesencephalic (midbrain), pontine, and medullary divisions are approximate. Phylogenetic variants on this theme exist. Because of longitudinal migrations of certain nuclear groups, embryonic origins may not correspond to final locations. For example, the trochlear nucleus (IV) has been shown to derive from the pontine division in lower mammals [redrawn and modified from Martin (1989), *Neuroanatomy*, with permission of the McGraw-Hill Companies].

underlies the fourth ventricle as its floor. The floor of the fourth ventricle and the ventral surface of the medulla oblongata show a relief of underlying longitudinal fiber tracts and nuclei. The lateral recesses of the fourth ventricle are bounded by a rim of neural tissue called the rhombic lip, which is continuous with a thin velum overlying the fourth ventricle. The caudal portion of the velum differentiates into choroid plexus. In the intact brain, the fourth ventricle is hidden by the cerebellum.

Eight of the 12 cranial nerves originate from the pons or medulla oblongata, issuing from specific sites on the ventral and lateral aspects (Fig. 1A). The trigeminal nerve issues from among the pontocerebellar fibers on the lateral aspect of the pons. The abducens, facial, and vestibulocochlear nerves issue from respectively medial to lateral positions at the pontomedullary border. The glossopharyngeal, vagus, and spinal accessory nerves issue from respectively rostral to caudal sites along the ventrolateral aspect of the medulla oblongata, dorsal to the inferior olive. The hypoglossal nerve issues from the ventral aspect of the medulla oblongata between the inferior olive and the pyramid.

The nuclei associated with the cranial nerves are organized into longitudinal motor and sensory columns that are subdivided according to which peripheral structures are innervated (Fig. 1B). The organization is similar to that in the spinal cord except for the presence of special columns that innervate structures specific to the head. The motor columns lie more medially and innervate either striated muscle (somatic and branchial columns) or parasympathetic ganglia (visceral column). The sensory columns lie more laterally and transmit tactile, proprioceptive, pain, or temperature signals (general somatic and visceral columns) or other specific sensory modalities such as audition and balance (special somatic column) and taste and olfaction (special visceral column). The sulcus limitans, a shallow longitudinal groove visible in the floor of the fourth ventricle, separates the motor from the sensory columns (Fig. 2).

The pons and medulla oblongata contain many fiber tracts that relay information between the cerebrum, cerebellum, and the spinal cord. The transversely oriented pontocerebellar projection is one of the largest of these and is the dominant external feature of the pons (Fig. 1A). Within the pons, longitudinal fiber tracts course internally to or intermingled with the pontocerebellar fibers. Within the medulla oblongata, most longitudinal tracts course at or near the outer (pial) surface. Some longitudinal tracts,

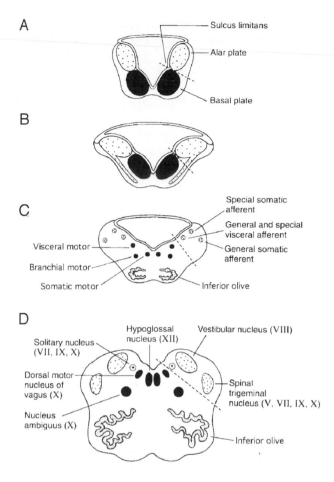

Figure 2 Series of transverse sections through the medulla oblongata at different stages of development. Different nuclei originate from basal and alar plates in a specific pattern. Motor and sensory cranial nerve-associated columns, for example, derive from the basal and alar plates, respectively. Note that inferior olive neurons derive from the alar plate but emigrate to the basal plate where they coalesce to form the nucleus [modified from Kandel *et al.*, (1992), *Principles of Neural Science*, 3rd ed., with permission from the McGraw-Hill Companies].

however, course at deeper locations near the ventral midline of the medulla oblongata. These include several important descending tracts to the spinal cord. The largest longitudinal tract, the corticospinal tract, is visible along the ventral medullary surface as the bilaterally paired pyramids, one of the dominant external features of the ventral medulla oblongata (Fig. 1A).

Like the cranial nerve nuclei, the longitudinal fiber tracts are differentially situated according to functional modality. Ascending tracts conveying sensory information from spinal and medullary centers to higher centers generally course at more dorsal and dorsolateral locations, whereas descending tracts generally course at more ventral and ventromedial locations. Exceptions to this general rule are the rubrospinal tract, which attains a lateral position within the medulla oblongata as it descends to the spinal cord; the medial lemniscus and ventral trigeminal tract, two sensory tracts that initially have a ventromedial course; and the spinal trigeminal tract, a sensory tract that descends along the dorsolaterally located spinal trigeminal nucleus.

Several well-defined nuclei exist within the pons and medulla oblongata in addition to those associated with the cranial nerve nuclei. The largest of these is the inferior olive, which produces a prominant bulge along the ventrolateral surface of the rostral medulla (Fig. 1A), and whose characteristically convoluted appearance in transverse sections makes it an unmistakable landmark (Fig. 2). The inferior olive is the source of climbing fiber afferents to the contralateral cerebellum.

The bulk of the pontine and medullary core is filled by a more diffusely organized population of neurons that make up the reticular formation, so named because it appears highly reticulated when stained nonspecifically for nerve fibers. This appearance, along with early physiological findings that demonstrated a lack of modality-specific activity in reticular efferents, led to the early notion that much of the reticular formation functioned as a distributed network involved in general activation and arousal. Recent anatomical and physiological studies, on the other hand, have demonstrated a higher degree of anatomical and functional mosaicism within the reticular formation than was previously appreciated. Anatomical subdivisions with characteristic patterns of connections and neurotransmitter profiles exist, and a number of well-defined premotor networks have been identified that organize and integrate specific goal-directed movements.

Certain reticular neuron populations are distinct enough anatomically to be defined as nuclei, even though most of these are not sharply delimited from the rest of the reticular formation. Two of the most distinct reticular nuclei are of special interest because of their neurotransmitter phenotypes. The raphe nuclei are clusters of neurons located within the ventral raphe, the majority of which are serotonergic. The locus coeruleus is a collection of noradrenergic neurons in the pons. The raphe nuclei and the locus coeruleus have exceptionally widespread projections and terminations and exert modulatory effects on a variety of neural systems.

B. Overview of Constituent Neuron Populations

1. Efferent Neurons

These include (i) motoneurons of cranial nerves V–VII and IX–XII that innervate striated muscle in the head and neck region (trigeminal motor, abducens, facial, ambiguus, and accessory nuclei), (ii) preganglionic neurons that innervate cranial parasympathetic ganglia (superior salivatory nucleus of cranial nerve VII and inferior salivatory nucleus of cranial nerve IX) and autonomic ganglia in the trunk (dorsal motor nucleus of nerve X), and (iii) cochlear and vestibular efferents from respectively the superior olive and reticular formation that innervate hair cells in the inner ear. All of these efferent populations are cholinergic.

2. Nuclei That Receive Cranial Nerve Sensory Afferents, and Some of Their Secondary Nuclear Targets

These include (i) sensory columns of the trigeminal system which receive inputs from nerves V, VII, and X; (ii) the vestibular and cochlear nuclei, which receive inputs from nerve VIII; and (iii) the solitary nucleus, which has subdivisions that receive afferents conveying taste via nerves VII, IX, and X, afferents from receptors in cranial skin and mucous membranes, and afferents from receptors in the gut, cardiovascular system, and lungs.

3. Other Relay and Integration Centers

These include the pontine nuclei, which relay primarily cortical inputs to the contralateral cerebellum; the inferior olive, which supplies climbing fiber inputs to the contralateral cerebellum, the nucleus prepositus, which is involved in regulating eye movements; the dorsal column nuclei, which integrate afferent information from the spinal cord and relay it to the thalamus; the deep cerebellar nuclei, which relay efferent information from the cerebellum; and various subdivisions of the reticular formation.

4. Sources of Descending Inputs to the Spinal Cord

These include the vestibulospinal, reticulospinal, and raphespinal populations and the locus coeruleus.

C. Functional Centers and Networks

In addition to being clustered into discrete nuclei with specific modalities, the neuron populations of the pons and medulla oblongata constitute interconnected networks that integrate somatic and autonomic sensory and motor functions. Many of these networks subserve reflex pathways that link the afferent inputs from certain cranial nerves with the motor output of others via interposed populations of interneurons within the reticular formation and specific relay nuclei. The complex coordination of the mouth, tongue, pharynx, and upper alimentary canal during the eating of a meal exemplifies the substantial degree of integration of different cranial nerve nuclei. The control of eye movements, the regulation of cardiovascular function, and a variety of autonomic reflexes, such as hiccuping, sneezing, and vomiting, are all examples of the interplay of different cranial nerve nuclei. The networks of interneurons that mediate these reflexes are not fully characterized, but some of them have been localized to specific sites within the reticular formation. Thus, in addition to functioning to some extent as a distributed integrative network, the reticular formation exhibits a substantial degree of functional compartmentalization.

Indeed, many of the regulatory functions exerted by the pons and medulla oblongata on other regions of the brain arise from specific, localized centers within the reticular formation. These include the regulation of pain impulses, the initiation of locomotion, and the control of cardiovascular function and respiration.

II. EMBRYONIC DEVELOPMENT

The development of the hindbrain has been the focus of intensive research during the past 10 years. Although the human hindbrain has been the subject of a few studies, most of our knowledge of the developmental programs and mechanisms that pattern the hindbrain is derived from animal studies. Since the hindbrain is an evolutionarily ancient brain structure, many of the key developmental features gleaned from other species are likely to be conserved throughout the vertebrate radiation, including primates. Nevertheless, species differences do exist, and the reader should note that some of the description that follows may differ in certain details from the developmental events occuring in the human embryo.

A. General Features

1. Morphogenesis

The brain and spinal cord originate from the embryonic ectoderm through the action of inductive signals from underlying mesoderm and within the ectoderm. During this process, a region of dorsal ectoderm called the neural plate is delineated, folds together at the midline to form the neural tube, and invaginates into the dorsal aspect of the embryo. Even before closure and invagination of the neural tube are complete, three initial subdivisions of the brain can be discerned, first by the appearance of indentations within the neural plate and subsequently by the expansion of the intervening regions into vesicles of the neural tube. These are the primary brain vesicles, the prosencephalon, mesencephalon, and rhombencephalon (Fig. 3). Within a short time (by about 4 weeks of development), further subdivisions of the neural tube, called neuromeres, can be seen. The neuromeres of the rhombencephalon are called rhombomeres (Fig. 3A).

During flexure of the developing neural tube, the rhombencephalon assumes a shape approximating a rhombus, hence the name (Fig. 4). This occurs at least in part because the mesencephalic and cervical flexures create constrictions in the neural tube, whereas the pontine flexure creates a lateral expansion. Initially, the wall of the rhombencephalic neural tube has approximately the same thickness around its entire circumference. As the flexures appear, however, morphometric changes occur that presage the mature structure (Fig. 2). The ventral portion starts proliferating extensively and eventually gives rise to the bulk of the pons and medulla oblongata. A specialized structure at the ventral midline known as the floor plate eventually gives rise to the raphe. The dorsal portion, also called the roof plate, becomes relatively much thinner and eventually gives rise to the velum of the fourth ventricle with its associated choroid plexus. No neurons differentiate within the roof plate and its derivatives. At pontine levels, the dorsal portion of the neural tube, on either side of the roof plate, develops into progressively thicker flaps of neural tissue that establish the major portion of the cerebellar primordium. A longitudinal indentation, called the sulcus limitans, appears in the floor of the fourth ventricle about midway between the floor plate and roof plate. This sulcus divides the wall of the neural tube into two longitudinal plates or columns, the basal plate and the alar plate.

Shortly after the hindbrain neural tube forms, and during the period when rhombomere and flexure formation is shaping the hindbrain, a population of progenitor cells at the dorsal aspect of the tube emigrates into the periphery. This population, a part of the cranial neural crest, contributes much of the mesenchyme of the cranium and branchial arches and

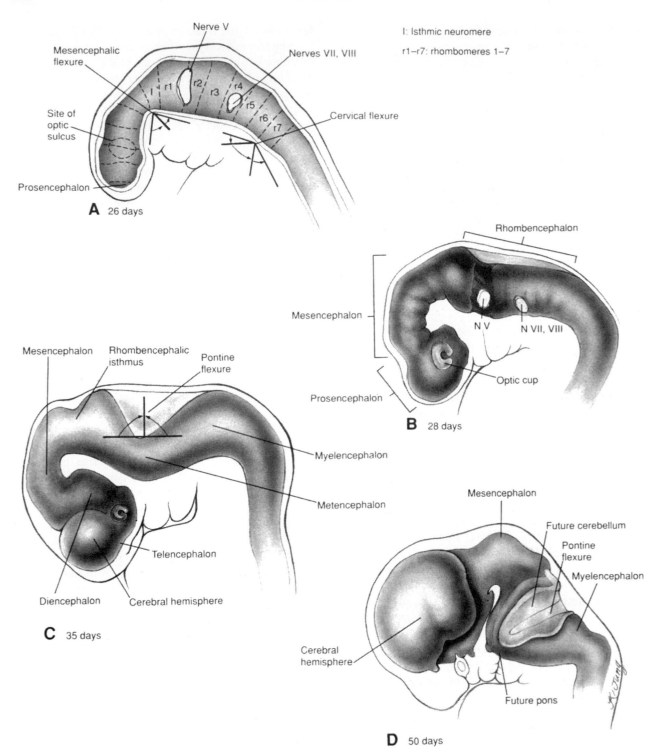

Figure 3 Important morphogenetic changes in the neural tube that shape the hindbrain [reproduced with permission from Larsen (1997), *Human Embryology*. Churchill Livingstone, New York].

of certain regions of the thorax including the developing thymus and heart. The neural crest cells proliferate and differentiate into a large number of cell types, including cartilage and other connective tissue structures, smooth muscle, melanocytes, peripheral neurons, and Schwann cells.

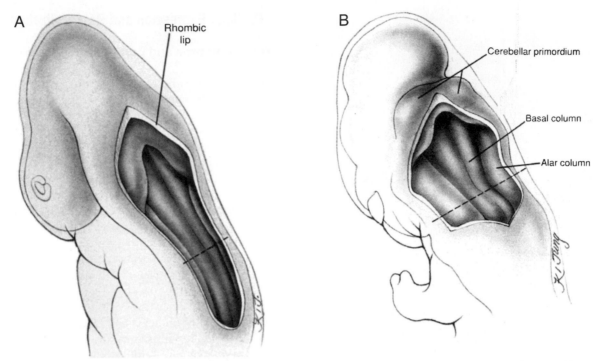

Figure 4 Dorsal views of the human embryo at approximately 4 weeks (A) and 5 weeks (B), showing the development of structural features in the floor of the fourth ventricle and the dorsolateral aspect of the hindbrain. The dotted line indicates the level of section shown in Fig. 2 [modified from Larsen (1997), *Human Embryology*. Churchill Livingstone, New York].

2. Neurogenesis and Migration

Neural progenitor cells of the neural tube proper are located and undergo mitosis near the inner (luminal) surface of the tube in a layer called the ventricular zone. As postmitotic neurons are generated, they migrate radially toward the outer (pial) surface, establishing a mantle zone where they begin to differentiate and aggregate into nuclei. Most neurons take up residence somewhere along this radial trajectory, but some turn to migrate circumferentially, either toward the floor plate or toward the roof plate, or longitudinally. Neurons generated in the alar plate, particularly the rhombic lip region, have a particular predilection for circumferential migration. Indeed, several nuclei, including the raphe nuclei and the inferior olive, are established within the basal plate through immigration from the alar plate (Fig. 2B).

By and large, the alar and basal plate domains maintain a coherent relationship to the sensory and motor divisions of the cranial nerve nuclei, respectively (Fig. 2), with the sulcus limitans persisting in the mature hindbrain as a landmark of this division. In general, motoneurons are generated within the basal plate, whereas the neurons of the sensory nuclei are generated within the alar plate. Some hindbrain cranial nerve nuclei, however, undergo circumferential migration, such as the trigeminal motoneurons, which migrate away from the floor plate, and the cochlear efferent neurons, which migrate toward the floor plate and cross the midline. The disposition of neuron groups in the mature hindbrain therefore does not necessarily accurately indicate their embryonic origins.

3. Axon Outgrowth and Tract Formation

Axon outgrowth is an early feature of neuronal differentiation and may be quite advanced even as neurons are migrating. Many axons are commissural, crossing the midline to course in axon tracts and innervate synaptic targets on the opposite side of the neuraxis. Once axons begin to project longitudinally, they tend to fasciculate into bundles that are located predominantly either near the pial surface or adjacent to the raphe. Two major axon bundles are present at early stages of hindbrain development: a medial longitudinal fascicle (mlf) and a lateral longitudinal

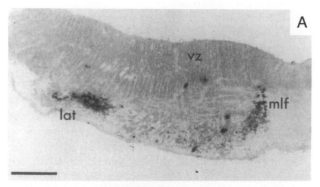

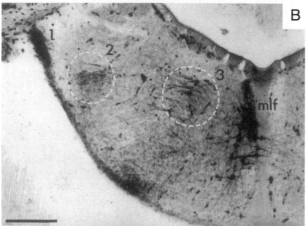

Figure 5 Transverse sections through the developing medulla oblongata of a chicken embryo illustrating the initial two longitudinal fiber bundles [A; medial longitudinal fascicle (mlf) and lateral longitudinal fascicle (lat)] and the splitting of the lateral longitudinal fascicle into separate tracts (B; 1, spinocerebellar tract; 2, spinal trigeminal tract; 3, lateral vestibulospinal tract) (modified from Glover and Petursdottir, 1991).

fascicle (llf) (Fig. 5). Each contains ascending and descending axons, which tend to be segregated into subfascicles containing axons of a given type. As the transversal area of the hindbrain expands, the mlf maintains its coherence alongside the raphe and remains as the tract of the same name in the mature brain. The llf, on the other hand, splits into several tracts, including various ascending sensory tracts, the spinal trigeminal tract, and the lateral vestibulospinal tract. This splitting is accompanied by intercalation of increasing numbers of neurons and other axons. Thus, the early formation of longitudinal axon tracts occurs on a simple scaffold that increases in complexity by a process of fission. Later formed tracts, such as the corticospinal tract and the pontocerebellar projection, are layered externally to the early formed tracts.

B. Gene Expression and Regionalization

1. Rhombomeres and Longitudinal Patterning

The rhombomeres are transient subdivisions that were described in the embryos of a number of species including the human starting in the late 1800s. Their analysis underwent a dramatic renaissance nearly 100 years later with the application of modern cellular and molecular techniques, spearheaded by the efforts of Andrew Lumsden and colleagues.

As many as eight rhombomeres have been described, and these are denoted r1, r2, r3, and so on from rostral to caudal (Fig. 3). The second through sixth rhombomeres (r2–r6) are similar in length and readily visible in most species. The first and last two rhombomeres may represent transitional neuromeres at the junctions between hindbrain and mesencephalon and hindbrain and spinal cord.

Rhombomere boundaries have several features that contribute to a physical segmentation of the hindbrain neural tube. The proliferation rate is lower at the boundaries, creating the indentations that mark their positions visibly. The pattern of intercellular communication via gap junctions is modulated at the boundaries, several extracellular proteins are preferentially expressed there, and cells in alternating rhombomeres have different cell adhesion properties such that they tend to segregate if mixed. All of this contributes to the formation of a physical barrier to cell movement over rhombomere boundaries. Indeed, in contrast to the extensive circumferential migration that occurs among certain hindbrain neuron populations, rostrocaudal migration is much more limited. This has led to the idea that the rhombomeres compartmentalize the hindbrain, confining progenitor cells and their offspring to specific rostrocaudal domains. Of course, longitudinal fibers penetrate the rhombomere boundaries, and some neuron populations breach the barriers as well, especially at sites of intersection by fiber tracts.

The rhombomeres appear during a period when many hindbrain neurons are being generated, and they fade away by the time most of the major nuclei of the hindbrain have appeared. The temporal concurrence with neurogenesis and differentiation suggests that the rhombomeres play a role in patterning that differentiation. Molecular correlates of rhombomeric compartmentalization strongly support this notion. In particular, the rhombomeric domains are correlated with the expression of a number of developmental regulatory genes that are involved in controlling the differentiation of neurons into specific phenotypes along the rostrocaudal axis.

One class of regulatory genes that figures prominently is the Hox gene family, which encodes transcription factors whose differential expression establishes regional patterns of differentiation in a variety of organisms and organ systems. Hox genes are ordered in a specific sequence within the genome, a relationship that is reiterated in their tissue expression pattern. Within the hindbrain, Hox genes have a sequentially overlapping pattern of expression that is strongly correlated with the rhombomeres and provides each of them with a unique combinatorial address (Fig. 6). Evidence that the Hox genes are important determinants of neuronal differentiation comes from a variety of manipulations that alter the pattern of Hox gene expression. These include transgenic knockouts of specific Hox genes, ectopic expression of Hox genes by retroviral gene transfer, heterotopic transplantation of rhombomeres, treatment with retinoids, perturbations of Hox gene promoter sequences that alter the region-specific expression pattern, and manipulation of other genes that regulate Hox gene expression. In parallel with alterations in Hox gene expression, these manipulations lead to changes in the regional pattern of neuronal differentiation, such that neuronal phenotypes

characteristic of a given rhombomere appear in a different rhombomere.

Hox genes are also expressed by the emigrating cranial neural crest cells and are involved in patterning the various mesenchymal derivatives of the cranium, branchial arches, and neural crest-derived thoracic structures.

How is the normal, longitudinally sequential pattern of Hox gene expression established? This appears to be a complicated issue that involves a number of factors. Hox gene expression is known to be regulated by retinoids, acting through nuclear retinoid receptors, which are ligand-dependent transcription factors that interact directly with Hox gene promoter sequences. This regulation is concentration dependent. Since retinoid synthesis has been shown to be high in the spinal cord but very low in the hindbrain, a diffusion gradient of retinoids from the spinal cord rostrally into the hindbrain could contribute to setting up the pattern. Hox gene expression is also regulated by the action of other transcription factors via specific promoter sequences that direct expression differentially according to tissue type and region. The pattern of expression of such transcription factors is therefore pivotal in setting up the pattern. Lastly, Hox gene expression is cross-regulated and autoregulated by Hox proteins, in cooperation with other transcription factors. An important feature that underscores the complexity of Hox gene regulation is the dynamic pattern of expression in the hindbrain. Hox genes do not merely pop up in specific longitudinal domains but may be expressed in broader domains that eventually become restricted and that are modulated over time also in the transverse plane.

The Hox genes are not the only genes that exhibit rhombomere-related patterns of expression, but they are the most extensively studied so far with respect to a role in regulating neuronal differentiation. Some of the other rhombomere-related genes are likely to be downstream targets of the Hox genes because they code for membrane receptors and signaling molecules that are involved in features of differentiation, such as directed cell migration and axonal outgrowth. Others, such as the *kreisler* and *Krox-20* genes, are also transcription factor genes that participate with the Hox genes in the network of gene activity that sets up the regional patterning of the hindbrain.

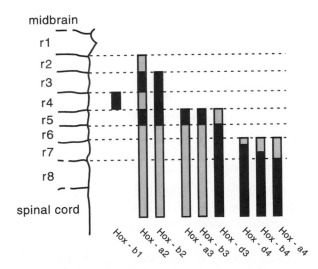

Figure 6 The relationship of rhombomeric domains to the longitudinal expression patterns of Hox genes in the mouse hindbrain. Black indicates strong expression, and gray indicates weaker expression (reproduced with permission from Keynes and Krumlauf, *Annual Review of Neuroscience*, Vol. 17, © 1994 by Annual Reviews, www.AnnualReviews.org).

2. Patterning in the Transverse Plane

In addition to the longitudinal patterning of the hindbrain exemplified by the rhombomeres, there is a

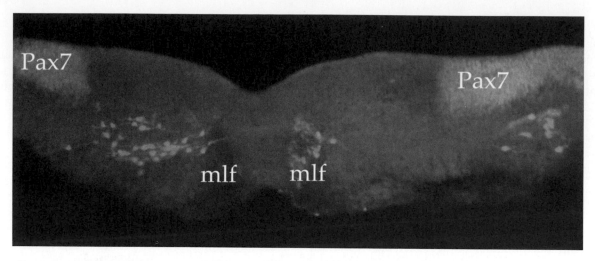

Figure 7   An example of hindbrain patterning in the transverse plane. Expression of the transcription factor *Pax7* by progenitor cells within the proliferative zone (immediately subjacent to the fourth ventricle) defines two zones with a sharp boundary at a specific site along the floor plate–roof plate axis. The hindbrain has been opened dorsally and laid flat prior to sectioning, such that the floor plate–roof plate axis runs medial to lateral on each side. Two different hindbrain neuron groups are retrogradely labeled from their axons in the right-side medial longitudinal fascicle (mlf). The group on the left side derives from the *Pax7*-negative progenitors, whereas the group on the right side derives from the *Pax7*-expressing progenitors.

systematic patterning along the floor plate–roof plate axis. This is not as obvious from the morphological standpoint because there are few related structural landmarks aside from the sulcus limitans. The organization of the cranial nerve nuclei into longitudinal columns, however, gives an immediate reflection of this transverse element of patterning. Transcription factors also figure prominently in setting up longitudinal domains within the hindbrain. Expression of Pax and Nkx genes within the progenitor cell population provides a good example. These genes, like the Hox genes, encode transcription factors known to regulate the regional differentiation of cells in a variety of tissues and species. They are expressed in overlapping longitudinal bands along much of the neuraxis, including the hindbrain, with very sharp boundaries of expression at specific levels along the floor plate–roof plate axis (Fig. 7). They can exhibit dynamic changes prior to boundary formation, and they can also exhibit modulations in expression intensity within the expression domain that becomes established. Thus, these genes provide a sequentially ordered combinatorial scheme of gene expression along the floor plate–roof plate axis in much the same way that the Hox genes pattern the longitudinal axis.

How is the normal pattern of gene expression in the transverse plane generated? This has been studied primarily in the developing spinal cord, but the emerging picture appears to be generally applicable to the hindbrain as well. Diffusible signals are released at or near the ventral and dorsal poles of the neural tube. Ventral signals derive from the notochord, a mesodermal structure that lies immediately ventral to the neural tube, as well as from the floor plate. Dorsal signals derive from the roof plate and overlying surface ectoderm. These signals establish opposing gradients that dictate which genes are expressed at different positions along the floor plate–roof plate axis. The way these signals work and the way the genes whose expression they regulate interact are complex issues that remain the subject of active research. The end result, however, is the establishment of overlapping, longitudinal bands of differential gene expression that, like the zones of differential Hox gene expression, can be correlated with the differentiation of specific neuron groups (Fig. 7).

3. From Gene Expression to Neural Networks

In combination, transcription factors encoded by these and other gene families are expressed in a kind of checkerboard pattern of intersecting rhombomeres and longitudinal bands. How does this relate to the regional pattern of neuronal differentiation? The spatial and temporal correlation of hindbrain neuron types to gene expression patterns is far from complete, but several conclusions can be made.

First, certain neuron groups are neatly delimited longitudinally by rhombomeric domains, and certain groups are neatly delimited along the floor plate–roof

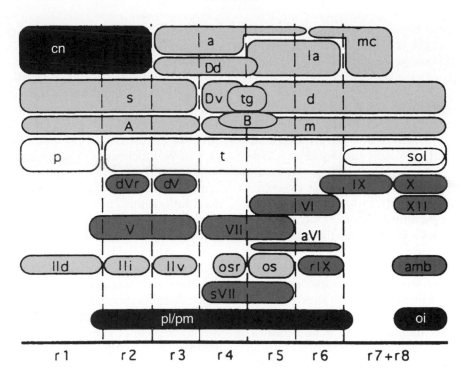

Figure 8 The relationship of hindbrain nuclei to rhombomeric domains in the chicken embryo. Nuclei are ordered roughly along the floor plate–roof plate axis from bottom to top. Different shades of grey indicate classes of related nuclei. Note that the rhombomeric pattern exhibits phylogenetic variants. cn, cerebellar nuclei; a, angularis; la, laminaris; mc, magnocellularis; Dd, Deiters dorsalis; s, superior vestibular; Dv, Deiters ventralis; tg, tangentialis; d, descending vestibular; A, vestibular cell group A; B, vestibular cell group B; m, medial vestibular; p, principal trigeminal; t, descending trigeminal; sol, nucleus of solitary tract; dV, dorsal trigeminal (r, rostral part); V, trigeminal motor; VI, abducens; aVI, accessory abducens; VII, facial; IX, glossopharyngeal; X, vagus; XII, hypoglossal; lld, nucleus of lateral lemniscus, (d, dorsal; i, intermediate; v, ventralis); os, superior olive (r, rostral part); rIX, retrofacial glossopharyngeal; amb, ambiguus; sVII, superficial facial; pl/pm, lateral and medial pontine nuclei; oi, inferior olive (modified from Marin and Puelles, 1995).

plate axis by longitudinal gene expression domains, whereas others are not (Fig. 8). There are several potential explanations for examples of noncongruity between neuron groups and these domains. For example, the pattern as described to date may be incomplete. Additional genes could subdivide the currently known expression pattern into additional domains; similarly, additional information about the phenotypic diversity of neuron groups may introduce novel group subdivisions. Alternatively, the noncongruity might result from the dynamic features of both gene expression and neuron group formation. As noted previously, gene expression patterns can change over time, and neurons can migrate, so correspondences may be evident only within very particular time windows and then disappear.

Second, the relationship between gene expression patterns and neuron groups is not necessarily applicable only to the classically defined cytoarchitectonic nuclei of the hindbrain. Rather, correlations may be stronger to neuron groupings defined by specific phenotypic characters, such as neurotransmitter profile or axon projection pattern. For example, within such populations as the reticulospinal neurons and the vestibular nuclear complex, subdivisions on the basis of axon projection pathway are more readily correlated to gene expression domains than are the classical nuclear divisions.

Third, it appears that the relationship between gene expression patterns and neuron groups can be extended to the connectivity patterns of hindbrain neurons. This feature has only been examined in a few instances, but there are compelling examples of neuron groups whose subdivision according to termination patterns onto synaptic targets can be correlated to gene expression domains. The vestibular nuclear complex provides an example. Here, the different subgroups connect in stereotyped patterns to target motoneurons, creating highly specific reflex pathways for eye and body movements. Although the action of particular genes in establishing this pattern of connectivity has not been experimentally tested, the striking correlation of the vestibular subgroups to gene expression domains suggests a direct link. Other functional systems within the hindbrain similarly appear to be constructed through the action of regional patterns of gene expression. For example, primordial respiratory activity is generated by a neural network with definable components localized to specific rhombomeres. Genetic manipulations that perturb the rhombomeric pattern lead to specific functional deficits in the network.

To summarize, hindbrain neurons are organized into distinct cranial nerve and other nuclei, with the reticular formation as a central core. The pattern of specific functional subdivisions within these nuclei and within the reticular formation is likely to be directly linked to the highly mosaic pattern of gene expression seen at early stages of hindbrain development. Moreover, this relationship likely contributes to establishing the basic pattern of synaptic connectivity within hindbrain networks. Identifying the gene combinations responsible for specifying the various neuron types and their synaptic connections is one of the major challenges of future research on the hindbrain.

III. BRIEF CONSIDERATIONS OF PATHOLOGY

Given the many critical functions of the pons and medulla oblongata, pathology in these hindbrain derivatives can have a wide variety of effects. Specific or diverse symptoms may result, depending on whether the pathology is focal, involving a particular nucleus or pathway, or more widespread. In either case, the pathological manifestations can be devastating and potentially life-threatening since so many areas of the pons and medulla participate in vital processes. Thus, contusions, tumors, and vascular lesions are often fatal. Several well-known pathological syndromes can be distinguished on the basis of particular combinations of symptoms, as these relate directly to the location of the lesion and the level at which fiber tracts decussate. For example, medial lesions typically present symptoms such as contralateral hemiparesis (corticospinal tract) and loss of proprioception (medial lemniscus). In contrast, lateral lesions typically present symptoms such as ipsilateral loss of facial cutaneous sensation (trigeminal sensory nucleus and tract), contralateral loss of pain and temperature sensation (spinothalamic tract), and Horner syndrome (ipsilateral descending autonomic fibers). In addition, each type of lesion will potentially affect the function of specific cranial nerves.

The different medial and lateral pontine and medullary syndromes lie within the basic diagnostic repertoire of the practicing neurologist. Hindbrain pathology reulting from genetic disorders is a less common class of diagnosis but almost certainly occurs more frequently than is currently recognized. Mutations in transcription factor genes have been established as the cause of a few pathological syndromes, such as Waardenberg's syndrome, that involve developmental defects in the cranial neural crest (cristopathies). Similar mutations in genes patterning the hindbrain neural tube could lead to catastrophic consequences if they disrupt major elements of the pattern, but they could also lead to more focal defects compromising the function of specific networks, with more subtle symptoms as a result. For example, nonlethal mutation of the *Krox-20* gene in the mouse, which disrupts rhombomeric patterning, perturbs the development of respiratory networks and leads to varying degrees of apnea. There are probably a large number of idiopathic conditions affecting the hindbrain that have a genetic basis, and it is not unreasonable to expect that as genetic analysis of hindbrain patterning progresses new syndromes will be classified for which mutation of identified patterning genes is the underlying cause.

See Also the Following Articles

BRAIN ANATOMY AND NETWORKS • BRAIN DEVELOPMENT • BRAIN STEM • CEREBELLUM • FOREBRAIN

Suggested Reading

Brodal, P. (1992). *The Central Nervous System: Structure and Function* (see Chapter 4). Oxford Univ. Press, Oxford.

Champagnat, J., and Fortin, G. (1997). Primordial respiratory-like rhythm generation in the vertebrate embryo. *Trends Neurosci.* **20,** 119–124.

Ericson, J., Briscoe, J., Rashbass, P., van Heyningen, V., and Jessell, T. M. (1997). Graded sonic hedgehog signaling and the specification of cell fate in the ventral neural tube. *Cold Spring Harbor Symp. Quant. Biol.* **62,** 451–466.

Glover, J. C. (1993). The development of brain stem projections to the spinal cord in the chicken embryo. *Brain Res. Bull.* **30,** 265–271.

Glover, J. C. (2000a). Neuroepithelial "compartments" and the specification of vestibular projections. *Prog. Brain Res.* **124,** 3–21.

Glover, J. C. (2000b). The development of specific connectivity between premotor neurons and motoneurons in the brain stem and spinal cord. *Physiol. Rev.* **80,** 615–647.

Keynes, R., and Krumlauf, R. (1994). Hox genes and regionalization of the nervous system. *Annu. Rev. Neurosci.* **17,** 109–132.

Larsen, W. J. (1997). *Human Embryology*, 2nd ed. (see Chapter 13). Churchill Livingstone, New York.

Lee, K. J., and Jessell, T. M. (1999). The specification of dorsal cell fates in the vertebrate central nervous system. *Cell* **96,** 211–224.

Lumsden, A. (1990). The cellular basis of segmentation in the developing hindbrain. *Trends Neurosci.* **13,** 329–335.

Lumsden, A., and Krumlauf, R. (1996). Patterning the vertebrate neuraxis. *Science* **274,** 1109–1115.

Marín, F., and Puelles, L. (1995). Morphological fate of rhombomeres in quail/chick chimeras: A segmental analysis of hindbrain nuclei. *Eur. J. Neurosci.* **7,** 1714–1738.

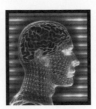

HIV Infection, Neurocognitive Complications of

Human Brain

IGOR GRANT

University of California, San Diego, and VA San Diego Healthcare System

GLOSSARY

acquired immune deficiency syndrome A disease resulting from collapse of cell-mediated immunity, resulting in infections, cancers, and other complications that lead to death. Human immunodeficiency virus is the causal agent.

antiretroviral drugs Drugs that interfere with various stages of the reproduction of human immunodeficiency virus.

CCR5 A type of chemokine receptor found on macrophages, dendritic cells, and certain other cells.

CD4 cells A type of lymphocyte that is important in coordinating numerous immune events. Infection and depletion of CD4 lymphocytes by HIV results in the evolution of acquired immunodeficiency.

cerebrospinal fluid Fluid surrounding the brain and spinal cord and also contained within the cavities of the brain. Analysis of cerebrospinal fluid may provide clues about pathological processes in the brain.

chemokines, chemokine receptors Chemokines are a family of molecules that are produced in the course of inflammation. Docking sites for such molecules (receptor sites) may be important for HIV entry into a host cell and also in HIV-mediated neural injury.

CXCR4 A type of chemokine receptor found predominantly on CD4 lymphocytes.

dementia, cortical A pattern of neurocognitive change similar to that seen in Alzheimer's disease.

dementia, subcortical Pattern of neurocognitive changes resembling those seen in Huntington's disease, Parkinson's disease, and certain "white matter" diseases of the brain.

gp120 A molecule in the envelope coating of HIV that may be neurotoxic.

human immunodeficiency virus The virus that causes HIV disease and AIDS.

integrase An enzyme of HIV necessary for the process whereby proviral DNA is integrated into the genome of the host cell.

neurocognitive Mental processes whose disruption strongly suggests reversible or irreversible brain injury. The neurocognitive functions (abilities) include attention, perceptual motor abilities, abstracting (including problem solving, planning, and executive functions), learning, remembering, and speeded information processing.

neurocognitive complications A spectrum of disturbances of neurocognitive functions ranging from asymptomatic impairment to frank dementia.

protease An enzyme contained in HIV that is involved in the late stages of HIV maturation.

protease inhibitors Drugs whose antiviral activity derives from their ability to interfere with the HIV enzyme protease.

reverse transcriptase An enzyme carried by HIV that allows it to form viral DNA from its RNA template.

reverse transcriptase inhibitors Drugs whose antiviral properties derive from their ability to interfere with the HIV enzyme reverse transcriptase.

virion A particle of HIV.

Acquired immune deficiency syndrome (AIDS) results from infection with human immunodeficiency virus (HIV). HIV infection is associated with destruction of certain immune cells, most notably the CD4 or "helper" T lymphocytes, leading ultimately to collapse of cell-mediated immunity and consequent susceptibility to various types of "opportunistic" infections and cancers. In the course of HIV disease, virus enters the central nervous system and this can result in disturbances in neurocognitive function—that is, deficits in mental processes such as attention, learning, remembering, problem solving, speed of information processing, and various sensory and motor abnormalities. In addition to the direct effects of HIV on brain function and structure, late complications that involve infection of the brain by other pathogens or development of neoplasia or vascular disturbances can also contribute to neurocognitive complications in late-stage HIV disease.

I. HUMAN IMMUNODEFICIENCY VIRUS

HIV is a member of the lentivirus subfamily of retroviruses. Retroviruses carry their genetic information on RNA (rather than DNA) but require the formation of viral DNA as a step in reproduction. This is accomplished by harnessing the machinery of the cell that the virus infects, wherein the viral enzyme reverse transcriptase facilitates forming DNA from the two strands of viral RNA within the infected host cell. The viral DNA so formed is integrated into the cell's genetic material and directs the host cell to manufacture new viral constituents. Essentially, these consist of a viral core surrounded by a glycoprotein envelope. Steps involved in viral replication are illustrated schematically in Fig. 1.

From a genetic standpoint, there are two types of HIV: HIV-1 and HIV-2. The predominant cause of AIDS worldwide is HIV-1, whereas HIV-2 remains limited to portions of western Africa. HIV-1, in turn, is classified on the basis of genetic analysis into a major group (group M) and an outlier group (group O). Again, the vast majority of infections worldwide are with group M viruses, with subtype B of group M

predominating in the industrial world. The greatest diversity of subtypes is found in Africa.

A. Transmission of HIV

In the industrialized world, transmission occurs most commonly through men having sex with men and through sharing of infected "works" by injection drug users. Heterosexual transmission is on the rise in industrialized countries, and it is the most prevalent form of transmission in Africa and India. Transmission also occurs from infected mother to fetus and through the administration of contaminated blood products. The latter is no longer an important risk in industrialized nations but poses a continuing hazard elsewhere. From the standpoint of sexual transmission, both unprotected anal and vaginal intercourse constitute the most risky circumstances, with orogenital sex representing a fairly small risk and other activities such as kissing regarded as essentially risk free.

B. Course of HIV Infection

Not all exposure to HIV, be it through unprotected sex or sharing of needles, results in infection. Whether infection occurs seems to depend on factors such as amount of inoculum, pathogenicity of virus, and host resistance. In terms of sexual transmission, the presence of sores, other venereal disease, and mucosal tears may all facilitate transmission.

Once HIV gains access to a tissue, its replication depends on its ability to enter host cells. Such entry appears to require at least two types of receptors (docking mechanisms on cell surfaces). Sections of viral envelope protein (gp120) are capable of attaching to CD4 receptor sites on host cells. However, full attachment leading to fusion of virus with cell requires a coreceptor of the chemokine type. Dozens of types of chemokine receptors are known, but the most important in terms of HIV infection appear to be CXCR4 [found predominantly on CD4 (T4) lymphocytes] and CCR5 (found on macrophages, dendritic cells, and other cells).

Once virus successfully enters host cells, replication begins. The presence of viral RNA can be found in the blood of infected individuals within 1 week of infection. Initially, there is a rapid proliferation of virus, with as many as 10 billion virions being formed every day, accompanied by massive destruction of CD4 lymphocytes of which millions must be replaced on a daily basis. Within several weeks to months, however, a "steady state" is reached wherein the host's defenses succeed in suppressing viral replication. At this point, viral load in the blood is significantly reduced or may even become undetectable. Antibody to HIV is present, however, and it is the basis for the commonly used HIV test (the enzyme-linked immunosorbent assay).

For reasons that are still incompletely understood, host responses are not ultimately effective in eradicating HIV. Chronically infected host cells (e.g., in lymph nodes) continuously seed HIV, which may gradually undergo further genetic variation (termed quasispecies formation) that may create genotypes that are increasingly more successful in eluding host defenses. Over the years, the host's capacity to mount an effective immune response diminishes, leading to a critical drop in CD4 lymphocyte concentration (normal CD4 counts are on the order of 1000 cells per cubic millimeter; persons with CD4 counts below 200 per cubic millimeter are diagnosed as having AIDS).

The collapse of cell-mediated immunity sets the stage for infection by organisms that are normally held in check by these mechanisms. These include various mycobacteria, fungi, yeasts, protozoa, as well as cancers stimulated by proliferation by other viruses (e.g., Kaposi sarcoma, which is linked to herpesvirus infection).

C. Classification of HIV Disease

AIDS represents the final stage of HIV disease. It is defined as the experience of certain major complications of HIV infection and/or the presence of CD4 cell counts below 200 (Table I). Although the course of HIV infection varies widely, it is typical for a person to experience HIV infection for 10 years before AIDS-defining events occur. Prior to that time, the individual may spend many years as an asymptomatic carrier (CDC stage A; Table I).

D. Scope of the Problem of HIV Infection

The World Health Organization estimates that approximately 33 million people are currently HIV infected worldwide. There are probably about 750,000 HIV-infected persons in the United States, and approximately 600,000 persons have died of the disease in the United States since it was first described

in 1981. In some countries of southern Africa, 25% or more of the population is HIV infected.

E. Treatment and Prevention of HIV Disease

In terms of prevention, some efforts have shown singular success (e.g., the virtual elimination of medical transmission in industrialized countries by ensuring the safety of blood supplies and use of universal precautions during medical treatments). On the other hand, the modification of sexual and drug use practices has been more difficult. Some successes have been achieved in selected high-risk groups (e.g., homosexual/bisexual men and some injection drug users participating in needle exchange programs). On a worldwide level, anti-AIDS campaigns have often been limited by political, cultural, socioeconomic, and education factors.

Progress toward developing a vaccine that might prevent the establishment of infection in the first place has been slow because of the great genetic diversity of HIV and its tendency toward rapid mutation. Several vaccines are in the process of being tested, but it remains to be seen whether such vaccines, usually based on the subtype B2 of HIV-1, will be useful in areas of the world where other subtypes predominate.

Considerable progress has been made in the development of antiretroviral medications that interfere at various stages of HIV replication. The earliest example was zidovudine [azidothymidine (AZT)], which interferes with HIV's ability to utilize reverse transcriptase (RT) to form viral DNA. There are now multiple examples of RT drugs of the nucleoside type, of which AZT is an example. Other types of RT inhibitors, termed nonnucleoside RT, have also been developed. Recently, drugs that interfere with another critical step in viral assembly, the protease inhibitors, have become available. The use of combination therapies that interfere at different stages of viral replication has proved effective in lowering plasma viral load to undetectable levels in many individuals that are treated. However, these drug combinations often have very significant undesirable and toxic side effects that may limit their tolerability; additionally, HIV's ability to rapidly mutate can eventually produce quasispecies that are resistant to various drug combinations. It is uncertain whether combination therapies can be effective in controlling viral replication on an indefinite basis. For a list of currently available drugs, see Table II. The U.S. federal guidelines for use of these drugs are shown in Table III.

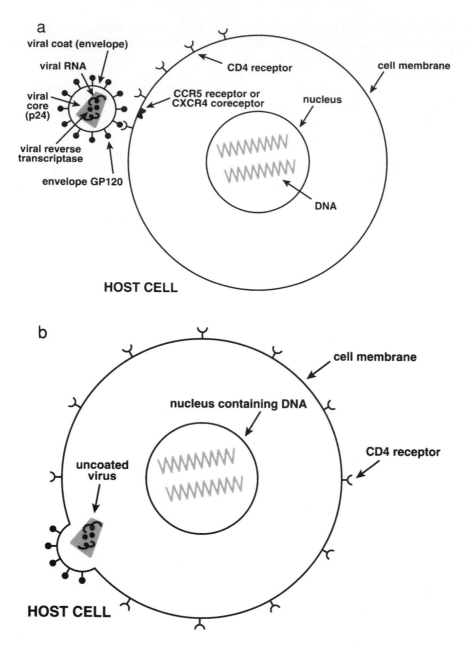

Figure 1   Stages of HIV replication. (a) HIV virion attaching to host cell. A segment of HIV envelope protein gp120 attaches to host cell CD4 receptor. Further process of attachment will involve linkage to a second host cell site, a chemokine coreceptor either of the CXCR4 (lymphocyte) or CCR5 (macrophage, dendritic cell) type. (b) After fusing with host cell wall, the uncoated HIV enters host cell cytoplasm. (c) Using its RNA template, HIV utilizes the viral enzyme reverse transcriptase to manufacture viral DNA within the host cell. This viral DNA ultimately enters the host cell nucleus and becomes integrated into host cell's DNA. (d) The viral DNA that is integrated into host cell's DNA directs formation of a viral RNA transcript, which leads to formation of viral RNA and genomic RNA. Through a translation process viral proteins are formed. (e) Viral constituents are assembled, virus particle buds off from host cell, and viral proteins are clipped into functional units by the viral protease enzyme.

II. HIV INFECTION OF THE BRAIN

There were reports of neuropsychiatric complications in AIDS even before HIV was determined to be the cause of the disease. Brain autopsies of persons dying with AIDS revealed a number of changes beyond those attributable to opportunistic infections or neoplasms. These HIV-related brain changes include

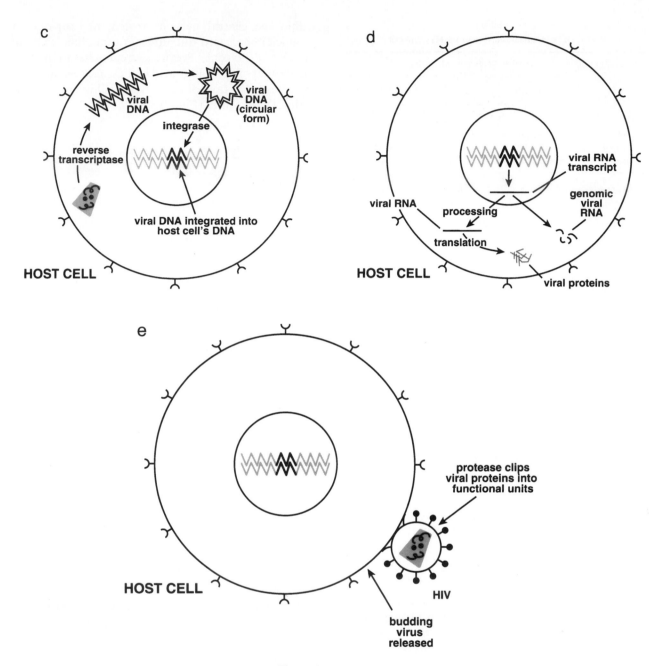

Figure 1 *(continued)*

inflammation, white matter abnormalities (vacuolar myelopathy), and nerve cell loss (poliodystrophy). The inflammatory process can be evidenced by perivascular lymphocytic infiltrates, accumulations of microglia into nodules, formation of multinucleated giant cells, as well as astrogliosis (Fig. 2).

Most persons dying with HIV infection have some detectable HIV in the brain. Although HIV can be found in any brain region, the greatest concentration of virus tends to be in subcortical gray structures (e.g., caudate nucleus) and surrounding white matter. HIV is localized within microglia and multinucleated giant cells but is not found in neurons. Despite this, the neurons of persons dying with HIV often display injury consisting of dendritic simplification and loss of synapses (Fig. 3). This has led to speculation that neural damage, and ultimately neuronal loss, may represent some combination of toxic factors and

Table I
1993 CDC Classification System for HIV Infection[a]

CD4+ cell count categories	Clinical categories		
	A[b] Asymptomatic or lymphadenopathy	B[c] Symptomatic but not A or C conditions	C[d] AIDS indicator conditions
>500/mm^3	A-1	B-1	C-1[e]
200–499/mm^3	A-2	B-2	C-2[e]
<200/mm^3	A-3[e]	B-3[e]	C-3[e]

[a] From CDC (1992).

[b] Category A includes acute HIV infection, asymptomatic infection, and progressive generalized lymphadenopathy.

[c] Category B includes conditions associated with HIV infection but that were not included in the CDC's 1987 case surveillance definition of conditions associated with severe immunodeficiency. Examples of "less severe" conditions include oropharyngeal candidiasis (thrush), persistent vulvovaginal candidiasis, severe cervical dysplasia or carcinoma, oral hairy leukoplakia, and recurrent herpes zoster involving more than one dermatome.

[d] Category C conditions are those associated with severe immunodeficiency identified in the CDC's 1987 surveillance definition for AIDS.

[e] CDC (1993) AIDS indicator conditions.

inflammatory mechanisms, balanced by protective mechanisms (Fig. 4).

III. MECHANISMS OF HIV NEUROPATHOGENESIS

A. Toxic Factors

It has been suggested that viral products, such as envelope protein gp120, may be neurotoxic. For example, gp120 causes cell death in neuronal cultures, and transgenic mice that constitutively overproduce gp120 show neuronal injury, with loss of dendritic spines and synapses. Lipton and colleagues suggested that gp120 may exert its effect by activating N–methyl-D-aspartate (NMDA) receptors, causing influx of calcium. Further evidence of this has been suggested by the fact that memantine, an NMDA antagonist, can block gp120-induced neurotoxicity. Recently, it has also been suggested that gp120 may bind to chemokine receptor sites on neurons, and this process may lead to activation of NMDA receptors and excitotoxicity.

Nonviral toxic products have also been implicated. For example, activated macrophages and astrocytes

within the central nervous system are capable of producing increased quantities of quinolinic acid, an excitotoxic molecule. Previous research has found that the amount of quinolinic acid in the cerebrospinal fluid increases with stage of disease and is highest in those with HIV dementia (Fig. 5).

B. Inflammatory Factors

HIV probably enters the central nervous system within macrophages from the periphery, thereby establishing an intracerebral focus of infection in closely related microglia. Microglia (immune cells within the brain closely related to macrophages) may become infected, and these two cell populations feature prominently in two of the hallmark changes found in the brain of persons dying with HIV encephalitis—microglial nodules and multinucleated giant cells (Fig. 2). Astrocytes may also become activated; in addition to producing abnormal quantities of various molecules

Table II
Currently Available Antiretroviral Medications

Medication	Generic name	Brand name	Usual abbreviation
Nucleoside analog reverse transcriptase inhibitors	Abacavir	Ziagen	ABC
	Didanosine	Videx	ddI
	Lamivudine	Epivir	3TC
	Stavudine	Zerit	d4T
	Zalcitabine	Hivid	ddC
	AZT+3TC	Combivir	
	AZT+3TC+ABC	Trizivir	
Nonnucleoside analog reverse transcriptase inhibitors	Delavirdine	Rescriptor	DLV
	Efavirenz	Sustiva	EFV
	Nevirapine	Viramune	NVP
Nucleotide analog reverse transcriptase inhibitors	Tenofovir	Viread	TFV
Protease inhibitors	Amprenavir	Agenerase	APV
	Indinavir	Crixivan	IDV
	Lopinavir+RTV	Kaletra	LPV
	Nelfinavir	Viracept	NFV
	Ritonavir	Norvir	RTV
	Saquinavir	Fortovase Invirase	SQV

Table III
U.S. Federal Guidelines for Initial Treatment of HIV Infection

One from group A (highly active protease inhibitors) and one combination from group B (NARTIs):

Group A	Group B
Indinavir	AZT + ddI
Ritonavir	d4T + ddI
Nelfinavir	AZT + ddC
Saquinavir SGC	AZT + 3TC
	d4T + 3TC

or

A combination of ritonavir + saquinavir

that may be neurotoxic (e.g., lymphokines and quinolinic acid), they may also alter their production of trophic factors that are necessary to sustain neurons. Examples of immune signaling molecules that can be damaging to neurons include tumor necrosis factor-alpha (TNF-α) and interleukin-6.

Masliah and colleagues suggested that different neuronal populations may be sensitive to differing types of injury. For example, pyramidal neurons may be particularly sensitive to NMDA-linked excitotoxic injury. However, interneurons, that are also damaged in HIV disease, contain proteins such as calbindin and parvalbumin that tend to protect against disruptions of calcium homeostasis. Masliah and colleagues argue that these neurons may be more vulnerable to damage by inflammatory mechanisms.

C. Protective Factors

Whether or not a neuron is injured may depend not only on the presence of inflammatory and toxic factors but also on protective mechanisms. For example, Sanders and colleagues recently reported that regions of the brain in which fibroblast growth factor (FGF) is expressed show less evidence of neural injury in the context of HIV infection. They suggested that FGF may be involved in altering intracellular signaling so that cascades leading to apoptosis (programmed cell death) are downregulated.

IV. DIAGNOSIS AND CLASSIFICATION OF NEUROCOGNITIVE COMPLICATIONS

The diagnosis of neurocognitive complications associated with HIV-1 infection requires the demonstra-

tion that there has been an acquired change in cognitive performance that has occurred since the person became HIV infected and that cannot be explained by other causes. Three levels of impairment have been described.

A. Asymptomatic Neuropsychological Impairment

This mildest form of neurocognitive complication is characterized by subtle changes in cognitive functioning that appear not to interfere in any obvious way in day-to-day functioning. Typically, a person will report feeling that he or she is not as "sharp" as he or she used to be and may complain of mild memory difficulties, difficulties in concentration, or some slight slowing down in mental functions. However, self-report alone is not sufficient to establish a diagnosis because this may be biased by mood disturbance (depression may lead to complaints that are unrelated to actual cognitive functioning) or lack of insight. The diagnosis requires demonstrating at least mild impairments in two different cognitive areas on comprehensive neuropsychological testing (Table IV).

B. Mild Neurocognitive Disorder

As described by the American Academy of Neurology, mild neurocognitive disorder, also known as minor cognitive motor disorder (MCMD), represents another mild form of cognitive abnormality that, however, is of sufficient magnitude that there is some impairment in at least one area of life functioning, such as inefficiency at work or management of domestic or financial affairs (Table V). As with asymptomatic neuropsychological impairment, comprehensive neuropsychological testing is necessary to establish that there are at least two areas of cognitive function in which performance is at least one standard deviation below that expected for persons of similar age, education, and sociodemographic background.

C. HIV-Associated Dementia

Dementia is diagnosed when there is impairment in at least two (and usually multiple) cognitive areas of sufficient severity to interfere markedly with day-to-day life (Table VI). Persons with HIV dementia are

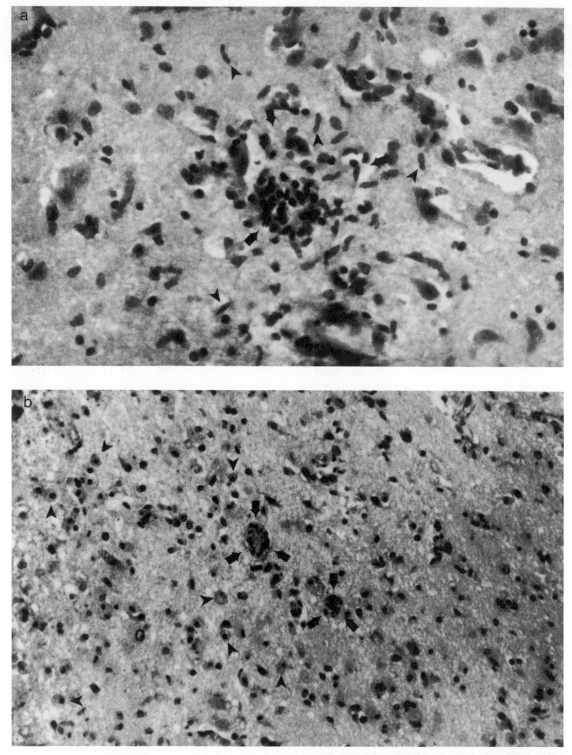

Figure 2   Microscopic anatomy of HIV brain disease. (a) Hematoxylin and eosin-stained, paraffin embedded section of AIDS brain tissue. A large microglial nodule is present in the center of the section (surrounded by three arrows). Numerous elongated microglial nuclei are present both within the nodule and in the surrounding tissue (arrowheads). Original magnification, × 600. (b) HIV p24 immunoperoxidase-stained, paraffin embedded section of AIDS brain tissue. Several large multinucleated giant cells (surrounded by arrows) contain black, amorphous immunoprecipitate of density similar to that of the oval nuclei. Numerous mononuclear macrophages (arrowheads) are distributed throughout the tissue. Original magnification, × 300 (courtesy of Clayton A. Wiley, University of Pittsburgh).

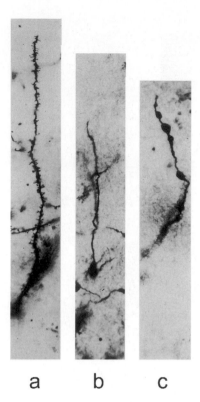

a   b   c

Figure 3 Dendritic pathology in HIV. Golgi-impregnated dendritic segments from control (a) and two cases with HIV dementia. There is loss of dendritic spines (b and c) and distortion and abnormal vacuolation of dendritic segment (c) (courtesy of Drs. Eliezer Masliah, University of California, San Diego, and Clayton A. Wiley, University of Pittsburgh).

typically unemployable and may have difficulty with independent living. The symptoms include significant psychomotor slowing and incoordination, marked inattention, slowness in information processing, difficulty in learning new information, and impairment in fluency. In some cases, the dementia may be accompanied by psychosis, including manic and paranoid phenomena. Some patients become markedly agitated, and others become apathetic and sometimes mute. The onset of frank dementia is a poor prognostic sign in HIV disease and is predictive of near future death in many instances.

V. EPIDEMIOLOGY OF NEUROCOGNITIVE COMPLICATIONS

Neurocognitive complications become more prevalent with progression of HIV disease. Thus, HIV dementia

almost never occurs in stages A and B of HIV disease, but it may be found in 4–7% of those with frank AIDS. In earlier stage disease, neurocognitive impairment, if it is seen, is typically mild and may have a relapsing–remitting course. Observers continue to disagree on the prevalence of these complications in earlier stage disease. Data from the San Diego HIV Neurobehavioral Research Center are presented in Fig. 6. It can be seen that the rate of impairment increases with stage of disease. In the medically asymptomatic form of disease, only the mildest form of neurocognitive impairment tends to be observed (i.e., asymptomatic neuropsychological impairment). Minor cognitive motor disorder becomes more prevalent in stage B and stage C disease.

VI. ASSOCIATED FACTORS AND CORRELATES OF HIV NEUROCOGNITIVE COMPLICATIONS

It is difficult to predict who will and who will not develop neurocognitive complications. Clearly, progression of disease is one factor, as the data in Fig. 6 illustrate. However, general markers of disease progression, such as a decrease in CD4 count and an increase in beta-2 microglobulin (a marker of immune activation), are not powerful predictors of future cognitive complications. Plasma viral load is associated with neuropsychological impairment, but measuring the concentration of HIV in the cerebrospinal fluid (CSF) may provide a more specific indicator. For example, Ellis and colleagues reported that in patients with AIDS there was an association between CSF viral load, but not plasma viral load, and likelihood of neurocognitive impairment.

Markers of immune activation in the CSF have also been associated with neurocognitive impairment (e.g., an increase in CSF neopterin and CSF beta-2 microglobulin). As noted previously, concentration of the

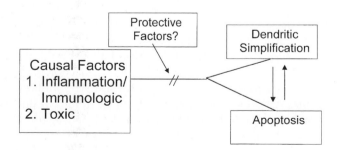

Figure 4 General model for HIV neural injury.

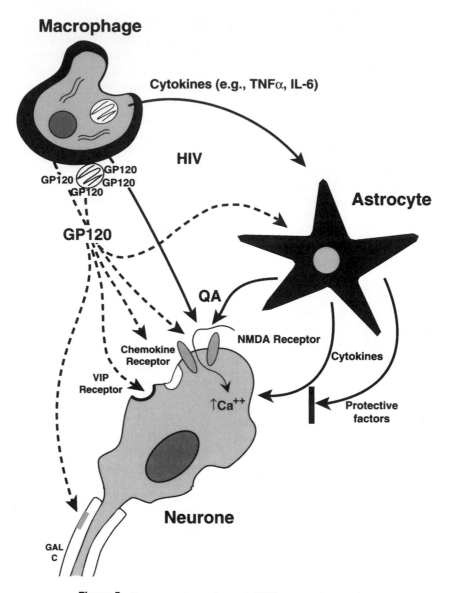

Figure 5   Some putative pathways in HIV neuropathogenesis.

excitotoxic compound quinolinic acid is also elevated in the CSF of those with HIV dementia; however, it is not clear whether quinolinic acid is another marker of immune activation or is somehow causally related to the neurocognitive impairment.

In terms of risk factors, contrary to expectation, there is no clear-cut association between injection drug use and heightened risk of neurocognitive complications. Although the rates of neuropsychological impairment tend to be higher among injection drug users generally, there does not seem to be an interaction between drug abuse and HIV status. An exception to this rule may be dependence on central stimulant drugs, especially methamphetamine. Preliminary observations suggest that history of methamphetamine dependence may enhance the likelihood of HIV-associated neurocognitive impairment perhaps because of some commonalities in mechanisms of neural injury that involve excitotoxicity.

There has been speculation that some of the subtle neuropsychological impairment found in HIV-infected persons might be due to depression, fatigue, or other nonspecific factors. This matter has received considerable exploration and the overall conclusion is that depression and medical symptoms generally do not explain the neuropsychological impairment. For

Table IV
Research Definition for HIV Neuropsychological Impairment

Performance at least 1.0 standard deviation below age–education norms in at least two different cognitive areas[a]

The impairment cannot be explained by comorbid conditions (e.g., substance abuse and medications)

The impairment does not occur solely as part of a delirium (e.g., due to CNS toxoplasmosis, lymphoma, or CMV)

[a]At least five of the following ability areas must be assessed: attention/information processing, language, abstraction/executive, complex perceptual motor, learning, recall/forgetting, motor skills, and sensory.

example, although depressive symptoms increase with frequency with disease progression, there is not a strong association between such symptoms and the likelihood of finding neurocognitive impairment. Similarly, Heaton and colleagues found that neuropsychological impairment could not be explained simply on the basis of fatigue and constitutional symptoms.

VII. COURSE OF NEUROCOGNITIVE COMPLICATIONS

HIV-related neurocognitive complications differ from those seen in degenerative disorders, such as Alzheimer's disease or Parkinson's disease. Most persons with mild impairments do not progress to develop dementia; indeed, many recover and some have a

relapsing–remitting course. This is illustrated by the data in Figs. 7 and 8, derived from research at the San Diego HIV Neurobehavioral Research Center (HNRC). In Fig. 7, it can be seen that after a period of 1 year only about half of the cases judged to have MCMD or asymptomatic neuropsychological impairment remain in the same category. About one-fifth improve, and a small proportion worsen. When data over a period of 5 years were considered, it was found that about one-fourth of HIV-infected persons had a "wobbly" or relapsing–remitting course. This pattern of waxing and waning symptomatology is consistent with the presumed underlying etiology, which is thought to be linked to periodic flare-ups of viral activity or immune activation within the central nervous system.

VIII. QUALITATIVE FEATURES OF NEUROCOGNITIVE COMPLICATIONS

HIV neurocognitive complications are often described as having "subcortical" features. This means that the pattern of impairment is somewhat reminiscent of that seen in neurological diseases that affect primarily the subcortical structures or white matter and possibly pathology involving frontostriatal circuits (e.g., Huntington's disease, Parkinson's disease, and multiple sclerosis). Persons with this pattern of neuropathology tend to have difficulties in psychomotor abilities, speed of information processing, initiation, divided

Table V
Criteria for Mild Neurocognitive Disorder[a]

Acquired impairment in cognitive functioning, involving at least two ability domains, documented by performance of at least 1.0 standard deviation below the mean for age–education-appropriate norms on standardized neuropsychological tests. The neuropsychological assessment must survey at least the following abilities: verbal/language, attention/speeded processing, abstraction/executive, memory (learning and recall), complex perceptual–motor performance, and motor skills.

The cognitive impairment produces at least mild interference in daily functioning (at least one of the following):

Self-report of reduced mental acuity or inefficiency in work, homemaking, or social functioning.

Observation by knowledgeable others that the individual has undergone at least mild decline in mental acuity with resultant inefficiency in work, homemaking, or social functioning.

The cognitive impairment has been present at least 1 month.

The cognitive impairment does not meet criteria for delirium or dementia.

There is no evidence of another preexisting cause for the MND.[b]

[a]As defined by Grant and Atkinson (1995).

[b]If the individual with suspected mild neurocognitive disorder (MND) also satisfies criteria for a major depressive episode or substance dependence, the diagnosis of MND should be deferred to a subsequent examination conducted at a time when the major depression has remitted or at least 1 month has elapsed following termination of dependent-substance use.

Table VI
Criteria for HIV Dementia[a]

Marked acquired impairment in cognitive functioning, involving at least two ability domains (e.g., memory and attention): typically, the impairment is in multiple domains, especially in learning of new information, slowed information processing, and defective attention/concentration. The cognitive impairment can be ascertained by history, mental status examination, or neuropsychological testing.

The cognitive impairment produces marked interference with day-to-day functioning (work, home life, and social activities).

The marked cognitive impairment has been present for at least 1 month.

The pattern of cognitive impairment does not meet criteria for delirium (e.g., clouding of consciousness is not a prominent feature) or, if delirium is present, criteria for dementia need to have been met on a prior examination when delirium was not present.

There is no evidence of another, preexisting etiology that could explain the dementia (e.g., other CNS infection, CNS neoplasm, cerebrovascular disease, preexisting neurological disease, or severe substance abuse compatible with CNS disorder).

[a]As defined by Grant and Atkinson (1995).

attention, learning difficulties, difficulties in retrieval of information but not accelerated forgetting, and some executive dysfunction. To the extent that there are language problems, these are more in the area of fluency rather than naming. In contrast, the so-called "cortical" dementias (Alzheimer's disease and multi infarct dementia) are characterized by severe memory impairment that includes difficulty in learning new information as well as rapid forgetting, problems in naming and comprehension, and disturbances of praxis.

Thus, HIV-infected persons with asymptomatic neuropsychological impairment or MCMD tend to have mild learning difficulties, some problems with attention, difficulties with speed of information processing, some psychomotor slowing, and occasionally, difficulties with fluency. Although this may be the most

typical pattern, it should be noted that since HIV-associated neurological injury can be widespread in the brain, there are some cases that have symptoms that are more cortical in nature, and others that have mixed features.

IX. SIGNIFICANCE OF NEUROCOGNITIVE COMPLICATIONS

Despite typically being mild and fluctuating in nature, HIV-associated complications can affect multiple aspects of life. For example, Heaton and colleagues demonstrated that those with impairment were twice as likely to be unemployed as persons without impairment. Also, even among the employed, those with mild impairment were performing at a level less

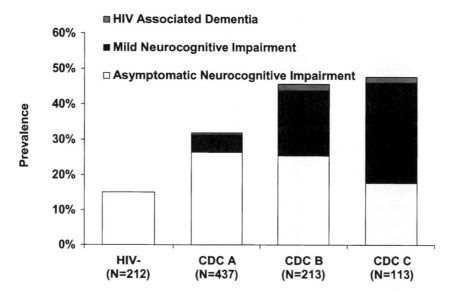

Figure 6 Prevalence of HIV neurocognitive complications at different stages of disease.

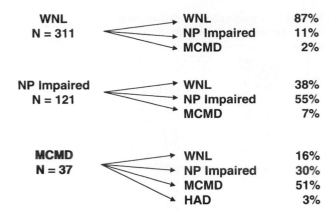

WNL	→ WNL	87%
N = 311	→ NP Impaired	11%
	→ MCMD	2%
NP Impaired	→ WNL	38%
N = 121	→ NP Impaired	55%
	→ MCMD	7%
MCMD	→ WNL	16%
N = 37	→ NP Impaired	30%
	→ MCMD	51%
	→ HAD	3%

Figure 7 One-year progression of neurocognitive complications. HAD, HIV-1-associated dementia; NP, neuropschological; MCMD, minor cognitive motor disorder; WNL, within normal limits.

than expected based on uninfected comparison groups and also on infected but not impaired controls. Neuropsychological impairment associated with HIV may also affect important life activities, such as driving and medication management. For example, Marcotte and colleagues, utilizing the driving simulator, noted that those with impairment had more simulated accidents than the unimpaired. Recent data suggest that such individuals also had more actual on-road accidents and incidents. Recent observation at the HNRC also indicates that those with neuropsychological impairment may have more difficulties with managing their antiretroviral medication regimens. For example, Fig. 9 shows that more of the mildly impaired patients fail to take their medications as scheduled or as directed.

The presence of neurocognitive complications also predicts earlier death. For example, Ellis and colleagues noted that patients with MCMD had a median survival of 2.2 years, and those with asymptomatic neuropsychological impairment 3.8 years, versus 5.1 years for those who were neurocognitively normal. Adjustment of the survival analysis for CD4 count and other disease indicators revealed an independent effect for neurocognitive impairment. The mechanism for this remains unclear, but similar data were also reported from the Columbia University cohort.

X. TREATMENT AND PREVENTION OF NEUROCOGNITIVE COMPLICATIONS

The extent to which antiretroviral therapy protects against neurocognitive complications remains uncertain. Historical data indicate that the advent of the first antiretroviral (AZT) was associated with reduction in diagnosis of AIDS-associated dementia. However, not all investigators have reached the same conclusion.

The advent of potent antiretroviral combination therapies holds with it the promise of reducing viral load to unmeasurable or very low levels. Studies are under way to determine whether such viral load reductions are associated with neurocognitive improvement. Preliminary observations indicate that reduction of viral load in the CSF may be more specifically associated with neurocognitive improvement than reduction in plasma load. If correct, this would raise questions about the differential efficacy of new antiretrovirals. In other words, the possibility arises that agents may be extremely potent in lowering peripheral viral load but, because of their poor

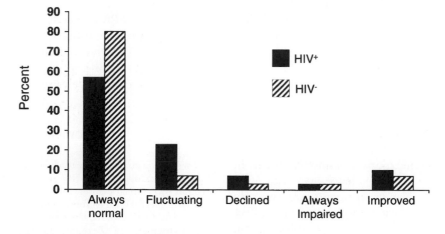

Figure 8 Neuropsychological course in participants with 5 years of annual assessments.

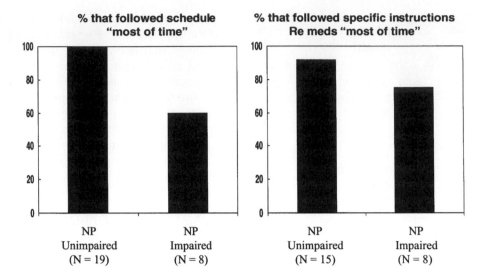

Figure 9   HIV neurocognitive impairment associated with worsened adherence to antiretroviral treatment.

penetration into the central nervous system, they may not be equally effective with regard to CNS complications.

Research is also ongoing to test drugs that may impact the putative mechanisms of neural injury. For example, a treatment trial is currently under way with the NMDA blocker memantine to determine whether reducing activity at glutamatergic receptor sites may be associated with neurocognitive improvement. A trial of peptide T, which putatively competes with viral envelope protein gp120 at neural receptor sites (e.g., receptor sites for VIP and possibly chemokine receptor sites), produced mixed results. Overall, it appeared that peptide T did not yield neurocognitive improvement; however, an analysis based on a subset of definitely impaired HIV-infected individuals did suggest some benefit. Thus, the question of peptide T's effectiveness remains unresolved. Pentoxyfylline, which blocks the action of TNF-α, was not promising in improving neurocognitive functioning in a preliminary trial.

XI. SUMMARY

Neurocognitive complications commonly occur in HIV disease, and their prevalence increases with disease progression. The impairments are typically mild in nature, often wax and wane, and affect primarily the capacity to learn new information, cognitive and psychomotor speed, and attention—a profile reminiscent of "subcortical" dementias such as those associated with Huntington's disease, Parkinson's disease, and white matter dementias. One of the fundamental substrates of the cognitive impairment is neural injury, including loss of dendritic spines and synaptic simplification. The mechanism of injury may involve the toxic effects of viral products such as gp120 as well as inflammatory mechanisms involving perhaps abnormal expression of various lymphokines. Protective factors may also be important, although the role of FGF and other trophic factors has yet to be established. Alhough they are usually mild in nature, HIV-associated neurocognitive disturbances can have substantial effects on day-to-day life, including employment, and day-to-day tasks such as medication management and driving skills. The presence of impairment is also associated with earlier mortality. Currently available antiretroviral drug combinations have increased survival of patients with HIV, but their potential to avert or improve neurocognitive complications is not conclusively established.

Acknowledgments

The work summarized in this article was performed in the context of the HIV Neurobehavioral Research Center (HNRC) (principal support by National Institute of Mental Health Grant MH45294). The San Diego HIV Neurobehavioral Research Center (HNRC) group is affiliated with the University of California, San Diego, the Naval Hospital, San Diego, and the San Diego Veterans Affairs Healthcare System and includes the following: director, Igor Grant, codirectors, J. Hampton Atkinson, J. Allen McCutchan; center manager, Thomas D. Marcotte; Naval Hospital, San Diego, Mark R. Wallace; neuromedical component, J. Allen McCutchan, Ronald J. Ellis, Scott Letendre, and Rachel Schrier; neurobehavioral component, Robert K. Heaton, Mariana Cherner, and Julie Rippeth; imaging component, Terry Jernigan, and John Hesselink; neuropathology component, Eliezer Masliah; clinical trials component, J. Allen McCutchan, J. Hampton Atkinson, Ronald J. Ellis, and Scott Letendre; data management unit, Daniel R. Masys and Michelle Frybarger, (data systems manager); statistics unit, Ian Abramson, Reena Deutsch, and Tanya Wolfson.

See Also the Following Articles

AUTOIMMUNE DISEASES • BORNA DISEASE VIRUS • CANCER PATIENTS, COGNITIVE FUNCTION • CERE-BRAL WHITE MATTER DISORDERS • COGNITIVE REHABILITATION • DEMENTIA

Suggested Reading

Centers for Disease Control (1992). 1993 revised classification system for HIV infection and expanded surveillance case definition for AIDS among adolescents and adults. *Morbidity Mortality Weekly Rep.* **41**, 1–19.

Ellis, R. J., Hsia, K., Spector, S. A., Nelson, J. A., Heaton, R. K., Wallace, M. R., Abramson, I., Atkinson, J. H., Grant, I., McCutchan, J. A., and the HIV Neurobehavioral Research Center Group (1997). Cerebrospinal fluid human immunodeficiency virus type 1 RNA levels are elevated in neurocognitively impaired individuals with acquired immunodeficiency syndrome. *Ann. Neurol.* **42**, 679–688.

Grant, I., and Atkinson, J. H. (1999). Neuropsychiatric aspects of HIV infection and AIDS. In *Kaplan and Sadock's Comprehensive Textbook of Psychiatry/VII* (B. J. Sadock and V. A. Sadock, Eds.), pp. 308–335. Williams & Wilkins, Baltimore.

Grant, I., Atkinson, J. H., Hesselink, J. R., Kennedy, C. J., Richman, D. D., Spector, S. A., and McCutchan, J. A. (1987). Evidence for early central nervous system involvement in the acquired immunodeficiency syndrome (AIDS) and other human immunodeficiency virus (HIV) infections: Studies with neuropsychologic testing and magnetic resonance imaging. *Ann. Intern. Med.* **107**, 828–836.

Grant, I., Olshen, R. A., Atkinson, J. H., Heaton, R. K., Nelson, J., McCutchan, J. A., and Weinrich, J. D. (1993). Depressed mood does not explain neuropsychological deficits in HIV-infected persons. *Neuropsychology* **7**, 53–61.

Heaton, R. K., Velin, R. A., McCutchan, J. A., Gulevich, S. J., Atkinson, J. H., Wallace, M. R., Godfrey, H. P. D., Kirson, D. A., Grant, I., and the HNRC group (1994). Neuropsychological impairment in human immunodeficiency virus-infection: Implications for employment. *Psychosom. Med.* **56**, 8–17.

Heaton, R. K., Grant, I., Butters, N., White, D. A., Kirson, D., Atkinson, J. H., McCutchan, J. A., Taylor, M. J., Kelly, M. D., Ellis, R. J., Wolfson, T., Velin, R., Marcotte, T. D., Hesselink, J. R., Jernigan, T. L., Chandler, J., Wallace, M., Abramson, I., and the HNRC group (1995). The HNRC 500 — Neuropsychology of HIV infection at different disease stages. *J. Int. Neuropsychol. Soc.* **1**, 231–251.

Heaton, R. K., Marcotte, T. D., White, D. A., Ross, D., Meredith, K., Taylor, M. J., Kaplan, R., and Grant, I. (1996). Nature and vocational significance of neuropsychological impairment associated with HIV infection [Published erratum appears in *Clin. Neuropsychol.* **10**, 236, 1996]. *Clin. Neuropsychol.* **10**, 1–14.

Lipton, S. T., and Gendelman, H. E. (1995). Dementia associated with the acquired immunodeficiency syndrome. *N. Engl. J. Med.* **332**, 934–940.

Marcotte, T. D., Heaton, R. K., Wolfson, T., Taylor, M. J., Alhassoon, O., Arfaa, K., Grant, I., and the HNRC group (1999). The impact of HIV-related neuropsychological dysfunction on driving behavior. *J. Int. Neuropsychol. Soc.* **5**, 579–592.

Masliah, E., Ge, N., Achim, C. L., DeTeresa, R., and Wiley, C. A. (1996). Patterns of neurodegeneration in HIV encephalitis. *NeuroAIDS* **1**, 161–173.

Masliah, E., Ge, N., and Mucke, L. (1996). Pathogenesis of HIV-1 associated neurodegeneration. *Crit. Rev. Neurobiol.* **10**, 57–67.

Masliah, E., Heaton, R. K., Marcotte, T. D., Ellis, R. J., Wiley, C. A., Mallory, M., Achim, C. L., McCutchan, J. A., Nelson, J. A., Atkinson, J. H., Grant, I., and the HNRC group (1997). Dendritic injury is a pathological substrate for human immunodeficiency virus-related cognitive disorders. *Ann. Neurol.* **42**, 963–972.

Mayeux, R., Stern, Y., Tang, M.-X., Todak, G., Marder, K., Sano, J., Richard, M., Stein, Z., Ehrhardt, A., and Gorman, J. (1993). Mortality risks in gay men with human immunodeficiency virus infection and cognitive impairment. *Neurology* **43**, 176–182.

McArthur, J. C., and Grant, I. (1998). HIV neurocognitive disorders. In *Neurology of AIDS* (H. E. Gendelman, S. Lipton, L. Epstein, and S. Swindells, Eds.), pp. 499–523. New York, Chapman & Hall, New York.

Sanders, V., Everall, I., Johnson, R., and Masliah, E. (2000). Fibroblast growth factor modulates HIV co-receptor CXCR4 expression by neural cells. *J. Neurosci. Res.* **59**, 671–679.

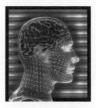

Homeostatic Mechanisms

PIERRE-MARIE LLEDO

Pasteur Institute

GLOSSARY

cybernetics A term introduced by the mathematician N. Wiener (1894–1964) from the Greek *kubernetes* ("steersman"). This term, which defines a theory of feedback systems (namely, self-regulating systems), could be applicable not only to living systems but also to machines.

emotion From the earliest philosophical speculations onwards, emotion has often been seen as interfering with rationality, as a remainder of our presapiens inheritance: Emotions seem to represent unbridled human nature "in the raw." Emotions are the product of an individual's own processing of occurrences on the basis of his or her own prior history and biology, and emotional response activates neural and neuroendocrine effector systems and leads to a variety of short- and long-term consequences that may or may not result in disease.

homeostasis The physiologist C. Bernard (1813–1878) introduced the concept of the constancy of the *milieu intérieur*. This internal milieu ensures the biological unity of the organism and confers a certain autonomy relative to the external milieu. The term homeostasis was coined some years later by W. B. Cannon (1871–1945). He developed the concept of homeostasis, which in modern terminology is the feedback control of servo-systems. This concept was not mathematically expressed until the 1940s, when it became the basis of cybernetics. Today, the term homeostasis refers to the adaptative response of an organism and tends to be substituted by a newer term, allostasis, which means "stability through anticipatory change"; the long-term consequences of continued demand on the physiologic response are referred to as allostatic load.

hypothalamus A brain area that encompasses the most ventral part of the diencephalon where it forms the floor and, in part, the walls of the third ventricle. The hypothalamus consists of several nuclei that form a neuronal continuum. It plays a central role in homeostasis by controling the autonomic nervous system, the neuroendocrine system through its control of both the anterior and posterior parts of the pituitary gland, and the motivational states.

limbic system In 1878, P. Broca was the first to describe an annular ring of tissue on the medial face of the cerebral hemisphere that represents the free edge of the cerebral cortex. He named this part of the brain *le grand lobe limbique* ("the great limbic lobe"), which led to the concept of the limbic system. This system includes the hippocampal formation, entorhinal area, olfactory regions, hypothalamus, and amygdala. Functionally, the limbic system is generally thought to be concerned with visceral processes, particularly those associated with the emotional status of the organism. In fact, the interaction of all the structures in the complex, from the entorhinal area to the hypothalamus, plays a major role in the elaboration of the final actions of an organism in a particular environment and in the formation of adaptive behavior patterns.

How does the body adapt to environmental conditions? How does it organize its reactions to the world and other people? What are desire, pleasure, and pain? Going beyond the traditional dichotomies of body and soul, or reasonable brain and passionate body, we shall deal with what is called the constancy of the internal milieu for a human being brought by homeostatic mechanisms. Are we reductionist when we decide to approach the molecular mechanisms of our emotions? It must be recognized that while we announce that being is not just the sum total of the parts of the machine, this very machine shows itself to be increasingly complex as it gradually yields the secrets of its inner workings. It is indeed astonishing that we can analyze networks of billions of interconnected elements of an extraordinary complexity and at the same time develop a single molecule capable of causing or correcting the most inextricable disorders of the mind. Therefore, the scientist is not the only one accused of reductionism: Nature provides an example of radical simplification.

Even a unicellular being has a certain degree of freedom between the information receptors on the cell surface and the effectors on the inside. The evolution of a species consists of a gradual increase in the number of intermediaries between information from the outside world and effectors responsible for actions. An animal's freedom increases in proportion to the number of these intermediaries. However, it is only because the liquid element and the substances it transports bring a solution of continuity to cell organization that this freedom is possible.

We shall therefore deal with the constancy of the internal milieu. The external milieu was a Greek invention, but the concept of internal milieu was introduced by C. Bernard (1813–1878). For Greek doctors and their disciples, man lived in harmony with nature. Temperament fixed the conditions of this harmony. However, the living being had no real identity or biological unity: The humors were nothing but a kind of reproduction, inside the animal, of the surrounding natural elements; there was no substantial difference between nutrients and living matter. The internal milieu ensures the biological unity of the animal and confers a certain autonomy relative to the external milieu. It is supposed to reconstitute around the cells the characteristics of the original marine environment.

In homeostasis, any departure from the norm draws mechanisms into play that tend to bring the trouble spot back to its initial state. Passions could thus be interpreted as a kind of neurosis of the normal, itself a fictitious immobile system of reference. In fact, behind the impassivity of the internal milieu a confused mesh of false constants is hidden, all of which are more or less dependent and variable from one species to the next, from one individual to the next, and, within each individual, from one situation to the next.

We can see the kind of safeguard that the constant agitation of the humors of the internal milieu offers the nervous system and its operational flexibility: Perhaps the brain runs the risk of falling victim (losing its soul?) to such a commotion. For its own protection, it can organize its own disorder: The brain–gland reveals itself as grand master of the humors by its multiple secretions of neurohormones. Like the brain–machine, the humoral brain simultaneously acts as the passionate victim and the orchestrator of its own passion.

I. THE INTERNAL MILIEU

Homeostasis is a widely and somewhat loosely used term for describing all kinds of responses following the principle of negative feedback control. The main concept of homeostasis is founded in the production of stability in dynamic systems by negative feedback. This concept is the basis of cybernetics, whose founding fathers were N. R. Ashby and G. Walter in the 1950s. However, the term homeostasis was coined years before cybernetics by the founders of modern physiology—C. Bernard, W. B. Cannon, and W. R. Hess. In Cannon's germinal book, *Wisdom of the Body*, the basic idea of feedback as a fundamental physiological principle is stated. In this context, constancy in the internal environment of the body is the result of a system of control mechanisms that limit the variability of body states. The internal milieu takes the form of a certain number of volumes called regulated variables. Without regulation, the changes in the external milieu and the functioning of the cells would make these volumes vary, when the very survival of the organism depends on their stability. Hence, stability is obtained as a result of a regulating system comprising several subsystems, each of which is subjected to control mechanisms and responsible for controlled variables. A regulated variable thus remains fixed within strict limits because of the intervention of controlled variables that have a much wider scope for variation. It is clear that this is an extremely important principle for almost all physiological processes as well as for the guiding of skilled behavior. Indeed, such a concept serves as a theoretical basis for the physiology of regulation. However, homeostasis, in the sense of constancy, does not adequately describe normal physiology, in which blood pressure, heart rate, endocrine output, and neural activity are continually changing—from sleeping to waking—in response to external factors and in anticipation of future events. At all times in the daily cycle, these parameters are maintained within an operating range in response to environmental challenges. The operating range, and the ability of the body to increase or decrease vital functions to a new level within that range upon challenge, particularly in anticipation of a challenge, has been defined as *allostasis* (or "stability through change"). The operating range for most physiological systems is larger in health than in disease, and it is larger in younger compared to older individuals. Exceeding this range can lead to disaster, as is the case when exertion leads to a myocardial infarction.

It is worth mentioning that the cell theory is inseparable from the concept of the internal milieu. The organism is composed of a host of cells that are scattered or grouped together in tissues. Each cell, individualized by its plasmatic membrane, plays out its fate under the genetic control of the nucleus. These cells are bathed with water-like fluid that forms the extracellular space, providing a medium for diffusion and homogenization around the cells. Bernard, comparing the weight of a mummy with that of a living human being of the same size, estimated the water content of the latter to be 90%—to be more precise, two-thirds water for one-third dry matter. This extracellular space, including the blood and lymph, is indeed a unifier of the organism. Unlike the external environment, which is subjected to uncontrollable change, the internal milieu oscillates slightly around normal values. Thus, the autonomy acquired by the organism relative to its external environment gives it an independent and free life since the constancy of the internal milieu does not mean fixity but rather a possibility to evolve.

The regulated variables define the constancy of the internal milieu. The most important are the gas content of the blood, acidity or pH, temperature, sugar content, blood pressure, and osmotic pressure. For example, we know that the more salty a solution, the higher its osmotic pressure. If for any reason an animals loses water, the salt concentration in the internal milieu (i.e., the osmotic pressure) increases. Because it is a regulated variable, osmotic pressure will be kept constant by regulating mechanisms: diminishing the outflow of water and/or increasing the intake. The outflow is reduced by slowing down the elimination process through the kidneys. Vasopressin, an antidiuretic hormone secreted by the brain, performs this function. The amount of this antidiuretic hormone circulating in the blood is a controlled variable that increases in responses to any increase in osmotic pressure. This is an example of hormonal regulation. The best way to increase intake is to drink. Beyond a certain level, the increase in osmotic pressure causes thirst and an urgent need to drink. Therefore, the regulating mechanisms can be of two kind: hormonal or behavioral. Despite the dry heat of the desert, a camel does not suffer from a much higher osmotic pressure than that of a bartender; it merely possesses more powerful regulating mechanisms that are adapted to the external milieu and that give the controlled variables, diuresis and water intake, a wider scope for action.

Nevertheless, there is a hierarchy to be respected. The most important constants must be maintained at all costs, even if this means sacrificing one of the lower orders. In case of need, a regulated variable can become a controlled variable. For example, blood pressure is constant, but if the oxygen content of the blood is endangered, because it is a hierarchical superior it will rise in order to provide a higher flow of gas and will thus temporarily become a controlled variable instead of remaining a regulated variable.

The internal milieu defined by Bernard—the blood and the fluids in which the cells are bathed—is thus the unifier of the organism. The cell draws from the extracellular fluid the nutrients its need, the fuel and oxygen that provide its energy, and the chemical factors that keep it in working order. It discharges into this milieu its waste and the produce of its activity. Here, we have Bernard's second idea, internal secretion, which is inseparable from the concept of the internal milieu. He discovered internal secretion while describing the glycogenic function of the liver. The hepatic cell draws from its reserves of glycogen the sugar that the organism needs and reintroduces it into the bloodstream. Internal secretion, which differs from excretion, demands a fluid medium that can receive the cell's outpourings. The term endocrinology, introduced by N. Pende (1909) to refer to the study of internal secretions, is now used only for the secretions of the so-called vascular glands, which are now called the endocrine glands. The function of these glands, which is much narrower than that of internal secretion, refers to a cellular secretion with no strictly metabolic function but that has a communicative role.

Although virtually all of the brain is involved in homeostasis, neurons controlling the internal environment are mainly concentrated in the hypothalamus, a neuronal structure located at the interface of the brain and peripheral functions. Here, I first focus on the anatomy of the limbic system and then on the anatomy of the hypothalamus, a small area that belongs to the diencephalon and that comprises less than 1% of the total brain volume. I then consider how the hypothalamus and other closely linked structures in the limbic system receive information from the internal environment and how they act directly to keep it constant by regulating endocrine secretion and the autonomic nervous system. Finally, other parts of the brain that may indirectly affect the internal environment by acting on the external environment through emotions and drives are described.

II. ANATOMY OF THE LIMBIC SYSTEM AND THE HYPOTHALAMUS

In 1953, J. Olds and P. Milner reported that the weak electrical stimulation of specific sites, most located in the hypothalamus or in its rostral continuation, the septum, could elicit in experimental animals an internal state of pleasure or in any case what psychologists describe as a state of reward. For the first time, this work provided a basis to the claim that the hypothalamus, and more generally a continuum of brain tissue in which the hypothalamus is central, is implicated not only in endocrine and visceral functions but also in affect and motivation. I first consider the structures and connections of the brain tissue related to the hypothalamus that belong to this neuronal continuum before examining the anatomy and numerous functions of the hypothalamus.

A. The Limbic System and Its Connections with the Hypothalamus

The neural continuum in which the hypothalamus is central is composed of a part of the brain stem and the limbic system. Part of the brain stem, the mesencephalic reticular formation, which receives inputs from spinoreticular fibers, possesses axons that ascend to the hypothalamus. There are also connections formed by axons directed upward to the hypothalamus from the nucleus of the solitary tract, a cell group in the medulla oblongata. These connections are quite revealing. The nucleus of the solitary tract is the only known case of a circumscribed secondary sensory cell group whose primary sensory input is from the visceral domain.

A second part of the continuum in which the hypothalamus is central lies rostral to it. It is largely interconnected with the phylogenetically primitive cortical tissue that surrounds the upper brain stem. A little more than a century ago, P. Broca observed an almost annular ring of tissue on the medial face of the cerebral hemisphere that represents the free edge of the cerebral cortex. This part of the brain, called *le grand lobe limbique* (the great limbic lobe) by Broca, has led to the concept of the limbic system. This "lobe" surrounds the diencephalon and the cerebral peduncles. He called it *limbique* from the Latin *limbus* because he conceived it as a threshold to the newer pallium. It is sometimes called the rhinencephalon to indicate that these regions of the brain derived during the course of evolution from structures previously associated with the sense of smell. However, the fact that the rhinencephalon is highly developed in animals such as the dolphin and man, in whom the sense of smell is nonexistent or limited, shows that it participates in other activities.

We shall retain only its key-ring structure opening upwards toward the neocortex and downwards toward the brain stem. Like the limbo of Christian mythology, the limbic system is the intermediary between the neomammalian brain heaven (represented by the neocortex) and the reptilian brain hell (including the reticular formation and the striate cortex). The limbic lobe includes the parahippocampal, the cingulate, and the subcallosal gyri. It also includes the underlying cortex of the hippocampal formation, which is composed of the hippocampus, the dentate gyrus, and the subiculum.

In the 1930s, it became evident to J. W. Papez that the limbic lobe formed a neural circuit that provides the anatomical substratum for emotions. He proposed that the hypothalamus is connected with higher cortical centers since it plays a crucial role in the expression of emotion. According to this idea, the neuronal circuit originally proposed by Papez consists of the cortex, which influences the hypothalamus through connections of the cingulate gyrus to the hippocampal formation. Information is then processed by the hippocampal formation and projected to the mammillary bodies of the hypothalamus by way of the fornix. The hypothalamus in turn provides information to the cingulate gyrus through a pathway from the mammillary bodies to the anterior thalamic nuclei and from the anterior thalamic nuclei to the cingulate gyrus (Fig. 1). P. MacLean's resynthesis of Papez's theory of emotions resurrected Broca's concepts and breathed new life into the concept of the all-pervasive limbic system. He included in the limbic system other structures anatomically and functionally related to those described by Papez, including parts of the hypothalamus, the septal area, the nucleus accumbens, neocortical areas such as the orbitofrontal cortex, and the amygdala (Fig. 1).

It is also noteworthy that all of the senses represented in the neocortex—vision, hearing, and the somatic sense—direct part of their information toward either one or both of two cortical districts: the frontal association cortex and the inferior temporal association cortex. The two are interconnected by a massive fiber bundle called the uncinate fasciculus. In turn, the inferior temporal cortex projects to the entorhinal area. The entorhinal area could be

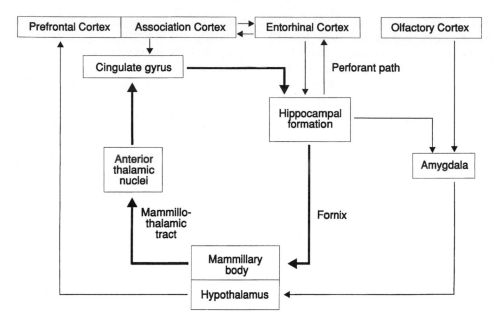

Figure 1 The neural pathways for emotion. The first circuit proposed by Papez is indicated by thick lines, whereas thin lines illustrate recently described connections.

considered as a cortical gateway for projections to the amygdala. In fact, in primates it gives the amygdala its single most important input. The projection is reciprocated; indeed, the amygdala directs its cortical projections to the inferior temporal cortex and to the frontal cortex (specifically the orbital surface of the frontal cortex). Therefore, the amygdala projects to the parts of the neocortex in which the final stages of the cascade of sensory information occur. Evidently, the amygdala also screens its neocortical input. Therefore, it has been tempting for many scientists to speculate that such a brain region could intervene in ideation and cognition. Ordinarily, one thinks of brain function as working inwards, i.e., sensory information being directed from sensory receptor organs over a sequence of synapses to the sensory cortex and from there (in what Papez called "the stream of thought") toward the limbic system. Here, we encounter the opposite: a set of connections directed outward. It is indeed as if the amygdala were participating in the brain's appreciation of the world.

The interoceptive and exteroceptive data reaching the neural continuum in which the hypothalamus is central are clearly distinguishable. The former consist of visceral sensory signals from the spinal cord and the brain stem. These data are unconditional stimuli pertinent to the maintenance of life. On the other hand, what enters the limbic system from the neocortex is fundamentally different. One might call it a repeatedly preprocessed, multisensory representation of the organism's environment. In this situation, the perception of the world is only biased by physiological needs.

It is also remarkable that among all the senses, olfaction possesses a particular link with the limbic system that was taken to be the "nose–brain". Today, it is clearly established that the primary olfactory cortex projects to the entorhinal area, which in turn contact the hippocampus. Thus, after years of fervent affirmation followed by years of fervent denial, the idea that the hippocampus receives olfactory signals was reintroduced. Indeed, the pathway that links olfaction with the limbic system is privileged. Hence, the path from the olfactory epithelium is more direct than the path from sensory surfaces such as the skin. Moreover, the primary olfactory cortex projects to the amygdala, in large part onto a particular cell group (the lateral nucleus of the amygdala), by bypassing the neocortex (Fig. 1). However, although it is clear that the main olfactory bulb (the first central relay for olfaction) projects to the amygdala in rodents, one wonders whether this connection is still present in humans. Indeed, the existence of a specialized area of the nasal mucosa called the vomeronasal organ, which sends information to a compartment of the accessory olfactory bulb, has been demonstrated in animals such as rats. The vomeronasal organ and the corresponding region of the accessory olfactory bulb are thought to form an apparatus dedicated to the processing of sexually significant odors, but in the fully formed human body none of these structures have been identified. Finally, to emphasize the privileged link between olfaction and the limbic system, it has to be mentioned that the primary olfactory cortex also projects to the hypothalamus.

B. Structure of the Hypothalamus

The hypothalamus in the mammalian brain encompasses the most ventral part of the diencephalon, where it forms the floor and, in parts, the walls of the third ventricle. Its upper boundary is marked by a sulcus in the ventricular wall, the ventral diencephalic or hypothalamic sulcus, which separates the hypothalamus from the dorsally located thalamus (Fig. 2). Caudally, the hypothalamus merges without any clear limits with the periventricular gray and the tegmentum of the mesencephalon. However, it is customary to define the caudal boundary of the hypothalamus as represented by a plane extending from the caudal limit of the mammilary nuclei ventrally and from the posterior commissure dorsally. Rostrally, the hypothalamus is continuous with the preoptic area, which lies partly forward to and above the optic chiasm.

By means of the previously mentioned external landmarks at the ventral surface of the brain, the hypothalamus can be subdivided in the anterior–posterior direction into an anterior part that includes the preoptic area, a middle part, and a posterior part. Another subdivision in the lateral–medial direction consists of three longitudinal zones recognized as the periventricular, the medial, and the lateral zones. The

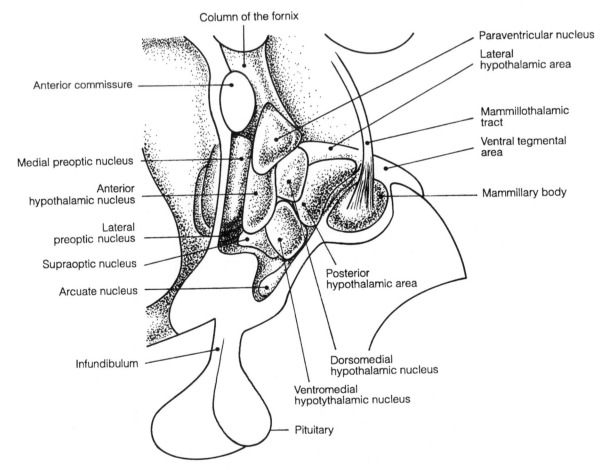

Figure 2 The location of the main hypothalamic nuclei shown in a medial view. The hypothalamus contains a large number of neuronal circuits that regulate vital functions, such as body temperature, heart rate, blood pressure, blood osmolarity, water and food intake, emotional behavior, and reproduction.

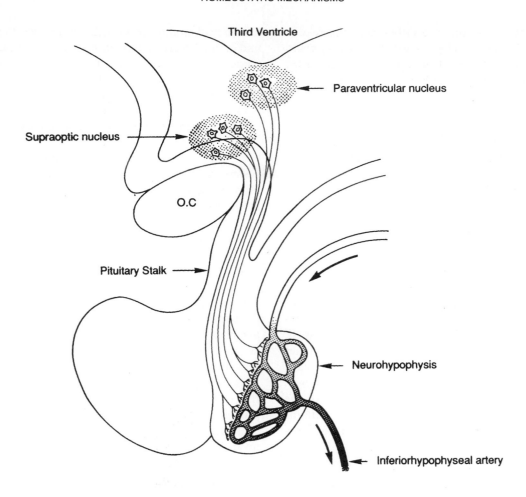

Figure 3   The posterior lobe of the pituitary gland. In the posterior lobe, axons from hypothalamic cell groups called supraoptic and paraventricular nucleus release vasopressin and oxytocin into the systemic circulation (inferior hypophyseal artery). OC, optic chiasm.

periventricular zone consists mostly of small cells that, in general, are oriented along fibers parallel with the wall of the third ventricle. The medial zone is cell rich, containing most of the well-delineated nuclei of the hypothalamus that include the preoptic and suprachiasmatic nuclei in the anterior region; the dorsomedial, ventromedial, and paraventricular nuclei in the middle region; and the posterior nucleus and mammillary bodies in the posterior region (Fig. 2). The lateral zone contains only a small number of cells interposed between the longitudinal fiber system of the medial forebrain bundle. This region possesses long fibers that project to the spinal cord and cortex as well as extensive short-fiber, multisynaptic ascending and descending pathways. The basal portion of the medial region and the periventricular region contain many of the small hypothalamic neurons that secrete the substances that control the release of anterior pituitary

hormones. Most fiber systems of the hypothalamus are bidirectional. Projections to and from areas caudal to the hypothalamus are carried in the medial forebrain bundle, the mammillo-tegmental tract, and the dorsal longitudinal fasciculus. Rostral structures are interconnected with the hypothalamus by means of the mammillo-thalamic tracts, fornix, and stria terminalis. However, there are two important exceptions to the rule that fibers are bidirectional in the hypothalamus. First, the hypothalamo-hypophyseal tract contains only descending axons of paraventricular and supraoptic neurons, which terminate primarily in the posterior pituitary (Fig. 3). Second, the hypothalamus receives one-way afferent connections directly from the retina. These fibers terminate in the suprachiasmatic nucleus, which is involved in generating light–dark cycles. The role of these rhythms in the control of motivated behaviors is discussed later.

The following section describes the interrelated functions of the hypothalamus and the pituitary gland as well as some of the major functions of the limbic system.

III. PARTICIPATION OF THE HYPOTHALAMUS AND THE LIMBIC SYSTEM IN HOMEOSTASIS

The internal environment of the body, a term embracing tissue fluids and organ functions such as blood pressure, heart rate, and respiration rate, is under the control of three independent processes. The autonomic nervous system plays an important role in homeostasis. Hence, in the brain, neurons that affect the activity of the preganglionic motor neurons of the sympathetic and the parasympathetic nervous systems are concentrated in the hypothalamus. The evidence is clear: When the hypothalamus of almost any animal, including man, is suddenly destroyed, the animal dies as a consequence of severe disruption of what Bernard called the internal milieu of the body. However, controling the autonomic nervous system is not the only means by which the hypothalamus maintains homeostasis. In addition, the hypothalamus governs the neuroendocrine system through its control of both the anterior and posterior parts of the pituitary gland, which in turn play a major role in the constancy of the internal milieu. Finally, the internal environment of the body is also regulated by motivational states; therefore, we shall also consider some of the hypothalamic funtions involved in a repertoire of voluntary behavioral responses.

In analyzing the nerve mechanisms involved in homeostasis, two centers, one an inhibitor and the other an excitator, are always involved in controlling the same function. This dualistic conception is in the traditon of C. Bernard and W. Sherrington. The former taught us that the centers come into play each time the internal milieu records an abnormal value, and the latter noted that these centers are linked by the principle of reciprocal innervation. The nervous control of eating behavior illustrates this mechanism perfectly when the hunger center is inhibited by the satiety center. An entire theory of paired centers could be built on the hypothalamus. Besides the centers of hunger and satiety, these are centers of pleasure and aversion, approach and retreat, a parasympathetic region opposed to the orthosympathetic region. This anatomical and functional Manicheism goes beyond the hypothalamus to other structures, especially the

limbic system and the amygdala, in which facilitating and inhibiting areas confront each other for each of the passions.

A. The Autonomic Nervous System

The autonomic nervous system is primarily an effector system that innervates smooth musculature, heart muscle, and exocrine glands. It is a visceral and largely involuntary motor system. Anatomical principles underlying the organization of both somatic motor and autonomic nervous systems are similar (Fig. 4) and the two systems function in parallel to adjust the body to environmental changes. Nevertheless, the two systems differ in several ways. Within the autonomic nervous system, two subsystems, the sympathetic and the parasympathetic, have long been distinguished by means of anatomical, chemical, and functional criteria. The sympathetic is the most extensive of the two systems. Its preganglionic motor neurons are located in the spinal cord, where they occupy a region called the lateral horn of the spinal gray matter. The preganglionic fibers employ the neurotransmitter acetylcholine, whereas the postganglionic fibers often must travel a substantial distance and employ the neurotransmitter norepinephrine. The sympathetic division of the autonomic nervous system promotes the organism's ability to expend energy (Hess called it ergotropic) and governs an endocrine gland, the adrenal medulla, considered to be a modified autonomic ganglion. It is indeed a universal mobilizing mechanism, valuable in emergencies, with postganglionic ramifications throughout the visceral realm.

In contrast, Hess described the parasympathetic nervous system as trophotropic to signify that it promotes the restitution of the organism. The parasympathetic nervous system in fact antagonizes the sympathetic's effects. The preganglionic motor neurons of the parasympathetic nervous system are in the brain stem and in a short stretch of the spinal cord near its caudal tip. Like the preganglionic motor neurons of the sympathetic nervous system, they employ acetylcholine as their transmitter, but the postganglionic transmitter of the parasympathetic is also acetylcholine. Their axons are long because the ganglia to which they project lie near the tissues of the viscera and sometimes even inside them (Fig. 4). The resilence of autonomic control is in good accordance with what is known about the conduction lines descending from the hypothalamus. Indeed, the hypothalamus emits axons

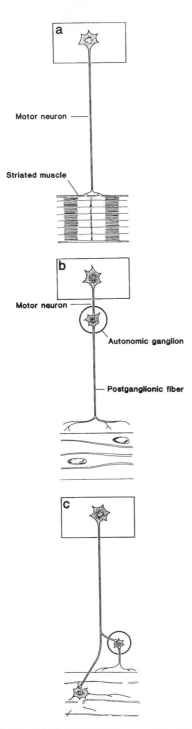

that descend toward both sympathetic and parasympathetic preganglionic visceral motor neurons, thus regulating the viscera. Hence, the hypothalamus may function as the so-called head ganglion of the autonomic nervous system that mediates conventional reflexes involving neural inputs and outputs. Fibers passing directly from the hypothalamus to the lateral horn of the spinal cord's gray matter, where the preganglionic motor neurons of the sympathetic nervous system are situated, have recently been found. However, these fibers seem to constitute a small minority of hypothalamic efferents; the hypothalamus has nothing similar to a pyramidal tract to carry its descending outputs. Instead, it appears in large measure to project no further than the midbrain, where neurons of the reticular formation take over. It is noteworthy that pathways descending to autonomic motor neurons are interrupted at numerous levels, at which further instructions can enter the descending lines.

Most of the regions of the brain that influence the autonomic nervous system's output (e.g., the cerebral cortex, the hippocampus, the entorhinal cortex, parts of the thalamus, basal ganglia, cerebellum, and the reticular formation) produce their actions by way of the hypothalamus, which integrates the information it receives from these structures into a coherent pattern of autonomic responses. The hypothalamus controls the output of the autonomic nervous system in two ways. The first one is direct and consists of projections to nuclei in the brain stem and the spinal cord that act on preganglionic autonomic neurons to control respiration, heart rate, temperature and blood pressure. Thus, stimulation of the lateral hypothalamus leads to general sympathetic activation (increase in blood presure, piloerection, etc.). Second, the hypothalamus that governs the autonomic nervous system by controlling the endocrine system, which releases hormones that influence autonomic functions is discussed in the following section.

B. The Neuroendocrine System

The Scharrers (1940) first hypothesized that the peptides of the neurohypophysis were in fact synthetized by specialized hypothalamic neurons and transported within their axons to the neural lobe to be released into peripheral blood. In the late 1940s, Harris and collaborators proposed the hypophysial portal chemotransmitter hypothesis of anterior pituitary

Figure 4 Three different motor innervations. (a) In the somatic motor pattern, a motor neuron from the spinal cord or in the brain stem animates striated muscles directly. In the visceral motor pattern, a two-neuron chain is required. (b) The sympathetic nervous system stations a "preganglionic" visceral motor neuron in the spinal cord. (c) The parasympathetic nervous system employs a two-neuron pathway. The first neuron is situated in the brain stem or toward the bottom of the spinal cord, and the ganglion is close or even inside the viscera.

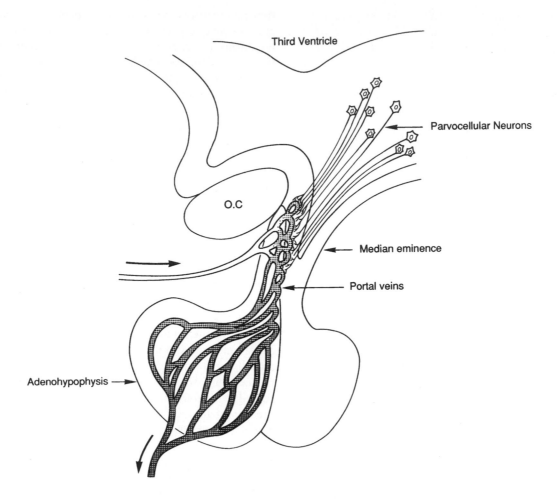

Figure 5   The anterior lobe of the pituitary gland. The anterior lobe synthetizes several hormones. Their release is induced by chemical signals, called releasing factors, that are secreted by hypothalamic neurons. These factors enter the hypothalamo-pituitary portal system, comprising first a capillary bed in the hypothalamus and then a venous drainage channel and, in the anterior lobe, a second capillary bed. OC, optic chiasm.

control, which stated that the factors regulating the anterior lobe are formed by hypothalamic neurons (later termed hypophysiotropic neurons) and transported to be released into the hypophysial portal circulation and carried to the anterior pituitary (Fig. 5), where they control the synthesis and release of anterior pituitary hormones into the general circulation. Both of these hypotheses have been confirmed and rationalized into a unified theory of neurosecretion in which the nervous system controls endocrine function. Neurosecretion is the phenomenon of synthesis and release of specific substances by neurons. Some neurosecretions are exported into the peripheral or hypophysial blood and act as true hormones; others, released in close apposition to other neurons, act as neurotransmitters or neuromodulators. Trans-

lation of neuronal signals into chemical ones has been termed neuroendocrine transduction and the cells have been called neuroendocrine transductors by R. J. Wurtman and F. Anton-Tay (1969). Two types of neurotransducer cells regulate visceral function: (i) neurosecretomotor cells, in which the neurosecretion acts directly through synapses on gland cells, and (ii) neuroendocrine cells, in which the neurosecretion passes into the blood and acts on distant targets.

Neurosecretory cells possess in common with other neurons the usual aspects of neuron functions. Most of the insight into the physiology of neurosecretory systems has been gained from studies of the hypothalamo-hypophyseal system. This system brings nervous and endocrine cells together in one anatomical entity in which the nervous system and the glandular cells of the anterior hypophysis communicate. These two structures share common properties. They both secrete peptidergic hormones (releasing and inhibiting hypothalamic factors and the hypophyseal stimulins), and both exhibit electrical properties such as excitability, with production of action potentials. Thus, electrophysiological techniques, which were previously reserved for studies of nerve and muscle cells, can be applied to the hypothalamo-hypophyseal system in both its nervous and endocrine structures. The electrophysiological properties of these cells reveal the existence of (i) stimulus-secretion coupling, particularly at the level of neurosecretory terminals in the posterior hypophysis, the median eminance, and the endocrine cells of the anterior hypophysis, and (ii) modifications in membrane electrical properties exerted by the binding of different regulatory factors to their receptors. These observations are used to explain the modulatory mechanism of membrane properties brought into play by each factor in order to enhance or inhibit hormonal release. Thus, the electrical properties play a central role in the regulation of endocrine secretion in the anterior hypophysis. These electrical properties, common to nervous and endocrine cells, are linked to changes in membrane permeability to different ions (i.e., Ca^{2+}, Na^+, K^+, and Cl^-).

The pituitary gland is divided into two main functional units—the neural (or posterior) lobe and the adenohypophysis (or anterior) lobe (Figs. 3 and 5). In many mammalian species an intermediate lobe (derived embryologically from the same tissue as the anterior lobe) is present, but in humans these lobe cells are dispersed throughout the entire pituitary gland.

In the neurohypophyseal system, hypothalamic neurons transmit action potentials along their axons in a similar manner to that used by unmyelinated neurons, and each action potential triggers the release of secretory granules from nerve endings by calcium-dependent exocytosis into the general circulation. The neural lobe is an anatomical part of the neurohypophysis that is commonly viewed as consisting of three portions—the neural lobe (infundibular process or posterior pituitary), the stalk, and the infundibulum. This latter portion forms the base of the third ventricle (Figs. 3 and 5). In fact, there is a fourth intrahypothalamic component of the neurohypophysial system that consists of the cells of origin of the two principal nerve tracts that terminate in the neural lobe—supraopticohypophysial and paraventriculohypophysial.

The neurohypophysial hormones secreted by the magnocellular neurons are vasopressin (antidiuretic hormone) and oxytocin, which are synthesized within the cell bodies in association with specific proteins, the neurophysins. Like most peptidergic hormones, vasopressin and oxytocin are cleaved from a larger prohormone. These prohormones are synthesized in the cell bodies of the magnocellular neurons and are cleaved within vesicles during their transport down the axons. Vasopressin, oxytocin, and at least two forms of neurophysins are secreted into the blood circulation; they are responsive to appropriate physiological stimuli and can be altered by stressful conditions.

Although the anterior lobe does not receive any direct nerve supply, its secretions are under control exerted by the hypothalamus. This control is mediated by chemical factors (hypophysiotropic hormones) secreted by the parvocellular neuroendocrine neurons located in several hypothalamic regions: the medial basal and periventricular regions and the arcuate, tuberal, preoptic, and paraventricular nuclei. Parvocellular neurons secrete peptides in the interstitial space of the base of the third ventricle and then diffuse into the capillary plexus of the median eminence that is interposed between the peripheral arterial system and the pituitary sinusoidal circulation (Fig. 3). By this anatomical arrangement, neurohormonal mediators synthesized and released by the hypothalamus are brought into direct contact with the adenohypophysis. The hormones released by the anterior lobe of the pituitary gland are called tropic (literally "switch-on") hormones. Each is the second and final messenger in a sequence of chemical signals leading from the brain to a particular endocrine gland. All the tropic hormones of the anterior lobe are simultaneously trophic hormones, in whose absence their target glands atrophy.

A different functional link leads from the neurons of the hypothalamus to the posterior lobe of the pituitary complex. This link is more direct since it does not include part of the circulatory system. It begins in two circumscribed magnocellular nucleus. They are the first hypothalamic nuclei whose function has been identified with some precision. All, or nearly all, of the axons originating in the supraoptic nucleus, along with approximately 30% of the axons originating in the paraventricular nucleus, pass through the pituitary stalk and reach the posterior lobe of the pituitary. The remaining 70% have several destinations, of which one is especially notable: The paraventricular nucleus is a substantial contributor to the pathway descending from the hypothalamus direct to the lateral horn of the spinal cord, which contains the spinal cord's preganglionic sympathetic motor neurons.

Unlike the anterior one, the posterior lobe is a part of the brain. Nevertheless, it contains no neurons; the terminations of the supraoptic and paraventricular axons make no synaptic contacts. Instead, they lie embedded in a tissue composed of modifed glial cells called the pituicytes and a dense plexus of capillaries. The glandular products of the supraoptic and paraventricular nuclei are synthesized in the cell body and packaged in neurosecretory vesicles in which some hormonal maturation may occur. These neurosecretory vesicles are transported down the axon to the neural terminal, where hormones are stored and released by secretion when the neuron is stimulated.

Recently, it has been demonstrated that a type of ependymal glial cell called tanycyte, which ensheaths the terminals of hypothalamic neurons, regulates the release of luteinizing hormone-releasing hormone (LHRH) from the hypothalamus and may therefore play a key role in the onset of puberty. LHRH axons that travel with the processes of tanycytes can be covered by slips of glioplasm. At the perivascular space level, the nerve terminals may be partially covered or exposed, potentially impeding or enhancing the secretion of LHRH into capillaries. Such observation, realized at a cellular level, illustrates the tremendous plasticity of the hypothalamus. Interestingly, it was found that these glial cells in the median eminence possess estrogen and epidermal growth factor receptors, whereas LHRH neurons apparently do not. Taken together, these observations provide strong evidence that, at puberty, glia is a crucial target for estrogenic action that may induce morphological changes accompanied by release of chemical signals that modulate hypothalamic neurons.

somatic responses. In line with this view, vasopressin, oxytocin, and other regulating hormones are not the only peptides of neurobiological interest that can be found in the hypothalamus. The opioid peptides, β-endorphin, and the enkephalins can also be detected in this structure, as can angiotensin II, substance P, neurotensin, cholecystokinin, and a host of other peptides known to be involved in multiple behavioral responses. Interestingly, almost every type of peptidergic neuron previously studied, including both parvocellular and magnocellular hypothalamic neurons, has been found to contain more than one type of peptide that could act synergistically. Furthermore, peptides released by the hypothalamic magnocellular and parvocellular neurons are not unique to these cells; they have also been found in other regions of the nervous system. Such peptidergic projections are well suited for coordinating neuroendocrine and autonomic responses. For example, regulatory peptides released at brain sites other than the median eminence may modulate behavior by actions independent of the release of pituitary hormones. The behavioral effects of regulatory peptides are thematically related to the type of endocrine effects produced by the same peptide acting on the pituitary. Corticotropin-releasing hormone (CRH) is an example of such a regulatory peptide. On the one hand, it acts on the pituitary to stimulate the release of adrenocorticotropic hormone in response to stress. On the other hand, when injected intracerebroventricularly, CRH evokes many of the behavioral and autonomic reactions normally seen in response to stress.

C. Behavioral Responses

When Hess succeeded in implanting electrodes in the brain and permanently fixing them to the skull of animals, he found that stimulation of different parts of the hypothalamus produced a array of behavioral responses. For example, electrical stimulation of the lateral hypothalamus in cats elicited autonomic and somatic responses characteristic of anger: increased blood pressure, raising of body hair, pupillary constriction, raising of the tail, and other characteristic emotional behaviors. Thus, the hypothalamus is not only a motor nucleus for the autonomic nervous system, as well as a neural part controlling the neuroendocrine system, but also a coordinating center that integrates various inputs to ensure a well-organized, coherent, and appropriate set of autonomic and

D. Limbic Functions

In 1937, Papez suggested that the limbic lobe formed a neuronal circuit that provided the anatomical substratum for emotions. Based on experimental results suggesting that the hypothalamus plays a critical role in the expression of emotions, Papez argued that since emotions reach consciousness and thought and, conversely, higher cognitive functions affect emotions, the hypothalamus must communicate reciprocally with higher cortical centers.

The representation of the outside world and the internal milieu are superimposed in the limbic system. All the sensory information about the perceiver's environment is inscribed in the neuronal network of the limbic cortex, the hippocampus, and the amygdala. The vegetative, nervous, and humoral functions that contribute to homeostasis are represented simultaneously in the limbic system. Moreover, the hippocampus has been described as a gatekeeper embodying the brain's ability to commit things to lasting memory. Evidence for such a role of the hippocampus is clear. For instance, the neurosurgical removal of the hippocampus on both sides of the human brain, as a treatment of otherwise intractable forms of epilepsy, leads to a central disorder called hippocampal amnesia. The patient retains the memories he or she collected well before the surgery but cannot collect new ones.

Other evidence suggests that the amygdala is not only essential for olfactory discrimination but also commands a number of adaptive responses. Lesions and electrical stimulations of the amygdala produce a variety of effects on autonomic responses, emotional behavior, and feeding. Consequently, the amygdala has been implicated in the process of learning, particularly learning those tasks that require coordination of information from different sensory modalities or the association of a stimulus and an affective response.

Finally, it has been extensively described that the interplay between the neural activity of the hypothalamus and the neural activity of higher centers results in emotional experiences that we describe as fear, anger, pleasure, or satisfaction. For example, the behavior of patients from whom a part of the limbic system (frequently the prefrontal cortex) has been removed supports this idea. Indeed, these patients are no longer bothered by chronic pain or, alternatively, when they do perceive pain and exhibit appropriate autonomic reactions the perception is no longer associated with a powerful emotional experience.

In summary, neurons from the limbic system form complex circuits that collectively play an important role in numerous behavioral responses, such as learning, memory, and emotions. Such a role played by motivational states in homeostasis is discussed in the next section.

IV. ROLE OF MOTIVATIONAL STATES IN HOMEOSTASIS

The role of the hypothalamus and the limbic system in the neuroendocrine and autonomic regulation of homeostasis was previously described. Here, I discuss the control of homeostasis by motivational states, the internal conditions that arouse and direct elementary

behavior. Motivational states (also called drives) are inferred mechanisms to explain the intensity and direction of a variety of voluntary behaviors, such as temperature regulation, feeding, consumption of water, and sexual behaviors. It is the internal state that creates drives by deviations from the norm that defines the conditions of equilibrium for the milieu. A drive is not the stimulus that triggers the behavioral response but rather the internal force that underlies it. However, a stimulus may cause a drive when it has been associated in the past with a particular internal state. Because of the flexibility of internal parameters that define a pseudoequilibrium for the internal milieu of a living organism, it would be more appropriate to refer to the internal state as a fluctuating central state.

Specific motivational states possess two components: *needs* and *rewards* participating in homeostatic drives. Drives represent urges or impulses based bodily needs that lead animals into action. This concept is central to Freudian psychology, which is related to needs and experiences of satisfaction. Needs are experienced as an intolerable internal situation that must be stopped. This internal state, called motivation by psychologists, induces a drive to accomplish the act that will relieve it. For example, a temperature-regulating drive is said to control behaviors that directly affect body temperature, such as rubbing one's hands together. Therefore, physiological deprivation may lead to the satisfaction of a need and this, in turn, will lead to response reinforcement. This means that this action will become more likely in similar future situations. Such a psychological process is considered by some behaviorists to be the basis of learning.

So far, I have dealt with the role of tissue needs in generating appropriate behaviors and physiological responses to fight against a bodily deficit. However, another component linked with motivated behaviors is reward, which may lead to a profit. For example, sexual responses do not appear to be controlled by the lack of specific subtances in the body but are rather oriented toward hedonic factors. In this case, drives, by producing goal-oriented behaviors, are defined by the goal to be reached and justified by the reward obtained. One form of reward is pleasure; therefore, the duality of profit and pleasure is the major component of drive. On the other hand, drive–reward constitutes one of the rules of learning.

Finally, in describing the factors that regulate motivated behaviors, I must also be noted out the role of ecological constraints and anticipatory mechanisms. The characteristics of most behavioral responses are determined by evolutionary selection, which retains only appropriate responses in a defined ecological surounding. In this context, one of the most determinant parameters that participate in keeping a specific behavioral response is the cost-benefit ratio. The other component that also controls motivated behaviors, namely anticipator mechanisms, gives to the homeostasis concept its temporal dimension. Sometimes, lack rather than need is able to activate drives. In the case of sexual arousal, a feeling of lack becomes a simulation of need. Accordingly, homeostatic regulation is often anticipatory and can be initiated before any physiological deficit occurs. Such a role is played by clock-like mechanisms that turn physiological behavioral responses on and off before the occurrence of any tissue deficits. The master clock mechanism that drives and coordinates many rhythms is located in the suprachiasmatic nucleus of the hypothalamus. One such common cycle is a daily rhythm called the circadian rhythm, which controls feeding, drinking, locomotor activity, and several other responses. After experiencing jet-lag due to long distances, travelers can confirm the important role played by circadian rhythms.

V. CONCLUSIONS

Homeostatic processes can be analyzed in terms of control systems or servomechanisms, comprising a set point, an error signal, controlling elements, a controlled system, and feedback detectors. This approach has provided a convenient and precise language to describe both concepts and experimental results. Moreover, it has been successfully applied to temperature regulation, feeding, and drinking. For example, in the temperature regulation system, the integrator and many controlling elements appear to be located in the hypothalamus. The normal body temperature is the set point and the feedback detector collects information about body temperature from two main sources—peripheral and central temperatures. The analysis of feeding and thirst behaviors can also be approached in terms of a control system, as for temperature regulation, although at every level of analysis the understanding is less complete than for the control of temperature.

The hypothalamus is concerned with the regulation of various behaviors directed toward homeostatic goals, such as consumption of food and water or sexual gratifications. Through its control of emotions and motivated behavior, the hypothalamus acts indirectly in maintaining homeostasis by motivating animals and human beings to act on their environment.

In regulating emotional expression, the hypothalamus functions in conjunction with higher control systems in the limbic system and neocortex. In addition to regulating specific motivated behaviors, the hypothalamus and the cerebral cortex are involved in arousal, namely the maintenance of a general state of awareness (the level of arousal varies from different degrees of excitement to coma, sleep, and drowsiness). However, because of its intimate relationship with both the autonomic and the endocrine systems, the hypothalamus appears to play a central role in regulating homeostatic behaviors. The hypothalamus contributes to these adaptive behaviors by integrating information from both external and internal stimuli that report on the homeostatic state of the animal.

See Also the Following Articles

AROUSAL • ARTIFICIAL INTELLIGENCE • BEHAVIORAL NEUROIMMUNOLOGY • BIOFEEDBACK • CIRCADIAN RHYTHMS • EMOTION • HYPOTHALAMUS • LIMBIC SYSTEM • NEUROTRANSMITTERS • PSYCHONEURO-ENDOCRINOLOGY • STRESS: HORMONAL AND NEURAL ASPECTS

Suggested Reading

Cannon, W. B. (1929). *Bodily Changes in Pain, Hunger, Fear and Rage*. Appleton, New York.

Damasio, A. R.(1994). *Descartes' Error: Emotion, Reason, and the Human Brain*. Grosset/Putnam, New York.

Ekman, P., and Davidson, R. J. (1994). The nature of emotion. Oxford Univ. Press, New York.

Papez, J. W. (1937). A proposed mechanism of emotion. *Am. Med. Assoc. Arch. Neurol. Psychiatr.* **38,** 725–743.

Sacks, O. (1987). *The Man Who Mistook His Wife for a Hat and Other Clinical Tales*. HarperCollins, New York.

Wurtman, R. J., and Anton-Tay, F. (1969). The mammalian pineal as a neuroendocrine transducer. *Prog. Horm. Res.* **25,** 493–513.

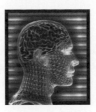

Humor and Laughter

JYOTSNA VAID

Texas A & M University

GLOSSARY

Duchenne display A characteristic facial display accompanying laughter in humans involving the joint contraction of lip and eye muscles.

gelastic seizure Typically unprovoked, stereotyped, and inappropriate laughter accompanying an epileptic seizure.

The ability to perceive and produce humor, highly valued across human societies, has been the subject of much philosophical interest but little sustained, empirical study. This article summarizes the variety of theoretical perspectives and available research relevant to the study of humor, including its nature, its origins in ontogeny and phylogeny, its behavioral manifestation in laughter, its psychological and evolutionary significance, and its hypothesized neural mediation. Although responding with humor may appear to be a way of evading a serious problem, it might also turn out to be a rather effective way of counteracting the

seriousness, or even danger, in a situation by deflecting its adverse effects and by offering an alternative to despair. Humor can provide a way for individuals to conceal or to reveal their vulnerabilities; it can also enable them to transcend a predicament. A person with a good sense of humor is viewed more favorably than one who is humorless. Humor is said to confer mental flexibility, openness to experience, playfulness, and maturity and, as such, is highly valued whether in a coworker, a leader, a friend, or a prospective mate. Indeed, the ability to be playful and humorous appears to be universally valued.

Although scholarly interest in the nature and functions of humor has a long history, empirical inquiry into the forms, uses, and biological bases of humor and laughter is fairly recent. This article addresses both well-researched and relatively unexplored questions pertaining to humor and laughter. The following are some of the questions that are considered here: What is humor? What is the role of laughter in humor? What are the ontogenetic and phylogenetic origins of laughter? How does humor work, cognitively? What is the functional significance of humor? What are the varieties of laughter and how are they perceived? What kinds of disorders of laughter have been documented and what do they suggest about the neural circuitry underlying laughter and humor?

I. DEFINING HUMOR

Humor normally requires at least two individuals (the humor initiator and the receiver) who cooperate in setting up what Gregory Bateson termed a play frame, in which the parties involved tacitly agree that what is inside the frame is not to be taken seriously. A play frame may also be set up by a single individual in response to a perceived incongruity in an event or situation. Verbal humor is a particular form of skilled language use in which at least two disparate meanings are interwoven into a text by making use of ambiguity, polysemy, intertextuality, or inconsistency in such a way that the listener is led to expect one meaning but actually experiences the other. The pleasure of humor is thought to arise upon the sudden recognition of the mismatch between the expected and the experienced meaning.

II. HUMOR AND LAUGHTER

In his 1872 monograph, *The Expression of the Emotions in Man and Animals*, Charles Darwin noted that "Joy, when intense, leads to various purposeless movements—dancing about, clapping the hands, stamping, etc., and to loud laughter." Laughter is indeed commonly seen as an expression of joy, happiness, or amusement. It typically occurs in informal social situations, usually in the presence of a close friend, sibling, caregiver, or intimate.

Although laughter is normally taken to be an indicator that the laugher is in a happy emotional state, it does not exclusively or necessarily signal such a state. One can clearly find something amusing without it actually making one laugh out loud. Similarly, one can feign laughter even when one is not actually amused. Other emotional states that give rise to laughter include scorn, embarassment, and nervousness. It remains to be determined whether the laughter in these different states is morphologically different. Under certain clinical conditions, laughter can be triggered in adults without their ability to control it. In such cases it occurs for no apparent reason and usually without accompanying positive affect. The occurrence of such dissociations between the motoric act of laughter and associated affective or cognitive states raises the possibility that laughter is under the control of a variety of different neural structures and systems at different levels and that these may be selectively disrupted in pathology.

III. ONTOGENY OF LAUGHTER

Laughter and crying both appear to be innate mechanisms in humans, although laughter's onset occurs later: whereas crying emerges at birth and smiling at approximately 2 or 3 weeks of age, the characteristic expiratory movement of laughter does not appear until approximately 4–6 months. However, cases of so-called gelastic (or laughing) seizures in neonates indicate that neural and physiological structures subserving laughter are in place at birth. Laughter's innateness is further suggested by the fact that it is observed in deaf–blind children, even those who could not have learned about it by touching people's faces. Although laughter initially occurs involuntarily, whether in response to tickling or peek-a-boo games or as a reaction to a sudden change in the sensory environment, such as an unexpected noise, over the course of development laughter becomes more regulated, under voluntary control, and elicited in response to cognitive and social stimuli rather than physical stimuli per se.

IV. PHYLOGENY OF LAUGHTER

Laughter is estimated to be 7 million years old. Like other vocalizations, such as moaning, sighing, and crying, laughing is thought to have preceded speech and, like these vocalizations, it may also have a communicative function.

Although laughter is often claimed to be unique to humans, behaviors similar to human laughter have been observed in other primates and something akin to laughter has even been argued to be present in rodents. In 1997, Signe Preuschoft and Jan van Hooff examined variations in the contexts and social functions of bonding displays in various primate species, including Old World primates, macaques, baboons, great apes, and humans. They noted a silent bared-teeth display (also called a grin, grimace, or smile) associated with inhibited locomotion, evasive and protective body movements and postures, and grooming and embraces. This display was observed in all macaque and baboon species and humans. A relaxed, open-mouth display ("play face"), marked by a widely opened mouth but without pronounced baring of the teeth, was observed in all macaque and baboon species, in each of the great apes, including the chimpanzee, bonobo, orangutan, and gorilla, in humans, and in more distant species such as vervets and squirrel monkeys.

One variant of the play face noted in some species was an open mouth, bared-teeth display with associated staccato breathing and bursts of vocalization. This latter display, which Preuschoft and van Hoof termed the "laugh face," appeared strikingly similar to human laughter. It was accompanied by boisterous body postures, brusque movements, mock biting, playful chasing, and evasive, repetitive glancing movements rather than a tense gaze. The laugh face was found only in certain macaques, mandrills, geladas, the orangutan, the bonobo, and, of course, humans, and it occurred primarily in social play contexts, although in some cases it was observed to accompany solitary play, but in these cases it occurred only when conspecifics were near. The presence of an audience thus appears to be at least facilitative, if not necessary, for releasing the laugh face display.

In 1987, Preuschoft and van Hooff proposed a functional significance of play that is relevant to the current analysis. They noted that in bonding behaviors (i.e., those involving care, sex, and affiliation), it is important to deemphasize competition and focus on shared interests. Play is one form of bonding behavior. An important element of play is the partner's unexpected performance of an expected behavioral act. Preuschoft and van Hooff suggested that the "essence of play seems to be to actively bring about incongruous and unexpected behaviors and to interpret them as nonthreatening." This, they argued, allows for affective and cognitive mastery of incongruous situations.

Whereas laughter in nonhuman primate species is found principally in play contexts and primarily occurs in the young of the species, laughter in humans occurs in a variety of social contexts throughout the life span. Moreover, there is no evidence that nonhuman primates have anything comparable to the human ability to produce, comprehend, and enjoy humor.

V. PRECONDITIONS FOR THE EMERGENCE OF HUMOR

Various factors have been proposed as preconditions for the emergence of humor perception in a species, including sociality, an exploratory drive, a system of communication (to allow for the members of the species to express and communicate beliefs and feelings), an ability to mentally represent and order the physical world, and an ability to construct possible imaginary worlds. Additional criteria proposed include a capacity to use logic and reasoning independently of affective or real-world constraints, a capacity to deceive or misrepresent the truth, a capacity for collaboration, reciprocity, compassion, and a theory of mind.

VI. WHAT MAKES SOMETHING HUMOROUS?

Speculating about the causes of mirthful laughter in human adults, Darwin noted that "[s]omething incongruous or unaccountable, exciting surprise and some sense of superiority in the laugher, who must be in a happy frame of mind, seems to be the commonest cause." In comparing laughter arising from actual tickling and that arising from the tickling of the imagination, he noted:

> From the fact that a child can hardly tickle itself, or in a much less degree than when tickled by another person, it seems that the precise point to be touched must not be known; so with the mind, something unexpected—a novel or incongruous idea which breaks through an habitual train of thought—appears to be a strong element in the ludicrous.

Darwin's insights anticipate many subsequent theoretical accounts of humor. With respect to its cognitive basis, an early formulation of the mechanisms underlying humor may be found in the work of a Gestalt psychologist, Norman Maier. Maier noted that a key element of humor is a sudden and unexpected restructuring of the elements of a configuration, not unlike that experienced during a flash of insight. A humorous narrative manipulates our expectations by leading us down a garden path only to present us with an altogether different conclusion than the one we were led to expect. Inasmuch as the conclusion disrupts the way in which we have been thinking about the events in the narrative, we are totally unprepared for it. After a momentary confusion of thought, we experience the newly restructured configuration with clarity; the amusement arises when we realize how we were misled. In 1992, Wyer and Collins proposed that diminishment is a key element in humor elicitation: For humor to be elicited, the new perception of the situation must in some sense be diminished in importance in comparison to the apparent reality that was first assumed.

Subsequent theorists have elaborated on these accounts. For example, cognitive approaches characterize humor perception in information processing terms as involving at least two and possibly three stages: a setup stage, a stage in which the incongruity is recognized, and a stage of incongruity resolution. Although there is debate regarding whether humor appreciation requires that the incongruity be satisfactorily resolved (with some arguing that incongruity recognition per se is sufficient to experience humor), theorists generally agree on the importance of the juxtaposition of two or more mental representations for humor to be perceived, following Arthur Koestler, who, in *The Act of Creation*, described humor as an example of bisociative thinking, which juxtaposes and brings together two disparate matrices of thought. Recent theoretical formulations in cognitive science have used concepts such as frame shifting and conceptual integration of mental spaces to formalize the processes underlying humor perception. To date, there has been little cognitively oriented experimental research on humor comprehension and even less on the processes underlying humor generation.

It has also been acknowledged that it is not enough to postulate incongruity as a prerequisite of humor because, in certain situations, incongruity may give rise to other emotional reactions, such as fear or apprehension, rather than humor. A humorous rather than apprehensive reaction is more likely when the receiver does not have too much invested in the content of the humor—that is, when the humor does not threaten the receiver's beliefs or feelings in any profound or disturbing way. Second, a humorous reaction is more likely when the receiver was led to expect something dangerous that turns out not to be. Indeed, Ramachandran suggests that laughter may have evolved as a false alarm signal—that is, as an immediate signal to conspecifics that some potentially threatening event has trivial rather than terrifying implications. This notion is similar to the diminishment view of humor developed by Wyer and Collins.

VII. FUNCTIONAL THEORIES OF LAUGHTER AND HUMOR

Theories about the uses of laughter and humor range from psychological and social/anthropological approaches to metaphysical and evolutionary ones.

A. Psychological

Among psychological theories, that of Sigmund Freud, as described in *Jokes and Their Relation to the Unconscious* (1963), is one of the earliest. For Freud, jokes allow a temporary expression of socially undesirable impulses from the subconscious. Freud notes that tendentious humor makes possible "the satisfaction of an instinct (whether lustful or hostile) in the face of an obstacle that stands in its way." The association

of humor with aggressive or sexual impulses has characterized subsequent accounts as well, although there is no current consensus as to whether hostility is inherent in humor.

Proponents of the so-called superiority theory (e.g., Aristotle, Plato, Hobbes, and Bergson) view laughter as reflecting a moral stance on the part of the laugher. For Bergson, laughter asserts the human values of spontaneity and freedom and therefore erupts whenever a person behaves rigidly, like an automaton: "Humor consists in perceiving something mechanical encrusted on something living." Hobbes described the passion of laughter as "nothing else but sudden glory arising from a sudden conception of some eminency in ourselves by comparison with the infirmity of others, or with our own formerly." Superiority is asserted not just by laughing at others' defects but also by showing that one can laugh at (and rise above) one's own imperfections.

In contrast to negative uses of humor, as in putdown or derisive humor, recent clinically based research has directed considerable attention to positive aspects of humor. Humor is increasingly viewed as a useful mechanism for coping with stress and regulating affect. In 1999, Galloway and Cropley proposed that laughter may reduce some existing mental health problems and a sense of humor may moderate the perceived intensity of negative life events.

B. Social/Anthropological

Social and ethological theorists (e.g., Martineau) have viewed laughter as a marker of group membership and solidarity (for those who share a joke) or exclusion (for those who are the "butt" of the joke) and as a means of maintaining social control and group cohesiveness.

Anthropologists have described "joking relationships" in various traditional societies; these refer to ritualized teasing between specific kin in which the receiver is required to take no offense. In an incisive analysis, anthropologist Mary Douglas suggested that joking is a subversive act in that it levels hierarchy and represents a triumph of intimacy over formality and of unofficial values over official ones. Not surprisingly, this subversive aspect of humor is particularly evident among members of minority groups who may use humor to portray reality in a way that exposes social inequities. Much feminist humor and political humor, particularly that found in Central and Eastern European countries while under authoritarian rule, is of this type. So-called "gallows" humor also has elements of this subversive aspect of humor.

C. Metaphysical

Although laughter appears to be associated with happiness and joy, some have taken the position that laughter arises precisely from the experience of suffering. The philosopher Nietzsche, for example, argued that humor was invented precisely because of the extent to which humans suffer. This view is echoed in existentialist philosophy. For the most part, though, humor has not been taken seriously in classical philosophical thought in the Western tradition, which has tended to regard it as irrational, irresponsible, and frivolous. In contrast, Eastern traditions, such as Hindu, Buddhist, and Sufi worldviews, regard humor as an appropriate reaction in the face of the vicissitudes of death, disease, and aging; humor here is seen as an insight that all human aspirations are ultimately comical and that wisdom ensues from that insight.

D. Evolutionary

Laughter is clearly an important aspect of human nature. All societies appear to value it. It has distinct facial and vocal manifestations. It emerges spontaneously in early childhood and persists through the life span and it is an intensely pleasurable social activity. All these aspects suggest that laughter may be a reasonable candidate for a psychologically adaptive characteristic. Indeed, it has been accorded a special place in several recent theoretical accounts of human evolution. Aside from the false alarm theory mentioned earlier, at least five different evolutionary accounts of laughter and humor may be distinguished.

1. Humor as a Temporary Disabling Mechanism

When we are truly amused by something, more often than not it takes us by surprise and distracts us from whatever it was that we were in the middle of doing or thinking. If we are heartily laughing, we quite literally cannot think of, let alone do, anything else. Wallace Chafe suggests that this disruptive effect of humor may be evolutionarily significant (i.e., that humor's basic adaptive function is a disabling one). Chafe proposes that the humor state may have arisen precisely in order to keep us from doing things that might be counterproductive; that is, things that our usual form of reasoning might lead us into but that, in a larger sense, would be undesirable. This view fits with a related notion of humor as a device for pointing out and sharing counterexamples, or providing disconfirmatory evidence, which in turn is useful in reasoning and problem solving. Chafe further suggests that the fact that laughter provides an audible signal to others may be significant because laughter signals to the receiver that the laugher is in a humor state and thus cannot be taken seriously; moreover, the laughter may in turn infect others present, rendering them temporarily disabled as well.

The notion that humor is a disabling device that is ultimately adaptive is an intriguing hypothesis and one that readily lends itself to empirical test. For example, one could ask whether the effect attributed to humor depends on the type of humor, the type of problem from which the laugher has been disrupted, the relevance of the humor content to the problem content, the presence of others, etc.

2. Humor as Social Learning

According to G. Weisfeld, humor provides exposure to fitness-relevant scenarios in a nonserious, playful context, motivating the practice of social skills that will be useful in serious contexts. In this view, humor is basically a form of social–intellectual stimulation that allows for the seeking and practicing of social skills that are fitness enhancing at some later point. Laughter, according to Weisfeld, conveys appreciation and gratitude to the humorist for having provided such stimulation.

3. Humor as Status Manipulation

The notion that mirthful laughter serves to create and solidify group boundaries forms the centerpiece of an evolutionary account of humor proposed by Richard Alexander in which humor is seen as a way of favorably manipulating one's status in a group to improve one's access to resources for reproductive success. Specifically, it is proposed that humor developed as a type of ostracism, a means of manipulating one's social status in a group (and thereby one's access to critical resources) by facilitating bonds with certain members and ostracizing others, through explicit or implicit exclusion.

Alexander's theory views humor primarily as a device for establishing dominance and thereby for being more competitive for critical resources. He suggests that humor, as a form of social scenario building, gives one an edge in learning how to negotiate in fitness-relevant domains. Humorous put-downs may be more successful than direct criticism or insults as a way of establishing dominance since they are indirect and therefore more face-saving ways of manipulating status than direct displays of hostility or strength. In Alexander's model, all humor, whether or not it has an ostensible butt or target, essentially developed in the service of status manipulation.

4. Humor as Vocal Grooming

An emphasis on vocal grooming characterizes an evolutionary view of language proposed by Robin Dunbar that has implications for humor. Dunbar speculates that human language evolved as a vocal extension of physical grooming, allowing, as it were, the simultaneous grooming across space of more than one partner and thereby the facilitating of social bonds with larger groups of animals. Language fosters social bonding by permitting the exchange of gossip, i.e., socially relevant information (specifically, who is doing what with whom), as well as the sharing of one's own experiences, actual or desired. The fact that laughter typically accompanies speech suggests that it facilitates and cements the social bonding process.

In this view, the pleasure in shared laughter is analogous to the pleasure of actual physical touch. Humor has in fact been characterized as a form of vicarious touch. The importance of touch for primate emotional development is well documented. Laughter may have served to attract like-minded others in the bonding process; as Konrad Lorenz noted, finding the same thing funny is not only a prerequisite to a real friendship but also very often the first step to its formation. Thus, just as language facilitates social bonding, laughter accompanying speech, and humorous discourse with or without laughter, could have evolved as a way of solidifying affectional bonds.

5. "The Wit to Woo": Humor as Mate Attraction

The most recent evolutionary proposal regarding humor emphasizes its importance in courtship and suggests that the creativity and unpredictability that is inherent in humor is seen as attractive to a prospective mate. In this account, proposed by Geoffrey Miller in *The Mating Mind*, creativity is seen as not just a random by-product of chaotic neural activity but also as something that evolved as an indicator of intelligence and youthfulness and as a way of playing into

our attraction to novelty. Creativity not only allows one to find unpredictable solutions to problems but also provides inherent pleasure because of its protean, unpredictable nature. Humor encapsulates these elements of creativity and it is therefore not surprising that a sense of humor is highly desired in a prospective mate. In this view, humor evolved because of its importance in courtship and mate choice.

The five evolutionary hypotheses emphasize different elements of humor. Humor is hypothesized to disrupt our routine for the better, to teach and reward us in our social interactions in fitness-relevant domains, to unify a group but also create group divisions, to create and strengthen affective bonds, and to attract and sustain a partner. Although there is evidence consistent with each of these views, research designed to examine the assumptions and claims of the different accounts is clearly warranted.

In the remaining sections we review theory and research on the expression and neural mediation of normal and abnormal manifestations of laughter and humor.

VIII. NORMAL LAUGHTER

A. Visuomotoric and Physiological Aspects

Laughter is a motoric and vocal activity requiring the coordinated action of 15 different facial muscles and associated clonic contractions of the thoracic cage and the abdominal wall. Laughter produces spasmodic skeletal muscle contractions, tachycardia, changes in breathing pattern, and increases in catecholamine production. Hearty laughter increases heart rate, blood pressure and respiratory rate, and muscular activity.

Physiologically, laughter is the opposite of crying. Although the upper half of the laughing face appears indistinguishable from the crying face, the lower half and the respiratory pattern in laughter are the reverse of those of crying. In laughter a characteristic facial display known as the Duchenne display is invoked. This display involves the joint contraction of the zygomatic major muscles (i.e., pulling the lip corners back and upwards) and the orbicularis oculi muscles (i.e., raising the cheeks and causing the eyes to wrinkle). Indeed, the movement of the eye muscles may serve as a marker for distinguishing emotional from voluntary (forced) laughter since the orbicularis oculi muscles do not contract during voluntary laughter. Laughter is also accompanied by the flaring of nostrils, mandible retraction, and brightening and sparkling of the eyes.

In terms of respiration, laughter typically begins with an abrupt exhalation followed by rhythmic expiration/inspiration cycles, which may or may not be phonated as "ha ha ha." No inspiration preceding the laugh is needed since laughter is produced at a low lung volume. The rhythmic pattern of laughter respiration is produced by contractions of muscles that are typically passive during normal expiration, i.e., the diaphragm, the abdominal (rectus abdominus), and the rib cage muscles (triangularis sterni). These muscles work together with the larynx. In crying, the saccadic contractions occur mainly with inspiration, whereas in laughing they occur with expiration; in both cases the contractions are accompanied by short, broken sounds. Autonomic correlates of laughter include arousal and muscle tension followed by relaxation of muscle tone, dilatation of cutaneous vessels of the face, neck, and hands, lacrimation, and fatigue.

In 2000, Niemitz, Loi, and Landerer examined specific visuomotoric aspects of the human laughing face and their affective interpretation by human raters. The expressive facial movements of 45 videotaped laughing adults and 13 children were shown to more than 100 adult raters. The results suggested that visual aspects of laughing faces that are judged as cheerful, winning, or generally positive were those in which (i) the laughs were fairly long, ranging from 3 to 6 sec; (ii) there were rapid eye and mouth movements during the first second of the expression of laughter; (iii) there was repetition of the mouth and eye movements; and (iv) there was almost complete closing of the eyelids, sometimes repeatedly, for 0.1–1.5 sec. There is a need for more such research quantifying how the various laughing expressions are decoded and interpreted, not just in the visual channel but also acoustically.

B. Acoustic Aspects

Willibald Ruch and Paul Ekman proposed a useful framework for describing the structure of laughter. They define a laughter bout as all the respiratory, vocal, facial, and skeletomuscular elements involved in a particular laughter event. A bout of laughter, in turn, consists of an onset (the prevocal facial component), an apex (involving vocalization or forced exhalation), and an offset (the postvocalization part, typically a smile that fades out). The apex contains laugh cycles, (i.e., repetitive laugh pulses); there are typically 4

pulses in a laugh cycle, although the number can range from 9 to 12 depending on lung volume. There are usually about 5 pulses per second. At the level of laryngeal movements, a laugh pulse can be further subdivided into the number and duration of vibratory cycles of the vocal cords. In one analysis, the duration of laughter pulses varied from 30 to 100 msec. Phonation in laughter pulses involves a series of stereotypic laryngeal adjustments that include four stages: an interpulse pause (a moment of quiet aspiration in the periods between voicing), adduction (closing) of the arytenoid cartilages, vibration of vocal chords, and abduction (opening) of the arytenoid cartilages.

Several features in the acoustic signal may serve to cue the degree of positive affect experienced by the laugher. Widening versus narrowing of the pharynx is known to affect voice quality and may signal friendly versus scornful laughter, respectively. Other cues may be provided by harmonics, melodic contour, and duration. The melodic contour, including the intonation and pitch contour, may be particularly informative of emotional state and meaning. The vocal ligaments are more likely to be tensed under conditions of arousal or anticipation, giving rise to laughter that has a rising melodic contour. The lips and the cheeks are typically elevated in joyful smiling or laughter; contraction of the muscles involved in the Duchenne display changes the form of the mouth opening, constraining the vowel sounds that can thus be produced. Indeed, one study showed that listeners can reliably infer a smiling from an unsmiling version of the same spoken message purely on the basis of the voice.

Fewer than a dozen studies have been conducted on the acoustic characteristics of laughter. Almost all have used adult participants. One study examined the acoustic characteristics of a group of 30 male and female adults from whom one laugh was elicited under each of four conditions: social, humor, tension release, and tickle. Significant differences in duration, intensity, and mean frequencies of three vowel formants above the fundamental frequency were found between the humor and social laughs and the tension release and tickle laughs. Moreover, listeners could reliably classify the laughs into the different types, suggesting a communicative aspect to the laughs. The mean fundamental frequency of laughter for males (175 Hz) was higher than that for females (160 Hz) and highest for the tickling condition. In another study, a group of 11 male college students were recorded while they viewed a videotape of comedic storyteller Bill Cosby. Analyses of 55 bouts of laughter showed that the mean peak fundamental frequency while laughing was more than twice as high as that when the subjects were counting. Moreover, an extended range of frequencies was exhibited during laughter, with a difference of 344 Hz between the lowest and the highest range observed. In general, there was considerable variability both within and between subjects on all the measures studied.

A limitation of existing studies with adults is the lack of naturalistic social interaction contexts. Studies with children fare better in this regard. One study recorded laughter among four 3-year-olds during three sessions of spontaneous free play between mother and child. An acoustic analysis revealed that the duration of laughter syllables in children was about the same as that found in adult laughter (i.e., about 200–220 msec). The total duration of the average laugh was also similar to that of adults. The main difference between adult and child laughter was in fundamental frequency, with most children's laughter having a frequency in the upper range of adult female laughter (400–500 Hz) or, in the case of one type of laughter (squeals), even higher (nearly 2000 Hz). Four distinct laughter types were noted in the child sample: (i) comment laughter (i.e., laughter occurring in conversational contexts that lasted about one-fifth of a second), which was subdivided into dull comment and exclamatory comment laughter; (ii) chuckle laughter, which lasted half a second and tended to occur in situations provoking more excitement than comment laughter; (iii) rhythmical laughter, which lasted 1–15 sec; and (iv) squeal laughter, which lasted half a second, had a very high fundamental frequency, and usually occurred without a break. The latter two kinds were more prevalent in the context of physical stimulation, anticipation, and fear.

It appears, therefore, that different types of spontaneous laughter have different acoustic characteristics. Moreover, laughter differs in different social contexts. Additional studies are needed with different kinds of communication dyads and with different age groups to examine in more detail the relationship between acoustic distinctions in laughter production and their affective interpretation by listeners. The specific ways in which spontaneous versus contrived laughter may differ, both structurally and neurobehaviorally, also warrant study.

C. Health Aspects

An implicit belief underlying most accounts of humor is that it confers psychological benefits. As reviewed by Martin, the benefits of humor may also extend to the physiological level. For example, laughter is known to increase respiratory rate and clear mucus. It is entirely conceivable that laughter may thus be beneficial to patients with chronic respiratory conditions such as emphysema. The increased heart rate and blood pressure accompanying laughter can exercise the myocardium and improve arterial and venous circulation, allowing a greater flow of oxygen and nutrients to tissues. This in turn may facilitate the movement of immune elements useful in fighting infections. Muscle relaxation following hearty laughter may break the spasm–pain cycle in patients with neuralgias or rheumatism. A reduction in laryngeal muscle tension accompanying laughter may help patients with vocal fold pathology to produce a more relaxed voice, and it may facilitate the recovery of phonation in patients with psychogenic dysphonia, an inability to phonate during speech despite intact articulation and the absence of any identifiable pathology of the larynx. Finally, the increased catecholamine levels associated with laughter may be responsible for the beneficial effects humor is thought to exert on mental functions, such as alertness and creativity. Many of these claims of the healthful benefits of laughter and humor have yet to be subjected to systematic study.

D. Neuroanatomical Hypotheses

There has been very little direct empirical investigation of neuroanatomical correlates of normal laughter. A hypothetical neural circuit was first theorized in 1924 by Kinnier Wilson. According to Wilson's model, laughter is produced by a medullary effector center that links the seventh nerve nucleus in the pons with the 10th motor nucleus in the medulla and with phrenic nuclei in the upper cervical cord. This center is modulated by the cerebral cortex and limbic structures by means of an integrative center in the mesial thalamus, hypothalamus, and subthalamus.

Activity of the laughter center is thought to be determined by a voluntary pathway (corticobulbar fibers) and fibers extending from the orbital surface of the frontal lobes through the bulbar nuclei. Input to these fibers comes from an involuntary pathway (the basal ganglia), which appears to be inhibited by the voluntary one. No single cortical area supplies the origins for the voluntary and involuntary fibers; the input derives from diffuse cortical regions including the frontal, premotor, motor, parietal, temporal, and hippocampal regions.

The notion of hypothalamic integration of cortical and limbic control on the brain stem laughter center remains to be substantiated, although it is consistent with clinical observations.

IX. DISORDERS OF LAUGHTER

Disorders of laughter and crying are very rare. Although strong emotional reactions are not uncommon following brain injury, the most common reaction described is fear. Medical research on laughing and crying disorders consists largely of case reports, with few systematic, large-scale investigations. Abnormal laughter, defined as laughter that is involuntary and inappropriate to the situational context, is most often seen in generalized affective or cognitive disturbances such as psychoses (e.g., schizophrenia). Individual cases of hysterical laughter spells, marked by silly, unrestrained, unmotivated, and unprovoked laughter, have been reported, as has epidemic hysterical laughter.

In many cases of abnormal laughter, the motor act of laughing may be dissociated from its emotional aspect. Such a condition has been termed pathological laughter. Kinnier Wilson defined pathological laughter and crying (PLC) as "a sequel to and consequence of a recognizable cerebral lesion or lesions in which attacks of involuntary, irresistible laughing or crying, or both, have come into the foreground of the clinical picture." This definition draws attention to the impaired control and the episodic aspect of the abnormal emotional expression.

In 1994, Shaibani, Sabbagh, and Doody proposed four criteria to distinguish pathological laughter and crying from normal laughter and crying. First, PLC is inappropriate to the situation since it occurs spontaneously or in response to nonspecific stimuli or inappropriate, arbitrary stimuli (e.g., one patient with a left cerellar hematoma showed pathological laughter following left hand tremor). Second, PLC is unmotivated; that is, there is no relation between the affect and observed expression, nor is there relief or mood change afterwards. Third, PLC is involuntary; that is, it has its own pattern and occurs against the patient's will. Neither the duration nor the content of PLC can be controlled, and patients do not gradually change from smiling to laughing but have a sudden, brief outburst without any warning. Fourth, PLC differs from emotional lability, which refers to an exaggerated emotional response to a normal stimulus. The latter characterizes patients with multiple sclerosis and Alzheimer's disease. These patients are overcome by uncontrollable laughter and crying that is usually appropriate to the situation and accompanied by mood alteration.

Very few patients actually meet the criteria for PLC. However, researchers do not concur on the ideal classification system and whether PLC must involve a dissociation between the expressed affect and the mood. It is acknowledged that the degree of volitional control of PLC varies from complete absence to some control.

The most common conditions associated with PLC are summarized in the following sections, subdivided into disregulatory and excitatory conditions.

A. Disregulatory Conditions

One disregulatory condition giving rise to abnormal laughter is amyotrophic lateral sclerosis (ALS). In 25% of ALS patients there is bulbar involvement; of these, 30–50% develop PLC. Patients without bulbar involvement do not develop PLC.

Multiple sclerosis is another condition that in 7–10% of patients leads to PLC, sometimes with euphoria. Characteristics of so-called pseudobulbar palsy associated with multiple sclerosis (as with bilateral strokes) include dysarthria, dysphagia, bifacial weakness, and weak tongue movements but preserved coughing, yawning, laughing, and crying.

In one large-scale study, PLC was observed in 15% of stroke patients 1 month after the stroke, in 21% at 6 months after the stroke, and in 11% a year following the stroke. Abnormal emotional reactions were particularly associated with lesions in the left frontal and temporal regions.

A rare syndrome of PLC is associated with acute infarction—the so-called "fou rire prodromique," first described in 1903 and in only a few cases since. In these cases, laughter lasts from between 15 minutes to 24 hours and is almost always followed by death. Lesions in this syndrome typically involve the left internal capsule-thalamus, left basal ganglia, or ventral pons. This syndrome contrasts with pseudobulbar palsy since it is not recurrent and, unlike epileptic laughter, it is not associated with electroencephalograph (EEG) changes or confusion.

A host of extrapyramidal disorders, including Parkinson's and Wilson's disease, are also associated with PLC. The syndrome of Angelman, a genetic disorder characterized by mental retardation and stiff puppet-like movements in children between the ages of

2 and 6 years, is also associated with frequent bursts of laughter. A variety of toxins, such as nitrous oxide and insecticides, have also been related to pathological laughter. Finally, various malignant brain stem tumors, such as clival chordoma and pontine glioma, have been implicated in pathological laughter.

B. Excitatory Conditions

The most common excitatory condition that is associated with pathological laughter occurs in epileptics. Laughter as part of an epileptic seizure was documented by the neurologist Trousseau in 1873 and was described in Dostoevsky's novel *The Idiot*. In 1957, the term "gelastic epilepsy" was coined to refer to epileptic fits in which laughter is the only or the most common symptom. More than 160 cases of gelastic epilepsy have been reported in the literature. Gelastic epilepsy often occurs in patients with hypothalamic hamartomas and precocious puberty, in patients with complex partial seizures and temporal lobe origin seizures, and in children with infantile spasms. The seizures usually begin in infancy or childhood and are associated with cognitive decline in later years. In patients with these seizures, involuntary, mechanical giggling typically occurs as the initial ictal behavior before an alteration in consciousness. The duration of the laughter in patients with hamartomas is usually less than 30 seconds and the seizures occur several times a day.

In a recent review of published reports of seizures involving laughter, Biraben and colleagues proposed the following neural hypotheses for the genesis of laughter:

1. Laughter arising as a reactional behavior (i.e., in response to a pleasant feeling or mirth: Only a few such cases have been observed, all involving seizures with a temporal focus. In one such case, involving stimulation of the left temporobasal region (fusiform and parahippocampal gyri), the individual experienced a change in the semantic connotation of stimuli (things became funny); in another case with stimulation in the same region, the modification experienced was perceptual (things changed in a funny way). Biraben *et al.* suggest that the laughter in these cases might be a physiological response to a modified cognitive process.

2. Laughter arising as a forced action or an automatism: Seizures with a frontal focus have characteristically produced laughter described as forced and unmotivated. Arroyo and colleagues describe one patient with a cavernoma of the anterior

cingulate gyrus whose laughter appeared to be an irrepressible motor behavior; resection of the lesion eliminated the laughing behavior. They suggest that the premotor mesial system acts as an interface between the limbic loop, which includes the anterior cingulate gyrus, and the motor loop, which includes the supplementary motor area. Biraben *et al.* propose that cases of gelastic seizure originating in the anterior cingulum involve a critical functional disconnection between the motor loop and the limbic loop within the mesial premotor system. The laughter arising in these cases reflects a behavioral output from a motor program separated from all motivation.

Laughter in one other epileptic patient reviewed, a nongelastic case, occurred after cortical electrical stimulation of the lateral border of the rostral part of the supplementary motor area. The laughter was natural, rather than forced, and was accompanied by a general feeling of amusement toward the environment at large. Biraben *et al.* suggest that such laughter may reflect an imbalance between the mesial and lateral premotor systems.

C. Neuroanatomical Hypotheses

Evidence for the neuroanatomy of pathological laughter and crying comes from the following sources: a limited number of autopsy reports; studies of congenitally malformed infants; case reports of patients with pathological laughter following neurological disease; EEG activity and electrical stimulation of the cortex; injection of a barbiturate to the right or left cortex, typically done in patients with epilepsy to determine the language-dominant hemisphere; and studies of humor comprehension in patients with left versus right hemisphere damage.

The autopsy data are of limited value in localizing laughter since the patients had suffered diffuse brain pathology. A review of such cases revealed no single cortical lesion as causing PLC. Together with clinical case reports, the autopsy data indicate that both unilateral and bilateral lesions that affect the descending tracts to the bulbar nuclei can cause PLC, as can lesions on either side in the anterior limb and genu of the internal capsule adjacent to the basal ganglia, thalamus, hypothalamus, and pons. Even localized brain stem lesions can cause pathological laughter. Case studies do not explain why some patients develop pathological laughter while others develop pathological crying or both. Studies of congenitally malformed newborns with severe anencephaly but with preserved pons and medulla indicate that newborns do not smile but can cry; those with intact midbrains can both cry and smile.

The predominant neuroanatomical account of pathological laughter and crying, first proposed by Wilson, regards it as arising from a loss of direct motor cortical inhibition of a laughter and crying center located in the upper brain stem. However, this explanation does not fully account for the range of phenomena observed in PLC. A recent alternative account, developed by Parvizi and colleagues, in light of new neuropathological findings, suggests that PLC is caused by dysfunction in circuits that involve the cerebellum (as well as the cortex) and influence brain stem nuclei.

There is evidence that the cerebral hemispheres may play different roles in the control of emotional states. In normal subjects the right hemisphere appears to be specialized for the perception and expression of emotion, particularly negative emotion. Lesions in the right hemisphere have been found to impair prosodic and lexical expression of emotion. Moreover, in epileptic subjects, injection of the right hemisphere with intracarotid sodium amytal has elicited unprovoked laughter, whereas left-sided injection has tended to produce bouts of crying. Patients with crying seizures tend to show right-sided foci, whereas those with gelastic seizures show mainly left-sided foci.

Patients with right hemisphere damage show a preserved sensitivity to the surprise element of humor but a diminished ability to establish narrative coherence. Disorders of humor, such as foolish or silly euphoria (so-called *moria*), and a tendency toward making inappropriate jokes (so-called *witzelsucht*), have been reported in patients with frontal lobe disorders including neurosyphilis. In 1999, a functional neuroimaging study by Shammi and Stuss determined that deficits in humor appreciation are restricted to patients with right frontal damage, supporting the view that the right frontal lobe serves an important role in integrating cognitive and affective information.

X. CONCLUSION

As may be evident from this overview, laughter and humor offer fertile ground for future investigation undertaken from a variety of theoretical and methodological perspectives, including ethological, cognitive, linguistic, clinical, and neuroscience. In a recent review, Jaak Panksepp observed that incisive research in this area has only just begun and that substantive research remains meagre. Many basic questions remain, such as the occurrence and significance of laughter in play and other social contexts; the role of laughter and humor in courtship, mate choice, and relationship maintenance; what different kinds of laughter communicate and to whom; and the neural circuitry responsible for normal laughter and feelings of mirth and joy.

See Also the Following Articles

CREATIVITY • DEPRESSION • EMOTION

Suggested Reading

Biraben, A., Sartori, E., Taussing, D., Bernard, A., and Scarabin, J. (1999). Gelastic seizures: Video-EEG and scintigraphic analysis of a case with a frontal focus; Review of the literature and pathophysiological hypotheses. *Epileptic Disorders* **1**(4), 221–228.

Brownell, H., and Stringfellow, A. (2000). *Cognitive perspectives on humor comprehension after brain injury.* In *Neurobehavior of Language and Cognition: Studies of Normal Aging and Brain Damage* (L. Connor and L. K. Obler, Eds.), Kluwer Academic, Boston.

Galloway, G., and Cropley, A. (1999). Benefits of humor for mental health: Empirical findings and directions for further research. *Int. J. Humor Res.* **12**(3), 301–314.

Goel, V., and Dolan, R. (2001). The functional anatomy of humor: Segregating cognitive and affective components. *Nature Neurosci.* **4**(3), 237–238.

Hull, R., and Vaid, J. (2001, July). *Cognitive basis of incongruity in verbal humor: An experimental inquiry.* Poster presented at the annual meeting of the Society for Text and Discourse, Santa Barbara, CA.

Martin, R. A. (2001). Humor, laughter, and physical health: Methodological issues and research findings. *Psychological Bull.* **127**(4), 504–519.

Mendez, M., Nakawatase, T., and Brown, C. (1999). Involuntary laughter and inappropriate hilarity. *J. Neuropsychiatr. Clin. Neurosci.* **11**(2), 253–258.

Niemitz, C., Loi, M., and Landerer, S. (2000). Investigations on human laughter and its implications for the evolution of hominoid visual communication. *Homo* **51**(1), 1–18.

Panksepp, J. (2000). The riddle of laughter: Neural and psychoevolutionary underpinnings of joy. *Curr. Directions Psychol. Sci.* **9**(6), 183–186.

Parvizi, J., Anderson, S., Martin, C., Damasio, H., and Damasio, A. (2001). Pathological laughter and crying: A link to cerebellum. *Brain* **124**, 1708–1719.

Provine, R. (2000). *Laughter: A Scientific Investigation.* Viking, New York.

Ruch, W., and Ekman, P. (2001). *The expressive pattern of laughter.* In *Emotions, Qualia and Consciousness: Proceedings of the International School of Biocybernetics Casamicciola, Naples, Italy, 19–24 Oct 98.* (A. Kaszniak, Ed.). World Scientific, Tokyo.

Shammi, P., and Stuss, D. T. (1999). Humour appreciation: A role of the right frontal lobe. *Brain* **122,** 657–666.

Vaid, J. (1999). *The evolution of humor: Do those who laugh last?* In *Evolution of the Psyche* (D. Rosen and M. Luebbert, Eds.), pp. 123–138. Praeger, Westport, CT.

Vaid, J., and Kobler, J. B. (2000). Laughing matters: Toward a structural and neural account. *Brain and Cognition* **42,** 139–141.

Vaid, J., and Ramachandran, V. S. (2001). Laughter and humor. In *The Oxford Companion to the Body* (C. Blakemore and S. Jennett, Eds.), pp. 426–427. Oxford University Press, Oxford.

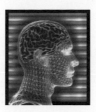

Hydrocephalus

CHIMA OHAEGBULAM and PETER BLACK

Children's Hospital/Brigham & Women's Hospital, Boston

GLOSSARY

basal cisterns The cerebrospinal fluid containing spaces on the undersurface of the brain, the largest of which is the cisterna magna in the angle between the cerebellum and the back of the brain stem.

cerebrospinal fluid (CSF) The fluid contained within the ventricles and surrounding the brain and spinal cord.

choroid plexus The structures within the ventricles that produce most of the CSF.

fontanelle The soft membranous gap between growing skull bones in the infant skull, the largest of which is the anterior fontanelle.

lumbar puncture The insertion of a needle between lumbar vertebrae in the midline of the back into the space around the spinal cord containing CSF.

shunts Systems, typically involving tubing and a valve, diverting CSF from the ventricles to another body site.

ventricles The system of interconnecting fluid-filled cavities within the brain.

Hydrocephalus is the abnormal accumulation of cerebrospinal fluid (CSF) within the ventricles of the brain. This always involves enlargement of ventricles, and there may or may not be increased intracranial pressure. Hydrocephalus is almost always a result of impaired CSF absorption or circulation.

I. INCIDENCE/PREVALENCE

The true incidence or prevalence of hydrocephalus is unknown. As an isolated congenital disorder, it probably occurs in about 1 in 1000 live births. There are no good data on the incidence of adult hydrocephalus.

II. HISTORY

A. Early Concepts/Myths

Early references suggest that Hippocrates was aware of the condition now described as hydrocephalus. In 1768, Whytt published "Observations on the Dropsy in the Brain," in which he cited other writers as far back as the 13th century. Numerous herbal remedies were recommended in those times, though success rates were described as very low. Other treatments included head binding, leeching or bloodletting, injection of strong iodine solution into the ventricles, and exposure to the sun.

B. First Therapies Based on Anatomy

CSF was given its name by Magendie in 1825, and he and others, including Key and Retzius, elucidated its circulatory pathways later in the 19th century. Better understanding of the location of CSF within the ventricles led to more direct surgical approaches such as ventricular puncture. In 1891, Quincke described lumbar puncture as a treatment for hydrocephalus, and this has evolved into the important diagnostic and therapeutic tool that it is today.

C. Early Shunts

As a better understanding of CSF circulation emerged, there were attempts to circumvent "obstructions" in the ventricular system in order to relieve hydrocephalus. Initial attempts to "shunt" CSF included external drainage in the late 19th century, invariably complicated by fatal infections. Other attempts were made using glass wool, gold tubes, catgut strands, and other materials to create conduits from the ventricles to the space beneath the scalp, the dura, and other areas. In 1908, Payr attempted the use of autologous vein to drain the ventricles into the sagittal sinus initially and later the jugular veins with some success. Others could not duplicate his results.

Cushing attempted bypass from the spinal subarachnoid space into the peritoneal cavity or retroperitoneal space by passing silver cannulae through the fourth lumbar vertebra. This had some success. The introduction of vulcanized rubber led to the availability of suitable conduit for the creation of shunts from the ventricular system to other body cavities. The first major innovation with the use of rubber catheters was by Torkildsen in 1939 to divert CSF from the lateral ventricles to the cisterna magna, but operative mortality remained high. It was eventually replaced by the more modern shunting procedures.

Numerous shunting procedures were created to other body cavities, notably the ureters. The ventriculoureteral shunt, reported by Matson in the 1950s, required a nephrectomy and had several infectious and metabolic complications. It also had a number of long-term survivors, however, and was the first effective shunt system used. Later shunts were developed to the atrial system, the pleura, and the peritoneum.

D. Other Operations

Walter Dandy, with Blackfan, identified the choroid plexus as the primary source of CSF production. On physiologic principles, in 1919, Dandy introduced choroid plexectomy as a treatment for hydrocephalus, in which the choroid plexus was ablated by cautery. This was initially performed as an open operation with a very high mortality rate but later was performed endoscopically by himself, Scarff, and others with a success rate of 70–80% and a mortality rate of approximately 15%. This procedure eventually fell out of favor with the subsequent discovery of significant extrachoroidal sources of CSF as well as the introduction of simpler shunting procedures.

Dandy also introduced open procedures for creating openings in the third ventricle into the basal cisterns on the undersurface of the brain. These were again developed into endoscopic procedures with success and mortality rates similar to those for choroid plexectomy. Patient selection for these was problematic before the modern imaging era because the optimal patient was one who had an obstruction in the aqueduct of Sylvius, which was the outflow tract for the third ventricle. There is a resurgence of interest in this procedure because of more sophisticated endoscopic techniques and equipment as well as the availability of appropriate imaging to select the right candidates.

E. Modern Era Shunts/Valves

The modern era of shunts owes its origin to the development of one-way valves by Spitz and Holter as well as by Pudenz. Polyvinyl chloride was initially used, but it was soon evident that silastic was better tolerated by the body.

The most popular shunting operation of this era was the ventriculoatrial shunt, in which the distal end of the catheter was introduced into the jugular vein and then to the right atrium. Numerous other sites for drainage have been reported, including the subdural space, mastoid air cells, thoracic lymphatic duct, fallopian tube, gall bladder, salivary ducts, stomach, and small intestine. Most of these sites are rarely, if ever, used today.

Ventriculoatrial shunting remained the most popular shunting procedure until ventriculoperitoneal procedures began to gain popularity at the end of the 1960s. The ventriculoperitoneal shunt was attractive for its simplicity, the absence of a permanent foreign body in the vascular system, and the reduced need for revision with inevitable growth of the patient.

III. CSF PRODUCTION AND ABSORPTION

A. Anatomy

1. Ventricular System

The foramen of Munro allows CSF to travel from the lateral ventricles to the third ventricle and the aqueduct of Sylvins connects the third and fourth ventricles. Much of CSF is produced by the choroid plexus of the ventricular system and leaves through the openings in the fourth ventricle (foramina of Luschka and Magendie) into the subarachnoid space that surrounds the brain and spinal cord. It then travels around the convexities up to the sagittal sinus.

2. Choroid Plexus

The choroid plexus is the source of 60% of CSF production: It is composed of villi, which secrete CSF. Hypersecretion of CSF is virtually never a source of hydrocephalus. It should be noted that 40% of CSF is probably derived from fluid from brain parenchyma.

3. Arachnoid Villi

Arachnoid villi are specialized clusters of arachnoid cells that appear to allow CSF absorption into the sinuses and perhaps along nerve roots. In dogs and some other animals, there are no villi: CSF is absorbed along nerve root sheaths. In humans, arachnoid villi seem to absorb about 60% of CSF; the rest may be absorbed by nerve root sheaths as well.

B. CSF

CSF is continuously produced at the rate of approximately 500 cc/day. The total volume of CSF is approximately 150 ml at any time. CSF is formed as an ultrafiltrate from the villi of the choroid plexus and production is partially regulated by the enzymes sodium potassium ATPase and carbonic anhydrase. One function of the CSF appears to be mechanical, serving as a kind of water jacket for the spinal cord and brain, protecting them from potentially injurious blows to the spinal column and skull and acute changes in venous pressure. CSF hydraulically balances the brain within the skull.

The CSF is also believed to serve to remove waste metabolites of cerebral metabolism and may act as a pathway for distribution of peptides and hormones within the nervous system. This possible function has never been adequately explored.

IV. CLASSIFICATION

Hydrocephalus may be classified as acute or chronic (in acute, there are symptoms for weeks; in chronic, there are symptoms for months); communicating versus noncommunicating (in communicating hydrocephalus, there is flow between the ventricular system and subarachnoid space; in noncommunicating hydrocephalus, there is a block to flow within the ventricular cistern); congenital (acquired at birth) versus acquired; and normal pressure versus high pressure, a distinction that depends on the symptom complex.

A. Congenital

Several congenital structural abnormalities can lead to obstruction of CSF flow and result in hydrocephalus.

1. Aqueductal Stenosis

Different conditions may obstruct the aqueduct, leading to CSF accumulation above the level of the aqueduct that may be congenitally stenosed, occluded by a septum, compressed by gliosis in the surrounding periaqueductal tissue, or "forked." It can also be compressed or kinked by structural abnormalities or masses.

In aqueductal stenosis, the fourth ventricle, which lies beyond the point of obstruction, is typically normal in size. The term triventricular hydrocephalus has been used for this condition, referring to the enlargement of the third and both lateral ventricles.

2. Dandy–Walker Malformation

In this abnormality, there is atresia of the foramina of Luschka and Magendie along with agenesis of the cerebellar vermis. A large posterior fossa cyst results that communicates with an enlarged fourth ventricle. Hydrocephalus results in most of these cases.

3. Neonatal Intraventricular Hemorrhage

This condition is acquired particularly in premature infants and is characterized by progressive ventricular enlargement.

B. Acquired

1. Mass Lesions/Tumors

Masses may compress CSF pathways. This is a potential cause of hydrocephalus in those portions of the ventricular system proximal to the obstruction. Any tumor along the CSF path may be involved. Colloid cysts of the third ventricle, pineal region tumors, and fourth ventricular tumors are examples. A tumor in the midbrain, for example, can cause critical aqueductal compression, resulting in hydrocephalus similar to congenital aqueductal stenosis. A cyst around the foramen of Monro can cause trapping of the lateral ventricle on that side. A posterior fossa tumor blocks aqueductal flow as well.

Tumors associated with abnormally high CSF protein concentrations impede reabsorption; ependymomas and other tumors of the spinal canal can do this. Diffuse spreading of tumor in the subarachnoid space can lead to hydrocephalus presumably due to both a higher CSF protein concentration and blockade of the arachnoid granulations.

2. Infection

Meningitis can result in fibrosis of the basal cisterns and arachnoid granulations that can lead to an obstruction of CSF around the brain stem. This includes tuberculosis meningitis, which is notorious for producing hydrocephalus.

3. Posthemorrhagic

Subarachnoid hemorrhage (most commonly from aneurysmal bleeding) and intraventricular hemorrhage can result in hydrocephalus because of the protein obstruction of arachnoid villi as well as inflammation of the aqueduct.

4. Idiopathic Normal Pressure Hydrocephalus

This entity was described by Hakim in 1965. It comprises communicating hydrocephalus with normal intraventricular pressures. Although a cause is not identified in most cases, it is usually believed to result from one of the obstructive causes described previously. An initial increase in pressure may lead to ventricular dilatation that reaches equilibrium, with pressures then returning to the normal range.

It is an important diagnosis because it is a treatable cause of dementia and gait disorder in the elderly. It is classically characterized by the triad of progressive gait disorder, dementia, and urinary incontinence. The gait disorder is usually shuffling with a broad base. Dementia is a recent memory disorder.

C. Pseudotumor Cerebri/Idiopathic Intracranial Hypertension

This diagnosis of exclusion is characterized by elevated intracranial pressure and papilledema in the absence of intracranial tumor or other recognized cause for increased pressure or hydrocephalus. Unlike hydrocephalus, most adults with this condition have normal or even "slit" ventricles on imaging studies. Headache is the cardinal syndrome. The mechanism of increased pressure is unclear in this condition but it appears to be a result of blockage at CSF outflow.

D. "Arrested" Hydrocephalus

This term refers to a condition of ventriculomegaly with no symptoms: The ventricles may sometimes be very large. It is not clear whether it is truly asymptomatic, as there may be very subtle problems associated with it.

V. DIAGNOSIS

A. Clinical

Infants may present with such symptoms as a large head, irritability, delayed development, and vomiting. Older children and adults may describe headaches, nausea/vomiting, or visual changes (diplopia, decreased acuity, or field cuts) as high-pressure symptoms. In normal pressure hydrocephalus the symptoms are gait difficulty, slowing of action, memory loss, and incontinence.

1. Exam

a. Infants Before the cranial sutures are "closed," the size of the head will enlarge in hydrocephalus. The fontanelles may be noted to be bulging and/or firm, with palpable separation of the suture lines between cranial vault bones. The scalp veins may be engorged and the eyes may not elevate above the meridian. The head circumference is increased when compared with standard growth charts.

b. Ophthalmologic Findings Infants may present with the "setting sun sign." This results from upward gaze palsy from pressure in the suprapineal recess.

There may also be an abducens nerve palsy that manifests as a weakness of sideways gaze. The long intracranial course of the abducens nerve makes it vulnerable to stretch injury in hydrocephalus.

These symptoms may also present in adults, but they are typically later or more unusual findings. More common is the presence of papilledema that results from transmission of CSF pressure along the sheath of the optic nerve to the optic disc.

2. Other Findings

Severe cases or those of rapid onset may be associated with reflex bradycardia or, in infants, apneic spells. Sudden death may occur from rapid decompression. A variety of endocrine abnormalities have also been associated with hydrocephalus, including infantilism and precocious puberty. These have been ascribed, at least in part, to the compression of the pituitary gland by ballooning and thinning of the floor of the third ventricle.

Memory loss, spastic paraparesis with mild spastic weakness of the upper extremities, and less often a mild dysmetria of the extremities may be signs and symptoms. Agitated state is sometimes a factor.

In adults and children older than 1 year, hydrocephalus may present with either a high-pressure or normal pressure syndrome. The high-pressure syndrome includes headache, nausea, and vomiting. The normal pressure syndrome includes gait disturbance with a broad base and small steps, memory loss, urinary incontinence, and slowing of action.

B. Imaging

1. Computed Tomography

Computed tomography (CT) scanning will show ventricular enlargement and may also help determine the cause of hydrocephalus (e.g., tumors/cysts, congenital anomalies, or the presence of blood). Asymmetry of the ventricular system or the pattern of ventricular enlargement may also suggest the cause, as in aqueductal stenosis. Periventricular hypodensity may be present in some cases, suggesting **extravasation** of fluid into the periventricular space. Besides their role in diagnosis, CT scans are also essential for assessing response to treatment as well as follow-up.

2. Magnetic Resonance Imaging

Conventional magnetic resonance imaging (MRI) provides similar information as that of CT scanning about ventricular size, but MRI has a higher yield in identifying or characterizing associated or causative abnormalities. Special sequences are useful for identifying or quantifying flow through the aqueduct, for example, and making the diagnosis of aqueductal stenosis as well as determining the efficacy of certain forms of treatment, such as endoscopic ventriculostomy.

3. Ultrasound

This imaging modality is practical only in infants who have a patent fontanelle. Its usefulness lies in its relative low cost (compared to CT and MRI) as well as its ease of application at the bedside or in restless infants. It is excellent at establishing ventricular size, symmetry, and even the cause of hydrocephalus (most commonly, intraventricular blood in this age group). It is also extremely useful for follow-up after treatment until the age of approximately 6 months, when the anterior fontanelle becomes too small.

C. CSF Pressure Monitoring

Monitoring of ventricular pressure is used occasionally in the context of normal pressure hydrocephalus. Lumbar puncture is an important tool in assessing CSF pressure but should be avoided in noncommunicating hydrocephalus. Measurement over several hours may result in the diagnosis of normal pressure hydrocephalus.

VI. TREATMENT

The treatment of hydrocephalus is largely surgical. Medical therapies are either obsolete or temporizing.

A. Medical Therapy

Abandoned therapies include glycerol, isosorbide, radioactive gold, and head wrapping. Diuretics are occasionally used for neonatal hydrocephalus secondary to intraventricular hemorrhage to temporize ICP control until enough blood is reabsorbed. Acetazolamide and furosemide are the drugs typically used, but both can cause significant electrolyte imbalance.

In neonatal IVH, spinal taps also serve as a temporizing measure to keep ICP in the "safe" range until CSF reabsorption resumes. In cases in which ventricular enlargement persists after the disappearance of blood and return of CSF protein to near normal levels, the patients must proceed to surgical therapy.

B. Surgical Therapy

The bulk of therapy for hydrocephalus is surgical. In an acute situation, CSF may be drained via a ventricular catheter to a sterile bag. Normally this is not done for longer than 2 weeks. Most hydrocephalus is treated by shunt placement. Shunts are permanently implantable devices for the diversion of CSF to one of several extracranial sites. They consist of a ventricular catheter, a valve, and tubing draining to a body cavity.

1. Temporary Diversion

Temporary diversion is sometimes sought when there is known infection in the CSF space precluding the implantation of permanent devices. This temporary diversion typically employs a catheter inserted into the ventricle that is tunneled underneath the scalp and connected to an external drainage bag. These systems are utilized for a few days until a permanent shunt can be placed if possible.

2. Routes of Diversion

The ventriculoperitoneal shunt is the most frequently employed route of diversion. Advantages include its relative simplicity and its complications are typically easier to manage than with other routes of diversion.

The ventricular catheter is inserted into the frontal horn of one of the lateral ventricles via frontal or occipital approaches. It is attached underneath the scalp to a valve, from which tubing passes subcutaneously down to the peritoneal cavity. This operation is often performed employing only two small incisions—the first for passing the catheter into the ventricle and the second for entry into the peritoneal cavity. The tubing is passed from one incision to the other using specially designed tunneling devices.

Ventriculoatrial shunting was the preferred route for shunting before ventriculoperitoneal shunting became popular. It is still widely employed primarily in some centers or where peritoneal shunting cannot be used.

The ventricular catheter is placed in the standard way, and the distal tubing is passed into the internal jugular vein and down to the right atrium, usually through the common facial vein, which is a small tributary of the jugular vein in the neck.

Other distal sites include the pleural cavity (a common option for diversion after the peritoneal cavity), the gallbladder, and ureter. These are rarely employed because of technical difficulty, much higher complication rates, and diversion to the ureters has typically required a nephrectomy.

Torkildsen preceded extracranial CSF shunting in its development. It involves the placement of a catheter from the lateral ventricle into the cisterna magna—the large subarachnoid space adjacent to the cerebellum and brain stem. It is useful only for aqueductal stenosis, a fourth ventricular pathology. It has been replaced by endoscopic ventricular fenestration.

There are two main valve types: differential pressure valves and variable resistance constant flow vavles. Different pressure valves provide a constant resistance and permit the flow of CSF when a certain hydrostatic pressure has been exceeded. This is the common basic valve design and includes slit valves, ball-in-cone valves, and diaphragm valves. Recently, a variable pressure valve has been created that controls the pressure of CSF release.

Variable resistance constant flow valves attempt to maintain more natural constant flow rates by varying the amount of resistance to flow in response to pressure changes and, indirectly, to posture. These valves are believed to lead to overdrainage less often than do differential pressure designs.

The use of lumboperitoneal shunts fell out of favor largely because of distal obstruction and the high incidence of kyphoscoliosis. Use of these shunts involved a laminectomy, and the tubing initially used had a propensity to cause a chemical arachnoiditis.

This technique has been repopularized with the introduction of less irritating Silastic tubing and due to the ability to place the tubing percutaneously, with specially designed needles, into the subarachnoid space without a laminectomy.

3. Endoscopic Therapy

The most common endoscopic technique in use today is the third ventriculostomy method. This is used when CSF absorption is believed to be normal but there is an obstruction to its egress from the third ventricle. In this procedure, an endoscope is introduced into the third ventricle (typically via a frontal approach) and a small hole is made in the floor of the third ventricle to permit the flow of CSF from this cavity into the subarachnoid space, thereby bypassing any mechanical obstruction in the ventricular system. The major indication for this procedure is aqueductal stenosis. Most surgeons, however, are not specifically trained in performing this procedure, and its widespread application is further limited by patient selection.

Newer endoscopic techniques include aqueductoplasty, which involves the endoscopic repair of short-segment strictures in the aqueduct, but experience is still limited with this procedure.

4. Lesion Removal

Occasionally, there are clinical situations in which a single lesion can be removed to cure, or at least improve, hydrocephalus. Certain tumors are amenable to removal. A choroid plexus papilloma, which over-produces CSF, can be resected, thereby obviating the need for a shunt. Another typical example is a colloid cyst, which commonly occurs around the foramen of Monro, obstructing CSF flow. Resection can lead to complete resolution of the obstructive hydrocephalus.

5. Choroid Plexectomy (Obsolete)

This procedure was performed as an open operation and involved the cauterization of choroid plexus. This carried a very high mortality early on, and it fell into disfavor. Later attempts were made to perform this endoscopically, and mortality rates decreased significantly, but it has not regained widespread use because of the relative safety and ease of other operations.

VII. COMPLICATIONS

Hydrocephalus, treated or untreated, results in a number of problems, some of which are described here. Untreated, hydrocephalus can result ultimately in death. Where its onset is relatively acute, the resulting increase in intracranial pressure will compress brain stem structures to the point at which neurovegetative functions are compromised. In more chronic courses, progressive neurological decline occurs, which will affect motor function, gait, and behavior.

Blindness may result from cortical lesions or damage to the visual pathways. Cortical blindness is caused by occlusion of the posterior cerebral arteries by downward pressure on them against the tentorial notch. Papilledema caused by increased CSF pressure may lead to optic atrophy and blindness.

Neurodevelopmental impairment can be attributed to both hydrocephalus and the initial condition that resulted in it. Hydrocephalus, where untreated, appears to cause sustained stretching of neurons and associated fibers, and this probably results in many of the clinical manifestations seen in the condition.

A. Shunt Malfunction

Shunt malfunction is typically the result of an obstruction in the shunt system. This may be proximal (in or around the ventricular catheter) or distal (in or around the peritoneal or other distal end). Occasionally, the valve may be obstructed by debris. These situations will often require surgery for replacement of the obstructed portion.

Proximal obstruction of the ventricular catheter is typically caused by adherent choroid plexus, debris, blood, or adherent brain tissue. Rarely, growing tumor or the inflammation resulting from infection can also result in proximal obstruction.

In the peritoneal cavity, obstruction is typically the result of low-grade infection that eventually causes formation of a pseudocyst around the tip of the catheter. Obstruction may also be caused by debris or malposition of the catheter from the initial surgery. Progressive growth of a patient who had a catheter placed early in childhood can lead to its withdrawal from the peritoneal cavity because it becomes too short for the patient's gradual increase in length. This previously common occurrence is relatively rare today because long redundant lengths of tubing are left in the abdomen at initial placement to account for expected growth. Disconnections, breaks, kinks, and other mechanical disruptions in the distal tubing may also occur.

B. Overdrainage

It is possible to "overdrain" CSF with a shunt. In the short term, this can result in symptoms similar to those of a "spinal headache," specifically headaches, nausea, and vomiting that tend to be postural and are relieved by recumbency. These symptoms will sometimes improve with time, but they may require shunt revision with a valve of higher pressure/lower flow rate or the addition of a so-called "antisiphon" device to the system to prevent overdrainage with upright posture. With variable pressure valves the pressure can simply be raised.

Overshunting of ventricles in the presence of thinned or atrophic brain can lead to collapsing away from the skull. This creates a subdural hygroma. This can result in tearing to bridging veins in the subdural space, causing bleeding, and the accumulation of a subdural hematoma.

Slit ventricle syndrome is a poorly understood complication of ventricular shunting characterized by collapsed or slit ventricles. It appears to occur when chronic overshunting of the ventricles results in a very low compliance state. The ventricles become slits and their walls may occlude the catheter impeding CSF drainage. The low compliance of the ventricular system then causes an abnormal increase in intraventricular pressure with small accumulations of CSF and symptoms of increased ICP result.

This problem is very difficult to treat. Options include replacing the ventricular catheter, changing to a higher pressure valve, or inserting an antisiphon device. Skull decompression is sometimes employed as a last resort on the principle that the miniscule increase in intracranial volume is enough to compensate for the changed compliance of the brain in this condition.

C. Shunt Infections

Shunt infections occur in about 10% of shunt procedures in children but are much less common in adults. They may occur at any time in relation to shunt placement and have been reported more than 10 years after shunt placement. The bacteria causing such infections are typically skin flora such as *Staphylococcus epidermidis* and *Propionibacterium* spp.

Most authorities recommend removing the entire shunt system in these circumstances, using an external diversion system during treatment with appropriate intravenous antibiotics, and placement of a new shunt after an interval from several days to a couple of weeks depending on a number of factors, including the virulence of the identified organism and the sterilization of CSF on serial cultures.

Other complications with shunts include the following:

- Occasional seizures (1%) that can result from the cortical irritation from catheter placement.
- Ascites (with peritoneal shunts) or pleural effusions (with pleural shunts) from poor local absorption of CSF.
- Bowel perforation, which can occur at the time of shunt insertion or even years later from gra-

dual erosion of the shunt tubing into the bowel lumen.
- Specific problems with atrial shunting, including bacteremia and endocarditis as well as shunt nephritis, which for poorly understood reasons appears to result from the deposition of antigen–antibody complexes in the renal glomeruli following shunt infection. Pulmonary emboli (which can be septic) can also occur, leading to pulmonary infarction.

Outcome in hydrocephalus is related to the increased ICP as well as the primary cause of the condition. Deaths from hydrocephalus in countries in which neurosurgeons and shunt are available are uncommon. One study cited an 80–90% 5-year survival rate in children with hydrocephalus. Most data on mortality are set in the context of treatment complications. Death from shunt failure is rare, with reported rates of approximately 1%.

Cognitive deficits are difficult to interpret in the context of underlying brain abnormalities. One study examining children with arrested (untreated) hydrocephalus found 25% with IQs below 50 and 45% with IQs higher than 85%. Another study examining children with treated hydrocephalus found 72% with IQs between 70 and 100 and 32% with IQs higher than 100. Only 4% had IQs below 70.

VIII. OUTCOME

Some patients have a higher likelihood of benefiting from CSF diversion than others, in terms of motor function. Up to three-fourths of patients with normal pressure hydrocephalus in which gait dysfunction is the primary symptom will improve after shunting. On the other hand, patients with dementia and no gait disorder will rarely benefit from surgery.

In children, shunt placement for high pressure hydrocephalus is likely to lead to complete reversal of high pressure symptoms.

See Also the Following Articles

BRAIN ANATOMY AND NETWORKS • VENTRICULAR SYSTEM

Suggested Reading

Scott, R. M. (Ed.) (1990). *Hydrocephalus*. Williams & Wilkins, Baltimore.

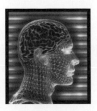

Hypothalamus

J. PATRICK CARD and LINDA RINAMAN

University of Pittsburgh

GLOSSARY

circumventricular organs Areas of the brain that lack a blood–brain barrier and are found on the midline surrounding the third and fourth ventricles. These regions are essential "windows" through which the brain exerts humoral control of peripheral systems and are also responsive to feedback humoral influences from the systems that they modulate.

fornix A well-defined myelinated fiber bundle that serves as an important histological landmark in the hypothalamus and is also the principle conduit through which neurons in the subiculum project to the mammillary bodies.

infundibular stalk The ventral evagination of the floor of the third ventricle that connects the hypothalamus to the pituitary gland. It contains the long portal vessels that transport release and inhibiting factors from hypothalamus to the anterior lobe of the pituitary gland and is also the conduit for axons of magnocellular neurons that terminate in the posterior (neural) lobe of the pituitary.

median eminence The highly vascularized portion of the tuber cinereum that is essential for hypothalamic regulation of the anterior lobe of the pituitary. The blood vessels in this region lack a blood–brain barrier and are therefore capable of transporting peptides and neurotransmitters from the hypothalamus to the anterior lobe.

stria terminalis A major fiber pathway through which the amygdala communicates with the hypothalamus.

tuber cinereum The protuberance on the ventral surface of the diencephalon that contains the median eminence and gives rise to the infundibular stalk.

The hypothalamus is a remarkable region of the central nervous system. This small subdivision of the ventral diencephalon communicates extensively with other regions of the neuraxis via classical synaptic interactions and also has profound influences on the hormonal regulation of peripheral organ systems. In essence, it is directly responsible for the regulatory control of homeostatic systems essential for survival of the parent organism. The ability of this region to exert such profound influence over behavioral state and physiology is reflected in both the properties of hypothalamic neurons and the mechanisms through which they communicate. Thus, the dynamic regulatory capabilities of the hypothalamus are defined by the unique properties (e.g., timekeeping capabilities) of its constituent neurons, the ability to influence peripheral systems by virtue of hormonal or "humoral" communication, and the responsiveness of hypothalamic neurons to feedback control by the peripheral systems that they regulate. This article reviews the basic organizational principles fundamental to hypothalamic function, focusing on well-studied hypothalamic systems that illustrate the functional parcellation of this small but influential region of the brain.

I. HYPOTHALAMIC ORGANIZATION

As its name implies, the hypothalamus is found below the thalamus in the diencephalon (Fig. 1). It is

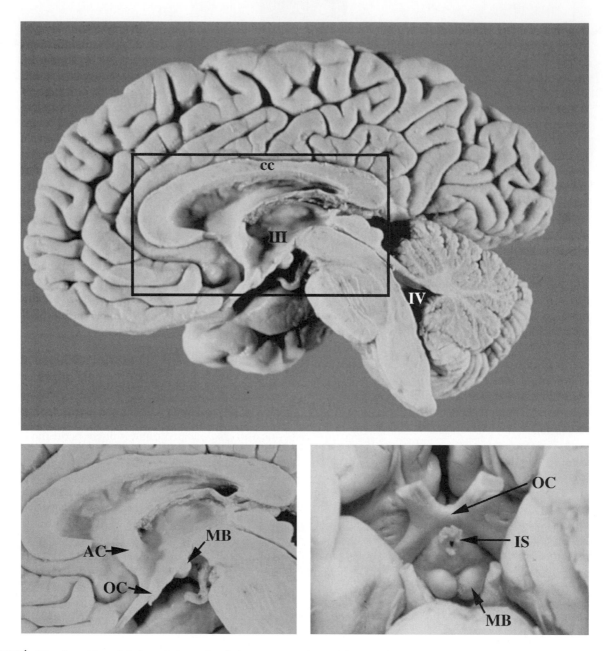

Figure 1 The disposition of the hypothalamus in relation to other regions of the central nervous system is illustrated in sagittal and ventral exposures of the human brain. In sagittal exposures of the brain the hypothalamus occupies a small region bounded by the anterior commissure (AC), optic chiasm (OC), and mammillary body. Ventral exposure of the brain reveals the three prominent landmarks that define the floor of the hypothalamus: the OC rostrally, the infundibular stalk (IS) arising from the tuber cinereum, and the paired spherical protuberances that constitute the MBs. III, third ventricle; IV, fourth ventricle.

distinguished by distinct external landmarks on the ventral surface of the brain that define its full rostrocaudal extent. These include the optic chiasm rostrally, the intermediate tuber cinereum marked by the prominent infundibular stalk, and the caudally placed mammillary bodies. Classic literature used these external landmarks to define internal subdivisions of the hypothalamus. Thus, it is still common to find references to the chiasmatic, tuberal, and mammillary subdivisions of hypothalamus. However, as our knowledge of the organization, connectivity, and function of hypothalamic cell groups has improved, the rationale for dividing the hypothalamus into three regions defined by external landmarks has become less compelling. Nevertheless, these landmarks remain useful designations for defining the general location of hypothalamic cell groups and are commonly found in the literature.

Coronal sections through the hypothalamus reveal prominent internal landmarks that have proven useful in defining the basic organization of hypothalamic cell and fiber systems. Among the most prominent is the third ventricle that separates much of the hypothalamus into identical halves. The fluid-filled reservoir is particularly prominent in the intermediate portion of the hypothalamus demarcated by the tuber cinereum. In coronal sections through this level, the lumen of the ventricle defines the dorsoventral extent of the hypothalamus. The floor of the third ventricle is formed by a thin bridge of tissue, commonly known as the median eminence, that is continuous with a stalk connecting the ventral hypothalamus to the pituitary gland. The median eminence is among the most important interfaces through which the hypothalamus exerts regulatory control over peripheral systems in that it is essential for regulation of hormone secretion from the pituitary gland. It is similar to another midline strip of tissue that contains the organum vasculosum of the lamina terminalis (OVLT) and that forms the rostral wall of the third ventricle in that it lacks a blood–brain barrier (BBB). The absence of the BBB at these sites provides the essential means for neurohumoral communication and will be considered in greater detail later.

The internal organization of the hypothalamus is characterized best in histological preparations of coronal sections. Classic Nissl preparations reveal three longitudinal zones that extend throughout the rostrocaudal extent of the hypothalamus. The location of each zone can be defined in relation to its proximity to the third ventricle and a prominent myelinated fiber bundle, the fornix, that enters the hypothalamus rostrally and then courses caudally to terminate in the mammillary bodies. The *periventricular* zone is a densely packed group of neurons immediately adjacent to the third ventricle. Occasionally, it contains well-demarcated cell groups, such as the suprachiasmatic, arcuate, or paraventricular nuclei. However, in the majority of its extent it is composed of a thin, densely packed group of neurons immediately adjacent to the ependymal lining of the ventricle. The *medial* zone is found between the periventricular zone and a vertical plane passing through the fornix. Nuclear groups in this region (e.g., the ventromedial

and dorsomedial nuclei) are among the most prominent and well-delineated cell groups in the hypothalamus. The *lateral* zone is found between the medial zone and the optic tract and internal capsule at the lateral extent of the diencephalon. Neurons in this region are more dispersed and do not form the distinct nuclear groups characteristic of the periventricular and medial zones. Nevertheless, immunohistochemical studies that have revealed distinct phenotypic parcellation of neurons in the lateral zone have contributed greatly to improving our understanding of the functional organization of this region.

II. MAJOR HYPOTHALAMIC CONNECTIONS

Connectional analyses have contributed greatly to our understanding of hypothalamic function and organization. Two well-known fiber tracts, the fornix and stria terminalis, provide major conduits through which the hypothalamus interacts with subdivisions of the limbic system. Each of these fiber tracts originates in the temporal lobe and pursues a looping trajectory over the thalamus to enter the hypothalamus dorsally and rostrally. An interesting new literature, particularly with respect to the fornix, has provided novel insights into the way in which axons traversing these pathways influence hypothalamic function. These advances have not only improved our understanding of how the hypothalamus functions within a larger ensemble of neurons but also provided a functional rationale supporting the aforementioned zonal organization of the hypothalamus.

As noted previously, early descriptions of hypothalamic organization established the intrahypothalamic course of the fornix as an important landmark separating the medial and lateral hypothalamic zones. Fibers traversing this tract divide into pre- and postcommissural bundles that pass either rostral or caudal to the anterior commissure. Individual axons of the postcommissural bundle leave the fornix along its course to terminate in hypothalamic nuclei while others continue caudally to terminate in the mammillary bodies. Axons in the precommissural fornix pass rostrally to terminate topographically within subdivisions of the lateral septum. The lateral septal neurons, in turn, project densely on the periventricular, medial, and lateral zones of the hypothalamus. Thus, the hippocampus provides a prominent topographically organized influence upon hypothalamic zones through parallel organized disynaptic projections involving the lateral septal nuclei. From the standpoint of sheer magnitude and number of hypothalamic neurons targeted by these disynaptic projections, it would appear that the precommissural fornix has a much more substantial influence upon hypothalamic function than the axons that course through the post-commissural branch.

Prominent limbic influences on hypothalamic function also arise from the amygdaloid complex and course into the hypothalamus through either the stria terminalis or the ventral amygdalofugal pathway. In contrast to the fornix, these afferents do not segregate within hypothalamic zones. Rather, evidence indicates that they provide more directed input to hypothalamic areas and cell groups. For example, axons that course through the stria terminalis terminate more densely in the rostral rather than the caudal hypothalamus and also provide dense input to subsets of nuclei within a zone.

The medial forebrain bundle (MFB) is another prominent fiber tract associated with the hypothalamus. The trajectory of this projection system brings it through the full rostrocaudal extent of the lateral hypothalamus. This pathway is more diffusely organized than the postcommissural fornix and carries both ascending and descending fibers. Many of the axons that pass through the MFB are simply traversing the hypothalamus in transit to other forebrain targets. The prominent dopaminergic projections from the substantia nigra and ventral tegmental area fall into this category. Brain stem noradrenergic and cholinergic neurons also project through the MFB to both diencephalic and telencephalic targets. Thus, whereas the MFB is an important conduit for axons innervating the hypothalamus, it is also a major projection pathway for axons projecting to and from forebrain nuclei. Loss of function in response to lesions that interrupted these fibers of passage confounded the interpretation of results from early studies that incorrectly ascribed functions to hypothalamic nuclei that were, in fact, subserved by axons passing through the hypothalamus in the MFB. Improvements in tract tracing and lesioning methods, as well as the development of other functional probes, have clarified many of these false interpretations.

III. THE HYPOTHALAMUS AND THE TEMPORAL ORGANIZATION OF BEHAVIOR

The hypothalamus has long been recognized as an important integrative area for the regulatory control of behavioral state and the temporal organization of behavior. Early evidence from lesion and stimulation paradigms implicated regions of the hypothalamus in the control of sleep and other rhythmic aspects of behavior and physiology. However, identification of the specific circuitry through which the hypothalamus coordinates internal homeostatic function with sensory stimuli of the environment only occurred with the advent of technical advances that permitted the identification and functional dissection of populations of hypothalamic neurons. Today, our knowledge of the neural systems that exert regulatory influence over these functions is far more precise, and in some instances the molecular mechanisms that contribute to this control are beginning to be unraveled. The following sections review the functional organization of hypothalamic systems that participate in the control of rhythmic functions, sleep, and arousal.

A. A Biological Clock in Hypothalamus

It has long been clear that mammals and other organisms exhibit daily cycles in physiology and behavior that persist in the absence of sensory input from the environment. These cycles are approximately 1 day in length (hence the term circadian) and in normal circumstances are synchronized with the environment. In essence, they are rhythms of behavior and physiology that are tightly coupled to the most pervasive signal in our environment, the daily rhythm of light and dark. The adaptive significance of such an endogenous timekeeping mechanism is obvious when one considers the practical benefits of synchronizing behavior to the light-dark cycle. Certainly, the restriction of the activity of nocturnal animals to nighttime has the practical advantage of reducing the possibility of predation, and the ability to precisely measure day length permits seasonal breeders to deliver their progeny during the portion of the year when nutrients are most prevalent. Thus, it is not surprising that this endogenous timekeeping system is among the oldest and most highly conserved systems of regulatory control in the animal kingdom.

Although circadian rhythms in both plants and animals have been long been recognized, determination that a "biological clock" resides in the hypothalamus of mammals is a relatively recent event that can be traced to anatomical studies conducted in the early 1970s. Recognizing that the entraining influences of light are essential to any timekeeping system, two research groups independently utilized new methods of defining neuronal connectivity to demonstrate that a circumscribed group of neurons overlying the optic chiasm receives dense retinal inputs. These neurons, comprising the suprachiasmatic nuclei (SCN), became the experimental focus of circadian biologists and there is now considerable evidence supporting the conclusion that a biological clock resides in the SCN of mammals. Specifically, animal studies have shown that the cells of the SCN exhibit a circadian rhythm of activity that is entrained by light, and that rhythmic aspects of physiology and behavior are abolished in animals in which the SCN have been destroyed. Importantly, it is also known that the rhythmicity of SCN neurons is genetically determined rather than the emergent property of a network, and "clock" genes that impart rhythmicity to SCN neurons have been identified. Thus, the hypothalamus contains a clock, the SCN, whose activity is synchronized to the external environment by virtue of sensory input transduced by the retina.

Elucidating the connections of the SCN has been an important component of understanding how this group of hypothalamic neurons imposes its temporal message on the physiology and behavior of the parent organism. One of the most well-characterized systems in this regard is the circuitry through which the SCN exerts regulatory control over the secretion of the hormone melatonin. Melatonin is secreted by the pineal gland in a circadian manner but is also responsive to light such that light stimulation during the dark phase of the photoperiod inhibits the normally high levels of melatonin secretion. This dynamic regulatory capacity renders the temporal profile of melatonin secretion a precise measure of day length. A large literature has established that the SCN controls both the circadian and photoperiodic aspects of melatonin secretion through multisynaptic pathways that sequentially involve the paraventricular hypothalamic nucleus, the intermediolateral cell column of the spinal cord, and neurons of the superior cervical ganglion that project to the pineal. Additionally, binding studies and localization of melatonin receptors have revealed that melatonin exerts feedback influence on the brain by binding to neurons in the SCN, paraventricular thalamic nucleus, and pars tuberalis of the infundibular stalk. Thus, the SCN not only regulates the secretion of melatonin but also is subject to feedback regulation by the hormone that it modulates. This is a common feature of the neurohumoral regulation exerted by the hypothalamus.

The SCN also imparts temporal organization to other systems and appears to do so through efferent projections that are largely confined to the hypothalamus. SCN neurons project to a relatively restricted group of nuclei in the hypothalamus that includes, but is not limited to, the region subjacent to the paraventricular nucleus (the subparaventricular zone), the preoptic area, and medial hypothalamic nuclei (e.g., arcuate and dorsomedial) involved in neuroendocrine regulation of pituitary function. These projections provide a substrate through which the SCN imparts temporal influences on a variety of systems.

B. The Hypothalamus and Sleep

Evidence that the hypothalamus is involved in the control of sleep emerged from a large literature dating to the early 1900s. Lesion studies correlating anterior hypothalamic damage with insomnia and caudal hypothalamic damage with somnolence were particularly informative. These and subsequent studies resulted in the concept of hypothalamic "sleep centers." A fascinating recent literature has demonstrated a cellular basis for hypothalamic influences on sleep and also provided insights into the means through which temporal organization is imparted on this behavior. It is now apparent that at least two distinct populations of neurons in the rostral and caudal hypothalamus are responsible for the hypothalamic effects on sleep. Using a creative experimental approach, it was demonstrated that neurons in a circumscribed region of the preoptic area [the ventrolateral preoptic nucleus (VLPO)] in rats express Fos, the protein product of the protooncogene *c-fos*, shortly following the onset of sleep. Since Fos expression reflects neuronal activation, this observation raised the possibility that VLPO neurons are involved in the initiation of sleep. A number of subsequent observations have validated this hypothesis and also revealed the larger network of hypothalamic neurons that participate in this function. Specifically, evidence now supports the conclusion that VLPO neurons inhibit arousal through projections to histaminergic neurons in the tuberomammillary (TM) nuclei of the caudal hypothalamus. In support of this conclusion, it was shown that GABAergic neurons in VLPO synapse on TM neurons and that pharmacological inhibition of TM neurons or blockade of histaminergic receptors promotes sleep. Those who recall the drowsiness that typically follows the use of early antihistamines (which act on central as well as peripheral histamine receptors) prescribed for the treatment of colds and allergies can appreciate the major influence of the diffusely project-ing neurons of the TM nuclei upon arousal.

Importantly, neurochemical lesions of VLPO and surrounding neurons have revealed greater functional parcellation of the anterior hypothalamic circuitry involved in sleep regulation. Cell-selective lesions that do not interrupt fibers of passage were shown to compromise different aspects of sleep based on the localization of the lesion. Lesions confined to the compact portion of VLPO dramatically reduce non-REM sleep and, in circumstances in which lesions are incomplete, the amount of non-REM sleep is linearly correlated with the number of Fos-expressing neurons in the portion of the VLPO that survived the lesion. Interestingly, lesions dorsal to VLPO that eliminate galanin-containing neurons that project to TM pro-duce sleep deficits more closely associated with REM than with non-REM sleep. Collectively, these obser-vations provide compelling evidence in support of a prominent role for the hypothalamus in sleep regula-tion and further indicate that there is functional parcellation in the neurons of the VLPO that partici-pate in this control.

It is also clear that the hypothalamus plays an important role in the temporal organization of the sleep–wake cycle. Sleep is a circadian function, and although the SCN is not essential for the generation of sleep, it is responsible for consolidation of sleep within cycles that occur within a circadian framework. Thus, if the SCN are destroyed, rats will sleep approximately the same amount of time but this sleeping time will be distributed in many short bouts throughout the light–dark cycle rather than in a consolidated period. The circuitry through which the SCN imposes this circa-dian influence on sleep remains to be established, but it is likely that it occurs via polysynaptic connec-tions that link the clock to nuclei involved in sleep regulation.

C. Hypothalamic Influences upon Arousal

Certainly, the aforementioned studies that have de-monstrated a role for hypothalamic nuclei in sleep indicate that the hypothalamus influences arousal states. However, recent studies have demonstrated that the influence of the hypothalamus on arousal is not restricted to the TM neurons in caudal hypotha-lamus. In particular, a prominent group of neurons confined to the lateral hypothalamus has recently been implicated in the sleep disorder known as narcolepsy. These neurons express novel neuropep-tides known as hypocretins or orexins and are differentially concentrated within the perifornical nucleus that surrounds the fornix in the tuberal hypothalamus. Mapping studies have shown that hypocretin/orexin neurons are similar to TM neurons in that they are confined to hypothalamus and give rise to extensive projections throughout the neuraxis. However, it is also clear that these neurons densely innervate areas (e.g., locus coeruleus) involved in the control of arousal, and there is good evidence that pathology of signaling pathways involving hypocretin neurons may be causal in narcolepsy. In this disorder, individuals exhibit daytime sleepiness and lapse un-expectedly into bouts of REM sleep. A dog model of the disease has identified a deletion in the gene encoding the hypocretin 2 receptor, and knockout mice lacking the hypocretin gene exhibit sleep dis-turbances similar to narcolepsy. Further, examination of postmortem human brains of narcoleptics has revealed substantial reductions in the number of hypocretin neurons, raising the possibility that the disease may be due to an autoimmune attack on the neurons. Thus, there is strong evidence that caudal hypothalamic neurons play an integral role in the regulation of arousal states.

IV. THE HYPOTHALAMUS AND NEUROENDOCRINE REGULATION

Neural regulation of pituitary secretion is one of the most important, well-characterized, and diverse func-tions of the hypothalamus. In fact, the demonstration that the hypothalamus exerts regulatory control over the pituitary is one of the landmark discoveries that tied the fields of neurobiology and endocrinology together. Recognition that hypothalamic control over the pituitary was humoral in nature resulted from structural studies that demonstrated a vascular link, or portal plexus, connecting these structures. Thus, the organizational features of the hypothalamic–pituitary axis are introduced below as a prelude to examining specific examples of hypothalamic control over pitui-tary secretion.

As noted earlier, the ventral diencephalon is con-nected to the subjacent pituitary via the infundibular stalk. Large-caliber magnocellular axons whose parent neurons reside in rostral hypothalamus traverse this stalk to terminate directly in the posterior lobe of the pituitary gland. This is the only direct neural connection between the hypothalamus and pituitary and represents only a small portion of the regulatory capacity of the hypothalamus over pituitary function. Control of the secretory activity of the anterior pituitary is achieved through a portal vascular plexus that arises in the median eminence and then pursues a directed course along the stalk to end in the anterior lobe of this gland. An important feature of this portal system is the absence of the BBB in the capillaries of the median eminence. Fenestrations in the median eminence vessels allow peptides and neurotransmitters released from axons in their vicinity to gain access to the portal plexus, whereupon they are transported to the anterior pituitary to influence the secretory activity of cells in that portion of the gland. This architecture forms the basis for the neurohumoral regulation of pituitary function that is the foundation of neuroendocrinology (Fig. 2).

The absence of the BBB is a defining feature of a group of structures known as circumventricular organs (CVOs). These regions, which include the median eminence, are found on the midline of the brain

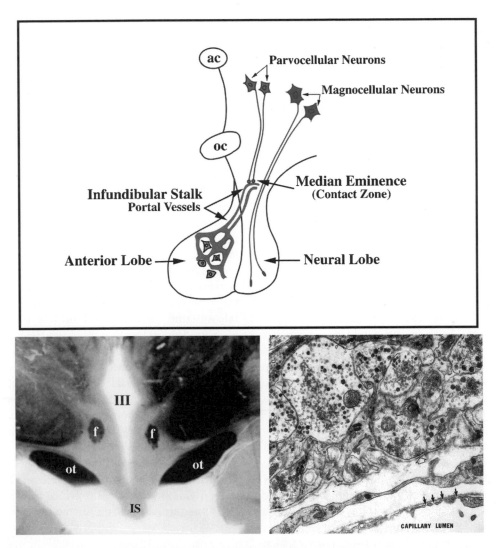

Figure 2   The basic organization of the hypothalamic–pituitary axis is illustrated in the schematic diagram. The anterior lobe of the pituitary is regulated by hypothalamic peptides and neurotransmitters that are released from parvocellular hypothalamic neurons into a vascular (portal) plexus and then travel to the anterior lobe to either stimulate or inhibit the release of hormones from cells in this portion of the gland. This is possible because the vessels at the neurohemal contact zone in the median eminence are fenestrated and large numbers of axon terminals terminate on the perivascular space adjacent to these vessels (bottom, right). Large magnocellular neurons project through the infundibular stalk (IS) to terminate in the posterior, or neural, lobe of the pituitary. ac, anterior commissure; f, fornix; OC, optic chiasm; ot, optic tract; III, third ventricle.

surrounding the third and fourth ventricles. Only two of the CVOs (the median eminence and OVLT) are found within the hypothalamus, but all are intimately associated with hypothalamic function by virtue of the connections that they maintain with various hypothalamic nuclei. For example, the absence of the BBB in the subfornical organ and area postrema allows neurons in these regions to respond to circulating cues and then modulate the activity of the hypothalamic–pituitary axis through classical synaptic connections with hypothalamic neurons. Thus, the absence of the BBB is essential not only for the ability of the hypothalamus to control the secretory activity of the pituitary but also for the feedback regulation of the hypothalamic–pituitary axis that imparts precision on endocrine regulation of peripheral systems.

The neurons that contribute to regulation of anterior pituitary secretion exhibit common features that are reflective of their function. First, they are confined to the hypothalamus and give rise to axons that terminate in the median eminence. Two hypothalamic nuclei, the paraventricular and arcuate, are particularly devoted to anterior pituitary regulation. Substantial numbers of parvocellular neurons in these nuclei give rise to dedicated projections to the external zone of the median eminence where their terminals abut on the perivascular space (contact zone) surrounding the fenestrated capillaries of the portal plexus. Neurons exhibiting the same organization are also dispersed in other areas of hypothalamus. For example, neurons involved in the regulation of growth hormone secretion are concentrated in the rostral periventricular and arcuate nuclei, whereas those that are important for regulation of ovulation in females are dispersed throughout the preoptic area. All these neurons project exclusively to the portal plexus in the median eminence and thereby exert their function in a neuroendocrine fashion.

A second feature of these neurons is their neurochemical diversity. Although they all have common structural features, the differing functions of these neurons are defined by their neurochemical phenotype. Many of the neurons manufacture and release small peptides that either stimulate or inhibit the secretory activity of cells in the anterior pituitary. Others utilize small molecule neurotransmitters such as dopamine toward the same end. These "releasing" or "inhibiting" factors impart another level of regulatory control over the hypothalamic–pituitary axis that is best illustrated by considering a specific example, such as growth hormone (GH) secretion. Peripheral metabolism is heavily influenced by release of GH from the anterior pituitary gland and this release, in turn, is regulated by two populations of hypothalamic neurons that produce opposite effects in the pituitary. Stimulation of GH release is under the control of neurons in the arcuate nucleus that produce growth hormone-releasing hormone, whereas inhibition of GH release results from the activity of somatostatinergic neurons in the rostral periventricular nucleus. Differential activation of these opposing systems permits precise regulation of GH secretion and emphasizes the importance of feedback regulation in activating the appropriate regulatory circuitry.

A role for hypothalamic timing mechanisms in neuroendocrine regulation is predicted by the rhythmic profiles of hormone release by the anterior pituitary and its target organs. This is clearly exemplified by the temporal profile of cortisol secretion by the adrenal gland. Release of plasma corticosteroids is under control of the hypothalamic–pituitary–adrenal (HPA) axis and exhibits a circadian profile, with peak levels occurring at the end of the dark phase in humans and the end of the light phase in rat. Although the temporal relations of these peaks differ between the two species, the temporal association of the peaks to activity is the same. Release of corticosteroids from the adrenal is under the control of corticotropin-releasing factor (CRF) neurons in the paraventricular hypothalamic nucleus. Release of CRF into the portal plexus at the median eminence elicits the synthesis and release of adrenocorticotropin hormone from the anterior pituitary, which subsequently stimulates corticosteroid release from the adrenal. Evidence suggests that the SCN modulates the activity of the HPA axis through a disynaptic pathway in which SCN neurons synapse on neurons in the dorsomedial hypothalamic nucleus that are presynaptic to CRF neurons in the paraventricular nucleus. Control of the HPA axis is also exquisitely sensitive to other sensory cues, such as feeding and stress. Thus, control of the HPA axis is a dynamic process in which the hypothalamus plays an important integrative role that defines the magnitude and temporal profile of corticosteriod release. It is probable that similar organizational principles account for the rhythmic release of other hormones.

V. HYPOTHALAMIC CONTROL OF AUTONOMIC OUTFLOW

As noted earlier, the hypothalamus plays an essential role in the maintenance of homeostasis. Neuroendocrine regulation of pituitary function constitutes one of the primary ways through which this is achieved. However, the autonomic nervous system (ANS) is also intimately involved in homeostatic regulation. A substantial body of work clearly indicates that the hypothalamus plays a major role in controlling the activity of the ANS. Extensive descending connections to brain stem and spinal preganglionic neurons of the ANS arise from hypothalamic nuclei, and these hypothalamic nuclei are the target of feedback regulation that is both synaptic and humoral in nature. However, it is important to emphasize that these hypothalamic nuclei function within a larger set of forebrain areas that influence autonomic outflow either indirectly by virtue of their connections with hypothalamus or directly via descending projections to autonomic nuclei in the brain stem and spinal cord. These areas include the visceral cortices (prefrontal and insular cortex) and components of the limbic system such as the amygdala.

The major hypothalamic efferents to autonomic nuclei arise in the paraventricular nucleus and the lateral hypothalamic area. Neurons in both of these regions give rise to descending projections to preganglionic neurons in both the sympathetic and parasympathetic subdivisions of the spinal cord and brain stem. The paraventricular nucleus (PVN) is a particularly important integrative center for both neuroendocrine and autonomic regulation of homeostatic function. As noted earlier, parvicellular neurons in the PVN are major contributors to the neuroendocrine regulation of anterior pituitary secretion by virtue of their projections to the portal plexus in the median eminence. Additionally, magnocellular vasopressinergic and oxytocinergic neurons in the PVN and supraoptic nuclei project through the median eminence to terminate in the posterior lobe of the pituitary gland. These peptidergic systems are important for the regulation of fluid homeostasis and lactation and are distinct from the large numbers of PVN parvicellular neurons that give rise to descending projections to autonomic nuclei. The latter projections arise from phenotypically distinct PVN neurons sequestered within subfields of the nucleus that are devoted to autonomic function (dorsal parvicellular subdivision) or to both neuroendocrine and autonomic regulation (medial parvicellular subdivision). This juxtaposition of neurons in the PVN that contribute to homeostatic regulation via neuroendocrine or autonomic pathways makes efficient use of the sensory feedback signals that are relevant to both modes of regulation. Defining the means through which this sensory information is integrated in the PVN to influence endocrine and autonomic function remains an active and important area of research. The complexity of the integrative capacities of the PVN is illustrated in the following section on the neural control of feeding.

VI. HYPOTHALAMIC CONTROL OF FEEDING

Our understanding of how the hypothalamus contributes to the regulation of feeding behavior has advanced substantially during the past decade. Identification and functional dissection of phenotypically distinct populations of hypothalamic neurons that are now known to influence ingestive behavior and energy metabolism have contributed greatly to these advances. Recent identification of peripheral signaling molecules that act centrally to modulate these hypothalamic circuits has also provided tremendous insights into how the hypothalamus participates in energy homeostasis.

Results from classic lesion studies carried out in the 1940s and 1950s led to a "dual-center" model for the hypothalamic control of hunger and satiety that drove scientific research in this area for more than 30 years. The model was based on profound and consistent changes in ingestive behavior observed in rats after bilateral mechanical or electrolytic lesions centered in the ventromedial nucleus of the hypothalamus (VMH) or lateral hypothalamic area (LHA). Rats with VMH lesions displayed an apparently insatiable hunger and would become quite obese when food was made freely available. Conversely, rats with LHA lesions displayed adipsia and anorexia, and they required careful nursing during the postlesion period to prevent fatal dehydration and starvation. The dual-center model of hunger and satiety enjoyed strong appeal as an organizing framework for understanding how the hypothalamus contributes to the central control of ingestive behavior. However, the model ultimately was undermined by demonstrations that the method commonly used to create the VMH and LHA lesions produced effects that were not specific to hypothalamic regulation of ingestive behavior but extended to other sensorimotor and metabolic control systems.

Although the original dual-center model of hunger and satiety eventually fell out of favor, it remains generally accepted that certain subregions of the hypothalamus play a key role in energy homeostasis, at least in part by influencing ingestive behavior. Recent findings have served to renew scientific interest in the role of the LHA in controlling ingestive behavior and energy balance. We now know that LHA neurons receive synaptic inputs from multiple sensory modalities relevant to ingestive control, and that their responses to these inputs vary as a function of nutritional status. Two distinct but partially overlapping populations of LHA neurons have been identified based on their content of unique neuropeptides (melanin-concentrating hormone and hypocretin/orexin) that appear to play important roles in the control of food intake and energy metabolism through distinct central neural pathways. LHA neurons that express these neuropeptides project to key areas of the brain stem and forebrain that mediate ingestive behavioral responses. Improved chemical methods for lesioning the diffusely scattered LHA neurons without damaging intermingled fibers of passage (including, most notably, the medial forebrain bundle) have demonstrated that the LHA is indeed necessary for normal feedback regulation of ingestive behavior.

Synaptic inputs to orexin/hypocretin- and MSH-containing neurons in the LHA arise from many regions of the central neuraxis. Perhaps most relevant to the control of ingestive behavior and energy balance is a recently discovered circuit that originates in the arcuate nucleus of the hypothalamus. Early studies indicated that neurotoxic damage to the arcuate nucleus (e.g., as produced by systemic administration of monosodium glutamate during early development) could produce syndromes of overeating and obesity in laboratory animals. New and exciting research findings have provided a possible explanation for this phenomenon. In 1994, a hormone called leptin was discovered that appears to exert tremendously potent inhibitory effects on feeding behavior. Leptin also produces significant physiological effects on thermoregulation and on the reproductive, thyroid, and adrenal axes. Leptin is released continuously from adipocytes and is present at a relatively high concentration in plasma (approximately 4 ng/ml). Leptin binds to receptors expressed in peripheral tissues and in a circumscribed set of brain regions, most notably the arcuate nucleus of the hypothalamus. Animals seem to adapt to their own unique circulating leptin levels (which are directly proportional to body adiposity), such that experimental perturbation of those levels will shift the animal's behavior and physiology toward either gaining or losing body weight in an apparent effort to restore normal leptin levels. For example, mice with genetic mutations that render them incapable of producing either leptin or leptin receptors become obese, whereas experimental elevation of circulating leptin levels causes animals to lose body

weight. A wealth of recent data indicate that circulating leptin provides a physiologically important negative feedback signal to constrain body weight by affecting both ingestive behavior and metabolic activity.

There is general consensus that the arcuate nucleus plays a major role in transducing the effects of leptin on both the behavioral and physiological components of energy balance. Arcuate neurons that express functional leptin receptors project to the LHA and to other hypothalamic areas implicated in energy homeostasis, including the dorsomedial and PVN nuclei. Arcuate projections to the PVN provide a basis for documented leptin effects on parvicellular neurosecretory neurons comprising the central limbs of the HPA and hypothalamo–pituitary–thyroid axes, the activities of which are regulated by leptin. The arcuate nuclei and PVN also provide important descending projections to autonomic neurons in the brain stem and spinal cord, and may play a role in leptin-mediated increases in energy expenditure through the stimulation of brown fat thermogenesis. Leptin-sensitive arcuate neurons that project to the LHA and PVN contain neuropeptides (including neuropeptide Y, proopiomelanocortin, and agouti-related protein) that exert potent effects on food intake and other relevant neuroendocrine and autonomic aspects of energy homeostasis. Thus, the arcuate nucleus can be viewed as a nodal point in the hypothalamic regulation of energy balance.

VII. CONCLUSIONS

There can be little doubt that our understanding of hypothalamic organization and function has improved dramatically during the past 25 years. Many of these advances can be traced directly to technical advances that have allowed the dissection of hypothalamic circuits from both organizational and functional perspectives. Thus, the ability to define the connectivity and phenotype of hypothalamic neurons and to assess the activity of anatomically defined circuits with functional probes such as Fos has proven to be enormously informative in defining the function of hypothalamic cell groups. Continued application of these experimental approaches promises to further illuminate our understanding of this small subdivision of the diencephalon that has long been recognized as a central integrative center for the control of homeostasis and behavioral state.

See Also the Following Articles

AROUSAL • CHEMICAL NEUROANATOMY • CIRCADIAN RHYTHMS • HOMEOSTATIC MECHANISMS • NERVOUS SYSTEM, ORGANIZATION OF • PSYCHONEUROENDO-CRINOLOGY • SLEEP DISORDERS • TIME PASSAGE, NEURAL SUBSTRATES

Suggested Reading

Card, J. P., Swanson, L. W., and Moore, R. Y. (1999). The hypothalamus: An overview of regulatory systems. In *Fundamental Neuroscience* (M. Zigmond, F. E. Bloom, S. C. Landis, J. L. Roberts, and L. R. Squire, Eds.), pp. 1013–1026. Academic Press, San Diego.

Iversen, S., Iversen, L., and Saper, C. B. (2000). The autonomic nervous system and the hypothalamus. In *Principles of Neural Science* (E. R. Kandel, J. H. Schwartz, and T. M. Jessel, Eds.), 4th ed., pp. 960–981. McGraw-Hill, New York.

Parent, A. (1997). Hypothalamus. In *Carpenter's Human Neuroanatomy* 9th ed., pp. 706–743. Willams & Wilkins, Baltimore.

Saper, C. B. (1990). Hypothalamus. In *The Human Nervous System* (G. Paxinos, Ed.), pp. 389–414. Academic Press, San Diego.

Sawchenko, P. E. (1998). Toward a new neurobiology of energy balance, appetite, and obesity. The anatomists weigh in. *J. Comp. Neurol.* **402**, 435–441.

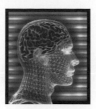

Imaging: Brain Mapping Methods

JOHN C. MAZZIOTTA

University of California, Los Angeles School of Medicine

RICHARD S. J. FRACKOWIAK

University College, London

Disorders of the human nervous system are among the most debilitating and devastating of all human illnesses. Such disorders not only affect the physical abilities of patients but often severely compromise the quality of life, the ability to function in society, family relations, and the ability to maintain gainful employment. As such, neurological, neurosurgical, and psychiatric disorders affect not only the patients but also their families and society at large because of the tremendous economic burden that results from their prevalence. Undoubtedly, this is one of the reasons brain mapping methods have advanced so rapidly and hold such promise for improved diagnostics, monitoring of therapeutics, and providing insights into the basic mechanisms of brain disease. Never before have so many methods been available to tackle these vexing problems. This article provides an overview of the methods and their applications in human diseases.

Throughout this article, it is important for the reader to keep in mind a number of important physical and

physiological factors when trying to understand the approaches of different brain mapping applications to the study of human cerebral disorders (Table I).

First, it is important to keep in mind that specific methods address only one or a few aspects of underlying cerebral physiology and pathophysiology. For example, electromagnetophysiological techniques, such as electroencephalography (EEG), event-related potentials (ERPs), and magnetoencephalography (MEG), provide information about large constellations of neurons and the net electromagnetophysiological vector that their firing produces. The electrical techniques are weighted toward surface structures, whereas the magnetic ones convey information about deeper brain structures with less distortion. This indicates another important aspect in assessing methods for the evaluation of disease states. That is, certain techniques are better suited to examination of particular sites in the brain than others.

Second, a number of techniques are devoted specifically to describing brain structure. These include X-ray computed tomography (CT), conventional magnetic resonance imaging (MRI), and blood vessel imaging using conventional angiography, magnetic resonance angiography (MRA), or helical CT. A number of techniques assess hemodynamic responses as a measure of function. These techniques include xenon-enhanced CT, functional MRI (fMRI), perfusion MRI, and cerebral blood flow or blood volume measurements using positron emission tomography (PET) or single photon emission computed tomography (SPECT). All the techniques that evaluate cerebral

This article has been reprinted from Mazziotta and Frackowiak (2000). The study of human disease with brain mapping methods. In *Brain Mapping: The Disorders* (Toga and Mazziotta, eds.) pp. 3–31. Academic Press, San Diego.

Table I
Advantages and Limitations of Current Brain Mapping Techniques of Use in the Study of Patients with Neurological, Neurosurgical, and Psychiatric Disorders

Method	Advantages	Limitations
X-ray computed tomography	Excellent bone imaging	Ionizing radiation
	~100% detection of hemorrhages	Poor contrast resolution
	Short study time	
	Can scan patients with ancillary equipment	
	Can scan patients with metal devices/ electronic devices	
Magnetic resonance imaging	High spatial resolution	Long study duration
	No ionizing radiation	Patients may be claustrophobic
	High resolution	Electronic devices contraindicated
	High gray–white contrast	Acute hemorrhages problematic
	No bone-generated artifact in posterior fossa	Relative measurements only
	Can also perform chemical, functional, and angiographic imaging	
Positron emission tomography	Can perform hemodynamic, chemical, and functional imaging	Ionizing radiation High initial costs
	Quantifiable results	Long development time for new tracers
	Absolute physiologic variables can be determined	Limited access
	Uniform spatial resolution	Low temporal resolution
Single photon emission computed tomography	Can perform hemodynamic, chemical, and functional imaging	Ionizing radiation Relative measurements only
	Widely available	Nonuniform spatial resolution
		Low temporal resolution
Xenon-enhanced computed tomography	Uses existing equipment	Ionizing radiation
		High xenon concentrations have pharmacologic effects
Helical computed tomography (CT angiography)	Provides high-resolution vascular images	Ionizing radiation
		Vascular and bony anatomy only
Electroencephalography	No ionizing radiation	Low spatial resolution
	High temporal resolution	Weighted toward surface measurements
	Widely available	
	Can identify epileptic foci	
Magnetoencephalography	No ionizing radiation	Low spatial resolution
	High temporal resolution	
	Can identify epileptic foci	
Transcranial magnetic stimulation	No ionizing radiation	Low spatial resolution
	Potential for therapy	Has produced seizures in certain patient groups
	Can be linked to other imaging methods (PET, MRI)	
Optical intrinsic signal imaging	No ionizing radiation	Complex signal source
	High temporal resolution	Invasive only (intraoperative)
	High spatial resolution	

function based on hemodynamic measurements are, by their very nature, at a physiological "distance" from the actual neuronal event. These methods assume that neuronal firing and blood flow increments or decrements are tightly coupled. In most cases, this holds true in the normal brain, but it may not always be true in pathologic states.

Third, the determination of chemical processes in the brain falls mainly in the domain of PET and magnetic resonance spectroscopy (MRS). The former can measure cerebral glucose metabolism, protein synthesis, amino acid uptake, pH, and other variables and does so in a quantitative manner reported in physiological units when appropriate rate constants and other factors are incorporated into mathematical models for their estimation. MRS provides relative measurements of chemical compounds relying primarily on hydrogen spectra but, at higher magnetic field strengths, can also estimate relative quantities of sodium fluorine-carbon, and phosphorus-containing molecules as well.

Fourth, the evaluation of receptor systems in the brain, both transmitter molecules and receptor complexes, has been an active area of research in both health and disease using PET and SPECT. Most information has been derived for the dopaminergic system but data also exist for the cholinergic, serotonergic, opioid, and benzodiazepine systems.

Last, there are interactive approaches. The most time honored, of course, is the direct observation of signs and symptoms in patients with cerebral disorders. Such information can be obtained in the traditional clinical setting or in the highly unusual circumstance of awake surgical procedures where recording from or stimulation of cerebral tissue can be correlated with behavioral states in a conscious patient. These latter methods, while in use for more than 50 years, still provide unique information about structure–function relationships in the human brain. Recently, such measurements have been augmented through the use of optical intrinsic signal imaging, in which changes in optical reflectance from the cortex are measured during surgery. Measurements can be made either in awake patients during behavior or with anesthetized patients receiving sensory stimulation or direct peripheral nerve stimulation. They provide measures of functional specificity for different brain regions in the operative field. The technique of transcranial magnetic stimulation allows the investigator to stimulate the cortex of the brain magnetically, resulting in an induced electrical discharge in the cortex and an observed or reported behavior from the subject. This technique has been used experimentally to map normal brain systems and in patients for experimental, diagnostic, and therapeutic purposes.

Each technique is capable of making measurements with a characteristic resolution in both the spatial and temporal domains. Tomographic imaging techniques produce the highest spatial resolution currently available, whereas the electromagnetophysiological methods provide the highest temporal resolution. Although knowledge of resolution is important, it must be matched to the question of interest in a particular patient population—a decision that also requires knowledge of the sampling characteristics of the technique. This latter term refers to the volume of brain tissue that can be assessed with a particular measurement. Thus, whereas fMRI may survey functional responses through out the entire brain, electrophysiological measurements from a depth electrode, despite producing data with exquisite spatial and temporal resolution, sample only a very small volume of brain tissue. As such, investigations aimed at trying to identify a functional disorder in a disease of unknown etiology (e.g., autism) would be better done with a global technique that surveys the entire cerebral landscape rather than with measurement at multiple sites with an electrophysiological method such as depth electrodes. The latter are better used to understand the local electrophysiology of a site that has a high probability of being abnormal and possibly also causative of a given disorder.

With these principles in mind, we now consider a more specific examination of the different strategies that can be employed with modern brain mapping methods to assess patients, either as individuals or as groups, with neurological, neurosurgical, or psychiatric disorders (Table II).

I. DIAGNOSTIC METHODS

A. Individual Processes

1. Structural Anatomy

a. Computed Tomography   X-ray CT was the first noninvasive imaging technique that allowed for direct visulization of the brain parenchyma. It revolutionized the evaluation of patients with neurological and neurosurgical disorders because it could image bone and provided the first opportunity to see the brain directly. It has a small dynamic contrast range so that

Table II
Brain Mapping Methods of Use in the Study of Human Disease along with the Types of Measurements They Provide and Some of the Clinical Situations in which They May Be of Use

Method	Measurements provided	Disorders
X-ray computed tomography (CT)	Brain structure	Acute/chronic hemorrhages
	Blood–brain barrier integrity	Acute trauma
		General screening of anatomy
		Focal or generalized atrophy
		Hydrocephalus
Magnetic resonance imaging	Brain structure	Acute ischemia
	Brain and cervical vasculature	Neoplasms
	Relative cerebral perfusion	Demyelinating disease
	Chemical concentrations	Epileptic foci
	Fiber tracts	Degenerative disorders
	Blood–brain barrier integrity	Infections
		Preoperative mapping
Positron emission tomography	Perfusion	Ischemic states
	Metabolism	Degenerative disorders
	Substrate extraction	Epilepsy
	Protein synthesis	Movement disorders
	Neurotransmitter integrity	Affective disorders
	Receptor binding	Neoplasms
	Blood–brain barrier integrity	Addictive states
		Preoperative mapping
Single photon emission computed tomography	Perfusion	Ischemic states
	Neurotransmitter integrity	Degenerative disorders
	Receptor binding	Epilepsy
	Blood–brain barrier integrity	Movement disorders
Xenon-enhanced computed tomography	Perfusion	Ischemic states
Helical computed tomography (CT angiography)	Vascular anatomy	Vascular occlusive disease
	Bony anatomy	Aneurysms
		Arteriovenous malformations
Electroencephalography	Electrophysiology	Epilepsy
		Encephalopathics
		Degenerative disorders
		Preoperative mapping
Magnetoencephalography	Electrophysiology	Epilepsy
Transcranial magnetic stimulation	Focal brain activation	Preoperative mapping
Optical intrinsic signal imaging	Integrated measure of blood volume, metabolism, and cell swelling	Intraoperative mapping

differentiation of gray and white matter is difficult (Fig. 1A). However, it is very sensitive for identifying cerebral hemorrhage and also lesions associated with an alteration in the blood–brain barrier, by virtue of leakage of iodinated contrast material in them. These abilities make X-ray CT ideal for direct and immediate assessment of patients with cerebral hemorrhage, multiple sclerosis, brain tumors, and traumatic

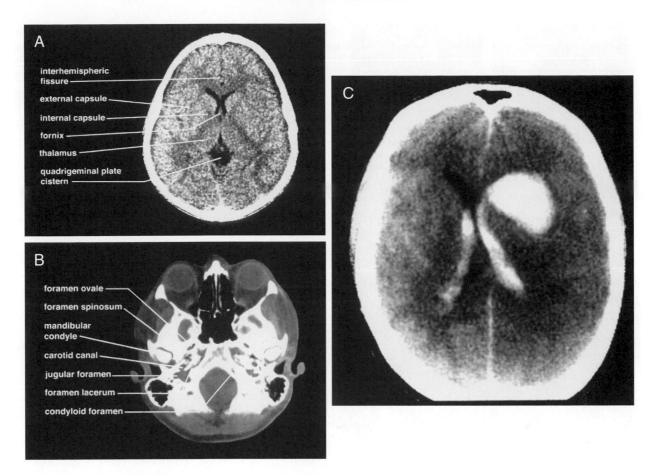

Figure 1 X-ray CT. (A) Images of the human brain from an X-ray CT device, demonstrating good anatomical detail, particularly of the skull and ventricular system as well as the subarachnoid CSF spaces. Note that there is less gray–white contrast than in MRI images (Fig. 2A). (B) X-ray CT provided very detailed images of bony structures that surround the central nervous system. This is particularly useful in evaluating pathologic states at the base of the skull, where conventional radiography is often difficult because of patient positioning and the overlap of bony structures in a two-dimensional radiograph. Furthermore, in situations in which trauma is a factor, often patients cannot be manipulated easily because of the possibility of fractures at the base of the skull or in the cervical spine. (C) Intracerebral hemorrhage demonstrated by X-ray CT. Sensitivity for detection of intracranial bleeds is effectively 100% with X-ray CT and it remains the imaging modality of choice in acute patients when identification of cerebral hemorrhage is urgent and important. This is typically the case in patients with an acute cerebral deficit when cerebral hemorrhage must be identified if thrombolytic or anticoagulant therapy is being contemplated.

injuries. Contrast sensitivity and the time needed for scanning have improved since X-ray CT was introduced, but with the advent of MRI technology many diagnostic studies that were formerly in the province of X-ray CT are now done with MRI. Nevertheless, X-ray CT continues to have an important role in resolving certain diagnostic questions and in particular patient circumstances.

X-ray CT has remained the imaging modality of choice for patients requiring urgent evaluation of suspected intracranial hemorrhage (Fig. 1C) and in patients with acute head trauma. In both these circumstances, the speed of the study and ease of patient access as well as availability of equipment are well matched to the ability of CT to evaluate such

patients. X-ray CT is also the procedure of choice when evaluating abnormalities of bony structures of the head particularly the skull base (Fig. 1B). Lastly, patients who cannot tolerate MRI because of claustrophobia or implanted ferromagnetic or electronic devices or that need to be attached to ancillary equipment such as is frequently encountered in critical care situations are also best scanned by X-ray CT if structural information is needed for clinical evaluation.

b. MRI Magnetic resonance imaging is the structural imaging modality of choice in all other situations. Its superior spatial resolution and contrast range, particularly useful in differentiating gray and white matter, are but two features of MRI that make it

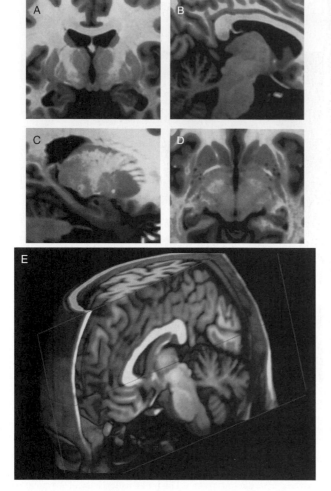

Figure 2 Magnetic resonance imaging. (A–D) Typical two-dimensional MRI images of the brain. Notice that the detailed anatomy of the brain parenchyma has better gray–white contrast than X-ray CT images (Fig. 1A). Notice also that there are none of the typical CT artifacts caused by the juxtaposition of dense bone and brain parenchymay. (A) Coronal view through the thalamus demonstrating the subnuclei of the thalamus, the mamillary bodies, and the internal, external, and extreme capsules as well as the two segments of the globus pallidus. Also note the detailed anatomy of the hippocampi. (B) Sagittal view demonstrating the colliculi of the midbrain, the midline of the thalamus, and the detailed anatomy of the midsagittal region of the cerebellum. (C) Sagittal view through the hippocampus and striatum. Note the fine bridges of gray matter between the caudate and the putamen. (D) Transverse section through the basal ganglia and upper midbrain. Note the periaqueductal gray matter, the detailed anatomy of the hippocampi, and the bilateral flow voids produced by the presence of the lenticulostriate arteries in the posterior portion of the putamen. (E) Three-dimensional reconstruction with cutaway of an MRI data set demonstrating the kind of anatomical detail that can be provided with three-dimensional MR images (courtesy of Colin Holmes and colleagues, UCLA School of Medicine, Los Angeles). [A–D from Holmes *et al.* (1998). Enhancement of magnetic resonance images using registration for signal averaging. *J. Computer Assisted Tomogr.* **22**(1), 139–152].

superior to CT for structural imaging (Fig. 2). The ability to image brain structures from any angle and avoidance of CT artifacts that result from soft tissue-dense bone boundaries in the field of view provide further arguments for the use of MRI in patients with cerebral disorders. This advantage is most notable in the posterior fossa, where artifacts from the dense petrous bones often obscure or obliterate relevant clinical information about the brain stem and cerebellum. Gadolinium and other paramagnetic contrast agents can be used with MRI to provide the ability to detect blood–brain barrier defects in a manner analogous to that used in X-ray CT with iodinated contrast agents.

2. Vascular Anatomy

a. MR Angiography The observation that protons leaving the field of view reduce the local signal in MRI studies has led to an entire field of MR angiography and associated flow-based MRI techniques. The so-called flow void occurs in the vascular system when blood that encounters a radiofrequency pulse leaves the field of view of the scanner and the resultant energy is therefore emitted outside the field of view. The result is a loss of signal within the lumina of blood vessels. When partitular pulse sequences are utilized to optimize this effect, an image of vascular anatomy results. Like most angiographic procedures, the image depicts the contents of the blood vessel (within the lumen) as opposed to the blood vessel wall and associated structures. However, unlike conventional angiography, in which arterial, capillary, and venous phases are distributed in time and images of each phase can be produced independently, MRA provides a composite image of all medium-to-large-diameter vessels, including arteries and viens.

Such studies have provided important opportunities for the evaluation of intracranial and cervical, medium and large vessels for abnormalities, including arteriovenous malformations, aneurysms, and occlusive disease. Smaller caliber vessels still require conventional angiographic or helical CT evaluation for the assessment of disorders such as vasculitis.

b. Helical CT In this technique, also called spiral CT or CT angiography, conventional CT technology is modified to produce very rapid sequential images of the head by having the relationship between the patient and the X-ray tube/detector system traverse a helical course through the tissue. This process is rapid and so

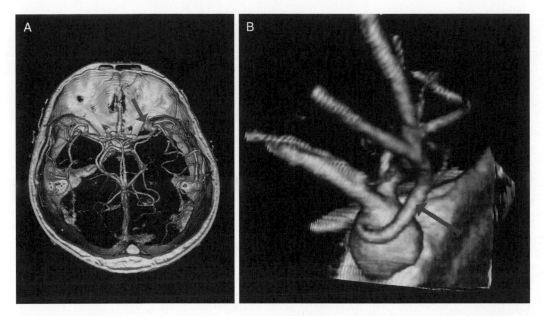

Figure 3 Helical CT angiography. (A) The cerebral vasculature is superimposed on this cutaway view of the skull seen from above. Note the line detail provided for the vascular structures, including the circle of Willis, the anterior, middle, and posterior cerebral arteries, and many of their branches. The arrow indicates an aneurysm arising from the middle cerebral artery at the anterior edge of the middle cerebral fossa. (B) Close-up view of the aneurysm demonstrated in A. Note that in this three-dimensional reconstruction, it is possible to see all of the blood vessels that contribute to or arise from the aneurysmal sack (left). Unlike conventional angiography, where the overlap of the aneurysm and the parent or daughter vessels can be obscured because of the two-dimensional projection required in this technique, full three-dimensional images are possible with helical CT angiography. By digital reconstruction and rotation of the data set from helical CT, these complex and important relationships can be evaluated prior to surgery, whereas with conventional angiograms multiple view would be required and still may not provide a sufficiently detailed view of these relationships. In addition, multiple views obtained with conventional angiography expose the patient to additional radiation and contrast risks. In this case, the angular artery (arrow) arises from the aneurysm sack. Endovascular coil placement might lead to obstruction of this important vessel, thereby making such a patient a candidate for surgical rather than endovascular treatment of this lesion (courtesy of Pablo Villablanca, UCLA School of Medicine).

arranged that it is coincident with the delivery of a bolus of iodinated contrast material into the cranial and cervical vessels from a peripheral vein. The resultant images are high-resolution depictions of the intracranial anatomy that can be reconstructed in three dimensions (Fig. 3A). Currently, limited information is available about the technique in terms of its clinical applications, but it is likely that there are circumstances in which it may be superior to conventional angiography. One of those is in the assessment of the local vascular anatomy of patients with aneurysms and arteriovenous malformations. In this case, conventional angiography, while high in spatial resolution, collapses the three-dimensional structure of such lesions into a two-dimensional projection. As such, the important relationship between aneurysm neck and a parent or daughter vessel may be difficult to ascertain or may require multiple intraarterial contrast injections and radiation exposure for the patient. Helical CT allows for a true three-dimensional reconstruction of local anatomy that can be manipu-

lated to assess such relationships in greater detail, while subjecting the patient to only a single radiation exposure and dose of iodinated contrast material (Fig. 3B). A similar situation exists when defining feeder vessels to arteriovenous malformations.

3. Blood Flow and Perfusion

a. PET The assessment of cerebral perfusion (i.e., cerebral blood flow per volume of tissue) can be determined quantitatively with PET using ^{15}O-labeled water, ^{11}C-labeled butanol, and potentially other agents. These agents are freely diffusible and knowledge of the time–activity relationship of the tracer compound in arterial blood and the tissue concentration over time in the brain permits a calculation of cerebral perfusion with approximately $5 \times 5 \times 5$-mm spatial resolution. These methods have been used extensively to evaluate increments in perfusion associated with underlying neuronal activity such as that

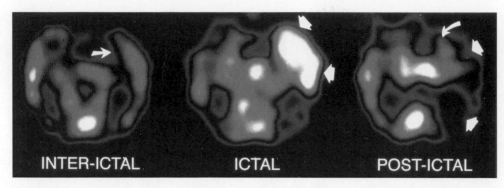

Figure 4 SPECT studies of a seizure focus in a patient with epilepsy, obtained using technetium-^{99}m-labeled HMPAO. By comparing the ictal study (hyperperfusion), obtained by injecting the tracer on a telemetry ward, with the postictal and interictal scans (hypoperfusion), it is possible, with a high degree of accuracy, to identify seizure foci responsible for focal epilepsies. Although such SPECT studies of relative perfusion may be confusing or misleading when evaluated in only one of these states, the composite information obtained from ictal, postictal, and interictal studies, particularly when the studies are aligned, registered, and subtracted, is useful in the presurgical evaluation of patients with focal or complex partial epilepsy [courtesy of Sam Berkovic, Austin Hospital, Melbourne, Victoria, Australia. From Berkovic, S. F., Newton, M. R., and Rowe, C. C. (1991). Localization of epileptic foci using SPECT. In *Epilepsy Surgery* (H. Luden, Ed.), pp. 251–256. Raven Press, New York].

associated with the performance of behavioral tasks, and as such can be used in patients to evaluate critical cortical and subcortical areas as part of the process of mapping brain regions adjacent to abnormalities that are under consideration for surgical resection.

Perfusion measurements are also of value in assessing patients with ischemic cerebrovascular disease not only to determine baseline conditions but also in the assessment of "cerebral perfusion reserve" by challenging such patients with cerebral vasodilation drugs such as acetazolamide.

b. SPECT Perfusion measurements with SPECT can be obtained in a semiquantitative way using xenon-133 or in a relative fashion using a host of technetium-99 m labeled agents (e.g., HMPAO). Studies have been used to evaluate patients with cerebrovascular disease in the assessment of patients with epilepsy. In the latter circumstance, ictal, postictal, and interictal studies are made using these agents and subtracted to identify foci of epileptic discharges that increase cerebral perfusion during seizures and reduce perfusion postictally and interictally (Fig. 4).

c. Xenon-Enhanced CT Nonradioactive xenon-133 alters the X-ray attenuation characteristics of the tissues that absorb it. Xenon-133 can be readily inhaled. Using strategies similar to those discussed previously, one can calculate changes in X-ray attenuation associated with the concentration of xenon in tissue to calculate an index of cerebral perfusion. This approach has been used to evaluate

patients with cerebrovascular disease and head trauma. One confounding factor with this approach is that relatively high concentrations of xenon are needed in brain tissue to produce accurate perfusion estimates. At these concentrations, patients experience pharmacological effects, including sedation and, ultimately, anesthesia. These direct neuronal effects of xenon can, in turn, affect cerebral perfusion and contaminate physiological measurements. Nevertheless, such studies have been used to assess patients in specific diagnostic categories when alternate techniques are not available.

d. MRI Relative and semiquantitative measurements of cerebral perfusion can be obtained with MRI using a variety of techniques. The basic difference among these techniques is whether exogenous agents are infused into the patient or whether changes in endogenous signals from the vascular system are monitored. With the former, bolus contrast agents such as gadolinium are delivered to a subject intravenously. Their local concentration in the cerebral vasculature estimates local cerebral perfusion, which in turn is proportional to neuronal firing rates. The change in MR signal, induced by a local change in concentration of a contrast agent, reflects a relative change in local perfusion that can be estimated. A refinement of this approach requires information about the concentration of the contrast agent in the blood over a period of time. This can be measured directly from an arterial source, although such a method is rarely employed, or from a large-diameter blood vessel in the scanner's field of view (e.g., arteries in the circle of Willis).

Alternatively, one can record endogenous local signal changes associated with alterations in cerebral perfusion induced by changing neuronal activity. When local neuronal firing increases, there is an increment in cerebral blood flow to an area. However, there is a proportionally smaller change in local tissue oxygen metabolism. As a result, more oxygen is delivered per unit volume of tissue (because of decreased fractional extraction) but there is little change in the amount of oxygen used. Thus, the oxygen content (i.e., the concentration of oxyhemoglobin) in venous blood increases. When compared to images in a state of "baseline" neuronal firing, this local change in venous oxyhemoglobin results in an alteration of the MR signal since deoxygenated blood is more paramagnetic than oxygenated blood (the difference is about 0.2 ppm). The change in signal provides an estimate of relative local cerebral perfusion changes associated with the change in underlying neuronal activity. This observation has resulted in the widespread use of the so-called blood oxygen level dependent technique in the evaluation of normal subjects performing behavioral tasks and in patients who are candidates for surgical resection of brain lesions such as tumors, vascular malformations, or epileptic foci. Such methods may ultimately supplant more invasive approaches to determining language dominance and memory function such as those employing the intraarterial injection of barbiturate compounds (e.g., Wada testing).

Diffusion imaging is also possible using MR scanning. Water, and hence protons, is freely diffusible. In the brain, however, the microscopic anatomy of the tissue compartmentalizes (with cells, along axons, etc.) this process. It is possible to obtain MRI images that are diffusion weighted (DW) and in which the signal is dependent on the ease with which protons diffuse in their local environment. Initially tested in cats, DW images were shown to demonstrate the boundaries of acute infarcts within minutes. Infarcted or ischemic areas are visible as regions of hyperintensity corresponding to local decreases in the apparent diffusion coefficient of water. The use of DWI in screening patients with early ischemia who are candidates for thrombolytic therapy is especially relevant (Fig. 5). When combined with MRI perfusion imaging, an assessment of the proportion of jeopardized and infarcted tissue can be made.

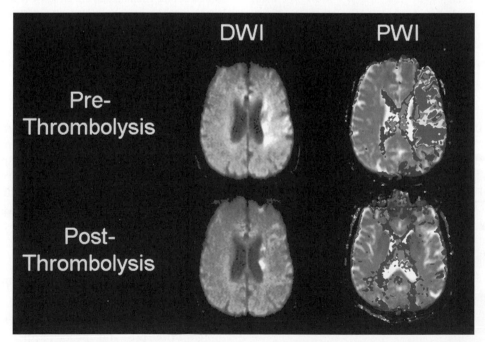

Figure 5 Diffusion-weighted (DWI) and perfusion-weighted (PWI) images from MRI are useful in selecting patients for cerebrovascular intervention therapies and monitoring their outcome. Here, a patient with a large region of hypoperfusion in the distribution of the middle cerebral artery already has some evidence of tissue ischemia as demonstrated by the white areas that border the ventricle in the prethrombolysis DW image (top left). Following thrombolysis (bottom row), note that perfusion has been reestablished to the area of the middle cerebral artery and the patient is left with only a small ischemia injury on the posterior border of the lateral ventricle (courtesy of Chelsea Kidwell, Jeffrey Saver, and Jeffrey Alger, UCLA School of Medicine).

4. Metabolism

a. PET Glucose and oxygen metabolism can be assessed using PET and ^{18}F-labeled fluorodeoxyglucose (FDG), ^{11}C-labeled glucose, and ^{15}O-labeled oxygen. A common approach has been to use FDG to evaluate glucose metabolism. Thought to be primarily an assessment of synaptic activity (i.e., deoxyglucose uptake is maximal i 1 the neuropil rather than in regions dominated by ce¹¹ ʰodies), scanning of patients using FDG has provided useful observations in a wide range of disorders. Hypometabolic regions are found interictally at epileptic foci and in specific cortical and subcortical regions in a wide range of degenerative and dementing processes and also appear to reflect the malignancy grade of cerebral neoplasms, particularly gliomas (Figs. 6–8). Oxygen metabolism and extraction measurements are of greatest utility in assessing patients with cerebrovascular disease, particularly that unique subset of patients for which extracranial–intracranial bypass or other surgical reperfusion approaches are contemplated.

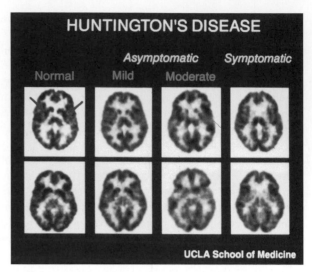

Figure 7 Glucose metabolism measured with PET in Huntington's disease. Two anatomical levels (rows) of a normal subject demonstrating glucose metabolism in the caudate and putamen as compared with three patients, two with mild or moderate asymptomatic Huntington's disease and one with frank symptoms. Note that in the symptomatic patient there is profound hypometabolism of the caudate and most of the putamen, whereas in the asymptomatic, gene-positive subjects, there is progressive loss of metabolism in the caudate. Such changes can be identified 5–7 years prior to the onset of symptoms in patients who carry an expanded triplet repeat sequence of the Huntington's disease gene. With advancing disease, hypometabolism extends throughout the striatum and can also involve the frontal cortices (courtesy of Scott Grafton and John Mazziotta, UCLA School of Medicine).

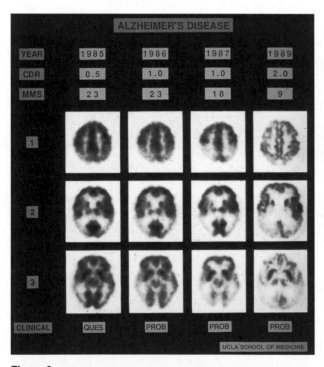

Figure 6 PET studies of cerebral glucose metabolism in a patient with Alzheimer's disease demonstrating the characteristic pattern of hypometabolism that occurs in the parietal and superior temporal cortices. As the disease progresses (from left to right), hypometabolism worsens in both spatial extent and magnitude, ultimately involving all neocortical structures.

b. MR Spectroscopy Concentrations of a wide variety of compounds can be estimated using MR spectroscopy. Proton spectra provide information about lactate as a measure of carbohydrate metabolism. Other chemical species as well as spectra obtained from other isotopes can provide additional clues about various chemical pathways. In addition, "tracer" techniques can be employed, e.g., using $^{17}O_2$, ^{13}C-labeled glucose, analogous to those used with PET or SPECT.

5. Ligands and Neuroreceptor Imaging

a. PET Ligands have been developed for PET to image both pre and postsynaptic neuroreceptors. Since one or both sides of a synapse can be affected by neuropsychiatric disease, the ability to image the integrity of both components of synaptic structure and function is useful. There are a large number of neurotransmitter systems in the human brain but

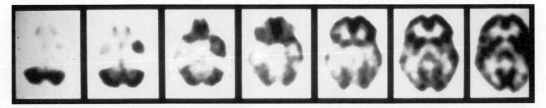

Figure 8 Interictal hypometabolism of the temporal lobe in a patient with complex partial epilepsy referable to that structure. Note the profound asymmetry of metabolism, particularly in the medical but also in the lateral portion of the temporal lobe, in six out of the seven axial images. Such studies are typically performed in the evaluation of patients who are candidates for surgical treatment of their epilepsy. In many patients, brain mapping techniques have obviated the requirement for depth electrodes and subdural grids in the presurgical evaluation of such individuals (courtesy of Jerome Engel, Jr., *et al.*, UCLA School of Medicine; J. Engel, P. H. Crandall, and R. Rausch (1983). The partial epilepsies. In *Clinical Neurosciences* (R. N. Rosenberg, Ed.), pp. 1349–1380. Churchill Livingstone, New York).

PET ligands have been developed for only some of these. Fewer still have been completely validated and are in clinical use.

The most extensively studied neurochemical system is the dopaminergic network. Presynaptic imaging of dopamine synthesis and reuptake have been evaluated with fluorinated (^{18}F) ligands. The uptake, metabolism, and flux of ^{18}F-labeled L-DOPA in presynaptic dopaminergic terminals have been used to evaluate movement disorders, particularly Parkinson's disease (Fig. 9), and a number of neuropsychiatric syndromes.

The same is true for the evaluation of presynaptic dopaminergic reuptake sites (e.g., with the WIN compounds). On the postsynaptic side, numerous ligands have been developed with a range of affinities for the different postsynaptic dopaminergic receptors. These tracers include raclopride, spiperone, and ethylspiperone. They have provided data for the movement disorders, schizophrenia, pituitary tumors, and other disorders of the brain. In addition, the labeling of drugs of abuse, such as ^{11}C-labeled cocaine, that bind to receptors in the dopaminergic system has

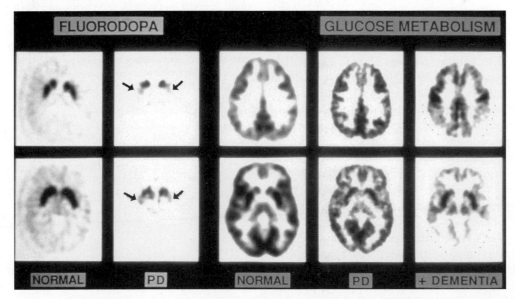

Figure 9 Evaluation of patients with Parkinson's disease using PET. Glucose metabolism in Parkinson's disease demonstrates a normal pattern in such patients (PD label) when compared to a normal control (middle column). When the dopamine-specific ligand [^{18}F]fluoro-L-DOPA is employed, however, a striking reduction in the uptake of this tracer is identified in the posterior putamen of patients with Parkinson's disease when compared to normals (columns 1 and 2). This is because the majority of the presynaptic dopaminergic terminals in Parkinson's disease are lost from the putamen at the onset of Parkinson's disease symptoms. Nevertheless, this population of synapses represents only a minority of all the synapses in this structure. As such, glucose metabolism remains normal but the uptake of fluoro-L-DOPA is dramatically reduced since this tracer images only that subpopulation of cells that have dopamine as their neurotransmitter. In patients with Parkinson's disease plus dementia, some patients also show hypometabolism of neocortex (+ DEMENTIA) similar to patients with Alzheimer's disease (see Fig. 6).

been helpful as a means of exploring the neurobiology of chemical addiction.

Cholinergic tracers are in use for the study of neurodegenerative disorders such as Alzheimer's disease and markers of the serotonin system and have been employed in the evaluation of psychiatric disorders. The central benzodiazepine system can be scanned with flumazenil labeled with carbon-11. Important findings have been made with this tracer in patients with epilepsy (Fig. 10A). Finally, opioid receptors have been studied with a host of ligands that bind with varying affinities to the many subclasses of opiate receptor. These compounds have been used in the exploration of eiplepsy, psychiatric disease, and movement disorders.

b. SPECT A number of iodinated compounds have been developed and serve as analogs of the PET tracers described previously. Used in a similar fashion, relative estimates of binding and receptor uptake can be obtained with SPECT (Fig. 10B). Although the number of compounds of this type is few compared to the inventory of PET ligands, interest in their development and use will result in an ever-increasing set of SPECT tracers.

6. Electrophysiology

a. EEG Electrophysiological techniques provide the best temporal resolution for studying neuronal activity in patients with neurosurgical, neurological, and psychiatric disorders. Although more limited in spatial resolution than the tomographic techniques, EEG data provide the investigator and clinician an opportunity to learn about the timing of events and their synchronicity. Particularly important in the investigation of patients with seizures, EEG has been the mainstay of diagnostic evaluation of such patients. The limited spatial resolution of scalp EEG can be overcome by the use of more invasive techniques when patients are surgical candidates. In that setting, subdural grid electrodes, depth electrodes, and cortical surface electrodes can be used to obtain local extracellular field potential recordings and electrocorticograms.

System-specific information can be obtained with EEG when recording is accompanied by specific sensory, motor, or cognitive stimulation, a technique known as ERP recording. The resultant ERP maps are used to identify the general location and relative timing of a cortical representation of such functions in the

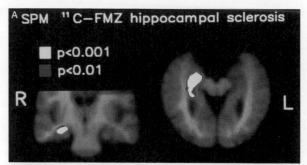

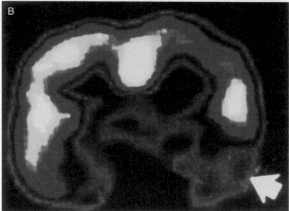

Figure 10 Benzodiazepine receptor imaging in patients with focal epilepsy. (A) PET evaluation with [^{11}C]flumazenil. In patients with focal temporal lobe epilepsy from hippocampal sclerosis producing complex partial seizures, flumazenil uptake is reduced in the medial temporal lobe. These changes are typically smaller in spatial extent than hypometabolism detected with FDG–PET. Comparison of the two studies may ultimately lead to more selective surgical resections of medial temporal lobe structures in such patients. [courtesy of John Duncan, National Hospital for Neurologic Disease, Queen Square, London. From *Brain* (1996), **119**, 1677–1687, with permission of Oxford University Press]. (B) Similar imaging can be performed using SPECT and the iodinated compound iomazenil. Although slightly lower in spatial resolution, such studies provide information comparable to that discussed for flumazenil PET imaging in patients with focal epilepsy [courtesy of A. C. van Huffelen, University of Utrecht (van Huffelen *et al.* 1990). From Berkovic *et al.* (1993). In *Surgical Treatment of the Epilepsies* (J. Engel, Jr., Ed.), 2nd ed., p. 238. Raven Press, New York].

brain. This approach has been used extensively to evaluate interruptions of the visual, auditory, or somatosensory systems (e.g., in multiple sclerosis) noninvasively and to provide more detailed cortical maps intraoperatively, or with subcortical or depth electrodes, in the evaluation of patients with seizure foci. Analysis of power spectra from scalp EEG and ERP recordings have also provided information of clinical use in neurodegenerative disorders and psychiatric syndromes.

b. MEG The measurement of minute magnetic fields in the brain with MEG is analogous to the measurement of electrical fields with EEG. Requiring far more complex equipment, the MEG method may have greater spatial resolution and greater accuracy in identifying electrophysiological dipoles, both at the surface and in the depths of the brain. Clinically, the method has been used to identify seizure foci and in a research setting has been employed for the experimental investigation of a wide range of neuropsychiatric disorders. Data with this technique are limited in number due to the fact that only a small number of MEG installations are currently operational and evaluating patients clinically.

c. Transcranial Magnetic Stimulation The creation of an intense focal magnetic field in the human cerebral cortex results in the induction of an electrical current that discharges cells lying tangentially within that volume of tissue. The discharge can result in a pseudophysiologic response. That is, if the motor cortex is stimulated, the appropriate contralateral muscle groups will contract. If the visual cortex is stimulated, a subject or patient will see a flash or phosphene in the contralateral visual field. Transient high-frequency stimulation of the cortex by magnetic stimulation will temporarily and reversibly deactivate it.

This approach has been used to create reversible lesions and has also been used as a therapeutic maneuver in the treatment of chronic depression, in a fashion analogous to electroconvulsive shock therapy delivered focally to the frontal cortex. When linked to a tomographic functional imaging technique, TMS can be used to map functional pathways directly in patients and normal subjects. There are guidelines for the safe use of this technique, which must be used with caution in epileptic patients.

7. Optical Intrinsic Signal (OIS) Imaging

The newest brain mapping technique to be used in a clinical setting is optical intrinsic signal imaging. This method provides information about cortical blood flow, blood volume, and metabolism in an integrated fashion. The approach is straightforward. White light is shone onto the exposed cortex and the amount of light of different wavelengths reflected from the cortex is measured. The reflectance and wavelength composition of light changes as a function of the neural activity of the illuminated tissue as a function of blood volume, blood flow, cell swelling, and the oxidative state of the

tissue (among other variables). An invasive technique, OIS is used in the operating room to provide functional maps in which neuronal activity is varied by stimulation of peripheral nerves or, in the awake patient, by the performance of behavioral (e.g., language) tasks. The method has the best spatial and temporal resolution of all the functional imaging techniques, approaching $50\,\mu m$ in the spatial domain and 50 ms in the temporal domain.

B. Multiple Modality Imaging

There are two types of multimodal integrative imaging studies that are important in the clinical evaluation of patients. The first is the within-subject integration of information from multiple brain mapping techniques, or the serial integration of multiple imaging studies in time using the same technique in the same individual. The second approach is the averaging or integration of information from multiple subjects, a much more difficult problem due to the great anatomical and functional variability that exists between individuals. The within-subject integration problem has yielded to a variety of excellent and elegant mathematical approaches for the alignment and registration of data. The between-subject problem is a more difficult one that is being resolved through the use of warping and morphing techniques.

1. Within-Subject Registration

A composite image of a patient derived from imaging using multiple imaging modalities or serial studies over time is a critical indicator of the clinical picture from an imaging perspective-for example, in a patient with a brain tumor in whom the natural history of the enlargement of the lesion can be evaluated quantitatively and objectively. Similarly, the integrated image of functional activation in cortical regions surrounding a lesion that is to be surgically resected can predict the relative risk of functional damage due to resection of normal cortex in the process of tumor ablation (Fig. 11).

Images of interictal spikes can be obtained by combining EEG and fMRI. Such images capitalize on the excellent temporal resolution of EEG and the complementary high spatial resolution of MRI. The relationship between hypometabolism in a seizure focus, determined with PET measurements of glucose metabolism, can be compared with benzodiazepine receptor binding, thereby increasing the specificity and

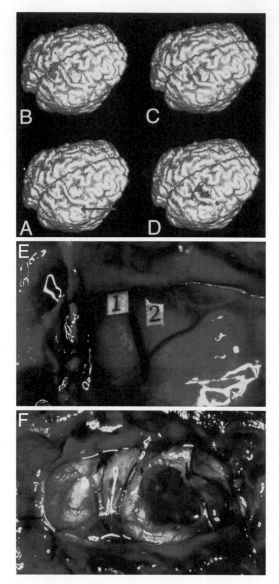

Figure 11 Within-subject registration techniques. (A) Three-dimensional reconstruction of a patient's brain with a cortical tumor in the region of the sensorimotor cortex (arrow). The structural data set, reconstructed from MRI, can then be combined with functional information about cerebral blood flow changes associated with motor tasks, derived from ^{15}O-labeled water PET studies when the patient moved the left leg (B), shoulder (C), or fingers (D). (E) Intraoperative view of the hand area of the motor cortex where the localization of sensorimotor hand function was identified intraoperatively with electrophysiologic techniques and labeled "1" and "2." (F) Operative view of site following resection of tumor. Because of the close proximity of the tumor to the activation site for finger movement, identified with preoperative PET imaging, it was predicted that this patient would have loss of fine motor control of the hand following complete resection of the lesion. This was in fact the case and is indicative of the accuracy and predictive power of preoperative mapping in patients with cortical lesions close to vital cortical structures (courtesy of Roger Woods, ULCA School of Medicine, and Scott Grafton, Emory University School of Medicine).

sensitivity of the combined result. One can also combine electrophysiologic data sets with tomographic data from PET, MRI, and MRS to provide a composite preoperative assessment of patients with epilepsy. PET measurements of cerebral blood flow, oxygen extraction, and oxygen metabolism in the same subject and comparison with diffusion-weighted MRI and MR angiography (or helical CT) provide a very complete picture of the supply–demand relationships of the brain parenchyma in patients with ischemic cerebrovascular disease. Such combined studies will undoubtedly become a clinical norm rather than an exception in the future.

Comparisons of scans between individual patients will become increasingly important. Such comparisons require that the scans be spatially normalized to account for individual differences in brain structure. The ability to normalize a scan to a standard brain space means that individual patient scans can be compared with a representative scan from a population of normal subjects that takes into account a realistic estimate of the anatomical variability in that population. In the structural domain, this ability may increase the sensitivity with which subtle heterotopias or other migrational abnormalities are identified in patients with focal epilepsy. Similarly, selected patterns of atrophy in neurodegenerative diseases should be detected in a more sensitive and specific fashion. The ability to compare representative scans across patient groups could also have importance for clinical trials where a patient group on an experimental therapy could be compared with a control group in an objective and quantifiable manner.

II. SURGICAL STRATEGIES

A. Preoperative

The preoperative investigation of patients with cerebral lesions falls into two general categories. The first is targeting areas for the purpose of stimulation or ablation. These circumstances occur in patients with movement disorders in which parts of the basal ganglia or other subcortical regions are selected for lesioning (e.g., pallidotomy) as a means of improving symptoms. Lesioning using stereotactic focal radiation or direct surgical ablation, by heating or freezing, are of interest for the treatment of cerebral neoplasms and vascular malformations. In a similar fashion, stimulating electrodes are now being employed in the treatment of Parkinson's disease and certain types of tremors.

The exact location for the placement of these electrodes requires knowledge of the structural anatomy and local electrophysiology or function to obtain maximal therapeutic benefit.

1. Targeting

Brain mapping techniques have already been employed for targetting. Currently, these approaches are limited to obtaining better definition of a patient's structural anatomy and developing better atlases to identify selected portions of the brain, given the individual variability among patients. With high-resolution structural imaging, specific locations for potential lesions can be identified anatomically and a frameless stereotactic approach can be used to direct an ablation probe or stimulation electrode. Once located, electrophysiological recordings can be used to verify the local functional environment of a given anatomical site.

Functional activation of deep brain sites (e.g., medial globus pallidus) is an important area of current investigation. Ideally, such sites should be located both structurally and functionally to identify a surgical target more accurately preoperatively. Such a facility would mean less retargeting and repositioning of electrodes and probes, thus reducing operating room time and morbidity, resulting in a higher success rate. Currently, there are no validated clinical examples of such an approach.

2. Differentiation of Normal from Abnormal Brain

Another important aspect of presurgical investigation of patients with brain mapping techniques is the identification of normal cortex or deep brain structures so that they may be avoided during surgical resection or ablation of cerebral lesions. The goal is to remove an abnormality in its entirety without removing normal brain tissue. Preoperative evaluation with PET, SPECT, fMRI, or transcranial magnetic stimulation may be employed to identify the functional anatomy of an individual's brain to determine the safety of surgery and a strategy for reaching an abnormal brain region to remove pathologic tissue.

Such functional imaging techniques may ultimately replace procedures such as the Wada test or reversible pharmacologic interruptions of brain function. The selective administration of barbiturates to brain regions that produce transient deficits has long been used to determine the relative safety associated with removal of a portion of the brain. Nevertheless, such tests are difficult to perform, particularly in younger children, and the exact distribution of the pharmacologic agent can be difficult to verify. If the same information can be obtained through presurgical use of functional imaging, it is hoped that both the accuracy and the ease of obtaining such data will be enhanced (Fig. 11).

The combined use of all of the noninvasive scanning methods, both current and experimental, resulting in integrated and composite images linked to interactive graphics stations in the operating room or the interventional neuroradiological suite, will surely become a part of such interventional procedures in the future. To be successful, these approaches need to be less costly, more accurate, and associated with lower eventual morbidity than conventional surgery without such ancillary noninvasive procedures.

B. Intraoperative Mapping

The most frequently used intraoperative brain mapping techniques are electrophysiological. These include electrocorticography for the identification of epileptic foci. Where cortical resections are indicated, evoked potential recordings with cortical electrodes are combined with peripheral nerve stimulation in anesthetized patients. Such an approach is frequently used to identify sensory and motor cortices. When more complex information is needed, particularly about language areas of the cortex, anesthesia is reversed and the patient is awakened during surgery. Direct electrical stimulation of the cortex is then used to reversibly disrupt local neuronal function while the patient performs behavioral tasks. In this setting, a patient must be psychologically able to accept the disturbing aspects of awake neurosurgery. Ideally, the examiner and the patient should have good rapport so that behavioral testing can proceed in an efficient and cooperative manner.

Optical intrinsic signal imaging, currently used in a research setting, may soon augment intraoperative electrophysiological measurements by directly providing visualization of cortical maps and functional responses seen ultimately through the operating microscope in real time. The high spatial and temporal resolution of this approach can be used to validate preoperative images of functional anatomy from individual patients. In addition, the functional brain maps can be updated as they become distorted from the preoperative state by changes in brain shape resulting from osmotic dehydration, ventricular drainage, or local edema during the course of the operation.

As more interventional neuroradiology and neurosurgery are performed within imaging devices, the reacquisition of structural and functional information as an invasive procedure unfolds will become possible and realistic. The most likely source of these data will be from MRI devices, where either patients are moved in and out of the device to update imaging data or the interventional procedure is performed within the magnetic field directly. In either case, direct updates of structural and, potentially, functional information can be provided to the clinical team performing the procedure.

III. ATLASES

The advent of modern mathematical and computational approaches to averaging imaging data across subjects has led to the generation of population-based probabilistic atlases. Such atlases are already in existence for the normal brain at different age ranges and for other regions of the body. Disease-based atlases may be useful for the differential diagnosis of human cerebral disorders.

The basic approach to generating such atlases is to obtain images from a large number of subjects (i.e., typically hundreds or even thousands) in a mathematical framework that produces a database that is probabilistic. Such an atlas allows the user to obtain relative information that takes into account the variance in structure and function in the human population (Fig. 12). Once established, such an atlas can interact with new data sets derived from individual subjects and patients or groups of subjects or patients. Thus, a clinician or investigator who performs an MRI scan of a single patient with focal epilepsy could call on a digital probabilistic atlas of normal subjects and compare the patient with the average normal atlas. The atlas will use the normal variance information estimated from the population of normals from which it is generated to determine whether a patient's scan falls within or outside normal morphometric limits. If the atlas is constructed from sufficient subjects, a subpopulation could be selected that more closely resembles a patient's demographic profile. In such a case, one might ask for only those normal subjects from the atlas who are right-handed, of a particular racial origin, and females ages 25–30. An increasing number of variables can be included in such a prior specification depending on the size of the data set constituting the atlas and the

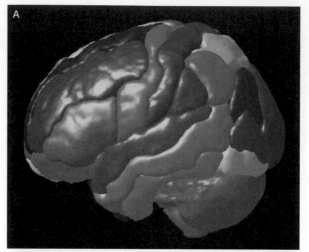

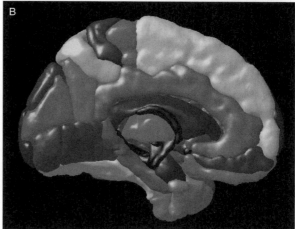

Figure 12 Probabilistic atlases. Population-based probabilistic atlas of the normal human brain derived from 67 subjects, ages 20–40 years, seen from the lateral (A) or midsagittal (B) views. The structures have been segmented to show cortical regions at a 50% confidence limit in the population [courtesy of Alan Evans and colleagues. Montreal Neurologic Institute].

range of demographic information collected about the contributing subjects. As a result, it would become possible to detect subtle abnormalities of diagnostic importance that would not be identified by the less sensitive conventional approach of qualitatively examining two-dimensional image sets by eye. In addition, such an atlas-based approach will give an objective and quantifiable magnitude to any detected abnormality. The scan data from any patient can be added to an atlas database, increasing its value with regard to particular patient groups.

Disease-based atlases, thus generated, are currently being assessed. It is possible to imagine morphometric or functional atlases for Alzheimer's (Fig. 13) and

Parkinson's disease, schizophrenia, and other disorders. Such atlases would also provide a population and disease-based opportunity to examine the natural history of morphometric or functional abnormalities as a function of disease progression, age of onset, or other variables. Such atlases could also be used to identify changes in natural course as a function of therapeutic intervention. Consider, for example, a clinical trial with a new drug for Alzheimer's disease. The Alzheimer's disease population atlas would provide estimates of morphometric changes in focal atrophy as well as, for example, alterations in crerebral glucose metabolism as a function of disease progression. A population of patients at a certain stage of the disease could be divided into two groups, one given an experimental therapy and the other given placebo. Serial imaging of both groups with the appropriate techniques would then provide longitudinal imaging data. Comparisons of morphometric and metabolic changes as a function of time between the two groups would be undertaken to detect objective and quantitative differences between the two groups. Any differences would represent a measure of the effect of the therapeutic intervention on progressive atrophy or

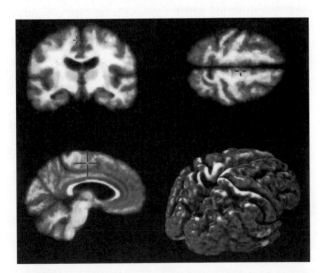

Figure 13 Probabilistic population atlas derived from nine individuals with Alzheimer's disease. This atlas is presented as a set of two-dimensional orthogonal views plus a three-dimensional rendering (bottom right) and is produced using a continuum-mechanical approach. Note the influence of atrophy on the composite image demonstrating widening of the major fissures of the brain as well as sulci in the neocortex. Such disease-based population atlases will be useful not only in tracking the natural history of cerebral disorders but also in providing objective and quantifiable information about structural and functional changes associated with experimental therapy for these disorders (courtesy of Paul Thompson and colleagues. UCLA School of Medicine).

glucose metabolism due to the natural history of the disease. It is probable, although currently unproven, that such an approach will be more sensitive in detecting differences between control and experimental groups, thereby requiring either fewer subjects or shorter time frames for therapeutic assessment, thus resulting in lower costs of clinical trials.

IV. PLASTICITY

One of the most exciting and dramatic observations to come from human brain mapping with a wide range of structural and functional techniques has been the dynamic plasticity of function in both normal brains and the brains of patients with neurological and neuropsychiatric disorders. Brain maps must therefore be viewed as dynamic, changing with development, disease progression, and normal learning and in the recovery of function after acute injury. The dynamic plasticity of functional brain maps provides an exiting opportunity to study these processes. It also means that the use of brain maps must take into account such variability in the design of brain mapping studies for patients with cerebral disorders.

For example, just as structural and functional studies must be normalized for spatial variability in the population, disease-based maps must be normalized in time to account for dynamic changes that occur with progression. Thus, a comparison of patients with Alzheimer's disease or other neurodegenerative disease should be stratified by time of onset or other variables that take into account the pattern of changing functional maps. The same is true after an acute brain injury, such as trauma or cerebral infarction. The complex interaction and highly variable changes in blood flow, blood volume, water diffusion, oxygen, and glucose extraction and metabolism will all be more appropriately interpreted if they are stratified by time from onset of cerebral injury. So too will plastic changes associated with recovery and reorganization after irreversible damage. Compensatory properties of the human nervous system have been clearly demonstrated in studies of patients following stroke who recover motor function (Fig. 14). The study of drug-induced, behaviorally associated and surgically promoted plasticity will, we predict, be an important part of brain mapping in the study of patients with neurological, neurosurgical, and psychiatric disorders.

The value of imaging data depends on an appreciation of the changing landscape of functional patterns.

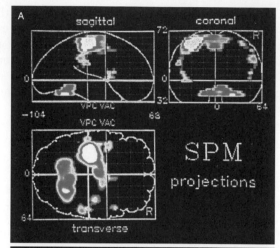

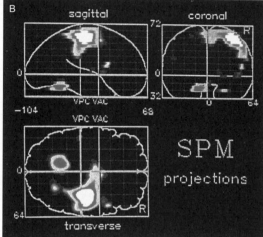

Figure 14 Compensatory reorganization of the brain after acute injury induced by cerebral infarction. (A) Normal response of a group of control subjects performing a motor task with the right upper extremity. Relative increases in cerebral blood flow derived from PET measurements demonstrating increased perfusion in the contralateral hand area of the motor cortex and the ipsilateral cerebellum. (B) The same motor task and methods were applied to a group of patients who had small subcortical cerebral infarctions associated with upper extremity paresis, all of whom recovered in the days to week following the acute ischemic injury. Note that when these subjects perform the same task, not only are there responses in the expected areas previously identified in the normal controls—that is, the contralateral hand area of the motor cortex and ipsilateral cerebellum—but also there are relative increases in cerebral blood flow in the ipsilateral hand area of the motor cortex and the contralateral cerebellum. Such studies provide useful insights into how the brain reorganizes following acute injury and can also be used to study compensation in more chronic states such as might be encountered in neurodegenerative disorders. These types of insights may be useful for designing more efficient, effective, and timely neurorehabilitation protocols employing behavioral, pharmacologic, or, potentially, surgical interventions for the restoration of function or its maintenance following acute or, chronic injury to the brain [courtesy of Francois Chollet and colleagues, Toulouse, France. From Chollet *et al.* (1991). *Ann. Neurol.* **29**, 63–71].

This is particularly true for techniques that make relative measurements. For example, relative cerebral blood flow measurements obtained with fMRI, SPECT, or PET may be misleading in patients with large cerebral infarctions. The evaluation of motor reorganization after cerebral infarction in a patient or group of patients must take into account a variable cerebral blood flow baseline in the setting of hemodynamically unstable tissue. Cerebral blood flow may be very low acutely, rise dramatically soon thereafter, and then reach some stable new level days, weeks, or months later. Currently, it is uncertain how increments or decrements in blood flow associated with neuronal firing changes that are task induced will behave under these different conditions of baseline blood flow. Is it valid to compare motor task activation in a cortical region when the "resting state" blood flow is altered from the normal value by 50–200%? Are there ceiling or floor effects in these responses? These issues need to be addressed before a proper interpretation of scans from such patients will be possible.

We predict that the ability to image plastic reorganization, both in normal and in pathologic states, will provide new insights, previously unavailable, about the constant reorganization of the human brain. Such information will be valuable in the design of behavioral, surgical, and pharmacological interventions in patients that facilitate and maximize the efficiency of the natural recovery processes. The imaging techniques should also provide a means to evaluate specific rehabilitation interventions, to determine their appropriateness, effectiveness, and timing, and to select patients for them. These abilities are currently lacking because the necessary information about the variables discussed has not been previously available.

See Also the Following Articles

CEREBRAL CORTEX • ELECTRICAL POTENTIALS • ELECTROENCEPHALOGRAPHY (EEG) • EVENT-RELATED ELECTROMAGNETIC RESPONSES • FUNCTIONAL MAGNETIC RESONANCE IMAGING (fMRI) • MAGNETIC RESONANCE IMAGING (MRI) • NEOCORTEX • NEUROIMAGING • PSYCHOPHYSIOLOGY

Acknowledgments

The authors thank contributing investigators for allowing their work to be reproduced in this article. This work was partially supported by a grant from the Human Brain Project (P01-MH52176-7) and generous support from the Brain Mapping Medical Research

Organization, The Ahmanson Foundation, the Pierson–Lovelace Foundation, the Jennifer Jones–Simon Foundation, the Tamkin Foundation, the Northstar Fund, and the Wellcome Trust. The authors thank Laurie Carr for the preparation of the manuscript and Andrew Lee for assistance with the illustrations.

Suggested Reading

Atlas, S. W. (1991). *Magnetic Resonance Imaging of the Brain and Spine*. Raven Press, New York.

Berkovic, S., Newton, M. R., and Rowe, C. C. (1992). Localization of epileptic foci using SPECT. In *Epilepsy Surgery* (H. Luders, Ed.), pp. 251–256. Raven Press, New York.

Chiappa, K. H. (1983). *Evoked Potentials in Clinical Medicine*. Raven Press, New York.

Chollet, F., DiPiero, V., Wise, R. J., Brooks, D. J., Dolan, R. J., and Frackowiak, R. S. (1991). The functional anatomy of motor recovery after stroke in humans: A study with positron emission tomography. *Ann. Neurol.* **29**(1), 63–71.

Daly, D. D., and Pedley, T. A. (1990). *Current Practice of Clinical Electroencephalography*, 2nd ed. Raven Press, New York.

Holmes, C. J., Hoge, R., Collins, L., Woods, R., Toga, A. W., and Evans, A. C. (1998). Enhancement of MR images using registration for signal averaging. *J. Computer Assisted Tomogr.* **22**(2), 324–333.

Luden, H. (Ed.) (1991). *Epilepsy Surgery*. Raven Press, New York.

Mazziotta, J. C., and Gilman, S. (1992). *Clinical Brain Imaging: Principles and Applications*, Davis, Philadelphia.

Mazziotta, J. C., Toga, A. W., Evans, A., Fox, P., and Lancaster, J. (1995). A probabilistic atlas of the human brain: Theory and rationale for its development. *NeuroImage* **2,** 89–101.

Newton, T. H., and Potts, D. G. (Eds.) (1981). *Radiology of the Skull and Brain: Technical Aspects of Computed Tomography*. Vol. 5. Mosby, St. Louis.

Shellock, F. (1997). *Pocket Guide to MR Procedures and Metallic Objects: Update 1997*. Lippincott–Raven, Philadelphia.

Toga, A., and Mazziotta, J. (1996). *Brain Mapping: The Methods*. Academic Press, San Diego.

Toga, A., and Mazziotta, J. (2000). *Brain Mapping: The Systems*. Academic Press, San Diego.

Williams, A. L., and Haughton, V. M. (Eds.) (1985). *Cranial Computed Tomography: A Comprehensive Text*. Mosby, St. Louis.

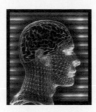

Information Processing

JOE L. MARTINEZ, Jr., STEPHEN A. K. HARVEY, ADRIA E. MARTINEZ, and
EDWIN J. BAREA-RODRIGUEZ

University of Texas, San Antonio

I. Learning and Memory as an Information
   Processing System

II. In Search of the Memory Trace (Engram)

III. Anatomical Basis of the Memory Information System

IV. Relationship between LTP and Learning

V. The Story of Arc: A Molecular Biological Exploration of
   LTP and Memory

GLOSSARY

amygdala A group of nuclei in the anterior–medial part of the brain that are involved in emotional memory.

declarative memory Memory that involves the conscious recollection of events.

DNA (deoxyribonucleic acid) The central library of an organism's genetic information.

DNA microarray Technique used to investigate thousands of genes from the same tissue sample.

engram The memory trace laid down in the brain. It is believed to be formed by changes in the synapse.

Hebbian synapse When a signal between two neurons is strengthened due to the simultaneous activation of the presynaptic and postsynaptic neurons.

hippocampus A structure located in the medial temporal lobe that is involved in spatial learning.

learning A change in behavior as a result of experience.

long-term potentiation A form of synaptic plasticity induced by brief high-frequency stimulation.

memory The ability to store and recall an experience.

nondeclarative memory Memory usually measured by performance, such as automatic motor skills.

RNA (ribonucleic acid) Short-lived molecule that contains information about the DNA.

transduction The change of physical energy into neural signals.

The neuron is the principal functional unit of the brain. Neurons both transform physical energy such as pressure and temperature into neural energy and conduct light and sound energy transformed by the eyes and ears. This transformation is the first step in information processing. Because we all have slightly different perceptual worlds and experiences, our individual identity is based on our memories of perceptions. This article presents learning and memory as an example of an information processing system. The article takes a cognitive and molecular biology approach in understanding how memories are formed.

*The world first exists, and then the states of mind;
and these gain a cognizance of the world which gets
gradually more and more complete.*

William James (1892)

Understanding movement of sensation from the external environment to the inside of one's head as useful information is a process that has consumed philosophers and scientists for hundreds of years. Think of the Challenger space shuttle explosion. In your mind's eye you can visualize the twin plumes of smoke streaking higher into the sky that represented the end of the mission. How did this image get into your brain and why will it be with you for the rest of your life? These are two questions this article seeks to address.

The human body exists in a sea of physical stimuli, only a tiny fraction of which we are aware. Consider the electromagnetic spectrum, which includes X-rays able to permeate solid objects and ultra-low-frequency radio waves with which we can contact submerged submarines thousands of miles away. We see only a tiny fraction, from 400 to 760 nm. We do not see cosmic rays or television transmissions. Perhaps our tiny range of vision allows us to focus on those external objects necessary for our survival. Our senses, then, are transducers that convert physical energy to neural energy. Ears convert sound, nerve endings convert temperature and pressure, the labyrinth converts gravity, the tongue converts acids and sugars, and the nose captures molecules from the air and gives them each a unique sensation. Consider the curious life of synasthets, people who hear light or see sound when their neural energies are crossed at the level of the thalamus so that hearing neural energy goes to the visual areas and *vice versa*.

We do not all perceive the same world because physical energy is transduced by biological systems that have many states and conditions. A person who walks into a darkened movie theater does not see nearly as clearly as the person who has been in the theater for a long time and who is dark adapted. At that moment their perceptual worlds differ. A person unable to distinguish red and green, a dichromatic, sees a different world, and a blind person does not see the world at all. Because we all have slightly different perceptual worlds and experiences, our individual identity is based on our memories of perceptions. As William James said, cognizance of the world is an iterative process that depends on perception and memory; together, perception and memory allow information processing. Everyone agrees that the brain is the organ that perceives the world and stores our individual memories, and the computational unit of a brain is the neuron (Fig. 1). As a cell, the neuron exhibits continuous metabolic activity but exists in only one of two transmission states, "on" and "off." Thus, it is analogous to a computer memory address, which contains a bit of information—either 1 or 0. Although the content of a computer memory address is set by a central processor, a neuron is much more complicated, gathering information from its dendrites and deciding whether and how many on states, called action potentials, it will generate. Neurons connect through special contacts called synapses at the end of axons. As depicted in the Fig. 1, a neuron connects with many other neurons, usually on a part of the neuron called a dendrite.

Figure 2 shows that neurons are organized into units called nuclei and these nuclei perform functions and communicate with other nuclei. Neuroanatomy is the study of the organization of nuclei. Continuing our computer analogy, nuclei function like integrated circuits. Note that in Fig. 2, neurons become more complex as one moves up the phylogenetic scale from mouse to human. Because it is more complex, the human neuron has more computational power. This is the basis of superior information processing in humans. Note that rat and human brains are similar in architecture. Both have cerebral hemispheres, both have a thalamus, and both have a cerebellum. Based on this similarity, we expect humans and rats to have similar functions, and both are capable of learning mazes, for example.

Now we can ask a difficult question: How can a perception become a memory and vice versa? Figure 3 shows a most intriguing result. In this experiment, a monkey was trained to look at a fixed point in the center of the circular pattern, and this was followed by

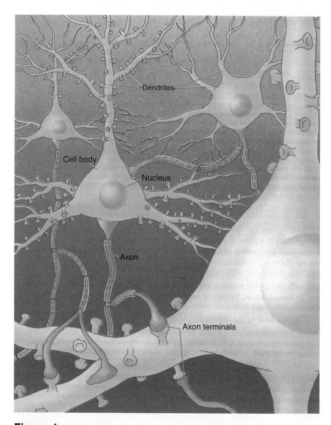

Figure 1 The neuron is the basic signaling unit of the nervous system. There are 10^{12} neurons in the brain and most have a cell body that gives rise to the axon, dendrites, and synaptic boutons or terminals [reproduced with permission from Rosenzweig, M. R., Leiman, A. L., and Breedlove, S. M. (1996). *Biological Psychology*. Sinauer Associates, Sunderland, MA].

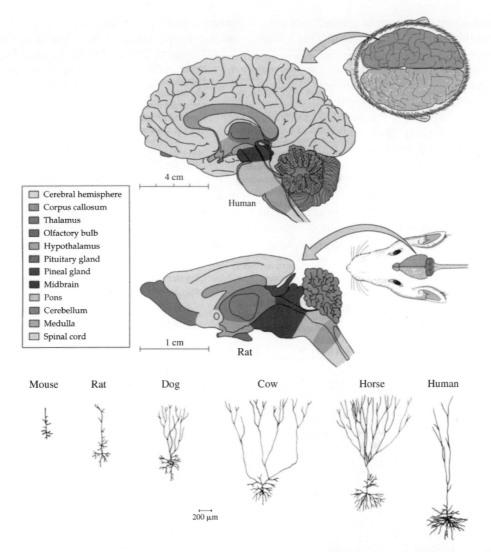

Legend:
- Cerebral hemisphere
- Corpus callosum
- Thalamus
- Olfactory bulb
- Hypothalamus
- Pituitary gland
- Pineal gland
- Midbrain
- Pons
- Cerebellum
- Medulla
- Spinal cord

Figure 2 Midsagittal view of human and rat brains. The structures observed contain neurons and each performs different functions [reproduced with permission from Rosenzweig, M. R., Leiman, A. L., and Breedlove, S. M. (1996). *Biological Psychology*. Sinauer Associates, Sunderland, MA].

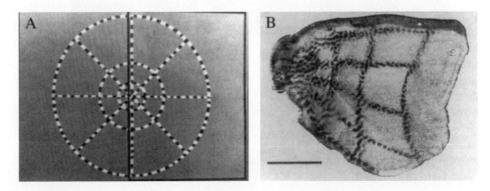

Figure 3 (A) A pattern of flickering lights shown in the visual field of a macaque monkey (B) Pattern is mapped in the striate cortex using 2-deoxyglucose (reproduced with permission from Tootell *et al.*, 1988. Deoxyglucose analysis of retinotopic organization in primate striate cortex. *Science* **218,** 902–904).

an injection with a synthetic form of glucose. Neurons that were metabolically active look darker. The circular pattern is recreated on the cortex of the monkey. A network of interconnected neurons represents the perception. The pattern can be stored in the monkey brain and made into a memory if the network that represents the circle can be made permanent. Hebb proposed this idea in 1949, but he called the network of neurons a cell assembly. In order for the monkey to re-experience the pattern, the network has to be reactivated in its brain.

Hebb proposed that the pattern could be made permanent if the connections between neurons were made stronger in a functional sense. That is, if neuron A, the first in the network representing the circle pattern, persistently fires neuron B, and so on, then some process takes place in either A or B and all the neurons that represent the pattern so that the efficiency of A firing B is increased. In other words, when neuron A fires the pattern is recreated. Today, the phenom-

enon by which one cell creates a larger response in the second by repeated stimulation is called long-term potentiation (LTP), and it is considered to be the best model of how the brain may store information.

Are there any nuclei in the brain whose function is to make memories? In the 1950s, a patient H.M. had his hippocampus removed on both sides of his brain to control his grand mal epilepsy. Following the surgery, H.M. could remember the past, but he could not remember anything new. He was said to have a deficit in his ability to consolidate or make permanent new memories. Interestingly, Fig. 4 shows that H.M. could learn a backward mirror drawing task, even though he did not remember the apparatus from day to day. It is thought that the hippocampus is a brain structure whose function is to lay down new declarative memories or "knowing that" (the apparatus) rather than "knowing how" (to draw backwards). In Section III.A, we take a closer look at the hippocampus and determine whether its organization or arrangement of

(a) The mirror-tracing task

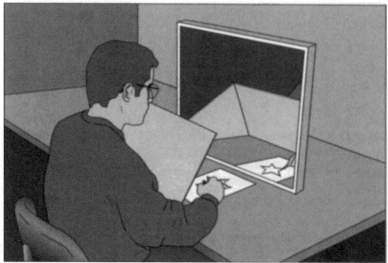

(b) Performance of H.M. on mirror-tracing task

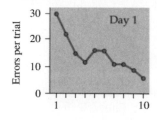
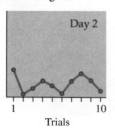
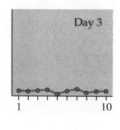

Figure 4   (a) The mirror-tracing task used to test memory in patient H.M. (b) Performance of H.M. on this task. Despite the improvement over days in this task, H.M. did not remember having performed this task in the previous days [reproduced with permission from Rosenzweig, M. R., Leiman, A. L., and Breedlove, S. M. (1996). *Biological Psychology*. Sinauer Associates, Sunderland, MA].

cells provide clues as to how it might lay down memories. In Section III.G, we examine the phenomenon of LTP in the hippocampus. If the hippocampus really is a nucleus designed to lay down memories, then LTP should abound in this structure. Finally, we examine an interesting phenomenon of memory: Many are permanent. What could possibly change in a neuron so that you remember the first time you rode a bicycle?

I. LEARNING AND MEMORY AS AN INFORMATION PROCESSING SYSTEM

In the morning an employee arrives to work and realizes that her usual parking spot is taken. She parks in another parking area, but before she leaves she inspects the area looking for landmarks that will help her find her parked car at the end of the day. At the end of the day she searches for her car in the parking lot by looking for specific landmarks. The ability to find the location of the car by searching for landmarks is possible because the person makes an association between the location of the parked car and the landmarks.

It is 12 noon, you are feeling hungry but still have work to do. You know that when the bell of the microwave oven sounds, your coworker, who is a great cook, is warming up food. Today, you hear the bell and your mouth waters. Sometime in the past an association was established between the bell and the food. In both the cases of using landmarks to one's car (declarative/spatial learning) and the sounding of the microwave oven bell causing one's mouth to water (nondeclarative/classical conditioning learning), it is said that learning occurred. Both visual and auditory stimuli were processed and associated in memory.

Using the spatial learning example (this also applies to auditory information), we can construct a model that explains how the person establishes an association between landmarks and the parked car. This model can be divided into a set of stages. The first stage involves the registration of the cues and the location of the car in the visual system. Thus, as described earlier, physical energy, light, which is used by the visual system to form the images (light pole, trees, or a sign with the lot number) that surround the car, is transformed by the sensory register into neural energy. Transduction is the first step in information processing—the transformation of physical energy into a type of energy that the brain understands. The second stage involves the processing of neural energy by the neural structures involved with establishing the association (the hippocampus). In the third and final stage, the information is retrieved as needed.

The information processing model constructed previously uses two approaches to explain the surrounding landmarks–parked car associations: cognitive psychology and computer science. The cognitive psychology approach seeks to understand the mental processes that take place during the time that a stimulus is perceived and the behavior that it elicits in an individual. The computer science approach helps us understand how information is processed so that it can be used at a later time. Interestingly, we can borrow many concepts from computer science. For instance, in order for perceived information to be used it needs to be encoded, stored, and retrieved. One major difference between the brain and a computer is that the brain uses billions of neurons in parallel fashion to process information. The computer has a main processor that allows the processing of a number of serial operations. You know that you have never seen the word "tedinu" (united backwards); you do not have to scan your memory from aardvark to zygote, as a computer does.

Humans are processors of information and human memory is an exemplar information processing system. In the past four decades we have learned a great deal about memory and the underlying mechanisms that subserve the encoding of information, and we are learning more about the mechanisms involved in the storage and retrieval of information. Next, we discuss the concept of the memory trace and current evidence that shows how a number of neural structures are involved in mediating the processing of information that leads to the formation of spatial and emotional memories.

II. IN SEARCH OF THE MEMORY TRACE (ENGRAM)

Curiosity in the understanding of the ability to remember information (memory) dates back as far as 800 BC, when memory was considered a virtue. Interestingly, even in those days teachers and philosophers recognized the importance of the sense of sight to develop strategies to remember information, also known as mnemonic techniques. The context became associated with all the information acquired in a place. Although an engram, the memory trace, was formed with a given experience, little was speculated about the localization of the engram.

III. ANATOMICAL BASIS OF THE MEMORY INFORMATION SYSTEM

Here, we focus on two types of learning presented previously—spatial (declarative) and classical conditioning (nondeclarative) learning that allow us to empirically understand the role of the brain in information processing. Interestingly, both humans and animals utilize these forms of learning. Furthermore, one type of learning may exist without the other. Before we discuss different types of learning, it is important to describe two structures believed to be involved in learning and memory—the hippocampus and the amygdala.

A. Anatomy of the Hippocampus and Amygdala

As noted earlier, the hippocampus was found to be involved in memory when H.M.'s hippocampi were removed and he exhibited anterograde amnesia. Figure 5 shows a view of the hippocampus and the amygdala using a transparent model of the human brain. The hippocampus was so named because it has a close resemblance to a sea horse ("hippo" means horse, and "kampos" is Greek for "sea monster"). The hippocampus is an elaborate infrastructure of computational systems. However, the complex basis on which the hippocampus functions can be understood in a simpler way by describing its trisynaptic structure.

The hippocampal formation is composed of the hippocampus proper and is formed by layers of neurons that form areas CA1–CA3 (cornu ammonis 1–3), the dentate gyrus, the entorhinal cortex, and the subiculum. The hippocampal formation has an internal circuit known as the trisynaptic circuit. First projection is from the entorhinal cortex to the dentate gyrus. Second, the dentate gyrus neurons give rise to the mossy fibers (axons) that project to CA3 cell fields. Third, the CA3 neurons give rise to the Schaffer collaterals (axons), which project to the CA1 cell field. In addition, the hippocampal formation receives projections from many subcortical structures (e.g., amygdala). Neuroanatomy is replete with nerve tracts that run from one physical location in the brain to another, but the hippocampus can be thought of as a loop that returns its signals to a location close to their cortical origin.

The amygdala, derived from the Greek word for "almond," is a collection of nuclei located in the temporal pole of the cerebral hemisphere rostral to the hippocampal formation. The amygdala comprises the lateral, medial, basolateral, and central nuclei. These nuclei have a number of functional roles, from receiving and processing olfactory information to sending projections to areas involved in autonomic responses. Studies suggest that the amygdala is directly involved in classical conditioning associated with fear.

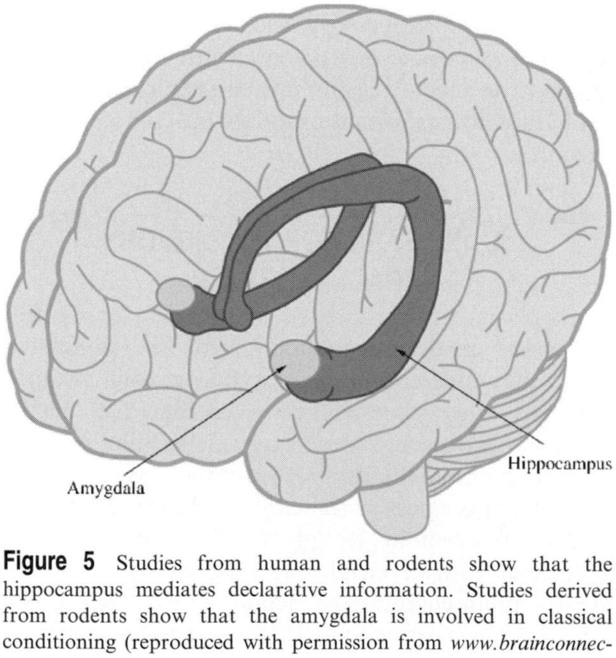

Figure 5 Studies from human and rodents show that the hippocampus mediates declarative information. Studies derived from rodents show that the amygdala is involved in classical conditioning (reproduced with permission from *www.brainconnection.com*).

B. Declarative Learning and the Hippocampus

Remember H.M.; imagine not being able to remember what you ate for breakfast, lunch, and dinner. Picture yourself at a dinner party unable to recognize any of the faces of the people whom you had met only minutes earlier. Recall that because H.M. suffered from epileptic seizures, doctors suggested that his hippocampus be removed. The result was both successful and unfortunate. H.M.'s seizures ended, but H.M. could not form any new memories. In addition to H.M.'s anterograde amnesia, he was unable to remember the 3 years of his life prior to the surgery (retrograde amnesia). Through endless studies and tests performed on H.M., many theories about learning and memory were revolutionized. Previous views focused on the concept of functional localization; this meant that specific brain regions were responsible for particular functions. This view (for some) was modified. Research from H.M. suggested that although functional localization is legitimate, there is a more complex circuitry associated with memory than once believed. It could have been hypothesized that because H.M. was incapable of transferring short-term memories into long-term memories, he could not have learned anything new. This was not entirely true. Remember that H.M. could learn skills such as the backwards mirror-drawing task. H.M. illustrated learning by improving at the task, despite his inability to recognize the test each day. This gave much insight into the process of converting short-term into long-term memory, a process called consolidation. H.M.'s ability to learn and improve at a task but to have no recollection of tracing the lines in the star gave novel insight into the role of the hippocampus in storing declarative memories.

C. The Role of the Hippocampus

Think of the hippocampus as the place where short-term memories are processed until they turn into long-term memories. Because H.M. lacked any ability to "remember" postsurgery, doctors and researchers deduced that the hippocampus was the locale where short-term memories turned into long-term memories. Keep in mind that H.M. could recall his life 3 years prior to the removal of his hippocampus. This illustrated the fact that long-term memories were not stored in the hippocampus; they were subsequently believed to be stored in another part of the brain called the neocortex.

D. Declarative Memory: One Type of Memory

Declarative memory is what we most often think of as memory. Remembering where you were when you first rode your bicycle or where you were when the Challenger exploded are examples of declarative memory. What defines declarative memory is the ability to consciously recollect the situation in which you learned something new. Declarative memory is context based. H.M. was able to recall experiences before his retrograde amnesia. H.M. had intact declarative memory to an extent, but he was unable to form any new declarative memories because he lacked the anatomical structure to do so.

E. The Animal Model

These findings provided an understanding about the hippocampus as a whole, but structurally there was much more to learn. Because of H.M. and considerable research on amnesic patients, we know now that the hippocampus is critical in transferring new memories into stored ones. How does this system work? Researchers needed to first find a model to test that was comparable to humans. Rats have similar nervous systems to humans, but unlike humans they are not able to verbally recall (declarative) what they have learned. They do use spatial cues to find their way in the environment (spatial learning). Spatial learning is mediated by the hippocampus, and thus used as a model for declarative learning in animals. The Morris water maze tests spatial memory by placing rats in a pool of opaque water. The rats have to find a submerged platform only by using cues (a large black star on the wall or an inflated beach ball) which are placed around the pool. Rats must first make a choice about what they did before (how they found the platform) and then use visual cues. Because the time spent finding the platform decreases with each new trial, it is believed that they have learned to find the platform by using the visual cues. Research on spatial information processing in the hippocampus shows that there are cells, known as place cells, that code for specific cues in the environment. Animal studies have shown that the dorsal hippocampus is specifically required for spatial learning, and the equivalent (posterior) part of the human hippocampus shows increased metabolic activity when navigational information is being recalled. Some species actually show an increased hippocampal volume during periods when they need to bury and retrieve cached food. Is there an equivalent change in humans? A professional requirement for London taxi drivers is a detailed knowledge of the tortuous streets of that large city. Interestingly, these taxi drivers have an increase in volume of the posterior hippocampus relative to a matched control population. Moreover, the longer they have been taxi drivers, the more pronounced is this change.

F. Nondeclarative Learning and the Amygdala

Previously, we used the example of a microwave bell and mouth watering to introduce nondeclarative learning. Physiologist Ivan Pavlov was the first to investigate classical conditioning. His studies showed that by repetitive pairing of a conditioning stimulus (bell) with an unconditional stimulus (food), dogs salivated at the sound of the bell. It was Pavlov's idea that the cerebral cortex was involved in classical conditioning.

Studies with animals show that the amygdala is involved in classical conditioning. In this case, the pairing of a tone with a foot shock elicits a freezing response when the tone is presented alone. That is, the tone predicts the presentation of the shock. Neurons in the amygdala respond to a shock-related tone only. Furthermore, damage to the amygdala eliminates the physiological changes associated with the freezing response. What is the circuit involved in this type of information processing? Studies by LeDoux and coworkers suggest that auditory information arriving at the auditory cortex travels to the basolateral nucleus and the central nucleus of the amygdala; first the auditory information arrives at the basolateral nucleus, then to the central nucleus. The central nucleus then sends information to the hypothalamus, which mediates autonomic responses (increased in heart rate); periaqueductal the gray area the brain stem, which mediates the actual emotional response (freezing); and the cerebral cortex, which mediate the emotional experience.

In the next section, we show that information processing can also be studied at the cellular and molecular level. Indeed, as suggested by Semon, Santiago Ramon y Cajal, and William James, the engram is formed by physiological changes in neurons. Neurons in both the hippocampus and the amygdala display physiological changes that are believed to mediate information storage.

G. Long-Term Potentiation Is a Form of Synaptic Plasticity That May Be Involved in Information Processing

As addressed earlier, Hebb increased our understanding of how information processing occurs in neurons by suggesting that activity in groups of neurons mediates memory formation. Because neurons communicate with each other only at synapses, changes in activity of groups of neurons likely occur at the synapses, and therefore memories are stored through LTP. The NMDA receptor is involved in forming LTP. Activation of the NMDA receptor requires both the release of the neurotransmitter glutamate and stimulation of the postsynaptic cell. That is, the NMDA receptor must be activated by glutamate and simultaneously there must be sufficient depolarization of the postsynaptic membrane to relieve a magnesium block in the NMDA-associated ion channel, which allows entry of the ion calcium (Ca^{2+}) into the postsynaptic terminal. Ca^{2+} activates a number of changes in the cells. Thus, this receptor acts as a coincidence detector, informing the neuron that it was activated in rapid succession. This is an example of a cellular mechanism that may be involved in information processing.

IV. RELATIONSHIP BETWEEN LTP AND LEARNING

The first evidence to associate LTP with learning was derived from studies that used drugs to block the activity of the NMDA receptor. The rationale behind these studies was that the blockade of the NMDA receptor would prevent changes in synaptic function. In the most comprehensive studies, the drugs were administered directly into the ventricles. This procedure allows the drugs to diffuse to the hippocampus in addition to other brain areas. The behavioral task investigated was the Morris water maze task, which is a spatial learning task. Blocking the NMDA receptor indeed affected spatial learning and also blocked LTP. Presumably, the blockade of changes in synaptic function prevented learning. As expected, LTP is also found in the amygdala, and NMDA receptor blockade in the amygdala prevents both nondeclarative learning and LTP.

A. LTP or Memory Formation Causes Changes in Gene Expression

Previously, we presented LTP as a model of information processing that leads to memory storage. We also considered the idea that information processing is associated with changes in synaptic function. However, changes in synaptic function alone cannot account for the permanence of memory storage. That is, there must be other mechanisms associated with information processing that allow for memories to remain for days to years. Many believe that the permanent storage of information involves a signal cascade that begins at the level of the synapse and includes the activation of a receptor and the activation of cellular changes known as second messenger systems. Then, at the level of the cell body, it involves the transcription of genes that have a short-lasting function (immediate early genes) and the activation of genes that have a longer lasting function. The activation of the latter may account for a more stable memory. The molecular biological revolution has taught us that long-term changes of cell function, as must occur in long-term memory storage, are controlled by gene expression and resultant protein production. Interestingly, almost every aspect of the signal cascade has been investigated in both learning and LTP.

How might changes in the synapse and then at the nucleus be involved in LTP and learning? If one accepts the hypothesis that long-term potentiation subserves memory, then one can alter information processing either by inducing LTP or by training an animal so that it forms a memory (task acquisition). After either of these experimental perturbations, electrophysiological and morphological responses are known to occur in the brain. For example, the electrical properties of a neuron could be changed by altered production of ion channel proteins, and dendritic morphology in neurons could be altered by changes in cytoskeletal and/or surface adhesion proteins.

Changes in gene expression can be measured in a number of ways. In "fishing" for the expression of genes that are unknown, two techniques have been used successfully: subtractive hybridization and differential display. Subtractive hybridization permits a mathematical subtraction of gene expression in control tissue from expression in treated or perturbed tissue, allowing isolation of mRNA specifically from genes that have been upregulated or downregulated. Differential display involves amplification of both control and perturbed sequences and subsequent separation of the amplified products, which permits one to determine directly which sequences have been increased. However, with the completion of the Human Genome Project and with other entire mammalian genomes in reach, a technique called DNA microarray analysis has become increasingly important. In principle, DNA microarray techniques can measure expression of all known genes at one time, and it likely will become the method of choice for some investigations. DNA microarray techniques have already been applied to studies of alcoholism, Alzheimer's disease, schizophrenia, and multiple sclerosis; they have examined the changes wrought in the brain by aging, sleep, environmental enrichment chemically induced seizures, and amphetamine.

Indications so far are that these conditions cause altered expression of a small subset of genes (approximately 12). One possibility is that this altered expression is sufficient to cause profound changes in a complex system such as the brain. Another possibility, which has yet to be examined, is that DNA microarray analysis of a relatively large piece of tissue containing millions of cells misses the changes that occur in a small subset of those cells. After all, neuroanatomy tells us that changes in highly localized nuclei or tracts within the brain will have profound effects. Other molecular biological techniques have been used to examine gene expression in a single cell, and it seems likely that DNA microarray analysis will be adapted to provide the same kind of specificity.

B. Restriction or Enhancement of Gene Expression Changes LTP and/or Memory Formation

Previously, we considered perturbing brain function and measuring the consequent changes in gene expression. Conversely, one can perturb normal gene expression and determine what effect this has on the ability of the brain to support LTP or the ability of the animal to acquire a task. For instance, single genes, controlling what are hoped to be specific events within cells, can be eliminated and the resultant effect can be studied simultaneously in whole animals minus one gene (so-called knockouts) for LTP and learning.

One reason to target genes is that these genetic procedures have the potential to overcome the current limitations of pharmacology. As mentioned previously, drugs used to block the NMDA receptors affected not just the NMDA receptors located in the hippocampus but also those all over the brain. In addition, drugs used to block second messenger systems are not specific. Thus, the idea of gene manipulation is to delete genes in local areas. Homologous recombination, a process that gives rise to natural diversity, is used to create knockout animals. To use this technique *in vitro*, one must know the DNA sequence bracketing the gene in question; also, the efficiency of recombination is low. In the first studies of genes related to LTP and learning, an area of focus was proteins known as kinases. Kinases are important because they activate other proteins (e.g., receptors). This presented a problem because the kinase family is composed of a number of subtypes, which appear to have varied functions. However, we can selectively impair the function of a specific kinase isoform by using knockout mutants.

The first kinase targetted was α-CaMKII, the type II α-calcium/calmodulin kinase. This kinase is important because it is activated when calcium enters through the NMDA receptor. Mice lacking this kinase had difficulty learning the Morris water maze. In the mutant mice, only the probability of LTP induction was altered; LTP induction was not abolished.

Protein kinase C is another kinase investigated using the knockout technology. In these mice the probability of LTP induction was reduced in the mutants much as it had been in previous studies employing knockouts. However, if the mutant mice were first treated with low-frequency stimulation, then the LTP was indistinguishable from that observed in wild-type controls. Regarding behavior, there were interesting findings in these mice. The mutant mice learned the Morris water maze at the same rate as did the normal mice; however, they had a deficit in contextual fear conditioning, a task that requires intact hippocampal function.

One potential function of kinases is to activate transcription factors, which are molecules that activate other genes and are found in the nucleus. Transcription factors are interesting because they mediate cellular and molecular mechanisms downstream of receptor activation (i.e., the cell body). One transcription factor involved in learning and memory is CREB. Previous studies indicated that better learning occurs when spaced trials are given as opposed to massed trials. One group used this finding to investigate learning in mice lacking CREB. Unique to these animals is impairment in long-term but not short-term memory. In this elegant study, it was found that in a number of behavioral tasks, including contextual conditioning, socially transmitted food preferences, and spatial learning, there was no impairment in learning when the animals were trained using spaced trials. The impairment observed with massed trials is explained by the fact that there is insufficient CREB to activate the long-term regulatory genes, whose proteins are essential for long-term memory. The use of spaced trials allows a limited amount of CREB to initiate sufficient transcription to allow long-term memory. These findings are important because they indicate the complexity that is inherent in the mechanisms involved in information processing in the brain. That is, since the deletion of CREB occurs throughout the entire animal, it is difficult to separate its primary effects in the central nervous system from effects outside the central nervous system. Since the animal's entire development occurs in the absence of the gene

product, a viable adult likely indicates that compensatory changes have been made in the levels of other gene products. DNA microarray analysis provides a means of measure for these compensatory changes.

Recently, second-generation knockouts have been created in which the gene deficiency can be localized to a specific region of the brain or can be turned on or off by treatment with a specific drug. Spatial localization within the brain is performed using two distinct genetically engineered animals. In one animal, part of the target gene is replaced by an identical sequence that is flanked by short, highly specific sequences of DNA (called lox sequences); these sequences do not affect gene function. In the second animal, the gene for a bacterial enzyme called Cre is inserted under the control of a promoter that is known to be activated in the brain. For example, the enzyme calcium/calmodulin kinase is highly expressed in the forebrain; therefore, inserting the promoter sequence for calcium/calmodulin kinase in conjunction will cause a high level of Cre expression. When these two mice are mated, some progeny will possess both the Cre enzyme and the lox-bracketed gene. The normal function of the Cre enzyme is to locate two lox adjacent sequences and join them together, excising the portion of the DNA that lies between them. In so doing, Cre inactivates the target gene. This inactivation will occur only in cells that express Cre, and since the expression of Cre is different among strains of engineered mice, workers were able to obtain a strain in which expression was highly localized to the principal cells of hippocampal region CA1. Studies accomplished with the first target gene—NMDAR1 or subunit 1 of the NMDA receptor—illustrate the elegance of this system. Conventional first-generation knockouts of NMDAR1 die shortly after birth. Since normal calcium/calmodulin kinase expression (and therefore Cre expression) does not occur until later in development, the second-generation knockouts have NMDAR1 present during critical early periods and are viable adults. However, the adults are deficient in long-term potentiation in area CA1 and have a greatly reduced ability to learn a spatial task.

The genetic techniques mentioned previously are all implemented in the mouse. Although behavioral training of mice is well established, the induction of LTP *in vivo* is technically more challenging in these smaller animals. The advantage of antisense oligonucleotides is that they can be used in the rat, which is the neurophysiologist's animal of choice. There is still no satisfactory explanation as to why this technique works, but it is particularly successful in the brain.

The target in this case is not the gene but the transcribed messenger RNA (mRNA), which directs protein synthesis. An oligonucleotide sequence approximately 20–25 bases long is synthesized that is complementary to part of the target mRNA. This antisense oligonucleotide is injected stereotaxically into the brain, where it enters the cells. Within the cytosol the antisense binds specifically to the target mRNA. The resultant nucleic acid duplex is vulnerable to cellular enzymes (e.g., RNase H) that cut both strands, inactivating the target mRNA. One disadvantage is that to "knock down" the levels of proteins that are constitutively expressed, a number of injections have to be given, often over several days. The antisense technique is best used against proteins that are expressed transiently, such as immediate early genes (IEGs). A further disadvantage is that to ensure that any effects seen are due to the specific antisense sequence used, it is useful to use more than one control sequence.

C. Transgenic Mice

As mentioned previously, the predominant form of LTP in the brain is dependent on the NMDA receptor. Functional NMDA receptors comprise more than one subunit and usually more than one type of subunit. For example, NMDAR1 subunits seem to be absolutely required for the survival of mice and are capable of assembling to form a working receptor. However, most receptors also contain NMDAR2 subunits, of which these are four different kinds (2A–2D). The NMDAR2 subunits do not form functional receptors on their own but modify the characteristics of NMDAR1 when they associate with it; each of the four subtypes combines with NMDAR1 to produce a receptor with slightly different characteristics. In the rat, NMDAR2A and NMDAR2B are strongly expressed in the hippocampus. The hippocampus has essentially no NMDAR2C (which is predominantly located in the cerebellum) or NMDAR2D (which is found in the thalamus and hypothalamus). Mice with targeted disruptions (knockouts) of NMDAR1 or NMDAR2B show no gross anatomical abnormalities in the brain but die after birth of respiratory failure and impairment of suckling response, respectively. Of the hippocampal NMDAR2s, electrophysiological studies suggest that NMDAR2B should be more effective than NMDAR2A in causing LTP. In a recent study, a transgenic mouse overexpressing the NMDAR2B was

created and evaluated; the researchers called their transgenic "doogie" after a precocious fictional medical student Doogie Hauser. These mice show enhanced retention of spatial memory and of both context (hippocampal-dependent) and cued (hippocampal-independent) fear conditioning, and they were dubbed "supermice" by the media. However, these mice show faster extinction (i.e., forgetting) of fear conditioning and enhanced novel-object exploratory responses, which are not traits likely to enhance survival in the wild. Between 20 days of age and adulthood, the amounts of NMDAR2A and NMDAR2B in the hippocampus decline slightly. A better name for this transgenic mouse might be Peter Pan since the decreased expression of the 2B subunit in adulthood is counteracted by overexpression, keeping the complement of 2B in a "child-like" state.

D. The Temporal Control of Gene Expression

Specialized proteins bind to the control regions of a gene (called promoters or operators) and increase or decrease the probability of transcription. In bacteria, genes to counter tetracycline antibiotics are kept switched off by the binding of a repressor protein to the appropriate operon (bacterial control sequence). Tetracyclines bind to the repressor and release it from the operon, permitting gene expression. A useful mutation of this system works in reverse: An activator of transcription does not bind the control region unless tetracycline is present so that antibiotic switches the system on. Insertion of these bacterial genes into mammals can be used to provide precise temporal control of gene expression. In one mouse, the activator protein (called rtTA) is placed under the control of calcium/calmodulin kinase, so it is expressed abundantly, but only in the forebrain. A second mouse has a transgene inserted that is under the control of tetO, the region of DNA to which rtTA binds. Progeny of these two mice will show elevated gene expression in the forebrain in response to a tetracycline-class antibiotic, such as doxycyclin. A proof-of-concept study used calcineurin as the transgene. Calcineurin is a protein phosphatase, and as a simplistic model it predicts that if protein phosphorylation by specific kinases is critical for the induction of LTP and for memory, then overexpression of phosphatases such as calcineurin should neutralize the kinase effects by dephosphorylating some of the critical proteins. This is indeed the case: The mutant progeny show normal LTP and a normal ability to recall their spatial training until doxycyclin is added to their food. Doxycyclin treatment significantly decreases both LTP and the ability to retrieve (recall) spatial training. When doxycyclin is withdrawn and the antibiotic clears from the animals' bodies, their LTP and ability to recall training revert to normal. Doxycyclin treatment does not alter the characteristics of the parental strains, which contain the individual components of the expression control system.

V. THE STORY OF ARC: A MOLECULAR BIOLOGICAL EXPLORATION OF LTP AND MEMORY

IEGs are expressed rapidly (within 30–60 min) after a stimulus. They include transcriptional factors, which act as intracellular signals, switching the expression of other genes on or off. However, IEGs also include proteins necessary for rapid extracellular signaling or for structural changes.

As an example of how molecular biology can be used to probe the processes underlying memory, consider the discovery and characterization of an IEG called *Arc* (activity-regulated cytoskeleton-associated protein) by Lyford and associates and Link and associates. Messenger RNA was extracted from the hippocampi both of control rats and of rats subjected to electroconvulsive stimulation. Subtractive hybridization was performed to isolate genes that were upregulated by stimulation. In order to confirm that the identified Arc DNA sequence could code for a functional protein, it was subjected to *in vitro* transcription/translation, which uses a mixture of the appropriate isolated cellular components to produce protein in a cell-free system. The predicted protein sequence of Arc indicated that it had no signal sequence for export outside the cell. Nor did it have long hydrophobic sequences or glycosylation sites, which are often diagnostic of a membrane protein; long hydrophobic sequences permit a protein to span the cell membrane, and glycosylation is a common feature of the extracellular domains of proteins. Sequence comparisons showed that one-half of Arc is closely related to α-spectrin, a cytoskeletal protein. The other half interacts with calcium/calmodulin-dependent protein kinase II. Measurement of Arc mRNA using Northern blot analysis showed that the unstimulated brain was enriched in Arc relative to other tissues, and that following electroconvulsive stimulation hippocampal

Arc was elevated between 30 min and 8 hr, returning to basal levels by 24 hr.

When a gene product shows increased expression, the following is one of the first questions asked: Where in the tissue of interest is this expression taking place? This question is answered by *in situ* hybridization: Tissue slices are taken and exposed to radioactive nucleic acid sequences that are complementary to the mRNA of interest and therefore bind to it specifically. Exposure to film results in an autoradiograph that localizes the mRNA to anatomic structures and even to subcellular regions. At 15 and 30 min after electroconvulsive stimulation, Arc was expressed principally in the cell bodies of the dentate gyrus granule cells. After 1 hr, Arc was also found in the dendrites (see Fig. 2).

In order to confirm that the expression of mRNA is paralleled by protein production, bacterial expression systems are used to generate large quantities of pure protein from the mRNA sequence. Immunizing animals with the protein yields antibodies that react specifically with the protein. These antibodies can be used to localize proteins in a tissue slice, a technique called immunohistochemistry. The general pattern of Arc protein localization in unstimulated tissue matched that obtained by *in situ* hybridization. Four hours after electroconvulsive stimulation the number of granule cells in the dentate gyrus that expressed Arc protein increased from 1–2 to nearly 100%. Moreover, protein was not expressed in axons or synaptic terminals but was expressed in cell bodies and also in dendrites. In these regions, Arc protein was subplasmalemmar (i.e., just inside the cell membrane), and this localization resembles that of spectrin and F-actin, important cytoskeletal components. Since Arc resembles a cytoskeletal protein in structure and localization, its ability to interact with other cytoskeletal proteins was measured. Arc did not interact with highly purified actin, but it did bind to a less purified preparation containing actin and actin-associated proteins.

The behavior of Arc, a protein rapidly synthesized in the nerve dendrites and capable of interacting with the cytoskeleton, would be interesting if it occured only in response to a pathological stimulus such as electroconvulsive stimulation. Does synthesis of Arc occur under conditions that more closely resemble normal physiology? Stimulation that leads to LTP induction *in vivo* causes changes in Arc mRNA expression similar to those seen in response to electroconvulsive stimulation. Blocking the induction of LTP in this model with an NMDA receptor antagonist also blocks the changes in Arc expression. Further analysis demonstrates that Arc is actually localized to the dendrites that are stimulated. As dentate granule cells extend into the molecular layer, they are contacted first (proximal to the cell body) by commissural/associational neurons, then (at an intermediate distance) by the medial perforant path, and finally (distal from the cell body) by the lateral perforant path. When electroconvulsive stimulation is used to generate Arc, there is no specific localization within the granule cell dendritic tree. However, when the afferent paths are stimulated separately, Arc mRNA is increased in the appropriate region of the dendritic tree. Immunohistochemistry confirms that Arc protein is localized in a similar way.

Are the increased expression of Arc and its subsequent localization distinct processes or are they related? Also, how is Arc targeted? As mRNA alone, with translation to protein occurring only at its dendritic destination, or as a polyribosome complex, with the newly synthesized protein required for localization? When Arc expression is increased by electroconvulsive stimulation (a process that causes no specific localization in the dendritic tree), subsequent high-frequency stimulation of the medial perforant path causes appropriate localization of the Arc mRNA within the dendritic tree, suggesting that localization is a process distinct from increased expression. Moreover, localization occurs in the presence of the protein synthesis inhibitors cycloheximide and puromycin, demonstrating that the signal sequence for localization is in Arc mRNA. An important negative control for all these data is that no other IEG so far discovered shows dendritic localization: mRNAs for these IEGs are retained in the cell body. A logical speculation is that Arc is required for the postsynaptic remodeling that occurs in the dendrite following high-frequency stimulation and that is necessary for synaptic plasticity.

It is known that the survival time of cellular mRNA is markedly decreased if it encounters a sequence that is complementary (antisense). The precise mechanism for this decreased survival time is incompletely understood, although it likely involves RNase H, an enzyme that specifically cleaves double-stranded RNA. If our speculation about the function of Arc is correct, treatment with oligonucleotide sequences (ODNs) antisense to Arc should change the pattern of LTP seen as a result of high-frequency stimulation. This proves to be the case: Direct injection of Arc antisense ODNs into the dorsal hippocampus significantly decreases the induction of LTP in the perforant path to dentate gyrus in the awake, behaving rat. In this experiment animals are injected in one hippocampus

with antisense ODN; as a control, a scrambled-sequence ODN is injected in the other hippocampus. Both sides show the same initial LTP, but from 4 hr up to 5 days a significant difference is apparent, with antisense-treated hippocampi showing only 30–60% of control LTP.

Given the likely correspondence between LTP and memory, it is interesting that the injection of Arc antisense ODNs also impairs the ability of rats to retain a spatial memory. In this experiment, rats receive bilateral injections of either Arc antisense ODNs or the scrambled control; three hours later, they receive training in the spatial Morris water maze for 1 hr. It is known that this spatial training, like the different forms of electrical stimulation mentioned previously, normally causes an increase in Arc expression in the hippocampus. Both sets of rats acquire the task successfully, but when they are tested 2 days later control animals can successfully distinguish the target location, whereas the rats treated with Arc antisense ODNs cannot. Since Arc-dependent consolidation of the memory likely occurs between 1 and 2 hr after training, antisense ODNs can actually be injected immediately after the spatial training and still interfere with the 2-day long-term memory; when injected 8 hr after training, the antisense has no long-term effect.

It is well-known from electrophysiological experiments that the hippocampus contains "place" cells, whose electrical activity increases when the animal is in a particular spatial environment. If Arc is involved in spatial memory, then whenever the animal is placed in a particular environment Arc expression should be increased in the corresponding place cells. Placing the animal in a different environment should activate Arc in a different set of place cells. As noted previously, microscopic localization of Arc in tissues can be achieved using *in situ* hybridization; if the visualization process uses fluorescent instead of radioactive probes, the acronym FISH (fluorescence *in situ* hybridization) is used. The method used to measure the increased expression of Arc very shortly after environmental stimulation is denoted compartmental analysis of temporal FISH (catFISH). Like all mRNAs, Arc originates in the nucleus but is rapidly exported to the cytoplasm of the cell body. Unlike other IEG mRNAs, Arc is then cleared from the cell body by targeting to the dendrites. By examining Arc's distribution relative to the nucleus, one can determine how recently a given cell was stimulated. For example, taking an animal from its home cage and placing it in a particular environment (e.g., environment A) 5 min before sacrifice yields a subpopulation of hippocampal cells with only nuclear labeling. If the sacrifice of the animal is delayed for more than 30 min, then there is a subpopulation of cells with only cytoplasmic labeling. How do we know that these subpopulations in different animals are comparable, or even that they are truly place cells? If an animal is exposed to environment A, returned to its home cage, and then reexposed to environment A immediately before sacrifice, a single subpopulation of cells shows both nuclear and cytoplasmic labeling—that is, the *same* subpopulation has been stimulated twice, at different times in the past. In hippocampal region CA1, this subpopulation represents about 40% of all cells. A completely different pattern is seen if the animal is exposed to environment A, returned to its home cage, and then exposed to environment B. Only 16% of cells in the CA1 show both nuclear and cytoplasmic labeling. If another 40% (fraction 0.4) of CA1 cells are activated by any given environment, then the number of cells stimulated in common by two different environments will be $(0.4)^2$ or 0.16 (i.e., 16%). We predict that 24% (40%−16%) of cells will be uniquely stimulated by environment A and the same number by environment B. The cells corresponding to environment A will show exclusively cytoplasmic labeling because of the delay prior to sacrifice. The cells corresponding to environment B will show exclusively nuclear labeling because no delay ensued. The experimentally determined values are 22 and 23%, respectively, showing the model to be internally consistent.

Given that the Arc story began in the dentate gyrus, it is interesting that although hippocampal regions CA1 and CA3 and the parietal cortex all show similar results using catFISH, the dentate gyrus shows essentially no Arc response to environmental change, or that ARC is not involved in storing spatial information in the dentate gyrus. This suggests that spatial data pass through the dentate gyrus without causing a change.

In summary, studies show that cellular and molecular events are the underlying mechanisms associated with the processing of information that leads to the permanent storage of memory. Interestingly, as suggested by Hebb, these cellular and molecular events are initiated by the activity between neurons.

See Also the Following Articles

ARTIFICIAL INTELLIGENCE • ATTENTION • CREATIVITY • HEURISTICS • INTELLIGENCE • LANGUAGE AND LEXICAL PROCESSING • LOGIC AND REASONING • MEMORY, OVERVIEW • NERVE CELLS AND MEMORY • NEURAL NETWORKS • NUMBER PROCESSING AND ARITHMETIC

Suggested Reading

Finger, S. (1994). *Origins of Neuroscience: A History of Explorations into Brain Function.* Oxford Univ. Press, New York.

Hebb, D. O. (1949). *The Organization of Behavior.* Wiley, New York.

Link, W., Konietzko, U., Kauselmann, G., Krug, M., Schwanke, B., Frey, U., and Kuhl, D. (1995). Somatodendritic expression of an immediate early gene is regulated by synaptic activity. *Proc. Natl. Acad. Sci. USA* 5734–5738.

Lyford, G. L., Yamagata, K., Kaufmann, W. E., Barnes, C. A., Sanders, L. K., Copeland, N. G., Gilbert, D. J., Jenkins, N. A., Lanahan, A. A., and Worley, P. F. (1995). Arc, a growth factor and activity-regulated gene, encodes a novel cytoskeleton-associated protein that is enriched in neuronal dendrites. *Neuron* 433–445.

Martinez, J. L., Jr., Barea-Rodriguez, E. J., and Derrick, B. E. (1998). Long-term potentiation, long-term depression and learning. In *Neurobiology of Learning and Memory* (J. L. Martinez, and R. Kesner, Eds.), pp. 211–246. Academic Press, San Diego.

Squire, L. R., and Kandel, E. R. (1999). *Memory: From Mind to Molecules.* Sci. Am., New York.

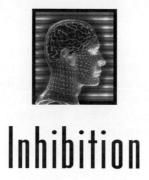

Inhibition

AVISHAI HENIK

Ben Gurion University of the Negev, Israel

THOMAS H. CARR

Michigan State University

GLOSSARY

anterior cingulate cortex A region of the medial frontal lobe involved in a variety of cognitive, motor, and emotional–motivational functions, including Brodmann's area 24 and perhaps the closely associated area 25.

attention A class of cognitive processes involving prioritization or selection among stimuli to be processed, tasks to be performed, or responses to produce.

frontal eye field A region centered at the intersection of the precentral sulcus with the superior frontal sulcus, that is, Brodmann's area 6. This region is involved in generation and control of eye movements.

reaction time The time elapsed from onset of the imperative stimulus to initiation of the subject's response.

saccade Rapid eye movement that changes the point of fixation from one location to another.

stimulus onset asynchrony The time elapsed from the onset of the first stimulus (or the cue) to the onset of the imperative stimulus.

Inhibition refers to mechanisms by which the nervous system suppresses information, restricts its use, or restrains its transmission from one place in the brain to another. This article addresses hypotheses about the role of inhibition at the systems level, considering the possible functional consequences of inhibitory processes for cognition and behavior. Ultimately, one might guess that at the neuronal level, inhibitory processes would be implemented via neuron-to-neuron communication in which release of inhibitory neurotransmitters reduces the probability of action potentials in postsynaptic target neurons of brain structures whose activity needs to be curtailed. As will be shown, however, reduction or suppression of activation is not the only way in which a systems-level inhibitory outcome can be achieved in cognition or behavior, although it is the most commonly proposed mechanism.

I. THE ROLE OF INHIBITION IN COGNITION AND BEHAVIOR

Cognition and the control of overt behavior rely on real-time orchestration of component cognitive processes or "mental operations." Each operation achieves a step in the sequence of steps leading from stimulus to response, intention to action, or thought to thought. A major distinction is made between reflexive or "automatic" operations and voluntary or "controlled" operations. The more automatic an operation is, the more able it is to occur without intention, needing only the appropriate stimulus conditions or information inputs to trigger it; to occur outside of conscious awareness, without being noticed phenomenologically; and to run in parallel with other mental operations.

Automatic operations gain these properties either from genetic hardwiring or, more frequently, from repetition under relatively unchanging conditions. Hence, they sometimes occur as reflexes, and they become quite prominent in familiar situations and well-practiced tasks. Controlled operations are the opposite. The more voluntary or controlled an operation is, the more its execution is intentional, conscious, and demanding of serial attention. Controlled processes become prominent when dealing with novel situations to which reflexes and habits are poorly adapted or when pursuing particular goals in situations that are likely to trigger reflexes and habits that would produce incorrect or inappropriate behavior if unrestrained.

To achieve flexibility in dealing with both the familiar, unchanging aspects of the world and with novel events, it is important to make automatic and controlled processes work in concert. Inhibition provides a tool for curbing or regulating automated responses in the service of controlled assessment and reaction.

Just how fundamental a role is played by inhibition of automated responses can be appreciated by thinking about the developmental trajectory of reflexes across the life span. One of the central principles of neurology is that disease processes affecting higher brain centers, especially the cerebral cortex, are revealed by reappearance of primitive reflexes. The knee jerk of a normal person is tonically inhibited, but it can become hyperactive after damage to the spinal cord that interrupts descending inhibitory pathways from the motor cortex. The sucking reflex of infants disappears after the nursing years but can reappear in a patient with Alzheimer's disease. Presumably, with the development of the nervous system, these primitive reflexes are inhibited throughout adulthood but may be disinhibited and reappear due to nervous system insult.

Other reflexes remain active throughout the life span. Among the most common are reflexive orienting reactions that involve the automatic deployment of attention to a suddenly appearing visual stimulus or a loud sound. Because these are very common occurrences, such attentional reactions are frequent and do not always occur at convenient times. When controlled deployment of attention is required by task performance, disruptive reflexive deployments may need to be inhibited.

Analogous problems can arise in controlling responses that are not reflexes but have become automated through practice. Attention deficit and hyperactivity disorder is a persistent individual difference characterized by an impulsive inability to resist engaging in prepotent or automated actions triggered by task-irrelevant stimuli in the environment or task-irrelevant thoughts in the mind. Intrusion of an unwanted or inappropriate automatic response occasionally occurs in normal children and adults as well. This can be seen in "slips of action" in which distraction of attention while carrying out a low-frequency task can result in inadvertently executing a different task that is higher in frequency given the situation and stimulus environment.

Other inhibitory functions are aimed at suppressing unwanted or incorrect perceptions and thoughts rather than controlling attention or inhibiting overt actions. These extraneous mental representations may become activated through relatively automatic processes of generalization because they are similar to correct perceptions and thoughts, or they may become activated because the environmental situation is ambiguous and admits multiple interpretations, only one of which is relevant to the task at hand. It is obvious that the wrong interpretation can be reached in an ambiguous situation, and if so it will need to be replaced. Less obvious, perhaps, is the possibility that all the interpretations of an ambiguous stimulus might be computed relatively automatically at an early stage of processing on every occasion, with one chosen for further processing at a later stage. In either case, contextually inappropriate interpretations will be active at some point in task performance and will need to be put aside or eliminated. This may involve inhibition. In this regard, Sir John Eccles wrote the following in 1977:

> I always think that inhibition is a sculpturing process. The inhibition, as it were, chisels away at the diffuse and rather amorphous mass of excitatory action and gives a more specific form to the neuronal performance at every stage of synaptic relay.

In this article, we present several examples representing the types of inhibitory function we have just described. Some are examples of inhibition regulating the deployment of attention. Others are examples of inhibition enabling disengagement from ongoing or automatically triggered responding so that overt behavior can be under voluntary and strategic control.

Still others are examples of inhibition tuning and sharpening the representation of the stimulus produced by perception or the interpretation of the situation produced by higher cognitive processes.

II. ATTENDING TO A SPATIAL LOCATION

Orienting of visual attention to a point of interest is commonly accompanied by overt movements of the head, eyes, or body. Attending may originate at will, such as when we decide to look at a particular location where something of interest is expected, or it may originate reflexively without intention when something captures our attention, such as when we orient to a flash of light in the dark or to a movement in the periphery of our vision. In everyday life there are constantly competing demands on attention by the outside world as well as from internally generated goals. The need for mechanisms to arbitrate between these competing demands is straightforward: This must be done so that they can be integrated, prioritized, or selected among to provide coherent and adaptive behavior.

Michael Posner developed a paradigm widely employed to study visual spatial attention. Figure 1 shows the basic features of this paradigm. In a typical experiment, the subject is first presented with three boxes on a computer screen. A trial begins with a fixation cross at the middle box. After a short interval, one of the boxes may flash briefly, and a target (an asterisk) appears in one of the peripheral boxes. The subject is asked to respond as quickly as possible, by pressing a key, to the appearance of the target. Reaction time (RT) is measured (in milliseconds) from target onset until the subject's response. It is possible to study covert attention by asking the participants not to move their eyes and by measuring keypress responses (rather than saccade latencies).

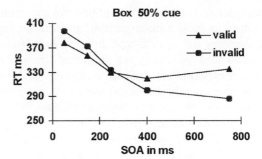

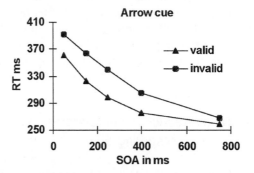

Figure 2 Typical time course for effects of a peripheral non-predictive luminance cue (box 50% cue) and a central predictive arrow cue. The task is a simple RT key press response to the appearance of the target. Mean detection RTs are presented as a function of cue–target interval (SOA) for valid and invalid cue conditions.

The cue may summon attention to the target location, in which case it is a *valid* cue, or it may summon attention to the wrong location, in which case it is an *invalid* cue. For volitional goal-directed shifts of attention, often called *endogenous* shifts of attention, a central arrow serves as a cue and predicts where the target is likely to occur in most trials. That is, in 80% of the trials the target will appear at the valid cue location and in 20% of the trials the target will occur at the invalid cue location. For reflexive stimulus-driven shifts of attention, often called *exogenous* shifts of attention, the peripheral luminance change that serves as a cue has no predictive value with respect to where the target will occur (e.g., in 50% of the trials the target will occur at the valid cue location and in 50% of the trials the target will appear at the invalid cue location). In order to measure the effectiveness of the cue in summoning attention, researchers have manipulated the time interval between cue onset and target onset [the stimulus onset asynchrony (SOA)]. The typical effects of the two types of cues are depicted in Fig. 2. The top panel of Fig. 2 shows the time course of a

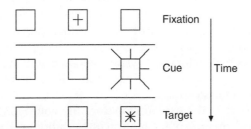

Figure 1 Basic paradigm for spatial attention, showing an exogenous cue and a valid trial.

nonpredictive peripheral luminance cue on summoning reflexive exogenous attention, and the bottom of Fig. 2 shows the time course of a predictive central arrow. These results were achieved in a covert attention experiment, with no movement of the eyes. The two cues are similar in the sense that in both types of cues the facilitory effects begin at 50 msec. However, there are differences. With endogenous cueing, the facilitory effect appears to be more sustained. With peripheral cueing, the advantage at the cued location changes, after a few hundred milliseconds, into an inhibition resulting in longer RTs for the cued location. No such inhibition is seen with endogenous cueing. These features of Fig. 2 will be discussed next, each related to a different mechanism of inhibition generated by the deployment of spatial attention.

A. Noise Reduction and Suppression of Competing Stimuli

Figure 2 shows that for about 200 msec after an exogenous cue and for 600 msec or longer following an endogenous cue, RT to detect the onset of a target is shorter when a target appears at the valid cue location compared to the invalid cue location. This RT effect indicates that attention has been drawn to the location of the cue, thereby facilitating the detection of the target at the valid location compared to the invalid location.

It is generally agreed that the presence of attention due to valid cueing increases the signal-to-noise ratio or sensitivity of information processing at the cued location. Of course, this could happen either if the signal from the attended location were enhanced (a facilitatory process) or if noise that might interfere with that signal were reduced or suppressed (an inhibitory process). The available evidence supports a combination of these two effects.

First, valid cueing can increase sensitivity even when a single target appears in an otherwise blank visual field. Since there are no other stimuli around to produce any noise or distraction, it would appear that attention is enhancing the signal from the attended location. However, the effect of cueing a target in an otherwise blank field is often small and sometimes disappears. The impact of cueing is usually greater when the target is accompanied by distracting stimuli at other spatial locations. From such evidence it has been argued that the primary contribution of spatial attention, especially in real-world visual environments, is to reduce noise or cross talk from unattended stimuli that if unsuppressed would interfere with processing the attended stimulus.

Direct evidence for inhibition of cross talk-based interference from unattended stimuli comes from single-cell recording in extrastriate cortical areas of the ventral object-processing pathway of monkeys. When two stimuli are present in the receptive field of a cell in one of these areas (e.g., V4 or TEO), the cell's response is less than if only one of them was present. This reduction in activity shows that the two stimuli interfere with each another's ability to activate the cell. However, if the monkey attends to one of the stimuli for the purpose of performing an experimental task, the cell's response returns to approximately the same level as if the attended stimulus were presented alone. This restoration of responsiveness shows that the unattended stimulus is being filtered out of the cell's receptive field and hence no longer interferes with processing the other stimulus. Analogous evidence that humans have a similar attention-driven mechanism of noise reduction through suppression of competing stimuli comes from functional magnetic resonance imaging (fMRI) experiments reported by Kastner and colleagues.

B. Inhibition of Return

A second important feature of Fig. 2, (seen only in the top), is that when SOA's following an exogenous cue are longer than 2–300 msec RT to detect a target is *longer* when a target appears at the valid location compared to the invalid location. That is, facilitation is transformed into inhibition. This is a standard outcome of experiments with nonpredictive cues, in which subjects have no reason to use the cue to guide attention and would prefer to keep attention focused at fixation or spread diffusely across the display.

Michael Posner and Yoav Cohen analyzed the effect of nonpredictive cues at the longer SOA durations, now known as the inhibition of return (IOR) phenomenon. Facilitation changes to inhibition (i.e., IOR) 200–300 msec after cue onset. IOR lasts for about 3 or 4 sec; it works in environmental rather than in retinal coordinates, it is not generated by endogenous cues unless the oculomotor system has been activated, and it declines as the distance from the original cued location increases.

What is the explanation for this counterintuitive transformation of facilitation into inhibition? Exogenous cueing commonly produces a reflexive shift of attention to the cued location or object (producing the early facilitation in Fig. 2). Even when people are asked not to pay attention to the cued location or it is in their favor to ignore the cued location, they find it difficult to avoid reacting to a peripheral luminance change and often cannot refrain from orienting to this kind of cue. As much as such efficient and rapid orienting is important for predatory and defensive behavior, voluntary control of reflexive orienting and the ability to strategically search the environment are also critical for survival. It appears that IOR is a mechanism that enables the organism to disengage from reflexive orienting and switch to the control of a more voluntary attentional system. How does it work? It seems that a location (or an object) that was recently cued or searched is tagged and IOR biases attention away from responding to events occurring at the tagged locations. Avoidance of tagged locations encourages search in new spatial locations. Accordingly, IOR seems to be a mechanism that supports efficient foraging behavior, which involves strategic search of the environment and use of knowledge about previous searched locations or objects.

Several lines of evidence point to the midbrain superior colliculus (SC) as the neural substrate for the implementation of IOR. IOR is abnormal in patients with damage to the SC. This has been shown in patients with midbrain degeneration due to progressive supranuclear palsy and in a patient with unilateral lesion to the SC. IOR is preserved in the presence of hemianopia, in which only the extrageniculate pathways are available to process visual information. It is present in newborn infants in whom the geniculostriate pathway is not yet developed. It is generated asymmetrically in the temporal and nasal visual fields. The temporal hemifield has stronger collicular representation than the nasal hemifield; accordingly, for monocular presentations of stimuli, IOR is larger for stimuli presented to the temporal than to the nasal hemifield. However, it seems that cortical structures play a role in the generation of IOR. In particular, the parietal lobe has been suggested as a structure that conveys the spatial coordinates of the tagged locations to the SC.

C. Inhibition of Reflexive Orienting

As suggested previously, other cortical structures in addition to the parietal lobes regulate activation of the SC. In 1966, James Sprague reported that occipitotemporal cortical ablation in cats produced stable hemianopia. However, visually guided behavior was restored by ablation of the dorsal midbrain contralateral to the cortical lesion. He noted,

This initial hemianopia is apparently due to depression of function of the colliculus ipsilateral to the cortical lesion, a depression maintained by influx of inhibition from the crossed colliculus. Thus, removal of the contralateral tectum, or splitting of the collicular commisure, abolishes this inhibition and allows the return of function in the ipsilateral colliculus, and with it the recovery from hemianopia.

This phenomenon is called the Sprague effect. A reversed version of the Sprague effect can be found with lesions to the frontal lobe, which will be described later.

The SC is involved in triggering reflexive saccades, whereas cortical mechanisms are needed for generating voluntary saccadic eye movements under strategic guidance. Early work showed that patients with frontal cortex lesions have difficulty executing saccades in response to verbal commands. When these patients scan pictures their eye movements are controlled by external stimuli rather than by instructions. In addition, lesions of the frontal lobes produce a deficit in inhibiting "reflexive glances." The patients seem unable to resist moving their eyes in the direction of a peripheral stimulus even when instructed to prevent such eye movements. It appears that the frontal eye fields (FEFs) are critical components of the frontal circuitry underlying inhibition of reflexive saccades and endogenous control of eye movements. Unilateral lesions of the FEF may shorten latencies of reflex saccades to targets in the contralesional field. Moreover, single cell recordings show that the FEF contains cells that respond in temporal correlation with purposive saccades even in the absence of an exogenous visual stimulus.

In line with these reports, Henik, Rafal, and Rhodes found that lesions to the FEF have opposite effects on endogenously activated and visually guided saccades to external stimuli. In a typical trial of an experiment examining saccades in FEF patients, subjects saw a visual cue ("get ready") followed by a target ("go"). The cue was informative (a small arrow) or neutral (a double-headed arrow). There were two types of target go signals: an asterisk appearing at the periphery (used to elicit reflexive, exogenously triggered saccades) or a large arrowhead in the center of the display pointing left or right (used to measure voluntary, endogenously generated saccades). The efficacy of saccade preparation was measured as facilitation in saccade latency in the informative cue condition compared to the neutral cue condition. Patients with FEF lesions presented slower endogenous saccades (in response to the central arrow) to the contralesional field, whereas exogenously triggered saccades (in response to the peripheral targets) were faster to the contralesional field (a reversed Sprague effect). These results indicate that the FEF is involved in generating endogenous saccades and therefore lesions in this region increase their latency. In addition, the FEF is involved in visually guided saccades through inhibitory connections to the SC. It seems that the FEF has the opposite effect on the extrageniculate visual system from occipital lesions. That is, whereas occipital lesions reduce activation of the ipsilesional SC (producing increased activation of the contralateral SC), FEF lesions disinhibit the ipsilesional colliculus, producing suppression of collicular function contralateral to the cortical lesion.

Taken together, this evidence indicates hierarchical control over eye movements. A relatively automatic system depending on SC is stimulus driven, responding to the appearance of new objects in the visual field and to movement, especially in the periphery. This system is also sensitive to sound via interactions between superior and inferior colliculus. Barry Stein and colleagues have shown that reflexive saccades and head turning are elicited when a movement that is subthreshold for triggering an orienting response is accompanied by a sound from the same spatial location that is also too weak by itself to cause orienting. The second level of control is cortical, depending on FEF. It exerts endogenous control rather than responding reflexively to stimulus inputs, implementing voluntary eye movements, and inhibiting the responses of the automatic system when such responses would conflict with the intended voluntary movement.

Interactions between automatic orienting and voluntary control have been studied extensively in the *antisaccade* task. This task requires subjects to move their eyes *away* from a stimulus that appears abruptly in the visual field—a stimulus that would ordinarily *attract* a reflexive saccade. Endogenous control is far from perfect in this difficult task. Errors occur in which the eyes move toward the abruptly appearing stimulus, and changes in error rate with experimental manipulations and subject characteristics can be used to diagnose the effectiveness of endogenous control. More evidence is provided by the latencies of correct responses away from the stimulus, which are slower than either reflexive saccades toward the same stimulus

or voluntary saccades toward stimuli that do not elicit reflexive saccades (either because they are already present in the visual field or because they are new but their onset is "ramped up" slowly to eliminate visual-onset transients). In general, factors that increase the perceptual salience of the stimulus, such as brightness, tend to increase errors and slow latencies, as do factors that reduce the subject's ability to concentrate on the task, such as attentional load, and factors that reduce the subject's ability to predict when effortful control will be needed, such as randomly varying foreperiods prior to stimulus onset. Furthermore, patients with frontal lobe damage have great difficulty with the antisaccade task.

III. "SELECTION FOR ACTION" AND CONFLICT RESOLUTION

The antisaccade task involves more than inhibiting the reflexive response toward the abruptly appearing stimulus. The subject must successfully implement another response at the same time the reflex is being inhibited. This second response is less well learned or less natural than the one that must be inhibited. Hence, the competition created by the automatic response is powerful, and resolving the conflict in favor of the less well-learned response is difficult. The antisaccade task is one example of a common method for studying the regulatory processes of cognitive control. This method involves creating a conflict situation in which the subject has to respond to one stimulus or to one aspect of the stimulus and ignore another stimulus or another aspect of the stimulus. In these situations, the subject needs to focus on the target (a stimulus or an aspect of a stimulus) and ignore all the rest of the display. Failures in attention are commonly revealed in two ways: (i) reduction in efficiency of responding to the target when the irrelevant features of the display are present and (ii) indications for processing of the irrelevant material, especially when it clearly interferes with processing of the target. The two most widely used paradigms for studying this type of selection are *Stroop color naming* and *negative priming*.

A. Stroop Color Naming

J. Ridley Stroop, a theologist with a side interest in psychology, sought an experimental method that would enable him to measure the interference of one stimulus dimension on attempts to process another. In

1935, he published a seminal paper describing three experiments. The second experiment asked subjects to name the color of the ink of color words (e.g., the word "red" printed in green ink) or the color of colored squares. The first condition is called "incongruent" and the second "neutral." Stroop found that the words interfered with naming the color. That is, RT to the incongruent condition was slower than RT to the neutral condition. Later, researchers added a congruent condition to the task (e.g., the word "green" printed in green ink). The congruent condition enabled one to look at facilitation, which is the difference in RT between congruent and neutral trials. It is commonly found that although facilitation in the congruent condition is small and on many occasions not significant, interference in the incongruent condition is robust and significant. Since 1935, this type of conflict has been studied extensively using variations of Stroop's color-naming task and in other Stroop-like situations with a wide variety of different stimuli and task demands. All studies converge on the conclusion that people cannot suppress the irrelevant dimension if it is heavily practiced and consequently overlearned (like reading words). Hence, the Stroop effect is considered a powerful example of automatic processing.

Nevertheless, several studies have shown that readers can modulate and partially control the impact of the word. Increasing the proportion of congruent trials relative to incongruent trials produces a larger Stroop effect. Moreover, even when the numbers of congruent and incongruent trials are kept constant while the proportion of neutral trials changes, the effect can be altered. It seems that the expectation to face a relatively large proportion of conflict trials prompts the adoption of a strategy that helps reduce interference. In addition, it seems that language competence may modulate the effect. When bilinguals are tested, under certain conditions they can reduce the effect in their first language but not in their second language. Note that they experience interference in both their first and their second language, but they are better able to control reading (i.e., reduce Stroop interference) in the language in which they are more competent.

Neuropsychological studies of brain-injured individuals suggest that the left frontal lobe is crucial to successful performance of the Stroop task. In particular, it has been reported that injury to the left dorsolateral prefrontal cortex results in enlarged Stroop interference. This result suggests that the Stroop interference presented by noninjured individuals is an underestimate of the potential interference.

Stroop interference presented by the noninjured individuals is the product of automatic intrusion of the irrelevant word and their ability (admittedly not perfect) to inhibit this reading. In addition, it points to the involvement of the left dorsolateral prefrontal cortex in the control processes by which Stroop interference is modulated. Consistent with this lesion evidence, neuroimaging studies of blood flow and changes in blood oxygenation during task performance show that the incongruent condition of the Stroop task activates left dorsolateral prefrontal cortex more than the neutral or congruent conditions. Even more noticeable in neuroimaging studies is differential activation of the anterior cingulate gyrus. Barch, Braver, Sabb, and Noll suggested that this medial–frontal structure is also active in a variety of other tasks in which selections must be made among competing stimuli, stimulus properties, and responses to them.

Of course, the crucial question in the present context is whether resolution of conflict in the Stroop task involves inhibition. Many theorists interpret the task in this way, although a well-known computational model of Stroop performance suggested by Cohen, Dunbar, and McClelland is able to account for many aspects of performance in the Stroop task by facilitation of the less automated process of color naming rather than inhibition of the more automated process of word reading. The phenomenon discussed next offers a more demanding and therefore more analytic test.

B. Negative Priming

In the incongruent or conflict condition of Stroop color naming, an additional slowing of performance is observed, over and above the usual interference, if the color name to be produced on any given trial is the same as the color word that had to be ignored on the immediately preceding trial. This effect, which has been dubbed *negative priming*, can be found in a wide variety of task situations in which two stimuli occur on each trial, one to be ignored and the other requiring a response. When a just-ignored distractor becomes the target on the next trial, responding is slowed relative to not having ignored the current target item in the recent past. Similar slowing occurs when there is just one stimulus on each trial to which subjects must produce a newly learned arbitrary response. Suppose that subjects must say "car" whenever they see "bike" or a picture of a bike, "plane" whenever they see "car" or a picture of a car, and "boat" whenever they see "plane" or a picture of a plane. Now suppose that as a prime the subject sees "car" and correctly says "plane." If the succeeding target is "bike," production of the correct response "car"—the overlearned response that had to be avoided when processing the prime—will be slower than if the prime was an unrelated stimulus that required an unrelated arbitrary response, such as "plane"–"boat."

The dominant interpretation of negative priming invokes a selective process that occurs while processing the prime. To respond appropriately, subjects must select against the distracter item that is the nonimperative component of the prime (or, in a task such as that of Shiu and Kornblum's just described, they must select against the overlearned but contextually inappropriate response that the prime tends to elicit). The act of selection leaves the distractor or the overlearned response in a state that makes it more difficult to process if it recurs as the target.

Two sorts of hypotheses have been offered about how this act of selection could be implemented. According to the distractor inhibition hypothesis, attentional operations actively inhibit either the prime's perceptually activated mental representation, in order to prevent it from competing for access to response selection operations, or the link between the prime's mental representation and the action ordinarily associated with the prime, in order to make that response unavailable. Inhibition takes time to dissipate. Therefore, if the inhibited representation or response link is needed soon thereafter for processing a target, more time and effort will be required for its activation. George Houghton and Steven Tipper constructed a simulation model embodying such processes.

According to an alternative proposal, the episodic retrieval hypothesis of W. Trammell Neill and colleagues, attentional operations mark the distractor item with a "do not respond to this stimulus" tag or the overlearned response with a "do not produce this response" tag. The tag provides an instruction that guides decision and response selection, and it remains a part of the experience of having processed the prime that is stored in episodic memory. When the target appears it acts as a cue to retrieve this memory. The tag that served the subject well when the tagged stimulus or response needed to be ignored causes confusion and interferes with performance when the tagged item becomes the target.

Note that the episodic retrieval hypothesis does not propose inhibition in the classic sense of reduction or suppression of activation. Its inhibitory process is "symbolic" rather than "analog," acting through an influence on a mental representation's informational content rather than its level of activity. Considerable effort has been expended attempting to distinguish these two underlying mechanisms by which an overtly inhibitory behavioral outcome might arise. Arguments have begun to appear that both mechanisms may be at work, and partly as a solution to the dilemma, in 1998 Milliken *et al.* made an important attempt to reinterpret negative priming in terms of the difficulty of deciding whether retrieved episodic memories of past processing should or should not be used to guide current performance rather than whether they have been inhibited or tagged with negative content. This debate illustrates a crucial point mentioned earlier. Inhibition of behavior (i.e., slowing of overt performance) does not necessarily signal inhibition of mental processing, if what one means by "inhibition of mental processing" is reduction or suppression of activation. Considerable theoretical analysis and empirical investigation are often required to make this determination.

IV. PRIMING AND RETRIEVAL FROM MEMORY

It is often possible to retrieve information from memory at will (though sometimes, of course, such intentional attempts at retrieval fail). At the same time, there are often occasions when thoughts come to mind without any apparent intention. Here again, we are dealing with two fundamental aspects of cognition: controlled and automatic processing. In the domain of retrieval of information from memory (general knowledge as well as specific episodes of experience), these two aspects of cognition have been investigated by exploiting *priming effects*. "Priming" consists of an alteration in the speed or accuracy of responding to a stimulus such as a word or object due to a previous encounter with that stimulus or with related stimuli.

A. Repetition Priming

Repetition priming refers to the change in responding to a word or an object as a result of a previous encounter with that same item, either in the same task or in a different task. Responding to words or objects is typically improved due to this previous experience (usually more so when the task as well as the stimulus item remains the same). For example, if a word appears for a second time in a task that requires reading the target aloud (naming task) or deciding whether the target is a word or a nonword (lexical decision task), responding is faster and more accurate than for words appearing for the first time at the same level of overall practice in the task. In addition, repetition priming can influence the probability of producing a previously encountered item as a response when a task allows multiple possible answers on each trial. For example, suppose that in the study phase of a two-phase experiment subjects are asked to study a series of words. After a delay that can range from minutes to hours they are given three-letter word stems and asked to complete each stem with the first word that comes to mind (e.g., gre_ for green). In this word stem completion task, the repetition priming effect appears when subjects respond more frequently with words that had been studied earlier than with words that were not encountered in the study phase.

As can be seen from the examples, repetition priming is commonly examined using tasks that do not require conscious recollection of past experience with the stimulus item to complete. Therefore, it potentially represents a nonconscious or unintended effect of that experience. Such effects are called implicit memory in the repetition priming literature. When it can be documented that repetition priming has occurred without conscious recollection, the priming is called implicit memory, and as such it represents another example of automatic processing.

Brain imaging studies using positron emission tomography (PET) and fMRI have shown that priming is accompanied by reduced neural activity within areas that were initially activated to perform the task. Reduced neural activity was found in occipital visual cortex (Brodmann's area 19), left frontal cortex, and inferior temporal cortex. Whereas the reduced neural activity in visual cortex is specific to visually presented stimuli, the activity reductions in left frontal cortex occur regardless of cue modality (visual or auditory). The reduced activity within the left frontal cortex suggests an amodal priming effect that represents access to the meaning of the word rather than to its visual or orthographic representation. Analogous modality-specific and amodal effects have been observed with objects.

Single cell recording in monkeys provides evidence about the neural mechanisms that might mediate these repetition priming effects, at least for nonverbal stimuli. Repeated experience with the same visual stimulus leads to suppression of neuronal responses in subpopulations of visual neurons. This "repetition suppression" was found in the delayed matching-to-sample task. In these studies a monkey was presented

with a sample stimulus followed by a sequence of test stimuli. The animal was rewarded for indicating which test stimulus matched the sample. For example, the monkey was presented with the sequence A ... B ... C ... A and was supposed to respond to the final A. Under these conditions, the common type of neural response was suppressive, and it was graded by similarity. The more similar the test stimulus was to the sample, the more the neural response was suppressed. Moreover, repetition suppression was associated with item repetition, whether the repeated item was the target or a distractor. Repetition suppression was found to be stimulus specific and long-lasting. In addition to visual cortex, this effect was recorded in the inferior temporal cortex and also in some regions of the prefrontal cortex.

Robert Desimone suggested that the reduction in cortical activation in human neuroimaging studies such as those described earlier was due to a repetition suppression effect such as that documented in monkeys. This repetition suppression effect at the neuronal level would result in a decrease in the total number of activated cells (and hence in a reduced demand for oxygenated blood, producing the signal change measured in PET and fMRI). This reduced population of neurons, according to Desimone, provides a sharpened stimulus representation. The prime tunes the population of neurons so that a selective subpopulation that carries the critical features of the stimulus gives a robust response when the stimulus recurs, whereas other neurons, which are probably related to other stimuli, are suppressed. The more selective representation allows for a more efficient responding upon the next encounter with the stimulus. Desimone's argument recalls the words of Sir John Eccles quoted earlier.

B. Semantic Priming

Semantic priming arises because the brain makes use of relations among similar or related stimuli in addition to using past experiences with the same stimulus. In the basic version of the semantic priming paradigm, subjects are presented with two successive stimuli called the prime and the target. They are usually asked to respond overtly only to the target. When words are the stimuli, the task may be naming or lexical decision. Supposing that the target is the word "nurse," the prime can be a related word (e.g., "doctor"), an unrelated word (e.g., "bread"), or a neutral stimulus (e.g., a row of X's). Under these conditions, the semantic priming or relatedness effect emerges. This effect can be described as a greater speed and accuracy of performance in the response to a target word when it is presented after a semantically related prime word than when it is presented after an unrelated prime word or after a neutral stimulus. This effect has been documented in a variety of situations. The semantic priming effect can occur when people are asked to pay attention to the prime and also when they do not pay attention to the prime, or even when they are unaware of its identity and do not phenomenologically realize that a prime has occurred. That is, semantic priming effects still exist when the target is presented very briefly and masked by visual noise presented immediately following the prime so that people believe they have seen only the visual noise and are not aware of the presence of the prime.

James Neely studied automatic and controlled processes by examining the ability of subjects to switch between semantic categories in an arbitrary fashion. He asked his subjects to think of parts of a building when the prime was the category name "body" (e.g., "body"–"door"). Subjects were able to follow the instructions when the time between the prime and the target (i.e., SOA) was long enough (e.g., 750 msec). That is, they responded faster to "door" following "body" relative to "door" following an unrelated prime (e.g., "tree") or even a neutral prime (e.g., XXXX). However, they were not able to switch from one category to another when the SOA was short (e.g., 250 msec). What was the fate of the rejected category? That is, when the prime was "body" and the subject made an effort to think of the category "building," what happened to parts of the body such as "arm"? "Arm" appearing after "body" was facilitated at short SOAs (<300 msec) and inhibited at long SOAs (between 500 and 2000 msec)—that is, RTs for related trials ("body"–"arm") were longer than RTs for neutral trials and equivalent to those for unrelated trials ("bird"–"arm").

Hence, priming can be achieved both by unintentional automatic activation, as shown by priming from masked words of which subjects are unaware, and from consciously perceptible words at short SOAs even when subjects are trying to think of unrelated words. However, priming can also be achieved by intentionally focusing on a concept and generating possibilities following some rule, even an arbitrary rule as in Neely's "switch condition," although such intentional focusing takes more time than automatic activation. Thus, these findings support the existence of two mechanisms of semantic priming. The first is

automatic, nonconscious, and can work without attention. By analogy to repetition priming, one might wonder if it is mediated by reduction of neural response in structures that store semantic knowledge. The second is voluntary, conscious, and occupies attention. One might expect that this mechanism would be associated with neural structures involved in the executive control operations of working memory, and that invoking this mechanism would increase neural activation in those structures. To date, however, we do not know of any neuroimaging studies of semantic priming.

C. Inhibitory Semantic Priming and the Center–Surround Theory of Retrieval Operations

Neely's evidence for inhibition of related words in his switch condition is one of the few instances in the literature in which semantic relatedness between successive stimuli harms performance in speeded tasks, such as naming or lexical decision. Another instance was reported by Dale Dagenbach and colleagues. They found that in certain circumstances lexical decisions following semantically related primes are slower than lexical decisions following unrelated primes—an absolute inhibition effect associated with semantic relatedness. This inhibitory priming occurs as a consequence of attempting to retrieve the meaning of a perceptually presented word when the meaning is weakly activated—either because the word is masked and hence perceptual input is easily confused with other input or because the word is newly learned and hence its representation in semantic memory is weak and easily confused with or overwhelmed by other representations. In either case, the weakly activated meaning is likely to suffer interference because other representations are activated that are similar but incorrect. Dagenbach and colleagues proposed that in such circumstances, the attempt to retrieve the weakly activated semantic code is accompanied by active inhibition of the related information that is producing the interference. This inhibition reflects the operation of a center-surround attentional mechanism, which works to facilitate a semantic code on which it is focused or "centered" while inhibiting "surrounding" codes. These are codes that are similar or related to but different from the desired code and are competing with it for retrieval. The center-surround hypothesis predicts that repetition priming should be facilitatory at the same time that semantic priming is inhibitory—a prediction that has been confirmed. Analogous findings have been reported by Steven Lehmkuhle and colleagues in the domain of spatial rather than semantic processing, suggesting that inhibition of similar or closely related representations may be a generalizable strategy for conflict resolution in the central nervous system.

V. EXECUTIVE CONTROL OF TASK PERFORMANCE: STOPPING AN ONGOING THOUGHT OR ACTION

Sometimes we start thinking about something or start to perform an action, only to realize it does not fit with our primary goal or our general plan at the moment or that our goal has changed and it is no longer appropriate. Such situations call for a change in the course of thought or action. We must stop the current thought or action in order to be able to switch to another one. An experimental method for studying this common example of executive control is the *stop signal paradigm* developed by Gordon Logan.

In this paradigm subjects are engaged in a primary task. In a relatively small proportion of trials they are signaled to stop before executing the response to the primary task. For example, participants can be asked to respond in each trial by pressing a button to an X and another button to an O. In addition, they are asked to withhold their response if a tone is presented at any point during a trial. The tone is presented in 25% of the trials at various delays after onset of the primary stimulus. Performance in this task can be successfully modeled as a race between a "go process" (perceiving and responding to the primary stimulus) and a "stop process." The stop process is conceived to be a separate sequence of mental operations that involves perceiving the stop signal and intervening in the ongoing sequence of operations involved in the go process or primary task. If participants finish the stop process before the go process, they inhibit their response to the primary stimulus. If they finish the go process before the stop process, they produce a response to the primary stimulus, failing to inhibit it. RT to the go signal can be measured directly, whereas stop-signal RT (the time needed to cancel the planned response) cannot be measured directly (since its behavioral signature is the absence of action and hence there is nothing overt to measure). However, Logan's race model provides quantitative methods for estimating the stop-signal RT.

Research applying this model shows that young adults can stop a wide variety of actions (key presses, hand movements, squeezes, and speech) very quickly, with an estimated latency from the stop signal of about 200 msec. Williams and colleagues reported that the ability to stop improves developmentally throughout childhood (i.e., stop-signal RT decreases) and then remains approximately constant across much of adulthood, falling off slightly but nonsignificantly in old age. Interestingly, speed of responding in most tasks that would be used as a primary task in this paradigm—the go process—also improves throughout childhood, but peak performance in young adulthood is followed by significant slowing beginning in middle adulthood. Thus, there appears to be a difference between the developmental trajectory of the execution of primary tasks and that of the type of inhibitory control represented by stopping. This supports Logan's hypothesis that processes governing inhibition are separate from those governing execution of speeded primary processing. Other research, however, shows that in old age the probability of stopping successfully does deteriorate, even if stop-signal RT remains fairly constant on those trials in which the stopping process succeeds. This suggests that old age may involve a loss of concentration in which inhibitory control processes are less likely to be implemented appropriately, even though they may still work effectively once deployed. Although this conclusion is consistent with the available data from the stopping paradigm, there is more to the relationship between age and inhibition. As will be discussed later, a major theory of cognitive aging proposes that most inhibitory functions decline in old age.

In addition to developmental changes, the ability to inhibit one's actions in the stopping paradigm is related to some personal characteristics and individual differences. Stop-signal RT varies with impulsivity, being longer for more impulsive individuals. Hyperactive children have trouble stopping. Their stop-signal RT is longer than that of normal controls and they fail to inhibit responding on many occasions. This pattern is not due to a failure to detect the stop signal itself but rather to a deficit in the inhibitory mechanism that implements stopping. Moreover, stimulant medication (methylphenidate) that improves behavioral symptoms of hyperactive children also improves their stopping performance.

Event-related potentials suggest two loci at which the stop process exerts its impact—a central locus in frontal cortex that acts on motor planning and execution operations and a more peripheral process that acts on descending motor commands after they have left cortex. Evidence on the frontal locus comes from application of the stop-signal paradigm to examine gaze control in the FEF of monkeys by Jeffrey Schall and colleagues. Recording from single neurons in FEF showed that movement-related activity, which began to increase when a signal to move the eyes was presented, decreased when a signal to cancel the saccade was presented. The activity associated with this inhibition began to decrease before the stop-signal RT was over. It seems that the preparation of a movement is a controlled process composed of both execution and inhibition processes. FEF is involved in the generation of saccades, as mentioned earlier; in addition, neurons in the FEF can specify saccade cancellation—a specific and well-documented example of inhibitory function.

VI. DEVELOPMENTAL ASPECTS

A. Development of Reaching and the "A Not B Error"

Studies of reaching behavior in human infants and monkeys suggest that development of such behavior involves both the ability to plan and execute sequences of action and the ability to inhibit certain reflexive actions or dominant response tendencies.

Piaget suggested that infants have difficulty in understanding objects and their properties, including spatial relations. However, it seems that infants, even as young as 5 months old, can understand the object concept but they have difficulty demonstrating this understanding by their reaching behavior. Reaching behavior of infants has been studied by Adele Diamond and colleagues using several paradigms. In one paradigm infants were presented with a Plexiglas box with a building block inside or outside the box. Infants were able to retrieve the object when a direct line of reach was possible (the object was in front of the box touching its front wall or in the middle of the box, away from its front wall). However, when the object was placed inside the box touching its front wall infants were unsuccessful in retrieving it. To retrieve the object in the latter situation there is a need to execute a sequence of two movements in order to avoid touching the front wall of the box—one away from the object and a second in the direction of the object. Moreover, when the infants touched the front of the box they reflexively grasped it or withdrew their hands. Seven-month-old infants rarely continued their reaching toward the object. In contrast, 10-month-old infants were much less likely to show these reflexive behaviors

upon touching the edge of the box. These infants were able to retrieve the object in these circumstances. It seems that the older infants developed the ability to execute a reach that requires a change of direction and to inhibit reflexive reactions of the hand.

Infants also have difficulty detouring around a barrier to retrieve an object. Here, the infant's task is to retrieve the object from a transparent box that has an open side. Infants 6.5–7 months old reach straight through the side at which they are looking at the object. If they see the object through the open side, they can retrieve it. Otherwise, they cannot retrieve the object and they do not try alternative reaching behaviors. Toward the end of the first year of life they can look through a closed side but retrieve the object from any open side of the box. In order to develop this ability infants need to inhibit the tendency to reach according to the line of sight.

In another paradigm the infant is presented with an object in one of two places, A or B. The locations are covered to hide the object from sight and the infant is then allowed to search for it by lifting the covers. After the infant retrieves the object, the object is again placed in one of the two locations and the search task continues. Suppose the object is first hidden at location A and the infant retrieves it successfully. If the object is then hidden at the second location B, the infant will often try to retrieve the object from A, even though the infant watched the experimenter hiding the object at B. This is the A not B error. Infants continue to make the A not B error from about 7.5 to 12 months of age, as long as the delay between hiding and retrieval is incremented as the infant gets older. Perhaps the most striking aspect of the phenomenon is that infants appear to know that the object is at B despite the fact that they reach toward A. Visual habituation and other visual memory tests indicate that infants remember the correct location. Sometimes, in the search task, the infant fixates B while he or she is reaching toward A. Moreover, infants show the A not B error even when the covers are transparent and the object can be seen. In order to prevent this type of error there is a need to hold details of the task and the situation briefly in short-term memory, and there is a need to inhibit the tendency to reach to A. The tendency to reach to A develops because reaching to A was reinforced earlier by successful finding of the object, and it increases with the number of times the infant has retrieved the object from location A before it is hidden at location B. The ability to meet both of these needs imposed by the task improves during infancy. Short-term memory improves as evidenced by the longer retention interval between hiding and allowing the infant to reach for the object needed to elicit the A not B error, and inhibition of the incorrect response tendency improves as evidenced by the eventual disappearance of the A not B error.

It seems from this evidence that during the second half of the first year of life infants begin to gain control over their reaching actions. They can inhibit interfering automatic tendencies and demonstrate planned and goal-directed control over manual behavior. The gradual ascendance of planned and goal-directed behavior over reflexive or practiced stimulus-action routines has been modeled both by Diamond and colleagues and Stuart Marcovitch and Philip Zelazo as changes with age in the relative strength or dominance of competing systems, one like working memory and the other like conditioned or procedural learning. Evidence from lesions and single-cell recordings suggests that the increase in dominance of the working memory-like system is achieved, at least in part, through the maturation of several components of frontal cortex: the supplementary motor area (SMA) and the dorsolateral prefrontal cortex. Reflexive grasping is released in adult humans following lesions of the SMA, and the same is true in the case of lesioned monkeys. Lesions of the dorsolateral prefrontal cortex in monkeys produce the A not B error and difficulties inhibiting the urge to reach straight ahead to retrieve an object.

B. Development of Selection and Conflict Resolution

It is possible to view the previously mentioned studies as conflict situations in which habitual or endogenous tendencies compete for control of behavior. Throughout early childhood there is development in the ability to resolve such conflict and select among competing stimuli, stimulus properties, and responses. Several researchers have suggested that central to this achievement is the development of the ability to effectively inhibit stimuli or associations that are irrelevant to the task. Moreover, it has been suggested that such a development relies on maturation of the frontal lobes.

The Stroop task and its many variations have played a major part in the study of this development. For example, when preschool children are asked to say "day" to a picture of a moon and "night" to a picture of a sun, their accuracy is reduced relative to a neutral condition (e.g., responding "day" or "night" to a checkerboard). In addition, their accuracy decreases across the experimental session. Older children are able to maintain above-chance accuracy throughout a session. Similar trends have been found in latency of responding. Other conflict situations present similar results and document continued development of inhibitory function during childhood. For example, when Stroop color naming is examined across the school years, intrusion of the irrelevant word in place of the color name decreases in the incongruent or conflict condition, as does the impact of the irrelevant word on latency of correct responding.

Combining this evidence on conflict resolution with the evidence on stopping discussed previously suggests a general improvement in the ability to inhibit prepotent and automated responses from infancy to adulthood. This ability frees the system from stimulus-driven control, enabling strategic control and planning to play a more dominant part in behavior. Moreover, it seems that such development is dependent on high levels of cortical maturation. Other trends in development are consistent with this idea that inhibitory function depends on cortical input. One example is IOR, discussed earlier. The SC, which seems to be the generator of IOR, is already developed in infancy. However, there appears to be a need for the parietal lobes to provide this system with the spatial coordinates necessary for producing IOR. Although in some circumstances IOR can be observed even in infants only a few days old, the appearance of robust and widespread IOR in the eye movement patterns of infants awaits parietal development, rather than depending only on maturation of the SC.

C. Cognitive Aging

Lynn Hasher, Rose Zacks, and colleagues have amassed a considerable body of evidence that inhibitory functions decline in old age. As a consequence, the cognitive processes of older adults are increasingly susceptible to interference from irrelevant or unwanted perceptions, thoughts, and tendencies toward action that are more successfully ignored by younger adults. Hasher, Zacks, and May suggested that the deleterious impact of interference appears to occur in addition to the generalized slowing observed in a wide variety of speeded task performances. Older adults produce more errors and slower correct responses in antisaccade tasks. They suffer greater interference in conflict resolutions tasks such as Stroop color naming, and they find it more difficult to inhibit primary task performance in the stopping paradigm. They suffer greater proactive interference in short-term memory tasks. They make more errors and retrieve answers more slowly in associative learning tasks when more than one response item is associated with a stimulus item (and in analogous "fan effect" fact-learning tasks in which multiple facts are learned about a single entity or topic item). They show less evidence of intentional or controlled forgetting in directed forgetting tasks, and they show less evidence of inhibiting irrelevant or inappropriate senses of ambiguous words and interpretations of ambiguous referring expressions in sentence reading and text comprehension. In many area of cognitive activity, older adults are susceptible to what Hasher, Zacks, and colleagues call "mental clutter."

Given the role played by prefrontal cortex in a number of the inhibitory functions reviewed in this article, one might wonder whether aging is particularly damaging to the integrity or efficiency of processing in frontal tissue. There is considerable evidence to support such an idea.

There are factors that moderate the impact of aging on cognitive activities with strong inhibitory components. One is practice, with task- and stimulus-specific practice being the most effective. Another is the level of circadian arousal. It is well-known that arousal levels vary systematically with time of day, and that individual differences in the time of occurrence of periods of optimal arousal create "morning people" and "evening people." These individual differences extend to task performance. Both younger and older adults perform a wide variety of tasks better during their optimal periods of arousal than during off-peak periods, and the impact of variation in circadian arousal is greater for older adults. Indeed, if testing is done in the morning when older adults are more likely to be in an optimal period and younger adults are more likely to be in an off-peak period, age differences in task performance are minimized and in some cases nearly eliminated. Testing in the evening, when older adults are likely to be in an off-peak period and younger adults in an optimal period, exaggerates age differences. Thus, circadian variation in locus coeruleus activity and right-prefrontal activity related to vigilance and preparation interact with other aging-induced changes in cortical efficacy.

Finally, there are a number of tasks in which performance does not appear to decline with age, at least in healthy adults free of nervous system insult such as stroke or Alzheimer's disease. Many of these are related to language use. Vocabulary scores continue to increase with age, although word-finding problems during real-time speech production and question answering may also increase. Sentence completion scores in fill-in-the-blank cloze tasks are not affected by age, nor is the accuracy of semantic categorization. All these language tasks that show little or no decline in old age are also affected little if at all by variation in circadian arousal. Perhaps the most surprising of the spared language functions is the ability to select one out of several possible and hence competing syntactic structures for application during real-time sentence production, which has been studied by Douglas Davidson in Zacks' laboratory. Here, the integrity of older adults' performance extends to speed as well as accuracy, violating both of the two best-established outcomes of cognitive aging—susceptibility to interference in conflict resolution situations and generalized slowing in speeded performances of many kinds. Thus, as has often been argued, language skills represent a domain-specific specialization whose operating principles seem to depart from those in many other areas of human cognition.

VII. CONCLUSIONS

Inhibitory functions are part and parcel of the cognitive processes that generate and control behaviors designed to provide specific solutions to dealing with environmental demands. In reviewing examples of inhibitory functions, we have seen that inhibition helps create coherent experience of the world along with the flexibility and efficiency required for skilled behavior.

The ability to inhibit prepotent or reflexive attentional and behavioral reactions and to stop unnecessary or inappropriate behavior develops throughout childhood. These developments free us from interference by otherwise dominant tendencies. This, in turn, enables us to exercise choice and intention over our actions. It seems that such changes are achieved through the development of various brain structures such as regions of the frontal lobes, including anterior cingulate, SMA, dorsolateral prefrontal cortex, and FEF. In doing their jobs, these control structures may interact or cooperate with regions of orbitofrontal cortex and amygdala involved in emotional regulation and sensitivity to delayed and long-term reinforcement contingencies. Note, however, that the ability of higher cortical structures to control reflexive behaviors by inhibiting them is not the only development that takes place. In some functional domains, inhibition already being produced by lower brain structures is made accessible to the influence of higher levels in the system.

An example of this type of development is IOR, which appears to occur in retinal coordinates early in development when SC alone is responsible for it, but it occurs in environmental and object-based coordinates once parietal cortex becomes sufficiently mature to contribute. Here, inhibition is already produced by certain brain structures but the development of cortical mechanisms allows this inhibition to be modulated by the higher brain mechanisms.

In addition, we presented results from memory and language processing suggesting that inhibition helps focus on an object or a concept by sharpening the activated representation. Moreover, it seems that this sharpening can sometimes proceed automatically, with no involvement of attention, and can be achieved without awareness, at least in some circumstances. In other circumstances, deployment of inhibitory tuning mechanisms appears to be under the control of intentions to process a particular kind of information.

In conclusion, inhibitory processes are ubiquitous in human cognition and vary in terms of the levels at which they operate and in terms of their relationship to various mental operations carried out in order to produce behavior.

See Also the Following Articles

ANTERIOR CINGULATE CORTEX • ATTENTION • COGNITIVE PSYCHOLOGY, OVERVIEW • CONSCIOUSNESS • EMOTION • HOMEOSTATIC MECHANISMS • NEUROFEEDBACK • NEUROTRANSMITTERS • STRESS: HORMONAL AND NEURAL ASPECTS • SUPERIOR COLLICULUS • UNCONSCIOUS, THE

Suggested Reading

Barch, D. M., Braver, T. S., Sabb, F. W., and Noll, D. C. (2000). Anterior cingulate and the monitoring of response conflict: Evidence from an fMRI study of overt verb generation. *J. Cog. Neurosci.* **12,** 298–311.

Cohen, J. D., Dunbar, K., and McClelland, J. L. (1990). On the control of automatic processes: A parallel distributed processing model of the Stroop effect. *Psychol. Rev.* **97,** 332–361.

Dagenbach, D., and Carr, T. H. (Eds.) (1994). Inhibitory Processes in Attention, Memory, and Language. Academic Press, San Diego.

Desimone, R. (1996). Neural mechanisms for visual memory and their role in attention. *Proc. Natl. Acad. Sci. USA* **93,** 13494–13499.

Desimone, R., and Duncan, J. (1995). Neural mechanisms of selective visual attention. *Annu. Rev. Neurosci.* **18,** 193–222.

Hasher, L., Zacks, R. T., and May, C. P. (1999). Inhibitory control, circadian arousal, and age. In *Attention and Performance XVII. Cognitive Regulation of Performance: Interaction of Theory and Applications* (D. Gopher and A. Koriat, Eds.), pp. 653–675. MIT Press, Cambridge, MA.

Henik, A., Rafal, R., and Rhodes, D. (1994). Endogenously generated and visually guided saccades after lesions of the human frontal eye fields. *J. Cog. Neurosci.* **6,** 400–411.

Kastner, S., De Weerd, P., Desimone, R., and Ungerleider, L. G. (1998). Mechanisms of directed attention in the human extrastriate cortex as revealed by functional MRI. *Science* **282,** 108–111.

Klein, R. M. (2000). Inhibition of return. *Trends Cog. Sci.* **4,** 138–147.

Marcovitch, S., and Zelazo, P. D. (1999). The A-not-B error: Results from a logistic meta-analysis. *Child Dev.* **70,** 1297–1313.

Milliken, B., Joordens, S., Merikle, P. M., and Seiffert, A. E. (1998). Selective attention: A reevaluation of the implications of negative priming. *Psychol. Rev.* **105,** 203–229.

Neely, J. H. (1991). Semantic priming effects in visual word recognition: A selective review of current findings and theories. In *Basic Processes in Reading: Visual Word Recognition* (D. Besner and G. Humphreys, Eds.), pp. 264–336. Erlbaum, Hillsdale, NJ.

West, R. L. (1996). An application of prefrontal cortex function theory to cognitive aging. *Psychol. Bull.* **120,** 272–292.

Wiggs, C. L., and Martin, A. (1998). Properties and mechanisms of perceptual priming. *Curr. Opin. Neurobiol.* **8,** 227–233.

Williams, B. R., Ponesse, J. S., Schachar, R. J., Logan, G. D., and Tannock, R. (1999). Development of inhibitory control across the life span. *Dev. Psychol.* **35,** 205–213.

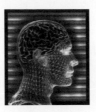

Intelligence

ROBERT J. STERNBERG and JAMES C. KAUFMAN

Yale University

GLOSSARY

biological approaches to intelligence Approaches emphasizing the anatomical and physiological substrates of intelligence.

cognitive approaches to intelligence Approaches emphasizing thinking and learning processes in intelligence.

intelligence The ability purposely to adapt to, shape, and select real-world environments.

psychometric approaches to intelligence Approaches emphasizing measurement operations for intelligence.

Intelligence can be defined as the ability purposely to adapt to, shape, and select real-world environments. However, most investigators of intelligence want to go beyond simple dictionary-like definitions to a deeper understanding of the construct.

I. DEFINING INTELLIGENCE

If you ask people what intelligence is, the answer depends on whom you ask and the answer differs widely across disciplines, time, and place. We begin this article by discussing the diversity of views regarding what intelligence is because empirical studies often assume rather than explore the nature of the construct they are investigating—in this case, intelligence.

A. Western Psychological Views

How have Western psychologists conceived of intelligence? Almost none of the Western views are adequately expressed by Boring's 1923 operationistic view of intelligence as what intelligence tests test.

For example, in a 1921 symposium on experts' definitions of intelligence, researchers emphasized the importance of the ability to learn and the ability to adapt to the environment. Sixty-five years later, Sternberg and Detterman conducted a similar symposium, again asking experts their views on intelligence. Learning and adaptive abilities retained their importance, and a new emphasis crept in—metacognition or the ability to understand and control one's self. Of course, the name is new but the idea is not because long before Aristotle emphasized the importance for intelligence of knowing oneself.

B. Cross-Cultural Views

In some cases, Western notions about intelligence are not shared by other cultures. For example, at the mental level, the Western emphasis on speed of mental processing is not shared in many cultures. Other cultures may even be suspicious of the quality of work that is done very quickly. Indeed, other cultures emphasize depth rather than speed of processing. They are not alone: Some prominent Western theorists have pointed out the importance of depth of processing for full command of material.

Yang and Sternberg reviewed Chinese philosophical conceptions of intelligence. The Confucian perspective emphasizes the characteristic of benevolence and of doing what is right. As in the Western notion, the intelligent person spends a great deal of effort in learning, enjoys learning, and persists in life-long learning with a great deal of enthusiasm. The Taoist tradition, in contrast, emphasizes the importance of humility, freedom from conventional standards of judgment, and full knowledge of oneself as well as of external conditions.

The difference between Eastern and Western conceptions of intelligence may persist even in the present day. A study of contemporary Taiwanese Chinese conceptions of intelligence found five factors underlying these conceptions: (i) a general cognitive factor, much like the g factor in conventional Western tests; (ii) interpersonal intelligence; (iii) intrapersonal intelligence; (iv) intellectual self-assertion; and (v) intellectual self-effacement.

The factors uncovered in both studies differ substantially from those identified in U.S. people's conceptions of intelligence—practical problem solving, verbal ability, and social competence—although in both cases, people's implicit theories of intelligence seem to go far beyond what conventional psychometric intelligence tests measure.

Another study varied only language. It explicitly compared the concepts of intelligence of Chinese graduates from Chinese-language versus English-language schools in Hong Kong. It was found that both groups considered nonverbal reasoning skills as the most relevant for measuring intelligence. Verbal reasoning and social skills were considered second in importance, followed by numerical skill. Memory was viewed as least important. The Chinese-language-schooled group, however, tended to rate verbal skills as less important than did the English-language-schooled group. Moreover, an earlier study found that Chinese students viewed memory for facts as important for intelligence, whereas Australian students viewed this skill as of only trivial importance.

A review of Eastern notions of intelligence suggested that, in Buddhist and Hindu philosophies, intelligence involves waking up, noticing, recognizing, understanding, and comprehending, but it also includes determination, mental effort, and even feelings and opinions in addition to more intellectual elements.

Differences between cultures in conceptions of intelligence have been recognized for some time. One study noted that Australian university students value academic skills and the ability to adapt to new events as critical to intelligence, whereas Malay students value practical skills as well as speed and creativity. Another study found that Malay students emphasize both social and cognitive attributes in their conceptions of intelligence.

The differences between East and West may be due to differences in the kinds of skills valued by the two kinds of cultures. Western cultures and their schools emphasize what might be called "technological intelligence"; thus, things such as artificial intelligence and so-called smart bombs are viewed, in some sense, as intelligent or smart.

Western schooling also emphasizes generalization or going beyond the information given, speed, minimal moves to a solution, and creative thinking. Moreover, silence is interpreted as a lack of knowledge. In contrast, the Wolof tribe in Africa views people of higher social class and distinction as speaking less. This difference between the Wolof and Western notions suggests the usefulness of examining African notions of intelligence as a possible contrast to U.S. notions.

Studies in Africa in fact provide another window on the substantial differences. Some psychologists have argued that in Africa conceptions of intelligence revolve largely around skills that help to facilitate and maintain harmonious and stable intergroup relations; intragroup relations are probably equally important and at times more important. For example, one study found that Chewa adults in Zambia emphasize social responsibilities, cooperativeness, and obedience as important to intelligence; intelligent children are expected to be respectful of adults. Kenyan parents also emphasize responsible participation in family and social life as important aspects of intelligence. In Zimbabwe, the word for intelligence, *ngware*, actually means to be prudent and cautious, particularly in social relationships. Among the Baoule, service to the family and community and politeness toward and respect for elders are seen as key to intelligence.

Similar emphasis on social aspects of intelligence has been found among two other African groups—the Songhay of Mali and the Samia of Kenya. The Yoruba, another African tribe, emphasize the importance of depth—of listening rather than just talking—to intelligence and of being able to see all aspects of an issue and to place the issue in its proper overall context.

The emphasis on the social aspects of intelligence is not limited to African cultures. Notions of intelligence in many Asian cultures also emphasize the social aspect of intelligence more than does the conventional Western or IQ-based notion.

It should be noted that neither African nor Asian notions emphasize exclusively social notions of intelligence. A current project is studying conceptions of intelligence in rural Kenya. The Kenyans that have been studied have variegated conceptions of intelligence, distinguishing school intelligence (*rieko*) from other nonschool kinds of intelligence (such as *luoro*, which has more of the quality of character). Near one village (Kisumu), many and probably most of the children are at least moderately infected with a variety of parasitic infections. As a result, they experience stomachaches quite frequently. Traditional medicine suggests the usefulness of a large variety (actually, hundreds) of natural herbal medicines that can be used to treat such infections. Children who learn how to self-medicate via these natural herbal medicines are viewed as being at an adaptive advantage over those who do not have this kind of informal knowledge. Clearly, the kind of adaptive advantage that is relevant in this culture would be viewed as totally irrelevant in the West and vice versa. Children who do better on tests of adaptive knowledge of this kind actually do worse on Western tests of intelligence and in Western schooling in English and mathematics.

These conceptions of intelligence emphasize social skills much more than do conventional U.S. conceptions of intelligence, while simultaneously recognizing the importance of cognitive aspects of intelligence. However, it is important to realize that there is no one overall U.S. conception of intelligence. Indeed, one study found that different ethnic groups in San Jose, California, had different conceptions of what it means to be intelligent. For example, Latino parents of schoolchildren tended to emphasize the importance of social-competence skills in their conceptions of intelligence, whereas Asian parents tended to heavily emphasize the importance of cognitive skills. Anglo parents also emphasized cognitive skills. Teachers, representing the dominant culture, emphasized cognitive more than social-competence skills. The rank order of children of various groups' performance (including subgroups within the Latino and Asian groups) could be perfectly predicted by the extent to which their parents shared the teachers' conception of intelligence. In other words, teachers tended to reward those children who were socialized into a view of intelligence that happened to correspond to the teachers' own view. However, as we shall argue later, social aspects of intelligence, broadly defined, may be

as important as or even more important than cognitive aspects of intelligence in later life. Some, however, prefer to study intelligence not in its social aspect but in its cognitive one.

II. COGNITIVE APPROACHES TO INTELLIGENCE

In 1957, Cronbach called for a merging of the two disciplines of scientific psychology—the differential and experimental approaches. Serious responses to Cronbach came in the 1970s, with cognitive approaches to intelligence attempting this merger. One team introduced the cognitive-correlates approach, whereby scores on laboratory cognitive tests were correlated with scores on psychometric intelligence tests. Another psychologist introduced the cognitive-components approach, whereby performance on complex psychometric tasks was decomposed into elementary information processing components.

In the 1990s, cognitive and biological approaches began to merge. A prototypical example is the inspection-time task. In this task, two adjacent vertical lines are presented tachistoscopically or by computer, followed by a visual mask (to destroy the image in visual iconic memory). The two lines differ in length, as does the amount of time for which the two lines are presented. The subject's task is to say which line is longer. However, instead of using raw response time as the dependent variable investigators typically use measures derived from a psychophysical function estimated after many trials. For example, the measure might be the duration of a single inspection trial at which 50% accuracy is achieved. Correlations between this task and measures of IQ appear to be about 0.4, slightly higher than is typical in psychometric tasks. There are differing theories as to why such correlations are obtained, but such theories generally attempt to relate the cognitive function of visual inspection time to some kind of biological function, such as speed of neuronal conduction. Next, we consider some of the biological functions that may underlie intelligence.

III. BIOLOGICAL APPROACHES TO INTELLIGENCE

An important approach to studying intelligence is to understand it in terms of the functioning of the brain, in particular, and of the nervous system, in general. Earlier theories relating the brain to intelligence tended to be global in nature, although not necessarily backed by strong empirical evidence.

A. Early Biological Theories

Halstead suggested that there are four biologically based abilities, which he called the integrative field factor, the abstraction factor, the power factor, and the directional factor. Halstead attributed all four of these abilities primarily to the functioning of the cortex of the frontal lobes.

More influential than Halstead has been Hebb, who distinguished between two basic types of intelligence: intelligence A and intelligence B. Hebb's distinction is still used by some theorists today. According to Hebb, intelligence A is innate potential; intelligence B is the functioning of the brain as a result of the actual development that has occurred. These two basic types of intelligence should be distinguished from intelligence C—intelligence as measured by conventional psychometric tests of intelligence. Hebb also suggested that learning, an important basis of intelligence, is built up through cell assemblies, by which successively more complex connections among neurons are constructed as learning takes place.

A third biologically based theory is that of Luria, which has had a major impact on tests of intelligence. According to Luria, the brain comprises three main units with respect to intelligence: a unit of arousal in the brain stem and midbrain structures; a sensory-input unit in the temporal, parietal, and occipital lobes; and an organization and planning unit in the frontal cortex.

B. Modern Biological Views and Research

1. Speed of Neuronal Conduction

Recent theories have dealt with more specific aspects of brain or neural functioning. For example, one view suggested that individual differences in nerve conduction velocity are a basis for individual differences in intelligence. Conduction velocity has been measured either centrally (in the brain) or peripherally (e.g., in the arm).

Some investigators tested brain nerve conduction velocities via two medium-latency potentials, N70 and P100, which were evoked by pattern-reversal stimulation. Subjects saw a black-and-white checkerboard pattern in which the black squares would change to white and the white squares to black. Over many trials, responses to these changes were analyzed via electro-des attached to the scalp in four places. Correlations of derived latency measures with IQ were small (generally in the 0.1 to 0.2 range of absolute value) but were significant in some cases, suggesting at least a modest relation between the two kinds of measures.

Other investigators reported on two studies investigating the relation between nerve conduction velocity in the arm and IQ. In both studies, nerve conduction velocity was measured in the median nerve of the arm by attaching electrodes to the arm. In the second study, conduction velocity from the wrist to the tip of the finger was also measured. Vernon and Mori found significant correlations with IQ in the 0.4 range as well as somewhat smaller correlations (approximately −0.2) with response time measures. They interpreted their results as supporting the hypothesis of a relation between speed of information transmission in the peripheral nerves and intelligence. However, these results must be interpreted cautiously because a later study did not successfully replicate these earlier results.

2. Glucose Metabolism

Some of the most interesting recent work using the biological approach has been done by Richard Haier and colleagues. For example, their research showed that cortical glucose metabolic rates as revealed by positron emission tomography scan analysis of subjects solving Raven matrix problems were lower for more intelligent than for less intelligent subjects, suggesting that the more intelligent subjects needed to expend less effort than the less intelligent ones to solve the reasoning problems. A later study showed a similar result for more versus less practiced performers playing the computer game of Tetris. In other words, smart people or intellectually expert people do not have to work as hard as less smart or intellectually expert people at a given problem.

What remains to be shown, however, is the causal direction of this finding. One could sensibly argue that the smart people expend less glucose (as a proxy for effort) because they are smart rather than that people are smart because they expend less glucose. Also, both high IQ and low glucose metabolism may be related to a third causal variable. In other words, we cannot always assume that the biological event is a cause (in the reductionistic sense). It may be, instead, an effect.

3. Brain Size

Another approach considers brain size. Investigators correlated brain size with Wechsler Adult Intelligence

Scale (WAIS-R) IQs, controlling for body size. They found that IQ correlated 0.65 in men and 0.35 in women, with a correlation of 0.51 for both sexes combined. A follow-up analysis of the same 40 subjects suggested that, in men, a relatively larger left hemisphere better predicted WAIS-R verbal ability than it predicted nonverbal ability, whereas in women a larger left hemisphere predicted nonverbal ability better than it predicted verbal ability. These brain size correlations are suggestive, but it is currently difficult to determine what they indicate.

4. Behavior Genetics

Another approach that is at least partially biologically based is that of behavior genetics. The literature is complex, but it appears that about half the total variance in IQ scores is accounted for by genetic factors. This figure may be an underestimate because the variance includes error variance and because most studies of heritability have been performed with children, but it is known that heritability of IQ is higher for adults than for children. Also, some studies, such as the Texas Adoption Project, suggest higher estimates: 0.78 in the Texas Adoption Project, 0.75 in the Minnesota Study of Twins Reared Apart, and 0.78 in the Swedish Adoption Study of Aging.

At the same time, some researchers argue that effects of heredity and environment cannot be clearly and validly separated. Perhaps, future research should focus on determining how heredity and environment work together to produce phenotypic intelligence, concentrating especially on within-family environmental variation, which appears to be more important than between-family variation. Moreover, peers seem to have a particularly large effect on the development of various personal attributes, probably including cognitive skills. Such research requires, at the very least, very carefully prepared tests of intelligence—perhaps some of the newer tests described in the next section.

IV. PSYCHOMETRIC APPROACHES TO INTELLIGENCE

The psychometric approach to intelligence is among the oldest of approaches and dates back to Galton's 1883 psychophysical account of intelligence, which attempts to measure intelligence in terms of psychophysical abilities (such as strength of hand grip or

visual acuity), and to Binet and Simon's 1916 account of intelligence as judgment, involving adaptation to the environment, direction of one's efforts, and self-criticism.

A. Theoretical Developments: Carroll's and Horn's Theories

Two of the major new theories proposed during the past decade are Carroll's and Horn's theories. The two theories are both hierarchical, suggesting more general abilities higher in the hierarchy and more specific abilities lower in the hierarchy. Carroll's theory will be described briefly as representative of these new developments.

Carroll proposed his hierarchical model of intelligence based on the factor analysis of more than 460 data sets obtained between 1927 and 1987. His analysis encompasses more than 130,000 people from diverse walks of life and even countries of origin (although non-English-speaking countries are poorly represented among his data sets). The model Carroll proposed, based on his monumental undertaking, is a hierarchy comprising three strata: stratum I, which includes many narrow, specific abilities (e.g., spelling ability and speed of reasoning); stratum II, which includes various group-factor abilities (e.g., fluid intelligence, which is involved in flexible thinking and seeing things in novel ways, and crystallized intelligence, the accumulated knowledge base); and stratum III, which is a single general intelligence, much like Spearman's 1904 general intelligence factor.

Of these strata, the most interesting is perhaps the middle stratum, which includes, in addition to fluid and crystallized abilities, learning and memory processes, visual perception, auditory perception, facile production of ideas (similar to verbal fluency), and speed (which includes both sheer speed of response and speed of accurate responding). Although Carroll does not break much new ground, in that many of the abilities in his model have been mentioned in other theories, he does masterfully integrate a large and diverse factor-analytic literature, thereby giving great authority to his model.

B. An Empirical Curiosity: The Flynn Effect

We know that the environment has powerful effects on cognitive abilities. Perhaps the simplest and most potent demonstration of this effect is the Flynn effect, named after its discoverer, James Flynn. The basic phenomenon is that IQ has increased over successive generations throughout the world during most of the past century—at least since 1930. The effect must be environmental because, obviously, a successive stream of genetic mutations could not have taken hold and exerted such an effect over such a short period of time. The effect is powerful—about 15 points of IQ per generation for tests of fluid intelligence. Also, it occurs throughout the world. The effect has been greater for tests of fluid intelligence than for tests of crystallized intelligence. The difference, if linearly extrapolated (a hazardous procedure, obviously), suggests that a person who in 1892 was at the 90th percentile on the Raven Progressive Matrices, a test of fluid intelligence, would in 1992 score at the 5th percentile.

There have been many potential explanations of the Flynn effect, and in 1996 a conference was organized by Ulric Neisser and held at Emory University to try to explain the effect. Some of the possible explanations include increased schooling, greater educational attainment of parents, better nutrition, and less childhood disease. A particularly interesting explanation is that of more and better parental attention to children. Whatever the answer, the Flynn effect suggests we need to think carefully about the view that IQ is fixed. It probably is not fixed within individuals, and it is certainly not fixed across generations.

C. Psychometric Tests

1. Static Tests

Static tests are the conventional kind in which people are given problems to solve and they solve them without feedback. Their final score is typically the number of items answered correctly, sometimes with a penalty for guessing.

Psychometric testing of intelligence and related abilities has generally advanced evolutionarily rather than revolutionarily. Sometimes, what are touted as advances seem cosmetic or almost beside the point, as in the case of newer versions of the Scholastic Assessment Test (SAT), which are touted to have not only multiple-choice but also fill-in-the-blank math problems. Perhaps the most notable trend is a movement toward multifactorial theories, often hierarchical ones, and away from the notion that intelligence can be adequately understood only in terms of a single general or g factor. For example, the third edition of the Wechsler Intelligence Scales for Children offers scores

for four factors (verbal comprehension, perceptual organization, processing speed, and freedom from distractibility), but the main scores remain the verbal, performance, and total scores that have traditionally dominated interpretation of the test. The fourth edition of the Stanford–Binet Intelligence Scale also departs from the orientation toward general ability that characterized earlier editions, yielding scores for crystallized intelligence, abstract visual reasoning, quantitative reasoning, and short-term memory.

Two new tests are also constructed on the edifice of the theory of fluid and crystallized intelligence of Cattell: the Kaufman Adolescent and Adult Intelligence Test and the Woodcock–Johnson Tests of Cognitive Ability–Revised. Although the theory is not new, the tendency to base psychometric tests closely on theories of intelligence is a welcome development.

The new Das–Naglieri Cognitive Assessment System is based not on fluid-crystallized theory but rather on the theory of Luria. It yields scores for attention, planning, simultaneous processing, and successive processing.

2. Dynamic Tests

In dynamic testing, individuals learn at the time of test. If they answer an item correctly, they are given guided feedback to help them solve the item until they either get it correct or the examiner runs out of clues to give them.

The notion of dynamic testing appears to have originated with Vygotsky and was developed independently by Feuerstein and colleagues. Dynamic assessment is generally based on the notion that cognitive abilities are modifiable, and that there is some kind of zone of proximal development, which represents the difference between actually developed ability and latent capacity. Dynamic assessments attempt to measure this zone of proximal development or an analog of it.

Dynamic assessment is cause both for celebration and for caution. On the one hand, it represents a break from conventional psychometric notions of a more or less fixed level of intelligence. On the other hand, it is more a promissory note than a realized success. The Feuerstein test, the Learning Potential Assessment Device, is of clinical use but is not psychometrically normed or validated. There is only one formally normed test available in the United States, by Swanson, which yields scores for working memory before and at various points during and after training as well as scores for the amount of improvement with intervention and the number of hints that have been given and a subjective evaluation by the examiner of the examinee's use of strategies.

3. Typical Performance Tests

Traditionally, tests of intelligence have been maximum-performance tests, requiring examinees to work as hard as they can to maximize their scores. Ackerman recently argued that typical performance tests, which, like personality tests, do not require extensive intellectual effort, should supplement maximal-performance ones. On such tests, subjects might be asked to what extent they agree with statements such as "I prefer my life to be filled with puzzles I must solve" or "I enjoy work that requires conscientious, exacting skills." A factor analysis of such tests yielded five factors: intellectual engagement, openness, conscientiousness, directed activity, and science/technology interest.

Although the trend has been toward multifaceted views of intelligence and away from reliance on general ability, some have bucked this trend. Among those who have are Herrnstein and Murray.

D. The Bell Curve Phenomenon

A momentous event in the perception of the role of intelligence in society occured with the publication of *The Bell Curve* by Herrnstein and Murray. The impact of the book is demonstrated by the rapid publication of a number of responses. A whole issue of *The New Republic* was devoted to the book, and two edited books of responses were quickly published. Some of the responses were largely political or emotional in character, but others attacked the book on scientific grounds. A closely reasoned attack appeared a year after these collections. The American Psychological Association also sponsored a report that although not directly a response to *The Bell Curve* was largely motivated by it.

Some of the main arguments of the book are that (i) conventional IQ tests measure intelligence, at least to a good first approximation; (ii) IQ is an important predictor of many measures of success in life, including school success, but also economic success, work success, success in parenting, avoidance of criminality, and avoidance of welfare dependence; (iii) as a result of this prediction, people who are high in IQ are forming a cognitive elite, meaning that they are reaching the upper levels of society, whereas those who are low in

IQ are falling toward the bottom; (iv) tests can and should be used as a gating mechanism, given their predictive success; (v) IQ is highly heritable and hence is passed on through the genes from one generation to the next, with the heritability of IQ probably in the 0.5–0.8 range; (vi) there are racial and ethnic differences in intelligence, with blacks in the United States, for example, scoring about one standard deviation below whites; (vii) it is likely, although not certain, that at least some of this difference between groups is due to genetic factors; and (viii) tests can and should be used as a gating mechanism, given their success.

Herrnstein and Murray attempted to document their claims using available literature and also their own analysis of the National Longitudinal Study of Youth data that were available to them. Although their book was written for a trade (popular) audience, it was unusual among books for such an audience in its use of fairly sophisticated statistical techniques.

It is not possible to review the full range of responses to Herrnstein and Murray. Among psychologists, there seems to be widespread agreement that the social policy recommendations of Herrnstein and Murray, which call for greater isolation of and paternalism toward those with lower IQs, do not follow from their data but rather represent a separate ideological statement. Beyond that, there is a great deal of disagreement regarding the claims made by these authors.

Our view is that it would be easy to draw much stronger inferences from the Herrnstein–Murray analysis than the data warrant and perhaps even than Herrnstein and Murray would support. First, Herrnstein and Murray acknowledge that, in the United States, IQ typically accounts only for approximately 10% of the variation, on average, in individual differences across the domains of success they survey. In other words, about 90% of the variation, and sometimes much more, remains unexplained.

Second, even the 10% figure may be inflated by the fact that U.S. society uses IQ-like tests to select, place, and, ultimately, to stratify students so that some of the outcomes that Herrnstein and Murray mention may actually be results of the use of IQ-like tests rather than results of individual differences in intelligence per se. For example, admission to selective colleges in the United States typically requires students to take either the SAT or the American College Test, both of which are similar (although not identical) to conventional tests of IQ. Admission to graduate and professional programs requires similar kinds of tests. The result is that those who do not test well may be denied access to these programs and to the routes that would lead them to job, economic, and other socially sanctioned forms of success in our society.

It is thus not surprising that test scores would be highly correlated with, for example, job status. People who do not test well have difficulty gaining access to high-status jobs, which in turn pay better than other jobs to which they might be able to gain access. If we were to use some other index instead of test scores (e.g., social class or economic class), then different people would be selected for the access routes to societal success. In fact, we do use these alternative measures to some degree, although less so than in the past.

Finally, although group differences in IQ are acknowledged by virtually all psychologists to be real, the cause of them remains very much in dispute. What is clear is that the evidence in favor of genetic causes is weak and equivocal. We are certainly in no position to assign causes at this time. Understanding of group differences requires further analysis and probably requires examining these differences through the lens of broader theories of intelligence.

V. BROAD THEORIES OF INTELLIGENCE AND KINDS OF INTELLIGENCE

In recent years, there has been a trend toward broad theories of intelligence. We consider some of the main such theories next.

A. Multiple Intelligences

Gardner proposed that there is no single, unified intelligence but rather a set of relatively distinct, independent, and modular multiple intelligences. His theory of multiple intelligences (MI theory) originally proposed seven multiple intelligences: linguistic, as used in reading a book or writing a poem; logical–mathematical, as used in deriving a logical proof or solving a mathematical problem; spatial, as used in fitting suitcases into the trunk of a car; musical, as used in singing a song or composing a symphony; bodily–kinesthetic, as used in dancing or playing football; interpersonal, as used in understanding and interacting with other people; and intrapersonal, as used in understanding oneself.

Recently, Gardner proposed one additional intelligence as a confirmed part of his theory—naturalist intelligence, the kind shown by people who are able to discern patterns in nature. Charles Darwin would be a notable example. Gardner has also suggested that there may be two other "candidate" intelligences: spiritual intelligence and existential intelligence. Spiritual intelligence involves a concern with cosmic or existential issues and the recognition of the spiritual as the achievement of a state of being. Existential intelligence involves a concern with ultimate issues. Gardner believes the evidence for these latter two intelligences is less powerful than the evidence for the other eight intelligences. Whatever the evidence may be for the other eight, we agree that the evidence for these two new intelligences is speculative.

In the past, factor analysis served as the major criterion for identifying abilities. Gardner proposed a new set of criteria, including but not limited to factor analysis, for identifying the existence of a discrete kind of intelligence: potential isolation by brain damage, in that the destruction or sparing of a discrete area of the brain may destroy or spare a particular kind of intelligent behavior; the existence of exceptional individuals who demonstrate extraordinary ability (or deficit) in a particular kind of intelligent behavior; an identifiable core operation or set of oeprations that are essential to the performance of a particular kind of intelligent behavior; a distinctive developmental history leading from novice to master, along with disparate levels of expert performance; a distinctive evolutionary history, in which increases in intelligence may be plausibly associated with enhanced adaptation to the environment; supportive evidence from cognitive experimental research; supportive evidence from psychometric tests; and susceptibility to encoding in a symbol system.

Since the theory was first proposed, a large number of educational interventions have arisen that are based on the theory, sometimes closely and other times less so. Many of the programs are unevaluated, and evaluations of others seem to be ongoing, so it is difficult to say at this point what the results will be. In one particularly careful evaluation of a well-conceived program in a large southern city, there were no significant gains in student achievement or changes in student self-concept as a result of an intervention program based on Gardner's theory. There is no way of knowing whether these results are representative of such intervention programs, however.

B. Successful Intelligence

Sternberg suggested that we should pay less attention to conventional notions of intelligence and more to what he terms successful intelligence—the ability to adapt to, shape, and select environments so as to accomplish one's goals and those of one's society and culture. A successfully intelligent person balances adaptation, shaping, and selection, doing each as necessary. The theory is motivated in part by repeated findings that conventional tests of intelligence and related tests do not predict meaningful criteria of success as well as they predict scores on other similar tests and school grades.

Successful intelligence involves an individual's discerning his or her pattern of strengths and weaknesses and then figuring out ways to capitalize on the strengths and at the same time compensate for or correct the weaknesses. People attain success, in part, in idiosyncratic ways that involve their finding how best to exploit their own patterns of strengths and weaknesses.

Three broad abilities are important to successful intelligence: analytical, creative, and practical abilities. Analytical abilities are required to analyze and evaluate the options available to oneself in life. They include identifying the existence of a problem, defining the nature of the problem, setting up a strategy for solving the problem, and monitoring one's solution processes.

Creative abilities are required to generate problem-solving options in the first place. Creative individuals are ones who "buy low and sell high" in the world of ideas: They are willing to generate ideas that, like stocks with low price–earnings ratios, are unpopular and perhaps even deprecated. Having convinced at least some people of the value of these ideas, they then sell high, meaning that they move on to the next unpopular idea. Research shows that these abilities are at least partially distinct from conventional IQ, and that they are moderately domain specific, meaning that creativity in one domain (such as art) does not necessarily imply creativity in another (such as writing).

Practical abilities are required to implement options and to make them work. Practical abilities are involved when intelligence is applied to real-world contexts. A key aspect of practical intelligence is the acquisition and use of tacit knowledge, which is knowledge of what one needs to know to succeed in a given environment that is not explicitly taught and that usually is not verbalized. Research shows that tacit knowledge is acquired through mindful utilization of experience, that it is relatively domain specific, that its possession is relatively independent of conventional abilities, and that it predicts criteria of job success about as well as and sometimes better than does IQ.

The separation of practical intelligence from IQ has been shown in different ways in different studies. Scribner showed that experienced assemblers in a milk processing plant used complex strategies for combining partially filled cases in a manner that minimized the number of moves require to complete an order. Although the assemblers were the least educated workers in the plant, they were able to calculate in their heads quantities expressed in different base number systems, and they routinely outperformed the more highly educated white-collar workers who substituted when the assemblers were absent. Scribner found that the order-filling performance of the assemblers was unrelated to measures of academic skills, including intelligence test scores, arithmetic test scores, and grades.

Ceci and Liker carried out a study of expert racetrack handicappers and found that expert handicappers used a highly complex algorithm for predicting post time odds that involved interactions among seven kinds of information. Use of a complex interaction term in their implicit equation was unrelated to the handicappers' IQ.

In a series of studies by Lave and colleagues, it was shown that shoppers in California grocery stores were able to choose which of several products represented the best buy for them, even though they did very poorly on the same kinds of problems when they were presented in the form of a paper-and-pencil arithmetic computation test. The same principle that applies to adults appears to apply to children as well: Carraher, Carraher, and Schliemann found that Brazilian street children who could apply sophisticated mathematical strategies in their street vending were unable to do the same in a classroom setting. In study by Grigorenko and Sternberg, practical intelligence was found to be a better predictor of everyday adaptation than was academic intelligence among adults in contemporary Russia.

One more example practical intelligence was provided by a study in which individuals were asked to play the role of city managers for the computer-simulated city of Lohhausen. Dorner and colleagues presented a variety of problems to these individuals, such as how best to raise revenue to build roads. The simulation involved more than 1000 variables. No relation was found between IQ and complexity of strategies used.

There is also evidence that practical intelligence can be taught, at least to some degree. For example, children in middle school given a program for developing their practical intelligence for school (strategies for effective reading, writing, execution of homework, and taking of tests) improved more from pretest to posttest than did control students who received an alternative but irrelevant treatment.

None of these studies suggest that IQ is unimportant for school or job performance or other kinds of performance, and indeed, evidence suggests the contrary. The studies do suggest, however, that there are other aspects of intelligence that are relatively independent of IQ and that are important as well. A multiple-abilities prediction model of school or job performance would probably be most satisfactory.

According to the theory of successful intelligence, children's multiple abilities are underutilized in educational institutions because teaching tends to value analytical (as well as memory) abilities at the expense of creative and practical abilities. Sternberg, Ferrari, Clinkenbeard, and Grigorenko designed an experiment in order to illustrate this point. They identified 199 high school students from throughout the United States who were strong in analytical, creative, or practical abilities, all three kinds of abilities, or none of these kinds of abilities. Students were then brought to Yale University to take a college-level psychology course that was taught in a way that emphasized memory, analytical, creative, or practical abilities. Some students were matched, and others mismatched, to their own strength(s). All students were evaluated for memory-based, analytical, creative, and practical achievements.

Sternberg and colleagues found that students whose instruction matched their pattern of abilities performed significantly better than did students who were mismatched. They also found that prediction of course performance was improved by taking into account creative and practical as well as analytical abilities. In the broader test of abilities they used, confirmatory factor analysis failed to reveal a general factor. In a separate study, Sternberg, Torff, and Grigorenko found that fourth-graders and eighth-graders taught either social studies or science in a way that emphasized analytical, creative, and practical thinking performed better on tests of achievement than did children taught in a way that emphasized primarily memory, even if the children's achievement was measured by memory tests.

C. True Intelligence

Perkins proposed a theory of what he refers to as true intelligence, which he believes synthesizes classic views

as well as new ones. According to Perkins, there are three basic aspects to intelligence: neural, experiential, and reflective.

Neural intelligence concerns what Perkins believes to be the fact that some people's neurological systems function better than do the neurological systems of others, running faster and with more precision. He mentions "more finely tuned voltages" and "more exquisitely adapted chemical catalysts" as well as a "better pattern of connecticity in the labyrinth of neurons," although it is not entirely clear what any of these terms mean. Perkins believes this aspect of intelligence to be largely genetically determined and unlearnable. This kind of intelligence seems to be similar to Cattell's idea of fluid intelligence.

The experiential aspect of intelligence is what has been learned from experience. It is the extent and organization of the knowledge base and thus is similar to Cattell's notion of crystallized intelligence. The reflective aspect of intelligence refers to the role of strategies in memory and problem solving, and it appears to be similar to the construct of metacognition or cognitive monitoring.

D. The Bioecological Model of Intelligence

Ceci proposed a bioecological model of intelligence, according to which multiple cognitive potentials, context, and knowledge are all essential bases of individual differences in performance. Each of the multiple cognitive potentials enables relationships to be discovered, thoughts to be monitored, and knowledge to be acquired within a given domain. Although these potentials are biologically based, their development is closely linked to environmental context; hence, it is difficult if not impossible to cleanly separate biological from environmental contributions to intelligence. Moreover, abilities may express themselves very differently in different contexts. For example, children given essentially the same task in the context of a video game and in the context of a laboratory cognitive task performed much better when the task was presented in the context of the video game. Part of this superiority may have been a result of differences in emotional response.

E. Emotional Intelligence

Emotional intelligence is the ability to perceive accurately, appraise, and express emotion; the ability to access and/or generate feelings when they facilitate thought; the ability to understand emotion and emotional knowledge; and the ability to regulate emotions to promote emotional and intellectual growth. The concept was introduced by Salovey and Mayer and popularized and expanded upon by Goleman.

There is tentative evidence for the existence of emotional intelligence. For example, researchers found that emotional perception of characters in a variety of situations correlates with SAT scores, with empathy, and with emotional openness. Full convergent–discriminant validation of the construct, however, appears to be needed.

Some scholars still hold a relatively simple view of intelligence not much different from the view proposed by Spearman in 1904. However, with the introduction of emotional intelligence and all the other kinds of intelligences, it seems like a simple view may fail to capture intelligence in all its richness.

See Also the Following Articles

ARTIFICIAL INTELLIGENCE • BILINGUALISM • CATE-GORIZATION • COGNITIVE AGING • COGNITIVE PSYCHOLOGY, OVERVIEW • CREATIVITY • EVOLUTION OF THE BRAIN • INFORMATION PROCESSING • LANGUAGE ACQUISITION • LANGUAGE AND LEXICAL PROCESSING • LANGUAGE, NEURAL BASIS OF • LOGIC AND REASONING • PROBLEM SOLVING • SPEECH

Acknowledgments

Preparation of this article was supported in part under the Javits Act Program (Grant R206R500001) as administered by the Office of Educational Research and Improvement, U.S. Department of Education. The opinions expressed in this article do not necessarily reflect the positions or policies of the Office of Educational Research and Improvement or the U.S. Department of Education.

Suggested Reading

Ackerman, P. L., and Heggestad, E. D. (1997). Intelligence, personality, and interests: Evidence for overlapping traits. *Psychol. Bull.* **121,** 219–245.

Ceci, S. J. (1996). *On Intelligence: A Bioecological Treatise on Intellectual Development* (expanded ed.). Harvard Univ. Press, Cambridge, MA.

Cole, M. (1996). *Cultural Psychology: A Once and Future Discipline.* Harvard Univ. Press, Cambridge, MA.

Fischer, C. S., Hout, M., Sanchez Janowski, M., Lucas, S. R., Swidler, A., and Voss, K. (1996). *Inequality by Design: Cracking the Bell Curve Myth.* Princeton Univ. Press, Princeton, NJ.

Gardner, H. (1999). Are there additional intelligences? The case for naturalist, spiritual, and existential intelligences. In *Education, Information, and Transformation* (J. Kane, Ed.), Prentice Hall, Englewood Cliffs, NJ.

Goleman, D. (1998). *Working with Emotional Intelligence.* Bantam, New York.

Grigorenko, E. L., and Sternberg, R. J. (1998). Dynamic testing. *Psychol. Bull.* **124,** 75–111.

Harris, J. R. (1998). *The Nurture Assumption.* Free Press, New York.

Jensen, A. R. (1998). *The g Factor.* Greenwood, Greenwich, CT.

Mayer, J. D., and Salovey, P. (1997). What is emotional intelligence? In *Emotional Development and Emotional Intelligence: Educational Implications.* (P. Salovey and D. Sluyter, Eds.), Basic Books, New York.

Neisser, U. (Ed.) (1998). *The Rising Curve.* American Psychological Association, Washington, DC.

Neisser, U., Boodoo, G., Bouchard, T. J., Boykin, A. W., Brody, N., Ceci, S. J., Halpern, D. F., Loehlin, J. C., Perloff, R., Sternberg, R. J., and Urbina, S. (1996). Intelligence: Knowns and unknowns. *Am. Psychol.* **51,** 77–101.

Sternberg, R. J. (1996). *Successful Intelligence.* Simon & Schuster, New York.

Sternberg, R. J., and Grigorenko, E. L. (Eds.) (1997). *Intelligence, Heredity, and Environment.* Cambridge Univ. Press, New York.

Sternberg, R. J., and Horvath, J. (Eds.) (1999). *Tacit Knowledge in the Professions.* Erlbaum, Mahwah, NJ.

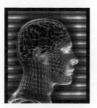

Ion Channels

B. ALEXANDER YI and LILY Y. JAN
University of California, San Francisco

I. Role of Ion Channels in Physiology

II. Principles of Ion Channel Mechanisms

III. Molecular Properties of Ion Channels

IV. Ion Channels by Family and Function

GLOSSARY

complementary DNA DNA that is synthesized from mRNA and therefore contains the coding sequence of the gene with no introns.

equilibrium potential The membrane potential at which there would be no net movement of ions across the membrane.

ligand A molecule that binds a protein.

neurotransmitter A chemical substance that is stored in vesicles at the nerve terminal and released to cause a change in the postsynaptic membrane, usually a change in the membrane to ions.

protease An enzyme that cleaves proteins.

resting potential The membrane potential of the cell in its quiescent state.

second messenger A molecule that is generated by the activation of surface receptors in response to hormones or neurotransmitters that lead to changes in the functional state of the cell.

In one sense, a cell is similar to a battery. Approximately one-third of the cell's metabolic energy is stored as an electrical potential in the form of ionic gradients across the plasma membrane. This energy is released at precise moments by "holes" in the membrane that allow ions to move down their electrochemical gradients across the membrane. These holes are ion channels. In the brain, a diverse array of ion channels coordinates their actions to generate complex waveforms that are used to transmit signals across long distances or between cells.

I. ROLE OF ION CHANNELS IN PHYSIOLOGY

Ion channels are membrane proteins that catalyze the transfer of ions down their electrochemical gradients across the plasma membrane. Ion channels are necessary because the plasma membrane is hydrophobic and thus by themselves they are impermeable to ions. In this article, we review what is known about the role of ion channels in physiology and their structure and function. More is known about some ion channels than others. In the last section, we introduce some of the major ion channel families that have attracted the interest of scientists who study ion channels.

There are two types of proteins that are able to move ions across the plasma membrane: ion pumps and ion channels. There are several features that distinguish them. Ion pumps are able to perform thermodynamic work (i.e., they are able to move an ion against its electrochemical gradient). This is accomplished by consuming energy in the form of ATP hydrolysis or the concentration gradients of other ions. Ion channels cannot perform thermodynamic work and the direction of ions traveling through an open channel is solely dependent on the electrochemical gradient. Sometimes ion pumps are said to carry out active transport, whereas ion channels carry out passive transport. Another major difference is the rate at which ions move through these proteins. Ion channels are essentially pores in the plasma membrane and the throughput of an ion channel can be fast—up to 100 million ions per second. The turnover rate of ion pumps is typically orders of magnitude slower.

Ion channels are found in nearly all cells in nature and play integral roles in a cell's basic physiology. It is likely that ion channels were among the proteins found in the earliest forms of life on this planet. Through millions of years of evolution, the number and diversity of ion channels have expanded to take on more complex functions such as those involved in learning and memory in the nervous system. Classically, ion channels are introduced via a discussion of neuronal action potentials that transmit signals down an axon. Beyond action potentials, ion channels play roles in other processes too many to enumerate. On a fundamental level, the activity of ion channels can change the membrane potential of the cell or alter the concentrations of ions inside the cell. These processes are basic to the cell's physiology; therefore, it is easily imagined that ion channels may be involved, directly or indirectly, in virtually all cellular activities. More directly, some of these activities may include setting the membrane potential, allowing the entry of ions for nutritive needs, allowing the entry of Ca^{2+}, which is used as a second messenger, and controlling cell volume.

In other cases, the physiological role of an ion channel is unknown. We have often learned about the function of ion channels by discovering instances when their activity goes awry—namely, disease states. It is becoming apparent that defective ion channels underlie the pathogenesis of many human diseases. The term channelopathy has been coined to refer to the expanding list of diseases in this class. For example, cystic fibrosis stems from a mutation in a chloride channel, cystic fibrosis transmembrane regulator (CFTR). In the lung, mutations in CFTR disrupt normal Cl^- efflux, which is necessary for the secretion of fluid that coats the airway epithelium. Consequently, patients with cystic fibrosis develop viscous mucus secretions that can obstruct the airways and are prone to acquiring life-threatening pulmonary infections. Another example is long-QT syndrome. Individuals with long-QT syndrome have abnormally prolonged action potentials in the heart and are at risk for ventricular arrhythmias that can lead to sudden death. Some individuals with long-QT syndrome have mutations in potassium channels that repolarize the cardiac muscle. The direct importance of ion channels in cardiac function is underscored by the effectiveness of antiarrhythmic drugs, many of which act on ion channels.

II. PRINCIPLES OF ION CHANNEL MECHANISMS

A. The Electrochemical Gradient

The electrochemical gradient determines the direction that ions will flow through an open ion channel and is a combination of two types of gradients: a concentration gradient and an electrical field gradient. We can consider these two gradients separately. Figure 1a shows two compartments that contain an aqueous solution of ions separated by a membrane. It is apparent that there is a concentration gradient, since the left side contains more ions than the right. Assuming the membrane is permeable to the ion, there will be a net movement of ions from the right to left side until the concentrations of ions on both sides are the same. In this case, when the concentrations on both sides equalize, the solution will have reached

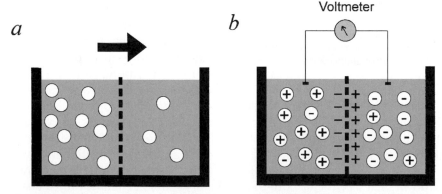

Figure 1 The electrochemical gradient is a combination of the concentration gradient and the electrical potential. The panels show two compartments that contain a solution of ions (circles). An ion-permeable membrane separates the two compartments. (a) There is a higher concentration of ions on the left side; therefore, ions will tend to diffuse from the left to the right (direction of arrow). It is also apparent that there is an osmotic gradient. Initially, water will tend to flow from the right to the left. At equilibrium, however, the two sides will be isoosmotic. (b) A voltage has been applied across the membrane. As a consequence, positively charged ions are drawn to the left and negatively charged ions to the right.

equilibrium. At equilibrium, an equal number of ions will diffuse across the membrane in both directions, and the concentrations of ions on either side will not change.

The electrical field gradient takes into account the charge on the ion. In Fig. 1b, an electrical potential has been applied so that the left side is negatively charged and the right side is positively charged. Ions that are positively charged will flow into the left compartment until it reaches a new equilibrium, in which the electrostatic forces that pull the cations into the left side are balanced by the tendency for the ions to move down its concentration gradient. Negatively charged ions will tend to flow into the right compartment. In this equilibrium, the final concentrations of ions on both sides are not equal.

The relationship between the electrical potential and the magnitude of the concentration gradient that is created is intuitive: The stronger the electrical potential, the greater the concentration gradient. The Nernst equation describes this relationship:

$$E_x = \frac{RT}{zF} \ln \frac{[X]_{out}}{[X]_{in}} \qquad (1)$$

where E_x is the electrical potential with units of millivolts, R is the gas constant, T is the temperature, z is the valence of the ion, and F is Faraday's constant. In words, the Nernst equation states that an electrical potential, E_x, will produce a concentration gradient with the ratio $[X]_{out}/[X]_{in}$ when the membrane is permeable to the ion. The converse is also true; a concentration gradient, $[X]_{out}/[X]_{in}$, will generate an electrical potential, E_x. Near room temperature (20°C), the Nernst equation simplifies to

$$E_x = \frac{58}{z} \log_{10} \frac{[X]_{out}}{[X]_{in}} \qquad (2)$$

E_x is also referred to as the equilibrium potential or the Nernst potential.

The cell is similar to the compartments in Fig. 1, only more ions need to be considered. The membrane potential is determined by the permeability of the membrane to a given ion. Figure 2 gives the concentrations of Na^+, K^+, Cl^-, and Ca^{2+} inside and outside a typical cell. Two processes work to maintain the concentration gradients of these ions. The action of ion pumps helps keep the cytoplasmic concentrations of Na^+, Cl^-, and Ca^{2+} low and the K^+ concentration high. Second, the presence of macromolecular anions inside the cell, such as proteins, tends to produce gradients of ions on their own. The redistribution of ions due to fixed charges in the cell is referred to as the Donnan effect.

At rest, the membrane is permeable to K^+; therefore, the resting potential of the cell is near E_K (in Fig. 2, approximately -84 mV). The flow of ions through the membrane is not large enough to affect changes in the ionic composition inside or outside the cell. Experimentally, currents can be elicited by changing the electrical potential across the membrane in short pulses. At membrane potentials of approximately -84 mV, there will be small K^+ currents since the membrane potential is near E_K, at which there is no net flow of K^+ across the membrane. Above E_K, there will be a net flow of K^+ outward because the electrical field gradient is not large enough to balance the concentration gradient. This results in an outward current (Fig. 3a). Below E_K, there will be a net inward current because the stronger electrical field gradient will tend to pull more K^+ into the cell. With the opening of sodium channels, the membrane becomes predominantly permeable to Na^+ rather than K^+. The low concentration of Na^+ inside the cell and the negative

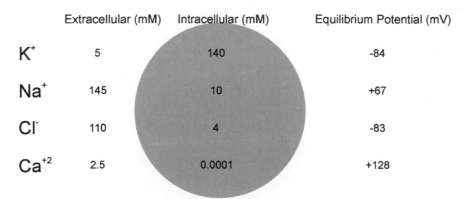

	Extracellular (mM)	Intracellular (mM)	Equilibrium Potential (mV)
K^+	5	140	-84
Na^+	145	10	+67
Cl^-	110	4	-83
Ca^{+2}	2.5	0.0001	+128

Figure 2 The concentration of ions inside and surrounding a typical mammalian cell. The equilibrium potentials were calculated using Eq. (2).

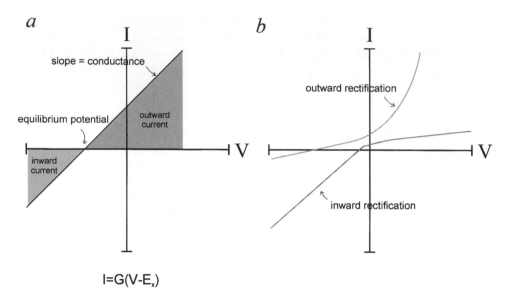

$$I = G(V-E_x)$$

Figure 3 Current–voltage plots of ion channels. (a) An *I–V* curve of an ion channel that conducts positively charged ions. Above the equilibrium potential, there is outward current; below the equilibrium potential, there is inward current. An ohmic ion channel has a linear *I–V* relationship. (b) Rectifiers pass more current in one direction. *I–V* curves of ion channels that rectify curve upwards or downwards.

membrane potential initially create a strong driving force for Na^+ to enter the cell and can cause the membrane potential to approach E_{Na}, (e.g., at the peak of action potentials).

B. Current–Voltage Relationships

Current is the movement of charge, and in cells the flow of ions through ion channels can be measured. By expressing cloned ion channels in heterologous systems or by silencing other channels with chemical blockers, the current from a single ion channel can be isolated. In these settings, it is often useful to apply different electrical potentials to the membrane and measure the magnitude and direction of the current as a function of voltage. If current through the ion channel is linearly related to the membrane potential as in Fig. 3a, then the ion channel is said to be ohmic because it behaves like a resistor and follows Ohm's law:

$$V = IR \tag{3}$$

where V is voltage, I is current, and R is the resistance. For the purposes of studying ion channels, it is useful to modify Ohm's law into the form

$$I = G(V - E_x) \tag{4}$$

Here, V is replaced with $(V-E_x)$ because $I=0$ at the equilibrium potential, and R is replaced with its

inverse, the conductance G. The conductance is the ease with which ions will flow through an ion channel, which is more intuitive since ion channels with a high conductance will conduct larger currents. $(V-E_x)$ constitutes the driving force, which together with the conductance determines the amount of current that flows through the ion channel. From Fig. 3a or Eq. (4), we can see that G represents the slope of the *I–V* curve. Ion channels with a higher conductance will have steeper *I–V* curves.

  I–V curves show the sensitivity of an ion channel to voltage. One should bear in mind that all ion channels are not ohmic. Ion channels that conduct more ions in one direction are said to rectify. For example, inward rectifier potassium channels preferentially conduct more K^+ into the cell than out of the cell (Fig. 3b). Other ion channels display outwardly rectifying currents.

C. Anatomy of a Typical Ion Channel

In the early 20th century, ion channels as we know them were considered nothing more than "holes in the membrane" that allowed ions to pass through them. We now know that ion channels are more complex than simple holes. In particular, there are two properties that distinguish them from simple holes: They exhibit selectivity for certain ions, and they open and close in response to stimuli.

All ion channels display many of the same basic properties. All ion channels are integral membrane proteins that form a pore in the lipid bilayer (Fig. 4). Like other membrane proteins, ion channels contain stretches of hydrophobic amino acids called transmembrane segments that anchor the protein within the lipid bilayer. These transmembrane segments pack against each other to stabilize the basic pore structure. Part of the pore is narrow and forms a barrier beyond which impermeant ions cannot cross. This region is lined with amino acid sidechains or backbone atoms that interact with the ion briefly as it crosses the pore. A flexible region of the ion channel forms a gate that acts to open and close access to the pore. The opening and closing of the ion channel is referred to as gating. The position of the gate can be influenced by regions that are modified by enzymes such as kinases or phosphatases. Finally, many ion channels extend processes that dock onto intracellular scaffolding proteins that are part of the cellular architecture. These interactions help direct those ion channels to specific locations within the cell such as the synapse or an intracellular organelle.

D. Ion Selectivity

All ion channels conduct certain ions over others—a property referred to as ion selectivity. Some ion channels are permeable to a class of ions; cation channels are one example, though most ion channels conduct a single type of ion. The selectivity of some ion channels is extraordinary. Voltage-gated calcium channels are 1000 times more selective for Ca^{2+} over other cations and pass Ca^{2+} almost exclusively. This is remarkable considering that the concentrations of other ions such as Na^+ can be much higher than that of Ca^{2+}. The mechanism by which ion channels pick and choose certain ions is still not fully understood.

At the molecular level, ions are little more than point charges with different valences. For ions with the same charge the only distinguishing feature is their ionic radius. Na^+ and K^+, which both have a charge of $+1$, have radii of 0.95 and 1.33 Å, respectively. Another feature is the water molecules that surround and interact with the ion. In solution, ions are surrounded by multiple layers of water molecules that are continuously exchanging with other "free" waters around it. Based on the mobility of ions in solution, Na^+ behaves as though they are larger than K^+. This is because its charge is concentrated in a smaller space and thus binds its waters of hydration more tightly.

The narrowest part of the pore has been termed by Bertil Hille as the ion selectivity filter. A filter with a fixed diameter is one way of explaining ion selectivity. In this view, ion channels are like sieves that allow small ions to pass but retain large ions. Although this mechanism is certainly at work in ion channels, an ion selectivity filter does not explain how an ion channel could be permeable only to large ions.

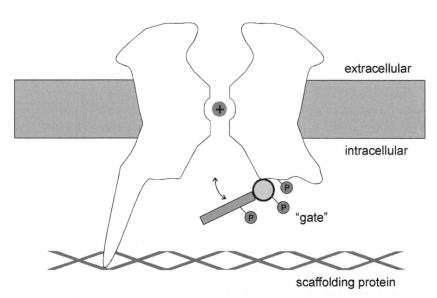

Figure 4 The "anatomy" of a typical ion channel. Ion channels are integral membrane proteins that sit in the plasma membrane. An ion is drawn sitting in a binding pocket in the ion selectivity filter (narrow part) as it passes through the ion channel. A gate (drawn as a door) swings open and closed.

It is likely that the permeant ion makes direct contact with the ion channel at some points during its passage. These interactions at specific binding sites may explain how an ion channel can be selective for large ions or discriminate between ions of similar radii. The binding sites can be depicted with the aid of an "energy landscape" diagram (Fig. 5a). Unfavorable locations are represented as regions of high energy, or peaks, whereas stable regions such as binding sites are represented by valleys. It is clear that some ion channels have more than one binding site within the channel. Multiple binding sites in close proximity may explain the high turnover rate of ion channels by setting up electrostatic repulsion between ions.

All potassium channel genes share a P region. The P region can be easily identified in potassium channel sequences since it contains the signature amino acid sequence GYG. The P region forms a part of the pore that is involved in ion selectivity since mutations in this region can alter the ion selectivity of potassium channels. The physical nature of the binding sites formed by the pore regions of most ion channels is unknown; however, it is likely that they are assembled from polar and charged amino acid sidechains or carbonyl oxygens from the protein backbone. These moieties could mimic the waters that may have been stripped away when the ion enters the pore. These interactions are likely to be transient and of low affinity given the high rate of turnover of an ion channel. One measure of the affinity can be obtained by measuring the current size at given ion concentrations (Fig. 5b). With no permeant ions present, an open ion channel will conduct zero current. As the concentration of ions is increased, the current will increase since the greater number of permeant ions will allow more ions to flow through the channel. Eventually, the current will reach a plateau or saturate. Plotted on a graph, the current can be fit with the Michaelis–Menton equation, and a constant (K_M), a measure of the affinity of the ion channel for the ion,

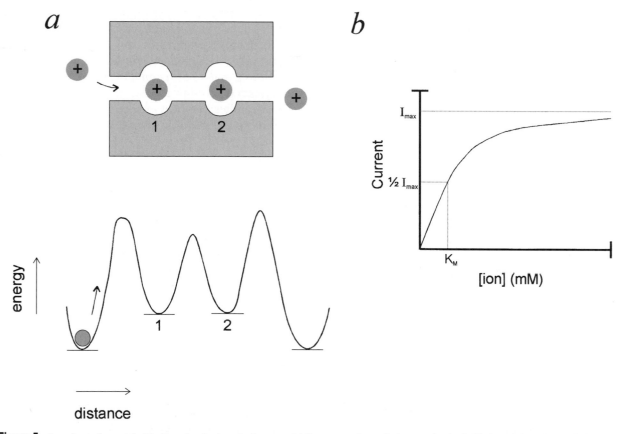

Figure 5 Ion channels contain binding sites for ions in the pore. (a) Ions move through the pore in single file from left to right. Binding sites 1 and 2 are places where the ions make interactions with the ion channel. The procession through the pore can be represented on an energy landscape diagram in which the binding sites are drawn as valleys. (b) The current amplitude eventually plateaus as the concentration of permeant ions is increased. This data can be fit using the Michaelis–Menton equation to derive the K_d, a measure of affinity.

can be obtained. Typically, ion channels show a K_M in the millimolar range.

E. Ion Channel Gating

Ion channels undergo a conversion between two types of states—closed and open—in a process referred to as gating. The gating behavior of an ion channel defines its functional role in physiology and is typically tied to the name of the ion channel. Ion channels are able to respond to a wide range of stimuli. The binding of a neurotransmitter (ligand-gated ion channels), a change in the membrane potential (voltage-gated ion channels), a physical pull on the ion channel protein (mechanosensitive ion channels), and heat are known to activate certain ion channels.

An ion channel with two states, one closed and one open, can be represented by a state diagram:

$$C \leftrightarrow O \qquad (5)$$

where C stands for closed and O stands for open. The $C \rightarrow O$ transition is referred to as activation; the reverse process, $O \rightarrow C$, is called deactivation. Since ion channels are metastable and can exist in multiple states, there is no way of knowing a priori which state a single ion channel will be in at any moment in time. After observing the activity of an ion channel for some length of time, however, one can collect statistics that describe the probability that an ion channel will be in the closed or open state, the average duration of each closing and opening, and the frequency of switching between states. These parameters are part of a set of fundamental variables that uniquely describe the activity of an ion channel. A stimulus can activate the ion channel by destabilizing the closed state or stabilizing the open state and thus increase the probability that an ion channel will be in the open state. A closed state that is accessed after the ion channel opens is referred to as the inactive state (I). An ion channel with three states may have the following state diagram:

$$C \leftrightarrow O \leftrightarrow I \qquad (6)$$

The $O \rightarrow I$ transition is referred to as inactivation. Often, the state diagrams of ion channels are complex and can contain multiple interconnecting closed, open, and inactive states.

The physical change in the ion channel structure that is responsible for gating remains an area of active research. Studies of several model ion channels have revealed a range of mechanisms by which ion channels may gate. For one channel, the nicotinic acetylcholine receptor (nAChR), scientists have been able to get a glimpse of the gating process with the use of the electron microscopy. Thus far, this has only been possible for the nAChR because the *Torpedo* electric ray produces abundant amounts of this protein that can form crystalline arrays in the membrane. These images revealed that this ion channel has an outer vestibule that makes it a great deal longer than the vertical height of the plasma membrane. Images taken before and after treatment with acetylcholine have been used to model the conformational changes that occurred after ligand binding. The binding site for acetylcholine lies on the outer vestibule, and the binding of ligand is transduced as a signal to the transmembrane segments that then undergo a concerted change in structure to open the pore. Unfortunately, the resolution of these images is too low to provide a detailed view of the gating process. One model postulates that the pore is lined by "kinked helices" whose vertices project into the pore in the closed state. After treatment with acetylcholine, the kinked helices appear to rotate away from the pore. This rotation may move hydrophobic residues that block the pore out of the way and replace them with polar residues.

Another well-studied gating mechanism is the inactivation gating of voltage-gated potassium channels (Fig. 6b). Inactivation can be eliminated, while other properties are left intact, by treating the inside of the channel with proteases. This and other experimental observations of the inactivation process can be explained by a "ball-and-chain" mechanism. In this model, part of the ion channel that binds the pore (ball) is tethered to the ion channel by a linker (chain) and blocks the pore once the channel has been activated. The region of the ion channel that forms the ball can be expressed by itself. As further evidence of this mechanism, when the ball is directly applied onto protease-treated ion channels, inactivation can be restored.

Inward rectifier potassium channels illustrate that the gate does not need to be an intrinsic part of the ion channel (Fig. 6c). Inward rectifying potassium channels pass larger currents into the cell than out of the cell. The channel alone, however, exhibits little or no rectification but displays rectification when it is brought near a cell, suggesting that a soluble factor is involved. In the case of inward rectifier potassium channels, it was discovered that Mg^{2+} and

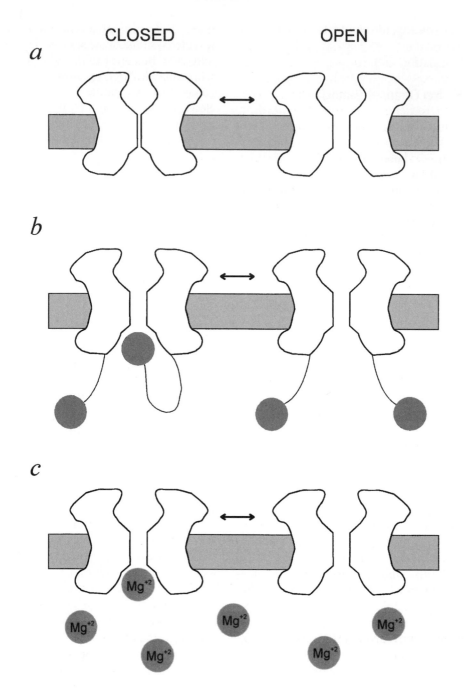

Figure 6 Three examples of ion channel gating mechanisms depicted as a cartoon. (a) Gating occurs via a generalized change in the structure in the region of the pore. The nicotinic acetylcholine receptor undergoes a conformational change of its M2 segment that closes the ion conduction pathway. (b) "Ball-and-chain" mechanism of inactivation gating in voltage-gated potassium channels. (c) Inward rectifiers are gated by extrinsic factors (e.g., Mg^{2+}) that block the pore. The block is voltage dependent; therefore, inward rectifiers conduct more current below E_K and little current above E_K.

polyamines, amino acid metabolites, produced rectification by binding to the pore of the channel at depolarized membrane potentials but not at hyperpolarized membrane potentials.

F. Ion Channel Modulation

Aside from the binding of a ligand or other stimuli that activate the ion channel, the gating of the ion channel can be affected by other factors that affect the ease of opening the ion channel. This process is loosely referred to as modulation and can occur through the binding of a second messenger or a covalent modification of the ion channel such as phosphorylation. The role of modulation is to tweak or fine-tune the gating of an ion channel, although in some instances the line between modulation and gating can be blurred. For example, the phosphorylation of CFTR is necessary for channel openings to occur.

In general, modulation events originate at receptors that are at a distance from the ion channel. The response is usually slower in onset because a second messenger needs to be generated and then diffuse to the ion channel. The signal transduction cascade also branches off to influence other effectors that produce major changes in a cell's functioning. The modulation of ion channels can be part of long-lasting changes in the cell.

III. MOLECULAR PROPERTIES OF ION CHANNELS

A. Primary Structure of Ion Channels

What do ion channels look like? Although ion channel currents have been measured for many decades, only recently with advancements in molecular biology have their structures been determined in any detail. The goal of understanding ion channel structure is a biochemical one. Usually, the initial step is to determine the primary structure of the ion channel protein. Currently, this is achieved by first cloning the ion channel gene and then reading the protein sequence from its cDNA. The nicotinic acetylcholine receptor was the first ion channel to have its sequence identified through the work of Shosaku Numa and colleagues in 1982. They first purified the ion channel protein from the *Torpedo* electric ray and obtained small bits of protein sequence. Then they designed short oligonucleotides that corresponded to their protein sequence and hybridized them to a cDNA library that contained genes from *Torpedo*. In this way, they obtained the entire cDNA sequence and read the entire amino acid sequence of nAChR.

Ion channels have also been identified using genetic methods. *Shaker*, a voltage-gated potassium channel from *Drosophila melanogaster*, was cloned by Lily and Yuh Nung Jan and colleagues in 1987. *Shaker* derives its name from the behavior of mutant flies when exposed to ether and was long suspected to be an ion channel based on biophysical studies. *Shaker* had already been localized to a region of the X chromosome. To identify part of the gene sequence, the Jan group performed Southern blots on a series of *Shaker* mutant flies with chromosomal rearrangements. Then, they were able to obtain the entire *Shaker* sequence by probing a *Drosophila* cDNA library with their partial DNA sequence.

Once a member of an ion channel family has been identified, other members of the same family can be identified by sorting through DNA libraries for genes that have related sequences. What was in the past done with petri dishes and nitrocellulose membranes is now being done using computers. With the growing information collected from genome sequencing projects, it is increasingly common for new ion channel genes to be identified through the Internet. Once a putative ion channel sequence has been found, a relatively straightforward sequence of steps can be used to clone the gene by amplifying from a sample of genomic DNA.

A great deal of information about what the ion channel looks like can be obtained from the primary structure. For example, it is known that membrane proteins contain discrete stretches of hydrophobic amino acids that span the lipid bilayer. These transmembrane segments can be identified with computer programs that search the protein for long stretches of hydrophobic residues. Combined with other information, one can derive a model of the membrane topology of the ion channel. The models that are generated, however, can be imperfect. There are several experimental methods by which scientists can test whether a region of the protein lies on the extracellular or intracellular face of the membrane. One is to identify sites that are glycosylated since they are known to be present only on the extracellular parts of a protein. Another is to raise antibodies against specific stretches of the protein and determine whether the antibodies bind from the inside or the outside surface of the cell.

The membrane topography is a useful scheme for classifying ion channels (Fig. 7). For example, there are three classes of potassium channels. The gene for voltage-gated potassium channels has six transmembrane segments, numbered S1–S6, and another hydrophobic region between S5 and S6 called the P region, which does not cross the plasma membrane. The P region contributes to the pore of the ion channel. The inward rectifier potassium channels have two transmembrane segments with a P region between M1 and M2. A third class of potassium channels is called two-pore channels because each gene contains two P regions. Two-pore channels have four transmembrane

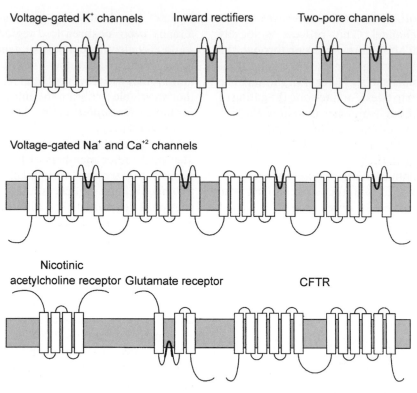

Figure 7 The membrane topology of ion channels. Voltage-gated sodium and calcium channels resemble four voltage-gated potassium channel subunits linked together. The nicotinic acetylcholine receptor and the glutamate receptor are both ligand-gated ion channels but have different membrane topologies. Two-pore channels look like two inward rectifiers fused together. Among ion channels, CFTR belongs to a unique class of membrane proteins.

segments, M1–M4. The membrane topology also gives clues about the function of different parts of the ion channel. For example, the binding site for acetylcholine in nAChR would be limited to those regions that faced the extracellular side.

Sequence analysis of different ion channel families suggests that ion channels are evolutionarily related. Two-pore channel genes resemble two inward rectifier potassium channel genes linked together, and voltage-gated sodium channels and voltage-gated calcium channels resemble four voltage-gated potassium channel genes linked in tandem.

The cloning of ion channels has revolutionized the study of ion channels by allowing scientists to make changes in the amino acid sequence and then test them. One particular strategy of making mutations—making chimeric ion channels—has been especially powerful in determining ion channel structure and function. In one well-known example, Numa, Sakmann, and colleagues used this method to conclude that M2 in the nicotinic acetylcholine receptor is important for determining the conductance of nAChR. In this strategy, one starts with two related ion channels that have

different properties. In this case, it was known that nAChR expressed with the δ subunit from calf has a conductance of 65 pS, whereas the δ subunit from *Torpedo* has a conductance of 87 pS. In order to identify the residues that were responsible, Numa and colleagues made hybrid genes by splicing parts of the gene for the calf δ subunit to the *Torpedo* δ subunit and measured their conductance. With successive chimeras that contained increasingly smaller parts of the *Torpedo* gene, they were able to determine that the M2 segment is the region that determines the difference in conductance between the calf and *Torpedo* δ subunits.

This approach has been instrumental in assigning functional roles to parts of ion channels. Using this approach, it has been revealed that ion channels are modular in design (Fig. 8). One caveat, however, is that one cannot exclude the involvement of other regions of the gene since replacement of those regions would not be detected if they shared a similar sequence or function.

Our understanding of ion channels has facilitated efforts to find more ion channel genes in computer

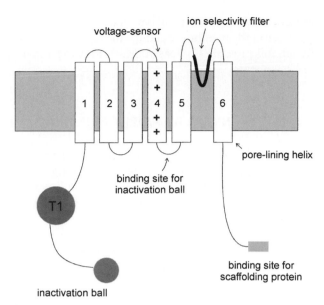

voltage-sensor

ion selectivity filter

binding site for
inactivation ball

pore-lining helix

T1

inactivation ball

binding site for
scaffolding protein

Figure 8 The modular design of voltage-gated potassium channels. Regions of the gene perform separate functions. Some of these functions can be transferred to other ion channels by transplanting that region alone.

databases. The parts of the ion channel that are functionally important are more likely to be conserved through evolution; therefore, database searches that are weighted to these residues are more likely to find homologs that may otherwise have little sequence conservation. The completion of the genomes of organisms with nervous systems, such as the fruit fly, *D. melanogaster*, or the worm, *Caenorhabditis elegans*, has ushered in a new set of more complex questions to be addressed. What are all the ion channels in a nervous system or in an animal? Given the redundancy of ion channel genes, what is the minimum set of ion channels needed for a functional nervous system?

B. Ion Channel Assembly

Ion channels are typically assembled from many subunits that form the pore-lining structure. The number of subunits that form ion channels varies from subfamily to subfamily. For example, four subunits of voltage-gated potassium channels assemble to form a single ion channel. Likewise, inward rectifier ion channels are tetramers. Most ligand-gated ion channels are pentamers, and gap junction ion channels are hexamers.

Ion channels that are members of the same subfamily can assemble with each other because they share

molecular determinants that allow them to interact. For example, there are four subfamilies of voltage-gated potassium channels, Kv1–Kv4, related to *Shaker*. It is known that members of one Kv subfamily can coassemble together, but not with members of the other subfamilies. By carefully designing chimeras between the different Kv genes, the Jan group identified a stretch of amino acids in the N-terminal cytoplasmic domain before S1 that determines whether two Kv channels can interact with each other. This region, called the T1 domain, appears to form a structural domain that by itself can form a stable tetrameric structure. The T1 domain has been solved by X-ray crystallography. Analysis of the structure of the T1 domain from different Kv subfamilies shows that the interface between the T1 domain from each subfamily differs structurally. This suggests that members of different Kv subfamilies cannot coassemble because their T1 domains are incompatible.

Ion channels assembled from different subunits will exhibit different functional properties. Because ion channels can assemble from several genes of a given subfamily, the number of potential ion channels is expanded combinatorially. The reason for this potential diversity is unknown. One possibility is that the incorporation of certain subunits is used to regulate ion channel selectivity, gating, or biosynthesis. The inclusion of a subunit with certain sequence motifs has been shown to be able to target an ion channel to specific compartments within the cell or alter the stability of an ion channel on the plasma membrane.

In vivo, ion channels are often part of a complex with accessory proteins that can modify its functional properties or stability in much the same way that mixing subunits can do so. These other proteins are often referred to as β subunits, with the ion channel being the α subunit. β subunits can be soluble or integral membrane proteins. In some cases, the ion channel cannot be expressed in heterologous systems without its accessory subunits, suggesting that the β subunit is an essential part of the functional ion channel complex.

C. The Three-Dimensional Structure of Ion Channels

The final frontier is to be able to visualize the three-dimensional structure of ion channels. In 1998, Rod MacKinnon and colleagues reported the three-dimensional structure of a potassium channel and Doug Rees and colleagues reported the structure of a mechanosensitive channel using X-ray crystallography. High-resolution structural studies of ion channels are difficult to perform because it is difficult to obtain sufficient quantities of ion channel protein for crystallization experiments and it is harder to coax membrane proteins into forming crystals than it is to coax soluble proteins. Both MacKinnon and Rees used bacterial ion channels that are easier to produce recombinantly.

Rod MacKinnon and colleagues determined the structure of the KcsA potassium channel from the bacteria *Streptomyces lividans* (Fig. 9a). KcsA has two transmembrane segments, which might place it in the same category as inward rectifier potassium channels. However, sequence analysis of KcsA suggests that it is more closely related to voltage-gated potassium channels than inward rectifiers. In support of this view, KcsA interacts with a peptide toxin, agitoxin2, that blocks *Shaker* but not inward rectifiers. One of the most satisfying aspects of the channel structure has been how well it agrees with predictions from functional studies of potassium channels. The structure is 45 Å long and the pore is narrow at the top, where the selectivity filter is predicted to be located. The helical structure resembles an "inverted teepee," and in the center of the ion channel there is a wide cavity that MacKinnon refers to as the "lake." As predicted by earlier experiments, the ion selectivity filter is formed from residues in the P region, and the carbonyl oxygens of GYG are held at a diameter that is optimal for allowing K^+ to pass. Previously we stated that ion channels catalyze the transfer of ions across an electrostatic barrier, the plasma membrane. The KcsA structure depicts two elegant mechanisms by which an ion channel overcomes the barrier. First, a water-filled lake reduces the electrostatic barrier by simply surrounding the ion in an aqueous environment. Second, the negative ends of the dipoles formed by four pore helices point toward the center of the lake, forming a point of negative electrostatic potential in the center of the membrane that is favorable for a cation.

Doug Rees and colleagues determined the structure of a mechanosensitive ion channel, MscL, from *Mycobacterium tuberculosis* (Fig. 9b). MscL is activated when lateral tension is applied to the lipid bilayer and is used by bacteria to rapidly release intracellular solutes when they are placed in a hypoosmotic environment. One motivation for studying MscL was to understand how mechanical stress could gate this ion channel. Since the open MscL channel has been shown to be able to pass a whole protein, thioredoxin, it is likely that the structure in Fig. 9b represents the closed channel. It is possible that normally lateral pressure in the membrane clamps the ion channel shut. When this pressure is released, MscL may expand into the open state.

IV. ION CHANNELS BY FAMILY AND FUNCTION

So far, we have discussed ion channels in the general sense. In the short time since the cloning of the nicotinic acetylcholine receptor, scientists have cloned and identified many ion channels, but it is clear that there are more ion channels that have yet to be discovered. An equally daunting task is to investigate the role that ion channels play in physiology. Although a complete review of the ion channel literature is beyond the scope of this articles in this section we introduce the major ion channel families and attempt to explain why some of these ion channels have attracted the interest of scientists.

A. Voltage-Gated Ion Channels

Broadly, voltage-gated ion channels are involved in the generation of electrical signals in excitable cells such as neurons (Table I). Voltage-gated sodium channels are activated when the membrane potential reaches a certain threshold potential, and they contribute to the rapid depolarization of the membrane potential. Some invertebrate species lack voltage-gated sodium channels. In these animals, voltage-gated calcium channels may partially fulfill the roles of voltage-gated sodium channels. Voltage-gated calcium channels also mediate the entry of Ca^{2+} in response to depolarization. In nerve terminals, activation of voltage-gated calcium channels by axonal action potentials is a critical step in the release of synaptic vesicles.

The voltage-gated ion channels are related in structure. Potassium channels contain one domain of six transmembrane segments per subunit, whereas sodium and calcium channels contain four domains in one large α subunit. The distinguishing feature of this group of ion channels is that they are sensitive to changes in the membrane potential. A remarkable feature of these ion channels is that they contain basic amino acids interspersed in the fourth transmembrane segment (S4). These charges could potentially sense the electric field across the membrane, and movement of S4 could transmit changes in the membrane potential to the gate. Although S4 is likely a part of the

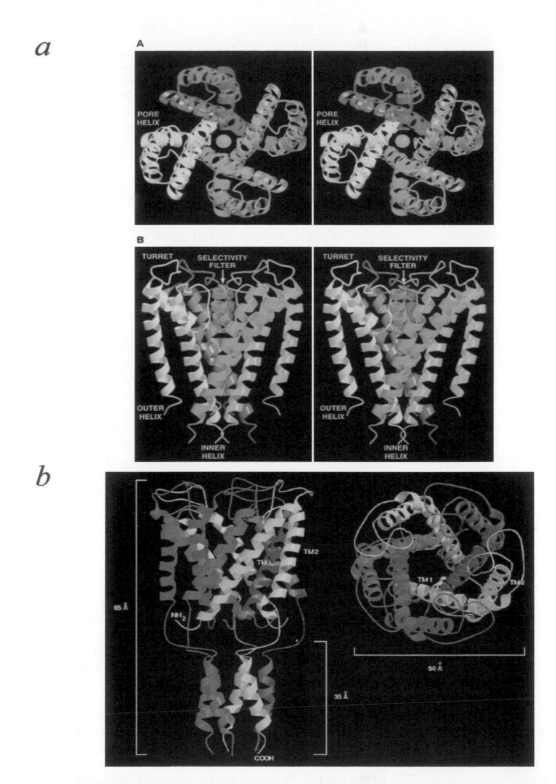

Figure 9   The three-dimensional structure of ion channels. (a) The top panels show stereoviews of the KcsA potassium channel as viewed from above the plasma membrane. KcsA is a tetramer and each of the subunits are shaded separately. The lower panel shows a side view (reprinted with permission from D.A. Doyle *et al.*, The structure of the potassium channel: Molecular basis of K conduction and selectivity. *Science* **280,** 73. Copyright © 1998 American Association for the Advancement of Science). (b) The side and axial views of the MscL mechanosensitive ion channel from *M. tuberculosis*. MscL is a pentamer (reprinted with permission from G. Chang *et al.*, Structure of the MscL homolog from *Mycobacterium tuberculosis*: A gated mechanosensitive ion channel. *Science* **282,** 2223. Copyright © 1998 American Association for the Advancement of Science).

Table I
Voltage-Gated Ion Channels

Ion channel	Ion selectivity	Function
Voltage-gated sodium channel	Na^+	Generates the upstroke in action potentials
Voltage-gated calcium channel	Ca^{+2}	Maintains the plateau of action potentials; allows the entry of Ca^{+2} in nerve terminals and muscle cells
Voltage-gated potassium channel	K^+	Generates the downstroke in the action potential; controls the frequency of action potentials; transports K^+ across membranes
Hyperpolarization-activated cation channel	Na^+, K^+	Mediates I_h and I_f; generates synchronous firing patterns in cells

mechanism by which ion channels sense voltage, precisely how voltage-gated ion channels respond to changes in the membrane potential and how this change is transmitted to the gate are still not completely understood.

Voltage-gated sodium channels and calcium channels are important targets of drugs used in the treatment of hypertension, cardiac arrhythmias, epilepsy, and pain. Voltage-gated sodium channels are famous for being the target of tetrodotoxin (TTX), a naturally occurring toxin most commonly associated with the pufferfish *Fugu* (it has been proposed that tetrodotoxin is actually synthesized by microorganisms living on the pufferfish). TTX blocks voltage-gated sodium channels with high affinity and thus inhibits action potentials, making it a potent neurotoxin. Marine species use TTX either to paralyze prey or to discourage natural predators. In Japan, fugu is treasured as a delicacy since low doses of TTX can produce paresthesia around the mouth when consumed (ironically, encouraging a predator). Fugu can only be prepared by licensed chefs; however, deaths from fugu poisoning are still reported.

In addition to their role in generating action potentials, voltage-gated potassium channels are involved in a wide array of other functions. This is reflected by the expression of voltage-gated potassium channels by cells outside the nervous system. The voltage-gated potassium channel family is much more diverse than the voltage-gated sodium and calcium channel families. Since the cloning of *Shaker*, the family of voltage-gated potassium channels has grown to include at least nine different subfamilies. One group, the calcium-activated potassium channels, is sensitive to changes in intracellular Ca^{2+} concentration as well as membrane potential. This feature allows them to help control the frequency of firing of action potentials. The entry of Ca^{2+} following repeated action potentials helps to activate these channels, which prolongs the duration of the undershoot of the

membrane potential following the spike. Longer afterhyperpolarizations can slow the rate of action potential firing or stop it.

A new class of voltage-sensitive ion channels that mediates a hyperpolarization-activated cation current was recently identified. This current, I_h or I_f, is also referred to as the pacemaker current because it is important in establishing the rhythmic oscillatory firing of action potentials. In the heart, I_f regulates the beat-to-beat variations in the heart rate, and in the brain it helps generate synchronous oscillations in neuronal networks that can be observed in electroencephalograms. The gene that encodes the pacemaker current appears to be a cousin of voltage-gated potassium channels; however, it is not apparent how this channel is activated by hyperpolarization while other voltage-gated ion channels are activated by depolarization.

B. Ligand-Gated Ion Channels

Ligand-gated ion channels are activated upon the binding of a neurotransmitter to the ion channel and are involved in fast synaptic transmisssion in the nervous system. Many of the ion channels in Table II have a wide tissue distribution outside of the nervous system and have other functions beyond synaptic transmission. These neurotransmitters include acetylcholine, γ-aminobutyric acid (GABA), glycine, glutamate, and serotonin (5-hydroxytryptophan), and the ion channels are more commonly referred to as receptors. Several of these neurotransmitters also activate a second distinct type of receptor. This second receptor type is a heptahelical receptor that produces intracellular second messengers through the modulation of G proteins. Most commonly in the context of glutamate receptors, the ligand-gated ion channel is referred to as an ionotropic receptor, whereas the G

Table II
Ligand-Gated Ion Channels

Ion channel	Ion selectivity	Function
Nicotinic acetylcholine receptor	Na^+, K^+	Fast synaptic transmission in the nervous system and at the neuromuscular junction
$GABA_A$ receptor	Cl^-	Fast inhibitory transmission in the brain
Glycine receptor	Cl^-	Fast inhibitory transmission, predominantly in the brain stem and spinal cord
Serotonin receptor	Na^+, K^+	Fast synaptic transmission
Glutamate receptor	Na^+, K^+, (Ca^{+2})	Fast excitatory transmission in the central nervous system; mediates ischemic neuronal cell death; involved in learning and memory?
P_{2X} receptor	Na^+, Ca^{+2}	Fast synaptic transmission; sensation of pain in the trigeminal system

protein-coupled receptor is referred to as a metabotropic receptor. A familiarity with the nomenclature is helpful in determing whether a neurotransmitter receptor is ionotropic or metabotropic.

On the basis of sequence similarity, it was originally assumed that these ligand-gated ion channels formed one superfamily. The current view is that glutamate receptors have a different transmembrane topology and belong to a distinct family of ligand-gated ion channels.

The nicotinic acetylcholine receptor is a pentamer, and each subunit contains four transmembrane segments with the N and C termini outside of the membrane. Among ligand-gated ion channels, the nicotinic acetylcholine receptor has been the most thoroughly characterized. This is due to the fact that the *Torpedo* electric ray has been a source of abundant amounts of the protein and this receptor mediates synaptic transmission at the neuromuscular junction, which is a synapse that has been amenable to biophysical studies. At the neuromuscular junction, acetylcholine is released from the motoneuron and diffuses across the synaptic cleft to activate the receptor. The opening of ion channels depolarizes the membrane and generates an action potential in the muscle that initiates muscle contraction.

The nicotinic acetylcholine receptor derives part of its name from nicotine, which is an agonist of this ion channel. The nicotine in tobacco products mediates the stimulatory and addictive effects of smoking and suggests that nACh receptors in the brain play a role in cognition as well as the activation of reward pathways. Along similar lines, experimental evidence suggests that patients with Alzheimer's disease have depleted levels of acetylcholine, indicating the importance of nicotinic acetylcholine receptors in normal cognitive functioning.

GABA is the major inhibitory neurotransmitter in the brain. $GABA_A$ receptors are ligand-gated ion channels, whereas $GABA_B$ receptors are G protein-coupled receptors. In the brain stem and spinal cord, glycine is also used as a neurotransmitter in inhibitory synapses. Both $GABA_A$ and glycine receptors are chloride channels that when activated hyperpolarize the cell and make it more difficult for excitatory neurotransmitters to depolarize the membrane. Clinically, $GABA_A$ receptors are the target of benzodiazepines, which are used as sedatives, muscle relaxants, and anticonvulsants. Benzodiazepines work by a distinctive mechanism. They do not activate $GABA_A$ receptors by themselves. Instead, they facilitate the action of GABA that is released by binding to an allosteric site on the ion channel.

Glutamate is the major excitatory neurotransmitter in the brain, and many scientists believe that glutamate receptors are involved in learning and memory. Under pathological conditions, glutamate receptors also mediate the neurotoxicity associated with cerebral ischemia. By analogy to the nicotinic acetylcholine receptor, glutamate receptors were originally believed to have four transmembrane segments. This model has since been revised so that the second transmembrane segment does not traverse the plasma membrane, leaving three membrane-crossing segments—M1, M3, and M4 (the numbering of the transmembrane segments was not changed). This moved the M3–M4 loop to the outside of the cell and the C terminus to the interior of the cell.

The glutamate receptors are heterogeneous and classified based on sequence and pharmacological profile into NMDA receptors, AMPA receptors, and kainate receptors. Many of the glutamate receptors have been cloned. The distinctive features of NMDA receptors versus non-NMDA receptors fit well with proposed mechanisms of neuronal plasticity. Near the resting potential, the majority of fast excitatory neurotransmission is mediated by AMPA receptors, which are permeable to Na^+ and K^+. NMDA receptors carry little current since they are blocked by Mg^{2+} at resting potentials. With a strong stimulus, however, enough AMPA receptors are activated to depolarize the cell and relieve the Mg^{2+} block of NMDA receptors. This is significant because NMDA receptors are highly permeable to Ca^{2+}. The entry of Ca^{2+} can initiate a signal transduction cascade that produces a long-lasting potentiation in subsequent synaptic potentials. Mechanisms of use-dependent enhancement of synaptic efficacy are often implicated in models of learning and memory.

Given the significance of Ca^{2+} permeability in glutamate receptors, the low Ca^{2+} permeability of AMPA receptors is achieved by a remarkable genetic mechanism. Sequencing of the gene and cDNAs of a particular AMPA receptor subtype (GluRB) revealed a discrepancy in the codon at a position in the second transmembrane segment. The gene contains a glutamine (Q) codon, whereas the cDNA contains an arginine (R) codon. It was later discovered that this codon is edited posttranscriptionally by the action of an enzyme in the nucleus that converts an adenine base into inosine. This single position, referred to as the Q/R site, also controls the Ca^{2+} permeability of AMPA receptors. In heterologous systems, AMPA receptors with Q in the Q/R site display high Ca^{2+} permeability, whereas AMPA receptors with R in the Q/R site display low Ca^{2+} permeability.

C. Inward Rectifiers and Two-Pore Potassium Channels

Inward rectifier potassium channels constitute another family of potassium channels distinct from voltage-gated potassium channels. Inward rectifiers are involved in maintaining the resting membrane potential near E_K or mediating the transport of K^+ across membranes (Table III). Some subfamilies of inward rectifiers respond to intracellular effectors that are produced by the activation of surface receptors. The activity of GIRKs (Kir3.0) is activated by the binding of the $G\beta\gamma$ subunits of G proteins. The activation of GIRKs is associated with the generation of slow inhibitory postsynaptic potentials in the brain and the slowing of the heart rate in response to vagal stimulation.

Inward rectifiers have the simplest structural plan of any ion channel. Like voltage-gated potassium channels, they are tetramers and contain a P region that forms part of the ion selectivity filter, but they contain only two transmembrane segments, M1 and M2. Inwardly rectifying potassium channels, as the name implies, allow more K^+ to enter the cell than to leave the cell. This property is a result of blocking of the pore from the intracellular side by polyamines or Mg^{2+} at depolarized potentials. Two acidic amino acid residues in M2 and the C terminus of inward rectifiers have been identified as part of the binding sites for the blocking particles.

Members of the Kir6.0 subfamily associate with the sulfonylurea receptor, a member of the ABC family, and form K_{ATP} ion channels that are sensitive to intracellular levels of ADP and ATP. Therefore, these ion channels link the membrane potential to the metabolic state of the cell. This property at work is best illustrated in the feedback regulation of blood glucose levels by the controlled release of insulin. In pancreatic β cells, the metabolism of glucose generates ATP, which inhibits K_{ATP}. This depolarizes the membrane potential and activates voltage-sensitive calcium channels that allow Ca^{2+} to enter the cell. The entry of Ca^{2+} then triggers the release of vesicles containing insulin, which stimulates glucose uptake by other tissues. Clinically, this pathway is utilized to help

Table III
Inwardly Rectifying Potassium Channels

Ion channel	Ion selectivity	Function
ROMK (Kir 1.0)	K^+	Salt reabsorption in the distal kidney
IRK (Kir 2.0)	K^+	Setting the resting membrane potential
GIRK (Kir 3.0)	K^+	Slowing the heart rate and slow inhibitory postsynaptic potentials in the brain
Kir 6.0	K^+	With the sulfonylurea receptor, forms K_{ATP}; regulates hormone release; cardioprotection during ischemia; regulates vascular tone

manage individuals with diabetes mellitus with oral hypoglycemics drugs that block K_{ATP} and stimulate the release of insulin.

Two-pore channels are a newly identified family of potassium channels. Their name derives from the presence of two P regions per gene. They have four transmembrane segments and resemble two inward rectifier subunits fused together. By analogy to inward rectifiers, it is believed that two-pore channels are dimers and not tetramers. Unlike inward rectifiers, two-pore channels display an outwardly rectifying current and are active at rest. Two-pore channels can be modulated by arachidonic acid or other unsaturated fatty acids, and inhibition of two-pore channels is a potential mechanism of excitatory neurotransmission. Evidence suggests that activation of two-pore channels may mediate some of the anesthetic effects of volatile gases such as chloroform or ether.

D. Chloride Channels

In addition to the $GABA_A$ and glycine receptors described previously, the chloride channels include the CLC family, CFTR, and other channel families that have yet to be identified. Chloride channels are involved in the regulation of cell volume, the transport of Cl^-, pH homeostasis, and membrane excitability. The CLC channels contain numerous hydrophobic stretches; however, the membrane topology of the CLC channels is unknown, with various models having 8–12 transmembrane segments.

The CFTR is a chloride channel that was cloned from molecular genetic studies of patients with cystic fibrosis. Its major role is in the transport of Cl^- across epithelial cells in many organs, such as the pancreas, lung, sweat glands, and kidneys. CFTR is a member of the ATP-binding cassette (ABC) family of ion transporters. ABC proteins are generally known for mediating the ATP-driven transport of substances; for example, the MDR protein pumps chemotherapeutic drugs out of the cell. Therefore, the CFTR ion channel is a unique member of this family.

Ion channels are fantastic molecular machines. Their functions are fundamental—they act as valves for ions to move into or out of the cell—and thus they play important roles in many physiological processes. The study of ion channels is challenging but rewarding since it ranges from exploring the function of ion channels on the cellular and systems level down to the atomic level to investigating how ion channels as proteins work. The first crystal structures of ion channels have ushered in a new era in ion channel research. With more structures and functional studies of ion channels and the cloning of ion channels involved in channelopathies, the next decade promises to be an exciting time for ion channel research.

See Also the Following Articles

ELECTRICAL POTENTIALS • GABA • NEUROTRANSMITTERS

Suggested Reading

Ackerman, M. J., and Clapham, D. E. (1997). Ion channels—Basic science and clinical disease. *N. Engl. J. Med.* **336,** 1575.

Aidley, D. J., and Stanfield, P. R. (1996). *Ion Channels: Molecules in Action.* Cambridge Univ. Press, Cambridge.

Ashcroft, F. M. (2000). *Ion Channels and Disease.* Academic Press, San Diego.

Dani, J. A., and Mayer, M. L. (1995). Structure and function of gluamate and nicotinic acetylcholine receptors. *Curr. Opin. Neurobiol.* **5,** 310.

Doyle, D. A., *et al.* (1998). The structure of potassium channel: Molecular basis of K conduction and selectivity. *Science* **280,** 69.

Foskett, J. K. (1998). CIC and CFTR chloride channel gating. *Annu. Rev. Physiol.* **60,** 689.

Hille, B. (1992). *Ionic Channels of Excitable Membranes,* 2nd ed. Sinauer, Sunderland, MA.

Jan, L. Y., and Jan, Y. N. (1997). Cloned potassium channels from eukaryotes and prokaryotes. *Annu. Rev. Neurosci.* **20,** 91.

Johnston, D., and Wu, S. M. (1995). *Foundations of Cellular Neurophysiology.* MIT Press, Cambridge, MA.

Nicholls, J. G., Martin, A. R., and Wallace, B. G. (1992). *From Neuron to Brain,* 3rd ed. Sinaver, Sunderland, MA.

Seeburg, P. H. (1993). The molecular biology of mammalian glutamate receptor channels. *Trends Neurosci.* **16,** 359.

Siegelbaum, S. A., and Koester, J. (2000). Ion channels. In *Principles of Neural Science* (E. R. Kandel, J. H. Schwartz, and T. M. Jessell, Eds.), 4th ed. Elsevier, New York.

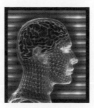

Language Acquisition

HELEN TAGER-FLUSBERG
Boston University School of Medicine

I. Prelinguistic Developments

II. Phonological Acquisition

III. Lexical–Semantic Development

IV. The Acquisition of Syntax and Morphology

V. Pragmatic Development

GLOSSARY

binding principles According to the syntactic theory, known as government binding theory, these are the rules of our grammar that dictate the relation between words, for example, pronouns and their referents.

communicative competence Linguistic competence and knowledge of the social rules for language use.

constraints Limits or biases that children bring to the task of language acquisition. A constraint may dictate a cognitive or pragmatic strategy in the interpretation of words.

grammar The finite set of rules shared by all speakers of a language that allows all possible sentences to be generated.

intentional communication Any communicative act that a person engages in purposefully.

language A symbolic system, based on syntactic, semantic, and phonetic features, that allows mutually intelligible communication among a group of speakers.

learnability Various models of language acquisition based on several assumptions concerning the nature of children, known learning mechanisms, the structure of language, and the logical inferences that can be drawn from these assumptions.

morphology The rules that govern the use of free or bound morphemes, the minimal meaningful units of language.

overregularization errors A common error among children that involves applying regular and productive grammatical rules to words that are irregular or exceptions.

parameter A type of linguistic switch that is set after children are exposed to particular forms in their native language; it is one of a finite number of values along which languages are free to vary.

phoneme A speech sound that can signal a difference of meaning in a language.

semantics The study of the meaning system of language.

speech acts Aspects of the pragmatic systems referring to different functions of utterances, such as requesting or promising.

theory of mind Knowledge about the mind and mental states of other people that is used to interpret their actions and the intended meaning of utterances.

universal grammar Hypothetical set of restrictions governing all forms that human languages may take.

Language acquisition refers to the process of achieving the ability to speak and understand the particular language or languages to which a child has been exposed. By the time most children reach the age of 5, they are highly competent speakers of their native language. During these early years of development, children acquire the ability to perceive and produce the speech sounds of the language to which they are exposed and the phonological rules for combining them to create words. They also acquire a large and varied vocabulary and the rules for combining them into complex grammatical sentences with correct morphology to mark tense, mood, number, and so forth. Finally, they become proficient users of this linguistic system to perform a range of different speech acts appropriate to varied social contexts. These remarkable achievements in the acquisition of language occur without explicit instruction or even significant feedback from others. Language is a complex, componential system composed of an abstract phonological rule system and lexicon, syntax, morphology, pragmatic, and discourse rules. These components depend on the development of different cognitive and neural mechanisms that interact over the course of acquisition.

I. PRELINGUISTIC DEVELOPMENTS

A. Speech Perception

Infants come into the world prepared to acquire language. At birth they are able to distinguish speech from other sounds and, indeed, to perceive and discriminate speech sounds in the same way as adults. They can discriminate between syllables that differ by a single phonetic feature (e.g., ba vs pa). Studies have demonstrated that during the first months of life infants discriminate all phonetic contrasts between speech sounds in their native language as well as those occurring in other languages to which they have not been exposed.

During the second half of the first year speech perception abilities undergo significant changes and reorganizations. As a result of continued exposure to the sound properties of their native language, infants show a reduction and eventual loss in the capacity to discriminate speech sound contrasts that are present only in foreign languages. At the same time, by the age of 6 months infants become more attuned to the sound structure of their native language, preferring the prosodic patterns of their own language as opposed to those found in languages they have not heard. By the age of 9 months, infants also prefer listening to word lists in which the words follow the constraints on ordering phonetic segments in their native language over those in which the words violate those constraints.

B. Social Developments

From the start, these sophisticated speech perceptual abilities are closely tied to the infant's social experience. Studies of newborns have shown that they distinguish their own mothers' voices from those of other mothers, which is most likely related to prenatal exposure to the acoustic properties of the mothers' speech. In the visual domain, newborns also show a preference for human faces and can even imitate facial expressions. Thus, from the beginning, the social niche for language is clearly established.

During the first few months of life, rapid changes take place. Mothers and their infants begin to interact in a finely tuned way with one another. They synchronize their patterns of eye gaze, movements, and facial expressions of affect in ways that resemble turn-taking patterns in conversations. By the age of 4 months, there is a marked increase in vocal turn-taking during these rich interactions between infants and their caretakers. Toward the end of the first year of life, vocalizations as well as other nonvocal behaviors again become genuinely integrated into social interaction as infants' developing social cognitive capacities lead to the onset of intentional communication. At this point, infants becomes capable of coordinating their attention to objects or events with other people through eye gaze patterns (joint attention), gestures, and vocalizations. This developmental achievement is generally viewed as a critical step in language acquisition, with the onset of communicative intent. Infants at this stage are able to communicate a variety of meanings, including protodeclaratives, which involve pointing or other gestures to draw another person's attention to an object of interest, and protoimperatives, meaning a gesture or vocalization to express a request or demand for an object. The significance of these communicative attempts is that they suggest the infant is capable of understanding the intentions of others (the beginning of a theory of mind), at least in a rudimentary or implicit form.

C. Speech Production

During the first year of life the infant's vocal abilities are also changing. Initially, because of anatomical limitations, newborns produce mostly cries or occasional gurgling. Infants begin producing sounds at approximately the age of 2 months, with the onset of cooing—vocalizations produced in the back of the mouth. By 4 months, most infants engage in vocal play, including a broad range of different kinds of sounds such as some rudimentary consonant–vowel (CV) syllables. By 6 months, infants produce canonical babbling, consisting of systematic CV syllables with adult-like timing. During this stage, infants are sensitive to the feedback they receive from their own babbling, and there are increases in the variety of consonants produced. By 10 months, infants babble in a conversational or modulated manner, with more complex strings of sounds that have varied intonation. These stages form the backdrop against which phonological development takes off during the second year of life.

One question that has been addressed in research on babbling is whether there is a connection between the sounds that an infant selects to produce and those in the target language in the infant's environment. A second question concerns the relationship between babbling and the onset of language. There is growing evidence suggesting that there is important continuity between prelinguistic babbling and the first words produced by infants. Not only do these stages overlap but also there is considerable overlap in sounds incorporated in babbles and early words. Furthermore, research on the development of vocal babbling in deaf infants suggests that the auditory feedback that infants receive from their own as well as others' sounds is crucial in shaping the course of development. Thus, recent studies have shown that deaf infants begin babbling later than hearing infants and in a more limited way. Even the sounds are somewhat different, presumably because deaf infants lack auditory feedback from their own sounds and have no access to the speech sounds in their environment. At the same time, deaf infants exposed to sign language during the first year of life begin manual babbling: They produce repetitive sequences of sign-language formatives that parallel the syllabic units of vocal babbling.

D. Mechanisms Underlying the Capacity for Language Acquisition

The development of the basic capacities that form the foundation of language acquisition in infancy is largely determined by the maturation of linguistic, motor (articulatory or manual), and social mechanisms that undergo developmental changes as a result of exposure to and feedback from particular language environments. Two distinct biologically based mechanisms are considered crucial for language acquisition: a domain-specific language system and a social mechanism that is dedicated to the development of understanding of other minds. Normal development of language depends on the integration of these distinct mechanisms, both of which depend on stimulation from the linguistic and social environment.

II. PHONOLOGICAL ACQUISITION

A. Stages of Development

As noted previously, it is generally agreed that there is essential continuity between prelinguistic babbling and the earliest stages of phonological development evidenced in the child's first words. The majority of sounds produced in the earliest words of children are the same as those preferred in their babbles. Initially, children's words are composed of simple CV syllable structures, using a relatively small inventory of sounds. Gradually, over time and with growth in the child's vocabulary, there is an expansion in the range of sounds produced by children. Although there is no universal order in the acquisition of phonological features, certain regularities have been found in the phonological sounds that are used across children. Mastery over vowels occurs before consonants. The main consonant classes that are used earlier in development include stops (e.g., b and d), nasals (e.g., m and n), and glides (e.g., w). Later developing consonants include fricatives (e.g., v) and liquids (e.g., l and r).

B. Systematic Error Patterns

As children begin producing more elaborated syllable structures and a wider range of sounds, they begin producing speech sound errors. The most striking feature of these errors is that although there are individual differences in the particular kinds of errors made, the errors are not random but instead fall into common patterns. In children with more severe articulation difficulties, words may be produced that involve combinations of different error patterns.

1. Omissions

Children will often omit syllables or specific sounds as they attempt to reproduce more complex adult words. Typically, unstressed syllables will be omitted—those occurring at the beginning of words (e.g., "mato" for "tomato") or in the unstressed medial position (e.g., "e'phant" for "elephant"). Consonant clusters will lead to omissions. For example, in English, one common error is to omit the /s/ in /s/ + stop consonant clusters (e.g., "top" for "stop"). Sometimes, final consonant sounds will be omitted (e.g., "go" for "gone").

2. Feature Changes

Another class of error patterns is the changing of sounds at the level of individual articulatory features. For example, voiced consonants may be changed to unvoiced consonants (e.g., bot for pot or gat for cat). Place changes also may be found in some children, with back consonants becoming more frontal (e.g., dame for game and bup for cup). These kinds of errors demonstrate the significance of features in children's phonological representations.

3. Assimilation Errors

A third class of errors illustrates how the child's representation of the target word may influence the kinds of sound substitutions that are made. Assimilation errors entail the change in one sound in the target word to make it more similar to another sound in that word. Such errors may involve assimilation in different feature classes, such as voicing (e.g., "doad" for "toad") or place ("gog" for "dog").

C. Theoretical Explanations

One of the main debates in the literature on phonological development has been between those advocating the view that very early phonological development is a discontinuous stage, which does not map onto the adult system, and those who argue that from the beginning young children's phonological systems share properties of the adult system. More evidence has accrued in favor of the latter view, called the continuity hypothesis, which suggests that the same underlying mechanisms are used in phonological acquisition as in the adult speaker.

One important piece of evidence for the continuity hypothesis is that infants are capable of perceiving speech in a mature, adult-like way before they even begin producing their first words. Furthermore, it is clear from the developmental and error patterns described here that children's attempts at producing target words are guided by abstract representations of speech sounds, including representations of syllable structures and distinctive articulatory features. At the earliest stages, the representations of syllable structures are very simple (e.g., simple CV structures referred to as minimal words), and these become more elaborate and complex over time. Similarly, children's earliest words may only include a small group of distinctive features that are considered marked (such as labials). Again, these expand over time, until by age 3 or so, the majority of children have mastered the phonology of their native language.

III. LEXICAL–SEMANTIC DEVELOPMENT

A. Stages of Development

Lexical development can be divided into three periods. The first period covers the acquisition of the initial 50 words or so, during which children are learning what words do. At this stage, some words appear to be tied to particular contexts and serve primarily social or pragmatic purposes. Word learning during this initial phase is relatively slow and uneven. A word may be equivalent to a child's holistic representation of an event. Especially in Western middle-class children, the child's vocabulary at this stage is dominated by names for objects, including animals, people, toys, and familiar household things. There will also be some social words (e.g., "hi" and bye), modifiers (e.g., "more" and "wet"), and relational terms that express success, failure, recurrence, direction and so forth.

By the middle of the second year, there is a significant increase in the rate at which children acquire new words. This new period is usually referred to as the vocabulary spurt, or naming explosion, and may be punctuated by many requests from children for adults to label things in the world around them. Words are learned very quickly, often after only a single exposure that may take place without any explicit instruction. This process of rapid word learning is referred to as "fast mapping." This phase of vocabulary growth is marked by a close relationship between lexical and grammatical development.

By the time children reach their third birthday, they begin to develop a more organized lexicon, in which the meaning relations among groups of words are discovered. For example, at this time children begin to learn words from a semantic domain, such as kinship, and they are able to organize the words according to their similarities and differences on dimensions of meanings. For nouns labeling concrete objects, children begin to organize taxonomies, also learning words at the superordinate and subordinate levels and understanding the hierarchical relations among terms such as dachshund, dog, and animal. Semantic developments at this stage will often lead to reorganizational processes as these kinds of relationships among words are realized by the child. The rate of word learning continues to be very rapid, with estimates suggesting that children acquired about 15–20 new words a day during the preschool years and beyond.

B. Developmental Processes

1. Conceptual Development

The fact that children can grasp the meaning of a word without explicit instruction, and in a variety of circumstances, suggests that there is a significant role played by preexisting or ongoing developing conceptual representations. During the early phases of word learning, studies demonstrate how specific conceptual developments at this stage are closely related to the acquisition of particular words. For example, infants develop the ability to retrieve hidden objects within a few weeks of acquiring words such as *"gone"* that encode the concept. In some children the words were acquired before the concept, in others the reverse was found. This suggests that at this early phase, while conceptual development can influence semantic development, it is also the case that semantic development can influence conceptual change. Thus, the relationship between language and conceptual development, or more generally between language and thought, is highly complex, with each system placing constraints on the other and both dependent on the social environment for their elaboration in development.

During the toddler years, objects tend to be named at the so-called basic object level (e.g., dog or car) rather than at the subordinate (e.g., dalmatian and Mercedes) or superordinate (e.g. animal and vehicle) levels. Objects within the same category at the basic object level tend to share perceptual and functional features, and they do not overlap with related semantic categories. Thus, this level may be the most useful for children for both functional and cognitive reasons. Parents also have been shown to name objects for children at the basic object level and this too might explain why this is the preferred level for children's early words.

Once a new word is learned it is quickly generalized to new contexts. Much of the focus of research on word meanings has been on the extension of a word. At this stage, children will sometimes overextend the meaning of a word, broadening the use of a term beyond its semantic boundaries. Typical examples include calling all women "Mommy" or using "ball" to name any round object. Overextension errors may be made on the basis of functional or, more frequently, perceptual similarity, or they may involve an associative complex of features. Another kind of extension error that is not so easily noticed occurs when the child *underextends* the use of word, not using a word to label an appropriate referent. Underextension errors tend to be noted at earlier stages of lexical development, whereas overextension errors are more typical of this period, after the naming explosion.

The most widely accepted view of what guides the acquisition of word meanings at this stage is the child's conceptual representations. The initial representation may be of a particular referent to which new examples are compared. Later, this semantic representation becomes more abstract and may be composed of a composite image or set of features for a prototype or best exemplar. This theory can explain both underextension and overextension errors; however, it is a theory of lexical development that is most usefully applied to the child's acquisition of names for concrete objects but not to other kinds of word classes.

2. Contextual Influences

Even during the earliest stages of word learning, children rarely make errors about the mapping between a word and its referent. Despite the fact that children may not have words for most concepts in the world, they almost always hone in on the correct meaning of a word learned in various social contexts. One important developmental process that makes this possible is that children understand other peoples' intentions and bring this knowledge of other minds to the task of word learning. Thus, they will carefully observe what a speaker is looking at or playing with when a new word is spoken. Children monitor the speaker's line of regard and assume that a novel word refers only to the object that is in the attentional focus of the speaker, indicating that they are sensitive to subtle cues to a speaker's referential intentions.

3. Constraints on Word Meaning

A number of researchers have argued that what makes word learning possible, especially when the child is capable of fast mapping, is a set of constraints that guides the child's hypotheses about the possible meanings of words. Eve Clark proposed a very general kind of constraint, called the *principle of contrast*, which states that every two words in a language contrast in meaning. This principle operates in conjunction with the *principle of conventionality*, which states that there are conventional words that children expect to be used to express particular meanings so that if a speaker does not use the conventional word, then the child assumes that the new word must have a somewhat different meaning. A different version of the principle of contrast is called the *mutual exclusivity constraint*. This constraint leads the child to assume that each object only has a single name, and that a name can only refer to one category of objects. When children hear a new word, they will look around for a referent for which they do not currently have a label. This explains why young children are reluctant to accept superordinate labels for individual objects. Other constraints that have been proposed include the *whole-object constraint*, which states that new words refer to whole objects rather than parts of objects (if, however, the child already knows the name of the object, then the word might be considered as labeling a part or property of the object), and the *taxonomic constraint*, which states that words refer to categories of objects.

Although some view these kinds of constraints as innate principles that are specific to lexical development, others view them as more general biases that may be an aspect of broader pragmatic or cognitive processes. Although there are still disagreements about how to characterize constraints on the child's hypotheses about the meanings of new words they encounter, most researchers agree that children use these heuristics to help them with the rapid mapping of words onto underlying meaning representations.

4. Syntactic Bootstrapping

Much of the research on semantic development has focused on the acquisition of nouns. Verbs, on the other hand, pose a different kind of problem because there is often not enough information in the context to help the child distinguish between related verbs such as "look" and "see." Children need to use syntactic information to help them figure out the meanings of verbs. The particular kinds of information that children can use include the number and kind of arguments that occur with the verb. Thus, transitive verbs take object arguments, whereas intransitive verbs do not. This kind of information is useful in helping the child interpret verb meaning. Syntactic bootstrapping is also useful for helping the child distinguish mass nouns (e.g., spaghetti) from count nouns (e.g., a potato) or common nouns from proper names, and very young children have been shown to be able to use this information when they hear new words in ambiguous contexts. As children's language progresses and they begin acquiring knowledge about the syntactic frames in which words occur, they begin to integrate syntactic and semantic information in this way. This process underscores the interrelationships that drive both semantic and syntactic development.

IV. THE ACQUISITION OF SYNTAX AND MORPHOLOGY

A. Stages of Development

Before the end of the second year, soon after the spurt in vocabulary development, children reach the next important milestone in language development: They begin to combine words together to form their first sentences. This is a crucial turning point because even the simplest two-word utterances show evidence of early grammatical development. The child's task in acquiring the grammar of her native language is complex. First, children need to segment the stream of language into morphemes (the minimal unit of language that carries meaning), phrases, and sentences. They must then discover the major word classes, such as noun, verb, and determiner, and map the appropriate lexical terms into these word classes. Children then learn how to grammatically encode tense, plurality, gender, and so forth, often using morphemes that are attached to verbs or nouns. At the same time, they acquire the major rules for organizing basic phrasal units such as noun phrase (e.g., article + adjective + noun—"*The tall man*") and verb phrase (e.g., verb + tense + prepositional phrase—"*walk-ed to the park*") as well as for organizing basic sentence structures for declaratives, questions, and negation. In the final stages, children figure out the syntactic rules for complex sentences involving coordinating and embedding multiple clauses.

B. Measuring Grammatical Development

1. Production

One of the obvious ways that children's sentences change over time is that they gradually grow longer. This fact is the basis for one of the most widely used measures of grammatical development, the mean length of utterance (MLU), which is the average length of a child's utterances as measured in morphemes. The assumption underlying this measure is that each newly acquired element of grammatical knowledge adds length to the child's utterances. Studies confirm that MLU increases gradually over time, and that it is a better predictor of the child's language level than chronological age. Nevertheless, it is only valid as a measure of development up to an average sentence length of four morphemes, and it may not be useful without significant modifications as a measure for languages other than English.

2. Comprehension

It is much more difficult to measure the child's comprehension of syntactic and morphological structures. Although in naturalistic contexts young children give the impression they understand significantly more that they say, this may reflect the child's use of nonlinguistic context and other cues rather than knowledge of abstract linguistic structure to compute the underlying semantic relations of sentences.

Methods to assess comprehension include a variety of paradigms, each of which has both advantages and disadvantages. The oldest method is the use of diary studies, which document the conditions and contexts in which a child understands or fails to understand a particular structure. Experimental procedures may include act-out tasks, in which an experimenter asks the child to enact a sentence or phase using a set of toys and props, or direction tasks, in which the child is asked to act out an event or command. Choice selection paradigms have also been developed, including picture-choice tasks, in which the child selects from a set of pictures the one that best represents the linguistic form presented by the experimenter, and preferential-looking tasks that have successfully been used with infants. In this kind of task infants listen to a linguistic message and have the choice of two videos to observe, only one of which matches the message. Infants who look reliably longer at the matching scene are credited with understanding the linguistic structure that was presented.

C. Early Word Combinations

When children begin to combine words to form the simplest sentences, most are limited in length to two words, although a few may be as long as three or four words. These early sentences are often unique and creative, composed primarily of nouns, verbs, and adjectives. In English, function words (such as articles or prepositions) and other grammatical morphemes, such as noun (e.g., plural –s) and verb inflections (e.g., past tense -ed or present progressive –ing), are usually omitted, making the child's productive speech sound "telegraphic"; however, this is less true for children learning other languages, such as Italian or Hebrew, that are rich in inflectional morphology.

1. Semantic Relations

Cross-linguistic studies of children at this stage have shown that there is a universal small set of meanings, or semantic relations, that are expressed, including agent + action, action + object, entity + location, entity + attribute, and demonstrative + entity. Children

talk a lot about objects by naming them and by discussing their locations or attributes, who owns them, and who is doing things to them. They also talk about people, their actions, their locations, their actions on objects and so forth. Objects, people, actions, and their interrelationships preoccupy young children universally.

2. Limited Scope Formulae

Initial studies of utterances produced in the two-word stage found that children used highly consistent word order. Indeed, the semantic relations approach assumed that the child uses a productive word order rule that operates on broad semantic rather than syntactic categories. This research was limited by focusing primarily on languages that make extensive use of order to mark basic relations in sentences and on a small number of children. It is now acknowledged that there is considerable individual variation among children learning different languages, and even for children learning English. Nevertheless, word order rules are used at this early stage of grammatical development, but they are more limited and more narrowly defined in semantic scope than is suggested by the semantic relations approach and therefore have been called *limited scope formulae*. For some children ordered combinations of words may even be based on specific lexical items rather than on semantic categories. Over time, these more limited rules expand to encompass broader semantic and later syntactic categories and begin to resemble the adult grammar.

3. Null Subjects

One characteristic of children's two-word sentences is that they often omit the subject. Recently, this has been interpreted from the perspective of current linguistic theory, which proposes a parameter-setting approach. Some theorists argue that all children begin with the subject parameter set in the null position (which holds for languages such as Italian or Spanish) so that children learning English must eventually switch the parameter setting to the position marked for required subjects.

Although this proposal is attractive because it connects early grammar to linguistic theory, there are several criticisms of this approach. Although English-speaking children do omit subjects, in fact they include them significantly more often than Italian-speaking children, which suggests that they know that subjects need to be expressed. Subjects are probably omitted because young children have limited processing capacity, and for pragmatic reasons subjects are more readily omitted than objects because they are often provided by the context.

D. Development of Grammatical Morphology

1. Invariant Order of Acquisition

As children progress beyond the two-word stage, they gradually begin to fill in the inflectional morphology and function words that are omitted in their early language. The process of acquiring the major grammatical morphemes in English is gradual and lengthy and some are still not fully controlled until the child enters school. Studies have found that the order in which English morphemes are acquired (e.g., articles, past tense, prepositions, or auxiliary verbs) is strikingly similar across children. The order of acquisition is not accounted for by frequency of use by the child or mother; instead, it is related to measures of both semantic and syntactic linguistic complexity.

2. Overgeneralization and Rule Productivity

One striking error that children make in the process of acquiring grammatical morphemes is the overregularization of regular forms to irregular examples. For example, the plural -s is frequently added to nouns that take an irregular plural, such as "*mans*" instead of "*men*" or "*mouses*" instead of "*mice*," and the regular past tense ending -ed is sometimes used on verbs that are marked with an irregular form, such as "*falled*," "*goed*," or "*teached*." These errors may not be frequent, but they can persist well into the school years and are quite resistant to feedback or correction. They are taken as evidence that the child is indeed acquiring a rule-governed system rather than learning these inflections on a word-by-word basis.

Other evidence for the productive use of morphological rules comes from an elicited production task introduced by Jean Berko Gleason called the Wug test. The child is shown drawings depicting novel creatures, objects, and actions and asked to supply the appropriate description that would require the inclusion of noun or verb inflections. For example, a creature was labeled a wug, and then the child had to fill in the blank for "*there are two ____.*" Preschool aged children performed well on this task, demonstrating their internalized knowledge of English morphological rules that can be applied productively.

Steven Pinker has argued that two different mechanisms are involved in acquiring regular and irregular forms. Regular forms involve a linguistic rule-governed mechanism, whereas irregular forms are retrieved directly from the lexicon and thus involve a memory storage system. This dual-mechanism hypothesis has been challenged by models developed within connectionist frameworks, in which only a single mechanism is needed to compute the correct form for regular and irregular examples, after being trained on mixed input. The debate between these camps continues.

3. Cross-Linguistic Evidence

There is a growing literature on the acquisition of morphology in other languages. Overgeneralization errors have been recorded in children learning many different languages suggesting this is a universal pattern for this aspect of grammatical development. However, the slow and gradual development of English morphology does not hold up for languages that have richer morphological systems. For example, children acquiring Turkish use suffixes on nouns that mark the noun as either the subject or object of the sentence, at even the earliest stages of language development, and children learning Italian acquire verb inflections marking person, tense, and number very rapidly and in a less piecemeal fashion than has been found for English morphology. These cross-linguistic variations seem to reflect differences among languages in the amount of inflectional morphology within a language and the degree to which inflections are optional. For example, English marks verbs only for the past tense, third person singular present tense (e.g., "*he walk-s*"), or progressive aspect (e.g., "*he is walk-ing*"), whereas Italian verbs are always marked in various ways. Children appear to be highly sensitive to these differences from the beginning stages of acquiring grammar.

E. The Acquisition of Sentence Modalities

1. Simple Declaratives

As children progress beyond the two-word stage, they begin combining words into three- and then four-word sentences. In doing so, they link together two or more basic semantic relations that were prevalent early on. For example, *agent + action* and *action + object* may be linked to form *agent + action + object*. These simple declarative sentences include all the basic elements of adult sentences. Gradually these may become enriched with the addition of prepositional phrases, more complex noun phrases that include a variety of modifiers, and more complex verb phrases including auxiliary and modal verbs. All these additions add length to the declarative sentences of young children.

2. Negation

Although children do express negation even at the one-word stage (e.g., using the word "*no!*"), the acquisition of sentential negation is not fully acquired until much later. There are three stages in the acquisition of negation in English: (i) The negative marker is placed outside the sentence, usually preceding it (e.g., "*not go movies*" and "*no Mommy do it*"); (ii) the negative marker is sentence internal, placed adjacent to the main verb but without productive use of the auxiliary system (e.g., "*I no like it*" and "*don't go*"); and (iii) different auxiliaries are used productively and the child's negations approximate the adult forms (e.g., "*you can't have it*" and "*I'm not happy*"). Although the existence of the first stage has been questioned by some researchers, there does appear to be cross-linguistic support for an initial period when negative markers are placed outside the main sentence.

Negation is used by children to express a variety of meanings. These emerge in the following order, according to studies of children learning a wide range of languages: "nonexistence," to note the absence of something or someone (e.g., "*no cookie,*"); "rejection," used to oppose something (e.g., "*no bath*"); and "denial," to refute the truth of a statement (e.g., "*that not mine*"). Some children show consistent patterns of form–meaning relations in their negative sentences. For example, one child used external negation to express rejection while at the same stage reserved sentence internal negation forms to express denial. These patterns may have had their source in the adult input.

3. Questions

There are several different forms used to ask questions, including rising intonation on a declarative sentence; yes–no questions, which involve subject–auxiliary verb inversion; *wh-* questions, which involve *wh-* movement and inversion; and tags, which are appended to declaratives and may be marked lexically (e.g., "*we'll go shopping, okay?*") or syntactically ("*we'll go shopping, won't we?*"). Children begin at the one- or two-word stage by using rising intonation and one or two fixed *wh-* forms, such as "*what that?*" Gradually, over the next couple of years syntactic forms of questions develop with inversion rules acquired simultaneously for both yes–no and *wh-* questions. Some data suggest that for *wh-* questions, inversion rules are learned sequentially for individual *wh-* words, such as "*what,*" "*where,*" and "*who,*" "*why,*" and may be closely linked in time to the appearance of those words used as *wh-* complements. Thus, syntactic rules for question formation may be *wh-* word specific in early child language.

Several studies of English and other languages have investigated the order in which children acquire various *wh-* questions and the findings have been consistent. Children generally begin asking and understanding "*what*" and "*where*" questions, followed by "*who,*" then "*how,*" and finally "*when*" and "*why*" questions. One explanation for this developmental sequence is that it reflects semantic and cognitive complexity of the concepts encoded in these different types of questions. Thus, questions about objects, locations, and people (i.e., *what, where,* and *who*) involve less abstract concepts than those of manner, time, and causality (i.e., *how, when,* and *why*). The early emerging *wh-* questions are also syntactically less complex in that they involve simple noun phrase replacement, whereas the later developing questions involve prepositional phrases or full sentence complements.

4. Passives

Despite the rarity of the passive construction in everyday conversations in English, a good deal of attention has been paid to how children use and understand passive sentences. Because the order of the agent and patient is reversed, this particular construction can reveal a great deal about how children acquire word order rules that play a major role in English syntax.

Elicited production tasks have been used to study how children construct passive sentences, typically using sets of pictures that shift the focus to the patient. Younger children tend to produce primarily truncated passives (e.g., "*the window was broken*") in which no agent is specified. These truncated passives generally have inanimate subjects, whereas full passives are produced by children when animate subjects are involved, suggesting that full and truncated passives may develop separately and be unrelated for the younger child. It has been suggested that truncated passives are really adjectival, whereas the later appearing full forms are complete verbal passives.

Numerous studies have used an act-out procedure to investigate children's comprehension of passive voice sentences. Typically, these studies compare children's comprehension of passive sentences to active sentences that are either reversible, in which either noun could plausibly be the agent (e.g., "*the boy kisses the girl*" or "*the boy is kissed by the girl*"), or semantically biased, in which one noun is more plausibly the agent than the other (e.g., "*the girl feeds the baby*" or "*the girl is fed by the baby*"). Studies find that children correctly interpret the plausible passive sentences before they do the reversible sentences. Preschoolers acquiring English tend to make errors systematically on the reversible passive sentences, suggesting the use of a processing strategy, called the word-order strategy whereby noun–verb–noun sequences are interpreted as agent–action–object. Children learning languages other than English may develop different processing strategies that closely reflect the canonical ways of organizing the basic relations in a sentence in their native language. For example, Japanese is a verb-final language that marks the agent with a suffix -*ga* rather than with a fixed word order, although there is a preference for an *agent–object–verb* order. Preschool-aged Japanese children tend to use a strategy that takes the first noun marked with -*ga* as the agent of the sentence. Thus, children's processing strategies are tailored to the kind of language they are acquiring and show that preschoolers have already worked out the primary ways that their language marks the basic grammatical relations.

Studies of the acquisition of other languages such as Sesotho, in which the passive construction is very frequent because subjects always mark sentence topic, have found that children acquire the passive much earlier and use it much more productively than do English-speaking children. Again, this suggests that children are sensitive to the typology of their language and that these factors influence the timing of development for the passive.

The semantic characteristics of the verb also influence the child's comprehension of passive sentences. Although 5-year-olds do correctly understand passive sentences that have action verbs, they find it more difficult to interpret passive sentences with nonaction verbs (e.g., "*Donald was liked by Goofy*"). Thus, the acquisition of passive voice continues into the school years as the child's knowledge becomes less constrained by semantic aspects of the verb.

F. Complex Sentence Structures

1. Coordinations

As early as 30 months of age, children begin combining sentences to express compound propositions. The simplest and most frequent method children use to combine sentences is to conjoin two propositions with "*and*". One question that has been investigated in numerous studies regards the order in which different forms of coordination develop. Both sentential (e.g., "*Mary went to school and Peter went to school*") and phrasal coordinations (e.g., "*Mary and Peter went to school*") tend to emerge at the same time in development, suggesting that these forms develop independently and are not, for young children, derived from one another. Children form phrasal coordinations by directly conjoining phrases, not via deletion rules.

Semantic factors influence the course of development of coordination. Children use coordinations first to express additive meaning, where there is no dependency relation between conjoined clauses (e.g., "*maybe you can carry this and I can carry that*"). Later, temporal relations (e.g., "*Joey is going home and take her sweater off*") and then causal relations (e.g., "*she put a Band-aid on her shoe and it maked it feel better*") are expressed, suggesting that children begin demonstrating greater semantic flexibility even while limiting themselves to the use of a single connective, "*and*."

2. Relative Clauses

Sometime after children begin using coordination, relative clauses emerge in their spontaneous speech. Initially, they are used to specify information exclusively about the object of a sentence (e.g., "*let's eat the cake what I baked*"), and often the relative pronoun is omitted or incorrect. The use of relative clauses in the spontaneous speech of young children is quite rare, perhaps because children avoid these syntactically complex constructions or because they lack the occasion to use them when the context is shared by the speaker and listener.

Elicited production techniques have been used successfully with preschoolers. These studies have also found that children find it easiest to add relative clauses to the ends of sentences rather than to embed them within the matrix clause. This suggests that some processing constraints operate on young children's productive capacities.

3. Anaphoric Reference

Children's knowledge of grammar continues to develop beyond the preschool years. One area that has received a good deal of attention from researchers is their knowledge of coreference relations within sentences, especially how anaphoric pronouns and reflexives link with referents. This research has been conducted primarily within a government-binding theoretical framework, investigating children's knowledge of the main binding principles. Spontaneous productions of pronominal forms suggest that quite young children use them correctly in their productive speech, however, the limits of their knowledge cannot be accurately assessed in naturalistic contexts.

Generally, children appear to develop knowledge of the main principles in the following order. By age 6 children know principle A, which states that reflexives are bound to referents within the same clause (e.g., "*John watched Bill wash himself*"; "*himself*" must refer to Bill, not John). Sometime later, knowledge of principle B emerges, which states that anaphoric pronouns cannot be bound to referents within the same clause (e.g, "*John asked Bill to hit him*"; "*him*" him must refer to John in the "*ask*" clause, not Bill in the "*hit*" clause). The last principle to emerge sometime during middle childhood is principle C, which states that backward coreference is only allowed if the pronoun is in a subordinate clause to the main referent (e.g., "*when he came home, John made dinner*"). Some researchers have argued that the grammatical knowledge of these principles is acquired much earlier that the research would suggest but that children's performance on tasks that tap this knowledge is limited by processing factors, pragmatic knowledge, or lexical knowledge. This debate continues in the developmental psycholinguistic literature.

G. Theoretical Explanations

1. Semantic Bootstrapping

Current theories in language acquisition attempt to address the central question of how the young child acquires the abstract and formal syntactic system of his or her language so rapidly, without formal instruction and with no feedback about whether he or she is using correct or incorrect forms. In the past two decades, one idea that has gained prominence in the literature is that children may use semantics or meaning to help break into the grammar of their language. Steven Pinker has been the main proponent to argue that children may use semantics as a bootstrap into syntax, particularly to acquire the major syntactic categories on which grammatical rules operate. Thus, children can use the correspondence that exists between names and things to map onto the syntactic category of noun, and they can use physical attributes or changes of state to map onto the category of verb. At the initial stages of development all sentence subjects tend to be semantic agents, and so children use this syntactic–semantic correspondence to begin figuring out the abstract relations for more complex sentences that require the category of subject.

2. Functionalism

A very different theoretical approach has been taken by those who view the central task of the child as gaining communicative competence. Much of the research conducted within this framework has focused on the acquisition of pragmatic aspects of language, including the functions of utterances and their use in discourse and other communicative contexts. Within research on grammatical development the functional approach does not take formal syntactic theory as its primary model. Instead, the structure of language is viewed from a functional or processing perspective. One example is the competition model of language acquisition proposed by Elizabeth Bates and Brian MacWhinney. In this model, the child begins by establishing the basic functional categories: topic–comment and agent. Different surface representations of these functional categories then compete for expression and initially the child may use a simple one form–one function mapping. Eventually, children move toward the adult system of form–function mappings.

3. Distributional Learning

At some point, all theories of acquisition need to consider how the child learns the major syntactic categories, even if they begin with a simple lexically specific, functional, or semantic approach. Thus, from the stream of words that children hear around them they must figure out which ones belong to the different major word classes, such as nouns, verbs, or adjectives. One important approach to this learning problem is the distributional learning view, according to which children not only use semantic mappings to acquire a category such as verb but also use distributional factors, such as it takes an *-ed* ending to express pastness or an *-ing* or *-s* ending in present tense contexts, it occurs with auxiliary verbs, and so forth. In this view, children come to know that a particular morpheme is a verb because they hear that morpheme cooccurring with inflections that mark tense, for example. This kind of approach argues that children are sensitive to all kinds of distributional patterns in the linguistic input to which they are exposed.

4. Parameter-Setting Theory

Linguists working within a government-binding framework who have taken an interest in the question of how children acquire the grammar of their language claim that the central task of acquisition is to set the parameters of universal grammar in the direction appropriate for the language that is being acquired. Some argue that the parameters are initially set in one position, which may then have to be switched. An alternative view holds that parameters start off neutrally—that is, they are not set in any position. As children are exposed to their native language, they use linguistic evidence present in the environment to set the parameters accordingly.

V. PRAGMATIC DEVELOPMENT

In recent years, there has been increased interest in investigating how children acquire the ability to use language to fulfill a range of functions and in a variety of communicative contexts. This emphasis reflects the notion that to become a competent speaker requires not only knowledge of the structural forms and meanings of a language but also the ability to communicate using those forms in a competent, flexible, and appropriate manner. Some researchers have argued that language forms develop to serve new communicative functions, not *vice versa*. This aspect of language development is closely tied to the child's developing theory of mind and related social knowledge.

A. Communicative Functions

1. Speech Act Theory

What are the communicative functions expressed in children's speech? This approach to the child's language is based on the theory of speech acts proposed by Austin and Searle, among others, and has been very influential in child language research. These philoso-

phers argue that many utterances do not simply make an assertion, but they also operate as *performatives*—that is, they perform an act (e.g., promise or refuse). Each utterance has three components: the *illocutionary intent*, or goal of the speaker; the *locutionary act*, or the actual form of the utterance; and the *perlocutionary effect*, the influence on the listener. In this way, we can account for the many different utterances that can be used, both direct and indirect, literal or metaphorical, to convey the same message. Thus, one of the questions that derives from this approach to language is how children come to use and interpret indirect and nonliteral uses of language.

2. The Development of Speech Acts

A number of researchers have focused on identifying and classifying the functions of early language, investigating the development of illocutionary intent and its relation to locutionary acts, and several systems have been developed. Children less than age 2 use language to fulfill a number of different functions, including getting people to do things, regulating their own or other's behavior, for social interaction, and as part of their imaginative play. By the time children are 3 years old, new functions emerge, including the use of language to describe objects or events and to assert an opinion, and also a range of conversational devices. At this point, children are also able to express each of these functions using a variety of different syntactic forms.

There is a more protracted period of development for indirect forms, such as indirect requests. Although 2-year-olds use terms such as *"want"* or *"need"* as a way of asking for something (e.g., *"I need new ball"*), genuine indirect requests do not emerge until approximately age 3 (e.g., *"Where is the truck?"*). By age 4, children can use polite forms, including modal verbs to make their request (c.g., *"Would you give me a cookie?"*), but hints or oblique indirect requests are not used until the early school years. Children aged 2 do not discriminate between requests for action and requests for information; however, throughout the preschool and early school years children gradually become able to understand increasingly more oblique levels of indirect speech acts.

B. Social Use of Language

A number of studies have focused on children's developing awareness of the perlocutionary effect of their utterances and the ability to modify locutionary acts to take into account their listeners' knowledge. Although 5-year-olds know when to use definite and indefinite articles ("*the*" and "*a*"/"*an*"), depending on the listener's presuppositional knowledge about an object, children younger than age 7 or 8 do not perform well on referential communication tasks, in which they are required to describe a scene or unusual object that is hidden from the listener's view. Using more naturalistic data, such as spontaneous speech, other studies have found that even 4-year-olds change the way they speak. For example, they use simpler language if they are talking to 2-year-olds, which shows some awareness of the distinct needs of a very young conversational partner.

C. Conversational Abilities

Communicative competence also entails knowing how to engage in conversations in appropriate and informative ways. A number of studies have focused on the development of conversational abilities, especially the ability to take turns and maintain the topic of conversation. From the earliest stages children are able to take turns in conversation, following their mothers' utterance with their own, usually, although not always, in a semantically related way. This ability to maintain topic increases during the preschool years and the child is now able to respond to his or her mother by expanding on the information in her utterances. This ability to add new information correlates highly with the child's developing linguistic skills, as measured by MLU, and leads to the ability to maintain a topic over longer chains of conversational turns.

The use of language in various contexts provides the interactive, communicative framework within which children acquire knowledge of the linguistic structures available in their native language so that they can express more fully the ideas that are generated by their developing cognitive and social systems.

See Also the Following Articles

ARTIFICIAL INTELLIGENCE • BILINGUALISM • CATEGORIZATION • CREATIVITY • EVOLUTION OF THE BRAIN • INFORMATION PROCESSING • INTELLIGENCE • LANGUAGE AND LEXICAL PROCESSING • LANGUAGE DISORDERS • LANGUAGE, NEURAL BASIS OF • READING DISORDERS, DEVELOPMENTAL • NEUROPSYCHOLOGICAL ASSESSMENT, PEDIATRIC • SEMANTIC MEMORY • SPEECH

Suggested Reading

Bloom, P. (2000). *How Children Learn the Meanings of Words*. MIT Press, Cambridge, MA.

Fletcher, P., and MacWhinney, B. (Eds.) (1995). *The Handbook of Child Language*. Blackwell, Oxford.

Jusczyk, P. (1997). *The Discovery of Spoken Language*. MIT Press, Cambridge, MA.

Locke, J. (1993). *The Child's Path to Spoken Language*. Harvard University Press, Cambridge, MA.

McDaniel, D., McKee, C., and Cairns, H. (Eds.) (1996). *Methods for Assessing Children's Syntax*. MIT Press, Cambridge, MA.

Pinker, S. (1994). *The Language Instinct: How the Mind Creates Language*. Morrow, New York.

Pinker, S. (1999). *Words and Rules: The Ingredients of Language*. Basic Books, New York.

Tomasello, M. (1998). *The New Psychology of Language: Cognitive and Functional Approaches*. Erlbaum, Mahwah, NJ.

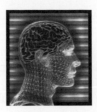

Language and Lexical Processing

RANDI C. MARTIN, MARY R. NEWSOME, and HOANG VU

Rice University

I. Lexical Processing

II. Sentence Processing

III. Higher Level Language Processing

IV. Conclusions

GLOSSARY

aphasia Disorder of language production and/or comprehension following brain damage.

Broca's area Area in the frontal lobe traditionally thought to contain the motor representations for words.

discourse processing Deriving meaning from conversation and text.

dissociation Preserved performance in one cognitive domain and impaired performance in another. A double dissociation occurs when one patient shows a disruption of one domain and preservation of the other, whereas another patient shows the reverse.

functional level First level of linguistic encoding in sentence production in which nonverbal conceptual information is used to select words and represent their relations.

immediacy of processing theory of comprehension Syntactic analysis and semantic interpretation are carried out on a word-by-word basis as each word is perceived.

lexicon The mental dictionary in which sound, spelling, meaning, and grammatical aspects of words are represented.

modularity hypothesis Hypothesis that different cognitive subsystems (i.e., modules) function independently.

orthography The written representations and rules for spelling of words.

parser A processing module that assigns syntactic structure to a sentence.

phoneme The basic unit of speech sounds.

phonological system The sound system of language.

positional-level Second level of linguistic encoding in sentence production in which the syntactic structure of the sentence is created and phonological representations are selected.

proposition Representation of part of a text that specifies the relations between actions and entities (people or objects) and between entities and their states or properties.

semantic system System that represents word and sentence meaning.

syntactic system System that represents grammatical information in the language.

thematic roles The roles that entities play with respect to a verb, such as agent, theme, or recipient.

Wernicke's area Area in the posterior temporal lobe traditionally thought to contain sound representations for words.

Within the realm of understanding and producing language, the brain is responsible for a wide range of tasks, from recognizing written words to understanding narrative. There is a fairly long history of behavioral studies of normal and brain-damaged populations that has delineated the organization of the component processes involved in various language tasks. Recently, lesion data have been supplemented by electrophysiological and neuroimaging data to reveal the regions of the brain that support language functions. A comprehensive view of language processing must take into account the theoretical developments from both behavioral and neuroimaging approaches.

The task of language comprehension is to transform written words or speech input into a conceptual representation, whereas that of language production is to translate a conceptual message into its spoken or written forms. Language processing can be examined at the word level, sentence level, or at higher discourse levels (e.g., text and narrative). Various models of language processing have been proposed to represent these levels of analysis. These models vary in scope and detail, but most assume that processing at a given level is carried out by a set of systems. For example, spoken sentence comprehension involves lexical, syntactic, and semantic systems. The lexical system includes the mental lexicon (or mental dictionary), which contains all the information about individual words. In the lexical subsystem, acoustic input is matched to a sound representation of a word (termed a lexical phonological representation). A match to a phonological representation then allows access to other aspects of a word's representation, including its meaning and its grammatical features (such as noun vs verb). A syntactic system uses the grammatical information from each word to construct a representation of the relationships among words within the sentence (i.e., syntactic relationships). The semantic system uses individual word meaning, syntactic information (e.g., which noun is the subject of the verb), and general world knowledge to construct an overall interpretation of sentence meaning.

Some researchers have hypothesized that the separate systems within a domain are modular—that is, they function independently. According to a strong version of the modularity hypothesis, once a module (i.e., system) receives input from another module (e.g., the syntactic system receives grammatical information about a word from the lexical system), the module carries out its computations (e.g., determines how the word fits into the syntactic structure) without further influence from any other modules (termed discrete processing). The output from the module is then passed on to the next module. According to a weaker version of the modularity hypothesis, each module may be represented independently in the brain; however, while a module is carrying out its computations, it may receive input from other modules that influences its processing (termed interactive processing). For example, compare the sentences "Mary saw the bird with binoculars" and "Mary saw the bird with red feathers." Both have the same syntactic structure but semantic information most likely causes listeners to assume that the prepositional phrase "with binoculars" modifies "saw" in the first sentence, whereas "with red feathers" modifies "the bird" in the second. The strong version of modularity would assume that this semantic information only comes into play after a syntactic decision has been made, perhaps leading to a reinterpretation of syntactic structure. The weaker

version of modularity would assume that semantic information influences the initial decisions that are made regarding syntactic structure (i.e., that the semantic and syntactic systems interact during early stages of processing). A completely nonmodular theory of language processing would assume that there is no distinction between syntactic and semantic representations—that is, both are represented in the same system, obey the same principles, and have been learned according to the same principles. As discussed later, the evidence from brain-damaged patients supports some form of modularity.

Many current models of language processing are instantiated in a network framework—that is, a network consisting of nodes that represent different types of units (e.g., letters, phonological representations, and concepts) and connections among these nodes. These network models are sometimes referred to as neural networks because the nodes and connections are argued to be analogous to neurons and their synaptic connections. The nodes of a certain type are all represented at the same level and the connections may be between levels or between units at the same level. For example, in written word recognition, there are layers of nodes representing visual features (e.g., straight line and curve), letters, and written word forms. In this type of model, processing is carried out via activation that spreads throughout the network. Stimulus presentation activates the first layer of nodes, and then activation spreads to subsequent layers. For example, if the word "bear" were presented, the visual features corresponding to each letter would be activated; activation would then spread along the connections between features and letters so that the appropriate letters would be activated. Activation of the letters would then lead to a spread of activation along connections between letters and words so that the appropriate word would be activated. In this type of model, partially consistent but incorrect letters and words would be activated, at least temporarily. For example, since "pear" shares features and letters with "bear," this word would be activated to some extent from presentation of "bear." In purely "feed-forward" network models, activation flows in only one direction (in this case, from visual features to words). In "feedback" models, activation flows in both directions. In a feedback version of this model, activation from letters would activate corresponding words; however, in addition, activation at the word level would flow back to the letter level, boosting the activation of letters consistent with activated words.

I. LEXICAL PROCESSING

A. Word Recognition

In visual word recognition, a whole word may be viewed at once (provided that it is short enough), and recognition is achieved when the characteristics of the stimulus match the orthography (i.e., spelling) of an entry in the mental lexicon. Speech perception, in contrast, is a process that unfolds over time as the listener perceives subsequent portions of the word. Upon hearing the first syllable of a spoken word such as the "un" in "understand," several words may be consistent with the input (e.g., "under," "until," and "untie"). As subsequent portions are perceived the pool (or "cohort") of words will be narrowed down, until only one word remains.

Despite these differences in the temporal course of processing, there are many commonalities in spoken and written word recognition. In both cases, the goal is to go from the perceptual information to the lexical form in order to access semantic and syntactic information about the word. In visual word recognition, a letter level intervenes between visual processing and lexical access. In auditory word perception, it is often assumed that a phoneme level intervenes between the acoustic input and lexical access. Phonemes are assumed to be the basic sound units of speech perception (and production). In English there are approximately 40 different phonemes, corresponding to the consonant and vowel sounds. The phonemes of other languages overlap those of English to a large degree, although some languages may lack some of the phonemes in English or may contain phonemes that do not exist in English. For example, Chinese does not distinguish between the "l" and "r" phonemes, and some African languages include clicking sounds as phonemes.

There is general agreement that spoken and written word recognition involve access to the same semantic and syntactic representations. There has been some disagreement, though, about whether there are separate lexical representations for spoken and written words. Some researchers have argued that written words have to be transformed into a sound representation in order to access semantic and syntactic information about the word. If so, then only a phonological representation (e.g., one that indicates the sequence of constituent phonemes and the stress pattern) is needed for each word. However, considerable neuropsychological evidence suggests that there are separate phonological and orthographic represen-

tations for words, and that access to word meaning can proceed for written words without conversion to a phonological form. Nonetheless, it is the case that for normal individuals the phonological representation of a written word appears to be computed automatically (through an implicit "sounding out" or "letter–sound" conversion process) when a written word is perceived. This derived phonological information can influence the time course of lexical access, making word recognition slower for words that have an unusual letter–sound correspondence, particularly if these words appear infrequently in print (e.g., "yacht"). Despite this slowing, the correct word is typically accessed, indicating that readers cannot be relying solely on letter–sound correspondences in accessing the meaning of written words.

B. Word Production

Spoken and written word production involve the reverse of the processing steps in word perception: conceptual processing to lexical to phonological or orthographic. Motor execution stages involved in articulation and writing would complete the output process.

More research has been devoted to speech production than to writing. In the domain of speech production, a distinction has been made between a nonverbal conceptual representation of the message to be expressed and a semantic representation that is specific to words. Speech production begins with the formulation of the nonverbal conceptual representation, followed by two steps of lexical access. In the first step, a lexical–semantic representation is selected (which also contains syntactic information about the word), and in the second step the phonological form corresponding to the semantic representation is accessed. In a strict modular approach with nonoverlapping stages, only one lexical–semantic representation is selected before processing proceeds to the phonological level. Other approaches assume what is termed "cascaded processing," in which activation spreads from the lexical–semantic level to the phonological level before a single lexical–semantic representation is chosen. Suppose that the speaker wishes to communicate the concept "cat." The conceptual representation for cat would serve to activate most highly the lexical–semantic representation for "cat" but would also activate related lexical–semantic representations to some extent, such as "dog" and "lion," because of shared conceptual features. In the cascaded model, the phonemes in "dog" and "lion" would also be activated to some extent, even though "cat" might eventually be the most activated at the lexical–semantic level. In a cascaded model with feedback, the activation of the phonemes in "cat" would cause backwards activation of words that shared phonemes with "cat," such as "mat," even though such words had no semantic relationship to "cat."

In writing, as in reading, some have argued that the orthographic forms are dependent on the phonological forms. That is, the writer is assumed to have followed similar steps in written word production as in spoken word production and has accessed a phonological form. This phonological form is then translated into a written form through a phoneme–grapheme conversion process. However, it is even clearer in writing than in reading that orthographic knowledge specific to individual words (i.e., a lexical orthographic representation) is needed for correct spelling. Even for a word with a regular correspondence between sounds and letters, there may be several alternative "regular" spellings (i.e., spellings that follow typical sound-to-letter conversion patterns in English). For example, "kat" or "cat" would be regular spellings for "cat," and "leaf," "leaph," "leef," and "leeph" would be regular spellings for "leaf." Thus, producing the correct spelling depends on having stored knowledge about the sequences of letters in words.

C. Neuropsychological Evidence on Lexical Processing

Evidence for independent modules in lexical processing can be obtained from individuals with brain damage due to a stroke or other injury who can competently produce or understand some types of linguistic information but not others. On the other hand, evidence that the same module is involved in performing two different tasks can be obtained by showing strong correlations between the factors affecting performance on each. In the domain of word recognition, double dissociations between written word and spoken word comprehension have been reported. That is, some patients who show a deficit in recognizing printed words can nonetheless recognize spoken words, whereas other patients show the reverse. For some of these patients, the deficit in spoken or written word perception cannot be attributed to difficulties with basic aspects of visual or auditory perception because the patient can recognize nonverbal materials in both modalities. Instead, the deficit is specifically in the phonological or orthographic processing systems. The existence of patients who can understand written words but who cannot understand spoken words because of disrupted phonological representations argues against the necessity of converting written words to phonological forms in order to access meaning. Evidence that the same lexical–semantic system is involved in comprehending spoken and written words comes from patients who show comprehension difficulties for certain words or certain semantic categories (such as animals or tools), and the same words are affected irrespective of whether the input is spoken or written. If there were separate semantic representations for spoken and written words, it would be highly unlikely that the same categories of words would be affected for both modalities.

Category-specific deficits have been noted for many patients and raise interesting questions concerning the nature of semantic representations in the brain. Although more specific deficits have been observed, these deficits tend to occur in the categories of animals, plants, and artifacts (i.e., man-made objects), with the most common deficit for animals or, more generally, for living things. One possible explanation of category-specific deficits is motivated by the fact that semantic properties of an object tend to be interrelated (e.g., having eyes usually occurs with having a nose) and that objects in the same superordinate category (e.g., tools or fish) share properties. If constellations of shared properties are organized together in the brain, then when damage occurs to a region in which semantic properties are stored, deficits that affect certain categories will result. The only difficulty with this account is that it does not explain why deficits tend to occur in three categories—that is, any constellation of shared properties should be subject to damage and we should observe patients with highly specific deficits such as a deficit for vehicles but not other artifacts.

Another possible explanation for category-specific deficits is that there are two separate semantic systems in the brain—one that represents sensory knowledge and another that represents functional knowledge (i.e., the functions that objects perform). Researchers have argued that knowledge of animals is mainly sensory, whereas knowledge of artifacts is mainly functional. Consequently, damage to the sensory knowledge system results in a deficit specific to animals, whereas damage to the functional system results in a deficit specific to artifacts. However, findings from some brain-damaged patients are problematic for this sensory/functional explanation. For example, some patients have been reported who have semantic deficits for only some subsets of living things (e.g., fruits and vegetables), and others have been reported who have a disruption of knowledge of both sensory and functional attributes of animals but a preservation of both sensory and functional knowledge for artifacts.

As discussed earlier, models of word production take either a discrete stage or interactive activation approach. Some data from speech errors in normal subjects (either spontaneous or experimentally elicited) support the interactive view. For example, sound exchange errors are more likely to occur if the exchange results in two words (saying "barn door" for "darn bore") than if the exchange results in nonsense words (saying "beal dack" for "deal back"). This effect of lexical status of the resulting error can be attributed to feedback from the phoneme level to the lexical level. The word production errors of aphasic patients can also be better accounted for by an interactive approach. Such an approach provides a means of accounting for some patients' tendency to produce words phonologically related to a target word (so-called "formal errors," such as saying "mat" for "cat") and for some patients' tendency to produce a large proportion of errors that are both semantically and phonologically related to a target (saying "rat" for "cat").

Double dissociations between deficits in written and spoken word production have been observed. Again, in many of these cases, basic deficits in the motor processes involved in speaking or writing can be ruled out, indicating that the modality-specific deficit is specific to phonological or orthographic output processing. Further evidence for the separation of phonology and orthography comes from patients who make semantic errors in only one output modality—for example, producing "pillow" as the name for a picture of a bed when speaking but producing "bed" correctly in writing. Such a pattern would not be expected if it were necessary to use the phonological form to guide spelling.

Evidence from speech production deficits provides information about the representation of grammatical information. Deficits specific to certain grammatical categories have been reported because some patients have selective difficulties in the production of function words (i.e., words such as prepositions, pronouns, and auxiliary verbs that play primarily a grammatical role in a sentence). Such difficulties are remarkable given that these grammatical words are often quite short and easy to pronounce (e.g., "to" and "will") and are the most frequently occurring words in the language. Some patients have demonstrated greater difficulty in producing nouns than verbs, and others have demonstrated the reverse. As with the semantic category deficits, there is no consensus on the explanation for these grammatical class deficits. In some cases, these apparent grammatical class effects have a semantic basis. For example, better production of nouns than verbs and better production of verbs than grammatical words may be observed because the patient is better able to produce more concrete words. However, for some patients, it appears that grammatical class effects cannot be reduced to a semantic basis; consequently, these deficits suggest that at some level in the production system words are distinguished neurally with regard to the grammatical role that they play in a sentence. The separability of grammatical information from other types of lexical information is supported by other findings showing that some patients with picture-naming deficits can provide grammatical information about a word, such as its gender (in a language such as Italian or French), even though they are unable to retrieve any of the phonemes in the word.

Neuropsychological research with brain-damaged patients, more so than research with normal subjects, has addressed the issue of the relation between the phonological processing systems involved in speech perception and production and the relation between the orthographic systems involved in reading and writing. Some patients show an excellent ability to recognize and remember input phonological forms (e.g., being able to decide whether a spoken probe word rhymes with any of the words in a preceding list but have great difficulty in producing output phonological forms (e.g., naming a picture). Other patients show the reverse pattern of great difficulty in holding onto input phonological forms (performing at chance on the rhyme probe task) but showing normal speech production. Similar double dissociations have been documented for orthographic processing. Thus, input and output forms in both speech and writing appear to be represented in different brain areas. However, although the input and output forms may be different, they are linked to each other. For example, individuals can repeat nonwords, converting an input to an output form. A close coupling between input and output forms appears to be involved in the development of speech production and in the maintenance of accurate speech production throughout adulthood.

D. Localization of Word Comprehension and Production

As we have seen, patient studies can be used to posit the nature of the functional components of language comprehension and production and their connections. Studies of localization reveal where in the brain those components may lie. Models of brain areas and their functions can be traced back to the late 1800s, beginning with Lichtheim and Wernicke. Wernicke's model assumed that language was represented in the left hemisphere. Findings since that time have indicated that although the left hemisphere is dominant for language in most individuals, the right hemisphere also plays some role. In addition, the right hemisphere is dominant in some individuals. The model incorporated a concept center that received input from sensory word images and provided output to motor word images. The sensory word images were thought to be represented in Wernicke's area, found in the superior (upper), posterior (near the back), left temporal lobe, and the motor images in Broca's area, found in the left frontal lobe near the motor cortex. Damage to Wernicke's area was thought to result in an inability to recognize and understand spoken words, although speech was thought to be fluent. Broca's aphasics were thought to have an impairment in articulating speech (i.e., "essentially mute, except for the repetition of the same few utterances"), but their comprehension was intact. Wernicke's and Broca's areas, though separate, were thought to be connected through a neural fiber tract (i.e., the arcuate fasciculus). This fiber tract was thought to be involved in translating an auditory word representation into a motor word representation. Based on Wernicke's model, one would predict that patients who had intact Broca's and Wernicke's areas but damage to this fiber tract should have good language comprehension and production but have difficulty repeating words and sentences. Patients were reported who showed this pattern (termed conduction aphasics), which seemed to provide a strong confirmation of the model.

There are a number of observations that cause difficulties for the classical model. For example, Broca's aphasics are not equally impaired on all types of words, typically being better able to produce nouns than verbs. Although they have difficulty producing function words, function words occurring in the middle of sentences are omitted less frequently than those that occur in the beginning of sentences. An additional complication for the Wernicke/Lichtheim models is that although Wernicke's aphasics' speech is

fluent it shows numerous aberrations, such as misordered phonemes, incorrect words, and nonsense words such as "tarripoi" in the statement spoken by one Wernicke's aphasic, "I can't mention the tarripoi." Moreover, current studies suggest that among individuals classified into any traditional syndrome category (Broca's, Wernicke's, and conduction aphasia), there are wide variations in the nature of their deficits. For example, within conduction aphasics, some patients produce fluent and appropriate speech output but make semantic substitutions or paraphrases in repeating sentences, suggesting that they have difficulty retaining phonological information on the input side. Other conduction aphasics make numerous phonemic errors in their speech output but do not make semantic substitutions in repeating, suggesting that they have difficulty constructing and maintaining phonological representations on the output side. Thus, localization of function on the basis of classical syndromes appears to be a misguided effort. However, careful examination of a series of individual cases who show similar behavioral deficits allows for the determination of the lesion site that is affected in all such individuals. On the basis of these data, one can look to behavior–lesion correspondences to draw conclusions about localization.

Recently, using methods that measure the physiological changes that occur in the brain, it has been possible to determine the brain areas activated in normal individuals while they are performing language tasks. Electrical activity occurring in the brain during various tasks [i.e., event-related potentials (ERPs)], can be measured. These ERPs show negative and positive electrical potentials that are time locked to the onset of the presentation of verbal stimuli. The brain distribution of these potentials can be plotted. The flow of blood into different regions of the brain can be detected through via positron emission tomography (PET) and functional magnetic resonance imaging (fMRI). The use of PET and fMRI for functional localization thus assumes that greater blood flow is observed in brain areas with greater neural activity. Although all these methodologies provide information about when and where activation occurs in the brain, ERPs are known for their good temporal resolution, whereas the strength of fMRI lies in its spatial resolution. The spatial resolution of PET is also substantially better than that from ERPs but worse than that of fMRI.

The traditional model of language processing predicts that processing of phonological information of heard words should occur in the posterior left temporal lobe (Wernicke's area) and phonological activation for spoken words should occur in left frontal lobe (Broca's area). Although the brain areas implicated in the traditional model have been confirmed by imaging studies, additional areas have been found to be active. That is, although neuroimaging studies show consistent evidence of Wernicke's area activation during phonological encoding, temporoparietal and frontal activation have been found as well. Similarly, studies have found activation both in Broca's area and in the lower portion of the posterior temporal lobe (Wernicke's area is the upper portion of the posterior temporal lobe) during language production. One caveat regarding the role of Broca's area is that it has been activated when research participants are asked to make hand and tongue movements, suggesting that activation of this area reflects general motor programming rather than motor programming specific to phonological output.

If visually presented words are converted into their phonological representations, then activation should occur in areas similar to those implicated for auditory word processing. Studies have found activation during reading of visually presented words in left temporoparietal cortex, which is also active during auditory word processing. The left posterior middle temporal gyrus, in addition to the occipital–temporal and left inferior temporal/fusiform regions, has also been shown to be active during word reading.

A variety of areas have also been implicated for semantic processing. Two tasks meant to measure semantic processing, categorizing words and generating actions that can be performed with objects, have shown activation in left frontal regions of Broca's and surrounding areas. Other research has suggested that the frontal cortex is involved in retrieving and maintaining semantic information rather than being the locus of representation of semantic knowledge. Recent studies with normal and brain-damaged research participants have suggested the role of temporal areas in semantic processing, including left posterior temporoparietal, inferior temporal, and anterior temporal cortex. Researchers investigating the localization of categorical knowledge with neuroanatomical and neuroimaging studies found a wide variety of brain areas to be involved during tasks that test knowledge of different categories. Even within a category, various brain areas have been activated. For example, the left temporal lobe, the right temporal lobe, and even the frontal and inferior parietal areas have all been reported to be active during processing of animals and living things. Areas responsible for

processing nonliving things also appear to be diverse. Despite the varied areas that have been reported to be involved in semantic function, one area that has shown activation across several different studies is the temporal lobe. Work with Alzheimer's patients who have semantic impairment suggests a further category distinction. Alzheimer's patients whose knowledge of the perceptual features of objects is disrupted tend to have temporal region damage, and those whose knowledge of how objects function tend to have frontoparietal impairment.

More consistent findings have been obtained regarding different localization for words of different grammatical classes. Neuropsychological and neuroimaging results suggest that nouns are represented in the temporal lobe and verbs in the frontal lobe. Some ERP studies have indicated that content words and function words elicit different timing of brain potentials and the involvement of different brain areas. For instance, one study showed early frontal activation from both word types with a similar pattern brain distribution at approximately 200–300 msec after the onset of the word. Approximately 150 msec later, however, differences for the word types were observed, with a different timing of the potential waveforms for the two word types and greater left hemisphere activation for the function words than for the content words. However, because this study measured processing of these word types in a sentence context, the different patterns may be due to the different roles that these words play in sentence processing rather than to different localization of lexical representations. For example, function words may lead to more predictions about the syntactic structure of upcoming words in a sentence.

Recent behavioral and neuroimaging data suggest that the right hemisphere may play more of a role in language processing than was previously assumed. Behavioral studies on this issue have used a priming paradigm in which word recognition (as measured by time to pronounce a word or to make a word–nonword decision) is facilitated by the prior presentation of a related word. To study hemispheric contributions, written words are presented to the left or right visual field, which engages processing in the contralateral cerebral hemisphere first. Priming studies have shown that priming occurs for only the most highly related words in the left hemisphere but for a broader range of related words in the right hemisphere. Also, for ambiguous words such as "bank" that have a dominant meaning (money) and a subordinate meaning (river), priming results indicate that immediately following presentation of an ambiguous word both meanings are activated in both hemispheres. However, within a short time, only the dominant meaning is available in the left hemisphere, whereas both meanings are still available in the right hemisphere. Taken together, the evidence suggests that the meanings of words are more coarsely coded in the right hemisphere. Neuroimaging studies of word processing have also often found activation in the right hemisphere in areas corresponding to the traditional language areas on the left, although the activation is often less than that obtained in the left hemisphere.

II. SENTENCE PROCESSING

A. Sentence Comprehension

Sentence comprehension processes involve more than combining the meaning of individual words in a sensible fashion. Even though the sentence "the girl chased the dog" has the same content words as "the dog chased the girl" and "the girl was chased by the dog," it is clear that the first sentence means something different than the latter two. Clearly, the grammatical roles that nouns play (e.g., subject vs object) and sentence structure (e.g., active vs passive) play a role in determining sentence meaning. Most models of sentence comprehension assume that in order to understand a sentence, the constituents (e.g., noun phrase, verb phrase, and prepositional phrase) of a sentence must be identified and related to each other structurally. The "parser" is the term used to describe the module that assigns syntactic structure to a sentence. Parsing allows the determination of the grammatical roles, such as subject, direct object, and indirect object. These grammatical roles are assumed to be mapped onto "thematic roles"—that is, conceptual roles that entities play with respect to a verb such as the agent (i.e., the entity carrying out the action), theme (i.e., the entity being acted upon), recipient, or location. The mapping between grammatical roles and thematic roles varies for different verbs and may vary for the same verb depending on the sentence. For example, the thematic roles of the subjects of the phrases "the boy received," "the girl opened," and "the key opened" are "recipient," "agent," and "instrument," respectively. Because of this variation in mapping, the lexicon needs to contain verb-specific information concerning the possible mappings between grammatical and thematic roles.

It is often the case that the syntactic structure to be assigned to a sequence of words is ambiguous. For example, for a sentence beginning with "The defendant examined," "examined" could be the main verb or could be part of a reduced relative clause construction (e.g., "The defendant examined by the lawyer was innocent"). A major issue in research on sentence processing has been whether a strict modular approach applies in which the parser assigns syntactic structure purely on the basis of syntactic rules of thumb (e.g., "choose the simplest structure") or whether an interaction between semantic and syntactic information affects parsing decisions. For example, if semantic information influences parsing, then "examined" should be less likely to be taken as the main verb in a sentence beginning "The evidence examined" since "evidence" is unlikely an agent of "examine." Current evidence supports the interactive view.

During comprehension, it is necessary to integrate different constituents of a sentence, sometimes over distances spanning several words. For example, in the sentence "The truck that the car splashed was green," it is necessary to retrieve "truck" as the direct object of "splashed" and to integrate "green" with "truck" rather than "car." Consequently, researchers have assumed that comprehension makes demands on working memory resources. The concept of working memory is similar to that of short-term memory, involving the temporary maintenance of information. The term "working" is used to signify that this capacity is used in carrying out computations in addition to maintaining information. Individual differences in working memory capacity of normal individuals have been found to correlate with aspects of sentence comprehension performance. However, neuropsychological findings suggest that there are different components of working memory that play different roles in sentence comprehension.

B. Sentence Production

In sentence production, as in comprehension, the mapping between thematic and grammatical roles and the construction of syntactic structure must be included in the processing stages. The processing stages in sentence production include the message level stage, in which a conceptual representation of the sentence is formed, two stages of linguistic encoding, and an articulatory stage. Thematic role relations between actions and entities are assumed to be represented at the message level. At the first level of linguistic encoding (termed the functional level), the message level information is used to select lexical representations (i.e., semantic–syntactic lexical representations) and to construct grammatical relations among these lexical representations based on the thematic role and other semantic information in the message. The prosodic structure of the sentence is also encoded during this stage. Prosodic factors such as word stress (the emphasis given to words) and intonation (using pitch to signify different meanings) are important methods of varying speech to facilitate communication. The second level of linguistic encoding (called the positional level) creates the syntactic structure for the sentence in terms of word order, function words, and grammatical markers (e.g., plural markers and past tense inflections). The phonological forms for the content words are also retrieved at this stage. Once the phonological representations have been retrieved, plans for articulation can be formed.

C. Neuropsychological Evidence on Sentence Processing

1. Sentence Comprehension

In the 1970s and 1980s, researchers demonstrated that some aphasic patients who understood the content words in a sentence might nonetheless show a failure of comprehension for the sentence as a whole if comprehension depended on the correct analysis of syntactic information. For example, these patients might have difficulty understanding "reversible" sentences—that is, sentences in which either noun could play the thematic roles of agent or theme, as in "The dog was chased by the girl" or "The truck that the car splashed was green." This comprehension difficulty could be demonstrated by asking the patient to choose between a picture depicting the correct thematic role relations and one depicting the reverse role relations (e.g., a girl chasing a dog vs a dog chasing a girl). Although the patients might perform at chance with such picture contrasts, they would do well if one of the pictures substituted an incorrect noun or verb (e.g., a girl chasing a cat or a girl walking a dog). One early hypothesis about the nature of such a comprehension deficit was that it derived from a general failure of syntactic processing because patients who showed this comprehension problem also produced "agrammatic speech." That is, their speech production was marked by simplified syntactic structure and the omission of function words and grammatical markers. However, recent findings have demonstrated that some patients may show only one side of this deficit (i.e., impaired

syntactic comprehension but not agrammatic speech, or the reverse). In addition, several studies have shown that patients who show this comprehension problem on sentence–picture matching may do well on judging the grammatical acceptability of sentences. Thus, rather than a global deficit in all aspects of syntactic processing, these patients may have a more restrictive comprehension deficit, such as a deficit in mapping between the grammatical structure of the sentence and the thematic roles that entities play in the sentence. For instance, for the sentence "The truck that the car splashed was green," the patient might be able to determine that "car" is the grammatical subject of the verb "splashed" but be unable to determine that the car is doing the splashing.

Other findings indicate that although agrammatic speakers may not provide the clearest evidence of a dissociation between syntactic and semantic knowledge, other patients do provide such evidence. Some patients with Alzheimer's dementia demonstrate very impaired knowledge of word meanings but show preserved grammatical knowledge. For example, they might be unable to realize that a phrase such as "The jeeps walked" is nonsensical but be able to detect the grammatical error in a phrase such as "The jeeps goes." Other case studies of aphasic patients show the reverse pattern of preserved semantic knowledge but disrupted grammatical knowledge. Thus, the findings indicate some degree of modularity in the sentence comprehension system, with separate modules for semantic and syntactic processing. However, other evidence from patients comports with the findings from normal subjects in showing that these modules do not typically operate in isolation but instead interact. That is, patients may use the grammatical structure of sentences when there are weak semantic constraints (e.g., understanding that "tiger" is the agent of "chased" in "The lion that the tiger chased") but fail to use the grammatical structure when there are strong semantic constraints (e.g., mistakenly interpreting the "woman" as the agent of "spanked" in "The woman that the child spanked"). These findings support the view that information from both semantic and syntactic sources typically combines during comprehension, but when one of these systems is weakened due to brain damage, the other system may override its influence.

As discussed previously, theories of comprehension often assume a role for a short-term or working memory system that is used to hold partial results of comprehension processes while the rest of a sentence is processed and integrated with earlier parts. Aphasic patients often have very restricted short-term memory spans, being able to recall only one or two words from a list compared to normal subjects' ability to recall five or six words. Many of these patients appear to have a deficit specifically in the ability to retain phonological information. Although it may seem intuitively plausible that restricted short-term memory capacity would impede comprehension, a number of studies have shown that patients with very restricted memory spans may show excellent sentence comprehension even for sentences with complex syntactic structures. Such findings support immediacy of processing theories of comprehension that state that syntactic analysis and semantic interpretation are carried out on a word-by-word basis, to the extent possible. Recently, some patients have been identified whose short-term deficit appears to be due to a difficulty in retaining semantic information rather than phonological. For such patients, their restricted ability to retain semantic information does impede comprehension for certain sentence types—that is, those that put a strain on the capacity to retain individual word meanings. Specifically, these patients have difficulty comprehending sentences in which the structure of the sentences delays the integration of word meanings into larger semantic units. One sentence type causing difficulty includes sentences with several prenominal adjectives, such as "The drab old red swimsuit was taken to the beach." In this example, the meaning of "drab" cannot be integrated with the noun it modifies until two intervening words have been processed. These patients do not have difficulty comprehending similar sentences in which word meanings can be integrated immediately. For example, these patients can understand sentences in which several adjectives follow the noun (e.g., "The swimsuit was old, red, and drab, but she took it along anyway"), because these sentences allow for the immediate integration of each adjective with the preceding noun.

2. Sentence Production

Sentence production deficits have also been a focus of research in aphasia, although in this domain much of the work has originated from a syndrome-based approach, concentrating on patients showing agrammatic speech. Agrammatism occurs predominantly in patients with articulatory disturbances who are typically classed as Broca's aphasics. However, several studies have documented that some features of agrammatism may appear in patients who are fluent speakers. Moreover, other studies have shown that the sentence structure and function word difficulties of agrammatic patients may dissociate, with some patients demonstrating reduced sentence complexity but accurate production of function words and inflections and others showing the reverse. In order to accommodate the dissociation between sentence structure and function word difficulties, deficits at different levels in the production process have been postulated. Several different suggestions have been made as to what these different deficits might be. An interesting recent approach relates deficits in sentence structure to deficits in the knowledge of verb representation. The verb plays a major role in structuring the roles of nouns (such as agents, patients, and recipients) with respect to the action in the sentence. The specific verb to be used dictates what grammatical role a noun with a specific thematic role will play (e.g., the recipient will be the subject of an active sentence using the verb "receive" but the indirect object of an active sentence using "give"). A deficit in knowledge of the relations of semantic and grammatical roles entailed by verbs could lead to a reduction in sentence structure, such as the failure to produce a required indirect object.

The disruption in the production of function words and inflections might be a result of a disruption at a different stage, specifically the stage at which the syntactic structure of the utterance is specified in terms of word order and grammatical markers (i.e., the positional level). Of course, many patients might have a disruption both in representing the relations of the verbs to the nouns and in constructing a syntactic specification, resulting in prototypical agrammatic speech.

D. Localization of Sentence Processing Mechanisms

Because of the association of Broca's aphasia with agrammatism and difficulties comprehending reversible sentences, some researchers have tried to link the frontal lobe, specifically Broca's area, to syntactic parsing. However, as discussed earlier, patients who are not Broca's aphasics have been shown to have difficulties understanding reversible sentences and to make grammatical errors in language production. With regard to comprehension, a study of lesion overlap among a group of aphasic patients with syntactic comprehension difficulties revealed that the critical area appeared to be in the anterior temporal lobe rather than Broca's area. ERP studies have revealed different patterns of brain potentials in response to semantic and syntactic errors in a sentence, supporting the independence of these processes. The semantic anomalies elicit negative-going waves approximately 400 msec after the onset of the anomalous word, whereas the syntactic anomalies elicit positive-going waves approximately 600 msec after the onset of the ungrammatical word. Both the negative semantic wave and the positive syntactic wave have central or posterior brain distributions, with a somewhat more posterior distribution for the positive syntactic wave.

There have so far been relatively few neuroimaging studies of sentence comprehension. All of the traditional left hemisphere language areas (i.e., areas surrounding the Sylvian fissure, including Broca's area and Wernicke's area) are activated; however, activation in the anterior temporal lobe is also observed in some studies. Given the many processing components involved in sentence comprehension (e.g., syntactic parsing, thematic role determination, semantic integration, and maintenance in working memory), it is unclear exactly what function is carried out in which part of this broad network of activation. Some studies have suggested a specific role for Broca's area in the comprehension of syntactically complex sentences; however, not all types of complex sentences induce activation in this area. It is possible that, instead, this area carries out a working memory function related to maintaining words that have not yet been assigned a thematic role. Only certain types of syntactically complex sentences would place a demand on such a working memory function.

With regard to sentence production, there have been few studies using lesion localization that have attempted to isolate different aspects of production. One well-established finding is that there are frontal areas involved in speech articulation. However, for more central linguistic encoding aspects of language production, the data are scarce. Some patients with frontal lesions who show difficulty comprehending sentences in which integration of meanings is delayed (i.e., sentences with several adjectives preceding a noun) also have difficulty producing similar sentence constructions. These findings suggest that the same frontal working memory area is involved in maintaining semantic representations in comprehension and production. Clearly, neuroimaging data would be useful in helping to localize aspects of language production. However, there are methodological difficulties in obtaining such data. If subjects move during PET and fMRI studies, this movement can induce the appearance of activation in brain areas that are in fact not activated. Thus, having subjects overtly produce speech could introduce movement artifacts in such

studies. Having subjects speak silently to themselves would prevent the experimenter from monitoring what the subject was saying. Future research may find means to obviate these difficulties.

III. HIGHER LEVEL LANGUAGE PROCESSING

A. Discourse Comprehension

The comprehension of continuous discourse involves more than word recognition, syntactic parsing, and deriving the meaning of individual sentences. Successful comprehension requires an understanding of the relationships among the various parts of the discourse context and is dependent on the reader's or listener's general world knowledge. Many researchers have argued that story comprehension implies the derivation of propositional representations. Propositions derived from a story specify relations between actions and participants in the actions, the states and attributes of the participants, the time and locations of the actions, etc. Propositions are specified in terms of entities (typically nouns) and predicates (such as actions or states) that apply to these entities. For example, consider a story titled "The Picnic," beginning with the following: "The sky was cloudy and the weather forecast was not encouraging. There was a 70% probability of showers. However, the Brown family had no intention of renouncing their plan." Propositions derived from these sentences might include time (past), sky (cloudy), forecast [not (encouraging)], and renounce (agent, family; object; plan). It is clear, however, that comprehension of the story depends not only on deriving propositions but also on relating propositions to each other and to world knowledge. Even for the first sentence in this example, not only are "sky" and "cloudy" linked, such that "cloudy" specifies the state of the sky, but also it is likely that this information would to be related to the title and to long-term knowledge that people prefer sunny skies for picnics. Moreover, this information is reinforced by propositions derived from the following sentences. Overlap among the propositions and their associations in long-term memory makes the text more easily comprehended and remembered.

Propositions can be related to each other by various means. A person or object mentioned earlier can be referred to again using an anaphor, such as a pronoun. For example, "she" is an anaphor for "The little girl" in the passage "The little girl wanted to play ball. She got the bat out of the car." Propositions can also be related via inferences. An inference is the drawing of a conclusion that is not explicitly mentioned in a discourse but, rather, is based on general world knowledge. In the picnic example discussed previously, someone hearing this story is likely to infer that it was the Browns who were planning the picnic mentioned in the title and that, contrary to usual expectations, they were not going to cancel because of the weather. In some cases, discourse or narrative texts (such as a mystery novel or an adventure story) may follow a familiar structure (termed a schema or script), and the presence of this structure may help the comprehender to organize the information.

B. Discourse Production

Narrative production requires that the speaker (or writer) produce a sequence of sentences that is coherent and comprehensible to the conversational partner (or the reader). The speaker has to be able to keep in mind what has already been stated and what remains to be stated and have some plan regarding the order in which information should be presented. Thus, in order to study narrative, measures beyond those of the individual phrase or sentence must be used in order to determine whether speakers are producing coherent narratives. Measures such as the overlap in propositions between utterances and the use of appropriate anaphors have been employed. Researchers may elicit target narratives by having the subjects view pictures or films and then asking the subject to tell the story of what happened. In such cases, the subjects' production can be assessed regarding whether the major elements of the story are present (such as introduction of people and situation, discussion of sequence of events and complication of the events, and resolution of the complication). Other measures can be used that assess whether the speaker uses vocabulary appropriate to the target audience and provides enough information, given the listener's knowledge, to allow for appropriate inferences.

C. Neuropsychological and Localization Evidence on Discourse Processing

As opposed to the dominance of the left hemisphere in carrying out single-word and sentence processing, the right hemisphere appears to play an important role in discourse comprehension and production. Research with right hemisphere-damaged patients demonstrates

an impaired understanding of various forms of discourse, including indirect requests ("Can you reach the bowl?"), jokes, ironic comments, and metaphors. This problem with discourse materials is not limited to verbal materials, but may be observed with stories that are told through cartoons or other pictures. Left hemisphere-damaged patients, in contrast, perform better than the right hemisphere-damaged patients and may even display normal levels of performance, particularly if the material is presented in a nonverbal format.

As discussed earlier, research on single-word and sentence processing indicates that multiple meanings or senses of words are activated and maintained by the right hemisphere. This has led to the proposal that semantic coding in the right hemisphere is coarse, allowing for a broad but weak activation of semantic representations that are distantly related to the word or context being processed. Weak activation of a broad semantic field may be of little use when the literal meaning of a word is required or when the most likely inference is the correct one. However, the activation and maintenance of multiple representations may allow the comprehension system to recognize and capitalize on distant semantic relationships in the comprehension of jokes or metaphors or in instances in which the comprehender has to revise an initial interpretation.

Like discourse and text comprehension, narrative production can be impaired even when production at the single-word or sentence level is preserved. That is, a speaker may fail to have an organized plan for communicating information, going off on topics tangential to the central one. The speaker might also fail to make coherent anaphoric reference between sentences or omit information that would be critical to the listener for drawing the appropriate inferences. Patients with right hemisphere brain damage and those with frontal damage have been shown to have discourse production deficits that are disproportionate to any deficits in vocabulary and grammar. Although relatively few studies have been carried out with right hemisphere-damaged patients, their deficits include an underspecification of information and a failure to take into account the listener's point of view. A larger number of studies have examined discourse deficits in individuals with closed head-injury (e.g., from a car accident). Individuals with closed-head injury often have frontal damage, and it has been assumed that the discourse deficits displayed by these patients are due to damage to this region. These individuals also display reduced information content and a lack of cohesion among the sentences in a story.

Some caveats should be kept in mind when considering the findings on discourse deficits. Much of this research has been carried out using group studies, even though researchers have found wide variation in the discourse deficits exhibited by right hemisphere-damaged or closed-head injury patients, with some patients showing no deficits. Clearly, the right hemisphere and the frontal lobes (both left and right) are very large cortical regions, and it is likely that only specific regions within these large areas are critical for discourse processing. Moreover, there are a variety of aspects of discourse processing that could be affected in different subgroups. Some individuals might have difficulty with the working memory demands involved in maintaining information across sentences during discourse comprehension or in planning a narrative to produce. Other patients might have difficulty taking into account other individuals' points of view, which makes their discourse production lack cohesion. Still others might have difficulty inhibiting irrelevant information that becomes activated during comprehension or production. Yet others might have subtle deficits at the level of lexical retrieval that become critical when several words have to be kept active simultaneously in planning discourse production. Carefully designed case studies testing for all these possibilities are necessary to delineate which components of discourse production are functionally isolable and which brain areas provide the cortical substrate for these functions.

IV. CONCLUSIONS

A substantial body of behavioral data has been amassed concerning language and lexical processing. Studies of brain-damaged patients indicate that considerable modularity of processing components exists in these domains. Although there is some knowledge concerning the brain areas involved in various aspects of language processing, the knowledge is currently at a broad rather than fine-grained level. Some of the same brain areas are implicated in a variety of language functions. For example, the temporal lobe appears to be involved in phonological, semantic, and syntactic processing. It is possible, however, that further study will reveal that nonoverlapping areas within the temporal lobe are involved in these different aspects.

Future research using series of case studies with well-identified functional deficits and neuroimaging studies with normal subjects should provide a better specification of the localization and interaction of brain areas involved in word, sentence, and discourse processing.

See Also the Following Articles

APHASIA • BILINGUALISM • BROCA'S AREA • CREATIVITY • EVOLUTION OF THE BRAIN • INFORMATION PROCESSING • LANGUAGE ACQUISITION • LANGUAGE DISORDERS • LANGUAGE, NEURAL BASIS OF • NUMBER PROCESSING AND ARITHMETIC • READING DISORDERS, DEVELOPMENTAL • SEMANTIC MEMORY • SPEECH • WERNICKE'S AREA

Suggested Reading

Ainsworth-Darnell, K., Shulman, H., and Boland, J. (1998). Dissociating brain responses to syntactic and semantic anomalies: Evidence from event-related potentials. *J. Memory Lang.* **38,** 112–130.

Berndt, R. S. (1991). Sentence processing in aphasia. In *Acquired Aphasia* (M. Sarno, Ed.), 2nd ed., pp. 223–270. Academic Press, San Diego.

Caplan, D., Alpert, N., and Waters, G. (1998). Effects of syntactic structure and propositional number on patterns of regional cerebral blood flow. *J. Cognitive Neurosci.* **10,** 541–552.

Dell, G. S., Schwartz, M. F., Martin, N., Saffran, E. M., and Gagnon, D. A. (1997). Lexical access in aphasic and nonaphasic speakers. *Psychol. Rev.* **104,** 801–838.

Eggert, G. H. (1977). *Wernicke's Works on Aphasia: A Sourcebook and Review*. Mouton, The Hague.

Joanette, Y., and Brownell, H. (1990). *Discourse Ability and Brain Damage: Theoretical and Empirical Perspectives*. Springer-Verlag, New York.

Linebarger, M., Schwartz, M., and Saffran, E. (1983). Sensitivity to grammatical structure in so-called agrammatic aphasics. *Cognition* **13,** 361–392.

Martin, R. C. (2001). Sentence comprehension deficits. In *Handbook of Cognitive Neuropsychology*. (B. Rapp, Ed.), Psychology Press, Philadelphia.

Mazoyer, B. M., Tzourio, N., Frak, V., Syrota, A., Murayama, N., Levrier, O., Salomon, G., Dehaene, S., Cohen, L., and Mehler, J. (1993). The cortical representations of speech. *J. Cognitive Neurosci.* **5,** 467–479.

Shelton, J. R., and Caramazza, A. (1999). Deficits in lexical and semantic processing: Implications for models of normal language. *Psychonomic Bull. Rev.* **6,** 5–27.

Tyler, L. (1992). *Spoken Language Comprehension: An Experimental Approach to Disordered and Normal Processing*. MIT Press, Cambridge, MA.

Neurologists and speech–language pathologists often describe aphasic patients as having one of a number of syndromes, which were first described in the second half of the nineteenth century. Because these syndromes are the foundation for contemporary descriptions of language impairments, and because they are still widely used by clinicians, I shall describe them here.

The paper that first led researchers to these syndromes was written by Paul Broca in 1861. Broca described a patient, Leborgne, with a severe speech output disturbance. Leborgne's speech was limited to the monosyllable "tan." In contrast, Broca described Leborgne's ability to understand spoken language and to express himself through gestures and facial expressions, as well as his understanding of nonverbal communication, as being normal. Broca claimed that Leborgne had lost "the faculty of articulate speech." Broca related this impairment to the neural tissue most badly damaged in Leborgne—the posterior portion of the inferior frontal convolution of the left hemisphere, which became known as Broca's area.

During the ensuing years, many cases of language impairments were described. In some, speech impairments were related to lesions in the left frontal lobe. Other speech impairments were associated with more posterior lesions. In 1874, Carl Wernicke, then a medical student, published a paper that appeared to reconcile many of these different findings. Wernicke described a patient with a speech disturbance, but one that was very different from that seen in Leborgne. Wernicke's patient was fluent; her speech, however, contained words with sound errors, other errors of word forms, and words that were semantically inappropriate. Also unlike Leborgne, Wernicke's patient did not understand spoken language. Wernicke related the two impairments—the one of speech production and the one of comprehension—by arguing that the patient had sustained damage to "the storehouse of auditory word forms." Under these conditions, speech would be expected to contain the types of errors that were seen in this case, and comprehension would be affected. Establishing the location of the lesion in this case was more problematic, however. Wernicke did not have the opportunity to perform an autopsy on his patient. However, he did examine the brain of a second patient, whose language had been described prior to her death by her physician in terms that made Wernicke think that she had a set of symptoms that were the same as those he had seen in his patient. The lesion in this second patient occupied the posterior portion of the first temporal gyrus, also on the left.

Wernicke suggested that this region, which came to be known as Wernicke's area, was the locus of the storehouse of auditory word forms.

These two seminal papers gave rise to a model of the relation of language processing to the brain. In this model, speaking involves activating the forms of words (in Wernicke's area) from concepts and transmitting these word forms to Broca's area to plan speech; Broca's area is also directly activated by concepts. Comprehension involves activating word forms from auditory input and then activating word meanings. Repetition involves transmitting the forms of words from Wernicke's area to Broca's area. Based on this model, researchers identified a number of aphasic syndromes, summarized in Table I.

The first two of these syndromes are Broca's and Wernicke's aphasia. Broca's aphasia, which affects primarily expressive language and leads to nonfluent speech, is due to lesions in Broca's area, the center for motor speech planning adjacent to the motor strip. Wernicke's aphasia follows lesions in Wernicke's area that disturb the representations of word sounds. Pure motor speech disorders arise from lesions interrupting the motor pathways from the cortex to the brain stem nuclei that control the articulatory system. These disorders differ from Broca's aphasic because they are not linguistic; they affect articulation, not the planning of speech. Pure word deafness affects the transmission of sound input into Wernicke's area. It therefore disrupts word recognition but not speech since words are intact and accessible for speech production purposes. Transcortical motor aphasia results from the interruption of the pathway from the concept center to Broca's area. This affects speech but not repetition or comprehension. Transcortical sensory aphasia follows lesions between Wernicke's area and the concept center. Repetition of words is intact, but comprehension is affected. Finally, conduction aphasia follows from a lesion between Wernicke's area and Broca's area. Repetition is affected, but comprehension is intact. Speech is also affected, in the same way as it is affected in Wernicke's aphasia, because the sound patterns of words, though activated, are not transmitted properly to Broca's area to be used to plan speech.

These syndromes have defined the domain of aphasia as a description of performances in the usual tasks of language use—speaking, understanding spoken language, reading, and writing. In terms of the linguistic elements, the disorders affect words, sounds of words, word endings, and classes of words such as function words that are produced, recognized, or understood. In this content, they contrast with other

---

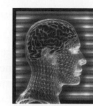

Language Disorders

DAVID CAPLAN
Massachusetts General Hospital

I. Language Structure and Processing
II. Classical Aphasic Syndromes
III. Problems with the Classical Aphasic Syndromes
IV. Psycholinguistic Descriptions of Aphasic Impairments
V. Conclusion

GLOSSARY

agrammatism Omission of function words, prefixes, and suffixes from speech.

agraphia Disturbance of writing.

alexia Disturbance of reading.

anomia Difficulty producing words, often nouns.

aphasia Disorders of language due to disease of the brain.

Broca's aphasia A type of aphasia with nonfluent speech and relative preserved comprehension.

paragrammatism Production of incorrect function words, prefixes and suffixes.

phonemic paraphasia Sound substitution in speech.

Wernicke's aphasia A type of aphasia with fluent error-containing speech and impaired comprehension.

Language is a code that relates different types of forms to semantic meanings. The forms of the code and their associated meanings are activated in the tasks of speaking, comprehension of spoken language, reading, and writing. Disorders of the brain can affect the ability to activate these representations in these tasks. Neurological and psychiatric disorders can also affect the use of language to accomplish tasks such as communicating ideas, storing information in long-term memory, reasoning, and solving problems.

Language disorders that have been most extensively studied neurologically are those that affect language processing in the tasks of language use.

I. LANGUAGE STRUCTURE AND PROCESSING

Human language can be viewed as a code that links linguistic representations to aspects of meaning. The basic types of representations of language (or language levels) are simple words (the lexical level), words with internal structure (the morphological level), sentences, and discourse. The lexical level of language makes contact with the categorial structure of the world. Lexical items (simple words) designate concrete objects, abstract concepts, actions, properties, and logical connectives. The basic form of a simple lexical item consists of a phonological representation that specifies the segmental elements (phonemes) of the word and their organization into metrical structures (e.g., syllables). The form of a word can also be represented orthographically. Words are associated with syntactic categories (e.g., noun and verb). The morphological level of language allows the meaning associated with a simple lexical item to be used as a different syntactic category (e.g., noun formation with the suffix -*tion* allows the semantic values associated with a verb to be used as a noun, as in the word "destruction" derived from "destroy") and thus avoids the need for an enormous number of elementary lexical items in an individual's vocabulary. The sentential level of language makes use of the syntactic categories of lexical items to build hierarchically organized syntactic structures (e.g., noun phrase, verb phrase, and sentence) that define relationships between words relevant

Encyclopedia of the Human Brain
Volume 2

to the propositional content of a sentence. The propositional content of a sentence expresses aspects of meaning, such as thematic roles (who did what to whom), attribution of modification (which adjectives go with which nouns), the reference of pronouns, and other referentially dependent categories. Propositional meanings make assertions that can be entered into logical and planning processes and that can serve as a means for updating an individual's knowledge of the world. The discourse level of language includes information about the general topic under discussion, the focus of a speaker's attention, the novelty of the information in a given sentence, the temporal order of events, causation, and so on. Information conveyed by the discourse level of language also serves as a basis for updating an individual's knowledge of the world and for reasoning and planning action.

The forms of language and their associated meanings are activated in the usual tasks of language use—speaking, auditory comprehension, reading, and writing. There is wide agreement among linguists, psychologists, and computer scientists that these different forms are activated by different "components" of a "language processing system." Components of the cognitive processing system are devices that accept as input a certain type of representation and operate on these inputs to activate another type of representation, where at least one of these representations is part of the language code. For instance, a component of the language processing system might accept as input the semantic representation (meaning) activated by the presentation of a picture and produce as output a representation of the sound pattern of the word that corresponds to that meaning.

The operations of the components of the language processing system are obligatory and largely unconscious. The obligatory nature of language processing can be appreciated intuitively by considering that we are generally unable to inhibit the performance of many language processing tasks once the system is engaged by an appropriate, attended input. For instance, we must perceive a spoken word as a word, not just as a nonlinguistic percept. The unconscious nature of most of language processing can be appreciated by considering that when we listen to a lecture, converse with an interlocutor, read a novel, or engage in some other language processing task, we usually have the subjective impression that we are extracting another person's meaning and producing linguistic forms appropriate to our intentions without paying attention to the details of the sounds of words, sentence structure, etc.

In general, cognitive processes that are automatic and unconscious are thought to require relatively little allocation of mental resources. However, many experimental results indicate that language processing does require the allocation of attention and/or processing resources. The efficiency of each of the components of the language processing system is thought to be a function of the resources available to that component, up to the maximum level of resource utilization of which the component is capable. Components of the system are remarkably efficient. For instance, it has been estimated on the basis of many different psycholinguistic experimental techniques that spoken words are usually recognized less than 125 msec after their onset (i.e., while they are still being uttered). Similarly, normal word production in speech requires searching through a mental word production "dictionary" of over 20,000 items, but it still occurs at the rate of about three words per second with an error rate of about one word misselected per 1 thousand and another one word mispronounced per 1 thousand. The efficiency of the language processing system as a whole reflects the efficiency of each of its components but also is achieved because of the massively parallel computational architecture of the system, in which many components of the system are simultaneously active.

Functional communication involving the language code occurs when people use these processors to undertake language-related tasks to accomplish specific goals—to inform others, to ask for information, to get things done, etc. The language code is remarkably powerful with respect to the semantic meanings it can encode and convey, and psycholinguistic processors are astonishingly fast and accurate. The ability to use this code quickly and accurately is critical to human success, both as a species and as individuals.

II. CLASSICAL APHASIC SYNDROMES

The language disorders that are best understood are those that affect the representation and processing of language in the usual tasks of language use. These disorders are known as "aphasia." By convention, the term aphasia does not refer to disturbances that affect the functions to which language processing is put. Lying (even transparent, ineffectual lying) is not considered a form of aphasia, nor is the garrulousness of old age or the incoherence of schizophrenia.

Table I
Classical Aphasic Syndromes

Syndrome	Clinical manifestations	Postulated deficit	Classical lesion location
Broca's aphasia	Major disturbance in speech production with sparse, halting speech, often misarticulated, and frequently missing function words and bound morphemes	Disturbances in the speech planning and production mechanisms	Posterior aspects of the third frontal convolution (Broca's area)
Wernicke's aphasia	Major disturbance in auditory comprehension; fluent speech with disturbances of the sounds and structures of words (phonemic, morphological, and semantic paraphasias)	Disturbances of the permanent representations of the sound structures of words	Posterior half of the first temporal gyrus and possibly adjacent cortex (Wernicke's area)
Pure motor speech disorder	Disturbance of articulation; apraxia of speech, dysarthria, anarthria, aphemia	Disturbance of articulatory mechanisms	Outflow tracts from motor cortex
Pure word deafness	Disturbance of spoken word comprehension	Failure to access spoken words	Input tracts from auditory system to Wernicke's area
Transcortical motor aphasia	Disturbance of spontaneous speech similar to Broca's aphasia, with relatively preserved repetition	Disconnection between conceptual representations of words and sentences and the motor speech production system	White matter tracts deep to Broca's area connecting it to parietal lobe
Transcortical sensory aphasia	Disturbance in single word comprehension, with relatively intact repetition	Disturbance in activation of word meanings despite normal recognition of auditorily presented words	White matter tracts connecting parietal lobe to temporal lobe or portions of inferior parietal lobe
Conduction aphasia	Disturbance of repetition and spontaneous speech (phonemic paraphasias)	Disconnection between the sound patterns of words and the speech production mechanism	Lesion in the arcuate fasciculus and/or corticocortical connections between Wernicke's and Broca's areas
Anomic aphasia	Disturbance in the production of single words, most marked for common nouns with variable comprehension problems	Disturbances of concepts and/or the sound patterns of words	Inferior parietal lobe or connections between parietal lobe and temporal lobe; can follow many lesions
Global aphasia	Major disturbance in all language functions	Disruption of all language processing components	Large portion of the peri-Sylvian association cortex
Isolation of the language zone	Disturbance of both spontaneous speech (similar to Broca's aphasia) and comprehension, with some preservation of repetition	Disconnection between concepts and both representations of word sounds and the speech production mechanism	Cortex just outside the peri-Sylvian association cortex

approaches to the description of aphasia. For instance, Hughlings Jackson described a patient, a carpenter, who was mute but who mustered the capacity to say "master's" in response to his son's question about where his tools were. Jackson's poignant comments convey his emphasis on the conditions that provoke speech rather than on the form of the speech:

The father had left work; would never return to it; was away from home; his son was on a visit, and the question was directly put to the patient. Anyone who saw the abject poverty the poor man's family

lived in would admit that these tools were of immense value to them. Hence we have to consider as regards this and other occasional utterances the strength of the accompanying emotional state.

Jackson and others sought a description of language use as a function of motivational and intellectual states and tried to describe aphasic disturbances of language in relationship to the factors that drive language production and make for depth of comprehension. This is a vital aspect of understanding language impairments. In many ways, it is more humanly relevant than a description of language impairments in terms of which phonemes are produced in spontaneous speech or repetition. Unfortunately, it is a very intractable goal, both in terms of psychological descriptions and in terms of relating these specific motivational states to the brain. The researchers who conceived and developed the framework of the classical syndromes focused aphasiology on the description of the linguistic representations and psycholinguistic operations that are responsible for everyday language use.

III. PROBLEMS WITH THE CLASSICAL APHASIC SYNDROMES

A major limitation of the classical syndromes is that they stay at arm's length from the linguistic details of language impairments. The classical aphasic syndromes basically reflect the relative ability of patients to perform entire language tasks (speaking, comprehension, etc.), not the integrity of specific operations within the language processing system. This is not to say that there are no linguistic or qualitative descriptions of language in the characterizations of the classical aphasic syndromes, only that they are incomplete and unsystematic.

A second problem with these syndromes is that they do not classify many aphasic patients very well. In practice, most applications of the clinical taxonomy result in widespread disagreements as to a patient's classification and/or to a large number of "mixed" or "unclassifiable." The criteria for inclusion in a syndrome are often arbitrary: How bad does a patient's comprehension have to be called a Wernicke's aphasic instead of a conduction aphasic or a global aphasic instead of a Broca's aphasic? Part of the problem is that patients can only be assigned to a single syndrome instead of being thought of as having multiple deficits.

A third problem that the classical aphasic syndromes face is that they are not as well correlated with lesion sites as the theory claims they should be. The correlations do not apply to many types of lesions, such as various sorts of tumors, degenerative diseases, and others. The classical syndromes are only related to lesion sites in cases of rapidly developing lesions, such as stroke; even in these types of lesions, they are not related to acute and subacute phases of the illness. Even in the chronic phase of diseases such as stroke, as many as 40% of patients have lesions that are not predictable from their syndromes according to some studies.

IV. PSYCHOLINGUISTIC DESCRIPTIONS OF APHASIC IMPAIRMENTS

Modern psycholinguistic analyses have greatly amplified the descriptions of aphasic syndromes. This work seeks to describe the aspects of language that are affected in individual patients. It differs from the syndrome approach in that a patient can have (and usually will have) more than one deficit. This work is far too extensive to review in detail here; I shall illustrate it with a few selective descriptions of analyses undertaken in this framework.

A. Disturbances of Word Meanings

Most recent research on disturbances of word meanings in brain-damaged patients has focused on words that refer to objects. Disturbances of word meanings cause poor performance on word–picture matching and naming tasks. However, the combination of deficits in word–picture matching and naming may be due to separate input- and output-side processing disturbances that affect word recognition and production. Cooccurring deficits in naming and word–picture matching are more likely to result from a disturbance affecting concepts when (i) the patient makes many semantic errors in providing words to pictures and definitions, (ii) he or she has trouble with word–picture matching with semantic but not phonological foils, (iii) he or she fails on categorization tasks with pictures, and (iv) the same words are affected in production and comprehension tasks.

Disorders affecting processing of semantic representations for objects may be specific to certain types of inputs. Elizabeth Warrington first noted a discrepancy between comprehension of words and pictures in two dementing patients. Dan Bub and colleagues described a patient who showed very poor comprehension of written and spoken words but quite good comprehension of pictures. These impairments have been taken as reflections of disturbances of "verbal" and "visual" semantic systems, although others have disputed this conclusion.

Semantic disturbances may also be category specific. Several authors have reported a selective semantic impairment of concepts related to living things and foods compared to man-made objects. The opposite pattern has also been found. Selective preservation and disruption of abstract versus concrete concepts, and of nominal versus verbal concepts, have also been reported.

Disturbances may affect the unconscious activation of semantic meanings or their conscious use. There are patients who cannot match words to pictures or name objects but who are unconsciously influenced by a word's meaning. For instance, in a word/nonword decision task, they will respond faster to the word "doctor" when it follows "nurse" than when it follows "house," indicating they are able to appreciate the relations between words unconsciously, even when they cannot indicate understanding of word meaning in conscious, controlled tasks such as word–picture matching. Conversely, some patients who appear to understand words well have abnormalities in tasks that examine unconscious processing of the meanings of words.

B. Disturbances of Oral Word Production

Disturbances affecting the oral production of single words are extremely common in language-impaired patients. There are three basic disturbances affecting word production (other than semantic deficits). They follow the stages of word sound production: accessing the forms of words from concepts, planning the form of a word for articulation, and articulation.

A disturbance in activating word forms from concepts is manifest by an inability to produce a word from a semantic stimulus (a picture or a definition), coupled with intact processing at the semantic and phonological levels (determined by answering questions about pictures, picture categorization tests, and repetition). The form of a patient's errors is not a good guide to whether he or she has an impairment at this level of the production process since disturbances in accessing word forms may appear in a variety of ways, ranging from pauses to neologisms (complex sequences of sounds that do not form words) and semantic paraphasias (words related to the meaning of the target item). Rarely, patients show an inability to name objects presented in one modality only (e.g., visually) even though they demonstrate understanding of the concept associated with that object when it is presented in that modality (optic aphasia). Because disorders of basic sensory and motor functions can be ruled out in these patients, these modality-specific naming disorders have been taken to reflect a failure to transmit information from modality-specific semantic systems to the processor responsible for activating the forms of words.

Disturbances of a patient's ability to convert the representation of the sound of a word into a form appropriate for articulatory production are usually manifest as phonemic paraphasias (substitutions, omissions, and misorderings of phonemes). Three features of a patient's performance suggest a disturbance in word sound planning. First, some phonemic paraphasias are closely related to target words (e.g., "befenit" for "benefit"). Second, some patients make multiple attempts that come increasingly closer to the correct form of a word. Third, some patients make similar phonological errors in word repetition, word reading, and picture naming. Because the form of a word is presented to the output system in very different ways in these three tasks, the errors in such patients most likely arise in the process of planning the form of the word that is suitable for articulation.

Patients with sound planning problems tend to be more affected on longer words and on words with consonant clusters. The frequency of occurrence of a word in the language has a variable effect on the occurrence of these types of errors. Planning disturbances only rarely affect function words compared to nouns, verbs, and adjectives. Some patients have trouble planning the sounds of words only when words are inserted into sentences, making phonemic paraphasias in sentence production but not naming or repetition tasks. In these cases, the errors probably arise when words are inserted into syntactic structures.

Patients often have disturbances of articulation, as shown by abnormalities in the acoustic waveform produced by a patient and in the movement of the articulators in speech. Investigators have identified two major disturbances of articulation—dysarthria and apraxia of speech. Dysarthria is marked by hoarseness, excessive nasality, and imprecise articulation, and it has been said to not be significantly influenced by the type of linguistic material that the speaker produces or by the speech task. Apraxia of speech is marked by difficulty in initiating speech, searching for a pronunciation, better articulation for automatized speech (e.g., counting) than volitional speech, abnormal prosody, omissions of syllables in multisyllabic words, and simplification of consonant clusters (often by adding a short neutral vowel sound between consonants). Both dysarthria and apraxia of speech result in sounds that are perceived as distorted. Apraxia of speech often cooccurs with dysarthria or with the production of phonemic paraphasias, and the relations between these disorders and the empirical basis for distinguishing one from another are the subject of active research.

C. Disturbances of Recognition of Auditorily Presented Simple Words

Disturbances affecting auditory comprehension of simple words have been attributed to impairments of semantic concepts, as discussed previously, and/or to an inability to recognize spoken words. The latter disturbances have, in turn, been thought to have two possible origins: disturbances affecting the recognition of phonemes in the acoustic signal and disturbances affecting the ability to recognize words despite good acoustic–phonetic processing.

Disturbances of acoustic–phonetic processing may affect the ability to discriminate or to identify phonemes. It is unclear, however, whether these disturbances lead to problems in recognizing or understanding spoken words. Several studies suggest that they do, but other researchers have found weak correlations between comprehension capacities and phoneme discrimination capacities in language-impaired patients.

Many researchers believe that patients can have disturbances of spoken word recognition despite good acoustic–phonetic processing. Such a disturbance was originally postulated by Carl Wernicke. However, there is no clear case of a patient who has intact acoustic–phonetic processing and who cannot recognize spoken words. In most cases, single-word comprehension problems are probably multifactorial in origin and result from a complex interaction of acoustic–phonetic disturbances, disturbances in recognizing spoken words, and disturbances affecting word meanings.

D. Disorders of Repetition of Single Words

Repetition of a word can be carried out in three ways: (i) nonlexically by repeating sounds without recognizing the word (as if one were imitating a foreign language), (ii) lexically by recognizing the stimulus as a word and uttering it without understanding it, and (iii) semantically by understanding the word and reactivating its form from its meaning. Any of these routes to repetition may be disturbed. For instance, one patient could only repeat by the semantic route; this patient made many semantic paraphasias in repetition and could not repeat nonwords. Patients with relatively isolated disturbances affecting the repetition of nonwords have been described, reflecting disruption of the nonlexical route. In most cases, patients have a more complicated picture, with lexical status (whether a stimulus is a word or a nonword), word frequency, and stimulus length affecting performance differently in different patients.

E. Disturbances of Processing Morphologically Complex Words

Disturbances affecting both the comprehension and the production of morphologically complex words have been described. With respect to recognition of morphologically complex words, researchers have observed that some patients who make derivational paralexic errors (e.g., "write" → "wrote," "fish" → "fishing," and "directing" → "direction") in the oral reading of complex words have particular difficulty with the recognition and analysis of written morphologically complex words compared to morphologically simple words. A patient with a disturbance affecting the auditory processing of words with inflectional but not derivational morphology has been described.

Disturbances affecting morphological processing also appear in single-word production tasks. In one study, patients had difficulties in producing plural, possessive, and third-person singular forms of nonwords. The fact that this disorder arose with nonwords that the patients were given by the experimenters suggests that the impairment affected the ability to construct new morphological forms. Such disturbances can arise in patients who perform well on tasks that require recognition and comprehension of written morphologically complex words.

Disturbances affecting the production of morphologically complex words are most commonly seen in sentence production, where they are known as "agrammatism" and "paragrammatism." The most noticeable deficit in agrammatism is the widespread omission of function words and affixes and the better production of common nouns. This disparity is always seen in the spontaneous speech of patients termed agrammatic, and it often occurs in their repetition and writing as well. Patients in whom substitutions of these elements predominate, and whose speech is fluent, are called paragrammatic. Recent observations have emphasized the fact that these two patterns cooccur in many patients. They may result from a single underlying deficit that has different surface manifestations.

Agrammatism and paragrammatism vary considerably, with different sets of function words and bound morphemes being affected or spared in different cases. In some patients, there seems to be some systematicity to the pattern of errors. For instance,

English agrammatic patients frequently produce infinitives (e.g., "to walk") and gerunds (e.g., "walking") because these are the basic forms in the verbal system. In other cases, substitutions are closely related to the correct target. Agrammatics' errors also tend to follow the tendencies seen in normal subjects with respect to errors that "strand" affixes (e.g., "I am going to school" → "I am schooling to go") and the "sonorance hierarchy" that establishes syllabic forms as easier to produce than simple consonants. Agrammatics generally produce real words, which makes for different patterns of errors in different languages that differ with respect to whether or not they require inflections to appear on a word. The fact that in almost all cases errors do not violate the word-formation processes of the language suggests that most agrammatic and paragrammatic patients retain some knowledge of the rules of word formation.

F. Disorders of Sentence Production

Disturbances at the sentence production level are the inevitable results of disturbances affecting the production of simple or complex words. In addition, many patients have problems in the sentence planning process.

Agrammatic patients usually produce only very simple syntactic structures. In one study, virtually no syntactically well-formed syntactic constructions were found in the utterances produced by one agrammatic patient. All the agrammatic patients studied in a large contemporary cross-language study showed some impoverishment of syntactic structure in spontaneous speech. The failure to produce complex noun phrases and embedded verbs with normal frequency were the most striking features of the syntactic simplification shown by these patients.

The ability to express the thematic roles of noun phrases requires the ability to use verbs. Many agrammatic patients have problems with verbs; in one, a category-specific degradation of the meaning of verbs resulted in almost no production of verbs in speech and limited the ability to convey thematic roles of nouns. In other studies, patients' inabilities to produce verbs were only partially responsible for the shortened phrase length found in their speech. It thus appears that in some patients a disturbance affecting the ability to produce verbs affects the production of a normal range of syntactic structures, whereas in others at least some syntactic structures are built despite poor verb production. Yet other patients cannot produce normal syntactic structures despite relatively good verb production.

Several studies suggest that syntactic errors in sentence production differ in paragrammatic and agrammatic patients. Five characteristic paragrammatic patients each produced many long and complex sentences, with multiple interdependencies of constituents, but tended to produce many types of syntactic errors, including errors in tag questions, illegal noun phrases in relative clauses, and illegal use of pronouns to head relative clauses. A type of error that has often been commented on in paragrammatism is a "blend," in which the output seems to reflect a conflation of two different ways of saying the same thing (e.g., "They are not prepared to be of helpful," which is a combination of "They are not prepared to be helpful" and "They are not prepared to be of help"). Some paragrammatic patients can solve anagram tasks according to syntactic constraints (whereas agrammatic patients solved them using semantic constraints). Because of the evidence that paragrammatic patients retain some ability to use syntactic structures, some researchers have suggested that the syntactic and morphological errors in paragrammatism result from the failure of these patients to monitor their speech production processes and their output.

The various disturbances that affect sentence production usually cooccur. A complex disturbance that results from the combination of the deficits in producing syntactic forms, disturbances in accessing and planning word forms, and impairments in producing morphologically complex words is known as "jargonaphasia."

Many patients have difficulty producing prosodic aspects of speech. These disturbances may be secondary to motor output disorders or associated with other sentence production disorders. However, these disturbances may occur in isolation. These are different from the aprosodias related to emotional display described after right hemisphere disease. They reflect a primary disturbance of production of intonation in right hemisphere-damaged patients that differs as a function of lesion location in the hemisphere.

G. Disorders of Sentence Comprehension

When a subject understands a sentence, he or she combines the meanings of the words in accordance with the syntactic structure of the sentence into a propositional content. There are many reasons why a patient might fail to understand the propositional content of a sentence. In addition to the carryover effect of disturbances affecting comprehension of simple and complex words, there are disturbances affecting the ability to understand aspects of propositional meaning despite good single-word processing.

The greatest amount of work in the area of disturbances of sentence comprehension has gone into the investigation of patients whose use of syntactic structures to assign meaning is not normal. The first researchers to show that some patients have selective impairments of this ability described patients who could match "semantically reversible" sentences such as "The apple the boy is eating is red" to one of two pictures but not "semantically irreversible" sentences such as "The girl the boy is chasing is tall." The difference between the two types of sentences resides in the fact that a listener can understand a sentence such as "The apple the boy is eating is red" via the lexico-pragmatic route, whereas understanding "The girl the boy is chasing is tall" requires assigning its syntactic structure since both boys and girls are capable of chasing one another.

Disorders of syntactic comprehension have since been examined in considerable detail. Patients may have very selective disturbances affecting the use of particular syntactic structures or elements to determine the meaning of a sentence. For instance, patients may understand sentences with reflexives ("himself") but not pronouns ("him") and vice versa. Some patients can understand very simple syntactic forms, such as active sentences ("The man hugged the woman"), but not more complex forms, such as passive sentences ("The woman was hugged by the man"). Many of these patients use strategies such as assigning the thematic role of agent to a noun immediately before a verb to understand semantically reversible sentences, leading to systematic errors in comprehension of sentences such as "The boy who pushed the girl kissed the baby." Other patients have virtually no ability to use syntactic structure. Most of these patients rely on inferences based on their knowledge of the real world and their ability to understand some words in a sentence.

Some patients can assign and interpret syntactic structures unconsciously but cannot use these structures in a conscious, controlled fashion. For instance, one patient's word-monitoring performances indicated that he was sensitive to certain syntactic anomalies but could not make judgments regarding these same anomalies at the end of a sentence. Some patients who have syntactic comprehension problems (e.g., who cannot match reversible sentences to pictures) can make judgments as to whether or not a sentence is grammatical. For instance, some patients can indicate that the utterance "The woman was watched the man" is ill formed and the utterance "The woman was watched by the man" is acceptable, despite not being able to match sentences such as "The woman was watched by the man" to one of two pictures. These results suggest that these patients can construct syntactic structures but cannot use them to determine propositional meaning (a so-called "mapping" problem). As with other areas of language functioning, it appears that patients may retain unconscious, on-line sentence comprehension processes but lose the ability to use the products of these processes in a controlled, conscious fashion in some tasks.

Some researchers maintain the view that short-term memory is used in comprehending more complex sentences and have pointed out a variety of sentence comprehension disturbances in patients with short-term memory limitations. Sentence length has been shown to affect certain comprehension tasks in some patients who do not show disturbances of syntactic comprehension. However, case studies show that patients with short-term memory impairments can have excellent syntactic comprehension abilities. Although many short-term memory patients have trouble in comprehension tasks, the relationship of these short-term memory disorders to sentence comprehension impairments remains unclear.

H. Disorders of Reading Single Words

The contemporary study of acquired dyslexias has largely focused on impairments in the ability to read single words aloud. One model of the mechanisms involved in reading a word aloud claims that there are three separate and partially independent routines in the brain for converting a written word into its spoken form: The first pathway (the semantic route) involves recognizing a word visually, gaining access to its meaning, and then activating the sound of the word from its meaning. The second pathway (the whole word route) translates the orthography of the entire word directly into a pronunciation, without first contacting the word's meaning. Finally, a third pathway (the sublexical route) decomposes the word into orthographic segments (graphemes and other spelling units) and derives a pronunciation by assigning each of them a spoken (phonemic) value. Other models of the reading-aloud process combine the second and third processes into one highly interactive system.

Brain damage can selectively affect a particular routine without impairing the function of the remaining branches of the system. Certain patients (phonological alexics) lose the operation of the sublexical route, which acts on subword units to assemble a response, leaving the semantic and whole word routes available. A patient with damage to the sublexical route is impaired in the reading aloud of nonwords, whereas legitimate words are mostly read correctly. Other reading disorders appear to be the outcome of severe damage to both the whole word route and the sublexical route. Patients with this pattern or impairment, termed deep dyslexics, are unable to pronounce written nonwords (indicating severe impairment to the sublexical route) but also make semantic paralexias (e.g., they read "chair" as "table") and are poor at reading abstract words aloud relative to concrete words. The failure to read nonwords combined with the presence of semantic errors and the influence of a semantic variable on the ability to read a written word aloud is consistent with the interpretation that the patient has lost the use of both the routines from whole words and subword units to sound and is forced to use a defective routine from the visual description of the word through meaning to pronunciation. Yet other dyslexic readers (surface dyslexics) have lost the ability to use both the semantically mediated reading route and the whole-word route but retain the translation of subword units into sound (the sublexical route). These patients can still read words aloud that obey regular correspondences between spelling and sound (e.g., "hint," "mint," and "stint"), but not those that do not (e.g., "pint"). Finally, some patients with dementia show the ability to use the whole-word reading route without the benefit of semantics. These patients can read irregularly spelled words correctly that they do not understand.

The fact that a patient has difficulties in reading words and/or nonwords aloud does not necessarily imply that he or she does not recognize or understand a printed word. Some patients have a severe disturbance of reading aloud known as "letter-by-letter reading" because they name each letter in a word before attempting (often with incomplete success) to pronounce the word. These patients take longer to read longer words, and it can take them many seconds to pronounce a printed word. Several of these patients have been tested for their abilities to recognize and comprehend words that are presented for short periods of time—far less than the time needed for them to read the words aloud. One such patient could recognize words and familiar letter strings as visual patterns, and

other letter-by-letter readers can extract at least some semantic information from briefly presented words. Most of these patients denied that they were able to recognize or understand these briefly presented words. These performances suggest that some reading problems arise after words have been recognized, and also that some alexic subjects, such as the patients with disturbances affecting auditory–oral processing described previously, may retain abilities to recognize and understand words without being aware that they do so.

I. Disorders of Writing Single Words

The acquired dyslexias have their counterparts in the acquired agraphias. Patients with phonological agraphia are severely impaired in their ability to spell or write nonsense words but are capable of very good performance on legitimate words, even words that are low in frequency and contain unusual spelling patterns (e.g., "leopard"). The deficit is these cases appears to lie in the ability to convert sublexical phonological units to orthographic units (graphemes and letters). The converse impairment—an inability to access the written forms of whole words with preserved ability to convert sublexical phonological units to orthographic units, termed surface agraphia or lexical agraphia—has also been described. A third disturbance, known as "asemantic writing," consists of the inability to write spontaneously but the retained ability to write to dictation. This suggests that the contents of the visual word-form system can be addressed from spoken input but not from the meaning of a word.

These disorders of writing can be strikingly different from patients' reading performances. For instance, one patient was unable to write nonsense words to dictation but read these items aloud without difficulty; another produced numerous misspellings when attempting to write orthographically irregular or ambiguous words but accurately read the majority of legitimate words perfectly. These dissociations have led researchers to infer that the orthographic knowledge necessary for word recognition in reading is different from the orthographic knowledge necessary for correct spelling in writing.

The abstract graphemic representation of familiar and unfamiliar words is ultimately converted by the writing mechanism into a sequence of rapid movements that generate letters on the page. A specialized working memory device is needed to maintain the graphemic code in a buffer zone while the spatial identity of each letter is chosen at the next processing stage. One patient made the same kind of errors in writing, oral spelling, and typing, a result that justifies the conclusion that the disturbance arose while these items were in the planning buffer and before the programming and execution of a particular motor act began.

Written production takes place by generating the spatial form of each letter (allographs) in the correct order. A few agraphic cases have been documented in which the impairment is plainly confined to the retrieval of elements in the allographic code. In these patients, adequate knowledge of the word's orthography can be demonstrated because oral spelling is carried out extremely well. When tested, other methods of forming a printed word that do not require a written response (typing or use of block letters) may also yield a high degree of accuracy. Writing, however, is characterized by numerous errors of omission, substitution, reversals, and insertions. The agraphia is not merely a disturbance in the production of a graphic motor pattern because patients can write single letters to dictation, and their writing of words, although flawed, is clearly legible.

Finally, the motor schema for a letter appears to distinguish between the movements denoting the shape of a letter and the parameters that govern scale factors such as magnitude and orientation. Cases of apractic agraphia reveal a loss of the motor programs necessary for producing letters. Written characters are poorly formed and may be indecipherable, although even severely affected patients maintain the distinction between cursive and printed letters and between upper- and lowercase. Evidence indicates that the disturbance need not be associated with limb apraxia. Certain patients with right hemisphere damage have no difficulty constructing written letters or words, but they exceed the correct number of strokes on letters that require repetitive movements.

V. CONCLUSION

This brief overview of the major acquired language disorders reveals their heterogeneity and specificity. It also highlights the fact that patients may have trouble with conscious, controlled use of the products of language processing, but retain the ability to compute certain language structures unconsciously on-line. Additional disorders, and further characterization of the impairments of the operating characteristics of psycholinguistic processors, continue to be documented in psycholinguistic aphasiological research. Most patients with language disorders have more than one primary language disorder and often have disorders of these processors due to other cognitive impairments as well (such as attentional deficits or problems with searching through semantic memory).

There is no simple, one-to-one relationship between impairments of elements of the language code or of psycholinguistic processors, on the one hand, and abnormalities in performing language-related tasks and accomplishing the goals of language use, on the other hand. Most patients who have disturbances of elements of the language code or psycholinguistic processors experience limitations in their functional communicative abilities. However, individuals with language processing disorders adapt to their language impairments in many ways, and some of these adaptations are remarkably effective at maintaining at least some aspects of functional communication. Time, rehabilitation, support, and a positive attitude can allow many aphasic patients to be productive and happy.

See Also the Following Articles

AGRAPHIA • ALEXIA • ANOMIA • AUTISM • BROCA'S AREA • DYSLEXIA • INFORMATION PROCESSING • LANGUAGE ACQUISITION • LANGUAGE AND LEXICAL PROCESSING • LANGUAGE, NEURAL BASIS OF • SPEECH • WERNICKE'S AREA

Suggested Reading

Caplan, D. (1992). *Language: Structure, Processing and Disorders.* MIT Press, Cambridge, MA.

Damasio, A. R. (1992). Aphasia. *N. Engl. J. Med.* **326,** 531–539.

Davis, A. (1999). *Aphasiology: Disorders and Clinical Practice.* Allyn & Bacon, New York.

Goodglass, H. (1997). *Understanding Aphasia.* Academic Press, New York.

Howard, D. (1995). Language in the human brain. In *Cognitive Neuroscience* (M. R. Rugg, Ed.), pp. 277–304. MIT Press, Cambridge, MA.

Lecours, A. R., Lhermitte, F., and Bryans, B. (1983). *Aphasiology.* Balliere Tindall, London.

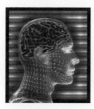

Language, Neural Basis of

DAVID CAPLAN

Massachusetts General Hospital

GLOSSARY

cortex The nerve cells along the outside edge of the brain; the most advanced part of the brain.

holism Models of the neural basis of cognitive functions that maintain that these functions depend on large areas of the brain (i.e., that they are not narrowly localized).

lateralization The fact that some cognitive functions rely on one hemisphere of the brain more than another.

localization The fact that sensory, motor, and cognitive functions are supported by small areas of the brain.

Perisylvian cortex The cortex around the Sylvian fissure in the brain.

Language is a distinctly human symbol system that relates a number of different types of forms to aspects of meaning. The forms of language and their associated meanings are activated in the processes of speaking, understanding speech, reading, and writing. Several types of data provide information about the way the brain is organized to represent and process language in these tasks. These include correlations between language processing deficits and brain lesions, regional cerebral blood flow and other hemodynamic responses to language processing in normal subjects, electro-

physiological and magnetoecephalographic responses to language processing in normal subjects, and the effects of electrocortical stimulation on language. These sources of data indicate that language is primarily represented and processed in perisylvian association cortex, with possible contributions from other brain areas. They indicate that different aspects of language processing are localized in different parts of the perisylvian cortex and lateralized differently in the two hemispheres. They also indicate that both localization and lateralization show some degree of variability across individuals.

I. LANGUAGE STRUCTURE

Language is a distinctly human ability that is vital to the cognitive and communicative abilities that underlie the success of humans both as individuals and as a species. Although many people think of language as a form of communication, it is more accurate to think of language as a code that can serve many functions, one of which is communication. The language code links linguistic representations to aspects of meaning. The types of representations of the language code include simple words, words with internal structure, sentences, and discourse. These types of representations are also called the lexical, word-formation, sentential, and discourse levels of language.

The lexical level of language consists of simple words. The basic form of a simple word (or lexical item) consists of a phonological representation that specifies the segmental elements (phonemes) of the word and their organization into metrical structures such as syllables. The form of a word can also be represented orthographically. Simple words are assigned to different syntactic categories, such as nouns, verbs, adjectives, articles, and prepositions. The semantic values associated with the lexical level primarily consist of concepts and categories in the nonlinguistic world. Simple words tend to designate concrete objects, abstract concepts, actions, properties, and logical connectives.

The word-formation level of language allows words to be formed from other words. In English, word formation can take place via affixation (e.g., the word "destruction" is derived from the word "destroy") and compounding (e.g., the word "paper tray" is formed from the words "paper" and "tray"). There are two basic types of affixation in English. Derivational morphological processes allow the meaning associated with a simple lexical item to be used as a different syntactic category without coining a large number of new lexical forms that would have to be learned (e.g., "destroy" → "destruction"). Inflectional morphological processes play roles in encoding syntactic relationships (e.g., subject–verb agreement: "destroy" → "destroys").

The sentential level of language consists of syntactic structures—hierarchical sets of syntactic categories (e.g., noun phrase, verb phrase, and sentence)—into which words are inserted. The meaning of a sentence, known as its propositional content, is determined by the way the meanings of words combine in syntactic structures. Propositions convey aspects of the structure of events and states in the world. These include thematic roles (who did what to whom), attribution of modification (which adjectives go with which nouns), and the reference of pronouns and other anaphoric elements (which words in a set of sentences refer to the same items or actions). For instance, in the sentence "The big boy told the little girl to wash herself," the agent of "told" is "the big boy" and its theme is "the little girl," "big" is associated with "boy" and "little" with "girl," and "herself" refers to the same person as "girl." Sentences are a crucial level of the language code because the propositions they express make assertions about the world. These assertions can be entered into logical systems and can be used to add to an individual's knowledge of the world.

The propositional meanings conveyed by sentences are entered into higher order structures that constitute the discourse level of linguistic structure. Discourse includes information about the general topic under discussion, the focus of a speaker's attention, the novelty of the information in a given sentence, the temporal order of events, causation, and so on.

Information conveyed by the discourse level of language also serves as a basis for updating an individual's knowledge of the world and for reasoning and planning action. The structure and processing of discourse involve many nonlinguistic elements and operations, such as search through semantic memory, logical inferences, and others.

II. LANGUAGE PROCESSING

Current models of language processing subdivide functions such as reading, speaking, and auditory comprehension into many different, semiindependent components, which are sometimes called modules or processors. These components of the language processing system perform highly specialized operations. For instance, the process of mapping the acoustic waveform onto phonemes and other phonological units involves a large number of highly specific operations that relate specific features of the acoustic signal to linguistically relevant units of sound. We may think of these operations as all being part of an "acoustic–phonetic" processor or module, or we may consider each of these operations as a distinct cognitive function. An analogy in the area of visual perception might be the claim that one function of the system is the identification of the three-dimensional shape of an object, which involves the identification of lines, surfaces, angles, and other geometric elements of shape; we may think of each of these more elementary perceptual operations separately or consider them as a whole with respect to their contribution to shape recognition. Different aspects of language involve different operations: The operations that have been postulated to be involved in constructing the syntactic structure of a sentence from words are different from those involved in recognizing linguistically relevant sounds. The visual system provides an analogy for this multiplication of different types of processors in that it has separate mechanisms for the perception of shape, color, texture, movement, and other visually perceptible elements. In the language system, as in the visual system, these different processing components, each composed of a variety of elementary operations, are semiindependent of the others in that each yields a particular type of representation. Each representation is finally integrated with others to achieve the overall goal of the processing system.

Information processing models of language can be expressed as flow diagrams (often called functional architectures) that indicate the sequence of operations of the different components that perform a language-related task. These models become extremely detailed and complex when all the operations and components used in a task are specified. For present purposes, it is adequate to identify the major components of the language processing system as those processors that activate units at the lexical, word-formation, sentential, and discourse levels of the language code in the usual tasks of language use—speech, auditory comprehension, reading, and writing. This approach to defining language processing components groups together different operations that all activate a similar type of linguistic representation in a given task into a single processor.

The major components of the language processing system that can be identified at this level of detail for simple words are listed in Table I, and those for the word-formation and sentence levels are listed in Table II. Figure 1 presents a model indicating the sequence of activation of components of the lexical processing system, and Fig. 2 presents a similar model of the processing system for word formation and sentences. These tables and figures are based on the results of experimental psychological research in both normal subjects and patient populations.

Table I
Components of the Language Processing System for Simple Words

Component	Input	Operation	Output
Auditory–oral modality			
Acoustic–phonological processing	Acoustic waveform	Matches acoustic properties to phonetic features	Phonological segments (phonemes, allophones, syllables)
Input-side lexical access	Phonological units	Activates lexical items in long-term memory on basis of sound; selects best fit to stimulus	Phonological forms of words
Input-side semantic access	Words (represented as phonological forms)	Activates semantic features of words	Word meanings
Output-side lexical access	Word meanings ("lemmas")	Activates phonological forms of words	Phonological forms of words
Phonological output planning	Phonological forms of words (and nonwords)	Activates detailed phonetic features of words (and nonwords)	Speech
Written modality			
Written lexical access	Abstract letter identities	Activates orthographic forms of words	Orthographic forms of words
Lexical semantic access	Orthographic forms of words	Activates semantic features of words	Word meanings
Accessing orthography from semantics	Word meanings	Activates orthographic forms of words	Orthographic forms of words
Accessing lexical orthography from lexical phonology	Phonological representations of words	Activates orthographic forms of words from their phonological forms	Orthographic forms of words
Accessing sublexical orthography from sublexical phonology	Phonological units (phonemes, other units)	Activates orthographic units corresponding to phonological units	Orthographic units in words and nonwords
Accessing lexical phonology from whole-word orthography	Orthographic forms of words	Activates phonological forms of words from their orthographic forms	Phonological forms of words
Accessing sublexical phonology from orthography	Orthographic units (graphemes, other units)	Activates phonological units corresponding to orthographic units	Phonological units in words and nonwords

Table II

Components of the Language Processing System for Derived Words and Sentences[a]

Component	Input	Operation	Output
		Processing affixed words	
Accessing morphological form	Word forms	Segments words into structural (morphological) units; activates syntactic features of words	Morphological structure; syntactic features
Morphological comprehension	Word meanings; morphological structure	Combines word roots and affixes	Meanings of morphologically complex words
Accessing affixed words from semantics	Word meanings; syntactic features	Activates forms of affixes and function words	Forms of affixes and function words
		Sentence-level processing	
Lexico inferential processing	Meanings of simple and complex words; world knowledge	Infers aspects of sentence meaning on basis of pragmatic plausibility	Aspects of propositional meaning (thematic roles, attribution of modifiers)
Syntactic comprehension	Word meanings; syntactic features	Constructs syntactic representation and combines it with word meanings	Propositional meaning
Construction of sentence form	Word forms; propositional meaning	Constructs syntactic structures; inserts word forms into structures	Sentence form (including positions of lexical items)

[a]Collapsed over auditory–oral and written modalities

Tables I and II and Figs. 1 and 2 outline the way information—in this case, sets of related linguistic representations—flows through the tasks of speaking, understanding spoken language, reading, and writing. The model depicted in these tables and figures simplifies this information flow in three ways: (i) It does not specify the nature of the operations in each of the major components of the system, (ii) it does not fully convey the extent to which the components of the system operate in parallel, and (iii) it does not convey the extent of feedback among the components of the system. Despite these simplifications, the model captures enough aspects of information processing in the language system to constitute an adequate starting place for a psycholinguistic approach to the neural basis of language.

The operations of the language processing system are regulated by a variety of control mechanisms, including both those internal to the language processor and those that are involved in other aspects of cognition. The first category, language-internal control mechanisms, probably consists of a large number of operations that schedule psycholinguistic operations on the basis of the ongoing nature of a given psycholinguistic task. The second category of control

mechanisms, those that are related to cognitive processing outside the language system, determines what combinations of processors become active in order to accomplish different tasks, such as reading, repeating what one has heard, and taking notes on a lecture.

Processing components are activated in serial and in parallel to accomplish language tasks such as reading a word aloud, producing a spoken sentence, and writing a word from dictation. Different tasks require different processors. For instance, referring to Table I and Fig. 1, reading a word aloud can be accomplished in several ways. All these "reading routes" begin with the processor that recognizes visual patterns as letters. One route then uses these letter identities to activate phonological units, which are assembled into a pronunciation. A second route uses letter identities to activate the orthographic forms of words, which in turn activate the phonological forms of words. A third route also activates the orthographic forms of words, which in turn activate meanings of words, and these then lead to the activation of the phonological forms of words. In all cases, the resulting phonological sequence is sent to the processor labeled "output phonological

COMPREHENSION

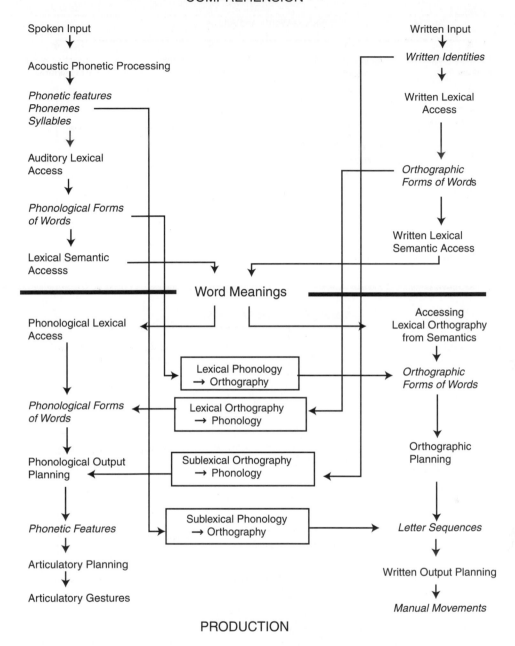

Figure 1 A model of the language processing system for single words. Processing components, indicated in boxes, activate linguistic representations in the sequences indicated by arrows. [from Caplan (1992). *Language, Structure, Processing, and Disorders*. Reproduced with permission of MIT press].

planning" to be turned into a form appropriate to activate motor speech activity. These three routes are thought to become active simultaneously. The processors used in reading aloud can be used in other language tasks. For instance, the processors involved

in activating the phonological forms of words from their meanings and in output phonological planning are also used in naming pictures.

Functional communication involving the language code occurs when people use these processors to

COMPREHENSION

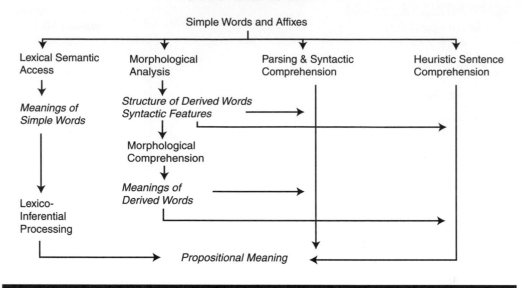

Simple Words and Affixes

| Lexical Semantic Access | Morphological Analysis | Parsing & Syntactic Comprehension | Heuristic Sentence Comprehension |

Meanings of Simple Words

Structure of Derived Words Syntactic Features

Morphological Comprehension

Lexico-Inferential Processing

Meanings of Derived Words

Propositional Meaning

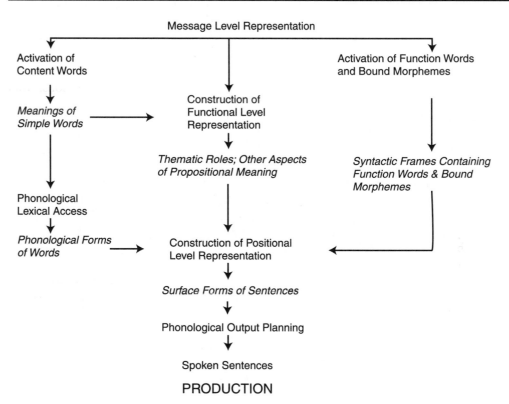

Message Level Representation

Activation of Content Words

Activation of Function Words and Bound Morphemes

Meanings of Simple Words

Construction of Functional Level Representation

Thematic Roles; Other Aspects of Propositional Meaning

Syntactic Frames Containing Function Words & Bound Morphemes

Phonological Lexical Access

Phonological Forms of Words

Construction of Positional Level Representation

Surface Forms of Sentences

Phonological Output Planning

Spoken Sentences

PRODUCTION

Figure 2 A model of the language processing system for derived words and sentences. Processing components, activate linguistic representations in the sequences indicated by arrows. [from Caplan (1992). *Language, Structure, Processing, and Disorders*. Reproduced with permission of MIT press].

undertake language-related tasks to accomplish specific goals—to inform others, to ask for information, to get things done, etc. It was previously noted that language is subject to control from other cognitive domains; conversely, one of the most important functions of language is to operate as a control mechanism for both intra- and interpersonal thought and action.

III. OVERVIEW OF NEURAL STRUCTURES SUPPORTING LANGUAGE

There is evidence that language processing involves the perisylvian association cortex—the pars triangularis and opercularis of the inferior frontal gyrus [Brodman's areas (BA) 45 and 44 (Broca's area)], the angular gyrus (BA39), the supramarginal gyrus (BA40), and the superior temporal gyrus (BA22: Wernicke's area)—in the dominant hemisphere. Data regarding the functional neuroanatomy of language processing were originally derived from deficit–lesion correlations and, recently, have been obtained from functional neuroimaging and electrophysiological studies in normal subjects. All these sources of data indicate that the perisylvian association cortex is involved in this function.

Patients with lesions in parts of this cortex have been described who have had long-lasting impairments of this function. Disorders affecting language processing after perisylvian lesions have been described in all languages that have been studied, in patients of all ages, with written and spoken input, and after a variety of lesion types, indicating that this cortical region is involved in syntactic processing, independent of these factors. Functional neuroimaging studies have documented increases in regional cerebral blood flow (rCBF) using positron emission tomography (PET) or blood oxygenation level-dependent (BOLD) signal using functional magnetic resonance imaging (fMRI) in tasks in associated with language processing. Event-related potentials (ERPs) whose sources are likely to be in this region have been described in relationship to a variety of language processing operations. Stimulation of this cortex by direct application electrical current during neurosurgical procedures interrupts language processing. From these data, it can be concluded that language processing is carried out in the dominant perisylvian cortex.

Regions outside the perisylvian association cortex might also support language processing. Working outwards from the perisylvian region, there is evidence that the modality of language use affects the location of the neural tissue that supports language, with written language involving cortex closer to the visual areas of the brain and sign language involving brain regions closer to those involved in movements of the hands than movements of the oral cavity and its contents. Some ERP components related to processing improbable or ill-formed language are maximal over high parietal and central scalp electrodes. This may suggest that these regions are involved in language processing, but two factors have to be considered before such a conclusion is drawn: The location in the brain of the tissue that generates an ERP wave is not easy to identify on the basis of the scalp location of that wave and may not be right below that wave, and some of these waves may reflect general processes related to detection of pragmatically implausible or unlikely events in general, not language processing per se.

Both lesion studies in stroke patients and functional neuroimaging studies suggest that the anterior temporal lobe, primarily in the dominant hemisphere, is involved in aspects of language processing. The leading candidate for such a function is the accessing of the sounds of words from their meanings in speech production. However, electrocortical stimulation studies and the effects of neurosurgical resections do not support this conclusion. On the other hand, both functional neuroimaging and electrocortical stimulation studies indicate that the inferior temporal lobe is involved in aspects of word processing, particularly the representation of meanings of nouns. Activation studies implicate the frontal lobe just in front of Broca's area in word meaning as well, although these activations may reflect switching sets rather than processing semantic representations. Injury to the supplementary motor cortex along the medial surface of the frontal lobe can lead to speech initiation disturbances; this region may be important in activating the language processing system, at least in production tasks. Activation studies have shown increased rCBF and BOLD signal in the cingulate gyrus in association with many language tasks. This activation, however, appears to be nonspecific because it occurs in many other, nonlinguistic, tasks as well. It has been suggested that it is due to increased arousal and deployment of attention associated with more complex tasks. The cerebellum also has increased rCBF in some activation studies involving both language and other cognitive functions. This may be a result of the role of this part of the brain in processes involved in timing and temporal ordering of events or because it is involved in many cognitive functions.

Subcortical structures may also be involved in language processing. Several studies report aphasic disturbances following strokes in the deep gray matter nuclei (the caudate, putamen, and parts of the thalamus), but studies of other diseases affecting the same nuclei fail to show significant language impairments. For instance, aphasias follow some caudate strokes, but language disorders are minimal in patients with Huntington's disease, even at the stage of the illness at which memory impairments are readily documented. It has been suggested that subcortical structures involved in laying down procedural memories for motor functions, particularly the basal ganglia, are involved in "rule-based" processing in language, such as regular aspects of word formation, as opposed to the long-term maintenance of information in memory, as occurs with simple words and irregularly formed words.

Some abnormal language behaviors seen after deep gray matter lesions probably reflect the effects of disturbances in other cognitive functions on language. An example of this is the fluctuation between neologistic jargon and virtual mutism seen after some thalamic lesions. This corresponds to a more general fluctuation between states of delirium and near akinetic mutism, and it most likely reflects the effects of some thalamic lesions on arousal, alerting, and motivational functions, some of which are seen in the sphere of language. Intraoperative stimulation studies of the interference with language functions following dominant thalamic stimulation also suggest that the language impairments seen in at least some thalamic cases are due to disturbances of attentional mechanisms. Perhaps the most important consideration regarding language disorders following subcortical lesions is the question of whether they result from altered physiological activity in the overlying cortex and not from disorders of the subcortical structures. In general, subcortical lesions cause language impairments when the overlying cortex is abnormal (often, the abnormality can only be seen with metabolic scanning techniques), and the degree of language impairment is much better correlated with measures of cortical rather than subcortical hypometabolism. It may be that subcortical structures serve to activate the language processing system but do not process language.

The other major component of the subcortical region of the cerebral hemispheres is the white matter. White matter tracts transmit representations from one area to another. Lesions of white matter tracts disconnect regions of the brain from others and make the operations performed in one region unavailable to others. This can cause language disorders. The best known such disturbance is a pure alexia, in which a patient can write but not read–not even his or her own writing. This can result from a lesion that destroys the primary visual cortex in the dominant hemisphere and extends forward in the white matter to cut off visual information coming to the nondominant hemisphere from the dominant hemisphere language area. In addition to these "disconnection" syndromes, lan-

guage disturbances of all sorts occur with lesions affecting many white matter tracts, whereas sparing of language functions can follow lesions in identical subcortical areas. The fact that multiple language processing disturbances occur following subcortical strokes affecting white matter is consistent with the existence of many information transfers carried out by white matter fibers, suggesting that many of the areas of cortex and/or subcortical nuclei that carry out sequential language processing operations are not contiguous.

In summary, a large number of brain regions are involved in representing and processing language. Ultimately, they all interact with one another as well as with other brain areas involved in using the products of language processing to accomplish tasks. In this sense, all these regions are part of a "neural system," but this concept should not obscure the fact that many of these regions appear to compute specific linguistic representations in particular tasks. The most important of these regions is the dominant perisylvian cortex.

IV. ORGANIZATION OF THE PERISYLVIAN CORTEX FOR LANGUAGE PROCESSING

Two general classes of theories of the relationship of portions of the perisylvian association cortex to components of the language processing system have been developed—one based on "holist" or distributed views of neural function and one based on localizationist principles. Although theories within each of these two major groupings vary, there are a number of features common to theories within each class.

The basic tenet of holist/distributed theories of the functional neuroanatomy for language is that linguistic representations are distributed widely and that language processing conmponents rely on broad areas of perisylvian association cortex. Karl Lashley identified two functional features of holist/distributed models that determine the effects of lesions on performance: equipotentiality (every portion of a particular brain region can carry out a specific function in every individual) and mass action (the larger the neuronal pool that carries out a particular function, the more efficiently that function is accomplished). The features of equipotentiality and mass action jointly entail that lesions of similar sizes anywhere in a specified brain region have equivalent effects on function, and that the magnitude of any functional deficit is directly proportional to the size of a lesion in this specified area. Recently, models of lesions in parallel distributed processing simulations of language and other cognitive functions have provided a mathematical basis for these properties of these systems.

All the traditional theories that postulate localization of components of the language processing system maintain the view that, discounting lateralization, the localization of components of the language processing system is invariant across the normal adult population. Thus, all the traditional localizationist theories have as a corollary that lesions in particular areas of the perisylvian association cortex interrupt the same language processing components in all individuals. Many localizationist theories also maintain that the specific localization of language processing components results from a computational advantage inherent in juxtaposing particular language processing components to each other or to cortex supporting arousal, sensory, and motor processes. Modern localizationist models relax these assertions, incorporating the ideas of individual variability and some degree of specialization wthin large-scale neural nets.

Because of the plethora of specific theories within each of these two general camps, it is impossible to critically review the empirical basis of all theories that have present-day adherents. I focus on the most widely cited theories as examples of each class.

A. Holist Theories

Unlike narrow localizationist theories, there is no one holist model that has emerged as the major example of this class of theories. However, several lines of evidence are adduced as evidence for holist theories, and all holist theories suffer from similar inadequacies in accounting for certain empirical findings.

The first line of evidence supporting holist theories consists of the ubiquity of general factors in accounting for the performance of aphasic patients. For instance, factor analyses of the performances of groups of patients both on general aphasia tests and on tests of specific language abilities almost always result in first eigenvectors (usually accounting for more than half of the variance in performance) that are approximately equally weighted for most of the subtests used to test the population. Such vectors are usually taken to reflect disruption of a single factor that affects performance on all measures, such as a limited amount of mental resources available for psycholinguistic computations. The existence of such factors would be the immediate consequence of a system in which functions were disruptable by lesions in a variety of locations, and they have therefore been widely taken as evidence for a distributed basis for language functions. A second finding supporting holist theories is the frequent observation of so-called "graceful degradation" of performance within specific language domains after brain damage. An example of such degradation is the strong tendency of certain dyslexic patients to read irregularly spelled words according to a regularization strategy (e.g., "pint" is read with a short "i"), a tendency that is inversely proportional to the frequency of the word. Graceful degradation reflects the preservation of the simplest (in many cases, the most commonly occurring) aspects of language processing after brain damage. Modern work with parallel distributed processing models, which provide formal models of holist concepts, indicates that such patterns of performance can arise following focal lesions in systems in which information is represented and processed in massively parallel, distributed forms. A third source of empirical support for holist theories comes from the finding of an effect of lesion size on the overall severity of functional impairments in several language spheres. This would follow from the principle of mass action. Therefore, these results therefore are consistent with some form of holism in the neural basis for linguistic representations and processes.

Against the complete adequacy of any holist model is the finding that multiple individual language deficits arise in patients with small perisylvian lesions, often in complementary functional spheres. For instance, studies of acquired dyslexia have documented patients who cannot read by a whole-word route (i.e., by using the entire form of a written word to gain access to the mental representation of that word) and others who cannot read by the application of spelling–sound correspondences at the letter and grapheme level. The existence of these isolated complementary deficits in different single cases indicates that at least one abnormal performance cannot result from the relative complexity of processing required by one of these tasks. Double dissociations of this sort abound in the contemporary psycholinguistic aphasiological literature. They indicate that the mode of organization of language in the brain must be one that allows focal lesions to disrupt specific aspects of psycholinguistic processing, not simply a mode of organization that produces complexity effects and degrades gracefully. Although some selective disruptions of function can occur when "lesions" are produced in simulated language processing systems that operate in parallel and distributed fashion, to date no mechanism of lesioning a distributed neural system has been shown to produce the range of specific patterns of language breakdown observed in patients.

B. Localizationist Theories

Although many localizationist models exist, the connectionist model of language representation and processing in the brain, revived by Norman Geschwind and colleagues in the 1960s and 1970s, is probably the best known localizationist model of the functional neuroanatomy of language, at least in medical circles in North America. This model is based on observations of aphasic patients and the interpretation of those observations that were first made more than a century ago.

Figure 3 represents the basic connectionist model of auditory-oral language processing and its relation to areas within the dominant perisylvian cortex. This model postulates three basic "centers" for language processing, all in cerebral cortex. The first (Fig. 3A), located in Wernicke's area, stores the permanent representations for the sounds of words (what psycholinguists would now call a "phonological lexicon"). The second (Fig. 3M), located in Broca's area, houses the mechanisms responsible for planning and programming speech. The third (Fig. 3C), diffusely localized in cortex in the 19th-century models, stores the representations of concepts. A major innovation proposed by Geschwind is in the location of one aspect of the concept center. Geschwind proposed that the inferior parietal lobule—the supramarginal and angular gyri—is the location at which the fibers projecting from somesthetic, visual, and auditory association cortices all converge and that as a consequence of this

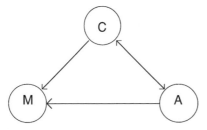

Figure 3 The classical connectionist model. A represents the auditory center for the long-term storage of word sounds. M represents the motor center for speech planning, and C represents the concept center. Information flow is indicated by arrows. The location of these centers in the brain is described in the text.

convergence, associations between word sounds and the sensory properties of objects can be established in this area. Geschwind argued that these associations are critical aspects of the meanings of words and that their establishment is a prerequisite of the ability to name objects.

Language processing in this model involves the activation of linguistic representations in these cortical centers and the transfer of these representations from one center to another, largely via white matter tracts. For instance, in auditory comprehension, the representations of the sound patterns of words are accessed in Wernicke's area following auditory presentation of language stimuli. These auditory representations of the sounds of words in turn evoke the concepts associated with words in the "concept center." Accessing the phonological representation of words and the subsequent concepts associated with these representations constitutes the function of comprehension of auditory language. In spoken language production, concepts access the phonological representations of words in Wernicke's area, which are then transmitted to the motor programming areas for speech in Broca's area. In most versions of this model, the proper execution of the speech act also depends on Broca's area receiving input directly from the concept center. Repetition, reading, and writing are modeled as involving similar sequences of activation of centers via connections.

Recently, these aphasic syndromes have been related to the brain using a series of neuroimaging techniques—first T^{99} scanning and then computed tomography MRI, and PET. All have confirmed the relationship of the major syndromes to lesion locations. Broca's aphasia is associated with anterior lesions; Wernicke's aphasia is associated with posterior lesions, centered in the temporal–parietal juncture; pure motor deficits of speech are associated with subcortical lesions; pure word deafness is associated with lesions in the auditory association areas and surrounding white matter tracts, often bilaterally; transcortical motor and transcortical sensory aphasia are associated with watershed infarcts between the anterior and middle cerebral arteries and middle and posterior cerebral arteries; and conduction aphasia is associated with smaller lesions that often appear to affect the arcuate fasciculus. However, despite these general correlations, the classical aphasic syndromes are not as well correlated with lesion sites as the theory claims they should be. Virtually all studies exclude many types of lesions, such as various sorts of tumors, degenerative diseases, and others.

The classical syndromes are best related to lesion sites in cases of rapidly developing lesions, such as stroke. Even in these types of lesions, the syndromes are never applied to acute and subacute phases of the illness and, in the chronic phase of diseases such as stroke, between 15 and 40% of patients have lesions that are not predictable from their syndromes.

Lesion-deficit correlations have been studied in patients with more specific functional impairments than are captured by the classic aphasic syndromes (e.g., semantic memory, whole-word writing and the conversion of sounds to their corresponding orthographic units, short-term memory, and word comprehension). For the most part, these studies have involved relatively small numbers of subjects because of the difficulty in obtaining large numbers of subjects with specific deficits. For instance, one study of disorders affecting semantic memory in stroke patients could only identify three patients with a selective deficit in this function from the many patients that were screened; many other patients had problems in naming objects or in matching spoken words to pictures but not with semantic memory.

These more focused studies have provided evidence for localization of function, but the picture that emerges is complex. The localizations found have often not been consistent with the classical connectionist model. For instance, semantic memory (word meaning) appears to be disrupted after temporal, not inferior parietal, damage, and auditory–verbal short-term memory appears to be disrupted after parietal, not temporal, lesions.

An important aspect of the database relating specific language functional deficits to lesions is the finding that individual components of the language processing system can be either affected or spared following lesions in particular parts of the perisylvian association cortex. This variability in the effects of lesions at particular sites ranges across all areas of the perisylvian association cortex and is true of components of the language processing system responsible for activating any of the linguistic representations described in Section I (i.e., lexical, morphological, and sentential representations). For instance, most studies have reported phoneme discrimination deficits after both anterior and posterior lesions, in both real words and in computer-synthesized stimuli. At the same time, some studies have found that most lesions producing these impairments occur with posterior lesions. Similar individual variability has been documented in the localization of the lesions responsible for the comprehension of single words, the production of morphological forms, aspects of sentence comprehension, the production of function words in sentence production, and the production of phonemic errors in spontaneous speech, picture naming, repetition, and reading, in some cases with "central tendencies" toward deficits following lesions in specific locations. This pattern has led some rsearchers to view the entire perisylvian cortex as a neural net that supports all aspects of language processing, with some degree of specialization of parts of this net for specific functions. Models of this type cannot account for severe impairments of a single langauge operation following small lesions in different parts of this region in different individuals, however.

The finding of variability in the effects of lesions on language functions also emerges from electrocortical stimulation studies, which have studied phoneme discrimination, picture naming, sentence comprehension, and other language functions. Each of these language tasks was most likely to be interrupted with stimulation in particular regions of the perisylvian cortex across all patients, but considerable variation in sites associated with interruption of each task was also noted. For instance, phoneme discrimination was interrupted by stimulation throughout the entire central region of the perisylvian association cortex in approximately 80% of cases and in sites within the language zone that are further removed from the Sylvian fissure (such as the more dorsal regions of the inferior parietal lobule) in the remaining 20% of cases.

This variability suggests that language operations are localized in small parts of the perisylvian association cortex, but that the areas in which they are localized are different in different people. The fact that lesions restricted to specific parts of the perisylvian cortex are each associated with all levels of performance of a language processing operation, from normal performance to the worst performances seen in aphasic patients, implies that for some individuals a lesion in each of these lobar regions does not affect the operation at all, whereas for others some or all of the operation is impaired by a lesion in the same region. It is difficult to understand how this could result from anything other than individual variability in the premorbid location of these operations.

On the other hand, to the extent that specific lesions tend to be associated with certain deficits, as may be the case for some impairments, these studies also support the view that there are central tendencies in the localization of these language processing components within the perisylvian cortex. A reasonable conjecture is that the functional neuroanatomy of language in the perisylvian association cortex has three features: (i) localization of language functions in individuals, (ii) tendencies for functions to be localized in specific portions of the perisylvian association cortex, and (iii) at least 20% of normal adults (and often many more) showing significant deviations from these central localizationist tendencies for each language processing component.

In the past 10 years, a considerable number of studies of the neural correlates of language processing have been published that employed PET, fMRI, and other "activation" techniques. As noted previously, some of these studies have led to the appreciation of possible roles for brain regions outside the perisylvian cortex in carrying out language operations. These studies also provide evidence about the organization of the perisylvian cortex for language. Many studies claim to find evidence for the localization of particular language representations, such as the phonological forms of words used in speech recognition, or language operations, such as transforming letters into their corresponding sounds, in particular parts of this cortex. Some of these localizations depend on specific tasks; for instance, the exact part of the perisylvian cortex in which blood flow changes during tasks that require comparison of sequences of phonemes has varied considerably in different studies in which different tasks were used. In other cases, there is more consensus about the areas that increase their vascular responses as a function of particular operations. Verbal rehearsal, which appears to involve Broca's area and adjacent parts of the frontal lobe, and maintenance of phonological representations in verbal short-term memory, which seems to activate the inferior parietal lobe, are examples of such functions; however, even here, different studies show some variation in the areas activated. Very few studies have examined patterns of vascular responsivity in individual subjects, which will be necessary to address the issue of variability. Much more work using these techniques can be expected, with consequent increases in the database relevant to our understanding of these issues.

V. LATERALIZATION

Most language processing occurs in one hemisphere called the "dominant" hemisphere. Which hemisphere is dominant shows considerable individual differences, which bear a systematic relationship to handedness. In approximately 98% of right-handed individuals, the left hemisphere is dominant, with the extent to which left hemisphere lesions cause language disorders influenced by the degree to which an individual is right-handed and the number of non-right-handeders in his or her family. Approximately 60–65% of the non-right-handed individuals are left hemisphere dominant, approximately 15–20% are right hemisphere dominant, and the remainder appear to use both hemispheres for language processing. The relationship of dominance for language to handedness suggests a common determination of both, probably in large part genetic (although the nature of the genetic effect remains unclear).

Although language was the first function known to be lateralized and is still the best example of a lateralized function, it is not completely lateralized. Although not as important in language functioning as the dominant hemisphere, the nondominant hemisphere is involved in many language operations. Evidence from the effects of lesions and split-brain studies, experiments using presentation of stimuli to one or the other hemisphere in normal subjects, and activation studies indicates that the nondominant hemisphere understands many words, especially concrete nouns, and suggests that it is involved in other aspects of language processing as well, such as syntactic processing. Some language operations may be carried out primarily in the right hemisphere. The best candidates for these operations are ones that pertain to processing the discourse level of language, interpreting nonliteral language such as metaphors, and appreciating the tone of a discourse as is manifest in, for instance, its being humorous. Some scientists have developed models of the sorts of processing that the right hemisphere carries out. For instance, it has been suggested that the right hemisphere codes information in a course way compared to the left hemisphere. This and other suggestions provide the bases for ongoing research programs on the nature of language processing in the right hemisphere.

Lateralization of language functions can be seen as a broad form of localization—the localization of a function in one of the two cerebral hemispheres. As noted previously, lateralization varies as a function of handedness and even within populations with similar handedness profiles. These facts suggest intriguing similarities between the phenomena of localization and lateralization of language. In both localization and lateralization, the location of a particular language processing component varies across the adult population as a whole. In both cases, however, there are central tendencies with respect to the location of particular language processing components: There appear to be preferred sites for particular language processing functions within the perislyvian region, and there is a strong preference for language processing components to be left hemisphere based. These patterns would result from any area of either perisylvian association cortex being capable of supporting any subcomponent of the language processing system at the initial stage of language development, and from different areas of cortex assuming particular language processing roles as a function of intrinsic, genetically determined, developmental patterns, modified by other factors such as the internal organic milieu and the nature of exposure to language.

VI. CONCLUSION

Our newly acquired abilities to identify specific language processing deficits in patients, to characterize lesions with modern imaging techniques, and to use technologies such as intraoperative electrocortical stimulation, event-related potentials, and metabolic scanning to study the neural basis for language position us to investigate the neural basis for language at a level of detail previously unattainable. Research

using these techniques is likely to continue to change our ideas of the way the human brain supports language functions.

See Also the Following Articles

APHASIA • BROCA'S AREA • INFORMATION PROCESSING • LANGUAGE ACQUISITION • LANGUAGE AND LEXICAL PROCESSING • LANGUAGE DISORDERS • LATERALITY • READING DISORDERS, DEVELOPMENTAL • SPEECH • WERNICKE'S AREA

Suggested Reading

Caplan, D. (1987). *Neurolinguistics and Linguistic Aphasiology.* Cambridge Univ. Press, Cambridge, UK.

Caplan, D. (1992). *Language, Structure, Processing, and Disorders.* MIT Press, Cambridge, MA.

Caplan, D. (1994). Language and the brain. In *Handbook of Psycholinguistics* (Gernsbacher, Ed.), pp. 1023–1074. Academic Press, New York.

Damasio, A. R., and Damasio, H. (1992). Brain and language. *Sci. Am.* **267,** 88–95.

Dronkers, N., Pinker, S., and Damasio, A. R. (2000). Language and the aphasias. In *Principles of Neural Science* (E. R. Kandell, J. H. Schwartz, and T. W. Jessell, Eds.), Appleton & Lange, Norwalk, CT.

Geschwind, N. (1979). Specializations of the human brain. *Sci. Am.* **170,** 940–944.

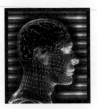

Laterality

JOSEPH B. HELLIGE

University of Southern California

GLOSSARY

corpus callosum Largest fiber tract that connects the left and right cerebral hemispheres.

handedness The tendency to prefer the use of one hand over the other and for motor performance to be better for the preferred hand.

hemispheric asymmetry Biological and functional differences between the left and right sides of the cerebral cortex.

hemisphericity Indication of the extent to which an individual is more reliant on the left or on the right cerebral hemisphere, inferred from measurement of the individual's cognitive skills and biases.

laterality Behavioral and biological manifestations of left–right brain differences or of hemispheric asymmetry.

manual praxis Purposeful, sequential actions in which spatial constraints imposed by the environment are minimal.

planum temporale Cortical area located on the superior surface of the temporal lobe posterior to the transverse auditory gyrus of Heschl.

split-brain patients Individuals whose left and right cerebral hemispheres have been surgically disconnected by severing the corpus callosum and other connecting fibers.

Sylvian fissure Deep groove on the lateral surfaces of the cerebral hemispheres that marks the boundary between the frontal and parietal lobes above and the temporal lobe below.

Laterality refers to the behavioral and biological manifestations of asymmetry between the left and right cerebral hemispheres. The cerebral cortex of the human brain is divided anatomically into two hemispheres, the left and the right. Although the two hemispheres are similar in appearance and structure, they are not biologically identical and they have different information processing abilities and propensities. This article provides an overview of this brain laterality and its consequences for perception, cognition, emotion, and action.

I. LEARNING ABOUT LATERALITY: TECHNIQUES AND TOOLS

Brain laterality has been studied in a variety of populations using several research techniques and tools. In fact, the existence of so many converging techniques is a very positive feature of research in this area. I begin by reviewing the major techniques on which later conclusions rest and, for the sake of example, indicate briefly how each technique provides information about laterality for aspects of human language. The oldest technique for studying brain–behavior relationships is the observation of behavioral deficits after localized brain damage. If the brain were completely symmetric in terms of structure and function, then injury to homologous areas of the two hemispheres should have equivalent effects. However, this is not the case. For example, specific language

Copyright 2002, Elsevier Science (USA).
All rights reserved.

deficits are more common and more severe after damage to certain temporal and parietal areas of the left hemisphere than after injury to corresponding areas of the right hemisphere. The deficits for which this is true include speech production and perception, phonetic analysis of printed text, the use of syntactic cues, and access to certain types of word meaning. As discussed later, certain other deficits (e.g., processing intonation cues) are associated more with right hemisphere damage. This is important because such double dissociations rule out the possibility that the left hemisphere is simply dominant for everything. Note that identification of deficits after localized brain damage can indicate the extent to which an area within one hemisphere is necessary for performing a particular task or executing a particular process. However, such studies do not indicate the extent to which one hemisphere is sufficient for performing the task or process or that the impaired process is localized within the damaged area.

Dramatic demonstrations of brain laterality come from the study of so-called split-brain patients whose hemispheres have been surgically disconnected in order to control the spread of epileptic seizures. This is done by cutting the corpus callosum, the largest fiber tract connecting the two hemispheres, as well as other connecting fibers. By using clever techniques of stimulus presentation and response measurement it is possible to examine the positive competence of each hemisphere in split-brain patients and thereby identify tasks and processes for which each isolated hemisphere is sufficient. These techniques take advantage of the fact that human sensory projections are organized so that input from one side of the body or one side of space is transmitted directly to the contralateral cerebral hemisphere. This includes sensory input from fingers of the left and right hands, the left and right halves of each retina (so that each visual half field projects directly to the contralateral visual cortex) and, under appropriate conditions, the left and right ears. With respect to certain aspects of language, the study of split-brain patients indicates that the isolated left hemisphere is far more competent than the isolated right hemisphere. For example, a split-brain patient can say the name of a common object (e.g., pencil) when it is placed into the right hand or when its picture or printed name is projected to the right visual field (i.e., to the left hemisphere) but not when it is placed into the left hand or when its picture or printed name is projected to the left visual field (i.e., to the right hemisphere). Of course, generalizing from such patients to neurologically intact individuals is tricky, in part because brain laterality may not operate the same way in the presence of extensive interhemispheric connections.

In neurologically intact individuals, it is not possible to test the competence of each hemisphere in isolation, but it is possible to measure speed and accuracy of performance as a function of which hemisphere receives information directly and must at least initiate processing. The techniques for studying this sort of behavioral laterality in neurologically intact individuals are the same as those used to lateralize stimuli for split-brain patients. When used with appropriate methodological care, such studies provide an important converging technique for learning about functional hemispheric asymmetry in the intact brain. Although often smaller, laterality effects in intact individuals are typically in the same direction as those found in split-brain patients. For example, there is a right visual field (left hemisphere) advantage for the identification of printed words and nonwords as well as a right ear (left hemisphere) advantage for the identification of spoken words and syllables.

In recent years there have been significant advances in brain imaging techniques that permit measurement of various structures in the living brain and of the relative amounts of neural activity in different cortical regions as individuals perform experimental tasks. The techniques include computerized axial tomography scans, magnetic resonance imaging (MRI) and functional MRI, measures of regional cerebral blood flow, positron emission tomography scans, event-related potentials, and magnetoencephalography. Among other things, brain imaging has provided a great deal of converging information about brain laterality. Later, I discuss certain well-established structural asymmetries as well as individual variation in the size of the corpus callosum. With respect to language, functional imaging techniques have shown greater activation in temporoparietal areas of the left hemisphere than in the right hemisphere when normal individuals speak, identify printed words, and so forth, with the specific areas of greatest activation depending on exactly which processes are relevant to the task. Furthermore, monitoring a list of words for semantic content also produces activation of frontal areas within the left hemisphere. In addition, verbal working memory tasks produce primarily left hemisphere activation, whereas spatial working memory tasks produce primarily right hemisphere activation. Of course, increased activity in a specific brain area does not indicate exactly what that area is doing or how well it is doing it. Nor is it possible to determine whether increased activation reflects excitatory or inhibitory neural processes. Nevertheless, functional imaging techniques have produced important results that are consistent with conclusions suggested by classical neuropsychology and clearly constitute a converging operation that will grow in importance.

II. BEHAVIORAL ASYMMETRIES IN HUMANS: LATERALITY FOR COMPONENTS OF ACTION AND COGNITION

The tools and techniques described in the preceding section have been used to identify and confirm a great many behavioral asymmetries in humans. Before summarizing a number of the most well-established asymmetries, it is useful to consider three general characteristics of laterality effects: ubiquity, subtlety, and complementarity. Ubiquity refers to the fact that the two cerebral hemispheres have different levels of ability and different processing propensities in a great many domains. In this section, I review examples in the domains of motor activity, language, perception, and emotion. Subtlety refers to the fact that it is rarely the case that one hemisphere can perform a task or accomplish a specific process quite well, whereas the other hemisphere cannot perform the task or process at all. Instead, both hemispheres typically have some ability, though they may go about a task in different ways and one hemisphere may do a better job than the other. A notable exception to this is speech production, which tends to be controlled exclusively by a single hemisphere (usually the left). Complementarity refers to the fact that in many domains, the roles for which each hemisphere is dominant can be described as complementary. Consequently, both hemispheres normally play a role in virtually all complex activities, such as understanding language or identifying faces, with their contributions fitting together like two pieces of a puzzle. Several examples of complementarity are given in the remainder of this article.

The most obvious behavioral asymmetry in humans is handedness, with approximately 92% of women and 88% of men favoring and being more proficient with the right hand for performing a variety of skilled activities, such as writing, drawing, eating, and using a needle to sew. Of the remaining non-right-handed individuals a few exhibit strong and consistent left-handedness, a few are truly ambidextrous, and others show hand preferences that vary from one skilled activity to another. In general, for both right-handed

and left-handed individuals, hand differences are weaker for unskilled activities such as picking up a small object. Furthermore, for tasks that require the coordinated activity of both hands, their roles are often complementary. In general, for right-handed individuals the left hand (controlled by the right hemisphere) performs movements of relatively low spatial and temporal frequency, whereas the right hand (controlled by the left hemisphere) performs movements of relatively high spatial and temporal frequency. An example of this complimentary arrangement is handwriting, during which the left hand arranges and steadies the paper while the right hand makes more frequent and smaller movements with the writing instrument. Though handedness is the most obvious example, there are also other motoric asymmetries. For example, for right-handed individuals the left side of the body is frequently preferred for postural support. In addition, the right side of the face (controlled by the left hemisphere) is superior for making certain oral movements associated with language and other precisely sequenced activities, whereas the left side of the face (controlled by the right hemisphere) is more emotionally expressive.

Left hemisphere dominance for many aspects of language is the most obvious and cited asymmetry outside of the motor domain. From clinical neurological data as well as other sources, it is estimated that speech production is limited to the left hemisphere in approximately 95% of right-handed individuals. As noted in the preceding discussion of research tools and techniques, the left hemisphere is also dominant for many aspects of language perception and for the verbal processing of stimulus material, although in these cases left hemisphere superiority is more a matter of degree than of the all-or-none asymmetry that is characteristic of speech production. In addition, when we consider understanding language for the purpose of communication, there is growing evidence that both hemispheres make important contributions. Whereas the left hemisphere is dominant for the perception of phonetic information, for the use of syntax and for certain aspects of semantic processing, the right hemisphere is dominant for processing the sort of intonation cues and prosody that communicate such things as emotional tone (e.g., anger versus surprise). The right hemisphere is also involved in processing narrative-level linguistic information. Some of these complementary, language-related asymmetries may be related to hemispheric differences in the efficiency of processing different aspects of acoustic signals. For example, identification of many spoken phonemes requires efficient processing of rapid changes in the acoustic signal over brief periods of time, a type of processing for which the left hemisphere is hypothesized to be superior. In contrast, identification of the emotional tone of voice requires efficient processing of much slower modulations of the acoustic signal over longer periods of time, a type of processing for which the right hemisphere is hypothesized to be superior. The two hemispheres also appear to access word meanings in complementary ways. When a word is presented, the left hemisphere restricts processing very quickly to one possible meaning, usually the dominant meaning or the meaning most consistent with the present context, whereas the right hemisphere maintains activation of multiple meanings and remotely associated words for a more extended period of time.

Neither hemisphere is uniformly superior for processing nonverbal perceptual information. Instead, both hemispheres contribute to perceptual processing and do so in ways that could be described as complementary. For example, in studies of the identification of visual patterns there is evidence of right hemisphere dominance for processing global aspects of stimuli (e.g., the outer contour of a face) and left hemisphere dominance for processing local details (e.g., small features of a face). Specifically, global and local processing are associated with the posterior superior temporal areas of the right and left hemispheres, respectively (though this may be affected by the relative sizes and perceptual clarity of the global and local levels within a stimulus). These effects may be related to hemispheric differences in the efficient use of information carried by visual channels tuned to relatively high versus relatively low spatial frequencies. Specifically, the left and right hemispheres are biased toward more efficient use of higher and lower frequencies, respectively, with at least three aspects of spatial frequency being relevant: the absolute range of frequencies contained in a stimulus, the range of frequencies that is most relevant for the task being performed, and whether the relevant frequencies are high or low relative to other frequencies contained in the stimuli used in the experiment. It has been hypothesized that analogous hemispheric differences extend to the processing of relatively high and relatively low temporal frequencies in audition and, perhaps, to movements of different temporal frequencies and spatial extent.

In the spatial domain, the brain computes at least two kinds of spatial relation representations—a categorical representation used to assign a spatial relation to a category such as "connected to" or "above" and a coordinate representation used to represent precise distances and locations. The right hemisphere makes more effective use of this latter coordinate system, whereas there is either no hemispheric difference or a left hemisphere advantage for processing categorical spatial relationships. Neural network simulations suggest that hemispheric asymmetry for making categorical versus coordinate judgments may be related to the nature of visual information that is most useful for processing categorical versus coordinate properties. For example, networks constructed to simulate relatively large overlapping receptive fields compute coordinate spatial information better than do networks constructed to simulate relatively small, nonoverlapping receptive fields. Exactly the reverse has been found for the computation of categorical spatial information. From this perspective, it is interesting that categorical spatial processing is disrupted by manipulations (blurring of stimuli) that selectively interfere with information carried by channels with small, discrete receptive fields, whereas coordinate spatial processing is disrupted by manipulations (use of a diffuse red background) that selectively interfere with information carried by channels with large, overlapping receptive fields. Additional neural network simulations have examined the possible importance of receptive field sizes for encoding information about shape. The same networks that favored coordinate spatial processing also favored coding the identify of specific shapes, whereas the same networks that favored categorical spatial processing also favored the assignment of shapes to categories. Interestingly, there is evidence of right hemisphere superiority for processing the sort of specific shape information that would be needed to distinguish among the exemplars of a single category but left hemisphere superiority for classifying the prototypes used to define different categories. Of course, it is possible to devise alternative ways of tying these different laterality effects together (e.g., in terms of left and right hemisphere attentional biases toward different ranges of spatial frequency) and more empirical as well as theoretical work is needed before we fully understand the mechanisms that underlie these complementary hemispheric specializations.

As noted earlier, the right hemisphere is superior to the left in using the intonation cues of speech to identify emotional tone of voice. The same tends to be true of identifying the emotion displayed on a face, though in both cases it is difficult to rule out interpretations in terms of the kind of auditory or visual information that is most useful for identifying emotion. With respect to the production or experience of emotions, hemispheric differences seem to be more complementary. For example, the balance of activation between the frontal lobes of the two hemispheres is related to the valence of an experienced emotion. Specifically, positive emotions are accompanied by relatively greater left hemisphere activation and negative emotions are accompanied by relatively greater right hemisphere activation. Emotions of negative versus positive valence (e.g., sadness versus happiness) are typically characterized by states of low versus high arousal, respectively, leading some researchers to suggest that it is the difference in arousal, rather than valence per se, that accounts for the observed hemispheric asymmetries.

These representative examples of behavioral asymmetries in humans are admittedly illustrative rather than exhaustive. Nevertheless, they illustrate that laterality is a pervasive characteristic of human behavior, that computational differences between the hemispheres are often subtle, and that each hemisphere makes important contributions to most aspects of behavior.

III. BIOLOGICAL ASYMMETRIES IN THE HUMAN BRAIN

At first glance, the left and right hemispheres appear to be biologically identical, leading one to wonder why there are so many functional asymmetries. However, postmortem studies of anatomy and structural imaging studies of the living brain have documented a number of consistent physical asymmetries. For example, in the majority of human brains the frontal region is wider and extends farther forward in the right hemisphere and the occipital region is wider and extends farther rearward in the left hemisphere, giving the brain a kind of counterclockwise torque. Because the temporoparietal areas of the left hemisphere are important for language, it may not be surprising that a number of anatomical and cytoarchitectonic hemispheric differences have been found in those areas. For example, consider the Sylvian fissure, which marks the boundary between the frontal and parietal lobes, which lie above the fissure, and the temporal lobe, which lies below the fissure. This fissure tends to be longer and straighter in the left hemisphere than in the right hemisphere, in which it tends to curl upward. In addition, the planum temporale, which is an extension of Wernicke's area in the left hemisphere (known to be

important for language), tends to be larger in the left hemisphere than in the right hemisphere.

There is evidence that individual variation in these structural asymmetries is related to individual variation in functional asymmetry. As noted earlier, handedness is the most obvious motoric expression of laterality. Therefore, it is interesting that the foregoing structural asymmetries are related to handedness. For example, for right-handed individuals the planum temporale is larger in the left hemisphere in approximately 65% of the cases, larger in the right hemisphere in approximately 10% of the cases, and approximately equal in 25% of the cases. The corresponding percentages for non-right-handers are approximately 25, 10, and 65%, respectively. Similar distributions characterize asymmetry of the Sylvian fissure. The ability to measure structure within the normal, living brain has also made it possible to search for relationships between structural asymmetry and a variety of other nonmotoric behavioral and perceptual asymmetries, but no clear-cut picture has emerged. Perhaps this is not surprising in view of the fact that structural characteristics revealed by contemporary imaging techniques are still relatively gross (e.g., the length of a fissure).

Despite the fact that structural characteristics such as length and size are difficult to interpret, some of the structural characteristics that have been observed are related to other aspects of individual variation. For example, the extent of leftward asymmetry of planum temporale size is greater in musicians with perfect pitch than in either nonmusicians or musicians who do not have perfect pitch. Also, although it is impossible to reach strong conclusions from the study of only one brain, there is something intriguing about the fact that neurons in areas that are known to be involved in spatial reasoning and mathematics received greater metabolic support in the brain of the great physicist Albert Einstein than in the brains of other individuals. However, it should be noted that attempts to relate structural asymmetries to other dimensions, such as sex, psychopathology, and cognitive deficit, have produced mixed results.

Though not as well established as the gross structural asymmetries, there are also indications of cytoarchitectonic and biochemical differences between the two hemispheres. For example, the extent of higher order dendritic branching seems to be greater in certain speech areas of the left hemisphere (e.g., Broca's area) than in corresponding regions of the right hemisphere. Conversely, lower order dendritic branches seem to be longer in the right hemisphere than in the left hemisphere. It has also been hypothesized that the distribution of two important neurotransmitters is asymmetric in the human brain, with dopamine being more prevalent in the left hemisphere and norepinephrine being more prevalent in the right hemisphere.

Structural imaging has also been used to study the correlates of more or less callosal connectivity between the two hemispheres by measuring such things as the midsagittal area of the corpus callosum. Although the size of the corpus callosum increases with the size of the brain, the relative extent of callosal connectivity (e.g., corpus callosum size relative to brain size) seems to decrease with increases in the size of the brain. Furthermore, there is some indication that fewer callosal fibers connect more asymmetric regions of the two hemispheres, although the functional significance of these relationships is not clear. Studies have also begun to examine the relationship between callosal connectivity as measured from brain images and various perceptual asymmetries. One hypothesis is that as the extent of callosal connectivity increases, interhemispheric transfer of information is facilitated, thereby decreasing the size of behavioral laterality effects. Despite a certain intuitive plausibility, the experimental evidence for this hypothesis is mixed, perhaps because increases in callosal connectivity also permit more inhibition from one hemisphere to the other.

IV. UNITY OF PROCESSING FROM THE LATERALIZED BRAIN: VARIETIES OF INTERHEMISPHERIC INTERACTION

One of the most striking and consistent observations in studies that involve functional brain imaging is that many areas within both brain hemispheres are activated by even very simple tasks. This reflects the fact that the behavior of neurologically intact individuals is virtually always the result of processing in both hemispheres as well as in a variety of subcortical structures. In this section, I consider a variety of ways in which the left and right hemispheres interact and the biological mechanisms that support those interactions.

The corpus callosum, with at least 200 million nerve fibers, is the largest fiber tract that connects the two cerebral hemispheres. Comparison of split-brain patients with intact individuals provides a clear indication that the corpus callosum is critical to normal interhemispheric interaction, especially interaction that requires the transfer of information about the identify or name of a stimulus. Although there are no

cortical landmarks that divide the corpus callosum, it is generally the case that different regions of the corpus callosum contain fibers originating in different cortical areas. That is, anterior portions of the corpus callosum contain primarily fibers that originate in premotor and frontal regions of the cortex, middle portions contain fibers that originate in motor and somatosensory, regions, and so forth. In addition, many callosal fibers are homotopic; that is, they connect homologous areas of the two hemispheres. An interesting hypothesis is that these fibers produce a type of homotopic inhibition at the computational level, thereby producing mirror-image patterns of activation and inhibition in the two hemispheres, which could be described as a kind of complementarity and that might contribute to the development of hemispheric asymmetry. However, the corpus callosum also contains fibers that originate in a specific region of one hemisphere and terminate in a completely different region of the opposite hemisphere, creating a mechanism whereby neural activity within one hemisphere could have more generalized excitatory or inhibitory effects on neural activity within the other hemisphere.

At a functional level, we have seen that the two hemispheres are often dominant for different task-relevant processing components. In such cases, each hemisphere is likely to take the lead for those components of processing that it handles best. In order for the two hemispheres to coordinate their activities effectively, the results of processing must be integrated across the two hemispheres. At the same time, many hemispheric asymmetries seem to involve complementary analyses of the sort that depend on incompatible neural computations, and it would seem useful to insulate those computations from each other in order for them to proceed efficiently at the same time.

With this in mind, it is not surprising that the corpus callosum has been hypothesized to play two important but very different roles: transferring information between the hemispheres and creating a kind of inhibitory barrier that minimizes maladaptive cross talk between the complementary processes for which each hemisphere is dominant.

Although the corpus callosum is certainly critical for certain forms of interhemispheric interaction, it is also clear that some types of information can be transferred subcortically. This includes information about the categories to which an object belongs, contextual information about an object, and certain aspects of information about spatial location. Subcortical structures can also play a role in producing unified individuals are likely to be rooted in early stages of ontogenetic development. In this section, I outline several promising developmental possibilities.

As noted previously, the emergence of laterality in the domestic chicken illustrates how laterality can result from the interplay of biological and environmental factors. During the last 5 days of incubation, the head of the chick embryo is turned so that the left eye is pressed against the body and the right eye is turned out toward the egg shell. If the egg (and, therefore, only the right eye) is exposed to light stimulation during this critical period, the chick becomes left hemisphere dominant for making visual discriminations and the right hemisphere becomes dominant for attack and copulation behavior. Lesley Rogers and colleagues have shown that it is possible to eliminate these population-level asymmetries by incubating the egg in darkness and to reverse them by experimentally manipulating the embryo so that only the left eye receives light stimulation. It is instructive to consider whether similar developmental scenarios might exist for humans.

During the course of fetal development in humans, certain areas of the right hemisphere seem to develop earlier than homologous areas of the left hemisphere. Various possibilities have been suggested as to the manner in which certain functional asymmetries could arise from the interaction of these maturational asymmetries and changes in the nature of environmental stimulation. One promising idea is that the earlier developing right hemisphere is initially more influenced than the lagging left hemisphere by the impoverished information that the developing brain encounters. This might include nonlinguistic intrauterine noises, global properties of visual stimuli in newborns, and coarse sensorimotor feedback before and for a few weeks after birth. By being more responsive to these early environmental influences, the right hemisphere may become dominant for perceiving various nonphonetic sounds, for processing global properties of visual stimuli, and for maintaining postural control. In contrast, by being on a later developmental trajectory, the left hemisphere may be saved for complementary specializations that involve processing of more detailed or finer-grained information and sensorimotor feedback and control. In addition, other asymmetric growth spurts during childhood may provide a mechanism for the continuing unfolding of functional hemispheric asymmetry. For example, between 3 and 6 years of age frontal and occipital areas of the left hemisphere appear to develop more rapidly than homologous areas of the right

hemisphere, coinciding with a developmental period that is also critical for the acquisition of several aspects of language for which the left hemisphere is dominant.

Psychologist Fred Previc has proposed that several additional prenatal asymmetries also influence later functional asymmetry. One hypothesis for which there is evidence is that certain craniofacial asymmetries that begin to appear as early as the first trimester of pregnancy lead to greater sensitivity of the right ear to sounds in the auditory frequency range that is critical for speech and that, as a result, the left hemisphere becomes more responsive to speech. It has even been suggested that this increased responsivity to speech may set the stage for the development of left hemisphere dominance for speech production. Asymmetries of fetal position during the last trimester of pregnancy have also been linked to later handedness. One ambitious hypothesis for which there is circumstantial evidence is that the typical position of the fetus during the last trimester favors enhanced development of the otolith on the left side, and this asymmetry in the organs of balance favors use of the left side for postural control and use of the right side for other more skilled activities. In view of the fact that there are neural connections between primary vestibular cortex and parietal areas, it has even been suggested that asymmetry in the organs of balance sets the stage for later right hemisphere dominance for spatial processing.

Additional research is needed to provide further tests of these hypotheses and others. Whatever the outcome, it is likely that asymmetries that are very small and subtle when they first appear can eventually have profound effects. As the developing organism encounters new and richer stimulation, the extent to which the brain's neural networks are responsive is likely to be influenced by how those networks have already been modified. It is reasonable to suppose that even a subtle difference can make one hemisphere more responsive than the other to some aspects of new sensorimotor information. In fact, neural network simulations illustrate the plausibility of such scenarios. As this process is repeated, laterality may snowball into the pattern characteristic of adults.

With the foregoing in mind, it is interesting that tasks and processes that are lateralized in adults seem to be lateralized from the time they can be accurately assessed. For example, there are indications that even in newborns there is a kind of left hemisphere dominance for speech perception and that activation of the left and right hemispheres is associated with positive and negative emotions, respectively. Also, in infants as young as a few months of age there appears

behavioral responses. Although the two hemispheres of the intact brain are capable of sharing many types of information, cooperation at all levels does not necessarily occur all the time. Studies of perceptual processing in normal individuals provide important insights about the factors that determine when it is more efficient for the two hemispheres to operate collaboratively than to operate independently. Laterality techniques described earlier have been modified to include trials that demand interhemispheric collaboration by presenting each hemisphere with only a portion of the total information needed to perform a task (the across-hemisphere condition) and comparing performance to conditions that present all the relevant information to one hemisphere (the within-hemisphere condition). One general conclusion suggested by this research is that distributing information across both hemispheres becomes more beneficial as the task becomes more demanding of attentional resources. That is, when the processing demands are minimal (such as indicating whether two letters are physically identical), there is often a within-hemisphere advantage. However, when the processing demands are increased (such as indicating whether two letters of different case have the same name or whether both are vowels), there is typically an across-hemisphere advantage. Dividing input between the two hemispheres is also beneficial when it permits them to engage in mutually inconsistent processes and at earlier compared to later stages of practice, although these may simply be additional ways of manipulating overall processing demand.

A somewhat different aspect of interhemispheric interaction has been studied in experiments that include bilateral redundant trials in which exactly the same information is presented simultaneously to both hemispheres. When normal observers attempt to identify printed consonant–vowel–consonant letter trigrams, there is a right visual field (left hemisphere) advantage, and the pattern of errors is different for the two visual fields (and hemispheres). On right hemisphere trials there are many more third-letter errors than first-letter errors, as if individual letters are processed in order one at a time. On left hemisphere trials this difference is reduced, even when the error types are normalized to compensate for the left hemisphere advantage. This may reflect the left hemisphere's ability to treat the trigram as a single pronounceable unit and thereby spread attention more evenly across the letters. When the same three-letter stimulus is presented simultaneously to both hemispheres, performance is even better than it is on left hemisphere-only trials, indicating the benefit of in-

cluding both hemispheres in processing. In view of the very good level of performance on redundant bilateral trials, one might expect the error pattern to be like that obtained on left hemisphere-only trials. In fact, the error pattern on redundant bilateral trials is intermediate between the left and right hemisphere patterns (and often more similar to the right hemisphere pattern), again suggesting processing contributions from both hemispheres.

The processing strategy on redundant bilateral trials is not always a mixture of the different strategies used on unilateral trials. In some cases, the bilateral strategy has been identical to the strategy associated with one hemisphere or the other. Interestingly, when this happens it is not always the strategy of the more efficient hemisphere that emerges on bilateral trials. In fact, it is not always possible to derive the processing strategy on bilateral trials from knowledge of the strategies utilized on unilateral trials. For example, in experiments that required normal observers to make rhyming judgments, certain effects of letter font and case on bilateral trials could not be predicted at all from the complete absence of such effects on unilateral trials. This suggests that interhemispheric collaboration can also have emergent properties that are impossible to deduce from the sum of the parts provided by the two individual hemispheres. It will be important in future studies to identify the factors that determine which of these different types of functional interaction will be observed and the biological mechanisms that underlie the different types of interaction. Uncovering the mechanisms of interhemispheric interaction may also have more general implications for how it is that unified processing emerges from a brain consisting of highly specific, modular subsystems.

V. LATERALITY IN NONHUMAN SPECIES

Behavioral and biological laterality is also ubiquitous in many nonhuman species, with many instances of asymmetry being at least analogous to asymmetries found in humans. At least some may also be homologous, in the sense of sharing common structures and developmental origins. Here, I review some of the most well-established laterality effects in other species and note their relationship to human laterality.

Motor asymmetries have been discovered for a number of species, with individuals sometimes showing very strong left–right preferences. However, population-level biases have been much rarer and none has matched the magnitude of right-handedness in the human population. Furthermore, preferences seem to depend on variables such as age and sex and on specific task demands. Despite these caveats, in several species of primates there tends to be a left-hand preference for reaching and maintaining postural control but a right-hand preference for manipulation and other high-level skilled activities. In addition to individual variation in paw preference, individual members of many species of mice and rats show a preference to turn in one direction or the other. Although an individual may exhibit a strong directional rotation bias, approximately equal numbers prefer each side. That is, there does not tend to be a population-level asymmetry. Individual rotation biases in rats have been related to asymmetries in distribution of the neurotransmitter dopamine, although the specific direction of the relationship differs for different populations.

There are also certain parallels between left hemisphere language dominance in humans and asymmetries in other species for the production and perception of vocalizations. In Japanese macaques, for example, the left hemisphere is dominant for the discrimination of species-specific vocalizations that are relevant for communication but not for the discrimination of other vocalizations. Also, in chimpanzees that have been trained to use certain visual symbols to communicate, there is evidence of left hemisphere dominance for processing those symbols but not for processing other, nonmeaningful symbols. There is even evidence that the ultrasonic calls emitted by rat pups are processed preferentially by the left hemisphere of their mother and it is well-known that there is left-brain dominance for the control of song in some species of song birds.

A number of asymmetries have been reported with respect to processing the identity and spatial characteristics of visual stimuli. In language-trained chimpanzees, for example, there is a right hemisphere advantage for processing the location of a line within a geometric figure and for identifying complex visual patterns that are not relevant for communication. In addition, rhesus monkeys have been reported to have right hemisphere superiority for recognizing monkey faces. In rats, there is evidence that the right hemisphere may be more involved than the left hemisphere in spatial exploration, although the asymmetry emerges only in rats that have been handled during the course of their early development. Pigeons and newly hatched chicks exhibit left hemisphere dominance for visual pattern discrimination. In chicks, this population-level bias occurs because light strikes only the right eye during a critical period of incubation

during which the visual system is developing rapidly. Finding effects of such variables as handling and light stimulation suggests that functional hemispheric asymmetries are likely to be shaped by the complex interaction of both biological and environmental factors.

Research with rats and chicks has also demonstrated asymmetry for emotional behaviors. For example, in both handled rats and chicks the right hemisphere tends to produce emotional activity, whereas the left hemisphere tends to inhibit emotional activity. In addition to providing interesting instances of laterality, effects such as these also illustrate the importance of reciprocal activity between the left and right sides of the brain.

There are also indications that some of the biological asymmetries found in the human brain characterize the brains of certain primates, although the nonhuman asymmetries are smaller and less frequent than those of humans. For example, the brains of both humans and apes show the kind of counterclockwise torque described earlier and in chimpanzees as well as humans the Sylvian fissure tends to be longer on the left side than on the right side.

As noted previously, it is difficult to know which laterality effects in other species are truly homologous to the effects found in humans. Nevertheless, the presence of so many asymmetries in other species provides a useful range of animal models that can be used to learn about the development of laterality across the life span of an individual and across evolutionary time. Among other things, laterality in other species indicates that the emergence of language is not a prerequisite for the emergence of other behavioral and biological asymmetries.

VI. LATERALITY ACROSS THE LIFE SPAN

The various functional aspects of laterality correlate with each other weakly or not at all. This is inconsistent with the hypothesis that there is but one fundamental processing dimension along which the hemispheres differ and from which all laterality effects are derived. Consequently, laterality is unlikely to be determined by any single developmental influence. Instead, the relative independence of different manifestations of laterality indicates that there are probably several different biological factors that interact with several different environmental influences to determine an individual's pattern of laterality. Furthermore, the laterality patterns that are characteristic of mature

opposite that which is considered prototypical. It is noteworthy that even though the relationship between handedness and other forms of laterality is only of weak to moderate strength, it has been demonstrated by all the various techniques and tools that are used to study laterality. This suggests that if the relationship of laterality to other variables such as biological sex were as strong as the relationship of laterality to handedness, it would be relatively straightforward for these techniques to uncover.

There are many effects of fetal hormone levels on brain development in other species, and in humans there are clear relationships between biological sex and cognitive ability. For example, women tend to outscore men on tests of verbal fluency, and men tend to outscore women on tests of spatial ability. Thus, it is plausible that there are sex-related differences in at least some aspects of brain laterality. This possibility receives modest support from the fact that the incidence of left-handedness is slightly higher in men than in women, consistent with the hypothesis that higher levels of fetal testosterone promote development of the right hemisphere relative to the left hemisphere. When handedness is controlled, however, evidence for additional sex-related changes in other forms of laterality is equivocal. The most encouraging indications of such relationships have come from the observation of deficits in patients with unilateral brain damage, with some studies finding evidence of greater functional hemispheric asymmetry in men than in women. However, not all studies have shown such sex differences and there may be alternative explanations for some of them. For example, it has been suggested that there is a lower rate of aphasia after left hemisphere damage in women than in men because of sex-related differences in the organization of language within the left hemisphere rather than because of differential lateralization per se. Behavioral laterality studies using neurologically intact men and women provide, at best, weak support for the hypothesis of greater functional laterality in men because the results have been quite variable. Also, even when sex-related differences are found, there are sometimes alternative explanations in terms of the tendency for men and women to prefer different cognitive strategies that may bias performance toward different hemispheres. Perhaps most clear is that if the laterality differences between men and women were as large as the laterality differences between right-handed and left-handed individuals, they would be well-known by now.

There are indications that individual variations in brain laterality may be related to individual differences

in cognitive ability. For example, relative performance on tests of verbal and visuospatial ability are related to handedness, but the relationship appears complex and is moderated by sex and by overall reasoning ability. There is also evidence that extreme intellectual precocity, especially for mathematical reasoning, is related to advanced development of the right hemisphere relative to the left, perhaps as a result of increased testosterone levels during fetal development. It also appears that some forms of dyslexia (impaired acquisition of reading) are related to subtle abnormalities within the language areas of the left hemisphere, perhaps leading to an overreliance on the less efficient mechanisms of the right hemisphere. Considerable additional work is needed, however, to substantiate these relationships and to discover the precise mechanisms that might account for them.

The existence of hemispheric asymmetry for emotion has led to consideration of the possible relationship of laterality to psychopathology. Among the more promising hypotheses is the idea that schizophrenia is related to dysfunction of an anterior region within the left hemisphere, an area that is believed to be important for language and for controlling parietal areas involved in attention. It has also been hypothesized that the corpus callosum, and therefore interhemispheric interaction, is dysfunctional in schizophrenics, but these hypotheses remain controversial and may apply to only a subset of schizophrenics. In a complementary way, depression has been linked to disturbances of the right hemisphere, but more work is needed to confirm this link and to understand its functional significance.

Popularized accounts of laterality have suggested that people can be classified as "right-brained" or "left-brained" depending on whether they prefer to use strategies and modes of cognition associated with one hemisphere or the other. Thus, left-brained people are said to be rational and analytic, whereas right-brained people are said to be intuitive, artistic, and creative. A few well-rounded individuals might even be lucky enough to be identified as "whole-brain thinkers." Various paper-and-pencil schemes have been proposed to achieve this sort of classification or measure of "hemisphericity," and exercises have been proposed to help more of us utilize whichever side of the brain we tend to neglect. To be sure, there is individual variation on the various dimensions of laterality, but there is no evidence that any neurologically intact individuals are functionally half-brained in the manner referred to as hemisphericity. Individuals do differ reliably in cognitive style, personality, creativity, and so forth. At the same time, however, we have seen that hemispheric asymmetries are subtle, with no indication that aspects such as rationality and creativity are the exclusive product of one brain hemisphere. Instead, both hemispheres contribute to virtually everything we do.

IX. CONSCIOUSNESS, MIND, AND THE DUAL BRAIN

The dual nature of the human brain has led to interesting discussion of the implications for consciousness and mind. Among other things, the discovery that both of the disconnected hemispheres of split-brain patients have a good deal of competence with respect to perception and motor control has led to speculation about whether or not the surgery has produced a doubling of consciousness or resulted in people with two minds. The neurobiologist Roger Sperry, who won the Nobel prize for his work with these patients, believed that this was the case. In part, he based his conclusion on the fact that the disconnected right hemisphere has its own perceptions, cognitions, and memories of which the disconnected left hemisphere is completely unaware. Others, however, have questioned whether the right hemisphere can truly think and whether its limited abilities include the same level of awareness and consciousness that seems typical of the left hemisphere. Certainly, the disconnected right hemisphere is usually incapable of speech and other forms of verbal communication that are uniquely human and that some have argued, are essential for the concept of "mind." Of course, there is much debate among philosophers and cognitive scientists about the extent to which language is essential for thinking, conscious reflection, or mental life.

An interesting hypothesis, advanced by Joseph LeDoux and Michael Gazzaniga, is that an important function of an individual's verbal left hemisphere is the construction of an internal, subjective reality or ongoing narrative based on its observations of his or her own overt behavior. In this view, observation of one's own behavior is necessary because many processes that influence behavior are not open to conscious experience. LeDoux and Gazzaniga emphasize this with respect to behavior and bodily sensations produced by the right hemisphere, of which the left hemisphere would have no direct knowledge. However, even within the left hemisphere there appear to be a great many modules whose processes may influence behavior but that are not themselves open to conscious

awareness. Thus, the need to create an ongoing personal narrative by making inferences about one's own behavior is likely to extend to covert processes performed by both hemispheres. More work is clearly needed, however, to test these and other hypotheses about the different roles played by the two cerebral hemispheres in the emergence of mind from brain.

See Also the Following Articles

BILINGUALISM • BRAIN DEVELOPMENT • CEREBRAL CORTEX • CONSCIOUSNESS • CORPUS CALLOSUM • EVOLUTION OF THE BRAIN • LANGUAGE, NEURAL BASIS OF • LEFT-HANDEDNESS • NEURAL NETWORKS

Suggested Reading

Banich, M. T., and Heller, W. (1998). Evolving perspectives on lateralization of function [Special issue]. *Curr. Directions Psychol. Sci.* **7**(1).

Beeman, M., and Chiarello, C. (Eds.) (1998). *Right Hemisphere Language Comprehension: Perspectives from Cognitive Neuroscience.* Erlbaum, Mahwah, NJ.

Christman, S. (Ed.) (1997). *Cerebral Asymmetries in Sensory and Perceptual Processing.* Elsevier, Amsterdam.

Corballis, M. C. (1997). The genetics and evolution of handedness. *Psychol. Rev.* **104**, 714–727.

Gazzaniga, M. S. (2000). Cerebral specialization and interhemispheric communication: Does the corpus callosum enable the human condition? *Brain* **123**, 1293–1326.

Halpern, D. F. (2000). *Sex differences in cognitive abilities.* Erlbaum, Mahwah, NJ.

Heilman, K. M. (1997). The neurobiology of emotional experience. *J. Neuropsychiatr. Clin. Neurosci.* **9**, 439–448.

Hellige, J. B. (1993; 2001 paperback). *Cerebral Hemisphere Asymmetry: What's Right and What's Left.* Harvard University Press, Cambridge, MA.

Hellige, J. B. (2000). Cerebral hemispheric specialization in normal individuals: Experimental assessment. In *Handbook of Neuropsychology* (F. Boller and J. Grafman, Eds.), Vol. 1, Part 1. Elsevier, Amsterdam.

Iacoboni, M., and Zaidel, E. (Eds.) (2002). *The Parallel Brain.* MIT Press, Cambridge, MA.

Ivry, R. B., and Robertson, L. C. (1998). *The Two Sides of Perception.* MIT Press, Cambridge, MA.

Kosslyn, S. M. (1996). *Image and Brain: The Resolution of the Imagery Debate.* MIT Press, Cambridge, MA.

Provins, K. A. (1997). Handedness and speech: A critical reappraisal of the role of genetic and environmental factors in the cerebral lateralization of function. *Psychol. Rev.* **104**, 554–571.

Rogers, L. J. (1997). Early experiential effects on laterality: Research on chicks has relevance to other species. *Laterality* **2**, 199–219.

Springer, S. P., and Deutsch, G. (1998). *Left Brain/Right Brain: Perspectives from Cognitive Neuroscience.* Freeman, New York.

Vallortigara, G. (2000). Comparative neuropsychology of the dual brain: A stroll through animals' left and right perceptual worlds. *Brain and Language* **73**, 189–219.

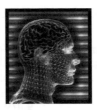

Left-Handedness

STANLEY COREN
University of British Columbia

GLOSSARY

Broca's area The location in the brain, typically the left hemisphere, that controls speech production.

diffuse control system This refers to control of a function or behavior that involves a number of brain centers and pathways.

genetically fixed traits Genetically determined traits that are characteristic of a particular species.

pathological handedness Handedness that results after some pathological event, such as birth stress-related events, disturbs the natural development of right- or left-handedness.

rare trait marker theory A theoretical and statistical model that explains why relatively rare, but apparently benign, traits in a species are often associated with pathological conditions.

sidedness The preferential use of the right or left hand, foot, eye, or ear.

soft sign A behavior or symptom that may suggest the presence of an underlying neurological or physiological pathology.

Wernicke's area The location in the brain, typically the left hemisphere, that controls speech comprehension.

Handedness refers to the fact that most people consistently use the same hand for tasks in which skill and dexterity are required and only one hand can be used. Thus, a person who almost always uses his or her right hand when writing, throwing a ball, cutting with a knife, or using a hammer would be defined as being right-handed. Estimates of the number of right-handers in the population are between 88 and 92%. Given such an overwhelming bias toward the right in humans, it is not surprising that researchers have asked the following questions: If, as a species, we appear to be programmed to be right-handed, then why are there any left-handers? Do left-handers differ from right-handers in any ways other than their handedness? Are there any advantages or disadvantages in being left-handed?

I. SIDEDNESS

Although everyone probably knows about the existence of handedness, most people are unaware of the fact that it is just one aspect of a group of lateral biases. In the same way that we are handed, we are also footed. One would demonstrate footedness in tasks such as habitually using the same foot to step on a bug or to kick a ball to hit a target. In footedness, humans also show a right-sided bias, with approximately 80–82% of the population being right-footed.

In addition to showing motor biases favoring one side, we also show sidedness in the use of our bilateral sense organs. We demonstrate eyedness by consistently choosing the same eye to sight down a telescope or to peep through a small hole. We would be showing earedness by usually choosing the same ear to listen to the faint ticking of a clock or to press against a door to hear noises on the other side. These manifestations of sidedness are also biased toward the right, although

of structures around the medial edge of the cerebral hemisphere. ("Limbus" means border or edge; e.g., to be "in limbo" is to be suspended between two states.) These structures include the amygdala, the hippocampus, the parahippocampal gyrus, and related structures, such as the orbital/medial prefrontal cortex, cingulate cortex, anterior and mediodorsal thalamic nuclei, the ventromedial corpus striatum (i.e., the accumbens nucleus and medial caudate nucleus), and the nucleus basalis of Meynert.

I. AMYGDALA

The amygdala is a complex of several nuclei in the rostromedial part of the temporal lobe (Figs. 1 and 2). There are several deep nuclei (lateral nucleus, basal nucleus, and accessory basal nucleus), which are

substantially interconnected with the temporal, insular, and frontal cortex, the striatum, and the mediodorsal thalamus. On the surface are a number of modified cortical areas, many of which are interconnected with the olfactory system. In the dorsal part of the amygdala are the central nucleus and medial nucleus, which have connections with the hypothalamus and autonomic brain stem nuclei.

The amygdala receives input from all the sensory systems. In lower mammals, these are dominated by inputs from the olfactory system, although there are also inputs from the taste/visceral afferent system and the visual and somatosensory systems. In primates the most prominent inputs are derived from higher order sensory association cortex, especially from the visual areas in the inferior temporal cortex (i.e., the temporal visual processing stream, important for analysis of form and color and recognition of complex stimuli

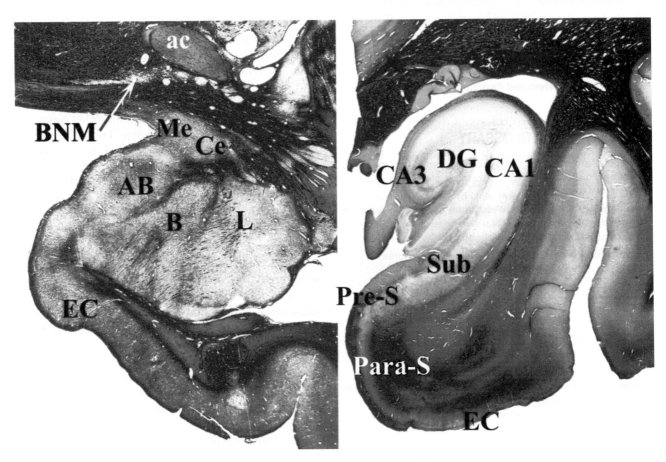

Figure 1   A photomicrograph of the amygdala, hippocampus, and parahippocampal gyrus from a human brain. BNM-basal nucleus of Meynert, ac-anterior commisure. The amygdala includes the lateral nucleus (L), basal nucleus (B), accessory basal nucleus (AB), central nucleus (Ce), and medial nucleus (Me). The hippocampus, located posterior to the amygdala in the medial temporal lobe, includes the parasubiculum (Para-S), presubiculum (Pre-S), subiculum (Sub), fields CA1 and CA3, and the dentate gyrus (DG). The entorhinal cortex (EC) occupies the parahippocampal gyrus ventral to the amygdala and hippocampus.

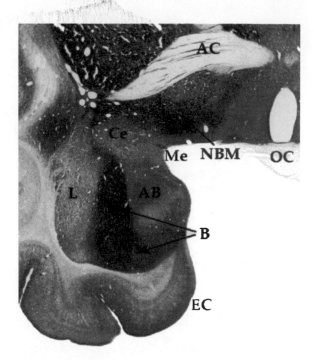
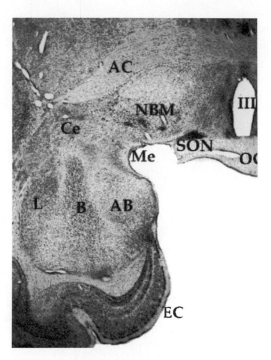

Figure 2 Photographs of the amygdala and entorhinal cortex (EC) of a macaque monkey, stained for acetylcholinesterase (left) and cells (Nissl method) (right). Note the component nuclei of the amygdala, including the basal nucleus (B), lateral nucleus (L), accessory basal nucleus (AB), central nucleus (Ce), and medial nucleus (Me). Also note the cholinergic nucleus basalis of Meynert (NBM), ventral to the anterior commissure (AC), the supraoptic nucleus (SON), the optic chiasm (OC), and the third ventricle (III).

such as faces) (Fig. 3). Recordings from the amygdala show that the neurons respond to complex sensory stimuli, including visual stimuli such as faces, as well as to other sensory modalities. In addition to the sensory aspects of the stimuli, the responses are influenced by the novelty of the stimulus or its affective sign (whether the stimulus is rewarding or aversive).

There is a complex system of intraamygdaloid connections that associate these inputs. These connect the deep amygdaloid nuclei (which interact with the cortex) with the central and medial nuclei (which connect to the hypothalamus and brain stem). There are also extensive connections to other limbic areas, including the hippocampus, parahippocampal gyrus, and the nucleus basalis of Meynert.

The outputs from the amygdala can be divided into three categories (Fig. 3):

1. Return projections back to the sensory areas that project into the amygdala: In the case of the visual system, these return projections even extend back to the primary visual cortex.

2. Descending projections to the visceral control centers of the hypothalamus and brain stem: The central amygdaloid nucleus projects to a wide variety of autonomic-related cell groups, including the lateral hypothalamus, the periaqueductal gray, the parabrachial nucleus, the nucleus of the solitary tract, the dorsal vagal nucleus, and the ventrolateral medulla. Through these projections, the amygdala can influence heart rate and blood pressure, gut and bowel function, respiratory function, bladder function, etc. For example, stimulation of the central nucleus can cause stomach ulcers as well as changes in cardiovascular function.

3. Interactions with the orbital and medial frontal cortex, both via direct amygdalocortical projections and via connections with the mediodorsal thalamic nucleus and the ventromedial parts of the basal ganglia: This circuit appears to be involved in determination of the affective "sign" of sensory stimuli (e.g., whether it is rewarding or aversive) and in setting mood.

Several additional observations may be used to illustrate the role of the amygdala in the control of emotional behavior. Bilateral lesions of the amygdala and adjacent medial temporal structures in monkeys

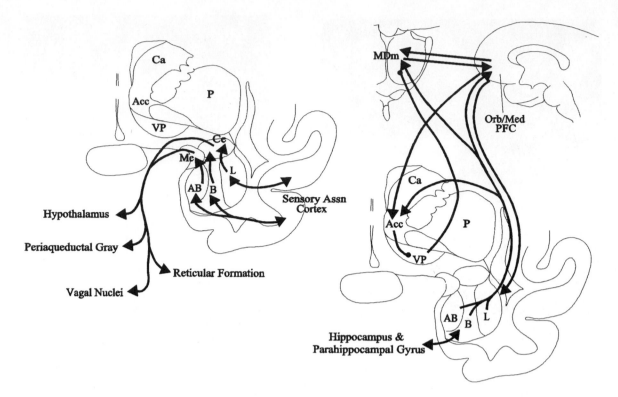

Figure 3 Schematic summary of the axonal connections of the amygdala. (Left) Inputs from sensory association cortical areas and output from the central and medial nuclei to the hypothalamus and brain stem. (Right) Connections are illustrated with the mediodorsal thalamus (MDm), the ventromedial striatum [accumbens (Acc) and caudate nuclei (Ca)], ventral pallidum (VP), and the orbital and medial prefrontal cortex (Orb/Med PFC) as well as with the hippocampal formation. The connections from Ca/Acc to VP and from VP to MDm are shown with arrowheads to indicate that they are inhibitory.

produce "psychic blindness" (Kluver–Bucy syndrome) in which the animals can see objects but are apparently unable to distinguish their significance. Such animals are not capable of appropriate social behavior, and in group settings they become isolated and solitary.

In rats, bilateral lesions of the amygdala block the acquisition of conditioned fear responses. For example, if a light is consistently coupled with a painful foot shock, the animal comes to associate the two stimuli, and the light becomes a "fearful" stimulus that can produce autonomic and behavioral responses characteristic of fear. After bilateral lesions of the amygdala, the shock produces the same response as before, but the light never becomes a fearful stimulus. Recent observations indicate that a similar deficit is present in humans who have a rare disease that results in bilateral amygdaloid destruction.

Stimulation of the amygdala in awake cats produces a defense reaction in which there are integrated behavioral and visceral changes that prepare the animal for fight or flight. Stimulation of the amgydala or hippocampus in human patients (during exploratory surgery for severe epilepsy) evokes complex sensory and experiental phenomena, often involving fear and including sensory hallucinations, feelings of deja vu, and memory-like episodes that resemble static dreams.

II. HIPPOCAMPUS

The hippocampus is a specialized part of the cerebral cortex, folded into the temporal horn of the lateral ventricle about the hippocampal fissure (Figs. 1 and 4). It is composed of several subregions, including (in order) the entorhinal cortex (in the parahippocampal gyrus), the parasubiculum, presubiculum, subiculum, fields CA1–CA3, and the dentate gyrus.

Like the amygdala, in rats the hippocampus receives strong olfactory inputs, but in primates it is dominated by multisensory inputs, mostly from higher order

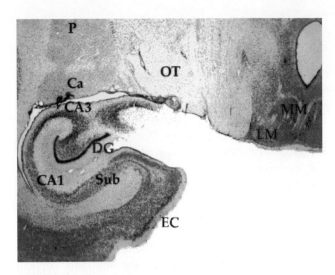

Figure 4 Photomicrograph of the hippocampal formation and the mammillary nuclei in a macaque monkey (stained with the Nissl method). Ca, caudate nucleus; EC, entorhinal cortex; DG, dentate gyrus; P, putamen; OT, optic tract; Sub, subiculum.

sensory association cortex. These inputs reach the hippocampus through a relay in the perirhinal and entorhinal cortex, which in turn receive inputs from multisensory association cortical areas. There is a relatively unidirectional set of connections through the hippocampus, beginning from the entorhinal cortex to the dentate gyrus, and then in turn to CA3, CA1, the subiculum, and back to the entorhinal cortex (Fig. 5).

Outputs to other parts of the brain mainly arise in the subiculum and entorhinal cortex. These resemble those of the amygdala:

1. Projections back to many sensory association cortical areas, including the visual and auditory areas of the inferior and superior temporal cortex.
2. Projections to the hypothalamus (but not to brain stem autonomic nuclei).
3. Connections with prefrontal and cingulate cortical areas, via direct projections and also via projections to the anterior and mediodorsal thalamic nuclei, and the mammillary nuclei, and projections to the ventral part of the basal ganglia.

The hippocampus and surrounding areas of the parahippocampal gyrus are critically involved in memory processing in general and spatial orientation in particular. Recordings in the hippocampus have demonstrated cells that fire when the animal is in a particular spatial location, as defined by characteristic

sensory and other experiential stimuli. This suggests that the hippocampus provides a neural mechanism for association of different parameters that are necessary for the moment-to-moment incorporation of experience into memory. Strikingly, bilateral lesions of the hippocampus and parahippocampal cortical areas produce amnesia, an inability to form new memories (although older memories may be intact). By comparison, amygdaloid lesions that produce emotional disturbances do not produce amnesia.

III. ORBITAL AND MEDIAL PREFRONTAL CORTEX AND CINGULATE GYRUS

Cortical areas on the ventromedial surface of the frontal lobe, in the cortex dorsal to the orbit and the region rostral and ventral to the genu of the corpus callosum, are substantially interconnected with all the limbic areas discussed previously and participate in many of the same functions. These areas vary from periallocortical agranular areas with a relatively simple cortical structure in the caudal part of the region to fully developed granular cortical areas more

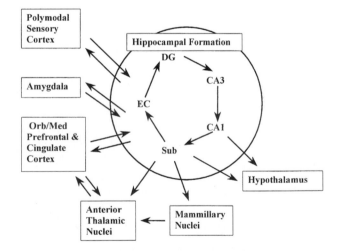

Figure 5 Schematic summary of major axonal connections of the hippocampal formation. Interactions with the polymodal sensory cortical areas occur primarily through the entorhinal cortex (EC). The amygdala, the orbital and medial prefrontal cortex, and the cingulate cortex interact with both the EC and the subiculum (Sub), whereas the Sub provides the primary output to the anterior thalamic nuclei, mammillary nuclei, and hypothalamus. Within the hippocampal formation, the principal flow of activity is from the EC to the dentate gyrus (DG), field CA3, field CA1, the Sub, and back to the EC.

rostrally. In rodents, the agranular areas dominate and the granular areas are almost nonexistent, whereas in primates and especially humans the granular areas are much larger than the agranular areas.

As a whole, the cortical areas can be divided into two relatively interconnected networks that appear to have related but distinct functions (Fig. 6). Sensory inputs from other cortical regions or the thalamus enter many of the orbital cortical areas, and these are integrated by corticocortical connections between these areas. Many of these are related to food or eating (e.g., olfaction, taste, visceral afferents, somatic sensation from the hand and mouth, and vision), and neurons in the orbital cortex respond to multisensory stimuli involving the appearance, texture, or flavor of food. In contrast, many of the areas in the medial prefrontal

cortex and a few related orbital areas provide output from the cortex to visceral control centers in the hypothalamus and brain stem. Therefore, the orbital and medial prefrontal cortex appears to be adapted to evaluate feeding-related sensory information and to evoke appropriate visceral reactions.

The function of the ventromedial frontal cortex is considerably wider, however. Food is a primary reward, and many of the orbital neurons respond to rewarding or aversive aspects of stimuli beyond their sensory characteristics. In this, the cortex is closely tied to the function of the related ventromedial striatum, in which reward-related neural activity has also been found.

In addition, lesions of the ventromedial frontal lobe produce dramatic behavioral deficits, which suggests that visceral reactions evoked through this cortical

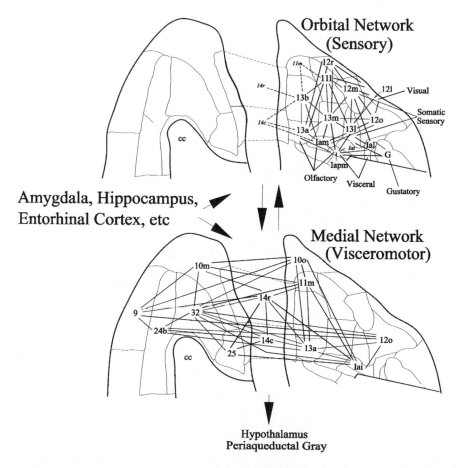

Figure 6 Diagram illustrating connections of architectonic areas in the ventromedial prefrontal cortex in macaque monkeys, drawn onto the orbital (right) and medial (left) cortical surfaces. Sensory input is particularly directed to an "orbital" network of areas (in the orbital cortex), whereas output to autonomic control centers in the hypothalamus and brain stem (especially the periaqueductal gray) arises from a "medial" network of areas (in the medial and orbital cortex). Corticocortical axonal connections between areas, which largely define the two networks, are indicated by lines connecting the areas. In addition to this sensory/visceromotor transfer, interactions with the amygdala, hippocampus, entorhinal cortex, and other limbic structure involve this cortical region in reward appreciation and affective behavior. The numbers and letters are designations of architectonic areas, modified from Brodmann; cc, corpus callosum.

area form a critical component in evaluating alternatives and making choices. As exemplified by the famous 19th-century case of Phineas Gage, individuals with damage to the ventromedial prefrontal cortex do not show deficits in motor or sensory function, or in intelligence or cognitive function, but have devastating changes in personality and choice behavior. Recent studies of such cases by Damasio and colleagues have shown that patients do not show usual visceral reactions to emotional stimuli, and this lack of response correlates closely with their difficulty in making appropriate choices. This has been explained by a somatic marker hypothesis, which postulates that visceral responses are monitored as a quick warning of choices to avoid.

In monkeys the cingulate gyrus is situated dorsal to the corpus callosum, but in humans it extends rostral and ventral to the genu of the corpus callosum and caudally around the splenium. The pre- and subgenual parts of the cingulate cortex are closely related to the medial prefrontal cortex in connections and presumably function, but more posterior cingulate regions appear to be distinct. Although the caudal pole of the cingulate gyrus is connected to the hippocampal formation, the central part of the cingulate gyrus has little relation to limbic structures.

IV. VENTROMEDIAL STRIATUM, VENTRAL PALLIDUM, AND MEDIAL THALAMUS

Although the ventromedial striatum, ventral pallidum, and medial thalamus are not part of the limbic system as traditionally defined, they have substantial connections with all the limbic structures discussed previously and are closely tied to them functionally. The amygdala, hippocampal formation, and the ventromedial prefrontal cortex all project onto the ventromedial part of the striatum, leading into a circuit that connects through the ventral pallidum to the mediodorsal thalamic nucleus (Fig. 4). Like other striato-pallidal-thalamic systems, this circuit involves two inhibitory (GABAergic) synaptic links, from the striatum to the ventral pallidum and from the ventral pallidum to the mediodorsal thalamus. In the mediodorsal nucleus, the inhibitory pallidal inputs interact with monosynaptic excitatory inputs from the amygdala, entorhinal cortex, hippocampus and other limbic structures.

Although it is usually assumed that the striatum is involved in motor functions, most of the motor-related activity is found in the dorsolateral part of the striatum, which is anatomically connected with sen-

sorimotor areas of the cerebral cortex. In contrast, the ventromedial striatum, in keeping with its limbic associations, has been shown to be related to reward and reward-related behavior. In both cases, the role of the striatum may be to inhibit or suppress unwanted patterns of activity in order to allow other patterns to be freely expressed. Specifically, the dorsolateral striatum and related areas of the globus pallidus appear to be involved in switching between different patterns of motor behavior, whereas the ventromedial striatum and pallidum may allow changing of stimulus–reward associations when the reward status of a stimulus has changed.

V. NUCLEUS BASALIS (OF MEYNERT) AND NUCLEUS OF THE DIAGONAL BAND (OF BROCA)

These nuclei consist of scattered groups of large cells in the basal part of the cerebral hemisphere, just ventral to the anterior commissure and the globus pallidus. The nucleus basalis (Figs. 2 and 3) is most prominent at the level of the anterior commissure, but some of its cell clusters extend caudolaterally toward the amygdala and dorsally around the edges of the globus pallidus. The diagonal band nuclei extend medially and dorsally (diagonally) into the septum. Because many of the cells utilize acetylcholine as their transmitter, the nuclei stain very darkly for acetylcholinesterase. Other cells in the complex use GABA as transmitter. As a group, they project axons widely to all parts of the cerebral cortex (and the olfactory bulb and amygdala), although individual neurons within the group appear to have very restricted projections.

The principal action of acetylcholine on cortical cells is to enhance the action of other synaptic inputs. The nuclei are situated along fiber pathways that connect limbic structures such as the orbital and medial prefrontal cortex and the amygdala with the hypothalamus and brain stem, and they receive major input from all of these. The magnocellular basal forebrain nuclei are therefore well situated to modulate cortical activity in relation to limbic activity. They have been implicated in the activation (desynchronization) of the cortex that is characteristic of the waking state, and they are presumably involved in many other functions as well.

VI. THE LIMBIC SYSTEM AND PSYCHIATRIC DISORDERS

Although lesions of limbic structures do not result in apparent sensory or motor deficits, dysfunction of these structures has been associated with a variety of psychiatric disorders, including depression, bipolar disorder, obsessive–complusive disorder, and schizophrenia. For example, structural changes have been noted in the hippocampal formation, medial thalamus, and prefrontal cortex in schizophrenic subjects. Observations from positron emission tomography indicate that the amygdala and related parts of the prefrontal cortex and medial thalamus are abnormally active in patients suffering from severe unipolar and bipolar depression. Cellular changes, especially in glial cells, have also been reported in the orbital and medial prefrontal cortex and amygdala in depressed subjects. Patients with lesions of these prefrontal areas have also been reported to have a relatively high incidence of depression. As noted previously, lesions of the ventromedial prefrontal cortex produce severe deficits in emotional reactions and in making choices.

See Also the Following Articles

CINGULATE CORTEX • ELECTRICAL POTENTIALS • HOMEOSTATIC MECHANISMS • MOOD DISORDERS • NEUROANATOMY • PREFRONTAL CORTEX

Suggested Reading

Aggleton, J. P. (Ed.) (1992). *The Amygdala: Neurobiological Aspects of Emotion, Memory, and Mental Dysfunction*. Wiley–Liss, New York.

Bjorklund, A., Hokfelt, T., and Swanson, L. W. (Eds.) (1987). Integrated systems of the CNS, part I: Hypothalamus, hippocampus, amygdala, retina. In *Handbook of Chemical Neuroanatomy*, Vol. 5, Elsevier, New York.

Broca, P. (1878). Anatomie comparée circonvolutions cérébrales: Le grand lobe limbique et la scissure limbique in la série des mammifères. *Rev. Anthropol. Ser. 2* **1**, 384–498.

Cavada, C., and Schultz, W. (Eds.) (2000). The mysterious orbitofrontal cortex [Special issue]. *Cerebral Cortex* **10**, 205–342.

Damasio, A. R. (1995). *Descartes' Error: Emotion, Reason, and the Human Brain*. Morrow, New York.

Fuster, J. M. (1997). *Prefrontal Cortex: Anatomy, Physiology, and Neuropsychology of the Frontal Lobe*, 3rd ed. Lippincott–Raven, Philadelphia.

LeDoux, J. E. (1994). Emotion, memory and the brain. *Sci. Am.* **270**, 50–57.

Papez, J. W. (1937). A proposed mechanism for emotion. *Arch. Neurol. Psychiatr.* **38**, 725–743.

Squire, L. R., and Zola, S. M. (1997). Amnesia, memory and brain systems. *Philos. Trans. R. Soc. London B Biol. Sci.* **352**, 1663–1673.

Vogt, B. A., and Gabriel, M. (Eds.) (1993). *Neurobiology of Cingulate Cortex and Limbic Thalamus: A Comprehensive Handbook*. Birkhauser, Boston.

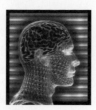

Logic and Reasoning

PHILIP N. JOHNSON-LAIRD

Princeton University

I. Logic

II. Deductive Reasoning

III. Implicit Inferences

IV. Reasoning and the Brain

V. Conclusions

GLOSSARY

deductive reasoning The process of establishing that a conclusion follows validly from premises (i.e., that it must be true given that the premises are true).

deontic reasoning Reasoning about actions that are obligatory, permissible, or impermissible.

formal rules of inference Rules that can be used to derive a conclusion from premises in a way that takes into account only the form, not the meaning, of the premises. Logical calculi rely on formal rules, and so do many psychological theories of reasoning.

implicit reasoning A fast, automatic, and largely unconscious process of making inferences in order to make sense of the world and of discourse (e.g., to select the appropriate sense of a word, or to establish the appropriate referent for a pronoun).

inductive reasoning The process of deriving plausible conclusions from premises.

logic The science of implications among sentences in a formalized language. Logical calculi are systems of proof based on formal rules of inference (proof theory); they have an accompanying semantics (or model theory).

mental models Representations of the world that are postulated to underlie human reasoning; each model represents what is true in a single possibility.

validity An inference is valid if its conclusion must be true given that its premises are true. A valid inference from true premises yields a true conclusion; a valid inference from false premises may yield a true or a false conclusion.

Logic captures the implications among sentences. A logical calculus consists of a precise definition of a language and a set of rules of inference that can be used to derive conclusions from premises. The rules are formal, that is, they operate on the form of sentences, not their meaning. The calculus, however, may have a semantics, which provides interpretations for all the sentences in the language. Modern logic lies at the heart of the development of computers and computer programming languages. However, logic is not easy to use in the evaluation of everyday inferences because no algorithm exists for translating such inferences into sentences in a logical calculus—a gap that the logician Bar-Hillel once referred to as the scandal of logic. Logic is also not a theory of how human beings reason. That topic is the province of psychology. Although psychologists studied deductive reasoning for almost the entire 20th century, they began to formulate theories of the process only in the past 25 years. Deductive reasoning is now under intensive investigation, and more is known about it than any other variety of thinking. The aim of this article is accordingly to outline the general principles of logic; to describe current theories of human reasoning, which owe much to logic; and to outline what is known about the role of the brain in reasoning.

I. LOGIC

From the founder of logic, Aristotle, onwards logicians have analyzed formal patterns of valid inference. A deduction is valid if its conclusion must be true given that its premises are true. The original aim of logic, as Leibniz remarked, was to replace rhetoric with calculation. Modern formal logic began during the last quarter of the 19th century, but nowadays logicians draw a sharp distinction between formal systems of logic, which they refer to as proof theory, and semantic systems of logic, which they refer to as model theory. The distinction is clearest in the case of the sentential calculus. This calculus concerns implications that depend on sentential negation, as expressed by "not," and various sentential connectives, such as "if," "and," and "or," which are treated in an idealized way. The following inference is an example of a valid deduction that can be proved in the sentential calculus:

> *If the brakes are on and the switches are on then the engine is ready to start.*
> *The brakes are on.*
> *The switches are on.*
> *Therefore, the engine is ready to start.*

The inference is based on three atomic sentences (i.e., sentences that contain neither negation nor any connectives): the brakes are on, the switches are on, and the engine is ready to start. The inference is valid and has the form

> *If A and B then C.*
> *A.*
> *B.*
> *Therefore, C.*

where A, B, and C, are variables that can take as values any sentences including those that in turn contain connectives.

Logicians can set up the proof theory for a calculus in various ways. They can formalize the sentential calculus, for example, using just a single rule of inference and a set of axioms, which are assertions that are assumed to be true. However, a more intuitive method, known as natural deduction, dispenses with axioms in favor of formal rules of inference for negation and for each of the sentential connectives. Certain rules introduce connectives into a proof, such as the rule that introduces "and," using it to conjoin two premises:

> *A.*
> *B.*
> *Therefore, A and B.*

Certain rules eliminate connectives from a proof, such as the well-known rule of modus ponens:

> *If A then B.*
> *A.*
> *Therefore, B.*

These two rules suffice to prove the conclusion about starting the engine:

1. If the brakes are on and the switches are on then the engine is ready to start.
2. The brakes are on.
3. The switches are on.
4. Therefore, the brakes are on and the switches are on [The rule for introducing "and" applied to sentences 2 and 3]
5. Therefore, the engine is ready to start. [Modus ponens applied to sentences 1 and 4].

Table I presents a set of formal rules of inference for the sentential calculus. With such rules, you can construct a formal proof, as in the preceding example, with each step in the proof warranted by one of the rules of inference.

Your knowledge of the meaning of the connectives helps you to understand the validity of the rules in Table I. However, the rules do not rely on these meanings. They work in a formal way, allowing you to write patterns of symbols given other patterns of symbols. A proof in a formal calculus is accordingly like a computer program. A computer predicts the weather, for example, but it has no idea of what rain or sunshine is or of what it is doing. It slavishly shifts "bits," which are symbols made up from patterns of electricity, from one memory store to another, and

Table I
Formal Rules of Inference for the Sentential Calculus[a]

A	Not (Not A)
∴ Not (Not A)	∴ A
A	A and B
B	∴ A
∴ A and B	
A	A or B, or both.
∴ A or B, or both	Not A
	∴ B
Rule for conditional proof	Rule for modus ponens
A (a supposition)	If A then B
...	A
B (i.e., B can be derived from A)	∴ B
∴ If A then B	

[a]The rules in the left-hand column introduce negation and the sentential connectives into inferences; those in the right-hand column eliminate them from inferences.

displays symbols that meteorologists can interpret as maps of weather. Indeed, proofs and computer programs are intimately related, and certain programs can prove inferences in logical calculi. Likewise, certain programming languages, such as PROLOG, are akin to a logical calculus.

Formal proofs establish that inferences are valid, but validity is not a concept that is defined within proof theory. Its definition hinges on truth, which underlies the semantics of the calculus (i.e., its model theory). In the model theory of the sentential calculus, the truth or falsity of compound sentences depends only on the truth or falsity of their constituent sentences. Thus, an assertion of the form, A or B or both, is true if A is true, B is true, or both of them are true. Otherwise it is false. Logicians lay out these definitions in truth tables, as shown in Table II. Each row in a truth table is a "model" of a possibility and presents the truth value of the compound sentence—in this case, A or B or both—in that possibility. The first row in the table, for instance, presents the case in which A is true and B is true, and so the disjunction is true in this possibility.

One problematic connective is "if." Its everyday usage sometimes departs from its idealized logical meaning in the sentential calculus. An assertion such as

If that patient has malaria then she has a fever

is, in fact, compatible with three possibilities: The patient has malaria and a fever, she has no malaria and fever, and she has no malaria and no fever. It is false in only one case: She has malaria and no fever. The assertion is therefore equivalent to

If that patient has malaria then she has a fever, and if she does not have malaria then she either has or does not have a fever.

Logical license exists just as much as poetic license: Logicians make simplifying assumptions about the meanings of logical terms.

The validity of an inference in the sentential calculus can be established using the model theory of the calculus. Table III shows how premises can be used to eliminate possibilities from a truth table. When you have eliminated the impossible then, as Sherlock Holmes remarked, whatever remains, however improbable, must be the case. In other words, an inference is valid if the conjunction of its premises with the negation of its conclusion is inconsistent (i.e., not a single row in the resulting truth table contains the entry "true"). For instance, if you conjoin the negation of the conclusion in Table III, "The engine is not ready to start," to the premises, then it would eliminate the last remaining possibility in the truth table. It is therefore impossible for the premises to be true and for the conclusion to be false: The inference is a valid.

Any conclusion that can be proved using formal rules for the sentential calculus is also valid using truth tables and vice versa. There is also a decision procedure for the calculus; that is, the validity or invalidity of any inference can be established in a finite number of steps. Unfortunately, sentential inferences are computationally intractable. It is feasible to test the validity of inferences based on a small number of atomic sentences. However, as the number of atomic sentences in an inference increases, its evaluation in any system —no matter how large or how rapid—takes increasingly longer and depends on increasingly more memory, to the point that a decision will not emerge during the lifetime of the universe.

The sentential calculus has a decision procedure, but it is intractable. The predicate calculus includes the sentential calculus, but also deals with quantifiers—that is, with sentences containing such words as "any" and "some," as in "Any electrical circuit contains some source of current." The predicate calculus does not even have a decision procedure. Any valid inference can be proved in a finite number of steps, but no such guarantee exists for demonstrations of invalidity. Attempts to show that an inference is invalid may, in effect, get lost in the "space" of possible derivations. The principal discovery of 20th century logic, however, is Gödel's famous proof that no consistent calculus is powerful enough to yield derivations of all the valid theorems of arithmetic. Arithmetic is thus incomplete. This result drives a wedge between syntax (proof theory) and semantics (model theory). Any attempt to argue that semantics can be reduced to syntax is bound to fail. Semantics has to do with truth and validity, whereas syntax has to do with proofs and formal derivability.

Table II

A Truth Table for the Disjunction *A or B or Both*, Which Shows Its Truth Value for the Four Possibilities Depending on the Truth or Falsity of A and of B

A	B	A or B or both
True	True	True
True	False	True
False	True	True
False	False	False

Table III
The Validity of an Inference Is Shown Using a Truth Table[a]

1. If the brakes are on and the switches are on then the engine is ready to start.
2. The brakes are on.
3. The switches are on.

All that remains is the first possibility, and so it follows validly: Therefore, the engine is ready to start.

Brakes are on	Switches are on	The engine is ready to start	Possibilities that are eliminated
True	True	True	
True	True	False	Eliminated by 1
True	False	True	Eliminated by 3
True	False	False	Eliminated by 3
False	True	True	Eliminated by 2
False	True	False	Eliminated by 2
False	False	True	Eliminated by 2
False	False	False	Eliminated by 2

[a]The premises are used to eliminate possibilities.

II. DEDUCTIVE REASONING

Logic tells us about implications among sentences, but it is not a theory of human reasoning. This topic is a concern of psychology. In the last 25 years of the 20th century, psychologists proposed a variety of theories of reasoning—that it depends on a memory for previous cases, on rules that capture general knowledge, on "neural nets" representing concepts, or on specialized innate modules for matters that were important to our hunter–gatherer ancestors. However, humans have the ability to reason about matters for which they have no specific knowledge. Even if you know nothing about brakes, switches, and engines, you can grasp the validity of the earlier inference about them. This ability lies at the heart of the development of mathematics and logic. Hence, a critical question is whether it depends on syntactic or semantic principles. The following sections describe psychological theories of both sorts.

A. Formal Rule Theories

The first theories of human deductive ability postulated that the mind tacitly uses formal rules of inference like those of a system of natural deduction. Such theories continue to have many proponents, notably Daniel Osherson, Lance Rips, and the late Martin Braine and colleagues. Philosophers have proposed similar theories, and computer scientists have implemented formal systems for the computer generation of proofs. What these proposals have in common is the idea that reasoning depends on applying formal rules of inference to the premises of an inference in order to derive the conclusion in a sequence of steps akin to a proof.

Rips's PSYCOP theory was the first formal rule theory in psychology to cope with connectives and quantifiers and to be implemented in a computer program (written in PROLOG). The system is otherwise typical of formal rule theories. It postulates that reasoning depends on a single deterministic process, that it relies on natural deduction, and that it makes use of suppositions—sentences that are assumed provisionally for the sake of argument, and that have to be "discharged" if a proof is to yield a conclusion. There are two ways to discharge a supposition. First, it can be incorporated within a conditional conclusion (see the rule for conditional proof in Table I). Second, if a supposition leads to a contradiction, then it must be false given that the premises are true (according to the rule of "reductio ad absurdum," which is not shown in Table I). As an example, consider the proof for an inference of a form known as *modus tollens*. There are two premises, such as

1. If the switches were not on then the engine did not start.

2. The engine did start.

The proof starts with a supposition:

3. Suppose: the switches were not on.

4. Therefore: the engine did not start. [Rule for modus ponens applied to 1 and 3]

There is now a contradiction between a sentence in the domain of the premises (The engine did start) and a sentence in the subdomain of the supposition (The engine did not start). The rule of reductio ad absurdum uses such a contradiction to negate, and thereby discharge, the supposition that led to the contradiction:

5. Therefore, the switches were on.

Like other formal rule theories, PSYCOP does not contain a rule for modus tollens, because the inference is more difficult for logically untrained individuals than modus ponens. Hence, it depends on the chain of inferential steps just given. In contrast, an inference of the following form, which we encountered earlier,

> If A and B then C.
> A.
> B.
> ∴ C.

could be derived in two steps, first conjoining A and B, and then using modus ponens to derive the conclusion. However, the inference is so easy that PSYCOP has a single formal rule for drawing the inference (a conjunctive form of modus ponens).

Formal rule theorists try to postulate psychologically plausible rules of inference and a mechanism for using them to construct mental proofs. One problem is that unless certain rules, such as the rule for introducing "and" (see Table I), are constrained, they can lead to futile derivations:

> The brakes are on.
> The switches are on.
> ∴ The brakes are on and the switches are on.
> ∴ The brakes are on and the brakes are on and the switches are on.
> ∴ The brakes are on and the brakes are on and the brakes are on and the switches are on.

and so on ad infinitum. One solution is to incorporate the effects of such rules within other rules. In computer programs, however, a rule of inference can be used in two ways: either to derive a step in a chain of inference leading forward from the premises to the conclusion or to derive a step in a backward chain leading from the conclusion to a subgoal of proving its required premises. PSYCOP allows the dangerous rules to be used only in such backward chains, and thereby prevents them from yielding futile steps. PSYCOP therefore has three sorts of rules: those that it uses only forwards, such as the conjunctive rule for modus ponens; those that it uses only backwards, such as the rule for conditional proof; and those that it uses in either direction, such as the rule for modus ponens. A corollary is that reasoners should make modus tollens inferences only when they are given the putative conclusion, or when they can guess the conclusion and then try to prove it.

Given an inference to evaluate, PSYCOP always halts after a finite number of steps either with a proof of the conclusion or else in a state in which it has unsuccessfully tried all its possible derivations. Hence, the theory implies that people infer that a conclusion is invalid only if they fail to prove it. They carry out an exhaustive search of all possible derivations, and only then do they judge that the conclusion does not follow from the premises. However, valid inferences exist that PSYCOP cannot prove. If its exhaustive search has failed to find a proof, then there are two possibilities. Either the inference is invalid, or it is valid but beyond the competence of PSYCOP to prove. A psychological corollary is that people should never know for certain that an inference is invalid.

Formal rule theories postulate that the difficulty of a deduction depends on the number of steps in its derivation and the availability and ease of use of the required rules of inference. Modus ponens is easy because it depends on a single rule; modus tollens is more difficult because it depends on a chain of inferences. Formal rule theorists have corroborated their theories in experiments using large batteries of deductions. They estimate post hoc the probability of the correct use of each rule of inference. When these empirical estimates are combined appropriately for each inference, they yield a satisfactory fit with the difficulty of the inferences in the battery.

B. The Mental Model Theory

The mind may not contain any formal rules of inference unless an individual has learned logic. Instead, inferences could be based on an understanding of the meaning of the premises. Consider the following inference:

> From where I stand, the peak of the mountain is directly behind the steeple. The old oak is on the

right of the steeple, and there is a flag pole between them. Therefore, if I move to my right so that the flag pole is between me and the peak of the mountain, the steeple is to the left of my line of sight.

Reasoners might rely on axioms and formal rules to make this inference, but it seems more likely that they imagine the relevant spatial layout. This idea lies at the heart of the theory of mental models.

The theory postulates that mental models have three principal characteristics. First, each model represents a possibility. For example, the disjunction "The switches are on or the brakes are on, or both" calls for a separate model for each of the three possibilities (shown here on separate lines):

> *switches*
>
> *brakes*
>
> *switches*   *brakes*

where "switches" denotes a model of the switches being on, "brakes" denotes a model of the brakes being on, and the third model combines the two.

Second is the principle of truth: Mental models represent only what is true and not what is false, and in this way they place a minimal load on working memory. Hence, the preceding models do not represent the row in the truth table in which the disjunction as a whole is false (Table II). Likewise, the first model represents that the switches are on, but it does not represent explicitly that in this possibility it is false that the brakes are on. People make a mental "footnote" about what is false, but normally they soon forget it. If they retain such footnotes, however, then they may be able to flesh out their mental models to make them fully explicit. Table IV presents the mental models and the fully explicit models for sentences based on each of the main sentential connectives. Mental models are accordingly like truth tables in which there are no "false" entries.

Third, the structure of a model corresponds to the structure of the situation that the model represents. A model is accordingly like a biologist's model of a molecule. The previous notation for the models fails to capture their rich internal structure. Visual images can be derived from some models, but models are often not visualizable. Early formulations of the theory concerned only the logical terms in the language, but recently the theory has been extended to deal with various sorts of nonlogical terms, such as spatial and temporal relations, and general knowledge about causal relations.

Table IV
Models for the Sentential Connectives[a]

Connective	Mental models		Fully explicit models	
A and B	A	B	A	B
A or else B	A		A	¬B
		B	A	B
A or B or both	A		A	¬B
		B	¬A	B
	A	B	A	B
If A then B	A	B	A	B
	...		¬A	B
			¬A	¬B
If and only if A then B	A	B	A	B
	...		¬A	¬B

[a]The middle column shows the mental models postulated for human reasoners, and the right-hand column shows fully explicit models, which represent the false components in true possibilities using negations that are true: "¬" denotes negation and "..." denotes a wholly implicit model. The footnote on the mental models for "if" indicates that the implicit model represents the possibilities in which A is false, and the footnote on the mental models for "if and only if" indicates that the implicit model represents the possibilities in which both A and B are false.

Reasoners use all the information available to them to construct models—discourse, perception, general knowledge, memory, and imagination. They formulate a conclusion that holds in their models but that was not explicit in the starting information. If a conclusion holds in all the models of the premises, then it is necessary given the premises. If it holds in at least one model of the premises, then it is possible given the premises. The probability of a conclusion depends on the proportion of models in which it holds, granted that each model is equiprobable, which is an assumption that reasoners make in default of evidence to the contrary. The theory accordingly unifies reasoning about necessity, possibility, and probability. They all depend on a semantic process rather than a formal one. They all depend on a grasp of meaning, which is used to imagine the possibilities compatible with the premises.

To illustrate the theory, consider the following inference:

> *The switches are on or the brakes are on, or both.*
> *The switches are not on.*
> ∴ *The brakes are on.*

The disjunctive premise elicits the models:

switches

                           brakes

switches   *brakes*

The second premise eliminates the models representing the possibilities in which the switches are on. The remaining model yields the conclusion that the brakes are on. This conclusion is valid because it holds in all the models—in this case, the single model—of the premises.

C. Five Empirical Phenomena

Psychological investigations have established five principal phenomena of deductive reasoning. The first phenomenon is that the more possibilities that reasoners have to envisage to draw an inference, the more difficult the inference—it takes them longer, and they are more likely to make a mistake. A simple example is that inferences based on a disjunction are more difficult when the disjunction is inclusive, as in the preceding example, than when it is exclusive and allows only two possibilities: "The switches are on or the brakes are on, but not both." The same effect of number of possibilities occurs in reasoning with other sentential connectives, in reasoning about spatial and temporal relations, and in reasoning with premises containing quantifiers, such as "all," "some," and "none."

The second phenomenon is that reasoners use counterexamples to establish invalidity. When reasoners draw conclusions for themselves, they may not consider counterexamples. However, when they reject a conclusion, they can do so by constructing a counterexample—that is, they envisage a possibility that satisfies the premises but refutes the conclusion. One experiment, for example, used problems, such as

> *More than half of the people in the room speak French.*
> *More than half of the people in the room speak English.*
> *Does it follow that more than half of the people in the room speak both French and English?*

Most people responded correctly, "no," and they typically reported having envisaged a situation analogous to the one represented in Fig. 1. They drew such diagrams when they were allowed paper and pencil.

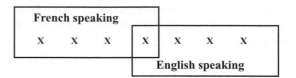

Figure 1 A counterexample used to refute an inference. Each x represents an individual: more than half of them speak French, and more than half of them speak English, but it is false that more than half speak both languages.

They also used counterexamples when they manipulated external models—cut-out paper shapes—in order to reason with quantifiers.

The third phenomenon is that human reasoners spontaneously develop a variety of different strategies in deductive reasoning. They do not use a single deterministic strategy. For example, in reasoning based on multiple premises containing sentential connectives, some individuals develop the strategy of translating each disjunctive premise into a conditional, some base their inferences on the most informative premise, and some make use of suppositions—even when there are categorical assertions among the premises. Many distinct inferential strategies occur, but the space of possible strategies has yet to be mapped.

The fourth phenomenon is the occurrence of illusory inferences. These inferences are compelling but invalid. The following is a typical example:

> *Only one of the following premises is true about a particular hand of cards:*
> *There is a king in the hand or there is an ace, or both. There is a queen in the hand or there is an ace, or both.*
> *There is a jack in the hand or there is a 10, or both.*
> *Is it possible that there is an ace in the hand?*

Most people respond "yes." The first premise is compatible with the possibilities:

King

                    Ace

King   *Ace*

They support the conclusion that an ace is possible. The second premise supports the same conclusion, and so reasoners are likely to respond affirmatively. However, this response overlooks the fact that when one premise is true, the others are false. Thus, if the first premise is true, the second premise is false. In which case, there cannot be an ace. Indeed, if there were an ace in the hand, then the first two of the premises would be true, contrary to the rubric that only one of the premises is true.

The rubric "only one of the premises is true" is equivalent to an exclusive disjunction, and a compelling illusion occurs in the following inference about a particular hand of cards:

> *If there is a king in the hand then there is an ace in the hand, or else if there isn't a king in the hand then there is an ace in the hand.*
> *There is a king in the hand.*
> *What, if anything, follows?*

Nearly everyone, experts and novices alike, infers that there is an ace in the hand. It follows from the possibilities that people envisage. However, given the disjunction of the two conditionals, it is an error. The disjunction implies that one or other of the conditionals could be false. If the first conditional is false, then even the presence of a king fails to guarantee that there is an ace in the hand. The fallacies arise from a failure to think about what is false. It follows that any manipulation that emphasizes falsity should alleviate them. This prediction has been corroborated experimentally.

The fifth phenomenon is that knowledge and beliefs affect both the interpretation of premises and the process of reasoning. Consider, for example, the following conditional assertion:

If she played a sport then she didn't play soccer. Conditionals are normally compatible with three possibilities (see the fully explicit models in Table IV):

> sport   ¬ soccer
> ¬ sport   ¬ soccer
> ¬ sport   soccer

where ¬ denotes negation. However, the meaning of the noun soccer entails that it is a sport, and so knowledge of this meaning automatically rules out the third of these possibilities. General knowledge and knowledge of the context of an utterance can also eliminate possibilities. Individuals often know what the different possibilities are, and such knowledge modulates the interpretation of assertions. As an illustration, consider the following conditional:

> *If you strike a match properly then it lights.*

Its interpretation includes the salient possibility:

> strike   lights

As often happens in discourse, however, the antecedent of the conditional fails to describe in complete detail the context in which the consequent holds. There are many circumstances in which a match will not light even if you strike it properly. You know, for instance, that if it is soaking wet it will not light. In fact, you have knowledge of the following explicit possibilities:

> soak   ¬lights
> ¬ soak   ¬lights
> soak   lights

Now, suppose you soak a match in water and then strike it. What happens? The conditional implies that it lights. Your knowledge implies that it does not light. Your knowledge, however, takes precedence over the possibilities that the conditional asserts.

Given the following premises in a form known as a syllogism,

> *All the Frenchmen are wine drinkers.*
> *Some of the wine drinkers are gourmets.*

the majority of reasoners draw the plausible conclusion:

> *Some of the Frenchmen are gourmets.*

However, with the next premises, which are identical in form,

> *All the Frenchmen are wine drinkers.*
> *Some of the wine drinkers are Spanish.*

few reasoners draw the conclusion

> *Some of the Frenchmen are Spanish.*

They envisage the possibility in which the wine drinkers are of both nationalities, but they search more assiduously—and successfully—for a counterexample because this conclusion is preposterous. Hence, the main effect of beliefs on the process of reasoning is that they influence invalid inferences far more than valid inferences: People refrain from drawing unbelievable invalid conclusions.

The difficulty of coping with falsity and the effects of content come together in a well-known reasoning problem, Wason's selection task, which has been studied experimentally more than any other paradigm of reasoning. Table V presents two versions of the task, one with a neutral conditional and one with a deontic conditional concerning what is permissible. The difficulty of the version with the neutral conditional, "If a card has an 'A' on one side then it has a '2' on its other

Table V
Two Examples of Wason's Selection Task

A	B	2	3

1. The participants know that each card above has a letter on one side and a number on the other side. Their task is to select those cards that they need to turn over to discover whether the following conditional is true or false about the four cards:

If a card has an "A" on one side then it has a "2" on its other side.

Most people correctly select the "A" card, and some select the innocuous "2" card too. They fail to select the 3 card. However, if it has an A on its other side, the conditional is false.

Drinking	Not drinking	21 years	16 years

2. The participants know that each card above represents a person. One side states whether or not the person is drinking alcohol, and the other side states the age of the person. The task is to select those cards that need to be turned over to discover whether or not a person is violating the following conditional rule:

If persons are drinking then they are over the age of 20 years.

Most people correctly select the "Drinking" card and the "16 years" card.

---

side," arises from the participants' inability to base their selections on the possibility that falsifies the conditional:

$$A \quad \neg 2$$

They need to choose those cards that could be instances of this case, i.e., A and 3 (which is an instance of ¬ 2). With neutral conditionals, reasoners appear merely to select cards on the basis of their mental models of the conditional rather than its falsifying instance.

When the selection task concerns what is permissible or impermissible, such as breaking a social contract, then reasoners tend to make the correct selections (Table V, problem 2). Some psychologists argue that this version of the task maps onto mental schemas with a content that concerns such deontic matters. Evolutionary psychologists propose that social contracts mattered to our hunter–gatherer ancestors, and so an innate module evolved for reasoning about cheaters. What appears to be the case, however, is that any experimental manipulation that helps reasoners to envisage false instances of conditionals improves their performance in the selection task. Knowledge of cheating is just such a cue, but there are others. Experiments have shown, for example, that instructions to check for violations or to envisage counterexamples improve performance. The context of a conditional can also exert such effects. One study

enhanced the participants' selections with a neutral conditional, "If A then 2." The participants were told that it was a rule followed by a machine that prints cards. The machine went wrong, and now the participants must check that it is printing out cards correctly.

Reasoners are sensitive to the likelihood of encountering potential counterexamples, and so some theorists have introduced probabilistic considerations into their analyses of the selection task. They defend a normative approach of this sort, arguing that participants rationally seek to maximize the expected gain in information from selecting a card. If they were testing in the real world, the following conditional:

If a creature is a raven then it is black.

it would make sense to examine creatures that are black because there are many fewer black than non-black creatures. Hence, the argument goes, people are rational in selecting 2 rather than 3 to test the neutral conditional. In one study, however, participants were each paid 1000 pesetas (about $7) before carrying out the selection task with a neutral conditional. They were charged 250 pesetas for each card that they selected, but they were told that they could keep whatever money they did not spend provided that their evaluation of the conditional was correct. This incentive failed to improve performance. Likewise, individuals with higher SAT scores tend to do better on the selection task than those with lower scores.

Whatever "rational" is taken to mean, it seems inappropriate to apply it to those who lose money rather than gain it and to those who score lower on tests of cognitive ability.

The five sorts of phenomena reviewed in this section were all predicted by the model theory, although readers will need to consult the literature for the derivation of the predictions. Formal rule theories allow that knowledge and beliefs can affect the interpretation of premises; otherwise, the phenomena are difficult for these theories to accommodate.

III. IMPLICIT INFERENCES

Psychologists distinguish between the deliberative thinking that underlies deduction and the implicit, automatic, and largely unconscious inferences that help people to make sense of the world and its descriptions. Consider, for example, the following passage:

> The pilot put the plane into a stall just before landing on the strip. He just got it out of it in time. It was a fluke.

Readers have no difficulty in understanding the passage, but every noun and verb in the first sentence is ambiguous. Also the search for the referents for the three occurrences of the pronoun "it" in the passage defeats even the most advanced computer programs for interpreting natural language. Humans have no difficulty with the passage because they are equipped with a powerful system that uses general knowledge to make implicit inferences. Readers should also have no difficulty in understanding the following passage:

> Apart from her husband, a hairdresser, Eve was the only woman among 52 men on the tour. As a costumier, she filled a much needed gap, because when a company of actors is putting on a play in a different town each night, no damage to the costumes is too trivial not to be mended.

In fact, most people do not notice that the passage contains three deliberate mistakes. It implies that Eve's husband is a woman. It states that what is needed is a gap rather than Eve. It also asserts that no damage to the costumes is too trivial not be mended instead of what it surely means—no damage to the costumes is too trivial to be mended. The system of implicit inferences overrides the literal interpretation of the sentences and makes sense out of nonsense. The inferences resolve the senses of words and determine the references of pronouns and other such expressions. They enable individuals to construct a single model of the situation described in a passage, and the implicit system does not attempt to search for alternative models unless it encounters evidence for them. The process is therefore rapid, and it becomes as automatic as any other cognitive skill that calls for no more than a single mental representation at a time. For the same reason, implicit inferences lack the guarantee that their conclusions are valid. They are inductions rather than deductions. However, the implicit system is not isolated from the mechanisms of deduction. Normally, the two systems work together in tandem.

One consequence of implicit inferences is that people often jump to a conclusion, which later they have to withdraw. In logic, if a conclusion follows validly from premises, then no additional premises can invalidate it. Logic means never having to be sorry about a conclusion. As new premises are added to existing premises, then increasing numbers of logical conclusions follow (i.e., logic is "monotonic"). However, in daily life, conclusions are often withdrawn in the light of subsequent information. These inferences are "nonmonotonic". The original conclusion may have been based on an assumption made by default that turned out to be false. For instance, I tell you about my cat Hodge, and from your knowledge of cats you infer that Hodge has fur and a tail. You withdraw your conclusion, however, when you learn that Hodge is bald and tailless. Your knowledge contains various assumptions that you can make in default of information to the contrary. The whole purpose of these default assumptions is to allow you to make useful inferences that you can withdraw in the light of contrary evidence.

A more problematic sort of nonmonotonic reasoning is illustrated in the following example. You believe the following premises:

> If Viv has gone shopping then she will be back in an hour.
> Viv has gone shopping.

It follows, of course, that Viv will be back in an hour. However, suppose that Viv is not back in an hour. You are in a typical everyday situation in which there is a conflict between the consequences of your beliefs and the facts. At the very least, you have to withdraw your conclusion. You also have to modify your beliefs, but in what way? Should you cease to believe that Viv went shopping or that if she went shopping she will be back in an hour, or both? Philosophers and students of artificial intelligence have made various proposals about these puzzles. Unfortunately, the understanding of nonmonotonicity in human reasoning lags behind.

Reasoning in daily life often calls for the generation of explanations and diagnoses. For example, in the case of Viv's failure to return, you do not merely modify your beliefs, you try to make diagnostic inferences about what happened:

Possibly, Viv met a friend and went for a coffee.
Possibly, Viv felt ill on the way to the shops.

One possibility leads in turn to further explanatory possibilities, for example,

Possibly, Viv couldn't get the car to start after shopping.
∴ Possibly, the car's battery is dead. Possibly, Viv left the headlights on.

You use your knowledge and any relevant evidence to generate possibilities. Human reasoners easily outperform any current computer program in envisaging putative explanations. Given two sentences selected at random from different stories, such as

Celia made her way to a shop that sold TV sets.
She had recently had her ears pierced.

they readily offer such explanations as Celia was getting reception in her ears and wanted the TV shop to investigate, or Celia had bought some new earrings and wanted to see how they looked on closed-circuit TV. This propensity to generate explanations underlies both science and superstition. The difference is that scientists test their explanations empirically.

Inferences in real life are often not deductively "closed"—that is, there is not enough information to draw a valid conclusion. Reasoners must therefore make inductions, that is, they use their knowledge to draw conclusions that go beyond the information given and that therefore may be false. There is no normative theory of induction and no comprehensive psychological theory of it, either. What does exist are a number of well-established heuristics, which were identified by two pioneers, Kahneman and Tversky. One heuristic is the availability of relevant knowledge. Most individuals, for example, judge that more people die in automobile accidents than as a result of stomach cancer. They are wrong, but the media publish more stories about auto accidents than about stomach cancer. Similarly, people rely on the representativeness

of evidence. If you are told that Bill is intelligent but unimaginative and lifeless, then you are unlikely to judge that he plays jazz for a hobby, though you may find it more likely that he is an accountant who plays jazz for a hobby. If so, you have violated the principle that a conjunction (being an accountant and playing jazz) cannot be more probable than one of its components (playing jazz). The description of Bill, however, is more representative of an accountant than of a jazz musician. It has therefore led you to overlook a simple principle of probability.

IV. REASONING AND THE BRAIN

The famous Russian neuropsychologist Luria once remarked, "The cerebral organization of thinking has no history whatsoever." Fodor, the distinguished philosopher of mind, predicted that it has no future either because thinking depends on general processes rather than separate brain modules, such as those that underlie perception or motor control. Nevertheless, a start has been made in the study of the neuropsychology of reasoning. The results so far have been largely at the level of "these areas of the brain underlie reasoning," and their interpretations are at best tentative.

A. Logical Reasoning and Personal Reasoning

Clinical studies in the early 20th century often reported the loss of "abstract thinking" as a result of brain damage. Such accounts, however, suffered from two irremediable problems. On the one hand, they never succeeded in characterizing a principled difference between abstract and concrete thinking. On the other hand, they failed to pin down the particular effects of lesions in different parts of the brain. This shortcoming is understandable given that many regions of the brain are likely to underlie reasoning. Modern neuropsychological investigations suggest that the real distinction is between logical reasoning with neutral materials and personal reasoning that engages individuals' beliefs and knowledge (Table V). Some studies suggest that logical reasoning depends on the left cerebral hemisphere, whereas personal reasoning implicates the right hemisphere and bilateral ventromedial frontal cortex. Positron emission tomography scans show greater left hemisphere activity when individuals evaluate syllogisms, such as

All men have sisters.
Socrates was a man.
∴ Socrates had a sister.

or judge the plausibility of inductive inferences, such as

Socrates was a great man.
Socrates had a wife.
∴ All great men have wives.

The control task was to judge how many of the sentences had people as their subjects. The effects of brain damage also appear to support the dissociation between logical and personal reasoning. For example, left hemisphere lesions impair simple relational inferences, such as

Mary is taller than John.
John is taller than Anne
Is Mary taller than Anne?

People who live in nonliterate cultures are happy to carry out personal reasoning, but they balk at logical reasoning when the content is outside their experience. Analogous effects have been obtained using electroconvulsive therapy (ECT), which suppresses cortical activity for 30 min or more. Before ECT, the patients (depressives and schizophrenics) tended to justify their responses to deductive problems on logical grounds. They also did so more rapidly and confidently after ECT had suppressed their right hemispheres. However, after the suppression of their left hemispheres, they tended to respond on grounds of personal experience in ways similar to members of nonliterate cultures, often rejecting a logical task based on unfamiliar content as impossible because it was outside their knowledge. Similar effects of brain damage occurred in a study of the selection task with a neutral conditional (Table V). Patients with left hemisphere damage, like control subjects, tended to err in the characteristic way. Surprisingly, however, half the patients with right hemisphere damage made the correct selections.

Perhaps the right hemisphere impedes logical reasoning because it allows knowledge and probabilistic considerations to influence performance. Certainly, the right hemisphere seems to play a role in automatic implicit inferences. Given the passage,

Sally approached the movie star with pen and paper in hand. She was writing an article about famous people's views about nuclear power.

normal individuals are likely to infer that Sally wanted to ask the star about nuclear power. Patients with damage to the right hemisphere infer that Sally wanted the movie star's autograph. They are misled by the first sentence and cannot make the implicit inference from the second sentence to revise their interpretation. Patients who have had a right-hemisphere lobectomy are also poorer at reasoning from false premises than those with a left hemisphere lobectomy. In general, right hemisphere damage seems to impair the ability to "get the point" of a story, to make implicit inferences establishing coherence, and to grasp the force of indirect illocutions such as requests framed in the form of questions.

It is tempting, but erroneous, to conclude that the left hemisphere is the seat of logic, whereas the right hemisphere is the seat of personal reasoning. Damage to the right hemisphere can lead to semantic difficulties in the interpretation of words, and so it may also impair the comprehension of discourse. For instance, it impairs the deduction of converse relations, such as

John is taller than Bill.
Who is shorter?

A recent functional magnetic resonance imaging (fMRI) study confirmed the existence of dissociable networks for logical and personal reasoning, which share circuits in common in the basal ganglia, cerebellum, and left prefrontal cortex. However, the activation suggested that personal reasoning recruits the left hemisphere linguistic system, whereas logical reasoning—even in inferences of an identical form—recruits the parietal spatial system. Also, when reasoning elicits a conflict between logic and belief, right prefrontal cortex becomes active, perhaps to resolve the incongruency. Another recent fMRI study established that deductive reasoning activates right dorsolateral prefrontal cortex whereas mental arithmetic from the same premises does not. This study also showed that when an inference depends on a search for a counterexample then the right frontal pole is activated.

Frontal cortex plays a crucial role in decision making, as shown in a major series of studies carried out by Damasio and colleagues. They also investigated the selection task in testing the consequences of their somatic marker hypothesis. This hypothesis postulates that ventromedial frontal cortex underlies the typical "gut reaction" on which implicit everyday decisions rely. Considerable evidence supports this hypothesis: For example, individuals with frontal lesions tend to go bankrupt in real life and in laboratory gambling tasks. Similarly, the investigators found that patients with lesions in ventromedial frontal cortex were unaffected by whether the selection task was based on familiar or unfamiliar neutral contents. However, patients with lesions in other areas, like normal individuals, showed the characteristic effects of content. Correct performance in the selection task depends on grasping what counts as a counterexample to the conditional assertion.

B. Imagery and Spatial Representations

Does deductive reasoning rely on visual imagery? Behavioral studies have produced little evidence to suggest this is the case. Readers might suppose that this lack of evidence counts against the model theory. This view, however, confuses models with images. The model theory distinguishes between the two: Mental models are structural analogs of the world, whereas visual images are the perceptual correlates of certain sorts of model from a particular point of view. Indeed, many mental models are incapable of supporting visual images because they represent properties or relations that are not visualizable, such as ownership, obligation, and possibility. Recent studies have sharpened the need to distinguish between the degree to which relations evoke spatial models as opposed to visual images. The studies examined three sorts of materials, as rated by an independent panel of judges:

1. Relations that are easy to envisage spatially and easy to visualize, such as above, below, in front of, and in back of
2. Relations that are not easy to envisage spatially but are easy to visualize, such as cleaner, dirtier, fatter, and thinner
3. Control relations that are neither easy to envisage spatially nor easy to visualize, such as better, worse, smarter, and dumber

The studies examined both conditional inferences and inferences about simple relations among entities. They showed that inferences were faster with contents that were easier to envisage spatially than with the control contents, which in turn were faster than contents that were easy to visualize but difficult to envisage spatially. It seems that a relation such as "dirtier", elicits a visual image, but one that is irrelevant to the construction of a mental model that allows reasoners to make the required inference. In

contrast, a relation, such as "in front of" elicits a spatial model that helps individuals to draw the inference. An fMRI study has also examined spatial reasoning. Given spatial problems, such as

The red rectangle is in front of the green rectangle. The green rectangle is in front of the blue rectangle. Does it follow that the red rectangle is in front of the blue rectangle?

significant activation occurred in regions of parietal cortex that are known to represent and to process spatial information. Moreover, there was no reliable difference in the degree of activation between the right and the left hemispheres. Clinical studies of how brain damage affects the use of imagery in reasoning have produced mixed results, perhaps because they have not separated the two sorts of contents—spatial and non-spatial—that are both easy to visualize.

In summary, clinical and imaging studies of the brain have yet to establish how reasoners make deductions. There is evidence for separate systems mediating logical inferences with neutral content and personal inferences with a content that engages knowledge and beliefs. Future studies may determine whether separate brain mechanisms underlie the control of different deductive strategies, the use of diagrams as opposed to verbal premises, and the construction and evaluation of multiple models.

V. CONCLUSIONS

Modern logic has developed both proof theory and model theory for systems powerful enough to cope with all the deductive inferences that human beings make. What is lacking is a systematic method for translating such inferences into formal logic. Psychologists continue to investigate deductive reasoning. Their two main theoretical accounts are based on rules of inference and on mental models, respectively—a distinction that parallels the one between proof theory and model theory in logic. Rule theorists emphasize the automatic nature of simple deductions and postulate rules corresponding to them. More complex inferences, they assume, call for sequences of simple deductions. In contrast, model theorists emphasize that reasoning is the continuation of comprehension by other means. The system for implicit inferences based on knowledge aids the process of constructing models of discourse. In deliberative reasoning, individuals tend to focus on possibilities in which the premises are true. However, they can grasp the force of counterexamples. The evidence suggests that people have a modicum of deductive competence based on mental models. Rules of inference and mental models, however, are not incompatible. Advanced reasoners may construct formal rules for themselves—a process that ultimately leads to the discipline of logic.

See Also the Following Articles

ARTIFICIAL INTELLIGENCE • CATEGORIZATION • CREATIVITY • INFORMATION PROCESSING • INTELLIGENCE • LANGUAGE AND LEXICAL PROCESSING • PROBLEM SOLVING

Suggested Reading

Baron, J. (1994). *Thinking and Deciding*, 2nd ed. Cambridge Univ. Press, New York.

Braine, M. D. S., and O'Brien, D. P. (Eds.) (1998). *Mental Logic*. Erlbaum, Mahwah, NJ.

Brewka, G., Dix, J., and Konolige, K. (1997). *Nonmonotonic Reasoning: An Overview*. CLSI Stanford Univ. Press, Stanford, CA.

Evans, J. St. B. T., and Over, D. E. (1996). *Rationality and Reasoning*. Psychology Press, Hove, UK.

Garnham, A., and Oakhill, J. (1994). *Thinking and Reasoning*. Blackwell, Cambridge, MA.

Jeffrey, R. (1981). *Formal Logic: Its Scope and Limits*, 2nd ed. McGraw-Hill, New York.

Johnson-Laird, P. N. (2001). Mental Models and deduction. *Trends in Cognitive Scien.* **5**, 434–442.

Johnson-Laird, P. N., and Byrne, R. M. J. (1991). Deduction. Erlbaum, Hillsdale, NJ.

Johnson-Laird, P. N., Legrenzi, P., Girotto, V., Legrenzi, M., and Caverni, J.-P. (1999). Naive probability: A mental model theory of extensional reasoning. *Psychol. Rev.* **106**, 62–88.

Kahneman, D., Slovic, P., and Tversky, A. (Eds.) (1982). *Judgment under Uncertainty: Heuristics and Biases*. Cambridge Univ. Press, New York.

Oaksford, M., and Chater, N. (1998). *Rationality in an Uncertain World: Essays on the Cognitive Science of Human Reasoning*. Psychology Press, Hove, UK.

Rips, L. J. (1994). *The Psychology of Proof*. MIT Press, Cambridge, MA.

Schaeken, W., De Vooght, G., Vandierendonck, A., and d'Ydewalle, G. (2000). *Deductive Reasoning and Strategies*. Erlbaum, Mahwah, NJ.

Stanovich, K. E. (1999). *Who Is Rational? Studies of Individual Differences in Reasoning*. Erlbaum, Mahwah, NJ.

Wharton, C. M., and Grafman, J. (1998). Deductive reasoning and the brain. *Trends Cognitive Sci.* **2**, 54–59.

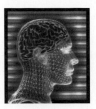

Lyme Encephalopathy

RICHARD F. KAPLAN

University of Connecticut School of Medicine

I. History and Background

II. Neurological Manifestations

III. Neuropsychological Studies

IV. Population Studies

V. LE in Children

VI. Post-Lyme Disease Syndrome

VII. Conclusions

GLOSSARY

fibromyalgia A chronic musculoskeletal rheumatological syndrome that is associated with muscular pain and fatigue. Symptoms include cognitive difficulties, mood change, and sleep disturbance. The etiology is unknown.

intrathecal antibody production Local production of specific antibody to *Borrelia burgdorferi* in cerebral spinal fluid.

Lyme disease A multisystem disorder of the skin, nervous system, heart, and joints caused by the tick-borne spirochete, *B. burgdorferi*.

neuropsychological assessment The use of procedures and tests that measure general intellectual abilities and specific cognitive functioning, such as memory, to aid in the diagnosis of brain dysfunction.

polymerase chain reaction A laboratory assay for *B. burgdorferi* DNA.

post-Lyme disease syndrome A condition characterized by fatigue, mood disturbance, and complaints of cognitive dysfunction that follow well-documented Lyme disease months to years after antimicrobial treatment.

single photon emission computed tomography A functional neuroimaging technique used to measure regional cerebral blood flow. Brain activity is recorded by externally placed gamma cameras, which detect a radiotracer such as t-HMPAO.

Lyme encephalopathy is a neuropsychiatric disorder beginning months to years after the onset of Lyme disease.

The symptoms are non specific and typically include fatigue, sleep disturbance, slowed thinking, memory loss, naming problems, and depression. The etiology remains controversial. This article defines the nature of the syndrome and offers possible explanations from a neuropsychological perspective.

I. HISTORY AND BACKGROUND

Lyme disease, originally termed Lyme arthritis, was first recognized in 1975 following an outbreak of arthritis in and around the rural community of Lyme, Connecticut. The association of the illness with a unique skin lesion, erythema chronicum migrans (ECM), and the close geographic clustering of these early cases suggested the disease might be an infection transmitted by an arthropod. Subsequent investigations revealed that the disease was transmitted by a newly identified tick *Ixodes dammini* or related ixodid ticks. A few years later, Willy Burgdorfer and colleagues isolated the spirochete, *Borrelia burgdoferi*, from a tick, *I. dammini*, and it was determined that this was the infectious organism. A disease similar to Lyme disease had been previously described in Europe and is now known to be caused by the same spirochete. Lyme disease is now recognized as a multisystem disorder. A skin lesion, ECM, is typically the first sign of infection, although not all patients infected with Lyme disease manifest this symptom. This can be followed by systemic manifestations involving the joints, heart, and nervous system. The diagnosis of active Lyme disease is not straightforward because, unlike some bacterial infections, *B. burgdorferi* is not easily cultured. Currently, the method recommended by the

Centers for Disease Control (CDC) for diagnosing the disorder includes physician-documented ECM or the detection of antibodies in blood serum, which indicate exposure to *B. burgdorferi*, and at least one late objective manifestation of the disease, such as musculoskeletal pain, chronic arthritis, myocarditis, cranial neuritis, or radiculoneuropathy. However, not all people who are infected have the typical clinical symptoms of Lyme disease, and for this relatively small group the diagnosis is sometimes questionable. This has made the diagnosis of some disorders that have been attributed to Lyme disease, such as Lyme encephalopathy, controversial. For most patients, Lyme disease can be successfully treated with antibiotic therapy. However, a small percentage of patients develop a mild to moderate chronic encephalopathy, a peripheral neuropathy, or both, which may occur months to years after disease onset.

II. NEUROLOGICAL MANIFESTATIONS

The classic neurological symptoms of early disseminated Lyme disease are meningitis, cranial neuritis, and radiculoneurotis. These occur alone or in combination in approximately 15% of untreated patients. A unilateral or bilateral facial nerve palsy is also a relatively common symptom of early disseminated disease. Symptoms usually last for weeks to months but can become chronic. Chronic neurologic manifestations of the disorder, which include encephalopathy, polyneuropathy, and leukoencephalopathy, usually occur late in the illness. Although there have been reports of cases with severe cognitive impairment, including psychosis and dementia, and vasculitic lesions, such cases are rare. A mild chronic Lyme encephalopathy (LE) is the most common neurologic symptom in patients with late-stage disease. Months to years after disease onset, sometimes following long periods of latent infection, a small percentage of patients develop a mild to moderate encephalopathy. The symptoms tend to be diffuse and nonspecific and can include memory loss, naming problems, sleep disturbance, fatigue, and depression.

The diagnosis of LE is difficult. It is generally believed that those with immunity to *B. burgdorferi* and abnormal cerebral spinal fluid (CSF) are more likely to have a neurological basis to their illness. Even if a patient is seropositive, it is difficult to know whether active infection is causing encephalopathy because serologic testing only indicates exposure to the *B. burgdorferi*, not active infection. The standard neurological examination is usually normal. The CSF examination may show a positive polymerase chain reaction to *B. burgdorferi* DNA, intrathecal production of antibody to *B. burgdorferi*, or increased CSF protein. Traditional brain neurophysiological and neuroimaging techniques have also not been shown to be highly sensitive to the pathophysiology of LE. The routine electroencephalograph is typically normal. Magnetic resonance imaging (MRI) abnormalities have been described in Lyme patients, but these are nonspecific and relatively infrequent. When MRI abnormalities are present they are usually white matter lesions, suggesting the possibility of an inflammatory process. Single photon emission computed tomography (SPECT) imaging has shown some promise in identifying brain abnormalities in Lyme patients. Because the spatial resolution of SPECT is relatively poor, it can be used together with MRI to provide information about metabolic activity in specific brain regions (Fig. 1). SPECT has proved sensitive in identifying pathophysiologic abnormalities in other neurobehavioral disorders such as Alzheimer's disease and other dementias. In 1997, Logigian and colleagues studied a series of LE patients using a quantitative SPECT technique. In their analysis, 10 transaxial slices were imaged from each brain and divided into 4320 macrovoxels (Fig. 2). Quantitative SPECT has an advantage over visual image analysis because regional radiotracer uptake is analyzed statistically for each macrovoxel using an analysis of covariance. Patient scans are compared macrovoxel by macrovoxel to normal subjects to determine which brain regions are hyperperfused.

The Lyme patients showed patterns of multifocal hypoperfusion, most notably in the subcortical areas including the basal ganglia and white matter of the cerebral hemispheres, which was not apparent in normal controls. Patients with more objective evidence of LE, including CSF abnormalities, demonstrated significantly lower cerebral perfusion than Lyme patients with encephalopathic symptoms without objective evidence of central nervous system (CNS) involvement. Studies using visual ratings to assess the reduction in regional uptake of radiotracer have similarly reported decreased perfusion in Lyme patients. The reduction of metabolic activity in frontal and temporal lobe structures may provide a clue to the neuroanatomic basis of LE. That these same white matter regions form the large-scale neurocognitive networks involved in mediating memory and attention also suggests a possible explanation for the cognitive

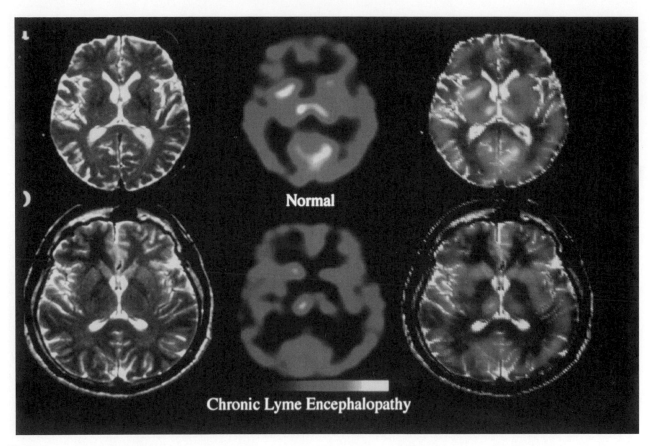

Figure 1 Representative MRI scan (left), SPECT image (center), and superimposed MRI/SPECT image (right) in a normal subject and in a patient with objective evidence of LE. The dark areas correspond to lower and the light areas to higher perfusion. (See color insert in Volume 1).

deficits described previously. Unfortunately, hypoperfusion in these brain regions is not specific to Lyme disease. Similar SPECT findings have been reported in other conditions that have symptoms similar to LE, such as depression and chronic fatigue syndrome. Although some investigators argue that the pattern of hypoperfusion in LE may differ from that seen in other disorders, current quantitative SPECT studies have not yet been done. Therefore, SPECT alone is not sufficient in diagnosing LE.

III. NEUROPSYCHOLOGICAL STUDIES

Although a number of studies that have attempted to define the relationship between positive serology, CNS infection, and cognitive dysfunction, few have used neuropsychological testing to characterize the nature of the cognitive deficits. Neuropsychological tests have an advantage over even comprehensive bedside mental status examinations in detecting cognitive dysfunction associated with LE because the deficits are often subtle. For most neuropsychological procedures, the presence or absence of functional impairment is made on a statistical basis. Ideally, performance on a given test is interpreted in comparison to normative data appropriate to the patient's age, sex, and education. Probable impairment on a specific cognitive test is inferred when performance falls below a designated cutoff score, usually two standard deviations below the normative mean. Whether or not a particular test will discriminate between normal and abnormal function for either individuals or clinical populations depends on a number of critical factors. Reliability and validity data are essential for understanding the limits of a given test. Additionally, the ability of a test to discriminate between groups depends on the purpose and population for which the test was developed. For example, tests such as the Mini-Mental State Examination that were developed to screen for dementia in elderly populations are relatively insensitive to cognitive deficits in patients with Lyme disease.

The traditional approach in neuropsychological assessment used to define cognitive deficits associated

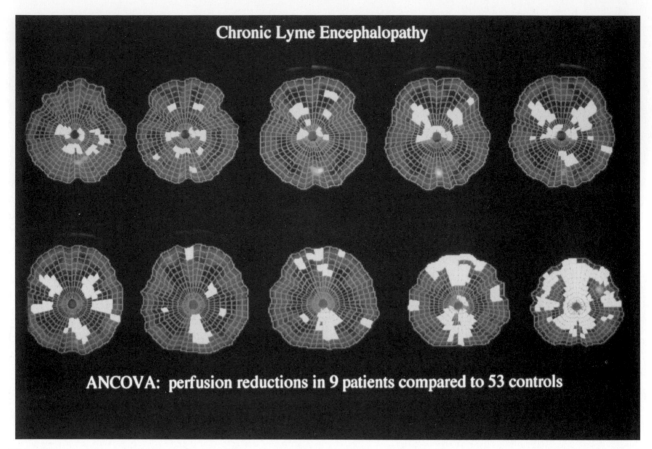

Figure 2 Quantitative SPECT analysis of nine patients with LE (mean data). Axial slices ascend from lowest (top left) to highest brain levels (bottom right). Macrovoxels whose mean perfusion is reduced at the $p < 0.001$ level below the mean of normal subjects ($n = 53$) are shown in white. The dark areas correspond to lower and the light areas to higher perfusion.

with brain disease is to administer a battery of tests. Often, differences in cognitive performance between two clinical populations, such as those with LE and those with depression alone, are best appreciated when the evaluation is based on an analysis of test score patterns. A pattern of scores not only indicates what is wrong with the patient but also what is right with the patient. The test battery usually includes both tests of general intellectual abilities, such as the Wechsler Scales, and tests developed to assess specific areas of cognitive dysfunction, such as attention, visual perception, construction, fine motor control, language, memory, and executive functioning. Test batteries also usually include measures of psychopathology in order to assess the patient's emotional state. The latter are often useful in interpreting other test results because psychological states such as anxiety and depression can impact a patient's cognitive abilities, particularly motivation and the ability to maintain and sustain attention. The importance of this cannot be overstated

because although the sensitivity of neuropsychological tests in identifying brain dysfunction is quite high (between 80 and 90%), the specificity may be considerably lower. For example, a memory test that discriminates traumatic brain-injured patients from normal subjects does not indicate how important variables such as attention or affective states may impact performance. It is also incumbent upon the clinician or researcher to interpret neuropsychological test data in the context of the patients' medical and psychosocial history as well as psychiatric status. Table I provides a list of neuropsychological tests that have frequently been used in assessing cognitive deficits in Lyme disease patients.

In comparison to other more well-known brain disorders such as Alzheimer's disease, for which there are large neuropsychological databases, the number of neuropsychological studies in LE is relatively limited. The following discussion presents the neuropsychological test data in considerable detail in an attempt to

Table I
**Neuropsychological Tests Frequently Used to Assess Deficits in
Lyme Disease**

Tested domain or function	Neuropsychological test
General cognitive abilities	Wechsler Intellignece Scales
	Shipley Institute of Living Scale
Attention/concentration	
Short-term auditory attention	Digit Span Test
Sustained attention	Stroop Test (Word and Color)
	Continuous Performance Tests
	Symbol Digit Substitution Test
Interference	Stroop Test (Color/Word)
Learning and memory	California Verbal Learning Test
	Selective Reminding Test
	Rey–Osterrieth Complex Figure Test
	Wechsler Memory Scale
Language and verbal output	
Naming	Boston Naming Test
Verbal fluency	Controlled Word Association Test
Executive functions	
Set maintenance and shifting	Trails A and B
Abstraction and set shifting	Wisconsin Card Sorting
Distractibility	Stroop Test
Problem solving	Halstead Category Test
Motor dexterity	Finger Tapping
	Grooved Peg Board
Neuropsychiatric symptoms	
Mood	Beck Depression Inventory
	Center for Epidemiologic Studies Depression Scale
	State Trait Anxiety Scale
Personality	Minnesota Multiphasic Personality Inventory
Anxiety	State Trait Anxiety Scale
Fatigue	Fatigue Severity Scale

demonstrate the nature and extent of cognitive dysfunction in LE.

In 1988, Halperin and colleagues published one of the earliest studies that included neuropsychological testing. They studied 17 Lyme patients before and after antibiotic treatment. All initially complained of memory deficits; however, only 4 had evidence of other neurological involvement and only 1 had abnormal CSF. The evaluation included tests of memory, visual spatial organization, conceptual thinking, and psychomotor and perceptual motor skills. The pretreatment results are difficult to interpret in part because these investigators failed to include a normal comparison group and also because there was no indication of the number of patients whose performance statistically fell outside the normal range. However, the authors report that there were pretreatment cognitive deficits in almost every area examined. Significant improvements following treatment were found on measures of recall memory on the California Verbal Learning Test (CVLT) as well as on tests of attention, concentration and motor speed, abstract problem solving, fine motor dexterity, and visual spatial organization. Improvement, however, was not evident on all tests. Patients' performances were unchanged on measures of tracking and sequencing, verbal fluency, auditory attention span, and recognition memory. Patients were also administered the Beck Depression Inventory (BDI), a self-administered questionnaire that measures the presence and severity of symptoms associated with depression. There was no evidence of significant depression either before or after treatment. However, the average score on the BDI, which reflects the overall severity of depression, was almost halved following treatment.

In a 1990 report, investigators at the New England Medical Center in Boston described 27 patients with chronic neurological abnormalities of at least 3 months duration following well-recognized manifestations of Lyme disease. Twenty-two of the 27 patients reported memory loss and 18 had CSF protein, evidence of intrathecal antibody to *B. burgdorferi*, or both. Each underwent a neuropsychological test battery consisting of tests of general cognitive abilities, memory, visual perception, construction, executive function, language, and fine motor dexterity. The patients were also administered the Minnesota Multiphasic Personality Inventory (MMPI) to assess emotional status. Standard scores were calculated from published, age-corrected normative data, and scores that were two standard deviations below the mean were considered as evidence of impairment on a particular test. Memory impairment was defined as two standard deviations below average on any one test or one standard deviation below average on two tests, according to a previously described system. All patients had IQ scores that were calculated or estimated to be average or above average. Twelve of the 22 patients reporting memory difficulty met the criteria for memory impairment, as did 2 patients who denied memory problems. Only 1 patient had a below average

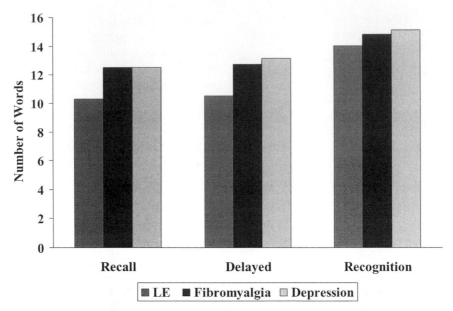

Figure 3   A comparison of memory scores for patients with LE, fibromyalgia, and depression on the CVLT.

performance on a test of abstract problem solving, the Wisconsin Card Sorting test, and 1 patient did poorly on a naming test. No patient had a below average performance on any of the other cognitive tests. Nine patients produced MMPI profiles consistent with depression. Of the 12 patients with objective evidence of memory impairment, 9 had abnormal CSF findings; however, it should be noted that 9 of 10 patients with normal memory scores also had abnormal CSF. The 4 of 24 patients with abnormal MRI scans, which were characterized as small round lesions in the periventricular white matter, all had impaired memory and 3 of the 4 had abnormal CSF.

In contrast to the earlier study by Halperin and colleagues that described a wide range of cognitive impairment, the only significant deficits in this study were in the area of memory impairment. However, unlike the patients in Halperin's study, more than half of the patients in this study had been treated with one or more courses of antibiotic treatment prior to testing. It is therefore possible that the discrepancy in results between the two studies reflects partial recovery.

Many of the symptoms of LE are similar to those reported by patients with depression. These include irritability, fatigue, emotional liability, poor concentration, impaired sleep, and memory disturbance. Depression is also common in late-stage Lyme disease. To examine the impact of psychological factors—particularly somatic concerns, depression, and anxiety

—on memory impairment in LE patients, my colleagues and I compared 20 patients with well-documented Lyme disease to patients with fibromyalgia and patients with mild to moderate depression. The rationale for comparing fibromyalgia and depressed patients with LE patients was that the cognitive symptoms in these illnesses are similar. Thirteen of the 20 Lyme patients had abnormal CSF and 2 had abnormal MRI scans. Memory was assessed using the three standardized memory instruments—the CVLT, the Wechsler Memory Scale (WMS), and the Rey–Osterrieth Complex Figure. Indices of psychopathology were obtained from the MMPI and BDI. The depression and fibromyalgia groups performed significantly better than the LE group on both the CVLT (Fig. 3) and a WMS visual memory subtest, whereas recognition memory on the CVLT did not differ. The depression group also performed better than the Lyme group on the WMS Verbal Paired Associate Learning test, another verbal learning test. In contrast, both the fibromyalgia and depressed groups showed greater evidence of psychopathology. On the MMPI, the Lyme group had significantly lower scores on the scales most sensitive to depression and anxiety compared to those of the depression group and significantly lower scores on scales sensitive to the somatic concerns compared to those of the fibromyalgia group (Fig. 4). The Lyme group also had lower BDI scores, but this did not reach statistical significance. These data strongly suggest that memory impairment in LE

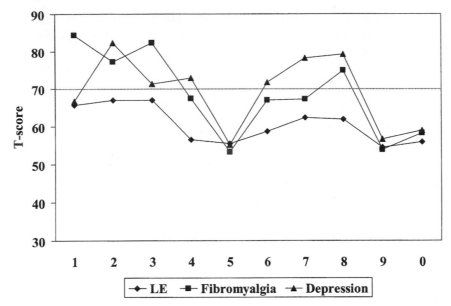

Figure 4   Composite MMPI for LE, fibromyalgia, and depression patient groups.

cannot be explained by affective symptoms alone, even though Lyme patients may report more symptoms of depression than normal controls.

If there is a pattern that emerges from the investigations outlined previously, it is that a memory disturbance appears to be the most common cognitive deficit found in LE patients. Other cognitive domains, such as attention, psychomotor performance, and executive functioning, were reported to be impaired in some but not all studies, even when observed problems in these other areas appeared to be of a lesser magnitude than the memory findings. Memory for verbal material appeared to be more affected than that for nonverbal material; however, this may be more a function of the type of test used because the verbal and nonverbal memory tests used are not of equal difficulty. The verbal list learning tests require acquisition of material over multiple trials and greater use of mnemonic strategy than the nonverbal learning tests (e.g., Rey–Osterrieth Complex Figure). It is also thought that tasks requiring sustained effort, such as the CVLT, may be more vulnerable to the effects of fatigue, and Lyme patients do report greater fatigue than controls. Furthermore, there is no anatomical reason why one would expect a material-specific memory deficit in this population. Recognition memory was spared relative to recall memory in every study. This is of interest because MRI and SPECT studies suggest that the pathophysiology of *B. burgdorferi* primarily affects CNS white matter. The

pattern of memory deficits in LE parallels that of another white matter disease, multiple sclerosis (MS). On list learning tests such as the CVLT, MS patients have been shown to have lower initial acquisition rates but similar rates of learning and forgetting when compared to healthy normals. The same pattern is true for LE.

IV. POPULATION STUDIES

In the laboratory studies of the LE described previously patients were selected on the basis of neurologic complaints. Although these types of studies have been helpful in understanding the nature and severity of neurologic deficits in Lyme disease, they tell us little about the prevalence of these symptoms. Nancy Shadick and colleagues studied the prevalence of persistent neurologic symptoms in a sample of unselected patients with a history of Lyme disease in Ipswich, Massachusetts, a community endemic for Lyme disease. These investigators initially studied 38 people who met CDC criteria for previous Lyme disease and 43 people who did not. There was a slight but statistically significantly difference between groups on the CVLT, with the Lyme disease group performing more poorly. Twelve of the 38 Lyme patients scored two or more standard deviations below mean on the word list test, compared to only 5 of the 43 controls. Patients with residual symptoms, neurologic and musculoskeletal, had longer duration of disease prior to treatment. These findings suggested that a small percentage of patients with previous Lyme disease may have permanent learning and memory deficits, albeit subtle. In a larger subsequent study on Nantucket, another community highly endemic for Lyme disease, these investigators compared 186 people with prior Lyme disease to 167 healthy controls using similar measures including the CVLT. Patients were studied an average of 6 years after infection. Although the patient group reported a higher incidence of nonspecific symptoms, including fatigue, difficulty sleeping, memory impairment, and poor concentration, there were no significant differences between groups on any of the objective tests of memory and concentration. At least two other population studies produced similar findings—namely, that the prevalence of objective measures of LE in previously infected patients who were treated for Lyme disese is very low. Thus, although patients previously infected with Lyme disease may report more neurologic symptoms than never infected controls, there is little evidence of any objective deficits. The relationship between reports of perceived memory dysfunction and performance on memory tests is discussed later.

V. LE IN CHILDREN

Although Lyme disease was first described in children, most studies of LE have involved adults. The incidence of Lyme disease is actually higher in children than in adults, but there are fewer reports of long-term problems. Even in children with Lyme arthritis, who were not treated or were treated years after the onset of infection, the incidence of encephalopathy was low. It has also been noted that children with Lyme disease almost never have the nonspecific symptoms of LE as the sole manifestation of the illness. Wayne Adams and colleagues studied 41 children, aged 6–17, with well-documented Lyme disease. All had been treated with antibiotics and the testing occurred about 2 years after disease onset. The children, 23 healthy sibling controls and 14 with subacute rheumatological diseases, were compared on a battery of standard neuropsychological tests, academic achievement tests, and parental rating scales. The neuropsychological test battery included measures of intelligence, information processing speed, fine-motor dexterity, executive functioning, and memory. The parents were also asked to complete a questionnaire rating perceived changes in their child's behavior in the areas of school, person-

ality, family, and friends since the onset of Lyme disease. Absentee records and the results of standard academic achievement tests were obtained from the schools. No significant group differences were found on any of these measures. Moreover, among children with Lyme disease, those with early neurologic involvement did not differ on any measure from those without any neurologic symptoms. The authors concluded that although there may be individual cases of Lyme-related cognitive abnormalities, children who are properly diagnosed and properly treated are unlikely to have any long-term negative consequences from Lyme disease. Since there is evidence that LE in adults may not occur for years after the onset of the illness, these same authors reexamined 25 of the their original sample and 17 sibling controls 4 years later. Again, there was no cognitive impairment in the Lyme disease children.

VI. POST-LYME DISEASE SYNDROME

The terms post-Lyme disease syndrome and post-treatment chronic Lyme disease are used to describe patients who were previously diagnosed with Lyme disease and develop persistent encephalopathic symptoms months to years after antibiotic treatment. Not all patients with a clinical history of Lyme disease who later present with encephalopathic symptoms are seropositive or have abnormal CSF. Most patients who are seronegative do not have Lyme disease, although it is possible to be seronegative and have post-Lyme syndrome. There are also reported cases of seronegative patients with CSF evidence of Lyme infection; however, this is rare. Most patients diagnosed with post-Lyme syndrome are seropositive for Lyme disease and develop symptoms after treatment.

In 1991, Krupp and colleagues compared a group of treated Lyme disease patients who continued to report memory problems after treatment, to a group of healthy controls. All subjects received a similar neuropsychological test battery to those described previously, with the addition of a fatigue rating scale. There were no differences between patients and controls on the any of the intelligence tests, tests of tracking and sequencing, and tests of abstract problems solving. The Lyme disease group performed significantly worse on the verbal fluency and two memory measures. Patients were also more depressed than controls. Neuropsychological test scores remained lower in the Lyme group, relative to controls, even when the presence of depression was controlled

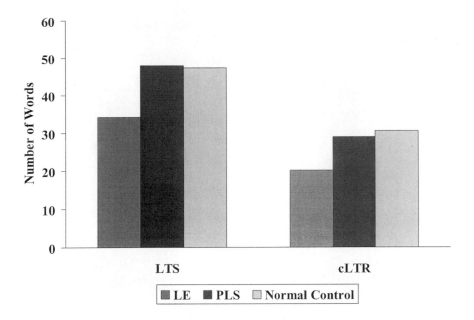

Figure 5 A comparison of memory scores for patients with LE, post-Lyme disease syndrome (PLS), and normal controls on the Selected Reminding Test. The two measures compared are total words recalled (LTS) and consistency of recall (cLTR).

statistically. Impairment was greatest for word recall on a verbal list learning test, the Selective Reminding Test (SRT). However, recognition memory did not discriminate patients and controls. The Lyme patients were also divided by the severity of neuropsychological impairment into mild, moderate, or severe categories based on the number of tests in which a patient's score fell below the published normative means (one or two standard deviations). On this basis, 9 of the 15 patients showed evidence of mild to moderate cognitive impairment, whereas 6 patients appeared normal despite complaints of memory trouble. Neither evidence of CSF infection nor MRI abnormalities correlated with the degree of cognitive impairment. However, fatigue was correlated with memory performance in the Lyme group but not the control group, with higher levels of fatigue associated with greater memory impairment. Interestingly, depressive symptoms were also correlated with memory scores. Paradoxically, however, more depressive symptoms corresponded to better memory scores.

Because it appeared that cognitive deficits exist in some Lyme patients independent of other evidence of neurological involvement, my colleagues and I studied the relationship between active infection and cognitive dysfunction. We compared 13 seropositive Lyme patients with evidence of inflammatory CSF to 20 seropositive Lyme patients without evidence of neu-

rological disease and 14 age-matched normal controls. Most patients in both Lyme groups described memory deficits as one of their symptoms. Eleven of 13 patients with abnormal CSF and 16 of 20 with normal CSF reported memory problems, versus none of the controls. On the SRT verbal memory measure, Lyme patients with abnormal CSF recalled significantly fewer words, were less consistent in their recall, and retrieved fewer items from memory than either Lyme patients with normal CSF or normal controls, who did not differ on any of these measures (Fig. 5). On the BDI, both Lyme disease groups endorsed significantly more symptoms than the normal control group, although no group's score was sufficiently high to meet the criteria for depression. Thus, although both groups of Lyme reported memory difficulties in our study, only the group with evidence of CNS infection performed more poorly on objective memory testing. However, both Lyme groups reported more symptoms of depression and anxiety than healthy controls (Fig. 6). These data suggest that depression may be a factor in perceived memory loss.

As a group, Lyme patients report significantly more symptoms of depression and fatigue than do controls, independent of evidence of CNS disease. In several studies the average depression scores for the Lyme patients were typically higher than for healthy controls but below the suggested cutoffs for clinical depression.

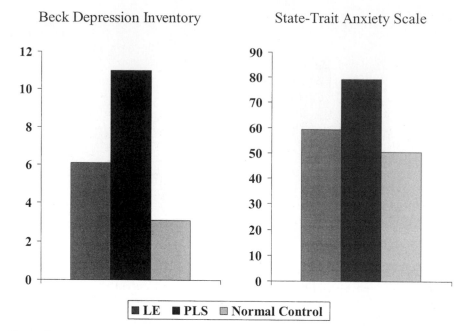

Figure 6 Depression and anxiety for LE, post-Lyme disease syndrome (PLS), and normal controls.

Moreover, although a significant proportion of Lyme patients meet the criteria for depression, depression scores and objective measures of memory loss have not been highly correlated. Fatigue, however, has been shown to be significantly correlated with poor memory in a number of studies.

In the study described previously, most Lyme patients complained of memory disturbance whether or not they had abnormal CSF. As such, the perception of memory loss was not a good predictor of objective impairment on neuropsychological testing. This finding has been replicated in several studies of Lyme disease patients. It is also not unique to Lyme disease. In most studies, self-reported poor memory is only weakly related to actual memory test performance, whereas it is strongly associated with conventional affective symptoms. Most studies have been done with elderly patients. These have shown that the relationship between subjective estimates of memory loss and objective measures of memory impairment is low. Instead, perceived memory loss tends to be related to psychological distress. As with many chronic illnesses, Lyme patients with late-stage disease often experience greater emotional distress, including depression and anxiety, than otherwise healthy people, although they do not meet the clinical criteria for psychopathology. It is therefore likely that the perceived memory disturbance in many Lyme patients

may be related to the stress and affective symptoms common to many chronic diseases.

VII. CONCLUSIONS

LE was originally used to describe mild confessional state—most commonly fatigue, sleep disturbance, memory loss, and depression—in patients with active systemic Lyme disease, particularly active arthritis. However, its meaning has become more general and is often used to describe patients with similar deficits but without laboratory confirmation of active Lyme infection. This has made the diagnosis of some disorders that have been attributed to Lyme disease highly controversial. In cases in which the patient has had the characteristic clinical picture, a positive serology to *B. burgdorferi*, and abnormal CSF, the symptoms are likely due to active infection. Moreover, there is evidence, from MRI and SPECT studies, that the infection preferentially affects white matter areas of the brain, although the mechanism is not known. Neuropsychological testing in these patients typically shows mild, but statistically significant, deficits on memory testing. After adequate antimicrobial therapy, most patients show significant improvements in their cognitive functioning and return to normal. In the one quantitative SPECT study, demonstrating a reduction of cerebral perfusion in patients with LE, there was also a partial reduction of hypoperfusion with antibiotic therapy.

The controversy regarding the diagnosis of LE stems from patients who report encephalopathic symptoms without clear evidence of an active Lyme infection, namely those with post-Lyme disease syndrome. Although some clinicians still attribute this to a subacute *B. burgdorferi* infection and recommend extended antimicrobial therapy, others question whether these symptoms are caused by active brain infection. Some neuropsychological investigations have shown these patients to perform more poorly than healthy normals, whereas others have not. Neuropsychological deficits in post-Lyme syndrome patients seem to be independent of a history of psychopathology but are correlated with concurrent fatigue. Lyme patients with independent evidence of CNS infection perform significantly worse on neuropsychological testing than post-Lyme disease syndrome patients. For patients without clear evidence of active Lyme disease, there is little efficacy to additional antimicrobial therapy. This has led some researchers to conclude that LE is probably overly diagnosed, and the lack of response to antibiotic therapy is the result of misdiagnosis. In addition to latent infection, other explanations for post-Lyme disease include the psychological consequences of chronic illness, residual deficits from past infection, and possibly an immune response. It has also been suggested that a fibromyalgia syndrome may be triggered by infection to *B. burgdorferi* after the infection is successfully treated since both disorders can result in similar cognitive complaints.

Patients with LE typically report memory problems independent of their performance on objective testing. The perception of cognitive difficulties may be common to a variety of physiological and psychological disorders. In chronic Lyme disease, patients with objective evidence of CNS infection, such as abnormal CSF, probably have a neurological basis to their reported cognitive decline. Other chronic Lyme patients are likely experiencing the stress and affective symptoms common to many chronic illnesses and similarly the perception of cognitive dysfunction.

Lastly, it is important to note that relative to the incidence of Lyme disease, the prevalence of chronic LE is quite low. Population studies have shown that only a small percentage of previously infected patients have neurological abnormalities, including objective evidence of memory impairment. Patients with residual deficits typically have had a longer duration of untreated disease prior to eventual treatment. Similarly, studies of children indicate that the chronic neurological deficits are rare when Lyme disease is adequately treated. Taken together, it is reasonable to conclude that the prognosis for returning to normal neurocognitive functioning after being infected with Lyme disease is good with adequate treatment.

See Also the Following Articles

BORNA DISEASE VIRUS • BRAIN LESIONS • CEREBRAL WHITE MATTER DISORDERS • PRION DISEASES

Suggested Reading

Adams, W. V., Rose, C. D., Eppes, S. C., and Klein, J. D. (1994). Cognitive effects of Lyme disease in children. *Pediatrics* 94, 185–189.

Halperin, J. J., Pass, H. L., Anand, A. K., Luft, B. J., Volkman, D. J., and Dattwyler, R. J. (1988). Nervous system abnormalities in Lyme disease. *Ann. N. Y. Acad. Sci.* 539, 24–34.

Kaplan, R. F., Jones-Woodward, L., Workman, K., Steere, A. C., Logigian, E., and Meadows, M.-E. (1999). Neuropsychological deficits in Lyme disease patients with and without other evidence of nervous system pathology. *Appl. Neuropsychol.* 8, 3–11.

Krupp, L. B., Masur, D., Schwartz, J., Coyle, P. K., Langenbach, L. J., Fernquist, S. K., Jandorf, L., and Halperin, J. J. (1991). Cognitive functioning in late Lyme borreliosis. *Arch. Neurol.* 48, 1125–1129.

Logigian, E. L., Kaplan, R. F., and Steere, A. C. (1990). Chronic neurologic manifestations of Lyme disease. *N. Engl. J. Med.* 323, 1438–1444.

Shadick, N. A., Phillips, C. B., Sanga, O., Logigian, E. L., Kaplan, R. F., Wright, E. A., Fossel, A. H., Fossel, K., Berardi, V., Lew, R. A., and Liang, M. H. (1999). Musculoskeletal and neurologic outcomes in patients with previously treated Lyme disease. *Ann. Intern. Med.* 131, 919–926.

Steere, A. C., Taylor, E., McHugh, G. L., and Logigian, E. L. (1993). The overdiagnosis of Lyme disease. *J. Am. Med. Assoc.* 269, 1812–1816.

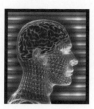

Magnetic Resonance Imaging (MRI)

JEFFRY R. ALGER

University of California, Los Angeles

GLOSSARY

longitudinal (T1) relaxation The process in which the nuclear spin magnetization recovers its orientation parallel to the applied magnetic field in characteristic time, T1, following a perturbation.

magnetic resonance imaging (MRI) A biomedical procedure that utilizes the magnetic resonance signal produced by the protons of tissue water to obtain vivid depictions of the internal macroscopic anatomy of soft tissues such as the brain.

nuclear spin magnetization The magnetic properties that result from the spinning behavior of a single atomic nucleus or an ensemble of atomic nuclei when placed in a magnetic field.

spin echo pulse sequence A frequently used procedure in MRI in which, for a variety of technical reasons, the appearance of the MRI signal is caused to be delayed for a defined time period after the excitation of the magnetization away from its equilibrium orientation.

transverse (T2) relaxation The process in which the nuclear spin magnetization loses its orientation perpendicular to the applied magnetic field in characteristic time, T2, following a perturbation.

time-to-echo The time delay between MRI signal excitation and the appearance of maximal signal when a spin echo pulse sequence is employed.

time-to-repeat The time between successive MRI signal excitations.

Magnetic resonance imaging (MRI) is a procedure that utilizes the magnetic resonance signal produced by the protons of tissue water to obtain vivid depictions of the internal macroscopic anatomy of soft tissues such as the brain. It has become the method of choice for nondestructive visualization of brain anatomy. The nuclear magnetic resonance (NMR) phenomenon on which MRI is based was discovered in the 1940s. NMR has become an indispensable tool in the fields of chemistry, biochemistry, and structural biology. In the 1970s, methods of forming images from the proton NMR signal produced by the water in living tissues were developed and became known as MRI. MRI is now a routinely used clinical tool and has growing utility for investigations involving brain structure. The purpose of this article is to familiarize the neuroscientifically inclined reader with key physical principles and fundamental technological aspects that underlie MRI.

I. MRI SIGNAL GENERATION

A. The Nuclear Spin

MRI is based on the fact that collections of atomic nuclei, when placed in a strong unchanging magnetic field, interact with an externally applied oscillating magnetic field when the frequency of the oscillating magnetic field meets certain specific criteria. Many texts inaccurately summarize this by saying that atomic nuclei absorb or emit electromagnetic radiation (i.e., radio waves). It is not accurate to infer an interaction between atomic nuclei and electromagnetic radiation because electromagnetic radiation requires the concurrent presence of electric and magnetic fields with specific spatial and temporal relationships. In

MRI one avoids use of oscillating electric fields because these do not interact with the atomic nuclei. Only the oscillating magnetic field interacts with the atomic nuclei. In MRI, it is the hydrogen nucleus (^1H), which is often referred to as "the proton," that is responsible for generating the signal from which the images are formed. Other atomic nuclei (e.g., ^{19}F, ^{31}P, and ^{23}Na) have been used in exploratory biomedical MRI studies. However, the use of nuclei other than protons is not widespread for brain MRI. The vast majority of the protons present in biological tissue are constituents of water molecules; therefore, water protons have the greatest relevance in MRI. However, the protons in the fatty acyl components of lipid molecules of fatty tissue can also be imaged. One of the reasons that MRI is a successful neuroimaging tool is that water, which is found at high concentration in soft tissues such as the brain, generates the signal from which the images are formed. MRI is distinct from conventional radiographic and computed tomographic approaches to brain imaging. In MRI, an intrinsic tissue signal is imaged, whereas X-ray techniques are based on attenuation of an X-ray beam by the tissue.

Figure 1 illustrates the fundamental properties of the proton that lead to MRI. Any particular volume element (voxel) of brain tissue contains a very large number of water molecules, each of which has two protons. A typical MRI voxel ($1 \times 1 \times 3\,mm^3$) of brain tissue contains about 10^{20} protons. Each proton behaves as a bar magnet because it acts as if it spins about an axis. The property of spin and the associated magnetism lead to the use of the terms "spin" or "nuclear spin" as synonyms for proton or hydrogen nucleus. In the foregoing, the verb "to behave" was used to reflect the fact that the magnetic and spin properties of the atomic nucleus are governed by the laws of quantum mechanics, the science that deals with the behavior of matter and energy at very small dimensions. A detailed discussion of quantum mechanical behavior of the nuclear spin is beyond the scope of this article. Accordingly, "real-world" descriptions will be used as an approximation for the behavior of the atomic nuclei in the quantum world.

B. Interaction of the Nuclear Spin with Magnetic Fields

MRI requires that the signal-generating protons be placed in a strong static magnetic field. It is conventional to denote the applied magnetic field by a vector quantity, B_0. The typical magnetic field strength used in brain imaging is 1.5 T (approximately 30,000 times stronger than the earth's magnetic field). The spatial

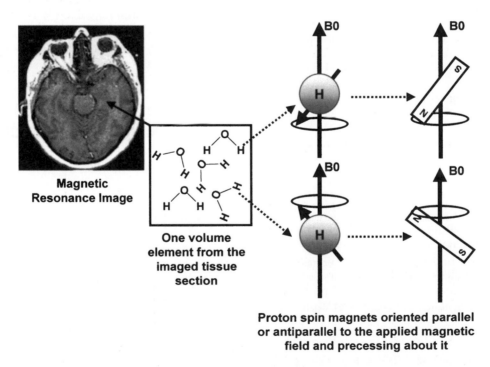

Magnetic Resonance Image

One volume element from the imaged tissue section

Proton spin magnets oriented parallel or antiparallel to the applied magnetic field and precessing about it

Figure 1 Key concepts related to MRI signal creation.

homogeneity of the magnetic field also plays an important role in defining feasibility of imaging. Typically, the magnetic field must vary less than 100 parts per million (ppm) over the entire brain volume and less than about 1 ppm over any particular imaging voxel. An important attribute of MRI is that the magnetic field readily penetrates bony structures, permitting MRI to "see" the brain through the bony cranium.

C. The Larmor Relationship

Figure 1 illustrates how the proton nuclear spins (equivalent to spinning bar magnets) behave in an imposed magnetic field. They tend to align parallel to (with) or antiparallel to (against) the magnetic field. Such behavior is readily appreciated when two magnets are manipulated in the macroscopic world. When a smaller magnet is placed inside a larger one, the smaller magnet's north pole tends to point toward the north pole of the larger magnet. "North to south" orientation has some stability, but a perpendicular orientation of the two magnets is highly unstable. In the quantum world, magnetic alignments are expressed in terms of their probabilities. Alignment in the parallel configuration is only slightly more probable compared to that of the antiparallel configuration. Furthermore, in the quantum world, the alignment is not perfect. The spin causes the nuclear magnet to "precess" about the applied magnetic field at a constant angle in each of the two allowed configurations. The precession frequency, v, (the number of precession cycles per second), is a linear function of the applied magnetic field

$$v = \gamma B_0$$

Precession characteristics such as these are found in everyday mechanical systems (e.g., gyroscopes). The relationship between the precession frequency and the applied magnetic field on the orbital motion of an electron was described in 1897 by Sir Joseph Larmor. Accordingly, even in the context of MRI, the expression that relates precessional frequency to magnetic field strength is known as the Larmor relationship. The Larmor relationship indicates that the precession frequency is directly proportional to the magnetic field strength, with γ (the gyromagnetic ratio) being a constant of proportionality that is a unique property of the type of nucleus. For the proton, γ is approximately 42 million cycles per second per Tesla. Therefore, the characteristic frequency at which the nuclear spins

precess about the commonly used applied magnetic field strength (1.5 T) is 63.8 MHz.

D. Behavior of Large Ensembles of Nuclear Spins

A single nuclear spin would produce a signal that is far too weak to detect. Therefore, it is necessary to consider how large numbers of nuclear spins behave in a collective sense to understand how a measurable MRI signal is produced. It is the 10^{20} protons in the typical MRI voxel that produce the signal used for image formation. Some of the spins are oriented antiparallel to the applied field, whereas others are oriented parallel to the applied field (Fig. 2). Nature tends to favor the parallel configuration because this represents an energetically more stable (lower energy) state. However, the two possible configurations do not differ to a great extent in their energy stability, and there are almost equal numbers of spins in the two configurations. The magnetic field from each of the spins in the antiparallel configuration is canceled by a spin in the parallel configuration, but there are spins in the parallel configuration that not canceled by antiparallel spins. These "uncanceled" parallel spins act cohesively as an ensemble. They collectively behave as a bar magnet oriented perfectly parallel with B_0. It is common practice to refer to the magnetic properties of the ensemble as the "bulk nuclear spin magnetization" or "magnetization." The angle between the magnetization and B_0 is lost because each nuclear spin precesses about the applied field independently of the others. Nature imposes no constraints on where along

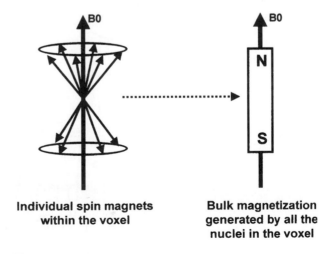

Individual spin magnets within the voxel   **Bulk magnetization generated by all the nuclei in the voxel**

Figure 2 Ensembles of nuclear spins create a magnetization parallel to the applied magnetic field.

each precession circle each spin happens to be, and the transverse component nuclear spin magnetization perpendicular to B_0 is zero. It is important to also emphasize that the bulk magnetization produced by an ensemble of many nuclear spins behaves differently than does the spin magnetization from a single spin. The bulk magnetization from an ensemble of nuclear spins can attain any arbitrary orientation relative to B_0. Its behavior is not "quantized" as is the case for a single spin's magnetization.

E. The Magnetic Resonance Signal

In MRI, images are formed from the electrical "signals" generated by each of the volume elements in the tissue. The bulk magnetization resultant from the ensemble of spins in each of the volume elements generates the MRI signals. In order to detect the MRI signal, it is necessary to first disturb the bulk magnetization away from the equilibrium configuration shown in Figure 2. This is done using a radiofrequency (RF) transmitter pulse (Fig. 3). The working part of the RF pulse is a second magnetic field, which is usually referred to as B_1. The B_1 magnetic field differs from B_0 in that it oscillates. In order to be effective, B_1 must oscillate at a frequency that is very near to the Larmor frequency (e.g., 63.8 MHz for 1.5 T). When this is the case, there is a coupling between B_1 and the nuclear spin precessions that causes the bulk magnetization to be rotated away from its equilibrium position toward the transverse plane perpendicular to B_0. Energy from the B_1 field is used to excite the magnetization to a nonequilibrium configuration. Figure 3 shows the result of a 90° pulse in which the magnetization is twisted through an angle of 90° into the transverse plane. Coupling between the bulk magnetization and a B_1 field having the appropriate oscillatory frequency is an example of the phenomenon known in physics as resonance. The oscillatory B_1 field is created by the flow of alternating electric current through a coil of wire (i.e., the RF coil) that is placed near the tissue being imaged. The alternating electric current frequency must be very near the Larmor frequency (typically 63.8 MHz) to create the appropriate oscillation frequency for B_1. Use of RF is a central part of radio and television broadcasting; therefore, one often hears that MRI results from an interaction between "radio waves" and nuclear spins. However, as has already been stated, only oscillating magnetic fields are used in MRI, and it is not correct to state that radio waves are used in MRI.

Once the magnetization has been disturbed as shown in Fig. 3, it precesses about the transverse plane

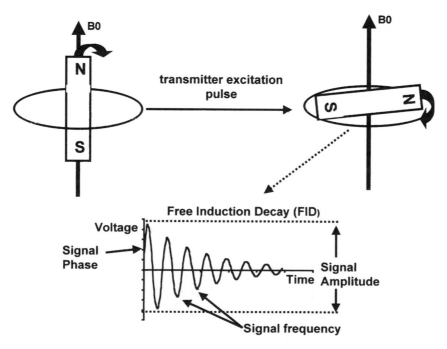

Figure 3 Perturbation of the magnetization with a radiofrequency pulse and the resultant free induction decay signal.

at the Larmor frequency. This precessional motion can be detected with a coil of wire (i.e., the RF coil) that is placed near the tissue of interest. The motion of the magnetization generates a voltage oscillating at the Larmor frequency in the coil. Therefore, one can describe the phenomenon by saying that the nuclear spins transmit a radio frequency signal on a characteristic radio "channel" that is detected by the MRI scanner. Note, however, that radio waves per se are not involved in this signal-generation process. The signal subsequently decays as illustrated in the graph shown in Fig. 3. The maximal signal amplitude (voltage) is proportional to the magnetization, which in turn is principally dependent on the number of nuclear spins in the ensemble, although other factors (described later) also play a role. The MRI signal that results immediately from a 90° pulse is known as a free induction decay (FID). It is often advantageous to cause the signal to appear sometime after the transmitter RF pulse is finished. One way of doing this is to form a spin echo. Spin echo MRI signals oscillate at the Larmor frequency just as FID signals do. However, they build up and then disappear at some defined period of time after the transmitter pulse is completed (Fig. 4). The time that elapses between the initial transmitter pulse and the formation of the echo is known as the time-to-echo (TE). The amplitude of the spin echo signal decays as the TE is progressively lengthened, as illustrated in the graph shown in Fig. 4. This will be discussed in more detail later.

Formation of a spin echo requires the use of two RF pulses given in a carefully prescribed manner. A series of pulses is referred to as a pulse sequence. In a broader sense, pulse sequences, which can be quite complicated, are frequently used in MRI to manipulate the magnetization in a defined manner so as to accentuate certain aspects of the MRI signal or for developing contrast. The spin echo pulse sequence is one of the simplest of a large and growing body of MRI pulse sequences.

II. IMAGING THE MAGNETIC RESONANCE SIGNAL

MRI visualization of structural anatomy requires measuring the MRI signal amplitude generated by each volume element within the tissue being imaged. Accomplishing this is more complicated than might be imagined. Because MRI does not use radio waves, it is not possible to focus "beams" of radio waves at suitable resolution to excite the MRI signal of only one volume element at a time and then sequentially sample all volume elements with this focused beam. Moreover, the sequential detection of the MRI signal from each volume element is highly inefficient and impractical.

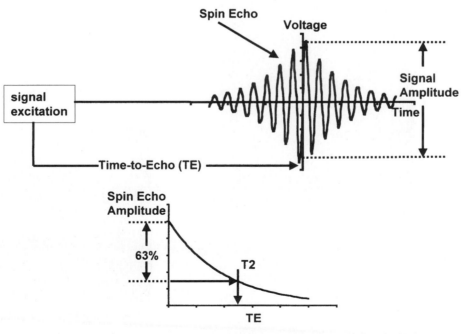

Figure 4 The spin echo signal and its dependence on TE.

Alternate ingenious methods based on the use of magnetic field gradients and precise frequency measurement are typically used for imaging entire sections or volumes of tissue.

A. Magnetic Field Gradients

A magnetic field gradient is a smooth (usually linear) variation in the static magnetic field (B_0) from one position to another position. Magnetic field gradients are purposefully applied in MRI as part of the imaging process. This is illustrated in Fig. 5. Application of a magnetic field gradient that varies smoothly in the inferior–superior direction causes B_0 in the neck to be relatively smaller compared to that in the brain. In the presence of this field gradient, the Larmor relationship ensures that there will be smooth linear dependence of the MRI signal frequency along the inferior–superior axis. Therefore, it is possible to know where along the superior–inferior axis a particular signal-generating volume element is located through precise frequency measurement. There is no strict requirement that a field gradient be oriented along any particular anatomic axis. Field gradients may be created that cause linear variation of B_0 along the left–right and the anterior–posterior axes or any arbitrary oblique axis

that lies at any angle between the principal anatomic axes. Furthermore, it should be understood that magnetic field gradients can be turned on and off (i.e., switched) during the pulse sequence. This permits the application of magnetic field gradients on different axes during different parts of the pulse sequence.

B. Slice Selection

In MRI, tomographic images of tissue slices having defined orientation, thickness and location are obtained. The slice selection process is accomplished by using a frequency-selective RF pulse during the application of a magnetic field gradient. A frequency-selective RF pulse permits the highly selective excitation of MRI signals having a narrow band of Larmor frequencies. The presence of a magnetic field gradient ensures that this narrow band of Larmor frequencies will correspond with a narrow tissue section. Protons that would generate signal outside of the narrow band of Larmor frequencies (i.e., those located beyond the edges of the narrow tissue section) are unaffected and do not produce signal. Figure 5 illustrates that an axial tissue section may be selected for subsequent imaging by using a frequency-selective RF pulse in the presence of a magnetic field gradient oriented along the inferior

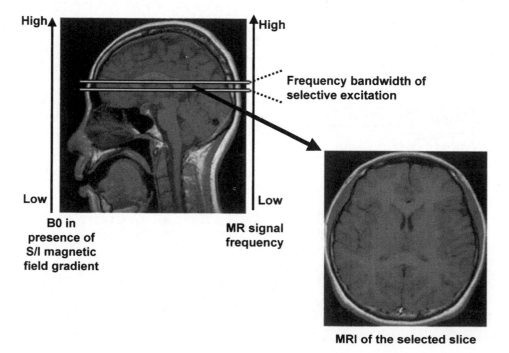

Figure 5   Slice selection in MRI.

to superior axis. Both the slice thickness and the slice location may be freely selected without physically moving the human subject or physically moving components of the scanning equipment relative to the subject. This is done by making suitable adjustments in the characteristics of magnetic field gradient or the frequency-selective RF pulse. Accordingly, the moving parts of MRI scanners tend to be limited to that needed for moving the subject into the appropriate part of the magnetic field at the beginning of the examination. Subsequently, neither the subject nor the scanning equipment moves during the image acquisition process. Furthermore, because a field gradient can be created along any arbitrary anatomic axis, it is possible to select slices in any of the three principal anatomic sectional planes (sagittal, axial, and coronal) or in any arbitrary oblique imaging plane without physically repositioning the subject or physically reorienting the imaging equipment (Fig. 6).

The obvious need to visualize anatomy in three dimensions is usually met through the use of mutlislice imaging. Figure 7 displays a series of 15 axial images that were obtained from tissue sections 3 mm thick. The conventional practice is to produce collages showing individual two-dimensional sectional images

as a means of visualizing three-dimensional (3D) anatomy. If the sections can be made sufficiently thin, it is possible to create a volume rendering that displays the cortical surface anatomy. Conventional multislice MRI for human subjects is limited to a slice thickness of about 3 mm. This is relatively thick for volume rendering purposes; therefore, when volume rendering is planned, special 3D acquisition techniques are employed in which more than 100 slices having slice thickness of about 1 mm are used. Figure 8 provides an example of volume rendered images that display brain surface anatomy from a variety of perspectives. In addition to viewing surface anatomy in the manner shown, it is also possible to section the digital representation of the brain volume and produce two-dimensional images in any chosen sectional plane. This is done retrospectively using purposely designed software that sections and displays images under user control. The volumetric nature of the image data also readily lends itself to studies in which it is desired to measure the volumes of specific neuroanatomical structures that can be visualized in the images. As a result, 3D acquisition techniques are often used in research studies in which quantitative evaluation of neuroanatomic volumes are sought. The volumetric

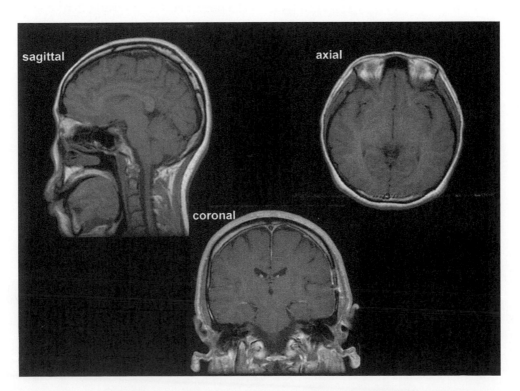

Figure 6   MRI slice selection can be in any chosen anatomic plane.

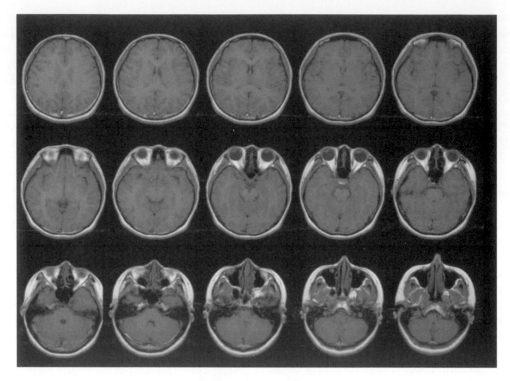

Figure 7   Multislice MRI.

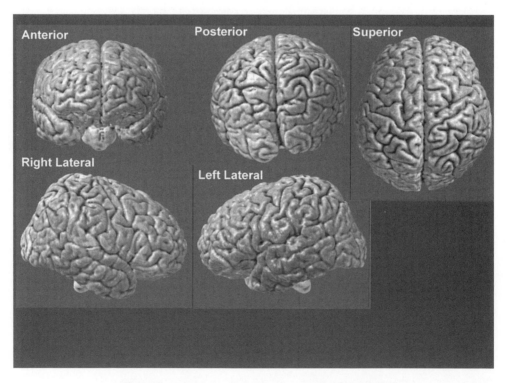

Figure 8   Volume rendering of three-dimensional MRI.

nature of the image data is also appropriate for the planning of neurosurgical procedures such as stereotactic biopsy. Accordingly, 3D volume MRI acquisition is often performed as part of the preoperative evaluation of patients for whom neurosurgical procedures are contemplated.

C. In-Plane Imaging: Frequency Encoding and Phase Encoding

Once the nuclear spins from a particular slice are excited, it is necessary to have methods of measuring how the MRI signal varies within the imaging plane. For two-dimensional imaging, two orthogonal coordinate directions are interrogated by application of magnetic field gradients that vary along these coordinate directions. Typically, frequency encoding and phase encoding gradients are used. To avoid confusing locations along the two orthogonal axes, the frequency encoding and phase encoding gradients are applied at different times during the pulse sequence. Figure 9 illustrates the general concepts. A magnetic field gradient is imposed such that the signal frequency is higher on the left compared to the right. (Note that it is customary in MRI to display the subject's left on the viewer's right.) This causes the signal frequency to depend on position along the left–right axis. A plot of signal amplitude versus frequency in the presence of this left–right frequency encoding gradient would give a one-dimensional image in which signal amplitude is projected down the columns along the anterior–posterior axis onto the left–right axis. The signal amplitude along this one-dimensional image defines the total amount of MRI signal generated by anterior–posterior columns. To obtain a two-dimensional image, a phase encoding gradient must also be used. In Fig. 9, the phase encoding gradient is applied along the anterior–posterior direction, causing the signal phase to depend on the position along the anterior–posterior direction. Phase encoding must be used because the signal frequency is already used for left–right encoding. Phase encoding is more complicated compared to frequency encoding. It is necessary to perform a number of phase-encoded signal measurements using different levels of the phase encoding to fully unravel the relationship between the position and phase. Typically, if it is desired to obtain a resolution of 256 image lines in the phase encode direction, then it is necessary to make on the order of 256 independent phase-encoded measurements.

The previous paragraph described the most commonly employed procedure for in-plane imaging. Several additional variant techniques have been

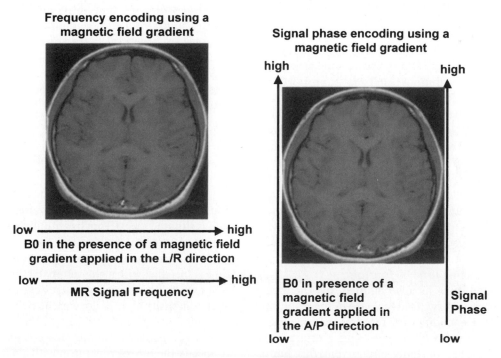

Figure 9 Frequency and phase encoding using applied magnetic field gradients with frequency measurement for in-plane imaging.

designed for specific purposes. The 3D acquisition techniques described previously use phase encoding in two dimensions and frequency encoding in one dimension without slice selection. This permits the slices to be made thinner than is typically possible when using conventional slice selection techniques. Another variant is known as echo planar imaging (EPI). In EPI, the frequency encoding and phase encoding are combined in a manner that speeds the imaging process considerably compared to conventional MRI. However, efficiency of EPI is partially offset by an increased susceptibility to artifacts arising from B_0 imperfections.

D. Resolution and Imaging Times

The typically attainable spatial resolution for brain MRI is approximately $1 \times 1 \times 3 \, mm^3$. Somewhat higher resolution can be attained in special circumstances (e.g., by using magnetic field strengths greater than $1.5 \, T$ or limited field-of-view RF coils). In general, the resolution is principally dependent on the signal-to-noise ratio (SNR) of the MRI signal produced by a single voxel. MRI "noise" results from the random movement of electric currents in the detection circuitry and in the subject. The noise level can generally be assumed to be a constant and only weakly dependent on the signal detection technique. Unfortunately, the MRI signal is relatively weak compared to that detected in many other forms of spectroscopy. It is often not appreciably larger than the noise. Reducing the size of the volume element to increase spatial resolution results in a proportional decrease in the SNR and this leads to an increased level of image "graininess," complicating visualization of subtle features. SNR may be increased through signal averaging (i.e., by spending more time at image acquisition), although this provides meager returns. In general, the SNR is directly proportional to the square root of the time spent at image acquisition. Doubling the image acquisition time leads to only a $\sqrt{2}$ (about 40%) improvement in SNR. If one wishes to improve the resolution by twofold without loss of image clarity (i.e., maintain the SNR), one must increase the imaging time by fourfold.

The imaging time is also limited by the phase encoding process. A twofold increase in the resolution along the phase encoding axis requires that one spend twofold more time at phase encoding. Certain rapid imaging techniques partially circumvent this limitation. EPI and fast spin echo imaging procedures are

examples. However, additional imperfections in image quality must be accepted as a consequence of more rapid imaging.

III. RELAXATION AND TISSUE CONTRAST

The process wherein the magnetization returns to its equilibrium configuration parallel to B_0 is known as nuclear spin relaxation. Typically, relaxation is conceptually separated into two separate processes: (i) relaxation of the magnetization component that is parallel to B_0 and (ii) relaxation of the magnetization component that is transverse to B_0. The former is known as longitudinal or T1 relaxation, and the latter is known as transverse or T2 relaxation.

Relaxation derives its energy from the random rotational and translational motion of the water (or lipid) molecules within the tissue. These motions are constrained by the tissue ultrastructure. It has not been possible to develop an exact theory of nuclear magnetic spin relaxation relevant to tissue due to the complex nature of the tissue ultrastructure. However, theories developed for simpler homogeneous materials can be extended to describe tissue nuclear spin relaxation. Moreover, tissue nuclear spin relaxation characteristics can be readily measured, so the absence of an exact theory is not a profound limitation. The practical utility is that different tissue types often display unique relaxation characteristics because of unique ultrastructural characteristics. Brain gray matter (GM), white matter (WM), and cerebrospinal fluid (CSF) each exhibit unique relaxation properties, and these may be used for developing image contrast between these tissue types.

A. T1 and Time-to-Repeat

T1 relaxation may be visualized as follows: At the conclusion of an excitation RF pulse, the magnetization is situated away from its equilibrium state. It takes a finite amount of time for the magnetization to recover to its equilibrium configuration. This recovery time is specified with a characteristic time constant that is known as T1. A series of image acquisitions produces signal intensity that is dependent on how rapidly the RF pulses are repeated relative to the rate at which the system is capable of relaxing. It is conventional in MRI to specify the rate of repetition with a parameter called time-to-repeat (TR). Figure 10 illustrates that repeated acquisitions done at short TR tend to produce a relatively weak signal (compared to longer TR) because the magnetization does not have sufficient time to reattain its equilibrium configuration. A series of measurements in which signal intensity is measured as TR is increased typically leads to results illustrated in Fig. 10. Increasing signal is observed as TR is lengthened and this generally follows an exponential mathematical function. Such a mathematical function can be completely described by a single "time constant," defined as the time at which some fraction (usually 50 or 63%) of the process is complete. Therefore, the relaxation time constant, T1, is defined as the TR at which 63% of the total available signal is measured. In other words, the T1 value is determined by locating the point along the curve where 63% of the total available signal is obtained and then projecting to the TR axis.

As indicated previously, the actual value of T1 depends on the extent to which the tissue ultrastructure constrains the molecular movement. Figure 11 illustrates general features of T1 relaxation in unique brain tissues. Tissues such as CSF in which the motion of water molecules is relatively unconstrained (and therefore rapid) tend to produce relatively long T1 values. T1 values in GM or WM are smaller than in CSF because the tissue ultrastructure constrains the water movement to a greater extent. Motional constants in WM are somewhat greater than in GM due to the presence of rigid myelin structures; WM T1 values are therefore shorter compared to GM T1 values. It is indeed fortuitous that the tissue T1 values are what they are. The TR must be on the order of T1 to realize an appreciable fraction of the total available signal. Brain T1 values are such that brain MRI may be performed with TR between 500 and 2000 msec. Therefore, a typical image acquisition (128 phase encodes) requires approximately 2 min. Were the brain T1 values to be significantly greater (as is the case for distilled water) the same acquisition would take 10 times longer.

B. T1-Weighted Imaging

Figure 11 illustrates the appearance of a T1-weighted (T1w) image. By definition, a T1w image is acquired using repetitive measures (for phase encoding and signal averaging) with full excitation (90° RF pulses) and TR that is between about 300 and 1000 msec. Image acquisition at this TR maximizes signal contrast between tissue types (Fig. 11). CSF shows the lowest (nearest to black on the gray scale) signal intensity. GM shows a somewhat stronger signal intensity (closer to white on the gray scale), but this is appreciably weaker than that produced by WM. The fatty tissue (not plotted on the graph) located around the orbits and in the superficial soft tissues shows a

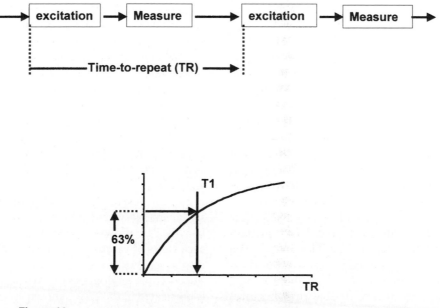

Figure 10   Longitudinal (T1) recovery and its relationship to the time-to-repeat (TR).

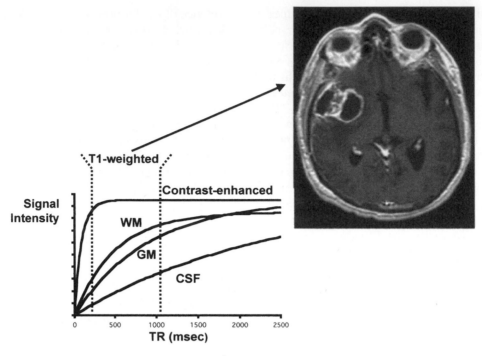

Figure 11   Contrast development through T1-weighted imaging.

very rapid T1 compared to brain tissues and this appears as intense signal in fatty tissues. The signal intensity differences in T1w imaging permit the reader to readily distinguish different tissue types and, thereby, to visualize the details of anatomic structure with great clarity.

Relaxation may be further enhanced by the use of relaxation agents, which are also called paramagnetic contrast agents. These materials have inherent magnetic properties arising from unpaired electron spins. They weakly associate with water molecules and through transient contact relax the water proton nuclear spins, making T1 very short. Intravenously infused paramagnetic contrast agents are commonly employed for clinical neuroimaging. The blood–brain barrier limits the access that such materials may have to normal brain tissue, and T1 of the normal brain tissue inside the intact blood–brain barrier is not altered. On the other hand, the agents tend to readily penetrate into tissue in which the blood–brain barrier is not intact (e.g., tumors). This leads to a relatively short T1 in tissues having a damaged blood–brain barrier and to very intense signal on T1w images. The image shown in Fig. 11 was obtained after intravenous administration of a commercially available contrast agent. It illustrates an intense double ring enhancement pattern produced by a tumor located at the right

(viewer's left) frontotemporal junction. The bright "ring" is generally thought to represent highly vascular living tumor tissue that does not have an intact blood–brain barrier.

Figure 12 illustrates that T1w imaging may also be used to obtain angiographic images showing the major intracerebral vessels. This is known as magnetic resonance angiography (MRA). Blood flow tends to accentuate T1 relaxation because flow is constantly moving new water into the tissue section that is being imaged. Therefore, intravascular water tends to show full signal intensity after each excitation because it was not in the slice during previous excitations. On the other hand, the brain water needs time to relax between excitations to produce strong signal. One MRA approach is to employ very heavily T1w contrast (i.e., very short TR) so that brain signal is very weak and the intravasular water produces a much stronger signal. This is illustrated in the image shown on the left in Fig. 12. One can appreciate spots and strings of high signal intensity that depict the major vessels in this heavily T1w (flow-sensitized) image. Although single-slice views of vascular anatomy such as this are useful, display of MRA results in a manner consistent with fluoroscopic angiography is typically employed. This is illustrated in the image shown on the right in Fig. 12. To construct an angiographic projection view,

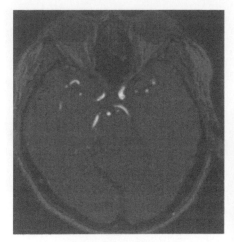

Flow Sensitized MRI

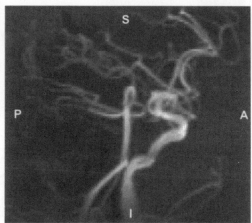

Maximum Intensity Projection

Figure 12   Magnetic resonance angiography.

flow-sensitized MRI is collected from many thin slices in a 3D format. This produces a 3D volume image in which the vessels are represented by relatively intense signal. Subsequently, the image intensities are projected onto a single viewing plane that may have any arbitrary orientation. In the example shown in Fig. 12, the angiographic information is being projected from a lateral perspective. From this perspective one can readily visualize the major feeding arteries of the corotid and basilar systems as well as many of the larger intracerebral vessels.

C. T2 and TE

Transverse (T2) relaxation is the process in which the finite components of the magnetization present in the transverse plane decay to zero (the equilibrium state). Often, T2 relaxation is discussed in terms of two separate processes. One of these is driven by molecular movements and is known as "pure" T2 relaxation. The other is the result of the presence of a magnetic field gradient within the voxel of interest and is known as T2* relaxation. To measure "pure" T2 relaxation independently of T2* relaxation, spin echo acquisitions (Fig. 4) are commonly used. The spin echo amplitude decays as the TE is lengthened, as illustrated in the graph in Fig. 4. This is generally found to be

described by a decaying exponential function that has a characteristic time constant. To determine the value of the characteristic time constant for transverse relaxation (T2), one finds the point at which 63% of the signal has decayed and then projects that point onto the TE axis.

As is the case for T1, the T2 value depends on motional constraints imposed by tissue ultrastructure. However, the functional dependence of T2 relaxation differs from that for T1 relaxation. Tissues in which the water molecule motion is unhindered (e.g., CSF) tend to produce a very long T2. Increasing constraints on water movement lead to progressively shorter values for T2. WM shows a shorter T2 compared to that of GM, and both of these show a shorter T2 compared to that of CSF. The T2 relaxation characteristics of the three tissues are illustrated in the graph shown in Fig. 13. Spin echo signals produced by each of the tissues decay as TE is lengthened, with the differences becoming more pronounced as progressively longer TE values are used.

D. Proton Density-Weighted and T2-Weighted Imaging

Figure 13 illustrates that spin echo imaging can be employed to obtain two different types of tissue

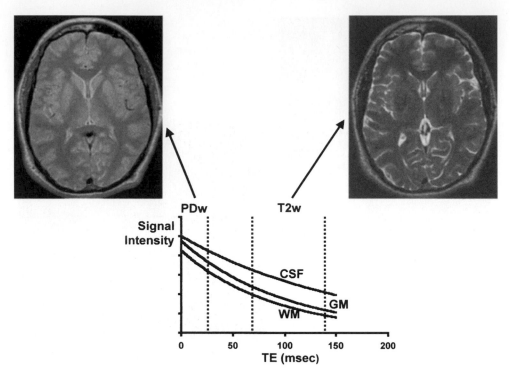

Figure 13   Contrast development through T2-weighted imaging.

contrast known as proton density contrast and T2 contrast. To obtain a proton density-weighted (PDw) image one uses a (relatively short) TE value of about 20 msec. Shorter TE values are desirable, but technical and engineering constraints usually prohibit their realization. In a PDw image the density of water protons is the predominant factor that defines what signal intensity is detected. Therefore, WM that has slightly fewer water protons per unit volume due to the presence of myelin tends to appear as lower (closer to black) signal compared to GM or CSF. CSF water density is slightly higher than in GM, causing the CSF to appear modestly more intense compared to GM. T2-weighted (T2w) images are typically obtained with TE values between 80 and 150 msec. This serves to maximize the contrast differences between the three tissue types as shown in the graph in Fig. 13. In the case of T2w images, the CSF shows the most intense signal, with GM and WM showing lower and almost equal signal intensities.

IV. MRI TECHNOLOGY

A typical MRI scanner is a complex system that utilizes advanced digital and analog electronics and expensive magnet technology. A simplified block diagram of a typical system is provided in Fig. 14. The system is centered around a computer system that interacts with a purposefully designed system controller. The system controller is responsible for coordinating each of the subsystems to produce pulse sequences and to acquire the MRI signal. The gradient system controller creates magnetic field gradient pulses by application of direct electric current to a set of gradient coils that are positioned around the subject within the magnet. The RF transmitter system is essentially a radio transmitter that is responsible for creating the RF pulses by appropriate application of alternating electric current to the RF coil. The RF receiver system is responsible for detecting the FID or spin echo signals induced in the RF coil by the movement of the magnetization.

The magnet is a relatively expensive system component. It often accounts for a large fraction of the system cost. The majority of current MRI systems use superconducting magnet technology because this provides adequate field strength, superior field homogeneity, and field stability with minimal operating costs. Despite the popularity of superconducting MRI magnets, permanent magnet technologies and conventional electromagnet technologies are also used in some commercial MRI scanners. The requirement for

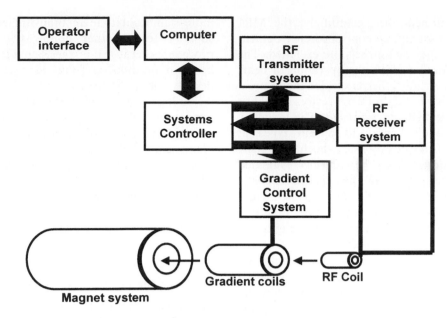

Figure 14   MRI scanner system design.

a strong magnetic field within the head necessitates that the subject be "inside" the magnet aperture (or bore). In addition, the subject's head must be placed within a RF coil, and this must be placed within a set of magnetic field gradient coils. Therefore, the RF coils and the gradient coils must also be placed within the magnet aperture (Fig. 15). In order to perform an imaging examination, the subject lies on the bed. The bed is raised to the level of the RF coil, and the RF coil is placed around the head. The subject is then moved into the magnet so the head is located approximately 1 m within the magnet bore.

V. SAFETY AND EXPOSURE

MRI is widely regarded as a safe, innocuous imaging procedure that can be repeated at virtually any desirable interval. It is generally deemed as being safe for use with normal subjects within the context of research studies. MRI is accomplished without the use of ionizing radiation (X-rays). In addition to exposing the subject to a static magnetic field of considerable strength, the imaging process also requires that the subject be exposed to magnetic fields that oscillate at a frequency used in radio and television broadcasting and also to switched magnetic field gradients. No studies have demonstrated that MRI exposure has any adverse affects on health in the short or long term. Of course, failure to detect an effect does not necessarily

mean that effects do not exist. The current negative findings, however, do suggest that any possible health effects are subtle at best. Because of the possibility of unknown effects on human development, MRI is generally not used during pregnancy.

The MRI environment does present some hazards. Probably the greatest potential hazard is being struck by a magnetic object while in the MRI scanner. MRI magnets create a fringe field around them that is capable of levitating and attracting (at great speed) iron and steel objects. The majority of MRI magnets use superconducting technology and these magnets are

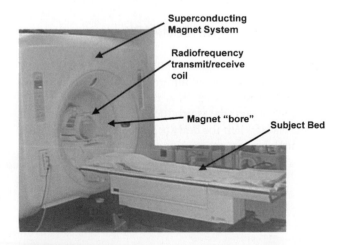

Figure 15   Photograph of a typical commercial MRI scanner.

rarely, if ever, turned off. Accordingly, the MRI scanner must be located in a controlled environment from which iron and steel objects are excluded. The magnetic field can also affect the operation of heart pacemakers and certain other electromagnetic prostheses. Individuals who rely on these devices should be excluded from the MRI environment. The magnetic field may also apply torque to certain types of aneurysm clips; therefore, subjects who have undergone vascular surgery must be carefully evaluated before being imaged with MRI. The switched magnetic field gradients used in MRI can induce electric current flow in the body and affect neuromuscular function. Accordingly, the limits of field gradient strength and gradient switching rates have been established by the appropriate regulatory authorities. Alternating RF electric currents can be induced in the body by the RF pulses used in MRI. Such currents dissipate energy in the form of heat and this can be a source of local tissue burns. This hazard becomes more probable when metallic objects (e.g., electrocardiographic electrodes) are located in or on the body in the vicinity of the RF coil. Therefore, the RF energy that can be used is regulated. With appropriate precautions, it is exceedingly rare for subjects to experience injury during MRI scanning.

Undergoing MRI is not necessarily a pleasant experience despite its innocuous health effects. MRI scanning is a relatively slow process during which the subject must remain motionless within the tight confines of the scanner hardware. Some subjects experience claustrophobia during MRI scanning. In addition, the magnetic field gradient pulses are accompanied by a high level of audio noise, which some subjects intensely dislike.

VI. SUMMARY

MRI provides exquisite images of the soft tissue structure of the brain at millimeter resolution from any viewing angle. It does this by detecting an intrinsic magnetic signal that is produced by the protons within tissue water when the body is placed in the appropriate magnetic environment. Nowhere are the uses of MRI more significant than in brain imaging. MRI is far superior to all other noninvasive brain imaging procedures because it images signal generated directly by the brain tissue and this signal is readily detected despite the presence of the bony cranium. The technology is sufficiently robust to routinely produce images at millimeter resolution with good tissue contrast. The signal detection process uses no form of ionizing radiation and is relatively innocuous. These properties permit subjects to be examined repeatedly. These attributes of MRI point to utility that extends well beyond the diagnosis and evaluation of disease. In recent years, neuroscientists have realized that MRI is a significant research tool that may be used for anatomic imaging in human and animal subjects.

See Also the Following Articles

ELECTROENCEPHALOGRAPHY (EEG) • FUNCTIONAL MAGNETIC RESONANCE IMAGING (fMRI) • IMAGING: BRAIN MAPPING METHODS

Suggested Reading

Brown, M. A., and Semelka, R. C. (1999). *MRI: Basic Principles and Applications*, 2nd ed. Wiley–Liss, New York.

Damasio, H. (1995). *Human Brain Anatomy in Computerized Images.* Oxford Univ. Press, New York.

Farrar, T. C., and Becker, E. D. (1971). *Pulse and Fourier Transform NMR; Introduction to Theory and Methods.* Academic Press, New York.

Gadian, D. G. (1995). *NMR and Its Applications to Living Systems*, 2nd ed. Oxford Univ. Press, Oxford.

Hashemi, R. H., and Bradley, W. G. Jr. (1997). *MRI: The Basics.* Williams & Wilkins, Baltimore.

Jackson, G. D., and Duncan, J. S. (1996). *MRI Neuroanatomy: A New Angle on the Brain.* Churchill-Livingstone, New York.

Lufkin, R. B. (Ed.) (1998). *The MRI Manual*, 2nd ed. Mosby, St. Louis.

Mitchell, D. G. (1999). *MRI Principles.* Saunders, Philadelphia.

Rajan, S. S. (1998). *MRI: A Conceptual Overview.* Springer, New York.

Toga, A. W., and Mazziotta, J. C. (Eds.) (1996). *Brain Mapping: The Methods.* Academic Press, San Diego.

Zimmerman, R. A., Gibby, W. A., and Carmody, R. F. (2000). *Neuroimaging: Clinical and Physical Principles.* Springer, New York.

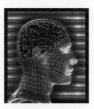

Manic–Depressive Illness

EDWARD H. TAYLOR

University of Minnesota

GLOSSARY

cycle length The time from the beginning of one depressive or manic episode to the start of a new episode. As episodes increase, cycle length decreases. Individuals tend to establish rather constant and individualized cycling patterns. The term rapid cycling is used when a patient has four or more episodes of depression or mania, in any combination, during a 12-month period.

cognitive information processing (also known as social cognitive information processing) The ability to appropriately identify, classify, assess, and correctly act upon or disregard significant environmental and social cues. Processing of information requires the brain to accurately observe or attend to the environment, select important cues while disregarding less meaningful data, compare the selected cues with facts stored in memory, label partial and incomplete data, and develop a cognitive schema for action or determine that no action is required. All of the bipolar disorders reduce a person's information processing skills during periods of depression, mania, or hypomania.

depressive episode An extremely decreased mood that remains symptomatic across all or most of the person's daily activities. Depression removes the capacity for experiencing pleasure and often the ability to find meaning in endeavors or interpersonal relationships that were previously positive and enjoyable. Approximately two-thirds of people in a depressive episode think about suicide, and 10–15% kill themselves.

hypersomnia An excessive experience of sleepiness during day hours. The symptom occurs in some patients with depression and bipolar disorders but is more commonly part of a nonpsychiatric medical problem such as sleep apnea or narcolepsy.

manic episode An abnormally euphoric, elevated, or irritable mood that is associated with impulsive behaviors, poor judgment, concrete and grandiose thinking, reduced sleep, and impaired problem-solving skills. In the beginning individuals in a manic episode may express feelings of elation, energy, and increased insight. These positive perceptions, however, often evolve into feelings of anger, confusion, and fear. Obsessive thoughts of persecution, religiosity, sexuality, fame, economics, or other life events preoccupy individuals who are in a severe manic state.

neurobiological disorders Psychiatric disorders that relate to disruptions or pathological changes in the brain's structure and chemical neural messenger system. Brain abnormalities often found in neurobiological disorders include enlargement of the lateral and third ventricles, reduced frontal cortex volume, cerebellar atrophy, frontal cortex and medial temporal lobe metabolic changes, and changes in the size–shape structure of the temporal lobe and hippocampus.

spectrum disorder A term denoting psychiatric disorders that are thought to have a common pathophysiology and overlapping symptoms and often, but not always, can be treated with identical or similar psychotropic medications.

I. INTRODUCTION

Manic–depressive illness belongs to a spectrum of neurobiological diseases that today are most often called bipolar disorders. The terms are often used interchangeably in popular and scientific literature and refer to an interrelated group of illnesses rather than a single disorder. The popular press and public speakers often use manic–depression and bipolar I disorder as synonyms for a single illness. This is understandable in that bipolar I disorder is one of the most severe forms of manic–depression illness. However, thinking of manic–depression as a cluster of similar mood disorders is more helpful. These illnesses, among other things, attack the brain, preventing individuals in varying degrees from willfully regulating their mood. Like all physiological and emotional problems, bipolar disorders can range in severity from mild to extremely disabling.

Definition of the disorders as simply shifts between high and low or depressed and manic moods misrepresents the affect, disabilities, and pain caused by these illnesses. People with bipolar disorders often report having moods and feelings that take control of their behaviors, motivations, thoughts, perceptions, and ultimately their lives. In a major depressive episode, feelings such as sadness, hopelessness, mental pain, and fatigue are amplified far beyond the normal human experience. Depression can create a pervasive and relentless sense of gloom, inadequacy, rumination, guilt, and worthlessness that the person is unable to dispel with logic, past experiences, or personal will. Mania swings an individual from an upward feeling of well-being, past exuberance, through a state of unexplained euphoria, and finally into a chaotic state of racing, incomprehensible, disconnected thoughts. Depressive and manic episodes are more than magnifications of everyday moods. They have the ability to decrease and control a person's cognitive information processing speed and accuracy, word retrieval, memory, motor speed and skills, concentration, abstract thinking and problem-solving skills, and perception of the social world. Whereas this article provides an overview of these disorders, readers should consult the American Psychiatric Association's *Diagnostic and Statistical Manual of Mental Disorders*, 4th ed., for specific diagnostic and assessment criteria.

Most authorities believe that bipolar I and II and cyclothymic disorders represent differing types, symptoms, and severities of bipolar disorders. A growing number of researchers and clinicians also consider schizoaffective disorder as part of the bipolar spectrum. Bipolar I disorder is a severe form of manic–depressive illness and always includes the occurrence of at least one manic or mixed episode. Most individuals who have bipolar I disorder will at some point experience a major depressive episode, even though this is not a required criterion for the diagnosis. The illness can start with an episode of either mania or depression. Bipolar I disorder can cause acute, severe problems requiring hospitalization to control symptoms like psychotic episodes, extreme manic behavior, immobilizing depression, or suicidal thoughts. Bipolar II is diagnosed if the person has one or more major depressive and hypomanic episodes, but no history of manic or mixed episodes. Hypomania is a milder, less severe form of mania that seldom leads to hospitalization. Mental health professionals are sometimes unable to identify the hypomania episodes and misdiagnose the illness as severe depression or a personality disorder.

Cyclothymic disorder is the mildest form of manic–depressive illness. The disorder causes low-grade chronic mood abnormalities. For 2 or more years the person has numerous periods of hypomanic symptoms alternating with numerous bouts of mild to moderate depression. Individuals with this disorder find that, particularly during periods of depression, it becomes difficult but possible to maintain their normal activities. When hypomania occurs, the person experiences an increase in activity and at least a slight decrease in judgment and problem-solving skills. Irritability may occur in both the hypomanic and the depressed states. Many individuals with cyclothymia appear fully functional, maintain their employment, and never seek professional help. What is not seen is their internal turmoil, decreased problem-solving skills, and the amount of energy required to complete required daily work tasks.

Schizoaffective disorder represents the other end of the spectrum. It is an extremely severe form of illness that incorporates symptoms found in both manic–depressive illness and schizophrenia. Schizoaffective disorder can produce a state of persistent psychosis along with episodes of mania and depression. Normally the psychotic symptoms continue after the mood episodes dissipate. Some individuals appear to have a schizomanic condition, whereas others have more symptoms of schizophrenia and depression. The fact that mood-stabilizing medications help people with schizoaffective illness but generally are not helpful for patients with schizophrenia argues for classifying the illness as part of the bipolar spectrum.

II. HISTORICAL OVERVIEW

Throughout history scholars have described the symptoms and effects of manic–depressive illness. Ancient Greek, Persian, and biblical writers recorded and attempted to explain the complexities of bipolar illness. In the second century AD Areteus wrote about patients who, in a state of euphoria, danced throughout the night, talked publicly, and acted overly self-confident then, for no apparent reason, shifted into a state of sorrow and despair. The fourth century BC Greek physicians lead by Hippocrates were perhaps the first to hypothesize that symptoms we now call bipolar disorder represented a neurological illness highlighted by major uncontrollable shifts in a person's mood. These early Greek scholars further taught that mental illness is caused by natural rather than spiritual forces, identified the brain as the major organ responsible for sanity and intellectual processes, attempted to classify major mental disorders, and developed crude medical treatments for mental disorders. Unfortunately, however, records from the ancient Egyptians, Greeks, Romans, Middle Ages, European Renaissance, and early American history indicate that this hypothesis gave way to assumptions of demoniacal possession, witchcraft, sinfulness, and other dehumanizing concepts. Nonetheless, traces of scientific and medical inquiries into bipolar disorders periodically appear throughout history.

The first person to identify the link between mania and melancholia or depression was Theophile Bonet. In 1686 Bonet described patients who cycled between high and low moods as having "manico-melancolicus." During the mid-1800s, French researchers Falret and Baillarger each independently observed that patients having manic and depressive episodes were not experiencing two different disorders, but rather two different presentations of the same illness. Falret described the disorder as "circular insanity" and listed the symptoms much as they appear in today's medical books and journals. He also (remarkably) hypothesized that the illness was hereditary and believed that through research a medication would be found for effectively treating the symptoms. The German psychiatrist Emil Kraepelin, building on Falret and Baillarger's work in the late 1800s and early 1900s, developed the definitive description and classification for manic–depressive illness that largely stands to this day. Kraepelin is credited with sensitizing past mood studies, clearly documenting that mania and depression are different symptoms of the same disorder, and with being the first researcher to assert that all mood disorders are neurologically related.

Kraepelin's basic concepts were challenged and widened by Eugen Bleuler in 1924. For Bleuler, mental disorders could not be classified into two major categories as Kraepelin claimed. Kraepelin believed that all mental illnesses fall into two basic, but separate groups. An illness was classified either as causing periodic recurring symptoms, such as manic–depression, or as a disorder characterized by ongoing neurological deterioration, such as schizophrenia. In his later work, Kraepelin did, however, clarify that it was impossible to neatly place everyone with mental illness into these two categories and that one cannot always discriminate among major disorders. Bleuler argued that manic–depressive illness and dementia praecox (schizophrenia) were not separate classifications, but rather a continuum. How a person was diagnosed and placed on the spectrum depended on the number of symptoms of schizophrenia that were found. More importantly, Bleuler broadened the manic–depression classification by identifying a number of subcategories and introducing the term affective illness. Between the early 1920s and mid-1980s, criteria independently developed by Kraepelin and Bleuler shaped most of the world's psychiatric diagnostic systems.

Between 1930 and 1940, mental health treatment providers largely abandoned the assumption that manic–depression and most other disorders, including schizophrenia and autism, developed from neurobiological abnormalities. Following World War II and until the early 1980s, mental health theory and treatment were mostly guided by psychoanalytic concepts proposed by Freud and his followers. Whereas psychoanalytic theory agreed that biological components played a role in affective disorders, practitioners insisted that early childhood parental or other environmental conflicts usually explained the onset and recurrence of manic–depressive episodes. As a result, it was thought that manic–depressive symptoms would resolve if individuals gained insight into their unconscious anger or other hidden emotional conflicts. Even though psychoanalysis and other forms of psychotherapy offered little help for most patients with severe manic–depressive problems, talk therapies nonetheless became the treatment of choice for decades. This preference continued for a number of years even after the introduction of lithium, the first drug found to successfully treat manic episodes.

Dr. John F. J. Cade, a doctor in the Mental Hygiene Department of Victoria, Australia, was dedicated to the belief that manic–depression was a biological, not an unconscious, psychological disorder. In the 1940s he was attempting to discover how urine toxicity levels from patients with various mental disorders differed. Cade wanted to inject guinea pigs with various concentrations of uric acid. However, uric acid is insoluble in water and difficult to inject. To resolve this problem Cade mixed uric acid with lithium. To Cade's surprise, guinea pigs injected with the lithium solution had less toxicity in their urine. The scientist next injected the animals with lithium carbonate and observed that the animals remained conscious but less active and responsive to their environment. On the basis of these findings, Cade administered a lithium salt preparation to several highly agitated manic patients. Each of the patients had a remarkable reduction in symptoms. After Dr. Cade successfully treated 10 additional patients with the solution, European doctors started to quickly accept lithium as an important advancement in treating bipolar disorders. Because of safety concerns documented by cases of hypertension and deaths resulting from a consumer salt substitute containing lithium, the drug was not approved for use in the United States until 1970.

III. EPIDEMIOLOGY AND CAUSE

Bipolar disorders usually start in late adolescence and young adulthood. These illnesses, however, can appear any time between ages 5 and 50 and in rare cases beyond the age of 50. Research indicates that between 25 and 30% of the people who develop manic–depression as adults had one or more related symptoms before their 6th birthday. The more severe forms of bipolar illness (bipolar I disorder) are considered to be rare in prepubertal children. Only about 0.6% of adolescents are thought to have a bipolar I diagnosis, but estimates of teens with bipolar II disorder have reached as high as 10%.

Estimates of the number of people with a bipolar disorder vary. This occurs in part because of diagnostic difficulties and because of the fact that many people who have mild symptoms either do not seek or do not receive professional attention. At any given time, about 8% of America's population is at risk for developing a mood disorder. Most studies estimate that between 1 and 2.5% of the U.S. population has a bipolar disorder. A representative number of studies estimate that the prevalence of bipolar disorders is 3–6.5% of the U.S. population. Unlike unipolar depression, bipolar disorders are found equally in females and males. Between 5 and 20% of adult cases that are first diagnosed as unipolar depression over time will receive a reevaluated diagnosis of bipolar disorder.

Science has gained a large amount of information about manic–depressive illness but has been unable to identify specifically how the illness starts. There are most likely several causes for this syndrome of disorders. Studies of families, twins, and adoptions suggest that most cases of manic–depression are genetically inherited. There is general agreement among researchers that genetic components play a more significant role in transmitting bipolar I disorder than major depressive disorder, but this perspective continues to be debated. Family studies report that having a first-degree relative with bipolar I disorder increases the chances of developing manic–depressive illness by 8–18 times over families with no first-degree members having a bipolar disorder history. The likelihood of developing bipolar I disorder is 1.5–2.5 times greater if a first-degree family member has a major unipolar depressive disorder. Perhaps more illustrative of the genetic relationship to manic–depression is the fact that 50% of all people with a bipolar I disorder have at least one parent with a mood disorder. Additionally, a 25% probability exists of a child developing bipolar I disorder if one parent has this form of manic–depressive illness, and a 50–75% chance exists if both parents have bipolar I disorder. There is only a limited amount of information from adoption studies on bipolar disorders. The available data document that children adopted as infants from biological parents with a major mood disorder remain at an increased risk for developing bipolar disorders. The link between genetics and manic–depression has also been established through the study of twins. Monozygotic twins show a concordance rate for bipolar I disorder of 75%, whereas the concordance rate for bipolar I disorder in dizygotic twins drops to 20%. In addition, scientists have hypothesized that some cases of bipolar disorder may not stem from a genetic transmission. Researchers have found indications that bipolar disorders may be caused by *in utero* neuroviruses that attack the fetus' forming brain. There is currently growing interest in the role neuroviruses and immunologic abnormalities play in the formation and development of major mental disorders, including manic–depressive illness and schizophrenia.

IV. MAJOR SYMPTOMS

The type of bipolar disorder a person has is largely determined by identifying the severity, number, type, and duration of manic and depressive symptoms the person has or is experiencing. Diagnosis of bipolar disorders is complicated by the fact that many symptoms of unipolar depression and manic–depression overlap. As an example, agitation and insomnia can occur in the depressed and in the manic state. Hypersomnia and psychomotor retardation, however, are observed more in bipolar than in unipolar depression.

Mania is one of the most dangerous of the abnormal mood states, but fortunately it is not present in all forms of bipolar disorder. Mania or manic behavior produces extreme and dramatic symptoms that can endanger the person's social and economic well-being and cause the individual to take life-threatening risks. The early stages of mania are experienced as pleasant and uplifting. The person feels energetic, creative, highly spirited, and capable. In the beginning of a manic episode, individuals are filled with a pleasant mood, ambitious thoughts, and self-confidence. They see great promise in their relationships, personal talents, skills, careers, and future. Goals are more clear, tasks seem less difficult, and life becomes magically filled with cosmic meaning and understanding. These exuberant and positive feelings, however, quickly pass and change into more pronounced psychiatric symptoms.

The person's cognitive information processing skills are disrupted by rapidly occurring thoughts that not only collide together but form incomplete and incongruent ideas. Additionally, the ability to screen and judge the appropriateness of one's thoughts, behaviors, productivity, and quality of work largely disappears. Furthermore, the previously elated mood filled with self-confidence, grandiosity, and positive symbolic meaning turns into unexplained, almost random anger and irritability. Whereas some individuals alternate between periods of elation and irritability, most slip into a state of mania dominated by dissatisfaction, frustration, intolerance, and an unsettling irritated mood. Some individuals also experience a constant internal rage that, with almost no provocation, can explode into verbal or physical violence. Mania also blunts and distorts learned social–cultural judgment while simultaneously stimulating a need for increased activity and excitement. In an attempt to alleviate these pressured feelings of desire, anxiety, anger, and grandiosity, the person behaves and makes decisions that are erratic and often dangerous. Without forethought or consideration of the consequences, individuals in a manic episode may run up large credit card debts, buy enormous quantities of a single and unusual item, engage in risky sexual activities with multiple unknown partners, drive recklessly, feel justified driving the wrong direction down a one-way street or disobeying traffic lights, indulge in large quantities of food and alcoholic drinks or go without eating and sleeping, drive aimlessly until the car runs out of gas, lose inhibitions and speak crudely or go nude in public, dress bizarrely, or verbally and physically lash out at others. Mania is always dangerous. As grandiosity is stimulated and judgment severely suppressed, the manic person can become extremely reckless and cause serious self-injury or death. The inability to foresee consequences and consider multiple solutions along with impulsive, agitated thinking and anger can induce rapid suicidal thoughts and behaviors. Depressed patients ruminate, plan, and deliberate the possibilities of suicide. For the depressed, death is often a means of ending mental anguish and hopelessness or stopping an unexplainable, but nonetheless constant drive and obsessive desire to die. In contrast, manic individuals kill themselves over poorly conceived, impulsive, almost momentary issues and feelings. Furthermore, severe mania often triggers physical violence and aggressive property destruction in people who have a more severe form of manic–depressive illness. People with a manic–depressive illness more often make death threats to presidents and other famous individuals than patients diagnosed with schizophrenia.

As the severity of a manic episode proceeds, thoughts can rush through a person's mind so fast that half-way through a sentence the beginning point is forgotten. This occurs when manic symptoms disrupt or block the brain's working memory. Under normal circumstances, working memory allows us to pull appropriate information from long-term memory, lock it in our mind, and manipulate the facts into interlinking complete thoughts and logical problem-solving models. In the most severe stages, mania can cause the person to experience psychotic hallucinations and delusions. Without medication, the person's manic hyperactivity and psychotic state will evolve into a stressful fatigue and loss of psychological orientation to time and place that causes the individual to appear completely confused, bewildered, and stupefied. In the past this was referred to as delirious mania. Fortunately today's modern medications and supportive treatment prevent most people with a manic–depressive disorder from reaching this level of severity.

Euphoria and hyperactivity that create difficulties but do not reach the level of severity of manic episodes is known as hypomania. This psychiatric condition was first described in the late 1800s by the German psychiatrist Mendel. A hypomanic mood produces behavior that resembles the first phase of a full manic episode. The person has an elated mood, increased energy, rapid thinking and speaking, and reduced information processing skills. Though thoughts occur quickly, information is processed in a more narrow, concrete, and restricted manner. As an example, one's abilities to form alternative solutions, empathize, consider input from others, or perform problem-solving tasks requiring an exact sequential sequence are substantially reduced. Additionally, hypomania causes problems perceiving, organizing, and analyzing fragmented social information and interpreting social cues that have multiple meanings. As a result, hypomanic individuals make impulsive decisions, fail to consider behavioral consequences, and seldom perceive how others experience their actions. The symptoms may also include an inability to screen verbal communications. That is, the person feels an actual need or urge to voice almost every thought. When this symptom occurs, the individual interrupts others, talks incessantly, and has little concern if his or her words insult and upset the listener. Furthermore, hypomania, like the first phase of mania, can cause grandiose self-perceptions. During periods of grandiosity individuals overvalue their skills, status, or personal magnetism and may engage in behaviors like risky investments and business decisions, overspending and credit card debt; sexual experimentation and excess, and careless and reckless activities. A hypomanic person often displays seductive and addictive behaviors that may first appear as spontaneity or personality characteristics. A closer examination, however, will show that the individual's actions extend beyond the boundaries that are acceptable for most people within the same age and cultural group. Many times individuals with hypomania are labeled by families, schools, and community agencies as immature or delinquent and neither receive a referral nor seek mental health treatment.

Only a brief overview of depression symptoms is provided in this section. Readers are directed, however, to the complete article on the subject that is included in this volume. Depression is different from sadness, grief and bereavement, feelings of loneliness and isolation, or disappointment. Each of these situations creates a normal, but nonetheless unpleasant mood reaction to a real or perceived event. More importantly, one is able to shift away from the reaction, receive relief, and often block the feelings by engaging in nonrelated activities. That is, normal depressive feelings are mood reactions that seldom pervade every domain of our life for an extended period of time. Even when one's mood is lowered by a specific event, most individuals continue to experience a range of positive thoughts and feelings.

Unlike reactive sadness, depression is a downward spiraling or narrowing of feeling and emotional range across most major life domains for an extended period. Dulling and despondent feelings relentlessly occur from depression and prevent one from experiencing pleasure, accepting solace and praise, and finding emotional relief. Rumination over issues like regret, guilt, personal loss, shame, incompetency, disappointment, and hopelessness is often experienced as emotional stress and pain. Severe depression can also create a numbing emptiness and an inability to care about oneself, family, others, or the future. Additionally, during a depressive episode most people with a bipolar disorder experience not only a feeling of gloom but also restrictions and deficits in their cognition, information processing, motor, and perceptual skills. Concentration and working memory are always reduced by depression. Abstract thinking along with simple social cognitive information processing is greatly slowed. Other common symptoms include social withdrawal, insomnia or hypersomnia, weight loss or gain, fatigue, headaches, constipation, loss of sexual drive, and loss of interest and enjoyment in past pleasures or life skills. In severe depressive episodes a bipolar disordered person may also develop delusional thinking, hallucinations, catatonic states, or other forms of psychotic symptoms. Approximately 50% of all people with a bipolar disorder will exhibit psychotic symptoms. Additionally, even without entering a psychotic state, severe depression can usher in and maintain paranoid thinking for an extended period. To stop the emotional pain stemming from hopelessness, lost cognitive skills, and hurt from burdening others or feeling unloved or undeserving of love, far too many bipolar disordered patients during a depressive episode make serious and deadly suicidal attempts. Approximately 15% of individuals with a bipolar disorder make a serious attempt to take their life.

Another cluster of manic–depressive symptoms forms the mixed affective mood states or simply mixed episodes. A small subgroup of individuals with bipolar disorders will, for a week or more, concurrently experience the symptoms required for diagnosing a major depressive and a manic episode. This is a highly torturous state that simultaneously inflicts the rushing frenzy of mania and the restrictive negative sensations of depression. Even though the mood abnormality was first described by a seventeenth century doctor, modern medicine continues to struggle with and debate the exact characteristics that define a mixed state. The prevailing symptoms can vary greatly for patients having a mixed episode. Some individuals, as an example, will feature psychotic symptoms, whereas others become highly irritable and yet others manifest more depressive behaviors. There is, however, growing evidence that a mixed state does not occur in all bipolar disorders. As a result, many experts believe that mixed episodes need to be thought of as a form of bipolar disorder or mixed mania that is separate from both depression and mania. Dysphoric mania is similar to mixed episodes, but the symptoms are less severe, often have a shorter duration, and do not qualify as full depressive and manic episodes. Patients who rapidly cycle between depressed and manic or hypomanic states can appear to be, but are not technically, in a mixed state.

The length of time between episodes of illness varies greatly among all patients with manic–depressive illness. For many people the cycle lengths shorten, causing more frequent episodes, then plateau at approximately 3–5 episodes per year, and finally shift to episodes that occur more or less annually. This appears to be the natural course of the illness. As the interval between psychiatric crises lengthens, most patients will have extended periods where their mood, and cognition, motor, and information processing skills return to normal. Unfortunately around 5–20% of bipolar patients have at least 4 manic or depressive episodes per year. This is known as rapid cycling, and episodes may take place in any combination and order.

Diagnostically, rapid cycling episodes do not differ in criteria from those that take place in non-rapid cycling. The symptoms must meet the criteria required for a manic, hypomanic, mixed, or major depressive episode. A smaller group of patients has ultrarapid cycling in which a depressive, manic, or a hypomanic episode may last for only a day or trigger multiple episodes within a 24-hr period. Unlike rapid and ultrarapid cycling, individuals with continuous cycling move through episodes without returning to their normal baseline or feeling normal for a significant period of time. With these individuals one depressive, manic, or hypomanic episode melts into another. Correct and prompt diagnosis of this illness is extremely important. Rapid cycling appears related to morbidity, is pharmacologically difficult to treat, and requires specific medication regimens. Studies show that these patients do not respond well to medications that are normally used with other bipolar disorders like lithium and antidepressants. Moreover, antipsychotic drugs may actually stimulate or exacerbate the cycling process.

V. CHILDHOOD ONSET

Even in the 1960s psychoanalytic theory hypothesized that children could not develop depression, let alone manic–depressive illness. This was founded on the assumption that depression results from unconscious superego conflicts. Because they thought children had not yet developed superegos, the assumption was that children also could not experience real depression. Today research documents that children, preteens, and adolescents can develop unipolar depression and bipolar disorders, but their course of illness and symptom patterns are often much different from these of adults. Manic–depression in children causes the general symptom categories found in adults but creates different patterns and behavioral problems. As an example, children have more chronic episodes distinguished by rapid and ultrarapid cycling. From the very beginning as infants many of these children behave differently from their peers. Mothers and nurseries report that the baby has long periods of crying, sleeplessness, and excessive activity.

As toddlers and preschoolers the children psychoanalytic theory destined for manic–depressive illness often are described as highly creative, bright, verbal, and intellectually ahead of most other children. Parallel to these positive developmental factors parents also recall that their children experienced severe separation anxiety and night terrors much longer than most youths. Additionally, many children who are developing manic–depressive illness have vivid, explicit dreams that typically focus on violent themes filled with blood and gore. This type of color-filled descriptive violence can also occur in the discourse of normal conversations. They may meet simple requests or instructive guidelines, such as gently requesting the child to remain in line, with an exaggerated physical threat. A parental "no" can send the manic–depressive child into a destructive rage for hours. During tantrums these children routinely cry, kick, hit, pull hair, bite, and attempt to punch holes in the wall or destroy other property. Discovery that the child has destroyed favorite personal items and damaged walls and furnishings when sent to a room for a time out punishment is a common experience among parents. Not only do many children rapidly cycle, often switching from one mood state to another within hours, but additionally high degrees of agitation, unhappiness, anxiety, and anger can accompany both depressive and manic episodes. Manic episodes may include obsessive silly behaviors that grate on others, including peers. As the child's grandiosity increases, the youth may make unrealistic claims and brag about current and future fame. Mania can also cause the child to steal or hitchhike and travel in a totally unplanned and unprepared manner. Many times children in a manic episode will not know where they are going or why they are traveling. Still others will break into a house and take off all clothing for no apparent or logical reason. Impulsive behaviors highlight childhood mania and greatly increase the risk for suicide and self-injury.

The onset of a bipolar disorder during childhood usually starts with a depressive episode. Both unipolar and bipolar early onset depression may feature a distinct loss of pleasure in activities that had been pleasurable, tantrums or crying for almost no known reason, lethargy and oversleeping, an increase in self-consciousness, previously unseen or greatly increased phobic anxiety, increased agitation, arguing, and physical fighting. In almost all cases the child's school behavior and academic performance decrease, and many children develop or experience increased separation anxiety symptoms.

VI. TREATMENT ISSUES

When symptoms first start in children and adults, an extensive physical exam from a qualified physician is immediately required. Both depression and manic symptoms can stem from problems ranging from vitamin deficiencies or excess to major autoimmune, cardiovascular, gastrointestinal, endocrine, hematologic, neurological, and pulmonary diseases or malignancies. Additionally, a long list of medications and drug interactions can cause manic–depressive behaviors. Commonly, bipolar symptoms caused by medical problems other than a neuropsychiatric disorder will improve as the person recovers from the primary physical illness. Once alternative medical problems are ruled out and the person is diagnosed with a bipolar disorder, psychotropic medications become the first and fundamental treatment method.

Lithium along with the anticonvulsant medications carbamazepine and valproic acid are widely used as mood stabilizers. Lithium continues to be the most widely used drug for combating manic episodes and has also been found to relieve depressive symptoms for some individuals. Approximately 70% of bipolar patients experience significant benefits from taking lithium. This, however, is not without a cost. Lithium can cause numerous transient cognitive and physiological side effects and become life-threatening if the amount accumulating in the blood becomes toxic. When taking lithium, blood must be drawn routinely to monitor the blood's drug level and insure that toxicity does not occur.

Depression in bipolar disorders can be difficult to treat. Standard antidepressant medications, especially those known as tricyclics, can induce mania and rapid cycling in bipolar patients. This presents a particular hazard for individuals with bipolar II. These individuals often present as having recurring severe depression. The hypomania component can be hidden and difficult to diagnose. When this occurs, the person is at risk of being incorrectly diagnosed, prescribed an antidepressant, and sent into a state of mania or rapid cycling. Therefore, best practice guidelines recommend that bipolar depression be treated first with one of the mood-stabilizing medications mentioned earlier. Lithium is reported to be effective for 30–79% of bipolar depressed patients. The other antimania drugs are significantly less effective in treating depression. When the depressive episode is not reduced by lithium treatment, the psychiatrist will add either an additional mood-stabilizing medication or an antidepressant. Because tricyclic medications are known to increase mania, physicians most often put the patient on a monoamine oxidase inhibitor (MOAI) or one of the newer serotonin re-uptake inhibitor (SSRI) antidepressants. MOAI have generally been found to be the most reliable class of antidepressant medications for bipolar patients, but the drug tolerance and effectiveness, as with other psychoactive drugs, vary from patient to patient. Reports on best practice methods for treating bipolar depression consistently emphasize that antidepressants generally must be coadministered with a standard antimanic medication. Furthermore, unlike unipolar depression, there is no evidence that maintaining a patient on an antidepressant after the bipolar depression ends prevents the recurrence of future episodes.

Psychotherapy is always part of the comprehensive treatment of manic–depressive illness. During severe depressive or manic episodes, therapy anchors the person offering support, assurance, hope, and reflections of reality. As episodes lift and normal moods and thinking emerge, psychotherapy assists in logical and systematic problem-solving, reinforcing positive behaviors and cognition, and understanding one's self and world. More specifically, psychotherapy can help individuals who have manic–depressive illness better understand their disorder, remain on prescribed medications, learn to predict and prevent or soften recurring episodes, learn to not be afraid when experiencing normal sadness, grief, or joy, how and when to let others take charge of their decision making, and how to better care for their significant others and friends. A combination of cognitive, behavioral, and supportive therapies can accomplish these goals with many individuals. An important part of psychotherapy is recording in a chart or journal how moods change over time, how they are affected by medication, and reactions in differing environments. Methods of this type are also used to identify internal thoughts or cognitive nonverbal self-talk. The messages we silently give ourselves can highlight strengths, fears, and oncoming depressive and manic episodes. By knowing that the patient's cognition and behaviors are changing dangerously, the treatment team can take steps for preventing or reducing the severity of an approaching illness. Prevention is accomplished by adjusting the person's medication, providing additional psychological support, and reducing stress in the person's home and work environment. Psychotherapy can help individuals make sense and meaning out of their physical and mental difficulties.

Families can provide important information concerning the patient's developmental history, illness onset, and current progress. Family members, however, also need support, understanding, and assistance from the treatment team. Living with an ill loved one is stressful and difficult. Psychotherapists or other treatment team members can offer families psychosocial education, guided problem-solving sessions, and methods for managing anxieties and organizing their thoughts. Psychosocial education provides the family information about the cause, treatment, care, and prognosis of bipolar disorders. Family members need to understand that manic–depression is a biological illness that can be treated. They also often need assistance in knowing how to relate with the ill family member and how to help with the on-going treatment. With the onset of illness, families not only must learn how to live together once again and redistribute work tasks but also concretely know how to respond to psychiatric emergencies. Family members, as an example, must know when and when not to call mental health professionals, police, clergy, and emergency rooms.

Treatment not only involves medication, psychotherapy, and education but also concrete support for the patient and the family. Comprehensive treatment must help patients and families gain real services and tangible resources. Bipolar disorders can greatly alter the patient's and the family's ability to earn money and provide transportation, housing, food, medication, and access to medical services. Family members and patients also need opportunities to separate and rest. Living daily with someone who is in the midst of a depressive or manic episode is extremely stressful. To prevent suicide or other hazardous behaviors, family members often remain with the patient continuously for an extended time. Other family members take on additional employment to pay for medical and rehabilitation expenses or spend countless hours coordinating services for the ill family member. Treatment teams need to not only understand the stressors experienced by families but substantially assist in the resolution of these problems.

VII. STRESS AND ONSET

Stress does not appear to be a major factor in explaining why individuals develop a bipolar disorder. Additionally, research does not support the idea that the number of depressive or manic episodes experienced by a patient relates to that individual's pre-onset stress level. There is also little or no scientific evidence that bipolar episodes are related to stress through the brain's kindling process. Kindling refers to the brain at the cellular level learning from repeated episodes to automatically trigger an event such as a seizure. Studies show that, after a number of electrically stimulated seizures, spontaneous epilepsy will occur without the introduction of electrical stimulation. The popular brain kindling and behavioral sensitization theory hypothesized that bipolar patients become highly aware of stress. Environmental and behavioral symbols for stress are then linked to repeated depressive and manic episodes. Eventually the brain will automatically trigger a relapse with only the slightest perception of a stressful stimulus. Whereas kindling has been shown to occur in laboratory animals, it has never been demonstrated in humans. No experimental or clinical research has shown that kindling occurs in the brain of individuals with a bipolar disorder.

There is some evidence that the onset of the first episode may partially be triggered by a stressful experience. This appears to be less true for depressive

of their brain that structurally differ from the neuroanatomy of individuals with no history of mental illness. Furthermore, there is growing evidence that differences in brain structure are also found among individuals with manic–depressive illness and other major diagnostic categories such as major depression and schizophrenia. University of Michigan researchers using positron emission tomography (PET) found that individuals with bipolar illness have a higher density of monoamine-releasing cells than people who do not have an affective disorder. These specialized cells are responsible for controlling the discharge of norepinephrine, serotonin, and dopamine. Magnetic resonance imaging (MRI) studies show that individuals with bipolar disorders have significantly enlarged lateral ventricles, frontal and temporal lobe sulci, and Sylvian fissures. Studies of third ventricular enlargement in bipolar disorders are at best mixed and often contradictory. This appears to be one of the anatomical differences between manic–depressive illness and schizophrenia. That is, there is strong evidence in schizophrenia, but not bipolar disorders, that lateral and third ventricular enlargement may be caused by a neuropathological process that is independent of sulcal changes. Furthermore, lateral ventricular enlargement and sulcal prominence have been found in many, but not all, patients with manic–depressive illness. Therefore, we currently cannot use neuroanatomical measurements as a means of diagnostically determining bipolar or other mood disorders.

Our understanding of how neuroanatomy differs between psychiatric diagnoses was greatly advanced by MRI studies of monozygotic twins discordant for either bipolar I illness or schizophrenia. Although these are genetically identical twins, one of each pair developed either manic–depressive illness or schizophrenia whereas the other twin remained well. The MRI study found a strong trend for the ventricular enlargement among twins affected with either bipolar I or schizophrenia disorders to be similar. When measured just within each discordant group, differences between right lateral, left lateral, and third ventricles were much more statistically significant. There was a greater difference, however, between the twins affected with schizophrenia and their well sibling twins than in the twins discordant for bipolar illness. Significant differences were also found between the schizophrenia-affected twins and their well sibling twins in the right and left hippocampus, amygdala, and basal ganglia areas of the brain. Interestingly, these differences did not significantly occur in the twins discordant for bipolar illness. This is at odds with numerous MRI nontwin studies of manic–depression. The lack of agreement may exist because the middle and posterior portions of the twins' hippocampus are yet to be studied.

X. CONCLUSION

Manic–depression is a spectrum of neurobiological illnesses that involve abnormal changes in the brain's chemistry and cellular structures. The neurotransmitters serotonin, norepinephrine, and dopamine appear to play key roles in triggering manic–depressive episodes. Anatomical damage or changes have been documented in the lateral ventricles, frontal and temporal lobe sulci, and Sylvian fissures. How bipolar disorders specifically start is yet to be explained. Evidence from family histories, adoptions, and twins strongly indicates that the disorders are genetically transmitted. There is, however, growing evidence that some individuals may develop manic–depressive illness from an *in utero* neurovirus. Environmental stress does not appear to play a major role in the causation of bipolar disorder or the number of episodes experienced by a person. Brain kindling and behavioral learning theories have not been helpful in explaining the cause or course of these disorders. Once individuals are in the midst of an episode, the reduction of environmental stress does appear to help reduce or soften the symptoms. Nonetheless, medications remain the principal treatment for bipolar disorders. Psychotherapy, psychosocial education, and environmental manipulation therapies serve as important adjuncts or additive components to treatment but are never the primary or sole intervention. This is particularly true for bipolar I and II and schizoaffective disorders. Approximately 70% of patients with bipolar I disorder significantly improve after taking lithium. Psychotherapy alone seldom has a meaningful impact on severe manic–depressive episodes. The future is extremely hopeful for individuals with bipolar disorders. New medications are currently being studied clinically, and our knowledge of how the brain functions is rapidly growing. Researchers are also learning to identify early risk factors and minor symptoms that signal the onset of illness. Unfortunately, manic–depression is an illness that cannot yet be prevented and continues, for many people, to be misdiagnosed. However, as our knowledge of medications, brain functioning, and early symptoms grows, science will be better positioned to effectively prevent and treat manic and depressive episodes.

See Also the Following Articles

AUTISM • BEHAVIORAL PHARMACOLOGY • COGNITIVE PSYCHOLOGY, OVERVIEW • DEPRESSION • DOPAMINE • MOOD DISORDERS • NEUROPSYCHOLOGICAL ASSESSMENT • NEUROPSYCHOLOGICAL ASSESSMENT, PEDIATRIC • NOREPINEPHRINE • PARKINSON'S DISEASE • SCHIZOPHRENIA • STRESS

Suggested Reading

Bearden, C. E., Hoffman, K. M., and Cannon, T. D. (2001). The neuropsychololgy and neuroanatomy of bipolar affective disorder: A critical review. *Bipolar Disorder* **3**(3), 106–150.

Beckham, E. E., and Leber, W. R. (1995). *Handbook of Depression*, 2nd ed. Guilford Press, New York.

Goodwin, F. K., and Jamison, K. R. (1990). *Manic–Depressive Illness*. Oxford University Press, New York.

Torrey, E. F., Bowler, A. E., Taylor, E. H., and Gottesman, I. I. (1994). *Schizophrenia and Manic–Depressive Disorder: The Biological Roots of Mental Illness as Revealed by the Landmark Study of Identical Twins.* Basic Books, New York.

Soares, J. C., and Gershon, S. (Eds.) (2000). *Bipolar Disorders Basic Mechanisms and Therapeutic Implications.* Marcel Dekker, New York.

Young, L. T., and Joffe, R. T. (Eds.) (1997). *Bipolar Disorder: Biological Models and Their Clinical Application.* Marcel Dekker, New York.

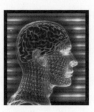

Memory Disorders, Organic

ANDREW R. MAYES

Liverpool University

I. Introduction

II. Working Memory Disorders

III. Deficits in Previously Well-Learned Semantic Information

IV. Organic Amnesia and Frontal Lobe Damage: Episodic and Semantic Memory

V. Priming Deficits

VI. Deficits in Other Kinds of Procedural/Implicit Memory

VII. Conclusion

GLOSSARY

amnesia Either a nonspecific term for any kind of memory disorder (usually one caused by brain damage rather than arising for psychological or motivational reasons) or the global amnesia syndrome in which an impairment of recall and recognition of postmorbid facts and episodes (anterograde amnesia) is accompanied by varying degrees of recall and recognition impairment for premorbidly acquired memories of facts and episodes (retrograde amnesia), together with preservation of intelligence and working memory.

declarative memory Memory for facts and personally experienced episodes that the subject is aware of remembering. As such, the memories can be declared either by verbal statements or by some non-verbal means such as drawing. It is contrasted with procedural or nondeclarative memory, in which subjects cannot typically indicate what they are remembering except in the broadest manner.

episodic memory Memory for particular incidents in personal life that have specific spatial and temporal contexts. It is often contrasted with semantic memory.

explicit memory A form of memory contrasted with implicit memory; the distinction between the two is very similar to that between procedural and declarative memory. Like declarative memory, explicit memory often involves intentional retrieval of factual or episodic information.

implicit memory A form of memory contrasted with explicit memory that corresponds closely with procedural or nondeclarative memory. The presence of memory is only indicated indirectly and the subject does not intentionally try to remember anything specific but tries to perform a task well, with changed performance indicating the presence of memory.

priming A form of information-specific implicit, procedural, or nondeclarative memory in which remembering is indicated by a change in the way that previously studied information is processed. In other words, studied information is processed faster, more accurately, or in some other way more efficiently, although subjects need have no awareness that they are remembering the information.

procedural memory Memory that is only accessible through performance in an indirect or implicit fashion and comprises skill memory, conditioning, priming, and simple forms of nonassociative memory. It is sometimes referred to as nondeclarative memory by those who wish to stress that it may be constituted of a heterogeneous collection of different kinds of memory, the only common feature of which is that they are not forms of declarative memory.

semantic memory Memory for facts or the kinds of information that can be stored in our mental dictionaries and encyclopedias. Unlike episodic memory, semantic memory contains no necessary reference to the personal context(s) in which it was acquired although some facts necessarily include reference to the non-personal contexts in which (for example, historical) events occurred. It is controversial, however, whether retrieving personal contextual information may nevertheless sometimes be important in remembering facts. Resolving this issue is difficult because a common but nonessential difference between semantic and episodic memory is that the former tends to be much more rehearsed than the latter.

working memory The temporary storage for a few seconds of information that is being processed in any of a range of cognitive tasks.

Damage to different parts of the brain impairs both short-term and long-term memory for different kinds of information often in very selective ways that leave basic processing intact. Lesions to association neocortex cause several different short-term memory disorders in which memory for phonological, visuospatial, color, or other kinds of information is selectively disrupted within approximately 1 sec of presentation. These immediate memory disorders occur in the presence of normal processing and are associated with longer term memory deficits for the same kinds of information. Several different kinds of long-term memory disorders exist. Posterior neocortical lesions disrupt semantic memory, but the deficit also seems to include episodic memories and to affect older memories much more severely than newer ones. Frontal neocortical lesions disrupt the ability to plan and organize processing in a variety of ways, and this causes impairments of long-term and perhaps (less severely) short-term memory for episodes and facts. At least in monkeys, there is some evidence that ventromedial frontal cortex lesions cause organic amnesia. This syndrome, which is known to be caused by lesions to the medial temporal lobe, the midline diencephalon, the basal forebrain, or their connections, involves pre- and postmorbid impairments of memory for facts and episodes but leaves intelligence and short-term, over-learnt semantic, and several forms of procedural memory intact. Processing of factual and episodic information seems to be relatively preserved. Priming of information already familiar at study is preserved in amnesia, but whether priming of previously novel information is preserved remains controversial. Perceptual priming has been shown to be impaired after posterior neocortical lesions. Other forms of procedural memory are disrupted by subcortical lesions. Thus, motoric classical conditioning is impaired by cerebellar lesions and skill learning is particularly disrupted by basal ganglia lesions. The range of distinct memory disorders has led to the view that there are several different memory systems, each dealing with a specific kind of information, dependent on different brain regions, and perhaps also dependent on qualitatively distinct kinds of memory processes.

I. INTRODUCTION

It has been known for more than 100 years that brain damage can impair memory in a relatively selective fashion. In the past 50 years, it has also become clear that damage to different brain regions selectively disrupts some kinds of memory, but leaves other kinds of memory intact. Since the 1970s, it has become increasingly possible to scan the brains of living memory-impaired subjects to better identify the location of damage that causes specific kinds of memory

deficit. In the 1990s, research exploring the effects of differently located brain lesions on memory was complemented by neuroimaging studies that have explored the brain regions that are activated when particular memory processes are engaged. These neuroimaging studies have helped clarify the normal role of brain structures that when damaged cause different kinds of memory disorder.

Memory depends on encoding (processing and representing) different kinds of information, which are then stored and later retrieved. The occurrence of selective memory disorders has several implications about the way in which the brain mediates these processes. First, the existence of selective memory disorders is surprising because it means that memory loss occurs although the information for which memory is impaired is still being processed (and hence encoded) relatively normally. This challenges a widely held assumption that information is stored in the same neural network that represents it during encoding because if the assumption is correct, then brain lesions that damage such networks should disturb not only storage but also the ability to process and represent the information. In other words, the assumption seems difficult to reconcile with the occurrence of selective memory deficits for particular kinds of information that are still processed normally at input. Because retrieval and encoding involve many overlapping processes, the assumption is still problematic even if it was postulated that a memory deficit was caused by a retrieval deficit. Therefore, care must be taken to determine the selectivity of memory disorders.

Second, the existence of different kinds of memory disorders is consistent with growing evidence that the whole central nervous system is, to varying degrees, plastic and thus capable of storing memories. The spinal cord, as well as the brain, should be regarded as a storer as well as a processor of information. That different kinds of memory should be disrupted by lesions in different brain areas should not be surprising because it is known that different kinds of information are processed and represented in different parts of the central nervous system.

Third, the existence of several different kinds of selective memory disorders caused by lesions in distinct brain regions has resulted in the view that there are several systems of memory organized in a hierarchical fashion. Memory systems differ from each other not only because they are mediated by distinct systems of neurons but also because they involve qualitatively distinct kinds of memory processes. Memory systems are organized hierarchically to the extent that certain kinds of memory share more qualitatively similar kinds of processes with each other than they do with other kinds of memory.

What is known about the range of short- and long-term memory disorders caused by brain damage and the selectivity of these disorders to memory are outlined before briefly considering what this reveals about how the brain mediates memory.

II. WORKING MEMORY DISORDERS

A. Impairments of Phonological and Visuospatial Working Memory

It has long been believed that memory that lasts for only a few seconds without rehearsal depends on different storage processes than does memory that lasts for minutes or longer without rehearsal. Short-term storage may depend on continued patterned activity in the neurons that represent information during encoding, whereas longer term memory may depend on structural changes between the same neurons that represent the information during encoding and short-term memory. If brain lesions can disrupt short-term memory for specific information, then this view would lead one to expect that long-term memory for that information would also be disrupted. Impaired processing of the poorly remembered information might also be expected.

Cortical damage can impair short-term or working memory while leaving processing relatively intact. This pattern of impairment has been explored most extensively with phonological short-term memory, for which the ability to hold sequences of phonemes in mind for several seconds has been found to be disrupted by lesions to the left parietal lobe, particularly in the left posteroinferior parietal lobe where it conjoins with the left temporal lobe. A patient with such damage may only be able to repeat one or two spoken digits when tested immediately after their presentation compared to the normal level of approximately seven digits, and spoken nonword repetition ability is lost with similar rapidity. Even the ability to hold one digit in memory is lost pathologically fast if rehearsal is prevented. Despite this rapid loss of phonological information, whereas some patients may be dysphasic, others show no other cognitive deficits, clearly understanding speech and seemingly processing phonemes normally when memory load is minimized. For example, some patients have been

shown to be unimpaired at making same–different judgments with spoken syllables. Therefore, impaired phonological working memory can occur in the presence of apparently normal processing of phonemes.

In his model of working memory, Baddeley postulated that there was a rehearsal loop as well as a short-term store for phonological information. There is evidence that the phonological short-term store and the rehearsal loop can be disrupted separately. Thus, although some patients have impaired phonological working memory despite normal rehearsal, there are other patients whose impaired phonological working memory is caused by deficient rehearsal. Interestingly, anarthria is not sufficient to cause an impairment of phonological working memory, which suggests that rehearsal of articulated information is mediated centrally and does not require overt speech.

Baddeley's model of working memory also postulated the existence of a visuospatial short-term memory store as well as a phonological one. There is evidence that working memory for visuospatial materials can be disrupted separately from phonological working memory. Thus, whereas some patients have impaired phonological short-term memory and intact visuospatial short-term memory, others have been found to show the reverse pattern of deficit sometimes following lesions in the region of the right Sylvian fissure. In other words, differently located cortical lesions can disrupt these two forms of working memory separately.

B. Other Kinds of Working Memory Disorder

Lesions also disrupt forms of working memory not postulated in the original working memory model of Baddeley. Thus, visual verbal short-term memory can be selectively disrupted, and there has also been a report of a patient with a selective short-term memory deficit for color information in the presence of normal processing of color when memory load was minimized. There is also evidence that relatively selective lexical semantic short-term memory deficits exist. Thus, a patient has been described who was more impaired than a second patient, who had a phonological short-term memory deficit, on tests dependent on lexical semantic short-term memory (e.g., word span tests) but performed better although not completely normally on tests primarily dependent on phonological short-term memory such as non-word span tests. This semantic short-term memory deficit was not caused by a semantic processing impairment because the patient's semantic processing was usually normal when memory load was minimized. The patient's lesion involved the left posterolateral frontal lobe and adjacent parietal regions anterior to where damage probably causes phonological working memory deficits.

Future work will examine the possibility that each sensory system and the motor system has one or more short-term memory systems by exploring whether the corresponding selective short-term memory deficits exist. This work will be guided in part by neuroimaging studies of working memory, which have already supported the implications of the lesion studies. For example, visuospatial and visual object working memory tasks have been found to activate distinct cortical regions. This leads to the expectation that there should be lesions that separately disrupt working memory for these two kinds of visual information.

C. Effects of Working Memory Disorders on Long-Term Memory

Until recently, it was widely believed that long-term memory is preserved in patients with short-term memory deficits because patients with impaired phonological short-term memory show normal long-term memory for spoken verbal materials. This finding was interpreted to mean that short-term memory processes do not trigger long-term memory processes, and the two are mediated by separable groups of neurons. These conclusions do not hold, however, because the preserved long-term memory shown by patients is almost certainly for semantic information, whereas their short-term deficit is for phonological information. Patients are able to recode phonological inputs into a semantic code very rapidly so that the recoding can be achieved even in the presence of very fast loss of phonological information. If care is taken to ensure that the phonological information cannot be recoded, then long-term memory might well be impaired. This has been shown in a patient with very impaired phonological short-term memory who was also found to be completely unable to learn spoken Russian words transliterated into her native Italian. In other words, she was impaired at both short- and long-term memory for meaningless spoken words, which she had to represent as phonological sequences. In a similar way, it has been found that another patient not only had impaired visuospatial short-term memory but also had severely impaired long-term memory for spatial lay-

outs and new faces. A third patient, who had a semantic short-term memory deficit, was also very impaired at long-term memory for lexical semantic information (e.g., word lists) but showed preserved long-term memory for any information for which he had normal short-term memory.

These results imply that short-term memory disorders are specific to particular kinds of information and can occur despite preserved processing of that information at input. Short-term memory for different kinds of information is mediated by distinct cortical systems of neurons, but it remains to be fully explored how these "working memory" neurons relate to the neurons that represent the information at initial coding. Short-term memory disorders are accompanied by long-term ones for the same information. This strongly implies that the same systems of neurons are involved in both short- and long-term storage for specific kinds of information such that damage to a specific system disrupts both short- and long-term memory for the information that it represents. The pattern of deficit, however, neither confirms nor refutes the view that short-term memory processes are necessary for *triggering* long-term ones.

III. DEFICITS IN PREVIOUSLY WELL-LEARNED SEMANTIC INFORMATION

A. The Relationship between Semantic and Episodic Memory Disorders

Memory for the kinds of fact that one might encounter in an encyclopedia or a dictionary (semantic memory) is often contrasted with episodic memory, which concerns personally experienced episodes. The two kinds of memory must interact closely, however, because the kinds of information they involve greatly overlap. Thus, memory for personally experienced episodes typically includes facts as well as perceptual information, and memory for facts may include memory for public episodes with their accompanying contextual markers (a key feature of episodic memory) and perceptual features. In comparing deficits of semantic and episodic memory, much attention needs to be paid to the information involved, and the amount of rehearsal that each kind of memory has received, because although this is not a defining feature, it tends to be greater for semantic memories. Semantic memory is certainly disrupted by brain lesions, but episodic memory may often be similarly disrupted when allowance is made for contaminating factors such as the amount of rehearsal.

Neocortical lesions, particularly to the anterolateral temporal cortex, cause impaired long-term memory for previously well-established semantic memories. These semantic memory deficits are found in dementing conditions, such as Alzheimer's disease and the variant of frontotemporal dementia known as semantic dementia, as well as following closed-head injury and herpes simplex encephalitis. Semantic dementia patients are impaired at naming, identifying, and describing the properties of objects, at defining spoken and written words, and at identifying semantic commonalities between pictures, but they show preservation of perception, non-verbal intelligence, and syntactical and phonological abilities. It is important to determine how selectively these deficits affect factual memory, how selective the dissociations between different kinds of factual memory deficits are; whether the location of cortical damage determines the specific factual memories disrupted; and whether the deficits reflect access or storage breakdowns.

There is an incomplete double dissociation between semantic dementia and organic amnesia. Semantic dementia has usually been regarded as a selective disorder of semantic memory, and amnesia has been regarded as a selective disorder of episodic memory because memory for premorbidly overlearned facts is preserved. Therefore, this dissociation has often been interpreted as evidence that memory for facts and memory for episodes are mediated by partially distinct brain mechanisms. The two memory systems clearly interact, however, although the nature of these interactions is poorly understood. Such interactions have been used to explain the incompleteness of the double dissociation between semantic dementia and organic amnesia. Thus, it is argued that semantic dementia patients typically acquire episodic memories relatively normally but do not show completely preserved episodic memory because new episodes will often involve factual information that they have forgotten (so that semantic dementia patients will not be able to make full sense of an episode). Failure to interpret new episodes in a normal semantic fashion reduces episodic memory because people show worse episodic memory when semantic encoding is minimal. Conversely, it can be argued that amnesics fail to learn new facts normally because their episodic memory impairment prevents the rapid acquisition of new fact memories although these eventually become independent of episodic memory. The implication is that facts can initially only be acquired rapidly as components of

episodic memories, which are selectively impaired in global amnesia.

There is evidence that suggests that "semantic dementia" is a misnomer. This is because the disorder does not seem to be selective to semantic memory; and it also involves an episodic memory deficit that is not secondary to the semantic memory impairment. It was found that semantic dementia patients have an inverted temporal gradient of deficit in which remote autobiographical memories (formed when semantic memory was normal) were more impaired than recent ones, which were sometimes preserved. Similarly, better recognition of famous faces and recall of information about them was found if these faces were encountered during the current time period rather than earlier.

These findings suggest that whether memories are semantic or episodic may not matter. Rather, the only thing that matters may be the memories' age. Thus, in semantic dementia, new facts and episodes seem to be learned as well as remaining semantic memory permits and such information is perhaps retained normally for a while. If memory depends minimally on encoding factual information, then in the short term it may be almost normal. For example, forced-choice recognition memory for recently studied real and chimeric animal pictures is relatively normal in semantic dementia patients. This kind of memory probably depends much more on perceptual than on factual information. However, very long-term storage even of information that can be mainly encoded in terms of perceptual features is very impaired in semantic dementia, because patients have damage to the neocortical structures, responsible for very long-term retention of facts and episodes, so that over a period of years both kinds of information are lost pathologically. This interpretation is consistent with the widely held hypothesis of medial temporal lobe (MTL) amnesia, which states that binding information for fact and episode memories is initially stored in the MTL but through processes such as rehearsal there is a gradual reorganization of storage that is transferred for very long-term maintenance to neocortical structures such as the anterolateral temporal cortex.

A few cases of very severe global amnesia have been reported in which very impaired episodic memory was accompanied by some ability to acquire postmorbid vocabulary and semantic facts, although memory for these things was also very impaired. Such findings can plausibly be regarded as evidence that there is a slow neocortical learning mechanism that gradually creates a long-term memory for semantic information over many learning trials. A disproportionate deficit for episodic memory relative to memory for postmorbidly encountered facts may arise simply because facts, but not particular episodes, are repeatedly encountered. In other words, it may be an artifact of the number of learning trials that facts and episodes typically receive. This would be true if the slow neocortical learning mechanism has the ability to slowly create memories for personally experienced episodes as well as facts. Whether different neocortical lesions can cause dissociable deficits for previously well-established semantic and episodic memories is currently unresolved. Dissociation seems likely to the extent that episodic information differs from semantic information, provided one assumes that memories are stored where they are represented and that different information is represented in different neural structures. In this assumption, semantic memories for different kinds of information are likely to be disrupted by different cortical lesions, and the same may apply to episodic memories of different kinds of episode. The different effects of cortical lesions on memory for different kinds of fact and episode may be much more striking than any general differences between semantic and episodic memory. This issue remains to be systematically explored. However, there is evidence that different cortical lesions do dissociably disrupt different subtypes of semantic memory.

B. Subtypes of Semantic Memory Disorder

There is good evidence that semantic memory for different categories of information breaks down in a dissociable manner although how such dissociations should be interpreted remains controversial. There are examples of dissociations, including ones between impairments of word and object knowledge and between knowledge of abstract and concrete words, respectively. Some semantic memory deficits can be extraordinarily specific. For example, following a stroke, one patient was found to have an impaired ability to name pictures and objects from the categories of fruits and vegetables. This patient could name other food objects and all nonfood objects without difficulty, so his difficulty with name retrieval was specific to the semantic categories of fruits and vegetables. The most explored semantic memory deficits have been those for animate category and inanimate category knowledge. Memory deficits for animate and inanimate categories of knowledge have frequently been shown to dissociate from each other. It

is still disputed by some whether this dissociation reflects uncontrolled differences between the categories tested in variables such as frequency, familiarity, and age of acquisition. Nevertheless, the dissociation might be expected if animate concepts primarily involve visual perceptual properties, whereas inanimate concepts primarily involve functional properties that are less visual in nature. The evidence is conflicting that this is the case. For example, this hypothesis has difficulty explaining why some patients with animate category knowledge deficits are impaired at identifying nonvisual as well as visual features of living things. One possibility that is supported by neuroimaging work is that visual information has to be retrieved even when nonvisual information about living things is retrieved (as revealed by activation of the left fusiform cortex), whereas this is not true about nonliving things. It remains to be seen whether this neuroimaging work can be reconciled with lesion evidence that suggests that more posterior temporal cortex lesions produce deficits in memory for man-made things, whereas more anterior temporal cortex lesions disrupt memory for animate things.

C. Evidence of Storage or Access Failure

In principle, deficits in semantic memory could occur because of degradation in storage, because of a disturbance in processes that access the stored information, or because both of these problems are present. In the 1980s, Shallice proposed five criteria for deciding whether a semantic memory deficit reflects a problem with keeping fact memories in store or with accessing them. The two most plausible of these criteria involve consistency of success or failure of retrieval and the presence or absence of priming or information-specific implicit (unaware) memory. Shallice argued that consistently unsuccessful retrieval of particular items on different occasions implies that storage has been degraded, whereas retrieval should be relatively consistently successful across occasions if storage is still intact. Conversely, if information is not recognized or recalled but is associated with normal priming, then the explicit memory deficit reflects an access problem selective to aware memory. This is because the same information is still available to unaware memory through the presumably distinct access mechanisms required for retrieving memories without awareness (priming). Minimally, Shallice's argument requires that consistent failure should not be found with intact implicit memory. The criteria currently lack a strong theoretical base, so it remains unclear whether they cover the effects of partial storage damage or even whether, for example, consistent failure might sometimes reflect access rather than storage deficits. Nevertheless, there is evidence that, in semantic dementia, when previously retrievable memories become inaccessible, they remain so consistently, so there is a reliable pattern of semantic memory breakdown that requires interpretation.

IV. ORGANIC AMNESIA AND FRONTAL LOBE DAMAGE: EPISODIC AND SEMANTIC MEMORY

A. Organic Amnesia

The most intensively studied of the organic memory disorders is the global organic amnesia syndrome, which was first characterized in the 19th century. In this syndrome, there is impaired recall and recognition of facts and episodes encountered both postmorbidly (anterograde amnesia) and (more variably) premorbidly (retrograde amnesia). These deficits often occur even when intelligence and shortterm memory are preserved. There is also preservation of overlearned semantic memories, of various forms of motor, perceptual, and cognitive skill learning and memory, and of at least some kinds of unaware memory for specific information (priming). The deficits can be produced by lesions to structures in the MTL, midline diencephalon, basal forebrain, and possibly ventromedial frontal cortex as well as to structures that link these regions, such as the fornix.

There is growing evidence that the syndrome is functionally heterogeneous. First, it has been claimed that retrograde amnesia can be produced relatively independently of anterograde amnesia. Several studies have found poor correlations in patients between severity of anterograde amnesia and deficits in more remote premorbid memory. There have also been several reports of relatively selective or focal retrograde amnesia in which patients had a severe and enduring deficit in premorbid memory but a relatively preserved ability to acquire new memories (so that old memories could be "relearned" to some extent). The location of lesions that cause this condition remains to be accurately resolved, but damage often includes the anterolateral temporal neocortex, particularly on the left. There have also been reports of patients with focal retrograde amnesia who had damage to their temporopolar and frontal cortices, mainly on the left. These patients showed extensive retrograde amnesia, but their new learning abilities were relatively intact. The results suggest that old memories about autobiographical and public information may be disrupted by lesions to parts of the temporal cortex. Damage to prefrontal cortex can also disturb these memories, but it is unproved that such lesions alone can disrupt premorbid memory relatively selectively. It needs to be determined more precisely which temporal (and possibly parietal) lesions disrupt remote premorbid memories and how these relate to the damage underlying semantic dementia. There is also a particular difficulty with these focal retrograde amnesia patients in proving that they are not malingering or suffering from a psychogenic deficit. In such cases, the premorbid memory deficit is not directly caused by brain damage but may reflect the patient's conscious wish to achieve financial gain or avoid something unpleasant or the patient's unconscious avoidance of something traumatic. These cases can appear very similar to those arising from brain damage.

Second, it has been argued that amnesia is heterogeneous because lesions to different MTL structures impair memory in distinct ways. It is generally agreed that amygdala damage does not usually cause anterograde amnesia, in contrast to other MTL lesions. However, the amygdala probably plays a role in emotional memory by modulating the effectiveness with which other MTL structures store memories when emotionally evocative information is encoded. This role of the amygdala would explain why events associated with marked emotional arousal are so well remembered (flashbulb memory). The effects of amygdala lesions on memory have been very little explored in humans because of the rarity of selective amygdala lesions.

Some researchers believe that lesions of either hippocampus or perirhinal cortex within the MTL disrupt memory in the same way, but that hippocampal lesions may have a lesser effect. This view implies that free recall and item recognition are equivalently disrupted after MTL lesions. In contrast, it has been argued that hippocampal and perirhinal cortex lesions cause dissociable deficits. This view is based on animal and human evidence. First, animals with perirhinal lesions have shown item recognition impairments but intact spatial memory, whereas the reverse effect has been found with hippocampal lesions. Second, meta-analysis of human recognition data has suggested that there is a single dissociation in which patients with damage to the hippocampus or other parts of Papez circuit, such as the fornix, mammillary bodies, or anterior thalamus, are relatively unimpaired on item recognition but as impaired as more generally lesioned global amnesics (who are also impaired at item recognition) on tests of free recall.

Several patients with apparently selective hippocampal damage were found to be clearly impaired on item recognition when an extensive battery of tests was given. However, patients with selective hippocampal sclerosis related to temporal lobe epilepsy were reported not to show impaired item recognition, and other patients with probable hippocampal damage caused by hypoxia showed a similar preservation. In addition, three patients with evidence of early selective hippocampal damage were shown to have completely selective free recall deficits because their item recognition was normal on a range of tests. Similar patterns of memory performance with relatively preserved item recognition have been found in patients with selective hippocampal damage acquired in adulthood, so it is unlikely that the pattern of selective free recall deficits reflects reorganizational processes following early brain damage.

Apparently selective hippocampal damage, sometimes causes severe item recognition deficits and sometimes leaves item recognition relatively or completely intact. Animal studies have shown that cerebral ischemia often produces damage that extends beyond the hippocampus. Because such damage may be both highly variable and difficult to identify either by structural imaging or by postmortem analysis, it is likely that those patients with more severe recognition deficits have damage extending into other brain regions important for item recognition, such as the perirhinal cortex. There is even evidence that extrahippocampal damage is exacerbated by abnormal processes in the hippocampus that are triggered by ischemia. Extrahippocampal damage is probably best detected by measuring whether blood flow is abnormal in nonhippocampal brain regions so that it can be determined whether such abnormalities are more striking in patients with severe item recognition deficits. This kind of abnormality, invisible to structural magnetic resonance imaging, has been identified using positron emission tomography in patients who suffered hypoxia following heart attacks. These patients showed reduced blood flow in regions that appeared normal in structural magnetic resonance imaging (MRI). It is possible, however, that less used and more sophisticated structural MRI procedures would identify abnormalities in these regions.

Selective damage to other parts of the Papez circuit has also been found to cause little or no disruption of item recognition. Thus, relatively selective free recall deficits have been reported after fornix lesions caused by colloid cyst surgery and also following relatively selective mammillary body lesions. Lesions that affect only the anterior thalamic nucleus within the thalamus are very rare, but one patient has been described whose thalamic damage was confined to the left anterior thalamic nucleus, although she also had damage to the head of the left caudate nucleus and the left fornix. This patient had completely normal recognition for items and a free recall deficit for verbal materials.

Some animal research supports the existence of another memory system that comprises the perirhinal cortex, the dorsomedial nucleus of the thalamus to which it is reciprocally connected, and possibly the orbitofrontal cortex to which the thalamic nucleus links. The interconnections of this system with the Papez circuit system are illustratred in Fig. 1. As indicated previously, in animals, selective perirhinal cortex lesions disrupt item recognition but not some kinds of spatial memory. They also disrupt associations between similar kinds of items. Little relevant work has been done in humans mainly because selective perirhinal cortex lesions are probably nonexistent and selective dorsomedial thalamic lesions are extremely rare.

However, total bilateral destruction of the perirhinal cortex (and other regions) in humans has been reported to show more severe impairments of recognition for complex patterns at delays of a few seconds compared to those of global amnesics without perirhinal cortex lesions. Interestingly, these patients performed normally at delays of 0 and 2 sec as well as when making judgments regarding when the stimulus was still present. This could mean that perirhinal cortex lesions selectively disrupt long-term memory because they leave short-term memory and visual perception intact. This interpretation is not undisputed because it has been argued, on the basis of animal research, that perirhinal cortex lesions disrupt the ability to represent complex conjunctions of stimulus features in perception, and that memory deficits may be secondary to these high-level perceptual deficits. If this argument is correct, then amnesia that is caused by perirhinal cortex damage does not constitute a pure memory deficit. In principle, the argument can also be extended to hippocampal lesions that might be causing disruption of the ability to represent other kinds of complex conjunctions (such as those between objects and locations or between faces and voices). Such high-level perceptual deficits would secondarily cause memory impairment, and they

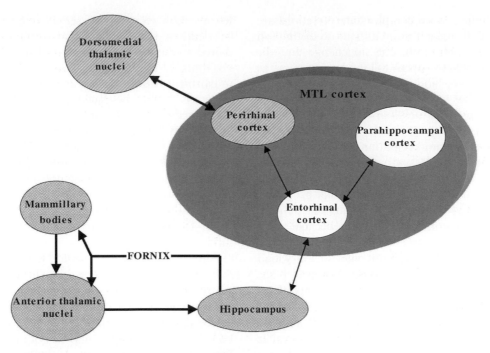

Figure 1 The connections between the structures that may constitute the two memory systems as well as interconnections between the systems and between the systems and neocortical regions. Shading with lines indicates structures that may form the perirhinal cortex–dorsomedial thalamic memory system, whereas pale gray shading indicates structures that may form part of the Papez circuit memory system. Arrows indicate that there is evidence that connections exist. Thick solid lines indicate connections that can confidently be related to the memory systems. Thin solid lines indicate connections that are known to link the two memory systems. Both systems connect to prefrontal association cortex, but it is uncertain what role this cortex plays in memory and it is also unclear whether the two memory systems interact in the prefrontal association cortex.

would be very difficult to detect because of the likelihood that affected patients would use compensatory strategies. It cannot therefore be confidently claimed that major forms of amnesia are unrelated to very specific forms of encoding failure.

The very severe long-term memory deficits that have been reported following perirhinal cortex lesions may be dependent on this damage being nearly total. Support for this possibility is provided by a subgroup of epileptic patients with selective damage that includes only part of the perirhinal cortex who show normal performance on standard tests of anterograde amnesia but accelerated forgetting over delays of weeks. By these delays, their memory is badly impaired. Partial perirhinal cortex damage may therefore cause a much less severe and much delayed item recognition deficit than does total damage to this cortex. The mnemonic effects of dorsomedial thalamic lesions may also critically depend on the extent of damage. Thus, patients with marked destruction of this nucleus show impaired item recognition as well as free recall, whereas patients with only a small portion

of the nucleus damaged show little evidence of memory deficits.

Papez circuit lesions and perirhinal cortex system lesions both cause retrograde as well as anterograde amnesia. Although severe retrograde amnesia can extend back to memories acquired decades before the causative brain damage, there often appears to be a temporal gradient in which earlier acquired memories are less disrupted. Considerable evidence suggests that Papez circuit lesions cause a less severe, more steeply temporally graded retrograde amnesia than do larger lesions that involve the whole of the MTL. This would be consistent with the hypothesis that the hippocampus (and perhaps other MTL regions) only stores facts and episodes for a limited time until reorganization results in neocortical storage in the sites that presumably represent the stored information. An alternative view that challenges this claim is that there is no reorganization of the location of long-term memories as a result of processes such as rehearsal, at least for some kinds of information (such as spatial). The simplest interpretation of this view is that it should predict no temporal gradient, although more complex interpretations are also possible that make it more difficult to distinguish between the predictions of the no change and the change views of what happens to long-term memory as it ages. Therefore, additional work is needed to determine whether memories cease to depend on the MTL as they age. Future work must also explore whether selective Papez circuit lesions minimally disrupt premorbid item recognition memory.

Exactly what processes are disrupted in patients with the amnesia syndrome? If the syndrome is heterogeneous, there must be several such processes. It is widely believed that many global amnesia patients process facts and episodes normally because their intelligence is preserved and normal kinds of information are available to them at input when memory load is minimized. As discussed previously, however, it has not been shown conclusively that subtle high-level perceptual processes may not be disrupted following MTL lesions. Evidence from transient global amnesia (TGA) indicates that it is unlikely that retrieval is impaired in global anterograde amnesia. TGA is a form of global amnesia that lasts for only a few hours and is usually caused by a reversible abnormality in the MTL, which has been revealed by showing that blood flow to the MTL (and sometimes other brain regions) is reduced during a TGA attack but usually returns to normal when tested later. Upon recovery, although all premorbid memories apart from those acquired in the few minutes or hours prior to the incident typically return, as does the ability to lay down new memories, no memories for the incident return. Because these memories do not return even when retrieval must be normal, global anterograde amnesia is probably caused by a failure to consolidate facts and episodes into long-term memory in the minutes following input.

If Papez circuit lesions do cause a selective amnesia, they will disrupt the consolidation of different kinds of information from those disrupted by perirhinal cortex lesions. The available evidence suggests that patients with selective hippocampal lesions can be relatively normal not only for recognition memory for single items (e.g., words or faces) but also for associations between the same kind of items (e.g., word–word or face–face associations). However, they are severely impaired at recognizing associations between components that would probably be processed in different cortical regions (e.g., object–location and face–voice). Similar and possibly more severe spatial memory deficits have also been reported following parahippocampal cortex lesions. The evidence is more conflicting about whether patients with selective hippocampal

lesions show relatively preserved remote memory for overlearned facts. Patients are unquestionably impaired at the initial acquisition of new facts (such as vocabulary) but it remains to be shown that their impairment does not occur because their factual memory cannot be facilitated by the retrieval of associated contextual information (which involves episodic memory and is disrupted). Also, some patients may learn to compensate for their learning deficit by rehearsing factual information much more frequently than people with normal memory. Probably, hippocampal and Papez circuit lesions disrupt consolidation of both factual and episodic associations, the components of which are represented in different cortical regions.

Although lesions that include the perirhinal cortex drastically impair item recognition, little is known about the effect of selective lesions of this structure in humans. Animal studies indicate that selective damage to this cortex disrupts recognition of items and associations between similar components but not memory for some kinds of spatial information. It is uncertain in humans whether perirhinal cortex lesions disrupt memory for all the kinds of information affected by hippocampal lesions and memory for some other kinds of information as well, or whether there are some kinds of memory (such as some forms of spatial memory) that are only disrupted by hippocampal lesions.

B. The Role of the Prefrontal Cortex in Memory

Prefrontal cortex damage sometimes disrupts long-term memory for post- as well as premorbidly experienced facts and episodes. Commonly, the deficits are of free recall, with item recognition being relatively normal. The ability to remember the temporal order in which items have been presented is also often impaired, as is the ability to remember the source (who said something or whether it was encountered via TV, the radio, or newspaper) of information. Prefrontal cortex lesions have also been found to disrupt various kinds of metamemory, such as being able to predict whether one will be able to recognize information one has failed to recall when it is presented later. However, recognition deficits have also been reported in the presence of free recall that is relatively good apart from the production of a pathological level of false positives.

Such memory impairments are probably secondary to the effect of frontal cortex damage on executive processes and perhaps working memory. If sophisticated encoding processes cannot be properly orchestrated, then memory will suffer, and the effect is likely (as is often found) to disrupt free recall, which is more dependent than item recognition on the storage of rich interitem associations. Similarly, if the organization of searching and checking operations during retrieval is disrupted, then free recall will probably be affected more than item recognition. Whether this kind of explanation accounts for the disruption of temporal and source memory in frontally damaged patients remains to be proved, but these kinds of contextual memory are likely to require considerable amounts of organization at both encoding and retrieval. Similarly, it remains to be determined whether the abnormal recognition shown by some patients with prefrontal cortex lesions is caused by the disruption of different executive processes from those affected in cases of free recall deficit or contextual memory deficit. Finally, it is believed by some that damage to the ventromedial prefrontal projections of the MTL causes a syndrome very similar, if not identical, to global amnesia.

Neuroimaging evidence indicates that the left and right prefrontal cortices are activated when verbal and difficult to verbalize information respectively are encoded into memory. This suggests that left and right prefrontal cortex lesions may respectively disrupt verbal and nonverbal memory. There is evidence that lateralized lesions do have this kind of material-specific effect, although it has been noted that laterality effects are weaker than with more posterior cortical lesions, and that verbal learning deficits are much more common after bilateral than after left prefrontal cortex lesions. Evidence for other kinds of dissociation between left and right prefrontal cortex lesions is weak. Although there may be a weak relationship between right frontal damage and retrograde amnesia for episodes, there is little evidence that right frontal cortex lesions disrupt retrieval for recently experienced episodes. However, a pathological tendency to make false alarms during recognition testing has been noted in some patients after both left- and right-sided frontal cortex damage. The manipulations that improve performance, however, are variable and include the use of a semantic orienting task at encoding and using foils that were in a different semantic category from all target items.

Long-term memory for episodes and facts involves a large network of neural structures interacting with each other. The network includes several frontal cortex regions interacting with both temporal and parietal cortices as well as subcortical structures. The precise characteristics of the memory impairments caused by lesions to specific parts of the network need further specification so as to test the functional deficit hypotheses more rigorously. Neuroimaging has provided evidence that the roles of the prefrontal and MTL cortices in memory are complementary. Thus, patients with amnesia caused by MTL lesions can show normal frontal activation patterns during encoding despite their impaired memory. If the frontal and MTL contributions to memory are complementary, then one would expect that temporal order memory deficits arise for different reasons in amnesia and following frontal cortex lesions. The impaired process is presumably different in the two cases, involving consolidation in the former and some kind of difficulty in executing effortful encoding and/or retrieval processes in the latter. It has been shown that the frontal deficit mainly occurs following intentional encoding, which indicates that the source of the problem is probably impoverished effortful encoding. If the deficit relates to poor consolidation in amnesia, amnesics should be impaired following both intentional and incidental encoding. This likely possibility remains to be tested.

V. PRIMING DEFICITS

Priming involves memory for specific information that people are typically unaware they are remembering. This kind of unaware memory is indicated by the enhanced fluency with which the remembered information is reactivated when cues that form part of the memory are encoded. Enhanced reactivation fluency of the remembered representation probably depends on storage changes at the synapses within the representing region so that the components of the memory are bound more tightly together. These changes should occur in different neocortical regions, depending not only on whether semantic or perceptual information is being implicitly remembered but also on precisely what kinds of such information are involved. Consistent with this, functional imaging has shown that whereas visual object priming produces reduced activation of visual cortex regions where the visual object information should be represented at encoding, semantic priming produces less activation in the left inferior frontal cortex where semantic information may be partially represented. This implies that perceptual and semantic kinds of priming occur in different cortical regions, although perceptual priming may not always be based in posterior cortex or semantic priming in frontal cortex regions. Lesions in these regions would be expected to disrupt the appropriate kinds of priming.

Amnesics, who do not have damage in these neocortical regions, might be expected to show preserved priming. However, if the priming involves retrieval of the kinds of association that amnesics fail to store normally, then deficits might be expected. The evidence is still incomplete. There is good evidence that amnesics show preserved priming for information that was already in memory prior to study (such as words or famous faces), but they are often impaired at priming for various kinds of information that were novel prior to study. Meta-analysis of available studies that involve priming of both novel and already familiar information reveals that although amnesic patients show completely normal priming for information that was already in memory at study, they are significantly impaired across studies at priming various kinds of novel information. One interpretation of such results is that normal people may effortfully be using explicit memory in those priming tasks at which amnesics are impaired, whereas the patients cannot do this. This interpretation, however, does not provide a principled explanation of why control subjects use or do not use explicit memory with similar priming tasks that differ merely with respect to whether studied information is novel or already familiar.

If perceptual information is processed in the posterior association cortex, then one might expect that lesions in this region will disrupt perceptual priming. This is consistent with evidence that Alzheimer patients typically show preservation of perceptual priming but impairment in more semantic kinds of priming. These patients have relative preservation of primary sensory processing regions in the posterior cortex but marked atrophy in the temporal association cortex, which together with the left frontal region plays a key role in processing semantic information. Thus, Alzheimer patients show preservation of priming for previously novel patterns but are impaired at a more semantic verbal free association priming task. There is disagreement about whether these patients are impaired at stem completion priming, which some argue may relate to this being a partially semantic priming task. A key requirement for preserved stem completion priming that may explain the inconsistent results is that patients have to explicitly process the words phonologically during study if they are to prime normally.

Alzheimer's patients are impaired not only at certain kinds of priming but also at explicit memory for facts and episodes, so they do not show evidence of impaired priming in the face of intact recognition and/or recall. However, selective impairment of perceptual priming has been shown in a patient with a right posterior neocortical lesion. This patient was impaired at certain kinds of visual repetition priming. In contrast, he was relatively normal not only at semantic priming but also at recognition of visually presented words for which visual repetition priming was impaired. A double dissociation was noted between this patient and amnesics who have disrupted recognition memory but normal visual priming of premorbidly familiar materials. A similar patient was found to be unimpaired in the familiarity component as well as in the recollection component of recognition.

Such a dissociation between perceptual priming of words and recognition of words might arise because visual word recognition usually involves familiarity as well as recollection for primarily semantic information rather than the kinds of visual information retrieved in the perceptual priming at which patients with right-sided visual cortex damage were impaired. However, it has been shown that recognition of modality and font of word presentation can also be preserved in the presence of impaired visual priming. If the perceptual information retrieved in the intact recognition and impaired priming tasks was truly matched, and the priming deficit was caused by a storage deficit, this finding would show that the perceptual fluency that underlies perceptual priming does not contribute to the familiarity component of perceptual recognition.

There has been little exploration of whether priming deficits can occur without accompanying, if subtle, processing deficits, so this remains an open issue. The priming deficits shown in the patients just described, however, are associated with some visual processing problems, so it remains possible that priming deficits are always accompanied by corresponding processing deficits. It could even be that a visual processing deficit produces the false appearance of a priming impairment, and that the memory underlying priming is preserved.

VI. DEFICITS IN OTHER KINDS OF PROCEDURAL/IMPLICIT MEMORY

Procedural memory comprises not only priming but also various forms of conditioning, various forms of skill memory, and nonassociative forms of memory such as habituation. The core feature of all these forms of memory is that remembering is not accompanied by a feeling of memory. They are probably much more functionally heterogeneous than semantic and episodic memory, but less is known about them. It is believed that they are mainly dependent on subcortical mechanisms, but neuroimaging evidence suggests that frontal and motor cortex regions are important in the early stages of skill acquisition.

Amnesics perform normally on nonpriming kinds of procedural memory such as classical conditioning as well as skill learning and memory. For example, they show preserved delay eye blink classical conditioning. Amnesics have also been shown to acquire normally the motor skill of mirror drawing, the perceptual skill of reading mirror reversed words, and the cognitive skill of intuitively grasping the relationship between variables to achieve a target value. Furthermore, amnesic performance has been shown to be preserved in the acquisition of adaptation-level effects with weights and in the acquisition of the ability to perceive depth using random-dot stereograms. This indicates that the forebrain regions critical for episodic and semantic memory play little or no role in these forms of procedural memory.

In contrast to amnesics, patients with Huntington's disease (HD), who have neostriatal damage, have been found to show impaired acquisition and retention of skills such as reading mirror-reversed words and relatively normal performance at verbal recognition tests. Similarly, Parkinson's patients, whose substantia nigra pathology also disrupts neostriatal function, have shown impaired acquisition of cognitive skills despite being normal at some explicit memory tasks.

With respect to motor skills, and unlike amnesics, patients with HD fail to show normal adaptation-level effects with weights. This is particularly interesting because although no correlation between motor dysfunction and motor skill acquisition dysfunction has been found in these patients, there is still uncertainty about what functional deficits underlie the motor skill acquisition deficit in HD. Because the adaptation-level task is much less dependent on overt movement than motor skill acquisition, it is likely that neostriatal damage disrupts the development of motor programs vital for both normal motor skill acquisition and adaptation-level effects. The neostriatum may be particularly involved in developing motor programs for sequences of motor acts because neurodegenerative diseases affecting the neostriatum disrupt serial reaction time performance. Cerebellar atrophy disrupts performance on the serial reaction time task, which suggests that the cerebellum is also involved in developing motor programs, perhaps because it indexes the temporal order of sensorimotor events.

The involvement of the striatum in perceptual and cognitive skills is supported by several reports of deficits in the development of such skills in patients with degenerative damage in the region. However, impairments are not always found because preserved acquisition of mirror-reading skill has been found in Parkinson's disease patients. Whether cerebellar damage impairs perceptual and cognitive skill acquisition is uncertain because although deficits have been reported, there is strong evidence that patients with selective cerebellar degeneration do not show deficits in learning to read mirror-reversed text or solving the tower of Hanoi difficulty. The difficulty is that many studies have included patients with degeneration that extended beyond the cerebellum.

Cerebellar lesions have, however, have been shown convincingly to disrupt the development of delay eye blink classical conditioning while leaving explicit memory intact. However, the same patients show unimpaired autonomic or emotional conditioning. Studies with animals indicate that fear conditioning, which typically involves autonomic as well as behavioral conditioning, is disrupted both by amygdala lesions and by lesions that disrupt sensory input to the amygdala. Therefore, the neural bases of motoric and emotional classical conditioning, appear to be very different, so it needs to be shown what these two forms of conditioning share apart from the name.

Whereas delay conditioning in which the conditioned stimulus is still present when the unconditioned stimulus appears is preserved in amnesics, more complex forms of conditioning may not be. Thus, amnesics are impaired at reversal discrimination conditioning (in which a response is first conditioned to one discriminative stimulus and inhibited to the other, after which the process is reversed) perhaps because normal performance depends partly on the use of aware (explicit) memory, which is impaired in amnesics. There is conflicting evidence about whether amnesics are impaired at trace motor conditioning (in which the conditioned stimulus ends before the unconditioned stimulus appears) although a growing body of evidence suggests that patients are unpaired. This conflict probably arises because measuring conditioned responses in the trace conditioning paradigm is difficult partly because fine grained features of the response's timing may indicate whether it is an automatic conditioned response or a voluntarily produced anticipation of the unconditioned stimulus. This difficulty may also relate to the dispute about whether trace conditioning depends on explicit memory for the contingencies between conditioned and unconditioned stimuli or is automatic and independent of explicit memory, as one would expect if it is a pure form of procedural memory.

VII. CONCLUSION

Differently located brain damage disrupts memory for different kinds of information despite often having little obvious effect on the processing of the poorly remembered information. Processing may not always be unaffected (as perhaps is the case with selective priming deficits) and it is sometimes difficult to show convincingly that it is not (as with skill memory and conditioning); however, insofar as it is unaffected, the view that information is stored in the same neurons that process and represent it is challenged. At least four explanations of this apparent challenge are possible. First, the damaged region may merely modulate storage in the neural system that represents the poorly remembered information. Basal forebrain structures may play this modulatory role. Second, partial damage to the representing neural system may be sufficient to disrupt its storage abilities while having a minimal effect on its representational processing abilities. This may apply to the short-term memory disorders. Third, there may be multiple representational–storage neural systems for the same information. In other words, the same information may be represented and stored in several different neural sites. Fourth, information is not stored exactly where it is represented.

The existence of multiple memory deficits has been used as evidence to support the claim that there are different memory systems for different kinds of information, each with its own neural system that may mediate memory through the use of qualitatively distinct processes. Two comments about such memory system views are warranted. First, if memory is organized as a set of systems, then these should be arranged hierarchically. This is true of the influential taxonomy that discriminates between declarative and nondeclarative memory, where the former involves all aware forms of memory and the latter all nonaware forms. If correct, all aware forms of memory should have more in common with each other than they do with any form of nonaware memory and vice versa. This would be untrue if amnesics have impaired priming for the same novel information for which they show impaired aware memory, as the available evidence suggests, and also if they are impaired at forms of conditioning that can be shown not to depend on aware memory, as some believe to be the case. The issue is very important and currently unresolved. Either memory systems are mainly organized around whether or not they produce aware memory or the kinds of information they store is more fundamental to their organization. Resolution will involve determin-ing the relationship between unaware and aware memory and how aware memory is produced.

Second, memory may be mediated by different brain systems, but they may work in the same way. Anatomical differences should not be regarded as equivalent to qualitative differences in processing. Although such qualitatively different memory processes may operate for memory of different kinds of information, the methods for showing this remain to be properly established. Indeed, one cannot even be sure for most organic memory disorders whether they are caused by encoding, storage, or retrieval failures. Thus, it is currently unknown whether radically different kinds of memory processing are mediated by distinct brain regions.

See Also the Following Articles

MEMORY, EXPLICIT AND IMPLICIT • MEMORY NEUROBIOLOGY • MEMORY, NEUROIMAGING • MEMORY, OVERVIEW • NERVE CELLS AND MEMORY • SEMANTIC MEMORY • SHORT-TERM MEMORY • WORKING MEMORY

Suggested Reading

Daum, I., Schugens, M. M., Ackerman, H., Lutzenberg, W., Dichgans, J., and Birbaumer, N. (1993). Classical conditioning after cerebellar lesions in humans. *Behav. Neurosci.* **105,** 748–756.

Jonides, J., and Smith, E. E. (1997). The architecture of working memory. In *Cognitive Neuroscience* (M. D. Rugg, Ed.), pp. 243–276. Psychology Press, Hove, UK.

Keane, M. M., Gabrieli, J. D. E., Mapstone, H. C., Johnston, K. A., and Corkin, S. (1995). Double dissociation of memory capacities after bilateral occipital-lobe or medial temporal-lobe lesions. *Brain* **118,** 1129–1148.

Mayes, A. R. (1988). *Human Organic Memory Disorders.* Cambridge Univ. Press, Cambridge, UK.

Mayes, A. R., and Downes, J. J. (Eds.) (1997). *Theories of Organic Amnesia.* Psychology Press, Hove, UK.

Patterson, K., and Hodges, J. R. (1995). Disorders of semantic memory. In *Handbook of Memory Disorders.* (A. D. Baddeley, B. A. Wilson, and F. N. Watts, Eds.), p. 167. Wiley, Chichester, UK

Schacter, D. L., and Tulving, E. (Eds.) (1994). *Memory Systems.* MIT Press, Cambridge, MA.

Troster, A. (Ed.) (1998). *Memory in Neurodegenerative Disease.* Cambridge Univ. Press, Cambridge, UK.

Vallar, G., and Papagno, C. (1995). Neuropsychological impairments of short-term memory. In *Handbook of Memory Disorders* (A. D. Baddeley, B. A. Wilson, and F. N. Watts, Eds.), pp. 135–166. Wiley, Chichester, UK.

Vargha-Khadem, F., Gadian, D. G., Watkins, K. E., Van Paesschen, W., and Mishkin, M. (1997). Differential effects of early hippocampal pathology on episodic and semantic memory. *Science* **277,** 376–380.

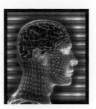

Memory, Explicit and Implicit

KATHLEEN B. MCDERMOTT

Washington University, St. Louis

GLOSSARY

explicit memory Intentional retrieval of the past as manifested on a test in which people are asked to recollect the past. Explicit memory is what laypeople typically mean by the term memory.

implicit memory The change in performance as a result of prior experience in the absence of intention to remember the prior event. Implicit memory is often facilitative, although it can cause interference.

generation effect The finding that requiring people to generate information (e.g., from a conceptual clue, "hot–c_____") leads to a higher likelihood of remembering the generated information (e.g., "cold") on a later explicit memory test than if the to-be-remembered item is simply presented to the person (e.g., they read the word "cold" or read "hot-cold").

level-of-processing effect The finding that on most explicit memory tests, events encoded with respect to their meaning are more likely to be retrieved at a later time than those processed only to a superficial level (e.g., in terms of visual features or sound).

picture superiority effect The finding that on most explicit memory tests, items previously presented as pictures are better remembered than those previously presented as words.

priming Change in performance on a current task caused by recent prior experience in the absence of intent to use that experience on the current task. This is the measure of memory on most laboratory-based implicit memory tests.

recall A type of memory test in which the subject must produce the previously encountered items, either from minimal cues (as in free recall: "Write down as many words as you can remember seeing in the previous study list") or in response to a cue (as in cued recall: "Tell me the word previously paired with "hot").

recognition A type of memory test in which the to-be-remembered items are presented to the subject, whose task is to decide whether he or she remembers having encountered the item previously (free choice recognition) or to decide which of several items he or she remembers having encountered (forced choice recognition).

Memory researchers typically discuss memory as being a three-stage process: encoding (or the acquisition of information), storage (or the retention of information over time), and retrieval (or accessing information previously encoded). Explicit and implicit memory refer to different ways that past events can be retrieved. Specifically, one can intentionally try to retrieve the past. This is what is commonly referred to as "memory" or memory retrieval and is what experimental psychologists call explicit memory. We "search our brains" for information previously encountered. For example, remembering where you parked your car, remembering your first day of school, and remembering the last time you ate at your favorite restaurant are all examples of explicit memory. Implicit memory, in contrast, refers to the unintentional manifestation of previous experience on a current task. Psychologists generally do not use the term "remembering" when discussing implicit memory; instead, they refer to "priming." If you recently heard an unusual word such as "perspicacious," you are more likely to use that word in conversation than you otherwise would be; You are "primed" to use the word. This is an everyday example of implicit memory. As will be seen, both explicit and implicit memory are typically studied by psychologists through controlled laboratory experiments in which people are given sets of materials (e.g., pictures or words) to remember, and retention of this information is assessed by one or more types of memory test.

I. EXPLICIT MEMORY

A. Definition

Explicit memory can be thought of as intentional retrieval. That is, explicit memory is the willful process of thinking back in time for the purpose of retrieving previously encountered events. It is also sometimes referred to as *episodic memory* because explicit memory involves memory for prior episodes in one's life (as opposed to memory for general knowledge of the world, e.g., who served as the first U.S. president, which is called *semantic memory*). In psychology experiments, explicit memory is usually defined operationally in terms of test instructions. That is, if participants are asked to retrieve a previous event, then the experiment is one that taps explicit memory.

B. Measures

Explicit memory is usually measured with tests of recognition or recall. *Recognition* refers to the case in which the memory test gives an answer and the person must decide whether or not it is correct (called *free choice recognition* or yes/no recognition) or choose from among possible alternatives (*forced choice recognition*). For example, imagine that subjects in an experiment were given a list of 100 words to remember. They might then receive a free choice recognition test in which 50 of these words are presented, mixed with 50 new words (the ratio need not be 50 : 50). The job of the participant is to determine for each word whether it had been presented in the study phase. Thus, they give a yes or no answer to each word. This test is similar to true/false tests often given in school. An alternative test would be forced choice recognition, in which people would be given a set of words, with each set containing at least 1 studied word and at least 1 nonstudied word. The subject's task would be to decide which of the words had been studied. This approach is analogous to what are called multiple-choice tests in educational settings.

Recall differs from recognition in that the answer is not presented to the person. There are several types of recall as well. In *free recall* and *serial recall*, no cues are given; people are simply told to think back to the study phase (in our example here, the word list) and write down (or say) everything they remember. Free recall differs from serial recall in that order of recall does not matter in free recall; in serial recall, however, people

are instructed to produce the studied items in the same order in which they were previously experienced. On a *cued recall* test, subjects are given cues to help them remember the list. For example, if the studied list contained the words "zebra," "lion," and "dog," they might be given the cue "animals" to help guide their recall. Perhaps they would be given the first few letters of the words (e.g., "ze___") to help them remember items in the list.

C. Typical Patterns of Results

As discussed previously, researchers generally conceptualize memory as having three stages (encoding, storage, and retrieval). The types of strategies that people use during the encoding (or acquisition) stage have a profound effect on what is remembered at a later time. Considered here are just a few of the classic variables shown to strongly affect performance on a later memory test.

1. Level of Processing

The *level-of-processing effect* is one of the most robust and well-known findings in the explicit memory literature. In two seminal papers on this topic in the mid-1970s, Fergus Craik, Robert Lockhart, and Endel Tulving showed that if people are encouraged to think about the meaning of words (from a list of words to be remembered later), they later recall and recognize those words with a higher probability than if they are encouraged to think about the sound (or phonology). For example, for the word "lizard", people could be asked "Is it an animal?" or "Does it rhyme with wizard?" The former question would lead to a higher probability of recall and recognition on average, across many words in the study list. Similarly, people remember words encoded with attention to sound better than words that are processed at a more superficial level (e.g., determining whether the word is in uppercase letters). This phenomenon is called *level of processing* because it was proposed that people must go through the more "shallow" levels (e.g., the letter level) to access the "deeper" levels (e.g., meaning-based processing). The level-of-processing effect is a very robust phenomenon; one of the primary principles of memory is that if one wants to remember something later, he or she will do well to think hard about its meaning and importance at the time of encoding.

2. The Generation Effect

The *generation effect* is similar to the level-of-processing effect in that it shows that the more meaningfully and effortfully items or events are processed, the better they will later be remembered on explicit memory tests (both recall and recognition). The way the effect is typically studied in the laboratory was popularized by Norman Slamecka and Peter Graf in the 1970s. People are either given antonyms to read (e.g., "hot–cold") or given the first word and asked to generate its antonym (e.g., "hot —"). Later, on recall and recognition tests, people remember "cold" better if they previously had to generate it themselves than if they simply read it. Consider the way children use flash cards to learn vocabulary words or the periodic table of the elements. Flash card techniques take advantage of the generation effect in that the information is generated by the user before looking at the answer. For example, the flash card user might see "mercury" on a card and try to generate its symbol (Hg) before checking the answer on the back of the card. Research has shown that even instances in which the generation attempt fails (e.g., the flash card user cannot successfully remember the item on the other side of the card), the generation effect occurs: Memory for the to-be-generated information can be facilitated relative to the condition of simply reading the information.

3. The Picture Superiority Effect

The *picture superiority effect* refers to the finding (made widely known through experiments by Allan Paivio in the late 1960s) that pictures are remembered better than words. This pattern occurs regardless of the type of explicit test—recall or recognition; it even occurs when the recognition test contains words (referring to pictures or words previously encoded). The source of this effect is thought to be that pictures access meaning more fully than words (and therefore are processed more "deeply" in level-of-processing terms); furthermore, pictures can often be accompanied by a verbal label. For example, if a picture of a fish is shown, people can easily think "fish" or "trout" to themselves when looking at the picture. Thus, pictures tend to access two types of codes (pictorial and verbal), whereas words tend to access only a single type of code (verbal). Of course, people could also form a mental image of a fish when given the word, in which case they would access both types of codes; indeed, when they do so, words are better remembered than when no imagery is invoked.

D. Neural Correlates

What parts of the brain contribute to our ability to remember the past? There are two primary ways of answering this question. The first and traditional way is to use unfortunate accidents of nature—naturally occurring brain lesions—to determine what cognitive processes break down when certain parts of the brain are injured due to stroke, accidents, or other insults to the brain. William Scoville and Brenda Milner described the memory impairments of a man known by his initials, H.M., who had his temporal lobes (including most of the hippocampi) surgically removed in the early 1950s in an attempt to cure intractable epilepsy (Fig. 1). The result was a profound loss of ability to remember anything that happened since the surgery (*anterograde amnesia*). However, H.M. was able to remember most things that occurred before the surgery and was able to converse somewhat normally. This pattern of results and similar outcomes exhibited by other patients with temporal lobe damage suggests that the temporal lobes (in or around the hippocampus) are necessary for the formation of new explicit memories. Interestingly, as will be discussed later, amnesic patients such as H.M. exhibit intact implicit memory (Fig. 2). The point to be taken from this study and other similar studies is that the medial temporal lobes play an important function in remembering the past; when they are removed or damaged, new explicit memories cannot be formed. One difficulty, however, lies in determining which stage(s) of the memory process (encoding, storage, or retrieval) this structure exhibits its effect. Does the information not enter the amnesic's brain properly? Is it encoded properly, with a breakdown in the storage or retrieval phase? Is it coded in one type of memory system (implicit) but not the other type (explicit)?

Recently, a new set of techniques has been developed that allows one to address these and similar questions. Specifically, *neuroimaging techniques* [e.g., *event-related potentials* (ERPs), *functional magnetic resonance imaging* (fMRI), and *positron emission tomography* (PET)] allow researchers to view the normal, living brain as it encodes and retrieves information (and while it processes information generally). By taking advantage of the fact that when specific brain regions are engaged in a task (e.g., a recognition memory test), these regions receive enhanced blood flow relative to their normal resting state (in the case of fMRI and PET) or the fact that electrical activity increases (in the case of ERP), these techniques can inform our understanding of the neural

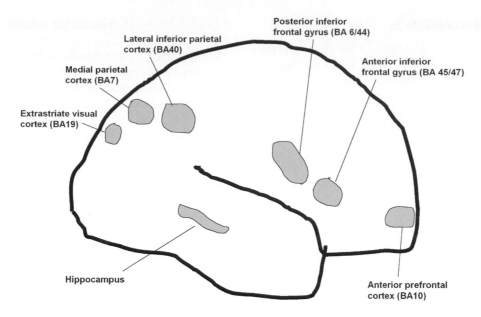

Figure 1   Schematically depicted brain regions involved in explicit and implicit human memory. The front of the brain appears on the right side of the figure. BA, approximate Brodmann's area.

underpinnings of memory. These approaches have shown that several regions are typically engaged during memory retrieval. Interestingly, although the hippocampus is sometimes shown to be active during

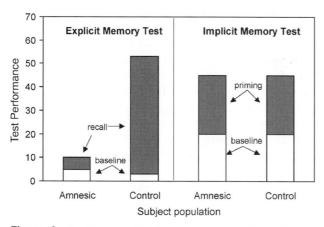

Figure 2   Explicit and implicit memory tests show different patterns of results. Data in this (and all) figures are idealized data demonstrating the general pattern observed across multiple studies. (Left) Patients with damage to the hippocampus and surrounding areas of the medial temporal lobes show profound impairments on tests of explicit memory. The baseline measure represents incorrect answers (or guessing). As shown here, amnesic patients show lower levels of recall than do normal control subjects. (Right) Patients with damage to the hippocampus and surrounding medial temporal lobes demonstrate intact priming. The baseline level represents performance in the unprimed state (e.g., completing a word fragment when the answer was not recently encountered).

encoding and retrieval on explicit memory tests, these techniques have pointed to other brain areas as also being important contributors to explicit memory. Some of these regions were relatively unanticipated from the literature on patients with brain lesions. Specifically, a region in the anterior portion of the frontal lobes [in or near Brodmann area (BA) 10] tends to be active when we try to think back to a previous point in time (Fig. 1). This region is sometimes active primarily on the right side and sometimes bilaterally; it is currently a topic of great interest to determine whether the two sides make different contributions and what those contributions might be. Some possibilities are that one or both sides represent the "mental set" or the fact that someone is trying to focus his or her attention to recollect an earlier point in time or that he or she performs reflective processing such as trying to recollect whether an item was seen previously as a picture or as a word. Recent findings demonstrate that these anterior prefrontal regions (in or near BA10) are more active when people successfully retrieve the past than when they try but fail to retrieve the past. A great deal of effort is currently being focused on these questions.

A second set of regions indicated by neuroimaging lie within parietal cortex. Regions within both medial parietal cortex (BA 7) and lateral parietal cortex (BA 40) have been shown to be active during retrieval (Fig. 1). Recent studies have shown that they tend to be more active during recognition for items studied before and correctly recognized by subjects (*hits*) than for nonstudied items correctly classified as such (*correct rejections*). These regions have thus far received less attention than the anterior frontal region, and their role in retrieval is uncertain.

Much more work needs to be done to determine the exact nature of the contribution of these memory-related regions, and such work is ongoing. The relatively new functional neuroimaging techniques will complement lesion studies in that the two techniques typically answer slightly different questions. Functional neuroimaging studies typically examine the normal human brain as it processes information. Functional neuroimaging can also be applied to patient populations, in which case patients are often compared with normal control subjects. Traditional lesion studies involve the study of people who have suffered brain damage; the goal is to determine which tasks they can no longer perform normally. Ultimately, both techniques will be important; if functional neuroimaging identifies a region implicated in performing a cognitive function, it will be important to show that this function breaks down when the region is damaged.

II. IMPLICIT MEMORY

A. Definition

As mentioned previously, explicit memory refers to intentional retrieval. In contrast, *implicit memory* can be thought of as unintentional or incidental retrieval. Implicit memory refers to the change in performance as a result of prior experience without intentionally trying to remember the prior, facilitating event. For example, if you were to read this entry a second time, you would read it faster than the first. This would happen even if you are not conscious of this difference or trying to produce it. What is important is that you are not attempting to draw on previous experience to aid you in the current task; instead, it manifests itself in the absence of your intent to use that information. As will be seen, implicit and explicit memory differ in many important ways.

B. Measures

Implicit memory is measured in terms of *priming*, or the amount of change (often facilitation) observed on an implicit memory test. In order to better understand how implicit memory works, psychologists have devised three main classes of implicit memory tests: perceptual implicit memory tests, conceptual implicit memory tests, and procedural learning.

Perceptual implicit memory tests require people to resolve a perceptually degraded object or word. For example, a word might be flashed very briefly (e.g., 30 msec) on a computer screen, and the task of the person is to try to guess the word. Accuracy in guessing the word is better if the word was recently read. Other types of tests involve completing word puzzles, such as those seen on game shows (e.g., "a _ r _ _ a r _" will be more readily recognized as "aardvark" if the intact word was recently read). Another popular test is to have people fill in the blanks to form the first word that comes to mind that begins with specified letters (e.g., "app_____"). If "apple" were previously seen, it would be primed; it would be used by subjects more often than if they had not previously seen this word. However, if "appendix" were previously seen, it would be the primed word. These tests are called word identification, word fragment completion, and word stem completion, respectively. Similar tests can be employed with pictures, unfamiliar objects, visual patterns, or sounds. For example in picture fragment identification, people are given line drawings of common objects (e.g., a lamp), but parts of the lines have been erased. Their task is to guess the name of the picture from its fragmented form.

The second type of implicit memory test, *conceptual implicit memory tests*, have received much less attention. They, too, use priming as the measure of memory, but they do so by observing how performance on a conceptual, or meaning-based task is influenced by the recent past. For example, if someone asked "What is the name of an airplane without an engine?" a person would be more likely to answer correctly with "glider" if he or she recently encountered that word. Similarly, if a person were asked to say the first word to come to mind when given "aviation", he or she would be more likely to say "glider" than he or she otherwise would if it had not recently been encountered. Peoples' thinking processes in the present are influenced by the recent past, even when there is no attempt to use that recent past to perform the task at hand.

Notice that unlike explicit memory tests, there are sometimes no correct or incorrect answers on an implicit memory test. For example, saying the first word that comes to mind when given another word (i.e., *word association*) or saying the first word that comes to mind that begins with "app____" have many "right" answers; priming, however, is measured in the enhancement of saying a word prespecified by the experimenter and recently studied. Specifically, researchers search for enhanced probabilities of producing whatever word was recently encountered (usually called the target word or the primed word) relative to the condition in which that word was not recently encountered.

Another example of a conceptual implicit memory test is a "liking" judgment. That is, the answer to "How much do you like this?" can be affected by recent experience. A song heard several times will sometimes tend to "grow on" a person, and this, too, is a form of conceptual implicit memory.

Procedural learning is a third index of implicit memory. The previous example of reading a passage of text faster the second time than the first is an example of procedural learning. Other examples include relearning mazes and recompleting jigsaw puzzles. People can perform complex procedural tasks more quickly and efficiently if they have had recent prior experience with the same materials.

C. Typical Patterns of Results

As mentioned previously, implicit memory tests tend to show different patterns of results from those of explicit memory tests. Perhaps the most dramatic difference is that patients with amnesia (e.g., patient H.M. described previously) perform normally on these tests, despite profound impairments on explicit memory tests (Fig. 2). Indeed, this finding was the spark that produced such great interest in these tests.

With respect to independent variables, perceptual implicit memory tests show patterns markedly different from those exhibited by most explicit memory tests. Conceptual implicit tests, however, tend to exhibit patterns similar (although not always identical) to many explicit tests. The following sections discuss the three patterns of effect of encoding tasks discussed previously with respect to explicit memory (the level of processing effect, the generation effect, and the picture superiority effect), as they relate to perceptual and conceptual implicit memory.

1. Perceptual Implicit Memory Tests

Perceptual implicit memory tests tend to show no (or a very small) difference in degree of priming as a function of level of processing. The explanation is that these tests are thought to be sensitive to the degree of overlap in perceptual features between study and test, and semantic (or meaning-based) processing does not modulate performance. If one sees "aardvark," view-

ing the visual form of that word will facilitate later reading of the same word because the visual system has an easier time identifying the incoming information. Therefore, verbal perceptual implicit memory tests are primed by verbal stimuli; picture-based perceptual implicit memory tests are primed by picture stimuli (Fig. 3). There is little cross-form priming; that is, if one makes contact with the concept but no visual features match, little or no priming occurs (e.g., seeing a picture of a windmill does not facilitate completion of its fragmented word; similarly, seeing the word "windmill" does not facilitate identification of a fragmented picture of a windmill; Fig. 3).

Similarly, level-of-processing effects and generation effects are typically absent (or very small) in perceptual implicit memory tests. In fact, the reverse pattern is often seen with a read/generate manipulation in that generating the word from a conceptual cue leads to less priming than does reading the word (Fig. 4, left). The explanation calls on whether there is perceptual overlap from the study and test phases; this overlap exists in the read condition, but there is no overlap of visual features in the generate condition.

The picture superiority effect that is seen in explicit memory tests also differs for perceptual implicit memory tests, as alluded to previously (Fig. 3). Because these tests are sensitive to the overlap in perceptual features, whether a picture superiority

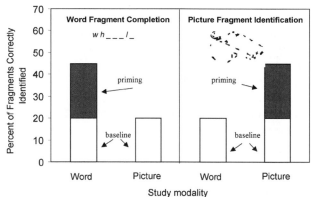

Figure 3 The picture superiority effect is not always seen on implicit memory tests. (Left) Overlap in perceptual features between the study and test phases influences priming on perceptual implicit memory tests. Robust priming occurs on a verbal perceptual implicit memory tests (e.g., word fragment completion) following visual presentation of words (e.g., seeing the word "whistle" primes solving the fragment "w h _ _ _ l _"). However, seeing a picture corresponding to the concept of interest (e.g., a picture of a whistle) does not facilitate performance on word fragment completion. (Right) The converse set of results is seen for picture fragment identification. Seeing a picture primes the identification of its later fragmented form, whereas seeing the corresponding word does not.

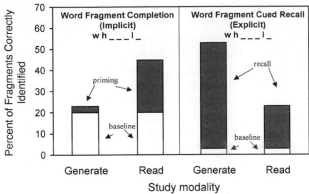

Figure 4 The retrieval intentionality criterion. The retrieval intentionality criterion is met here because the same test cues are used (word fragments) with two different sets of test instructions, and different patterns of results are observed for the implicit and explicit tests. (Left) A reverse generation effect is seen on word fragment completion. Less priming results from generating a word from a clue relative to reading the word. The explanation for this pattern is that there is transfer with respect to the visual features of the word in the read condition but not the generate condition (i.e., the word is seen in the read case, but not the generate case). (Right) The typical generation effect is seen on word fragment cued recall (an explicit test in which people are given a word fragment and asked to complete it with a word from a previously studied list).

effect is present depends on the exact type of test. If a picture-based test is given, the perceptual overlap between study and test will be enhanced for a picture study condition (relative to a word study condition). However, the opposite is true for a verbal perceptual implicit memory test: Encountering words in the study phase primes these more than pictures.

When different patterns are obtained on explicit and implicit tests, the tests are said to have been *dissociated*. The most convincing dissociation occurs when the only feature that differs between the implicit and explicit test is the instructions; when this occurs, it is said that the *retrieval intentionality criterion* is met, as described in the late 1980s by Dan Schacter, Jeffrey Bowers, and Jill Booker. For example, word stems ("whi____") could be given either with implicit instructions (fill in the blanks with the first word that comes to mind— word stem completion) or with explicit instructions (fill in the blanks to form a word that you encountered earlier in the experiment—word stem cued recall). The only feature that differs between the two cases is instructions: One instructional set requires that people intentionally retrieve, whereas the other does not.

When different patterns of results are obtained on different memory tests, one can argue that different forms of memory underlie the different tests. For example, examine Fig. 4. People either read words

during the study phase (e.g., "whistle") or generated the word from conceptual cues (e.g., "blow-w____"). As discussed before, explicit tests exhibit a generation effect such that the generate condition enhances later retrieval relative to the read condition. This pattern is found for the explicit test of word fragment-cued recall in which people are given cues (e.g., "w h ___ l _") and asked to use the cue to create a word from the study list. However, if the same cues are given with a different set of instructions, in which people are simply asked to fill in the fragment with the first word that comes to mind, the opposite pattern is observed. The read condition leads to more priming than does the generate condition. In this case, the retrieval intentionality criterion is met; the only procedural difference between the word fragment-cued recall and word fragment completion tests is instructional; Instructions for the former ask subjects to recollect the past, whereas instructions for the latter ask people simply to perform a task to the best of their ability and no mention is made of the relevance of the recent past.

2. Conceptual Implicit Memory Tests

As discussed previously, conceptual implicit memory tests show many of the same patterns exhibited by most explicit memory tests. For example, they show greater priming following meaning-based processing relative to superficial processing (a level-of-processing effect), and they also demonstrate a generation effect. One surprising finding is that a picture superiority effect is not observed on these tests, and the reasons for this unexpected finding are not well understood. In general, however, conceptual priming demonstrates the same patterns of results seen on most explicit tests.

D. Neural Correlates

As alluded to previously, damage to regions in the medial temporal lobes does not produce a general impairment on perceptual implicit memory tests. Whether general impairments occur on conceptual implicit memory tests is more controversial. The finding of intact perceptual priming in patients with damage to the hippocampus and surrounding structures within the medial temporal lobe was reported by Elizabeth Warrington and Lawrence Weiskrantz in the late 1960s. This finding spurred interest in the phenomenon of priming. Prior to this finding, it had been thought that the medial temporal lobes were globally important in memory; however, this finding demonstrated that this was not the case.

If the medial temporal lobes are not critical for producing perceptual priming, then what brain regions are? The brain mechanisms that underlie priming effects differ as a function of the type of implicit memory test. In general terms, brain regions that are critical for performing a task in the unprimed state are *less active* in the primed state. This makes sense if one thinks about priming as facilitation; the brain regions critical to performing the task have to put forth less effort in the primed (facilitated) state.

Consider first perceptual implicit memory tests. Reading a visually presented word taxes the visual system. However, regions in extrastriate visual cortex (Fig. 1) show less activity in the primed state relative to the unprimed state, consistent with the idea that less neural effort is required to perform the task; the neural pathways necessary to accomplish the goal are facilitated. Although less well studied, on the basis of this logic we would expect auditory implicit memory tests (e.g., identifying an auditory word stem) to show less activation in regions of the brain responsible for auditory processing (relative to the unprimed state).

Conceptual implicit memory tests, however, are not sensitive to the match or mismatch in perceptual features between the study and test phases; hence, the neural manifestation is not at the perceptual level. Rather, facilitation is observed at higher level regions of the brain, which are concerned with the task at hand. Consider the case of generating an associate to a presented word (e.g., given the word "elephant," the person would respond with a related word, such as "tusk"). This task calls on many brain regions, and two critically important regions lie within the left inferior frontal cortex (Fig. 1, anterior and posterior inferior frontal gyri). These regions show diminished activation in the primed condition. Again, it can be seen that regions that are important for performing the task have to put forth less effort to accomplish the task at hand in the primed condition. The brain is more efficient in the primed case.

III. IMPLICATIONS

As previously reviewed, implicit and explicit memory differ as a function of:

1. Subject populations: The finding that amnesic patients exhibit intact implicit memory despite grossly impaired explicit memory spawned a great deal of interest in characterizing implicit memory tests.
2. Independent variables: Many standard findings in explicit memory do not hold up (and often are reversed) for perceptual implicit memory tests. Explicit and implicit memory seem to be fundamentally different types of memory.

3. Neural substrates: Explicit memory tests show *increased* activity in a network of brain regions, including regions within anterior prefrontal cortex and lateral and medial parietal cortex. Implicit memory tests show *decreased* activity in regions critical for performing that task (e.g., in visual cortex as seen for word stem completion).

In the late 1980s, there was a debate over the question of whether different memory "systems" were responsible for performance on implicit and explicit memory. This hotly contested question was argued before the tools to observe localized brain activity relatively directly (via PET and fMRI) had become widely available. The availability of these techniques has allowed researchers to go beyond debating whether there is a system or network of regions in the brain responsible for implicit memory (or explicit memory) and instead to focus on the precise role of various specific brain regions to specific memory tasks. The general conclusion is that no single brain region is solely responsible for implicit (or explicit) memory. We do now have an emerging understanding of the network of brain regions underlying implicit memory and explicit memory tests, and there are marked differences between the two. However, differences also exist among various explicit tasks as well as among different implicit tasks. Whether one wants to refer to the networks underlying performance as brain systems is largely a matter of taste. One suggestion advocated here (in collaboration with Henry Roediger and Randy Buckner) is that it makes sense to put the question of systems aside until the individual components of the systems (i.e., individual brain regions) are better understood, with the eventual goal being to understand the entire network of brain regions contributing to implicit and explicit memory in their multiple instantiations.

IV. TERMINOLOGICAL CONSIDERATIONS

I consider here a few difficult issues involving terminology. First, implicit and explicit memory tests have been defined here according to instructions. However, consider the case in which the instructions given to subjects are for an implicit test, but people choose to ignore the instructions and decide to think back to the past in an effort to enhance performance on the test. Is the test still implicit? Conversely, what if people decide that an explicit memory test is too difficult and therefore begin responding with whatever first comes to mind? Is the test explicit simply because the instructions asked people to think back in time? The approach advocated here is that safeguards can (and in some situations should) be built into experiments to ensure that subjects do indeed follow instructions; this is as true of explicit memory experiments as of implicit memory experiments, however. Thus, instructions to subjects define the test type to a first approximation, but it is desirable to have some behavioral evidence documenting that people did follow those instructions.

A second issue that researchers have wrestled with is the concept John Gardiner termed *involuntary conscious recollection*. This term refers to the situation in which a person vividly recollects some aspect of the past even though he or she is not trying to do so. Consider the case in which, for example, you are walking down the street when seemingly out of nowhere you recall going to the circus as a child. You did not intentionally recall that memory; it simply "popped to mind," perhaps sparked by the unconscious association to some cue in the environment. Does such an experience tend to happen on implicit memory tests—a subject recognizes a word as studied after it has been retrieved—and, if so, does it contaminate the results? Although such phenomena sometimes do occur on implicit tests, research indicates that it need not affect the implicit test results. As long as people do not alter their strategy on the implicit test (i.e., as long as they do not adopt a strategy of attempting to recollect the recent past to aid performance on the test and instead continue to follow instructions), such involuntary conscious recollection does not contaminate the results.

A third difficult issue is that implicit and explicit have been referred to here as representing test types as defined by instructions and have also been referred to as representing different manifestations of memory, which underlie performance on the two types of test. This confounding of terms is pervasive in the field but can lead to confusion. One approach (advocated here) is to apply the terms to the type of test (implicit or explicit memory test) because test type can be defined (at least approximately) by instructions, whereas "implicit memory" and "explicit memory" cannot be observed directly. However, the title of this article referred to implicit and explicit "memory," and these concepts are widely discussed in the literature; therefore, implicit and explicit are used in both senses throughout this article.

V. SUMMARY

Perceptual implicit tests of memory and traditional, explicit tests of memory demonstrate fundamentally different types of memory. The former is preserved in amnesia, sensitive to the overlap in perceptual details between the study and test phases of experiments but relatively insensitive to higher level strategies. Conversely, explicit tests of memory demonstrate profound decrements for amnesic patients. Also, they are relatively insensitive to mismatches in perceptual features between the study and test phases, but are highly sensitive to the types of study strategies invoked during the study phase. Understanding both types of memory and the brain regions contributing to them will provide a more complete understanding of the workings of human memory.

See Also the Following Articles

ALZHEIMER'S DISEASE, NEUROPSYCHOLOGY OF • CATEGORIZATION • COGNITIVE AGING • MEMORY NEUROBIOLOGY • MEMORY, NEUROIMAGING • MEMORY, OVERVIEW • NERVE CELLS AND MEMORY • PRIMING • SEMANTIC MEMORY • SHORT-TERM MEMORY • WORKING MEMORY

Suggested Reading

Gardiner, J. M., and Java, R. I. (1993). Recognising and remembering. In *Theories of Memory* (A. Collins, M. A. Conway and P. E. Morris, Eds.), pp. 163–188. Erlbaum, Hillsdale, NJ.

McDermott, K. B. (2000). Implicit memory. In *The Encyclopedia of Psychology* (A. E. Kazdin, Ed.), pp. 231–234. Oxford Univ. Press, Oxford.

Richardson-Klavehn, A., and Bjork, R. A. (1988). Measures of memory. *Annu. Rev. Psychol.* **39,** 475–543.

Roediger, H. L. (1990). Implicit memory: Retention without remembering. *Am. Psychol.* **45,** 1043–1056.

Roediger, H. L., and McDermott, K. B. (1993). Implicit memory in normal human subjects. In *Handbook of Neuropsychology* (F. Boller and J. Grafman, Eds.), Vol. 8, pp. 63–131. Elsevier, Amsterdam.

Roediger, H. L., Buckner, R. L., and McDermott, K. B. (1999). Components of processing. In *Memory: Systems, Process, or Function?* (J. K. Foster and M. Jelicic, Eds.), pp. 31–65. Oxford Univ. Press, Oxford.

Schacter, D. L. (1987). Implicit memory: History and current status. *J. Exp. Psychol. Learning Memory Cognition* **13,** 501–518.

Schacter, D. L., and Buckner, R. L. (1998). Priming and the brain. *Neuron* **20,** 185–195.

Tulving, E., and Schacter, D. L. (1990). Priming and human memory systems. *Science* **247,** 301–306.

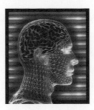

Memory Neurobiology

RAYMOND P. KESNER

University of Utah

GLOSSARY

event-based memory system This system provides for temporary representations of incoming data concerning the present, with an emphasis on data and events that are usually personal or egocentric and that occur within specific external and internal contexts.

knowledge-based memory system This system provides for more permanent representations of previously stored information in long-term memory and can be thought of as one's general knowledge of the world.

language attribute This attribute involves memory representations of phonological, lexical, morphological, syntactical, and semantic information.

response attribute This attribute involves memory representations based on feedback from motor responses (often based on kinesthetic and vestibular cues) that occur in specific situations as well as memory representations of stimulus–response associations.

reward value (affect) attribute This attribute involves memory representations of reward value, positive or negative emotional experiences, and the associations between stimuli and rewards.

rule-based memory system This system receives information from the event-based and knowledge-based systems and integrates the information by applying rules and strategies for subsequent action.

sensory-perceptual attribute This attribute involves memory representations of a set of sensory stimuli that are organized in the form of cues as part of a specific experience.

spatial (space) attribute This attribute involves memory representations of places or relationships between places.

temporal (time) attribute This attribute involves memory representations of the duration of a stimulus and the succession or temporal order of temporally separated events or stimuli.

Memory neurobiology is defined as the organization of memory systems in terms of the kind of information to be represented, the processes associated with the operation of each system, and the neurobiological substrates including neural structures and mechanisms that subserve each system.

I. INTRODUCTION

Memory neurobiology is defined as the organization of memory systems in terms of the kind of information to be represented, the processes associated with the operation of each system, and the neurobiological substrates including neural structures and mechanisms that subserve each system. Because it is assumed that memory is highly complex and distributed across many neural systems, the overall organization of memory systems can take many forms, with different emphases on the nature of memory representation and different operations associated with processing of mnemonic information.

For example, the most widely accepted view of memory is based on the idea that memory can be divided into a declarative component based on conscious recollection of facts and events and mediated by the hippocampus and interconnected neural regions, such as the entorhinal cortex and parahippocampal and perirhinal cortex, and a nondeclarative

Copyright 2002, Elsevier Science (USA).
All rights reserved.

component based on memory without conscious access for skills, habits, priming, simple classical conditioning, and nonassociative learning mediated by a variety of brain regions, including the striatum for skills and habits, the neocortex for priming, the amygdala for simple classical conditioning of emotional responses, the cerebellum for simple classical conditioning of skeletal musculature, and reflex pathways for nonassociative learning. Others have used different terms to reflect the same type of distinction, including a hippocampal-dependent explicit memory vs a nonhippocampal-dependent implicit memory and a hippocampal-dependent declarative memory based on the representation of relationships among stimuli vs a nonhippocampal-dependent procedural memory based on the representation of a single stimulus or configuration of stimuli.

According to these models, the key difference in memory representation across different brain regions is based on conscious access to the information to be processed or stored. Support for this distinction comes from studies with human amnesic patients. For example, Korsakoff patients, with presumably diencephalic damage, and patients receiving electroconvulsive shock treatments, which presumably produce major disruptive effects in the temporal lobe, can acquire and retain (for at least 3 months) a mirror reading skill as easily as normal subjects (nondeclarative memory). However, when asked to remember the words they read in this task, they were severely impaired (declarative memory). Patient H.M. with bilateral medial temporal lobe damage, including hippocampus and amygdala, can learn and remember a set of complicated skills associated with solving the Tower of Hanoi problem, but this patient cannot recall any contextual aspect of the task or the strategies involved in solving the task. Thus, it appears that amnesic patients can acquire skills necessary for correct mirror reading performance but cannot remember the specific facts or events associated with the experiment. Further support for a problem with conscious awareness associated with declarative information is based on a patient with bilateral damage to the hippocampus who was impaired in learning which stimuli were paired with an unconditioned response but learned very readily a conditioned autonomic response to the critical visual and auditory stimuli. In contrast, a different patient with a bilateral lesion of the amygdala was impaired in learning a conditioned autonomic response to visual or auditory stimuli but learned very readily which stimuli were paired with the unconditioned response. Also, amnesic subjects with damage to the hippocampus are not impaired on a variety of tests that measure implicit memory for a number of stimulus patterns using the nondeclarative memory system, but they are impaired in explicitly remembering the same stimulus patterns using the declarative memory system. Finally, amnesic subjects can learn a complex probability classification task, but they perform poorly on multiple-choice tests that attempt to measure the training experience.

Others have suggested that memory can be divided into a short-term, working or episodic memory system defined as memory for the specific, personal and temporal context of a situation and mediated by the hippocampus and a reference or semantic memory defined as memory for rules and procedures (general knowledge) of specific situations mediated by nonhippocampal brain regions, such as the neocortex. According to these models the key difference in memory representation across different brain regions is not necessarily based on conscious access to the information to be processed or stored but rather on differential processing of short-term vs long-term memory representations.

A more comprehensive view of memory organization based on multiple processes and multiple forms of memory representation is based on the neurobiology of a multiple attribute, multiple process, tripartite system model of memory that will be presented later. The tripartite attribute model of memory is organized into event-based, knowledge-based, and rule-based memory systems. Each system is composed of the same set of multiple attributes or forms of memory, characterized by a set of process-oriented operating characteristics and mapped onto multiple neural regions and interconnected neural circuits.

II. TRIPARTITE MEMORY SYSTEM

On a psychological level, the event-based memory system provides for temporary representations of incoming data concerning the present, with an emphasis on data and events that are usually personal or egocentric and that occur within specific external and internal contexts. The emphasis is on the processing of new and current information. During initial learning, great emphasis is placed on the event-based memory system, which will continue to be of importance even after initial learning in situations in which unique or novel trial information needs to be remembered.

The knowledge-based memory system provides for more permanent representations of previously stored information in long-term memory and can be thought of as one's general knowledge of the world. The knowledge-based memory system would tend to be of greater importance after a task has been learned given that the situation is invariant and familiar. The organization of these attributes within the knowledge-based memory system can take many forms and they are organized as a set of attribute-dependent cognitive maps and their interactions that are unique for each memory.

The rule-based memory system receives information from the event-based and knowledge-based systems and integrates the information by applying rules and strategies for subsequent action. In most situations, however, one would expect a contribution of all three systems with a varying proportion of involvement of one relative to the other.

The three memory systems are composed of the same forms, domains, or attributes of memory. Even though there could be many attributes, the most important attributes include space, time, response, sensory perception, and reward value (affect). In humans, a language attribute is also added. A spatial (space) attribute within this framework involves memory representations of places or relationships between places. It is exemplified by the ability to encode and remember spatial maps and to localize stimuli in external space. Memory representations of the spatial attribute can be further subdivided into specific spatial features, including allocentric spatial distance, egocentric spatial distance, allocentric direction, egocentric head direction, and spatial location. A temporal (time) attribute within this framework involves memory representations of the duration of a stimulus and the succession or temporal order of temporally separated events or stimuli. A response attribute within this framework involves memory representations based on feedback from motor responses (often based on kinesthetic and vestibular cues) that occur in specific situations as well as memory representations of stimulus–response associations. A reward value (affect) attribute within this framework involves memory representations of reward value, positive or negative emotional experiences, and the associations between stimuli and rewards. A sensory-perceptual attribute within this framework involves memory representations of a set of sensory stimuli that are organized in the form of cues as part of a specific experience. Each sensory modality (olfaction, auditory, vision, somatosensory, and taste) has its own memory representations and can be considered to be part of the sensory-perceptual attribute component of

memory. A language attribute within this framework involves memory representations of phonological, lexical, morphological, syntactical, and semantic information. The attributes within each memory system can be organized in many different ways and are likely to interact extensively with each other even though it can be demonstrated that in many cases these attributes operate independent of each other.

Within each system attribute information is processed in different ways based on different operational characteristics. For the event-based memory system, specific processes involve (i) selective filtering or attenuation of interference of temporary memory representations of new information, labeled pattern separation; (ii) short-term memory or working memory of new information that is partly based on pattern associations; (iii) consolidation or elaborative rehearsal of new information; and (iv) retrieval of new information based on flexibility, action, and pattern completion.

For the knowledge-based memory system, specific processes include (i) selective attention and selective filtering associated with permanent memory representations of familiar information, (ii) perceptual memory and long-term memory storage based on pattern associations, and (iii) retrieval of familiar information based on flexibility and action. For the rule-based memory system, the major process includes the selection of strategies and rules for maintaining or manipulating information for subsequent action.

III. EVENT-BASED MEMORY SYSTEM

On a neurobiological level each attribute maps onto a set of neural regions and their interconnected neural circuits. For example, within the event-based memory system it has been demonstrated that in animals and humans the hippocampus supports memory for spatial and temporal attribute information, the caudate mediates memory for response attribute information, the amygdala subserves memory for reward value (affect) attribute information, and the perirhinal and extrastriate visual cortex support memory for visual object attribute information as an example of a sensory-perceptual attribute (Fig. 1).

Evidence supportive of the previously mentioned mapping of attributes onto specific brain regions is based in part on the use of paradigms that measure the short-term or working memory process based on performance within matching or nonmatching-to-

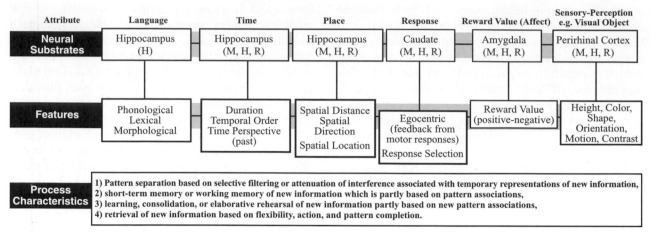

Key: **M**=Monkeys, **H**=Humans, **R**=Rats

Figure 1   Representation of the neural substrates, features, and process characteristics associated with the event-based memory system for the language, time, place, response, reward value (affect), and sensory-perception attributes.

sample, delayed conditional discrimination or continuous recognition memory of single-item or lists of items tasks; the consolidation and retrieval process, based on learning and retention of a variety of behavioral tasks; and the pattern separation process based on performance within category memory or discrimination tasks.

A. Spatial (Place) Attribute

With respect to short-term or working memory, the data indicate that animals and humans with damage to the hippocampus are severely impaired in working memory for spatial information, including spatial features such as allocentric spatial distance, egocentric spatial distance, head direction, and spatial location. In contrast, rats, monkeys, or humans with damage to the hippocampus are not impaired in working memory for response, reward value (affect), or visual object attribute information. Similar patterns of results have been reported for the involvement of the hippocampus in mediating spatial but not response, reward value, or visual object information during new learning (consolidation).

In the context of the pattern separation process, it has been shown that the hippocampus responds to all sensory modalities, suggesting that a possible role for the hippocampus is to provide the opportunity for using sensory markers to demarcate a spatial location

so that the hippocampus can more efficiently represent spatial information. It is thus possible that one of the main process functions of the hippocampus is to encode and separate spatial events from each other. This would ensure that new highly processed sensory information is organized within the hippocampus and enhances the possibility of remembering and temporarily storing one place as separate from another place. It is assumed that this is accomplished via pattern separation of event information so that spatial events can be separated from each other and spatial interference is reduced. This process is akin to the idea that the hippocampus is involved in orthogonalization of sensory input information, in representational differentiation, and indirectly in the utilization of relationships.

Since pattern separation paradigms are new and have been developed only recently, a more detailed description of the paradigms is presented. In this task, rats are required to remember a spatial location dependent on the distance between the study phase object and an identical object used as a foil. Specifically, during the study phase an object that covers a baited food well is randomly positioned in 1 of 15 possible spatial locations on a cheese board. Rats exit a start box and displace the object in order to receive a food reward and are then returned to the start box. On the ensuing test phase rats are allowed to choose between two objects that are identical to the study phase object. One object is baited and positioned in the previous study phase location (correct choice), and the other (foil) is unbaited and placed in a different location (incorrect choice). Five distances (min = 15 cm; max = 105 cm) are randomly used to separate the foil from the correct object. Following the establishment of a criterion of 75% correct averaged across all separation distances, rats are given either large (dorsal and ventral) hippocampal or cortical control lesions dorsal to the dorsal hippocampus. Following recovery from surgery the rats are retested. The results indicate that whereas control rats match their presurgery performance for all spatial distances, hippocampal lesioned rats display impairments for short (15–37.5 cm) and medium (60 cm) spatial separations but perform as well as controls when the spatial separation is long (82.5–105 cm). The fact that the hippocampal lesioned group is able to perform the task well at large separations indicates that the deficits observed at the shorter separations are not the result of an inability to remember the rule. The results suggest that the hippocampus may serve to separate incoming spatial information into patterns or categories by temporarily storing one place as separate from another place. It can be shown that the ability to remember the long distances is not based on an egocentric response strategy because if the study phase is presented on one side of the cheese board and the test originates on the opposite side, the hippocampal lesioned rats still discriminate the long distances without difficulty. Furthermore, the hippocampal lesioned group has no difficulty discriminating between two short distances. It is clear that in this task it is necessary to separate one spatial location from another spatial location. Hippocampal lesioned rats cannot separate these spatial locations very well, so they can perform the task only when the spatial locations are far apart. Subsequent experiments have shown that lesions of the dorsal dentate gyrus result in the same spatial pattern separation problem, but lesions of the dorsal CA1 region do not produce an impairment, suggesting that pattern separation mechanisms might reside in the dentate gyrus. Similar deficits have been observed for new geographical information in patients with hippocampal damage due to an hypoxic episode.

Does spatial pattern separation play a role in the acquisition (consolidation) of a variety of hippocampal-dependent tasks? One example will suffice. Because rats are started in different locations in the standard water maze task, there is a great potential for interference among similar and overlapping spatial patterns. Thus, the observation that hippocampal lesioned rats are impaired in learning and subsequent consolidation of important spatial information in this task could be due to difficulty in separating spatial patterns, resulting in enhanced spatial interference. Evidence in favor of this idea comes from the observation that when fimbria–fornix lesioned rats are trained on the water maze task from only a single starting position (less spatial interference), there are very few learning deficits, whereas training from many different starting points results in learning difficulties. In a similar study it was shown that total hippocampal lesioned rats learned or consolidated rather readily that only one spatial location was correct on an eight-arm maze.

Response, reward value, and visual object pattern separation are not processed by the hippocampus but involve the caudate for response pattern separation, amygdala for reward value pattern separation, and perirhinal cortex for visual object pattern separation. With respect to associations, the hippocampus does not mediate all arbitrary associations, not even all stimulus–stimulus associations, but only associations that involve spatial or temporal information, such as object–place and odor–place associations or trace classical conditioning, but not, for example, odor–odor or odor–object associations or delayed classical conditioning.

B. Temporal (Time) Attribute

With respect to short-term or working memory, the data indicate that animals and humans with damage to the hippocampus are severely impaired in working memory for temporal information, including duration and temporal order. It has been suggested that trace conditioning requires memory for the duration of the conditioned stimulus. Thus, it is of importance to note that rabbits with hippocampal lesions and humans with hypoxia resulting in bilateral hippocampal damage are impaired in acquisition (consolidation) of trace but not delayed eye-blink conditioning.

Based on ample evidence that almost all sensory information is processed by hippocampal neurons, perhaps to provide for sensory markers for time, and that the hippocampus mediates temporal information, it is likely that one of the main process functions of the hippocampus is to encode the temporal order of events. This would ensure that newly highly processed sensory information is organized within the hippocampus and enhances the possibility of remembering and temporarily storing one event as separate from another event in time. On this basis, it has been shown that the hippocampus is involved in temporal pattern separation for spatial, visual object, odor, or language information.

C. Language Attribute

With respect to language attribute information, it can be shown that with the use of the previously mentioned paradigms to measure short-term memory there are severe impairments for lists of words for humans with left hippocampal or bilateral hippocampal damage, suggesting that the hippocampus plays an important role in short-term memory representation of word information as an important feature of language attribute information. There is much evidence supporting the idea of lateralization of hippocampal function in humans, with the right hippocampus representing spatial information and the left hippocampus representing linguistic information. For example, patients who had left or right temporal lobectomies that included the hippocampus were tested on a task of recall for a visual location. In this task subjects made a mark on an 8-in line in order to reproduce as close as possible the exact position of the previously shown circle. Subjects with right temporal lobe lesions were impaired on this task, whereas subjects with left temporal lobe lesions were not significantly different from control subjects. In contrast, recall of a list of words resulted in an impairment for subjects with left, but not right, temporal lobe resections. Additional support for the idea that the right hippocampus mediates memory for temporal order for novel spatial information and the left hippocampus mediates temporal order for novel linguistic information comes from the demonstration that subjects with right temporal lobe lesions are impaired relative to controls for temporal order for novel spatial location information but not for the temporal order of novel linguistic information. In contrast, subjects with left temporal lobe lesions are impaired relative to control subjects for the temporal order of novel linguistic information but not the temporal order of novel spatial information. Even though hypoxic subjects or left temporal resected patients are impaired in remembering the order of presentation of words in nonmeaningful sentences requiring the processing of new event-based linguistic information, they are not impaired in remembering the order of presentation of words in syntactically or syntactically and semantically meaningful sentences requiring the processing of knowledge-based linguistic information.

D. Response Attribute

With respect to short-term or working memory, data indicate that animals and humans with damage to the caudate are severely impaired in working memory for response information, including memory representations based on feedback from motor responses (often based on kinesthetic and vestibular cues) that occur in specific situations as well as memory representations of stimulus–response associations. For rats with caudate lesions there are profound short-term memory deficits for a right or left turn response, for an egocentric distance response, for head direction, and for response-based sequential learning. For humans with caudate damage due to Huntington's disease, there are short-term memory deficits for reproducing a hand movement, remembering a list of hand motor movement responses, or learning the sequence of motor movements. Furthermore, rats, monkeys, and humans with caudate lesions have deficits in tasks such as delayed response, delayed alternation, and delayed matching to position. One salient feature of these tasks is the maintenance of spatial orientation to the baited food relative to the position of the subject's body often based on proprioceptive and vestibular feedback. These data suggest that the caudate plays an important role in short-term memory representation for the feedback from a motor response feature of response attribute information. The memory impairments following caudate lesions are specific to the response attribute because these same lesions in rats do not impair short-term memory performance for spatial location or visual object attribute information. Similar patterns of results have been reported for the involvement of the caudate in mediating response, but not spatial or reward value, information during new learning (consolidation) and response-based pattern separation. With respect to associations, the caudate mediates associations that involve the response attribute, thereby supporting primarily stimulus–response-type associations.

E. Reward Value (Affect) Attribute

With respect to short-term or working memory, data indicate that animals and humans with damage to the amygdala are severely impaired in working memory for affect information including reward value (affect) associated with magnitude of reinforcement or for a liking response based on the mere exposure of a novel stimulus. The memory impairments following amygdala lesions are specific to the affect attribute because these same lesions in rats do not impair short-term memory performance for spatial location, visual object, or response attribute information. Similar results have been reported for the involvement of the amygdala in mediating affect, but not spatial, response or visual object information during new learning (consolidation) and to some extent reward-based pattern separation. With respect to associations, the amygdala mediates associations that involve the reward attribute, thereby supporting primarily stimulus–reward-type associations.

F. Sensory-Perceptual Attribute

With respect to sensory-perceptual attribute information, I concentrate on visual object information as an exemplar of memory representation of this attribute. In the context of short-term or working memory, data indicate that animals and humans with damage to the extrastriate or perirhinal cortex are severely impaired in working memory for visual object information. The memory impairments following perirhinal cortex lesions are specific to the visual object attribute because these same lesions in rats do not impair short-term memory performance for spatial location attribute information. Similar patterns of results have been reported for the involvement of the perirhinal cortex in mediating visual object information during new learning (consolidation) and visual object-based pattern separation. With respect to associations, the perirhinal cortex mediates associations that involve visual object information, thereby supporting primarily visual–visual-type associations.

Thus, it appears that the neural systems that support different attributes within the event-based memory system can be dissociated from each other, suggesting that they can operate independent of each other. However, it is clear that many interactions can occur between the proposed brain regions (e.g., between hippocampus and amygdala, between hippocampus and perirhinal cortex, or between hippocampus and caudate nucleus). Furthermore, there are interactions that are based on convergence onto other brain regions (e.g., hippocampus and amygdala projections to the

same neurons in the nucleus accumbens). Each neural system subserves a different attribute but engages the same set of processes and is therefore part of the same event-based memory system.

The event-based memory system is more akin to episodic memory; however, it also maps to some extent onto declarative memory, but without the emphasis on the need to use conscious processing and the need to require only the operation of the medial temporal cortex. Instead, the attribute model suggests that there are additional brain circuits that mediate multiple attributes or forms of memory and specifies to a much greater extent the operation of specific multiple processes. Finally, this event-based memory system incorporates rather well White's three- system model that includes the hippocampus for stimulus–stimulus associations, the caudate for stimulus–response associations, and the amygdala for stimulus–reward associations.

IV. KNOWLEDGE-BASED MEMORY SYSTEM

Within the knowledge-based memory system, it has been demonstrated that in animals and humans (i) the posterior parietal cortex supports memory for spatial attributes; (ii) the dorsal and dorsolateral prefrontal cortex and/or anterior cingulate support memory for temporal attributes; (iii) the premotor, supplementary motor, and cerebellum in monkeys and humans and precentral cortex and cerebellum in rats support memory for response attributes; (iv) the orbital prefrontal cortex supports memory for reward value (affect) attributes; and (v) the inferotemporal cortex in monkeys and humans and TE2 cortex in rats subserve memory for sensory-perceptual attributes (e.g., visual objects) (Fig. 2).

Evidence supportive of the previously mentioned mapping of attributes onto specific brain regions is based in part on the use of paradigms that measure the perceptual memory process based on performance within a repetition priming or a discrimination performance paradigm, the attention process by measuring performance within selective attention and stimulus-binding tasks, and the long-term storage and retrieval process by measuring learning and retention in a variety of behavioral tasks. Due to of space constraints, I discuss only the role of the parietal cortex in processing spatial information and that of the inferotemporal cortex in processing visual object information.

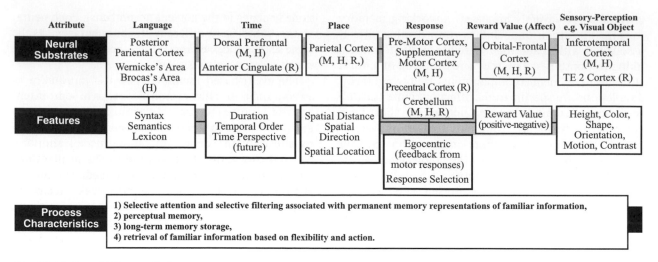

Key: **M**=Monkeys, **H**=Humans, **R**=Rats

Figure 2 Representation of the neural substrates, features, and process characteristics associated with the knowledge-based memory system for the language, time, place, response, reward value (affect), and sensory-perception attributes.

A. Spatial (Place) Attribute

Monkeys with lesions of the parietal cortex show deficits in place reversal, landmark reversal, distance discrimination, bent-wire route finding, pattern string finding, and maze-learning tasks. Similarly, rats with parietal cortex lesions cannot perform well in mazes. Furthermore, rats with parietal cortex lesions display deficits in both the acquisition and retention of spatial navigation tasks that are presumed to measure the operation of a spatial cognitive map within a complex environment. They also display deficits in the acquisition and retention of spatial recognition memory for a list of five spatial locations. In a complex discrimination task in which rats have to detect the change in location of an object in a scene, rats with parietal cortex lesions are profoundly impaired, but on less complex tasks involving the discrimination or short-term memory for single spatial features including spatial location and allocentric and egocentric spatial distance, there are no impairments. Similarly, there are no impairments in discriminating between visual objects in terms of either new learning or performance of a previously learned visual discrimination. When the task is more complex, involving the association of objects and places (components of a spatial cognitive map), parietal cortex plays an important role. Support for this comes from the finding that rats with parietal lesions are impaired in the acquisition and retention of

a spatial location plus object discrimination (paired associate task) but show no deficits for only spatial or object discriminations.

Humans with parietal cortex lesions have difficulty in drawing maps or diagrams of familiar spatial locations. They also have problems in using information to guide them in novel or familiar routes, to discriminate near from far objects, and to solve complex mazes. There is also spatial neglect and deficits in spatial attention. There is a general loss of "topographic sense," which may involve loss of long-term geographical knowledge as well as an inability to form cognitive maps of new environments. Using positron emission tomography (PET) scan and functional magnetic resonance imaging (fMRI) data, it can be shown that complex spatial information results in activation of the parietal cortex. Thus, memory for complex spatial information appears to be processed by the parietal cortex.

The parietal cortex is probably not the only neural region that mediates long-term memory for spatial information. For example, topographical amnesia has also been reported for patients with parahippocampal lesions and spatial navigation deficits have been found following retrosplenial and entorhinal cortex lesions. Thus, other neural regions (e.g., parahippocampal cortex, entorhinal cortex, and retrosplenial cortex) may also contribute to the long-term representation of a spatial cognitive map.

B. Sensory-Perceptual Attribute

With respect to sensory-perceptual attribute information, it can be shown that lesions of the inferotemporal cortex in monkeys and humans and temporal cortex (TE2) in rats result in visual object discrimination problems, suggesting that the inferotemporal or TE2 may play an important role in mediating long-term representations of visual object information. Additional support comes from PET scan and fMRI data in humans, in whom it can be shown that visual object information results in activation of inferotemporal cortex. In a different study, it was shown that neurons within the inferotemporal cortex responded more readily after training to a complex visual stimulus that had been paired with another complex visual stimulus across a delay, suggesting the formation of long-term representations of object–object pairs within the inferotemporal cortex. Finally, it has been shown in rats that based on a repetition priming paradigm, perceptual memory for spatial location information is mediated by the parietal cortex but not the TE2 cortex, whereas perceptual memory for visual object information is mediated by TE2 cortex but not the parietal cortex, suggesting support for independent mediation of spatial location and visual object attribute information within the knowledge-based memory system.

V. INDEPENDENCE OF THE EVENT-BASED AND KNOWLEDGE-BASED MEMORY SYSTEMS

Even though the two systems are supported by neural substrates and different operating characteristics, suggesting that the systems can operate independent of each other, there are also important interactions between the two systems, especially during the consolidation of new information and retrieval of previously stored information. It is thus likely to be very difficult to separate the contribution of each system in new learning tasks since each system supports one component of the consolidation process. However, there are a few examples based on tasks in which the major consolidation processes have already taken place. Olton and Papas ran animals in a 17-arm maze with food available in 8 arms and no food available in 9 arms. In order to solve this maze, an animal should not enter unbaited arms, activating knowledge-based memory, but should enter baited arms only once utilizing event-based memory. After learning the task to criterion performance, animals were given fimbria–fornix lesions. The lesioned animals had a deficit only for the event-based memory memory component of the task. In a different study, it was shown that in an 8-arm maze parietal cortex lesions placed in rats after training on 4 unbaited and 4 baited arms resulted in a deficit in the knowledge-based but not event-based memory. If one assumes that the presentation of unbaited arms reflects the operation of the knowledge-based memory system and that the presentation of baited arms reflects the operation of the event-based memory system, then it appears that lesions of the hippocampus disrupt only the event-based memory system, whereas lesions of the parietal cortex only disrupt the knowledge-based memory system. Similarly, in humans there is evidence that patients with hippocampal damage do not have difficulty remembering knowledge-based information, whereas they have difficulty remembering event-based information. For example, hypoxic subjects or left temporal resected patients are impaired in remembering the order of presentation of words in nonmeaningful sentences requiring the processing of new event-based linguistic information, but they are not impaired in remembering the order of presentation of words in syntactically or syntactically and semantically meaningful sentences requiring the processing of knowledge-based linguistic information.

In a different series of studies a double dissociation between perceptual memory (a measure reflective of the operation of the knowledge-based memory system) and short-term memory (a measure reflective of the operation of the event-based memory system) was reported in human subjects. It was shown that patients with a right occipital cortical lesion displayed impaired performance for perceptual memory tests of visual priming for words but intact performance on short-term tests of recognition and cued recall of words. In contrast, the reverse pattern was present for amnesic subjects with hippocampal damage. Furthermore, for patients with parietal lesions resulting in spatial neglect, there was a deficit in spatial repetition priming (perceptual memory) without a loss in short-term or working memory for spatial information. In a different study, it was shown that, like humans with parietal cortex lesions, rats with such lesions are impaired in a spatial repetition priming (perceptual memory) experiment but perform without difficulty in a short-term or working spatial memory experiment, suggesting that the parietal cortex plays a role in spatial perceptual memory within the knowledge-based memory system but does not play a role in spatial memory within the event-based memory system.

In a different set of studies it was shown that patients with temporal lobe lesions that did not involve hippocampus or perirhinal cortex had difficulty in naming familiar objects (semantic dementia) but had no difficulty in recognizing the same familiar objects, whereas amnesic subjects with hippocampal damage had no difficulty in naming objects, but were impaired in recognizing those objects. If one assumes that naming is a process that is supported by long-term memory and thus a characteristic of the knowledge-based memory system, then these data provide further support for a dissociation between the knowledge-based and event-based memory systems.

The knowledge-based memory system is akin to semantic and reference memory, but it also maps to some extent onto nondeclarative memory but without the emphasis on the need to use unconscious processing and the need to require only the operation of the medial temporal cortex. The nondeclarative memory system has a large memory representation, and compared to the tripartite attribute model it includes the knowledge-based and rule-based memory systems as well as some components of the event-based memory system. It is therefore very difficult to characterize the operations that are necessary for efficient functioning of the nondeclarative system. Instead, the tripartite attribute model suggests that for the knowledge-based memory system there are specific brain circuits that support a set of processes that differ from the brain circuits that support a different set of processes within the event-based memory system. Furthermore, it appears that the knowledge-based memory system and the event-based memory system can operate independent of each other and that information can be processed by distinct neural regions, even though there are also important interactions between the two systems, especially during the consolidation of new information and retrieval of previously stored information.

VI. RULE-BASED MEMORY SYSTEM

Within the rule-based memory system it can be shown that different subdivisions of the prefrontal cortex support different attributes. For example, the dorsolateral and ventrolateral prefrontal cortex in monkeys and humans and the infralimbic and prelimbic cortex in rats support spatial, visual object, and language attributes; the premotor and supplementary motor cortex in monkeys and humans and precentral cortex in rats support response attributes; the dorsal, dorsolateral, and mid-dorsolateral prefrontal cortex in monkeys and humans and anterior cingulate in rats mediate primarily temporal attributes; and the orbital prefrontal cortex in monkeys and humans and agranular insular cortex in rats support affect attributes. (Fig. 3).

Evidence supportive of the previously mentioned mapping of attributes onto specific brain regions is based in part on the use of paradigms that measure the use of rules within short-term or working memory based on performance within matching- or nonmatching-to-sample, delayed conditional discrimination or continuous recognition memory of single-item or lists

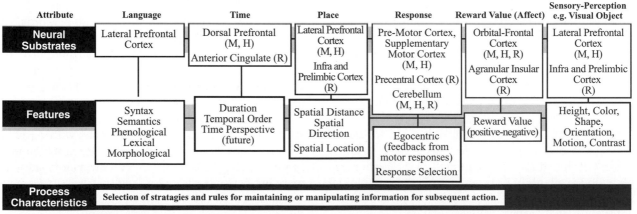

Key: M=Monkeys, **H**=Humans, **R**=Rats

Figure 3 Representation of the neural substrates, features, and process characteristics associated with the rule-based memory system for the language, time, place, response, reward value (affect), and sensory-perception attributes.

of items tasks, temporal ordering of information, and sequential learning. It is also based on paradigms that measure the use of rules in cross-modal switching, reversal learning, paired-associate, and problem-solving tasks. Here, I concentrate only on the data reported in the context of short-term memory or working memory.

A. Spatial (Place) and Sensory-Perceptual Attributes

The dorsolateral and ventrolateral prefrontal cortex in monkeys and humans and infralimbic and prelimbic cortex are involved whenever there are rules associated with working memory for spatial and visual object attribute information. Evidence for this idea comes from the finding that rats with lesions of the infralimbic and prelimbic cortex disrupt working memory for spatial information and working memory for object information. In monkeys lesions of the dorsolateral and ventrolateral regions disrupt performance on delayed response, delayed alternation, delayed occulomotor, spatial search, and visual object recognition tasks. Furthermore, in monkeys, for working memory there are delay-specific cells in the dorsolateral and ventrolateral prefrontal cortex in spatial tasks, such as delayed response, delayed alternation, and delayed occulomotor tasks, and in visual object delay tasks. In humans, based on a meta-analysis of multiple studies using neuroimaging techniques, both the dorsolateral and the ventrolateral cortex are activated during object and place working memory tasks. Thus, the data indicate that the infralimbic and prelimbic cortex in rats and dorsolateral and ventrolateral cortex in monkeys and humans play a very important role in processing visual object and spatial attribute information, suggesting a possible contribution of this region in supporting the use of working memory rules associated with object and spatial attributes. The working memory impairments following infra- and prelimbic lesions are specific to the object and place attributes because these same lesions in rats do not impair working memory performance for response or affect attribute information.

B. Temporal (Time) Attribute

The dorsal prefrontal cortex, dorsolateral prefrontal cortex, and mid-dorsolateral prefrontal cortex in monkeys and humans and anterior cingulate cortex in rats are involved whenever there are rules associated with working memory for temporal attribute information. Evidence for this idea comes from the finding that in rats, monkeys, and humans, following lesions of this region, there are deficits in working memory for temporal order information and memory for frequency information. Furthermore, using fMRI, it was shown that the dorsolateral prefrontal cortex is activated in a memory for a temporal order task. All the previously mentioned results suggest that this region plays an important role processing temporal attribute information. The working memory impairments following anterior cingulate cortex lesions in rats are specific to the temporal attribute because these lesions do not impair working memory performance for spatial, visual object, or affect attribute information.

C. Response Attribute

The premotor and supplementary motor cortex in monkeys and humans and precentral motor cortex in the rat are involved whenever there are rules associated with the processing of response attribute information. Support for this idea comes from the observation that lesions of the precentral cortex in the rat disrupt rules associated with processing of response information such as working memory for a motor (right–left turn) response. Also, in humans prefrontal cortex lesions result in a deficit for memory for a motor movement and memory for a list of motor movements, supporting a role for this region in processing response attribute information.

D. Reward Value (Affect) Attribute

The orbitofrontal cortex in monkeys and humans and agranular insular prefrontal cortex in the rat are involved whenever there are rules associated with working memory for affect attribute information, especially based on odors and tastes. Evidence for this idea comes from the findings that in both animals and humans, following lesions of this region there are deficits in working memory for taste or odor (affect attribute) information. The working memory impairments following the agranular insular prefrontal cortex lesions are specific to the affect attribute because these same lesions in rats do not impair working memory performance for spatial attribute information.

the prefrontal cortex is not specified in the declarative–nondeclarative model.

E. Language Attribute

The lateral prefrontal cortex in humans is involved whenever there are rules associated with working memory for language attribute information. This is based on evidence demonstrating activation of the lateral prefrontal cortex in verbal learning tasks and impairments in working memory for verbal information in patients with lateral prefrontal cortex lesions.

Various subregions within the prefrontal cortex also play a role in the use of rules associated with other tasks besides working memory, such as tasks that measure the use of rules in cross-modal switching, reversal learning, paired associate, and problem solving.

It is assumed that there are important interactions between the rule-based and event-based memory systems across specific attributes. In support of this assumption, it was shown based on a disconnection experiment that there are interactions between prefrontal cortex and perirhinal cortex but not between perirhinal cortex and amygdala or hippocampus in supporting short-term memory for visual object attribute information. It should be noted that the role for

VII. INTEGRATION

The overall tripartite attribute model of memory is shown in Fig. 4. Different forms of memory and its neurobiological underpinnings are represented in terms of the nature, structure, or content of information representation as a set of different attributes, including language, time, place, response, reward value (affect), and visual object as an example of sensory perception. For each attribute, information is processed in the event-based memory system through operations that involve pattern separation or orthogonalization of specific attribute information, short-term memory processing, encoding of specific pattern associations into long-term memory, and retrieval of stored information via flexibility and pattern completion. In addition, for each attribute, information is processed in the knowledge-based system through operations of long-term storage, selective attention, perceptual memory, and retrieval of pattern associations. Finally, for each attribute, information is processed in the rule-based memory system through the integration of information from the event-based and knowledge-based memory systems for the selection of strategies and rules for maintaining or

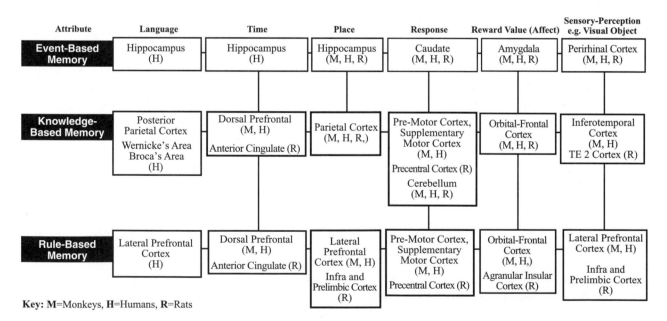

Figure 4 Representation of the neural substrates associated with the event-based, knowledge-based, and rule-based memory systems for the language, time, place, response, reward value (affect), and sensory-perception attributes.

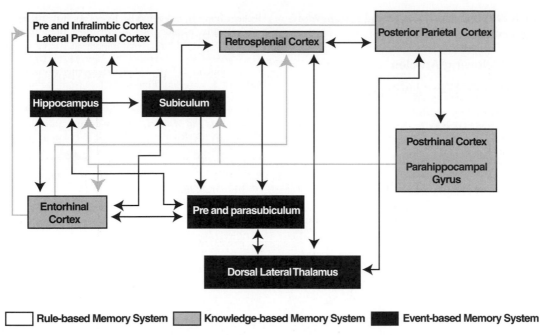

☐ Rule-based Memory System	▨ Knowledge-based Memory System	■ Event-based Memory System

Figure 5 Representation of the spatial attribute neural circuit incorporating neural regions that mediate rule-based, knowledge-based, and event-based memory.

manipulating information for subsequent action. The neural systems that subserve specific attributes within a system can operate independent of each other, even though there are also many possibilities for interactions among the attributes. Although the event-based and knowledge-based memory systems are supported by neural substrates and different operating characteristics, suggesting that the two systems can operate independent of each other, there are also important interactions between the two systems, especially during the consolidation of new information and retrieval of previously stored information. Finally, because it is assumed that the rule-based system is influenced by the integration of event-based and knowledge-based memory information, there should be important interactions between the event-based and knowledge-based memory systems and the rule-based memory system. Thus, for each attribute there is a neural circuit that encompasses all three memory systems in representing specific attribute information. Space only allows for the presentation of one neural circuit as an example. Figure 5 depicts the neural substrates and their interconnections associated with the spatial (place) attribute across all three memory systems. Note that the dorsal lateral thalamus, pre- and parasubiculum, hippocampus, and subiculum represent neural substrates that support the event-based memory system; the entorhinal cortex, parahippocam-

pal gyrus or postrhinal cortex, posterior parietal cortex, and retrosplenial cortex support the knowledge-based memory system; and the lateral prefrontal cortex or pre- and infralimbic cortex support the rule-based memory system. This circuit provides anatomical support for a possible independence in the operation of the hippocampus as part of the event-based memory system and posterior parietal cortex as part of the knowledge-based memory system in that spatial information that is processed via the dorsal lateral thalamus can activate both the hippocampus and the posterior parietal cortex in parallel. Also, information can reach the lateral prefrontal cortex or pre- and infralimbic cortex as part of the rule-based memory system via direct connections from the posterior parietal cortex as part of the knowledge-based memory system and hippocampus as part of the event-based memory system. Finally, spatial information can interact with other specific attributes via a series of direct connections, including an interaction with reward value attribute information via hippocampal–amygdala connections or lateral prefrontal cortex–orbital frontal cortex connections or an interaction with response attribute information via hippocampal–caudate or lateral prefrontal–premotor or supplementary motor connections. In general, the tripartite attribute memory model represents the most comprehensive memory model capable of integrating the extant knowledge concerning the neural system representation of memory.

See Also the Following Articles

INFORMATION PROCESSING • LANGUAGE AND LEXICAL PROCESSING • MEMORY, EXPLICIT AND IMPLICIT • MEMORY DISORDERS, ORGANIC • MEMORY, NEUROIMAGING • MEMORY, OVERVIEW • SEMANTIC MEMORY • SHORT-TERM MEMORY • WORKING MEMORY

Suggested Reading

Burgess, N., Jeffery, K. J., and O'Keefe, J. (Eds.) (1999). *The Hippocampal and Parietal Foundations of Spatial Cognition.* Oxford Univ. Press, New York.

Eichenbaum, H. (1999). The hippocampus and mechanisms of declarative memory. *Behav. Brain Res.* **103,** 123–133.

Kesner, R. P. (1998). Neurobiological views of memory. In *Neurobiology of Learning and Memory.* (J. L. Martinez and R. P. Kesner, Eds.), pp. 361–416. Academic Press, New York.

LeDoux, J. E. (1995). Emotion: Clues from the brain. *Annu. Rev. Psychol.* **46,** 209–235.

Martinez, J. L., and Kesner, R. P. (Eds.) (1998). *Neurobiology of Learning and Memory.* Academic Press, San Diego.

Roberts, A. C., Robbins, T. W., and Weiskrantz, L. (Eds.) (1998). *The Prefrontal Cortex: Executive and Cognitive Functions.* Oxford Univ. Press, New York.

Schacter, D. L., and Buckner, R. L. (1998). Priming and the brain. *Neuron* **20,** 185–195.

Squire, L. R. (1994). Declarative and nondeclarative memory: Multiple brain systems supporting learning and memory. In *Memory Systems 1994* (D. L. Schacter and E. Tulving, Eds.), pp. 203–231. MIT Press, Cambridge, MA.

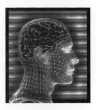

Memory, Neuroimaging

JOHN JONIDES, TOR D. WAGER, and DAVID T. BADRE

University of Michigan

GLOSSARY

declarative memory Information stored in memory that can be retrieved explicitly.

encoding The set of processes that transform some physical event into a memory representation.

episodic information Information in memory that is tied to the time and/or place of occurrence, such as being tied to one's autobiographical past.

executive processes The set of operations that allows one to shift attention from one task to another, plan a set of operations, tie information to its context, and generally modulate the operation of other mental processes.

long-term memory The system of storage that is the large repository for information that is stored for very long periods of time.

procedural memory Information that allows one to engage in some skill, including motor and cognitive skills.

retrieval The processes responsible for extracting information from memory for some purpose. The most frequent kinds of retrieval are recall and recognition.

semantic information Information that is generic in form without being tied to some time or place of occurrence, such as knowledge of facts about the world.

storage The processes responsible for holding information in memory for some period of time.

working memory The system of storage that is responsible for small amounts of information for short periods of time.

The study of memory has been remarkably facilitated by the use of neuroimaging tools in recent years. As we now know, memory is not a unitary function or set of processes; rather there are multiple systems of memory that underlie our cognitive life. This article examines the full taxonomy of memory in humans, and reviews what we know about the brain basis of memory from neuroimaging studies. Beyond this, the purpose of the article is also to illustrate how knowledge of the brain mechanisms of memory can help inform us about a proper psychological view of how memory works functionally.

I. SOME INTRODUCTORY CONCEPTS

A. Types of Memory

One of the critical properties that makes the human mind so extraordinarily suited to understanding and dealing with the world is its ability to shift in time—to model the future and reconstruct the past. Reconstruction of the past requires memory, and memory is fundamental to nearly any cognitive skill. It is involved in complex processes such as problem-solving, and it is involved in even what seem to be the simplest skills, such as recognizing a familiar face. The role played by memory in cognition is complex enough that not just a single memory system will do. Humans and other animals have several memory systems with different characteristics and different neural implementations, and these systems, acting in concert, contribute to the human mind's tremendous adaptability.

At the broadest level, one can distinguish between "working memory" and "long-term memory." Working memory refers to the system that stores a small amount of information for a brief span of time. Information stored in working memory is then used in the service of other cognitive tasks. For example, if we were solving an arithmetic problem such as $817 + 723$ without the benefit of writing anything on paper, working memory would be used to store the problem, store the intermediate steps in the addition, and store the final solution. In addition to temporary storage, an important component of working memory is what is called "executive processing:" the set of operations that permits one to manipulate the contents of working memory. In the previous example, executive processes would be involved in switching attention from one column of addition to another and in organizing the order of steps to arrive at a final sum. Whereas there is as yet no overall agreement about a full list of executive processes, they generally can be thought of as operations that regulate the processes operating on the contents of working memory, processes such as selective attention to relevant information (more about this shortly).

In contrast to the short duration and small capacity of working memory, long-term memory is a system with very long duration memory traces and a very large storage capacity. In our previous mental arithmetic example, long-term memory would be the repository of the facts of addition that would be needed to solve the mental arithmetic problem. Of course, long-term memory stores much more than that. For example, it is the repository of all the words we know in our language, of the sensory information that we all have stored for untold numbers of events (e.g., the taste of a good chocolate), of the spatial information we have stored for navigating around our world, and so on. In addition, many pieces of information are stored that we normally do not retrieve consciously but that nevertheless guide our everyday behavior, such as the rules of language or habitual actions in which we engage every day.

Larry Squire of the University of California and Endel Tulving of the University of Toronto have proposed schemes that summarize the various forms of long-term memory. One way of synthesizing and expanding these schemes is shown in Fig. 1. The figure shows that there are two broad divisions of long-term memory: declarative and procedural. Declarative memory refers to the facts and events that we can retrieve at will, often consciously. By contrast, procedural memory refers to stored information that has an impact on our behavior but that is not willfully retrieved. Consider, for example, the concept of a bicycle. A declarative memory you might have of a bicycle is that it is blue and that it has 21 gears, mountain terrain tires, two handbrakes, and so on. These are all facts that can be willfully retrieved from memory. By contrast, you also have stored information that allows you to ride your bicycle—a task that any 6-year-old child will tell you is not easy. This information is not consciously retrievable; indeed, it is a nontrivial problem in physics and kinesiology to describe just how people are able to ride a two-wheeled bicycle without falling over. The contrast between these two sorts of memory is a contrast between declarative and procedural memory. Perhaps the most compelling evidence that procedural knowledge is different from declarative knowledge is that patients with damage to their hippocampi and surrounding medial temporal lobes can learn new procedural skills, even though they cannot encode where they learned

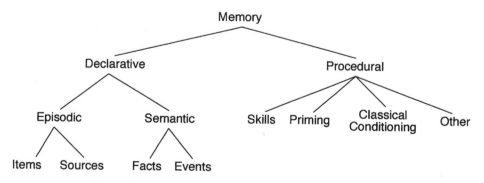

Figure 1 A taxonomy of various forms of long-term memory.

the skill or remember any details of having practiced it, even when that practice occurred very recently. Other patients with cerebellar damage can remember the practice sessions, but their skills on most motor tasks do not improve. This pattern of deficits, called a double dissociation, helps to define procedural and declarative processes as distinct types of memory.

Declarative memory itself comes in two forms. One is called episodic memory, or memory for specific events, and it consists of memory traces that are accompanied by memory for the context in which they were formed. Each piece of episodic memory has a source tag associated with it, possibly including the time and place of memory formation and other details about the context. When retrieving an episodic memory, one can retrieve either the item itself, given information about the source, or the source, given information about the item. For example, you may recall where and when you purchased your current bicycle or, given the time and place, you may recall the features of the bicycle that you purchased. The other category of declarative memory is semantic. This type of memory consists of the vast store of facts and events that you have in long-term memory, regardless of whether you can retrieve when and where you learned them. For example, you may remember the fact that bicycles can be mountain bikes, racing bikes, hybrid bikes, and so on, yet you may not be able to recall when or where you learned this semantic fact.

Procedural memories also are of various sorts. There are skills, for example, such as riding a bicycle. There are classically conditioned responses, which entail a previous pairing of an unconditioned with a conditioned stimulus to yield a conditioned response. And there are cases of priming, in which a previously learned piece of information facilitates processing of some new piece of information. Psychological measures of priming, such as decreases in response time to recognize a previously viewed word, indicate that a trace of the previously learned piece of information is affecting current cognitive processing—even if there is no conscious recollection of having seen the word before.

Another important dimension of memory, whether working or long-term, is the type of information being stored. As we shall see later, the brain circuitry involved in a memory task honors the type of information that is stored and retrieved. Perhaps the most frequently studied case of this concerns the distinction between linguistic information (such as letters, words, sentences, and stories) and visual or spatial information (such as a scene, an object, a face,

or a spatial environment). By now ample evidence exists that the two hemispheres of the brain are differentially activated by these two types of information, with the left hemisphere specialized for verbal information and the right for visual or spatial information in most humans.

B. Types of Processes

Memory entails three cognitive operations: encoding, storage, and retrieval. These terms refer to the sequence in which memory processes are thought to occur. Entering information is first put into the proper internal code and a new memory trace is formed (encoding). Encoding is followed by storage of the information for some period of time. This stage may include consolidation or alteration of memory traces to make them last longer and ease retrieval. Retrieval is the process of reporting information from storage.

The nature of encoding depends on two factors: the type of material that is involved in the memory task and the task that is performed with that material. The type of material exerts a strong influence on the path of activity in the brain early in the processing sequence. The best example of this is the visual system. Spatial information about a visual stimulus is selectively routed to a dorsal stream of information processing that mainly includes the parietal lobes, whereas information about shape and other nonspatial object features of the same stimulus is processed by a ventral stream in the occipital and inferior temporal lobes. To generalize from this example, we can say that the nature of incoming information will influence the path of processing that the information takes in the brain. Beyond this, though, there is also an influence of the task with which a person is faced, as many different operations may be performed on any given type of material. For example, one can process a word by noting its meaning or by noting whether it is printed in uppercase or lowercase letters. These very different types of processing on the same stimulus yield different patterns of activation in the brain, as we shall see later.

Once encoded, information is retained for some period of time. Consistent with the fundamental distinction between working and long-term memory, the length of the retention interval in large part will determine which of these systems is most heavily involved. Retrieval after short retention intervals—up to, perhaps, intervals as long as 30 sec to 1 min—uses working memory. Retrieval of information stored for longer periods will, under most circumstances, necessitate the involvement of long-term memory storage. Which memory system is engaged will be revealed by the circuitry that is activated. Working memory engages circuitry in frontal and parietal cortices most prominently, whereas long-term memory requires the involvement of frontal and parietal circuitry as well as hippocampal and parahippocampal mechanisms.

Just as encoding different types of material engages different mechanisms, storage of different types of material also requires different mechanisms. This has been demonstrated most handsomely in the contrast between verbal and visual material, which predominantly activate left and right hemisphere structures, respectively. This distinction has been demonstrated for both working memory and long-term memory, as we shall see later.

Once encoded and stored, information in memory can then be retrieved as needed. Suppose, for example, that we ask a person to memorize a list of words. Retrieval can be accomplished in several ways. We might simply ask the person to recall as many of the words as possible (free recall). Or we might guide recall by giving some of the words on the list as hints and asking the person to recall the others (cued recall). Or we might present the person with a longer list of words, some of which were presented on the original list and some not, and ask the person to decide which is which (recognition). Any of these procedures requires the person to access the stored information in memory and produce an explicit response that depends on that stored information. For this reason, these are often called explicit tests of memory. However, there are also implicit tests. Suppose, for example, that we presented someone with a list of words and later flashed the same words and new words, one by one, so briefly that they were difficult to identify. If the person were more accurate in identifying words that had been presented on the original list than ones that had not (which is what happens in this perceptual identification situation), then we could conclude that the original words were stored in memory even though no explicit retrieval of them was ever demanded. The process of storage and use of information without explicit memory is called priming. Evidence from positron emission tomography (PET) and functional magnetic resonance imaging (fMRI) suggests that implicit and explicit tests of memory recruit different brain areas, as reviewed later.

With these preliminaries about memory in place, we are now in a position to review what neuroimaging evidence has contributed to understanding basic mechanisms of human memory.

II. WORKING MEMORY

The canonical model of working memory is due originally to Alan Baddeley, and it is this model that has been investigated in detail using neuroimaging methods. The model claims a fundamental distinction between short-term storage of information and the executive processes that manipulate this information. This general view is supported by the existence of patients who have intact short-term storage but deficits in executive processes; this pattern of impairments contrasts with that of other patients who have deficits in executive processing but intact short-term storage. Such a double dissociation suggests that the circuitries of storage and executive processing are separable, and imaging studies have confirmed this separability.

A. Short-Term Storage

The short-term storage of information in working memory appears to be accomplished via two mechanisms: one that retains information and another that "rehearses" that information in order to keep the memory traces active during a retention interval. This is perhaps best illustrated for verbal information. A task that has been used frequently to study the mechanisms of verbal working memory in neuroimaging experiments is the item-recognition task. In this task, participants are presented with a small number of target items, typically randomly selected letters, to store for a retention interval of several seconds. Following this interval, a single probe item is presented and participants must decide whether this item was a member of the memorized set. When participants engage in this task in PET and fMRI settings, a number of easily replicable sites of activation exist compared to a control condition that does not require memory at all or in which the memory requirement is minimal. One frequent site of activation is in the posterior parietal cortex, typically more prominently in the left hemisphere than the right. In addition, a set of activations appears in frontal areas, including the inferior frontal gyrus on the left, premotor cortex (more prominently on the left than on the right), and supplementary motor cortex. These brain regions, and all other major regions discussed throughout this article, are shown in Fig. 2.

The frontal cortical areas that are activated in this task are quite similar to those activated in a task that requires one to make judgments of rhyming, a task that

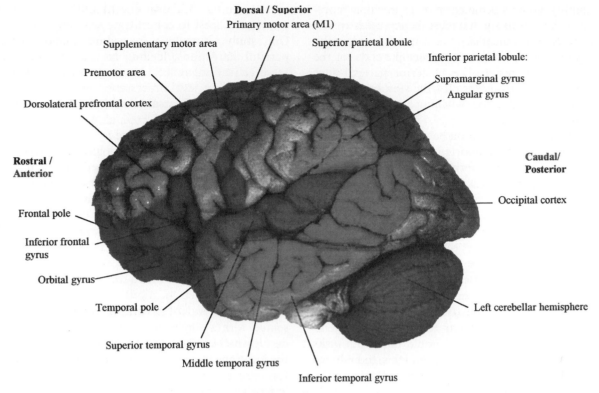

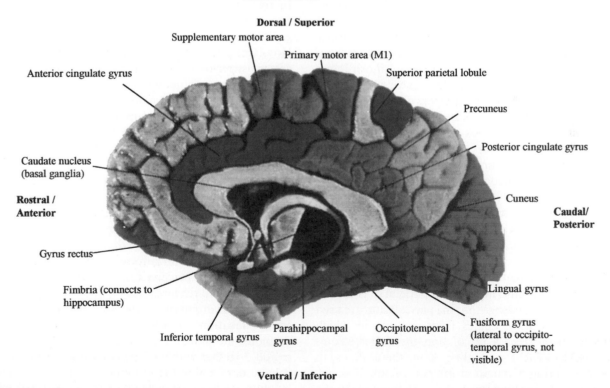

Figure 2 Brain diagrams highlighting the major structures discussed in the text. The upper figure shows a lateral view of a left hemisphere of the human brain, and the lower figure shows a view of the right hemisphere as seen from the midline of the brain. Major structures of relevance to memory are labeled.

presumably requires production of a speechlike representation. So, it is likely that these frontal areas are the ones involved in rehearsal, which involves internally generating and regenerating a speechlike code for the stored verbal material. The posterior parietal sites have been suggested as sites for the storage of verbal information as well as for switching attention between one item and another.

The purported dissociation between the frontal and parietal sites is nicely supported by a study that used a different task involving verbal working memory, the two-back task. In this task, participants see a series of letters presented at a pace of one every 2.5 sec, and they must judge whether each matches in identity the one that appeared two letters back in the series. This task clearly requires storage and rehearsal of each letter, as well as other processes that we discuss next. Compared to a task in which participants must simply judge whether each letter in the series matches a single target (say, the letter "P"), the two-back task produces activations in regions similar to those in the item-recognition task. This is as it should be if both tasks involve storage and rehearsal. Beyond this, though, the two-back task has also been compared to another condition, one in which participants had to silently rehearse letters to themselves with little storage requirement (e.g., say the letter "P" for 3 sec, followed by silently saying the letter "M," and so on). Subtraction of the activation in this rehearsal condition from that in the two-back condition revealed much lower activation in the frontal areas. The rehearsal condition is presumed to involve the explicit production of silent speech. Subtraction of the activations in this condition from those in the two-back condition reduces frontal but not parietal activation; therefore, one can conclude that the frontal activations in the two-back and other verbal working memory tasks must reflect an inner rehearsal process as part of those tasks. These same frontal regions are also activated in tasks that require a recall response, so they are not unique to the peculiarities of the item-recognition task or the two-back matching task.

Just as we can identify the frontal sites used in verbal rehearsal, we can also identify the parietal sites used in verbal storage. Evidence that the parietal sites are used in part for storage comes from a study in which subjects memorized a set of nonsense letter strings (e.g., "MAVER") and then kept these items in memory during a retention interval of some 50 sec, during which they underwent PET scanning. After the scan, they had to retrieve the items to be sure that they had been stored accurately. Scanning during just the

retention interval allows one to isolate storage processes or at least to concentrate scanning on storage. One study using this procedure found posterior parietal activations, leading to the conclusion that these activations reflected storage processes and not encoding or retrieval processes.

Storage and rehearsal should not be restricted to verbal information, of course, if they are general properties of working memory as Baddeley has supposed. Indeed, many studies have investigated the storage and rehearsal circuitry used for spatial information as well. The clearest result of these studies is that the circuitry activated by spatial information in a working memory task is quite different from that activated by verbal information, even when the tasks are quite similar and only the material differs. For example, in an analog to the item-recognition task, subjects are presented with a set of dots on a screen and asked to store their locations in memory. Following a retention interval of several seconds, they are presented with a single probe dot, and their task is to decide whether it appears at the same location as one of the locations they have stored. This task has the same formal structure as the item-recognition task for letters, yet it yields activations that are quite different. In common are activations in the posterior parietal and premotor cortex, although with a tendency for greater activation in the right than the left hemisphere. However, quite different are activations in the occipital cortex, superior frontal cortex, and inferior frontal cortex, most prominently in the right hemisphere.

The common activations in parietal and premotor cortex between verbal and spatial versions of the task suggest that there are some processes in common between the tasks, possibly having to do in part with allocating attention to several items in memory. However, the differences in activations suggest that the mechanisms by which information is stored and rehearsed may be different. Indeed, there is evidence of a similarity in circuitry between processes mediating spatial working memory and those mediating shifts of attention to various locations in the visual field when stimuli are being perceived. This leads to the conclusion that spatial rehearsal may amount to a successive allocation of attention to internal representations of spatial locations, a process possibly mediated by premotor mechanisms near the frontal eye fields. This region, together with parietal cortex, may also play a role in maintaining the representations of the spatial locations as well, a conclusion that is consistent with lesion studies and electrophysiological studies of monkeys in spatial working memory tasks. So, we can see that, although storage and rehearsal are common features of spatial and verbal working memory, they appear to be implemented in the brain in different ways.

Of course, visual information that is stored need not be spatial in nature. Features such as the shape of an object or its color are not spatial, even though they are visual. As described earlier, the brain honors this distinction in simple visual processing, and indeed neuroimaging research suggests that spatial memory and memory for other visual information are processed differently in the brain as well. One experiment that demonstrates this used pictures of three faces presented sequentially in three different spatial locations. After a retention interval, a probe picture was presented in one of the locations. When subjects were tested on their working memory for objects, they had to decide whether the probe face was the same as any of the previous three; when they were tested on spatial working memory, they had to decide whether the probe was in the same location as one of the original faces. The elegance of this design is that it involves the very same stimuli, and only the nature of the memory task changes. The results show that this change in task produces an important difference in brain activation: The object task activated regions of dorsolateral prefrontal cortex, whereas the spatial task activated a region posterior to this in the premotor cortex. Beyond this, a meta-analysis of several spatial and object working memory tasks suggests that there is also a dorsal–ventral difference in activation in the posterior cortex. Spatial working memory tasks activate more dorsal structures in the posterior cortex, whereas object working memory tasks activate more ventral structures.

B. Executive Processes

In addition to storage components, the model of working memory proposed by Baddeley includes a component due to executive processes. Although there is not yet a clear taxonomy of executive processes in hand, descriptions of them typically include the following: (a) focusing attention on relevant information and inhibiting attention from irrelevant information; (b) scheduling processes in tasks that require multiple processes; (c) planning and prioritizing a sequence of steps to meet some goal; (d) updating and checking the contents of working memory; and (e) coding internal representations for time or place of occurrence. All of these processes involve the manipulation of information that is temporarily stored in working memory. Research on executive processes using neuroimaging techniques has revealed a heavy contribution of frontal mechanisms regardless of the executive process in question.

As an example, recall the verbal item-recognition task. In that task, subjects are presented with a set of letters that they have to retain for several seconds, after which they have to decide whether a probe letter matches one of the letters in memory. Several studies have introduced an inhibitory component in this task in the following way. Trials were included in which the distractor probes (probes that did not match an item in the current memory set) were letters that did match a letter in the memory set from the previous trial. Thus, these probes were relatively familiar because they had been memorized recently. This design creates a situation in which participants have a sense of familiarity about the probe item, but they must remember that it does not match the memory set on the current trial. On such trials, subjects take longer to give a "no match" response. Both PET and fMRI studies show that there is a site in the left lateral prefrontal cortex that is activated on these trials, and the activation occurs most prominently at the time the probe is presented. Furthermore, older subjects, who show a greater interference effect on these trials, also show less activation at this left lateral site, and patients with damage to this area show a dramatically increased interference effect compared to patients with damage elsewhere in the frontal cortex. Taken together, this evidence suggests that the left lateral site is involved in resolving the conflict between familiarity and source memory that arises on these trials.

Another example of a task in which executive processes interact with storage processes is the two-back task described earlier. Recall that, in this task, single letters are presented in succession and subjects must judge whether each letter matches the one two earlier in the sequence. To succeed at this task, one not only has to store the recent stream of letters but also has to update this stored set as new letters are presented, dropping older letters and adding newer ones. This task is similar to the item-interference task in that it includes an inhibitory component, as described earlier. In addition to this executive process, the letters that are stored in memory also have to be tagged by their order of appearance so that the subject can keep in mind which one is two back, which is one back, which is three back, and so on. Thus, the two-back task must recruit an executive process responsible for temporally tagging information, a sort of short-term episodic memory requirement. Indeed, the two-back task shows evidence of activations in the dorsolateral prefrontal cortex in addition to other sites that may well be responsible for temporal tagging. The dorsolateral prefrontal activation that arises in this task seems to be a common broad site of activation in many tasks that require manipulation of the information stored in working memory, and so this leads to the general conclusion that prefrontal mechanisms may be responsible for a wide array of executive processes.

C. Summary of Working Memory

Overall the neuroimaging research concerned with working memory has reliably revealed a set of structures that may be important for storage, rehearsal, and executive processes. Posterior parietal mechanisms have been implicated in the storage of verbal material, and prefrontal ones concerned with language processing have been implicated in the rehearsal of stored verbal material. For spatial material, the sites of storage and rehearsal are different; nonetheless, one can conclude that there are storage and rehearsal processes for nonverbal material as well, but that these may be implemented via nonlinguistic mechanisms. Finally, various sites in the prefrontal cortex, most prominently dorsolateral prefrontal areas, have been documented in the mediation of executive processes. Thus, the psychological architecture proposed by Baddeley in his model of working memory seems to be amply supported by a brain architecture that may honor the same distinctions among processes.

III. EPISODIC MEMORY

As described earlier, episodic memory can be defined as memory for information that is associated with a time and place of occurrence. Take, as an example, a semantic fact: one may know that the turn of the century French impressionist painter Claude Monet lived and worked for many years in his provincial home at Giverny. This fact is in the domain of semantic memory. However, one's memory of learning this fact in an art history course would be an episodic memory. Episodic memory is often studied in a controlled laboratory setting using recognition or recall tasks, described in the introduction to this article. These tasks require memory for a source code (e.g., time or place of occurrence) that is the essence of episodic memory. In

the context of neuroimaging, the encoding and/or retrieval phases of these tasks are scanned using PET or fMRI and then compared to a control task with a diminished or absent demand on memory.

These studies have identified a set of regions underlying episodic memory. These include medial temporal structures, such as the hippocampus and parahippocampal areas, prefrontal cortex, anterior cingulate cortex, cerebellum, and parietal and superior temporal association cortices (shown in Fig. 2). Important hemispheric, regional, and functional differences exist, however, between the encoding and retrieval phases of episodic memory. In addition to exploring these differences, neuroimaging studies have also begun to examine cases in which this system performs inadequately.

A. Episodic Encoding

As discussed earlier, memory entails three important general stages: encoding, storage, and retrieval. At the encoding stage, processes must be involved that create an internal code for a piece of information and then attach a context (a place or time) to the new memory.

Several neuroimaging studies have scanned participants while they perform some task to encode a set of items. For example, participants might be asked to make a judgment about whether a word represents an animal or vegetable, an encoding task that requires access to the semantics of the word. Alternatively, a subject might simply be asked to memorize a set of items and be tested on them later. Subsequent testing of the items confirms whether subjects have effectively encoded the items. These studies show that encoding involves the left prefrontal cortex, hippocampus, parahippocampal cortex, anterior cingulate, and some superior temporal cortex. Further experimentation, including converging evidence from neuropsychology and other experimental paradigms, has begun to examine the role of each of these regions and their relationships to one another.

The hippocampus and surrounding areas have long been associated with memory. Evidence from both animal studies and studies of brain-damaged patients has shown that damage to the hippocampus can result in amnesia, one form of which is caused by damage to medial temporal structures such as the hippocampus and parahippocampal gyrus. Though amnesics typically are able to retrieve memories from their distant past, they show a profound deficit in the ability to form new memories, a phenomenon known as anterograde amnesia. For this reason, the hippocampus is thought to be involved with the encoding and consolidation of long-term memories.

In line with this, many neuroimaging studies using the encoding paradigms described earlier have shown hippocampal activity. Neuroimaging evidence has shown, however, a selective response of the hippocampus to novelty. In one experiment, participants were shown pictures of indoor and outdoor scenes while in the MRI scanner. They were required to judge whether each scene was an indoor scene or an outdoor scene and remember the pictures for a later test. In some scans, the same two pictures were repeated many times so that participants became very familiar with them. During other scans, the scenes were entirely novel and unfamiliar. Comparison of the unfamiliar scans to the familiar scans showed activity in the parahippocampal gyrus bilaterally. Given this fact, it would seem that the medial temporal lobe is particularly responsive to novel stimuli—a finding consistent with the intuition that most episodic memory encoding occurs on the first presentation of new material.

The function of the left prefrontal cortex appears to involve processing the context (or source) in which new information is learned. An event-related fMRI experiment has studied the different functions of left prefrontal and hippocampal mechanisms in episodic memory. Event-related fMRI allows the examination of areas of the brain that are active in response to different events occurring within the context of a single cognitive task. In this experiment, participants were required to learn word pairs in which the first word served as semantic context for a second word, for example, "athlete–boxer." Participants were presented with several of these word pairs during each scan. Sometimes the context for a word would change, as in "dog–boxer." Other times the word would change as in "dog–labrador." Both word and context could also be new or both could be old. This design permitted independent manipulation of the novelty and the context of the item to be learned during encoding. The hippocampus was active when either the context word or the related word was new, and it was most active when both were new. This corroborates the idea that the hippocampus is involved in processing novel items. The left prefrontal cortex was most active when an old context was attached to a new word or a new context attached to an old word. This finding suggests that the prefrontal cortex is involved in representing the context of the item to be remembered, a function that is critical for episodic memory.

We can test whether the effectiveness of encoding is related to the brain activations that reflect encoding by varying what is called the depth of processing participants apply to material. It is well-known that evaluation of the semantic content of material (deep encoding) leads to more elaborate processing and a longer lasting memory trace than evaluation of the physical features of material (shallow encoding). One experiment that takes advantage of this effect required subjects to judge whether a word was abstract or concrete (deep encoding) or whether it was printed in upper- or lowercase characters (shallow encoding). Deeply encoded words were remembered better than words encoded shallowly, replicating previous behavioral results. When the two conditions were compared, it was found that there was greater activity in the hippocampus and left prefrontal cortex for deep encoding, suggesting that both areas are more vigorously involved with deep than with shallow encoding.

This result by itself does not indicate that more activity in the prefrontal cortex and hippocampus produces better behavioral performance; it only indicates that depth of encoding and activation are correlated. To address the performance question, several studies have directly examined the relationship between performance on retrieving an individual item in memory and brain activation while encoding that item. After being scanned, the participants had to recognize the encoded items, and they were grouped by whether the items were retrieved correctly or incorrectly, an indication of good or poor encoding, respectively. This comparison revealed activity bilaterally in the hippocampus and in the left prefrontal cortex. Hence, it would seem that for effective encoding not only must the information be consolidated effectively by the hippocampus but the prefrontal cortex must also assist in processing the context.

To summarize, encoding recruits a set of regions that includes the left prefrontal cortex, hippocampus, parahippocampal gyrus, parietal cortex, and anterior cingulate (as shown in Fig. 2). These regions appear to be involved in transforming information into a mental code in the brain that can later be retrieved. Two processes entailed by this task are the consolidation of a novel item by the hippocampus and the processing of its context by the left prefrontal cortex. The extent to which the information being encoded can be effectively recovered at a later time is strongly dependent on the depth of encoding, which seems to have an effect on the activity of the hippocampus and left prefrontal cortex.

B. Episodic Retrieval

Retrieval of episodic memory is mediated by regions that generally are functionally and anatomically distinct from those used in encoding. Most neuroimaging studies of retrieval use a task design similar to that used in studies of encoding, in which participants must study a set of items and are subsequently tested for their memory of the items. The difference is that participants are scanned while they retrieve (recall or recognize) rather than while they encode the material. In recognition tasks, an item is shown, and it is the task of the participant to indicate whether that item was presented during the study phase. Hence, it is necessary only to access the source and not the item. In recall tests, it is necessary to generate the item as well. Neuroimaging studies of both recall and recognition typically show activity in the right prefrontal cortex, hippocampus, medial as well as inferior parietal cortex, anterior cingulate, and cerebellum. There are some important variations in this pattern, however, that are discussed next.

The hippocampus is typically considered to be involved in the consolidation of long-term memories, as discussed earlier. Although this function implies that the hippocampus should not be involved in retrieval, some studies *have* found it to be activated during retrieval tasks. To test whether the effort required for retrieval might influence activation of the hippocampus, one study varied the amount of effort required to search memory. In a "high-recall" condition, words were deeply encoded and, hence, less effortfully retrieved. When the recall phase was scanned, this manipulation revealed activity in the hippocampus bilaterally, supporting the view that the hippocampus is involved in effortless, conscious recall. In a "low-recall" condition, words were encoded more superficially and, hence, required more effortful retrieval. Scanning during this more effortful recall phase showed bilateral prefrontal but not hippocampal activation. The finding that the prefrontal cortex is involved in effortful retrieval is consistent with the view that one function of the prefrontal cortex is to implement retrieval strategies. The hippocampus, by contrast, may be involved in relatively more automatic retrieval.

Certain neuroimaging studies of episodic retrieval have found not only increased activity in the right prefrontal cortex but also decreased activity in other areas such as the left prefrontal cortex. On the basis of this effect, some have suggested that episodic retrieval is not just an active process of search and retrieval but involves the active inhibition of certain regions of the brain by other areas of the brain. By this model, the right prefrontal cortex could be actively inhibiting left frontal regions as well as inferior temporal regions, areas that sometimes show deactivations in retrieval tasks. In the case of the temporal regions, for example, this might indicate the suppression of language processes during episodic retrieval. This effect has been termed "ensemble inhibition" and suggests that episodic retrieval may be carried out, in part, by inhibitory processes.

Retrieval processing involves an interplay between the right prefrontal cortex and the hippocampus in the implementation of search strategies and conscious, effortless retrieval, respectively. The involvement of other areas of the brain such as the precuneus, parietal cortex, anterior cingulate, and cerebellum has yet to be fully elucidated, so much further research is required on this problem.

C. Synthesis: The HERA Model and Its Extension

Stable differences appear to exist in the activations accompanying encoding versus retrieval. The most striking pattern is in the activity of the prefrontal cortex. Most studies of encoding have shown activity in the left prefrontal cortex at a more anterior site, whereas most studies of retrieval have shown activity in the right prefrontal cortex, also at a more anterior site. This hemispheric difference in prefrontal activity in episodic memory is typically referred to as the Hemispheric Encoding–Retrieval Asymmetry model or HERA.

Other areas of the brain have also come to be included in the HERA model. For example, the left cerebellum seems to be more active during retrieval than during encoding. The cerebellum's anatomical connections are predominantly with the contralateral prefrontal cortex (via the thalamus), so that the coupling of right prefrontal and left cerebellar activations is not surprising. What function the cerebellum might be serving in the context of episodic retrieval is unclear. The cerebellum has long been associated with motor coordination and visuomotor skill learning. It is possible that the cerebellum is serving one of these general roles in effortful retrieval, but its exact role remains to be elucidated.

The association cortices have also gained some attention in regard to the HERA model. The left temporal cortex has been found to be activated in some studies of encoding, whereas activation in the right or bilateral parietal cortex has been documented during retrieval. These findings, though not entirely uncontroversial, seem to follow the HERA pattern, with encoding being a left hemisphere function, in this case in the temporal lobe, and retrieval being a right hemisphere function, in the parietal cortex. There is a great deal of speculation as to exactly what these areas are doing. Some accounts claim that they are involved in some way in the execution of special encoding or retrieval strategies. In the case of the temporal cortex, this might be attaching some kind of mnemonic code to items to ease retrieval later on. Others suggest that the parietal cortex is involved in perceptual aspects of retrieval, such as mental imagery. Further study is necessary to fully understand the functions subserved by these regions, as well as the way that they interact with the other areas of the brain that are active during episodic encoding and retrieval.

It must be noted that there are important exceptions to the HERA model's general description of the patterns of brain activity during tasks of episodic memory. The model does not do well in predicting patterns of activation in the hippocampus. Hippocampal activation has been found unilaterally on the right and left and bilaterally in tasks of both encoding and retrieval. The pattern of activity in the hippocampus is best described as being dependent on the type of material being encoded or retrieved, not on encoding and retrieval by themselves. This is shown by systematic patterns of activation depending on whether verbal or nonverbal stimuli are used in an experiment. Most experiments using verbal information have shown predominantly left hippocampal activity. In contrast, the right hippocampus or both hippocampi may be more active in encoding visual information. For example, a study in which people retrieved information about a spatial route through a town activated bilateral hippocampi. It should be noted as well that the material specificity of activations extends to the prefrontal cortex. One area of prefrontal cortex often observed in studies of episodic memory does not follow HERA but rather depends on whether the stimulus material is verbal or visuospatial, the former producing activation on the left and the latter on the right. So, even within the prefrontal cortex, one region obeys the description given by the HERA model and another does not.

Overall, it does appear that many patterns of activity demonstrated in tasks of episodic memory follow an asymmetric hemispheric pattern in regard to encoding and retrieval. In the prefrontal cortex and in temporal and parietal association areas, activity in the left hemisphere is associated with encoding processing and activity in the right hemisphere is associated with retrieval processing. The cerebellum also shows a hemispheric asymmetry, but it is the reverse pattern with the left cerebellum engaged during retrieval. There are exceptions to this pattern, and these are seen in the hippocampus, posterior regions, and some anterior regions of prefrontal cortex as well. The patterns of activity in these regions are dependent on the modality of the information being processed—verbal information lateralized to the left hemisphere and visuospatial lateralized to the right—rather than encoding and retrieval processes.

D. False Memories

Memories of our personal experiences are extremely vulnerable because memory often is not *reconstructive* but *constructive*. When retrieving an episodic memory, we try to reproduce the event as closely as possible, constructing the most plausible approximation. Consequently, we often incorporate aspects of the event that are close to the original but not exactly it, and we can even insert information that never occurred at all. This vulnerability can even go so far as to produce elaborate situations that never actually happened, though the person might swear that they did.

Neuroimaging studies have begun to examine differences in brain activation, comparing retrieval of a true past event from false memory for an event that did not occur. Most of these studies have used a task in which participants are shown lists of words to study. After a long retention period, the participants are asked to perform a recognition task, indicating which words on a second list were present on the first list. Some of the words on the second list that were not present on the first list, called foils, are semantically related to the words on the first list. For example, the words "pajama, bed, night" might have appeared on the first list, but the word "sleep" might appear at the time of the recognition test. Semantically related foils often were falsely recognized as having appeared on the originally studied list. Furthermore, participants often rated their confidence that the words had been on the original list as highly as they rated their confidence that actual words had appeared. Thus, it appeared as if the participants had created false memories of semantically related foil words.

Neuroimaging studies have compared activations due to falsely recognized words to activations due to correctly recognized words. One difference that emerges is activation in the frontal cortex during true recognition. This is consistent with other retrieval studies, as reviewed earlier. Another feature of activation is that words on the recognition test that had actually been presented sometimes caused activation in the primary sensory cortex of the modality in which they had appeared. For example, a word presented aurally, when tested at the time of recognition, might show activation in the superior temporal cortex. By contrast, words that did not appear showed no such sensory cortex activation. Thus, a neural signature apparently exists that permits one to distinguish actually presented words from semantically related foils, even if one does not access this signature in the recognition judgments.

IV. SEMANTIC MEMORY

Episodic memory is distinguished by the fact that it requires not only the retrieval of an item from memory but also a source or context for that item. But many times, we retrieve a fact with no knowledge of its context, as when we can identify various types of bicycles without knowing when and where we learned about the various types. Semantic memory can be defined as memory for facts about the world, naked of their source context. This kind of knowledge plays a critical role in all forms of cognition, from language to reasoning to problem-solving. Hence, semantic memory is an important topic for study. Most studies of semantic memory have focused on the retrieval of semantic information from memory because this is studied most readily and because it is more difficult, given the normal course of learning, to study encoding or storage of semantic memory.

A. Verbal Semantic Memory

Many of the concepts that make up our semantic knowledge are coded in the form of language, probably because we are such intensely linguistic creatures. These concepts come from various categories, of course, such as living things and nonliving things, distinctions that we can readily make for many concepts. Evidence from patients with focal brain injury shows that the brain seems to honor some of these categorical distinctions among concepts. For example, there are patients who appear to have lost

their ability to identify living things, such an elephant or a flower, even though they are still capable of identifying nonliving things, such as tools. One interpretation of this result is that the brain's organization of semantic memory is, in part, organized by broad categories. To test whether this is so in normal adults as well as brain-injured adults, one study used PET to examine what areas of the brain are active during the retrieval of three different semantic categories. Participants were given several scans during each of which they were asked to name photographs of either famous people, animals, or tools. As predicted, different brain activations resulted from naming each kind of stimulus. Naming famous people produced activity in the most anterior part of the temporal cortex, called the temporal pole. Naming animals produced activity in a more posterior area of the temporal cortex in inferior and middle temporal gyri. Naming tools showed activity in an even more posterior portion of the inferior temporal gyrus. In general, the more specific the item that had to be named, the more anterior the activation in the temporal cortex. These findings are consistent with the notion of a visual processing stream that spreads from occipital cortex into temporal cortex, moving from general classification to more specific categorization in the anterior temporal cortex.

A related PET study of object and face naming provides corroborating evidence for these findings and further distinguishes between activations involved in the identification of specific faces versus the simple recognition of stimuli as faces. In one condition, participants were asked to make gender discrimination judgments of familiar and unfamiliar faces. Relative to a control condition, this task produced activations broadly in the extrastriate occipital cortex. Only when participants identified faces of famous people, and so had to make a specific face identification, were the temporal poles activated. Also activated were other structures in the temporal cortex (fusiform gyri, right lingual and parahippocampal gyri, and left middle temporal gyrus) as well as the orbitofrontal cortex.

Object naming in this study shared some common areas of activation with face naming, including the orbitofrontal cortex, left middle temporal gyrus, and left fusiform gyrus. Converging evidence from animal and lesion studies may shed light on the roles of these regions. Neuropsychological data suggest that the left middle temporal gyrus may be necessary for naming, but not recognizing, objects and faces. Lesions of orbitofrontal cortex have been related to visual memory impairments in animals. Finally, the fusiform gyri appear to be involved in the recall of both faces and objects, with face recognition activating the right gyrus and object recognition the left. Interestingly, the fusiform gyrus has also been implicated in the *perception* of faces and objects, so the region responsible for semantic memory for this type of information may be similar to the region used to perceive it. This hypothesis is supported by intracortical electrode studies done on patients in preparation for possible surgery to treat epilepsy. These recordings showed that face recognition elicited electrical activity in the fusiform gyrus and that electrical stimulation in this same region resulted in an inability of the patients to name a face for the duration of stimulation.

These complementary results suggest that face perception and recognition share a common substrate and that the boundary between perception and semantic memory may be indistinct for this type of material. Studies of object naming more generally show that semantic memory about concrete objects appears to be organized, at least to some degree, in cortical modules devoted to particular types of remembered material, and these become more specific moving from posterior to anterior brain regions.

Semantic memory for words must take on more than just a simple recognition and naming function. Indeed, when faced with an object it is often more useful to know what can be done with that object rather than just its name. This type of information, as well as information about constructs that are not concrete, is within the domain of semantic memory and has been directly studied.

To examine this sort of semantic memory, a PET experiment was designed that required participants to generate an associated verb for each word in a list of nouns. For example, when shown a picture of an apple, a participant might respond "eat." This experiment revealed a preferential role of lateral and inferior frontal cortex in the generation of verbs associated with visually presented objects. It has been suggested that verbs are at the core of semantic structure, and hence activation in frontal cortical areas might be an indication of which areas are critical in mediating the generation of semantic concepts. Further study of this verb-generation situation compared a task in which participants had to name a verb for each noun presented to two control conditions—reading words and passively viewing words. Multiple subtraction conditions were used to identify areas related to the motor execution of speech (motor cortex), word reading (left insula), and verb generation (left frontal cortex, anterior cingulate, and right cerebellum). This

study also revealed changes in activation with practice on this task, as reviewed later. The constellation of regions that were activated in this study probably included a complex combination of areas involved in attention, inferential reasoning, willed action, episodic encoding, and working memory, but most prominently, significant activation occurred in the left prefrontal cortex and elsewhere that could be attributed to semantic retrieval.

V. COGNITIVE SKILL LEARNING

Investigation of practice-related changes in the verb-generation task provides a convenient segue into a discussion of skill acquisition—another vital aspect of memory. After 15 min of practice on the verb-generation task, 90% of the verbs that participants generated were rote responses that had been consistently associated with the nouns. Participants no longer had to search through memory for a novel association; instead, they could quickly recall a response they gave previously. Analysis of the difference between the PET images early and late in the verb-generation task showed that, with practice, activity decreased in the anterior cingulate, left prefrontal cortex, bilateral inferior frontal gyri, left temporal cortex, and right cerebellum—the very areas that were active when verb generation was compared to word reading. In fact, after practice the PET images were indistinguishable from those of word reading. Increases in activation with practice were observed in the precuneus and cuneus on the medial wall of the posterior cerebrum and in the right superior parietal cortex. These shifts in activation could be due to decreased demand on attention and effort, decreased searching of semantic memory, or some other factor.

Without further evidence, it is hard to distinguish among these causes. Certainly evidence exists that some of these areas are involved in other cognitive processes. For example, the left prefrontal cortex is activated in verbal working memory tasks and in the encoding of long-term memories, as we reviewed earlier. The anterior cingulate is also activated in some overpracticed motor tasks, particularly when they might require attending, making inferences about a pattern, or anticipating future stimuli or feedback. One region that may have a clearer role in the practice effect seen in the verb-generation task is the insula, an area located anatomically near the region responsible for speech output and an area that showed increased activation in the verb-generation task with practice.

This activation may be an indication of increasing automaticity in producing verb associations given nouns as stimuli, a kind of stimulus–response connection that developed even over the course of relatively little practice.

Of course, one might ask whether skill in the verb-generation task is a good example of cognitive skill learning in general. The shifts in activation in this task seem to result not from an improved ability to generate *novel* verbs, but rather from the ability to call up from memory the same verb the subject gave on the last trial, a kind of automatic stimulus–response mapping. It is not yet understood how true cognitive skills, such as the ability to make inferences and manipulate abstract concepts, are learned, except that their appearance in children seems to parallel development of the frontal lobes. However, a great deal of what we normally consider to be cognitive skills, such as expertise in chess, can be explained as the formation and retrieval of ever larger and more complex sets of associations in semantic memory.

A final example of cognitive skill learning comes from a PET study of categorization. Experimental studies have shown that people learn to categorize objects in several ways: through the application of rules, learning of specific exemplars of a category, and implicit learning of an average or "prototype" of the category. Patients with medial temporal damage, who have virtually no remaining episodic memory, fail on rule- and exemplar-based categorization but learn prototype-based categorization as readily as do normal participants. In the study, people classified pictures of contrived animals based on previous practice with similar (but not identical) animals. One practice group learned to categorize animals by a rule, and the other group learned the categories by trial and error. The rule group categorized the new animals presented during scanning by applying the rule. The trial-and-error group categorized animals during PET scanning on the basis of their similarity to the animals they saw during training, an exemplar-based strategy. Only rule-based categorization activated the bilateral parietal cortex, right prefrontal cortex, and bilateral supplementary cortex, possibly reflecting greater working memory demands, attention shifting, and retrieval and application of the rule. Exemplar-based categorization activated the left extrastriate cortex and left cerebellum. The extrastriate activation may reflect greater use of a perceptually based memory trace in the exemplar-based strategy, consistent with the involvement of extrastriate visual cortex in studies of implicit memory. This study suggests that different learning regimens may have a profoundly different effect on the brain circuitry recruited to the task, at least for a task requiring categorization processes.

VI. LEARNING PROCEDURAL SKILLS

Procedural knowledge, as described earlier, consists of knowledge of how to do something. It includes all the behaviors shown as examples of procedural knowledge in Fig. 1, common to all of which is the fact that they do not require explicit retrieval of information; rather, they require the person to tap memory in the service of some other task, such as riding a bike taps memory to coordinate the muscles in various ways so that balance can be maintained. This is often called "implicit" memory. Viewed this way, it is clear that a vast number of motor skills are mediated by procedural memory. Of course, procedural memory must develop over the course of practice, and the changes that occur with practice are often highly specific, improving performance on precisely those tasks we practice. Although this may seem to limit our behavioral repertoire, in fact, once we have learned a sequence of motor movements, we can quickly learn to adapt these movements to similar situations.

Skill learning occurs when a new movement or sequence of movements is acquired, and performance becomes both faster and more accurate with training. Sometimes this learning might involve the acquisition of new sensory–motor mappings. Studies of motor skill learning have focused on either the acquisition of some new sequence of motor movements, such as a sequence of finger taps, or the acquisition of some sensory–motor mapping, such as guiding a visual cursor with joystick movements.

A note: it is often difficult to separate the brain areas involved in learning a skill from those involved in other aspects of processing that change along with skill learning. As people learn a skill, for example, they devote less attention to the task, so that neural circuitry responsible for focusing attention is less involved. At the same time, the incidence of errors decreases, so the brain activity related to error detection and correction will decrease. The brain regions responsible for mediating task performance may also change as skills become automatic. All of these changes obscure the interpretation of neuroimaging studies of the learning process by making it difficult to determine which activations are due to skill learning per se and which are due to other processes.

A. Motor Skill Learning

Execution of motor tasks such as tapping fingers in a particular sequence or maintaining contact between a target moving in a circular pattern and a hand-held marker activates large regions of cerebral cortex and subcortical structures, including sensory motor cortex (primarily the primary motor cortex), supplementary motor area (SMA), premotor area (PMA), putamen, cerebellum, and sensorimotor thalamus (see Fig. 2). Traditionally, and consistent with data on the anatomical layout of the motor system, neuroimaging studies have found activations in these areas on the side contralateral to hand movement (with ipsilateral activation of the cerebellum because of its crossed connections to the cortex). However, evidence indicates that complex movement of even one hand can activate motor areas bilaterally. For example, in one experiment, participants rotated two metal balls at a constant rate in either their right or left hand. These complex movements activated the regions mentioned previously, including significant bilateral activations in the postcentral gyrus, traditionally considered primary somatosensory cortex, and intraparietal sulcus. Notably missing from this list of activations is the basal ganglia, which appear to be preferentially activated during the performance of learned sequences of movements.

Areas involved in the learning of motor skills are largely the same areas as those used during task performance. However, some regions become active only during initial learning or only after performance has become automatic and requires little effort. These changes are specific to the type of task—they vary depending on whether automatic performance involves increased or decreased use of sensory cues and whether the task involves learning a new movement, a sequence of movements, or a sensory–motor association.

B. Sequence Learning

Among the first motor learning tasks studied is the sequential tapping task, in which participants must tap the fingers of their dominant hand (all studies reviewed here used right-handed subjects) in a prespecified sequence. An early study scanned participants doing sequential finger tapping at three stages in the learning process. The three levels corresponded to an initial learning phase when a skill is first being learned, the phase when a skill becomes automatic after significant practice, and skilled performance after performance level has reached its asymptote. The ipsilateral (right) cerebellum was activated in all three conditions, and the activation per movement in the cerebellum decreased as training progressed. The striatum was also activated during advanced practice, suggesting a role for the basal ganglia in the development of automaticity.

Subsequent studies of sequential finger tapping have examined the role of the cerebellum and other structures, including changes in primary motor cortex, in more depth. Unpracticed performance activated a network of areas often associated with the planning and execution of movements: contralateral primary motor cortex and putamen, bilateral PMA and SMA (with more activity on the contralateral side), and cerebellum. With practice, activity decreased in the lateral portion and deep nuclei of the cerebellum, supporting the view that the cerebellum is important in sequence learning and may be less important in the execution of highly learned sequences.

Subsequent studies examined activations during a sequential finger-tapping task in which participants had to learn the correct sequence by trial and error. The first study compared activations between new sequences, learned sequences, and a resting control. Similar to the earlier studies, the performance of learned sequences with some degree of automaticity activated the contralateral (left) primary motor cortex, PMA, SMA, putamen, bilateral cerebellar hemispheres, vermis, deep cerebellar nuclei, anterior cingulate, parietal cortex, and ventrolateral thalamus. Of course, because sequence performance was compared with a resting condition, this network includes areas responsible for processes irrelevant to sequence learning. When compared to rest, the performance of new sequences showed, in addition to these areas, increases in prefrontal cortex and more extensive activation of the cerebellum. When compared to the practiced sequence directly, learning of a new sequence produced activations in the bilateral PMA, cerebellum, anterior cingulate, prefrontal cortex, and medial thalamus. It seems likely that the requirement that the participant infer the correct sequence on the basis of feedback was responsible for the activation of the anatomically interconnected prefrontal–anterior cingulate–medial thalamus network. However, as we will see later, it is possible that the cerebellum also contributes to error detection and correction.

In another revealing manipulation, participants were asked to pay attention to their finger movements while performing a highly learned sequence. Attention resulted in the reactivation of the anterior cingulate and prefrontal cortex. By comparing learning of a new sequence with a control condition that required a similar level of attention and similar decision and motor processes, the researchers found activation of the caudate nucleus and cerebellum. This result indicates that these two structures may be important in learning a new sequence, as opposed to other task-related processes. Together, these studies suggest that the basal ganglia and cerebellum, and possibly the PMA, are involved in skill learning, whereas anterior cingulate and prefrontal areas are involved in attention and higher level control processes.

A more controlled version of the tapping task is the Repeated Sequence Task. In this task, participants see a cue appear above one of four squares, and they must touch that square as quickly as possible. As a particular sequence appears more frequently, participants become faster in pressing the appropriate squares. The faster responses for the learned sequence indicate that implicit learning of the sequence has occurred, even though participants have no explicit, declarative memory for the sequence.

Doyon and co-workers, using this paradigm, compared PET activation among several conditions, including different amounts of learning, and included a condition in which subjects were given explicit knowledge of the sequence prior to scanning. Performance on highly learned versus random sequences resulted in increased activation in the right (ipsilateral) ventral striatum, right cerebellum, bilateral anterior cingulate, right medial parietal cortex, and right extrastriate cortex. Decreases were found in the ventrolateral frontal, frontopolar, and lateral parietal cortices, all on the right side. As with previous studies, basal ganglia activity increased when performance was highly learned. These changes are consistent with animal models suggesting a role for the basal ganglia in the performance of movement sequences.

When compared with newly learned sequences, highly learned sequences showed increased activity in the cerebellum, suggesting a role for the cerebellum in sequence performance or in the development of automaticity. This finding contrasts with previous sequence learning studies, which found that cerebellar activity decreases as performance becomes automatic. Thus, further research is necessary to investigate the role of the cerebellum. It is possible that the cerebellum has multiple roles and plays a part both in initial learning and in later retrieval of sequences. An alternative explanation for cerebellar activity in the learned–unlearned comparisons in these studies is that the cerebellum is required for speeding up movements while maintaining a criterion level of accuracy. In the early stages of training, it may be difficult to keep movements speedy, resulting in cerebellar activation that decreases as it becomes easier to perform the task at the requisite speed. This hypothesis highlights the fact that neuroimaging results may be interpreted in multiple ways.

Newly and highly learned sequences in the Repeated Sequence Test were also examined before and after participants were given explicit knowledge of the sequence. Explicit knowledge of highly learned sequences relative to implicit performance decreased activation in the right (ipsilateral) cerebellum and increased activation in the right ventrolateral frontal cortex. Explicit versus implicit knowledge of newly learned sequences resulted in increased activation of the right cerebellum and left ventrolateral frontal cortex.

The sequence learning studies reviewed here implicate the cerebellum and basal ganglia in initial learning and automatization of new skills. Three studies found significant activity in the basal ganglia with practiced, but not novel, sequences. Two other studies found basal ganglia activity in newly learned sequences, one relative to a resting control and the other relative to a free-selection tapping task. The cerebellum appears to be involved in early learning of the sequence, but it is also active during skilled performance relative to rest. Its activity may increase as participants gain skill, if that skill involves making speeded responses to visual cues.

Notably, none of these PET studies showed changes in the primary motor cortex as a function of practice. However, some researchers have shown that skill learning produces nonmonotonic changes in the strength and spread of activation within the primary motor cortex. These researchers scanned participants learning one of two similar finger-tapping sequences using fMRI. Initially, a habituation effect to sequence performance was found: activity in the primary motor cortex was lower when it was performed later in the scanning block. After 30 min of practice, activity in the primary motor cortex was higher when it was performed later in the scanning block, but only for practiced sequences, possibly reflecting fast learning processes that set up later consolidation of a new motor sequence. After 4 weeks of daily practice, more areas in the primary motor cortex were recruited during performance of the learned sequence, showing that practice resulted in a true expansion of the cortical area recruited in the primary motor cortex.

C. Learning Sensory–Motor Associations

What are strikingly missing from analyses of sequence learning, but apparent in other motor learning tasks, are changes in activation of the premotor and supplementary motor cortices. Studies of sequential finger tapping primarily require the learning of associations between movements that form a sequence. This kind of learning may be fundamentally different from learning that requires improvement in coordination or learning an altogether new motor movement. In addition, the finger-tapping task requires a series of internally generated movements rather than movements elicited by sensory cues. We have already seen that learning in the Repeated Sequence Test, which involves visuomotor associative learning, may produce a different pattern of cerebellar activity than learning of internally generated movement sequences. Perhaps examination of nonsequence motor learning, including studies of rotor pursuit, trajectory movements, joystick movements, and maze tracing, may help resolve discrepancies.

Rotor pursuit involves maintaining contact between a hand-held stylus and a target moving in a circular pattern. Several studies have compared rotor pursuit with visual tracking of the stylus, identifying changes due to skill learning of the appropriate hand movement. An initial study showed increases with practice in the primary motor cortex, SMA, and pulvinar nucleus. In a later study, PET scans over 2 days of learning revealed a similar pattern of activation on day 1, this time including practice-related changes in the ipsilateral cerebellum, cingulate, and inferior parietal cortex. On day 2, after an extensive practice period, the rotor pursuit–visual tracking subtraction revealed changes in the putamen and parietal cortex bilaterally and the left (contralateral) PMA. Improvement on the task was correlated with increased activity in the premotor, prefrontal, and cingulate areas and decreased activity in visual processing areas.

An opposite pattern of changes in the PMA and SMA were observed in a series of studies of maze tracing. In the maze-tracing task, participants practiced tracing cutout maze patterns with their eyes closed. Tracing a novel maze with the right hand in a clockwise pattern (relative to a control) resulted in increases in the right PMA and left cerebellum. Practice diminished both of these loci of activity: PET scanning after 10 min of practice produced increases in SMA and decreases in the right PMA and left cerebellum. Contrary to expectations, training affected activity in the ipsilateral cerebrum and

contralateral cerebellum. A follow-up study examined maze tracing with the left hand in a counter-clockwise pattern and, strikingly, produced the same results. A third study confirmed that only the primary motor cortex and anterior cerebellum showed activation depending on which hand was used, suggesting that learning and performance in the maze-tracing task require an abstract representation of movements and patterns not directly tied to motor activity.

Contradictory effects of practice in similar tasks, such as that found in PMA and SMA in the studies reviewed earlier, may reflect something of the underlying functions of premotor brain regions. It has been suggested that the SMA is active in the internal generation of responses, and PMA is preferentially active when responses are contingent upon sensory cues. That distinction can be applied to neuroimaging studies of human skill learning. In the rotor pursuit studies, learning of a new motor skill resulted in increased activity in SMA. After the movement was automatic, PMA and basal ganglia were activated in adapting the movement to the motion of the stylus. In the maze studies, initial performance relied heavily on somatosensory feedback from the cutout maze, and so the PMA was heavily recruited. After the maze was well-learned, a coordinated, internally generated movement could be used to trace the maze successfully without reliance on sensory feedback. This type of internally generated movement appears to be the domain of the SMA. Consistent with this view, neuropsychological evidence shows that patients with PMA damage are impaired in sensory-cued motor learning.

A study in which participants had to write the letter "R" found increases in the right PMA and right parietal cortex, possibly indicating enhanced attention to sensory feedback. Again, the activation was unexpectedly ipsilateral to the hand used. When participants wrote the letter as quickly as possible, a network including the left primary motor, PMA, SMA, and right putamen was activated. These experiments also compared writing novel ideograms with the right hand to a baseline in which participants watched the figures being drawn. Novel ideograms, as compared to baseline, activated the left primary motor cortex and right cerebellum. Practiced ideograms minus baseline activated the right PMA, left SMA, and right cerebellum. Once again, cerebellar activity appeared during the initial learning and automatization phases of new visuomotor patterns, but was not apparent when writing the letter "R," a highly practiced ideogram.

These studies show increases in PMA when sensory feedback or external cues are critical for task performance. Right PMA increases appear to be modulated by task demands, e.g., asking participants to be accurate, and independent of the hand used. In the study of unilateral two-ball rotation mentioned earlier, positive correlations were found between unilateral PMA activity during movements of either hand and skill improvement for the ipsilateral hand. Skill improvement was measured during nonscanning intervals by comparing the maximum rotation speed of the balls just after the first scan and just before the last scan. The strongest correlation was between right PMA activity and skill improvement for the right hand. Correlations between left PMA and skill improvement for the left hand were also positive and significant.

The cerebellum appears to play a particular role in the learning of new visuomotor associations. In a classic study, participants made joystick movements to align a cursor with a visual target in one of three joystick–cursor mappings: normal mapping, reversed mapping in which joystick movements caused the cursor to move in the opposite direction, and random mapping with no relationship between joystick and cursor movement. The PET camera in this study was centered on the cerebellum to allow maximum sensitivity to changes in this structure. When the mapping between joystick movements and cursor movements was reversed, cerebellar activity was high during initial learning and decreased as performance improved. When the mapping between joystick movements and cursor movements was random, no learning occurred and cerebellar activity remained high. The authors concluded that the cerebellum contributes to visuomotor skill learning by participating in the detection and correction of errors. It should be noted, in closing, that the cerebellar contribution to skill learning may be primarily in sensory–motor association tasks. Patients with cerebellar atrophy can improve on some motor skill tasks, but they fail to coordinate and adapt movements to environmental contexts.

D. Learning Perceptual Skills

Research on the psychophysics of perceptual learning suggests that long-term learning of skills is not limited to motor areas. This research suggests three striking findings: learning to detect a visual stimulus is specific to a retinal location, it only occurs if the stimulus is behaviorally relevant, and effects of learning remain robust after nearly 3 years without practice.

Although there has been relatively little neuroimaging research on perceptual learning, the research that has been conducted is illuminating. Perhaps the first study was an fMRI experiment of mirror reading. Participants viewed words and matched nonwords printed backward and decided whether the stimulus was a real word. Improvement in mirror reading is still detectable after 2 months of practice, and changes in performance are evident after 1 year without practice. The researchers compared mirror reading with normal reading and practiced, mirror words with unpracticed ones. Mirror reading compared to normal reading produced increases in blood flow in a number of areas, including the medial and lateral occipital cortex, right superior parietal cortex, bilateral fusiform gyrus, pulvinar, and cerebellum, particularly on the right side. Decreases were found in nearby regions of some of the same areas, including the medial occipital and right superior parietal cortices, as well as in the precuneus and bilateral middle–superior temporal gyrus. The occipital, fusiform, and pulvinar areas form an anatomically interconnected network associated with visual processing, object recognition, and visual attention. The authors suggested that these activations were due to visual transformation of the letters in unpracticed mirror reading.

With practice, mirror reading activation increased in the precuneus, left superior parietal cortex and fusiform, and right cerebellum and superior temporal gyrus. Decreases were found in a number of areas, including left lingual gyrus, bilateral occipital cortex, right cerebellum, superior and inferior parietal, inferior temporal, and pulvinar. The deactivation of right superior parietal cortex and occipital cortex could reflect decreased involvement of attention, which is associated with right parietal activation in a number of studies, or it could result from a decreased need to rely on visuospatial transformations. Increases in the left fusiform gyrus, activated in at least one other letter recognition study and in studies of object recognition, could reflect a shift to direct letter recognition processes. Overall, the results are consistent with a shift in strategy from sensory transformation to direct recognition of mirror words.

E. Implicit Memory

All of the studies of skill learning discussed earlier involved both explicit and implicit memory for motor activity. Although procedural in nature, in most of the tasks participants were allowed to develop conscious recognition of the sequences and movements to be learned. In one study, explicit awareness of a sequence was associated with changes in the cerebellum, ventrolateral frontal cortex, and medial frontal cortex. The remainder of the changes with skill learning, found prominently in parts of the cerebellum, primary motor cortex, SMA, PMA, and basal ganglia, presumably reflect changes in procedural motor processes: the kind you can do, but cannot describe—and, if you are amnesiac, may not remember that you ever learned.

Implicit memory is not limited to motor and perceptual learning, however. Exposure to words, pictures, faces, and other stimuli influences later processing of this information, even though subjects may not remember any of the trained items. This unconscious memory is independent of explicit recollection, meaning that the amount of explicit memory one has for a stimulus does not predict the amount of implicit memory. Also, implicit memory is not affected by depth of encoding as is explicit memory. The two forms of memory appear to be separate species that operate independently of one another. Neuroimaging results support the conclusion that explicit memory and implicit memory are mediated by separate circuits in the brain—explicit memory by the hippocampus, prefrontal cortex, and related circuitry, and implicit memory by perceptual areas similar to those discussed in the previous section.

One of the most common ways to study implicit retrieval is the word stem completion task. In the encoding phase of the task, participants are given a list of words and asked to make some judgment, semantic or otherwise, about the words. Subsequently, the participants are given a list of incomplete words, such as the first three letters, and asked to complete the fragments with whatever word comes to mind. If the fragments match words that they viewed before, participants are more likely to complete the stem with the previously viewed word, whether or not they consciously remember it.

Daniel Schacter and co-workers predicted that, when only implicit memory is involved in a task, stem completion will not activate the hippocampus, the structure critical to explicit episodic memory. They asked participants to count the number of "T" junctions in a list of words and compared activation during stem completion of words from the list with novel words. Participants did not explicitly remember the words, but their performance showed priming effects. Their PET scans revealed no hippocampal activation, but did show decreases in extrastriate (visual) cortex. In another study, Schacter *et al.* compared stem completion when participants had encoded words deeply (when they were required to make semantic judgments) or superficially (when they counted T junctions). Explicit memory and hippocampal activation during stem completion were greater for the deeply processed words. Other studies have replicated this basic finding with object naming and categorization tasks. Taken together, these results indicate a dissociation between explicit and implicit memory; explicit memory involves the activation of hippocampal structures, whereas implicit memory involves the deactivation of posterior neocortex.

Studies in other domains of semantic knowledge, such as object categorization and object naming, show similar priming-related reductions in activation. One explanation of the decrease in activation is that repeated presentations lead to more efficient perceptual processing and lower levels of activation. However, in an auditory word stem completion task studied by Schacter and colleagues, auditory presentation of words and auditory stem completion produced the same regional cerebral blood flow (rCBF) decreases in bilateral extrastriate cortex, as well as decreases in the right anterior medial prefrontal cortex, right angular gyrus, and precuneus. Thus, priming effects on the extrastriate cortex appear to be modality-independent.

VII. SOME CONCLUDING REMARKS

There has been remarkable progress in the study of memory during the last half of the twentieth century. The development of neuroimaging techniques has contributed in no small part to this progress. These techniques have provided a source of evidence about the relationship between brain structure and psychological function that complements evidence from the study of human patients with brain injury, behavioral evidence from normal human subjects, and evidence from animal models. Taken together, these sources of evidence have sketched the outlines of complex memory systems. These systems, in their interaction, form a seamless whole capable of dealing with a variety of cognitive problems. Our memory apparatus has multiple components (working memory, long-term memory), multiple representations of information in different formats (e.g., verbal versus spatial), multiple retrieval schemes (explicit versus implicit), multiple circuitries, and multiple processes (encoding, retention, and retrieval). We are far from getting our arms around a complete description of this system, but continued use of the full array of investigative tools promises much new progress in the current millenium.

See Also the Following Articles

INFORMATION PROCESSING • MEMORY DISORDERS, ORGANIC • MEMORY, EXPLICIT AND IMPLICIT • MEMORY NEUROBIOLOGY • MEMORY, OVERVIEW • NERVE CELLS AND MEMORY • NEUROIMAGING • SEMANTIC MEMORY • SHORT-TERM MEMORY • WORKING MEMORY

Acknowledgment

Preparation of this manuscript was supported in part by a grant from the National Institute of Mental Health to the University of Michigan.

Suggested Reading

Anderson, J. R. (1995). *Learning and Memory: An Integrated Approach*. Wiley, New York.

Baddeley, A. (1990). *Human Memory Theory and Practice*. Allyn and Bacon, Boston.

Campbell, R., and Conway, M. A. (1995). *Broken Memories*. Blackwell, Cambridge.

Gordon, B. (1995). *Memory: Remembering and Forgetting in Everyday Life*. Mastermedia, New York.

Reisberg, D. (1997). *Cognition*. W. W. Norton, New York.

Schacter, D. (1996). *Searching for Memory: The Brain, the Mind, and the Past*. Basic Books, New York.

Schacter, D. (2001). *The Seven Sins of Memory: How the Mind Remembers and Forgets*. Houghton Mifflin, Boston.

Squire, L. R., and Kandel, E. R. (2000). *Memory*. Scientific American Library, New York.

Vallar, G., and Shallice, T. (1990). *Neuropsychological Impairments of Short-Term Memory*. Cambridge University Press, UK.

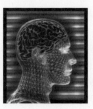

Memory, Overview

JOHN A. LUCAS

Mayo Clinic

I. Classification of Memory

II. Neurobiological Bases of Memory

III. Neuroanatomy of Memory

IV. Summary

GLOSSARY

Alzheimer's disease A gradually progressive degenerative dementia of insidious onset that is characterized by early, prominent memory dysfunction and loss of the ability to perform activities of daily living.

amnesia Loss of memory.

dementia A behavioral description of any acquired disorder that involves amnesia plus impairment of at least one other cognitive ability, such as language, visuospatial function, attention, or problem solving. The degree of cognitive impairment must be severe enough to interfere with social functioning, occupational functioning, or activities of daily living.

Korsakoff syndrome An amnesic disorder resulting from severe thiamine deficiency, most often seen in patients with chronic alcoholism.

neocortex In evolutionary terms, the newest, most highly evolved region of the brain, containing six neuronal layers and forming the outer surface of the brain.

Memory is the ability to maintain previously learned information within an internal storage system so that it may be accessed and used at a later time. Memory may be observed in overt behavior, such as when a student recalls information from previous readings in order to answer questions on a test, or in less readily observable events, such as neuronal development and change. This article reviews the behavioral components of memory as well as the neurobiological bases and underlying neuroanatomical substrates believed to be important to memory functioning.

I. CLASSIFICATION OF MEMORY

Memory is not a unitary construct but instead reflects a number of distinct cognitive abilities that can be categorized along a number of different dimensions. For example, one can characterize memory based on the amount of time that elapses between presentation and recall of information (e.g., short- vs long-term memory) or the nature of the information that is remembered (e.g., visual vs verbal). Memory behaviors can also be characterized by task demands (e.g., recall vs recognition) or by the cognitive processes that underlie these demands (e.g., retrieval vs retention). These and other conceptual divisions of memory are reviewed in this section.

A. Short- and Long-Term Memory

In 1890, William James distinguished between memory that endured for a very brief time and memory that lasted after the experience had been "dropped from consciousness." The former, known as short-term (or primary) memory, refers to one's ability to recall material immediately after it is presented or following uninterrupted rehearsal. The latter, known as long-term (or secondary) memory, refers to the ability to remember information at a later time without the need for intervening rehearsal.

Short-term memory is of limited capacity, holding an average of seven pieces of information at any one time. This information can be maintained for up to several minutes, but it is lost or replaced by new information if not sustained by active rehearsal. A common example of short-term memory is the act of looking up an unknown telephone number in a directory and dialing that number. The number is held briefly in short-term memory as one looks away from the directory and dials the number. If the telephone is across the room, one can maintain the number in short-term memory by repeating it continuously until it is dialed. Soon after dialing, however, the number is usually forgotten.

In contrast, long-term memory has an extraordinarily large capacity, with the potential for holding information indefinitely without the need for continued rehearsal. For example, one can recall his or her own telephone number, as well as a myriad of other facts, experiences, and personal information, without needing to reference an external source or rehearse the information continuously.

The clinical significance of the distinction between short- and long-term memory has been exemplified in patients with amnesic disorders. One of the most famous case studies in the neuropsychological literature describes a patient (H.M.) who became amnesic following surgical treatment for epilepsy. After surgery, H.M. was unable to retain any new information that he learned, such as the names of new staff in his doctor's office or information that he read each day in the newspaper. His ability to repeat information immediately following presentation or hold onto new information with active rehearsal, however, was normal. This dissociation underscores the distinct nature of the processes required to create new short- and long-term memories.

A second notable dissociation of memory functions demonstrated by H.M. was that although he was unable to form new long-term memories, he could recall previously learned information normally. This discrepancy suggests that the cognitive processes required to retain and access stored information differ from those required to encode new information.

B. Encoding, Retention, and Retrieval

Encoding, retention, and retrieval refer, respectively, to the processes by which information is acquired and transformed into a stored mental representation, maintained over time without active rehearsal, and brought back into consciousness from storage. Successful encoding occurs when an individual demonstrates acquisition of more information than would normally be possible to hold in short-term memory alone. For example, if someone is presented a list of 16

words, he or she might be able to recall only 6 or 7 of those words after seeing the list for the first time (e.g., a normal amount of information that can be held in short-term memory). If the list is repeated, however, a neurologically intact individual will remember increasingly more words with each subsequent repetition. The ability to remember more words than could normally be held in short-term storage indicates that the information has been encoded into a more permanent, long-term storage.

Once information is encoded, it must be retained for later use and accessed when needed. Failure to remember encoded information may indicate a problem with either retention or retrieval mechanisms. These are distinct memory processes that can be distinguished by examining the relationship between free recall and recognition. Free recall of information places maximum demands on retrieval processes because an individual must actively search memory to find and access the information. Recognizing the correct answer among multiple choices, however, is a less difficult memory task because it minimizes search and retrieval demands. If information is retained successfully but cannot be retrieved, free recall will be impaired but recognition of the correct information will be disproportionately better. In contrast, if information is not retained in long-term storage, both recall and recognition of information will be equally poor. The differences in memory performances among individuals with selective deficits in encoding, retention, and retrieval are presented in Fig. 1.

C. Retroactive and Proactive Interference

Memory can be disrupted by events or information encountered at approximately the time of encoding. This disruption is known as an "interference effect."

1. Retroactive Interference

Retroactive interference (RI) refers to the disrupting effect that new learning has on the ability to recall previously learned information. For example, a student studying several text chapters for an exam will be able to recall a greater amount of information from a chapter that he or she has just finished reading than from a chapter that was read earlier in the evening. In this example, information read in the most recent chapter interferes with memory for information from previous chapters.

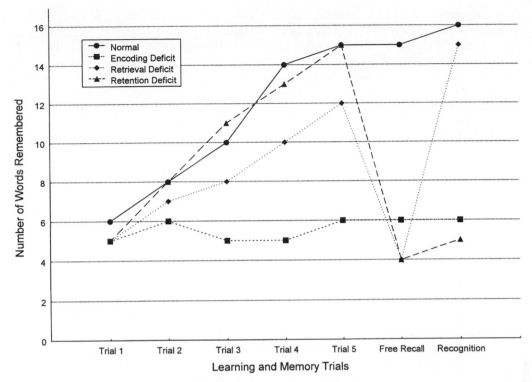

Figure 1 Memory test profiles expected in neurologically intact individuals and patients with primary deficits of encoding, retrieval, or retention. A list of 16 words is presented over five learning trials, with memory for the list assessed immediately after each trial. Memory for the word list is again assessed after a 20-min delay by means of free recall and recognition. Compared to individuals with no memory disorder, patients with encoding problems do not recall more words with repeated exposure to information. Patients with retrieval problems show poor delayed memory when assessed by free recall but normal memory when assessed by recognition. Patients with retention problems do not benefit from recognition testing.

The effect of RI is a function of the amount of new information encountered and the degree to which the interfering information and target information are similar. If a large amount of similar material is presented between initial learning and eventual recall of target information, recall will be poorer than if small amounts of dissimilar information had been presented during the intervening time.

2. Proactive Interference

Proactive interference (PI) occurs when information presented at an earlier time interferes with one's ability to learn and recall new information. For example, suppose one is asked to learn several lists of different words. After the first list is presented and memory for the words is assessed, a new list of words is presented and memory for the new words is assessed. As more lists are presented, memory for the new words declines because previously learned words produce interference.

As with RI, the effect of PI on recall also increases with the amount of interfering information and the degree of similarity to the target information. If one were presented five successive word lists, the effect of PI would be greater after the fifth list was presented than after the second list was presented. In addition, if the lists all contain similar words, such as animal names, memory for each new list will be worse than if each list contained a variety of different words.

One interesting aspect of PI is that presenting dissimilar interfering information can facilitate memory. Using the previous example, suppose a group of individuals are asked to learn four successive word lists, all of which contain different animal names. Now suppose a fifth trial is given. Half of the individuals are presented another list of animal names, whereas the other half are presented a list of words belonging to an unrelated category (e.g., clothing). Results of such an experiment are presented in Fig. 2. Individuals who are presented more animal names on trial 5 continue to demonstrate PI, whereas those presented with a

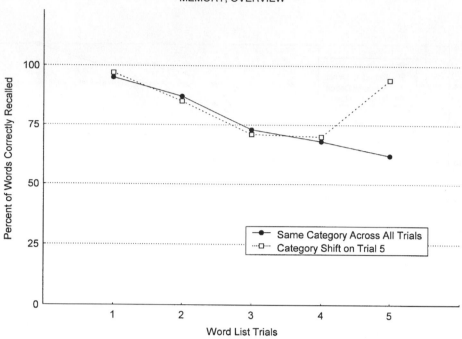

Figure 2 An illustration of proactive interference (PI). On four consecutive trials, study participants are asked to recall different lists of words from the same semantic category (e.g., animals). The effect of PI can be seen in the decline in performance over these trials. On the fifth trial, participants who are asked to recall another set of words from the same category continue to demonstrate PI, whereas those who are asked to recall words from a new semantic category (e.g., clothing) show improvement, known as "release" from PI.

dissimilar list of words demonstrate improved recall. This phenomenon is commonly known as "release" from PI.

D. Anterograde and Retrograde Memory

Anterograde memory is the ability to learn new information and to form new memories from a given moment forward. In contrast, retrograde memory is the ability to recall or recognize information or events that occurred prior to a specific moment in time.

Anterograde and retrograde amnesias are often seen in patients with brain injuries. Patients who are injured in motor vehicle accidents, for example, may not recall the events leading up to the accident (i.e., a retrograde deficit) or the events that occurred immediately following the accident (i.e., an anterograde deficit). The degree of anterograde and retrograde amnesia following a head injury is highly correlated with the severity of brain damage sustained. Anterograde and retrograde amnesias can also occur independently. It is common for patients with certain disorders to have intact memory for past events but poor ability to lay down new memories. The reverse pattern, however, is rare. Individuals who present with complete loss of

past memories, personal history, and personal identity typically are found to have psychological rather than neurological disorders.

1. Recent and Remote Memory

The temporal dimension of retrograde memory is often divided into recent versus remote time frames. Recent memory typically refers to information that has been acquired within a relatively short period of time prior to an event (i.e., injury or time of evaluation), whereas remote memory refers to information about events or experiences that occurred years or decades before.

Patients with retrograde amnesia often demonstrate a temporal gradient in which memory for more recent events is disrupted to a greater extent than memory for remote events. This gradient is illustrated by the case of patient P.Z., a distinguished scientist who became amnesic secondary to alcoholic Korsakoff syndrome. Several years prior to the onset of his amnesic syndrome, P.Z. completed an autobiography. Investigators used this information to assess P.Z.'s memory for his own past life events. A temporally graded retrograde amnesic disorder is illustrated in Fig. 3, as this patient demonstrated significantly greater

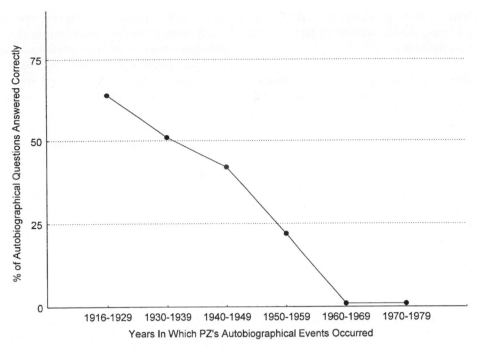

Figure 3 Temporally graded retrograde amnesia for autobiographical information as seen in patient PZ. Information from earlier decades in PZ's life was recalled better than information from recent decades.

impairment of memory for recent experiences and events compared to his memory for events from his early life.

E. Declarative versus Nondeclarative Memory

Declarative memory (also called explicit memory) refers to the acquisition of facts, experiences, and information about events. It is memory that is directly accessible to conscious awareness and thus can be "declared." In contrast, nondeclarative memory (also called implicit memory) refers to various forms of memory that are not directly accessible to consciousness. These include skill and habit learning, classical conditioning, priming, and other situations in which memory is expressed through performance or skill rather than through conscious recollection.

1. Types of Declarative Memory

a. Episodic Memory Episodic memory refers to information that is linked to a particular place and time. The ability to answer questions regarding what you ordered at a restaurant the night before or what information was presented at a meeting you attended are examples of episodic memory. That is, in order to recall the target information correctly, the individual must access information regarding the time and place the information was acquired.

b. Semantic Memory Semantic memory refers to general knowledge that is not linked to a particular temporal or spatial context. For example, defining the word "restaurant" or reciting the alphabet do not require knowledge of where or when that information was originally learned. Both episodic and semantic memories are declarative, however, in that retrieval of information is carried out explicitly, on a conscious level.

2. Types of Nondeclarative Memory

a. Procedural Memory Procedural memory is the process of retrieving information necessary to perform learned skills. These skills may be movement based, such as tying a shoe or riding a bicycle, or they may be perceptual in nature, such as learning to read mirror-reversed text. Although some aspects of skills can be declared, the skills are most often performed automatically, without conscious retrieval of information regarding the procedure. Amnesic patients such as H.M. can learn how to perform several complex tasks and will demonstrate normal retention of these new skills despite not being able to remember having ever learned how to do the tasks.

b. Conditioning Classical conditioning is one of the most basic forms of learning. A stimulus that naturally produces a certain response is paired with a neutral stimulus. After repeated pairings, the neutral stimulus alone will elicit the response. For example, a dog will naturally begin to salivate when presented food but not when presented with the sound of a bell ringing. If, however, a bell is rung repeatedly along with presentation of food, bell ringing alone will eventually produce salivation. As with procedural memory, patients with very poor declarative memory can demonstrate normal conditioning despite being unable to recall any of the training sessions that led to the conditioned response.

c. Priming Priming is the phenomenon by which prior exposure to information influences performance on later tasks even without conscious awareness. Priming effects are demonstrated by presenting a stimulus on one occasion and measuring its influence on performance on a subsequent occasion. Depending on the level of processing, priming can be perceptual or conceptual in nature. Perceptual priming occurs when exposure to the *form* of a stimulus influences later behavior. Two examples of perceptual processing are priming for picture identification and verbal information. In picture identification tasks, an individual looks at pictures or line drawings of different objects. Later, the individual is presented a series of "degraded" pictures (i.e., pictures in which much of the visual information is masked or missing) and asked to identify them. Identification of degraded pictures is faster and more accurate if the individual had previously seen the complete picture than when a novel picture is presented, indicating some form of memory for the information.

Perceptual priming for verbal information is commonly demonstrated in word-stem completion paradigms. During the first phase of the paradigm, individuals perform tasks designed to expose them to different words. For example, they may be shown a series of words and asked to judge whether each word has a "pleasant" or "unpleasant" connotation. Later, during the test phase, a new task is introduced in which the first three letters of words (i.e., word stems) are presented and the individuals are asked to complete each stem with the first word that comes to mind. Study participants are more likely to complete word stems with words seen during the exposure phase of the study, even if they are less commonly used words. For example, individuals who participate in the exposure task and see the word "motel" will be more likely to use that word to complete the word stem "mot__" than individuals who did not participate in the exposure task. When not previously exposed to the word "motel," the more common completion of this stem is the more frequently used word, "mother."

Although the previous example involves verbal stimuli, it is the perceptual aspect and not the meaning of those stimuli that is primed. When processing the meaning of a stimulus influences later behavior, *conceptual* priming has occurred. The exposure phase of conceptual priming experiments is similar to that of the word-stem completion paradigm. During the test phase, however, participants engage in word-association tasks or other activities that require the processing of word meanings. Suppose, for example, the word "crown" is presented during an exposure task. Individuals who were primed by exposure are more likely to respond with the word "crown" when asked for the first word that comes to mind in response to the word "king," whereas naive (i.e., "unprimed") study participants more often respond with the word "queen."

Patients with impaired episodic memory typically perform normally on perceptual priming tasks even though they have no memory of having previously seen the words or pictures that have been primed. Conceptual priming, however, may be reduced in patients with declarative memory dysfunction.

II. NEUROBIOLOGICAL BASES OF MEMORY

Early investigators hypothesized that learning and memory might occur through growth of new neurons in the brain, much in the same way that strength is increased through growth of muscle tissue. It soon became clear, however, that the central nervous system was limited in its ability to generate new cells. Investigators eventually showed that existing neurons possessed the ability to form new processes and connections, and that learning and memory reflected modification of neuronal signal processing, interneuronal communication, and functional relationships among brain systems. There is now a rapidly growing and exciting literature suggesting that generation of new neurons may indeed be possible in adulthood. Although this avenue of exploration holds much promise, to date evidence suggests that neuronal modification remains the primary mechanism underlying memory formation.

A. Memory as Change of Synaptic Structure and Efficacy

A complete discussion of neuronal function and synaptic transmission of information is beyond the scope of this article. Briefly, a synapse is a functional juxtaposition of two or more neurons (Fig. 4). When a neuron is stimulated to a sufficient degree, chemicals known as neurotransmitters are released from its axon terminal into the microscopic space that separates it from its neighboring neuron. The presence of neuro-

transmitters within this region produces characteristic changes in the membranes of neighboring neurons.

Each neuron in the brain interconnects with many other neurons in this fashion, forming a series of networks and feedback loops. In the first half of the 20th century, D. O. Hebb proposed that psychologically important events such as memory were manifestations of the flow of activity within a given network of neurons that were acting together as a single unit. He suggested that when an event or experience caused a set of neurons to be excited together, the synapses involved in that pathway became functionally connected.

Although some of the specific neuronal mechanisms that Hebb proposed were not supported by subsequent research, the basic hypothesis of memory as structural

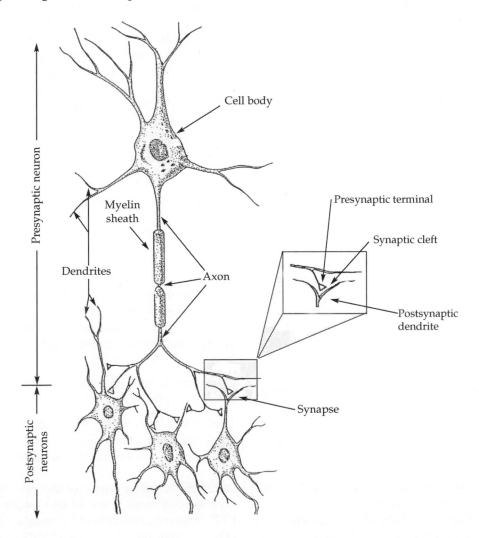

Figure 4 Illustration of the basic structure of neurons and neuronal synapses. Modified from Kandel, E. "Principles of Neural Science," 3rd ed. (1992), The McGraw-Hill Companies. Reproduced with permission of The McGraw-Hill Companies.

and functional change involving neuronal activity and synaptic transmission has endured. Research has shown that when animals are trained to perform specific tasks or are exposed to enriched environments, new synapses grow and preexisting synaptic connections become better developed. Synaptic change in response to new learning is observed in both young and adult animals and can occur subsequent to a single learning experience.

B. Neuronal Processes Underlying Short- and Long-Term Memory

A distinction can be made between the neuronal processes underlying short- versus long-term memory. Although temporary changes in the dynamics of neuronal functioning can maintain information for up to several minutes, more permanent structural changes are believed to be necessary to retain information for days or longer.

1. Neuronal Processes Underlying Short-Term Memory

Studies show that a neuron's function can be modified by intense activity. High-frequency stimulation by a presynaptic neuron, for example, tends to increase the responsiveness and efficiency of postsynaptic membranes, a phenomenon known as potentiation. Some neurons can demonstrate increased responsiveness lasting for several minutes to more than 1 hr after active stimulation has ceased. This temporary increase in synaptic effectiveness is known as posttetanic potentiation (PTP) and reflects one possible way that recently learned information can be remembered. PTP may cause neurons activated during learning to remain active for a brief time after learning has ceased, thus allowing that information to remain available.

Another possible mechanism by which neuronal activity associated with recently learned information may be maintained for a brief period of time is by means of a feedback loop. Specifically, excitatory input from exposure to information could theoretically be maintained after active input ceases if neurons within a closed loop excite each other (Fig. 5). Excitatory neuronal feedback systems such as these are known as reverberatory circuits.

The amount of time that elapses before information in short-term memory degrades is believed to be a function of PTP strength and/or the level of neuronal excitement in reverberatory circuits caused by the

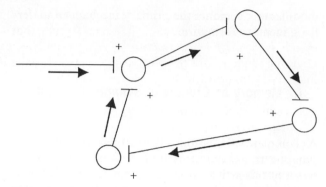

Figure 5 Schematic of a reverberatory circuit. Neuronal responses are prolonged by reexcitation of excitatory neurons.

learning experience. More intense changes in these neuronal dynamics are typically associated with more persistent memory, whereas weaker changes are associated with more rapid forgetting. Are short- and long-term memories, then, different ends of a single graded continuum of neuronal dynamics, with long term-memory reflecting a chronic state of persisting neuronal activity?

If both types of memory relied on dynamic mechanisms such as PTP and reverberatory circuits, then interrupting those dynamics should interfere with both short- and long-term memory. Studies of patients undergoing electroconvulsive therapy (ECT), however, show that this is not the case. ECT is a treatment for medically refractory depression that works by delivering low-voltage electric current to the brain. Neuronal activity in the brain is briefly "short-circuited" by this procedure, thus interfering with all electrical activity, including PTP and activity within reverberatory circuits. Following recovery from ECT, patients demonstrate memory loss for information immediately preceding treatment; however, memories in long-term storage remain intact.

2. Neuronal Processes Underlying Long-Term Memory

The ability to encode information into a more permanent long-term storage system is believed to be a function of long-term potentiation (LTP). LTP is similar to PTP in that high-intensity stimulation increases the effectiveness of the neuronal synapse. LTP is much more powerful and longer lasting than PTP, however, and it cannot be produced by activation of only a single presynaptic neuron in a single pathway. Instead, a minimum number of inputs must be present to produce an effect.

Another difference between LTP and PTP is that LTP is associated with the activation of genes that direct the growth and structure of synapses. These neuronal changes are believed to underlie long-term memory formation and are not observed in short-term memory.

It is unlikely that every neuronal synapse is modified by each learned experience, nor is it likely that each memory corresponds to changes in a single neuron in a one-to-one fashion. So where in the brain are long-term memories formed and stored? The first neurons to be discovered that were capable of LTP were found in the hippocampus and surrounding structures, although it has since been recognized that neurons in other brain areas also demonstrate LTP. Similarly, behavioral studies of memory function and dysfunction in humans and animals indicate that a number of different brain regions are important for memory.

III. NEUROANATOMY OF MEMORY

The cumulative literature of learning and memory in humans and nonhuman animals provides a broad outline of the major neuroanatomical structures and connections believed to be important for memory functioning. In the following sections, the neuroanatomical substrates of declarative and nondeclarative memory are reviewed.

A. Neuroanatomical Correlates of Declarative Memory

Several brain regions are believed to be important to encoding and storage of long-term declarative memories. These include structures in the medial temporal lobes, medial diencephalon, basal forebrain, and prefrontal cortex. In addition, certain subcortical nuclei and white matter pathways are important for retrieving acquired information from storage. The gross anatomy of the lateral and medial surfaces of the brain is illustrated in Figs. 6 and 7, whereas some of the more important structures related to memory are illustrated in Fig. 8.

1. The Temporal Lobes

Recall from the beginning of this article the case of H.M., who suffered a profound long-term memory

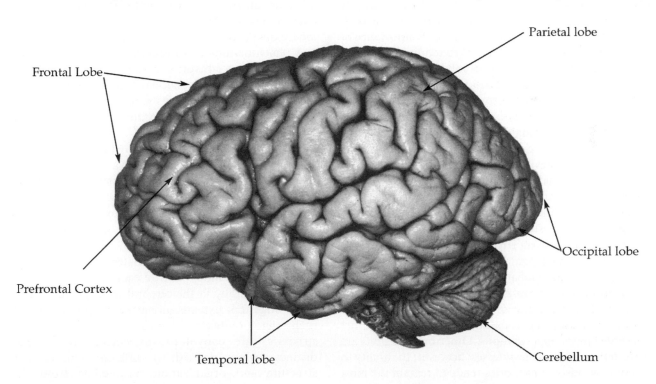

Figure 6 Lateral surface of the brain. From "Structure of the Human Brain: A Photographic Atlas," 3rd ed. by S. J. DeArmond, M. M. Fusco, and M. M. Dewey, copyright 1974, 1976, 1989 by Oxford University Press, Inc. Used by permission of Oxford University Press, Inc.

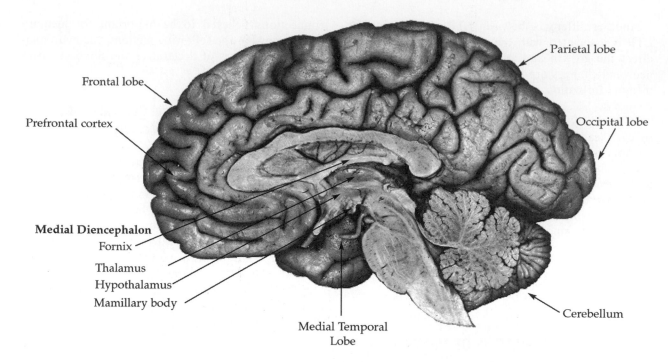

Figure 7 Medial surface of the brain. From "Structure of the Human Brain: A Photographic Atlas," 3rd ed. by S. J. DeArmond, M. M. Fusco, and M. M. Dewey, copyright 1974, 1976, 1989 by Oxford University Press, Inc. Used by permission of Oxford University Press, Inc.

disorder following brain surgery. H.M.'s surgery involved the removal of the medial portion of both temporal lobes, thus demonstrating the importance of this region to long-term memory functioning. Patients with bilateral medial temporal lobe dysfunction typically demonstrate a global anterograde memory deficit. Although short-term memory for newly presented information may be unaffected, these patients cannot encode information into long-term storage. On memory tests, they demonstrate poor recall and poor recognition of previously presented information. Patients with medial temporal lobe damage, however, demonstrate intact memory for information that had been acquired prior to their injury, semantic knowledge, and previously learned skills. They also demonstrate normal priming effects.

Patients with bilateral medial temporal lobe dysfunction demonstrate global declarative memory deficits. The most common cause of this type of brain dysfunction is Alzheimer's disease, a progressive degenerative disorder in which neuropathological changes are first observed in the hippocampus. Other brain regions are affected as dementia progresses; however, the ability to form new episodic memories tends to remain the most significant behavioral symptom.

Patients with focal brain diseases such as stroke or tumors may demonstrate unilateral temporal lobe dysfunction. In such cases, material-specific memory deficits may be observed. Patients with left temporal lobe damage typically have more difficulty learning and remembering verbal material, such as stories or word lists, than nonverbal material, such as abstract geometric patterns, faces, tonal patterns, or the spatial location of objects. Patients with right temporal lobe damage tend to demonstrate the opposite pattern of memory impairment.

The temporal lobe is a relatively large brain region with several anatomically distinct areas. Most investigators agree, however, that the structures in the medial portion of the temporal lobes—specifically the hippocampus, its surrounding cortex, and the amygdala—are most important for memory (Figs. 8–10).

a. The Hippocampus and Related Structures The human hippocampus and associated cortices are located bilaterally in the cerebral hemispheres, forming a ridge that extends along the temporal horn of each lateral ventricle. As illustrated in Fig. 9, these structures are convoluted in shape, with several distinct regions defined by differences in cellular structure and organization. Proceeding from the collateral sulcus, the parahippocampal gyrus curves dorsally, transitioning into the subiculum, which curves medially and transitions into the hippocampus

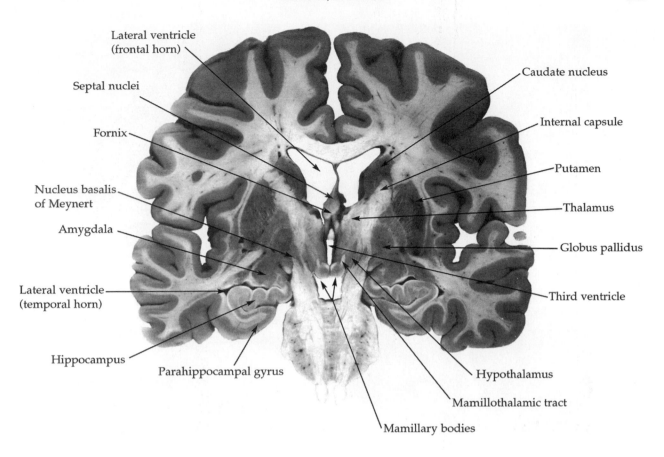

Lateral ventricle
(frontal horn)

Septal nuclei

Fornix

Nucleus basalis
of Meynert

Amygdala

Lateral ventricle
(temporal horn)

Hippocampus

Parahippocampal gyrus

Caudate nucleus

Internal capsule

Putamen

Thalamus

Globus pallidus

Third ventricle

Hypothalamus

Mamillothalamic tract

Mamillary bodies

Figure 8   Coronal section of the brain at the level of the anterior portion of the temporal lobes illustrating many of the structures believed to be important to memory. From "Structure of the Human Brain: A Photographic Atlas," 3rd ed. by S. J. DeArmond, M. M. Fusco, and M. M. Dewey, copyright 1974, 1976, 1989 by Oxford University Press, Inc. Used by permission of Oxford University Press, Inc.

proper. The hippocampus curves inward again, forming the hippocampal fissure. When the hippocampal fissure is opened, a narrow layer of cortex can be observed, known as the dentate gyrus. Axons arise from neurons comprising the hippocampus proper, converge to form the fimbria, and continue into the fornix, which is the major white matter tract out of the hippocampal formation.

b. The Amygdala   The amygdala is a collection of nuclei and specialized cortical areas situated in the dorsomedial portion of the temporal lobe rostral and dorsal to the tip of the temporal horn of the lateral ventricle (Fig. 8). Although early investigators believed the amygdala was primarily an olfactory structure, later studies revealed substantial inputs from brain regions responsible for processing many different types of sensory information, including visual, auditory, somatosensory, and autonomic stimuli. Outputs from the amygdala project to many brain regions believed to be important to memory,

including the hippocampal formation, thalamus, hypothalamus, prefrontal cortex, basal forebrain, and corpus striatum.

The amygdala is important to emotional, autonomic, reproductive, and feeding behaviors. Electrical stimulation of the amygdala in animals typically results in a constellation of aggressive and fear-related responses. Bilateral lesions to the amygdala in humans result in Klüver–Bucy syndrome, a disorder characterized by excessive docility, lack of fear response, hypersexuality, hyperorality, and changes in dietary habits.

c. Relative Contributions of the Hippocampus and Amygdala to Memory   Given the close proximity of the hippocampus to the amygdala, both structures are typically damaged in clinical cases of amnesia, thus leading to the question of which structure is more important to memory. The preponderance of case studies reported in the literature suggest that when damage is restricted to the hippocampus proper,

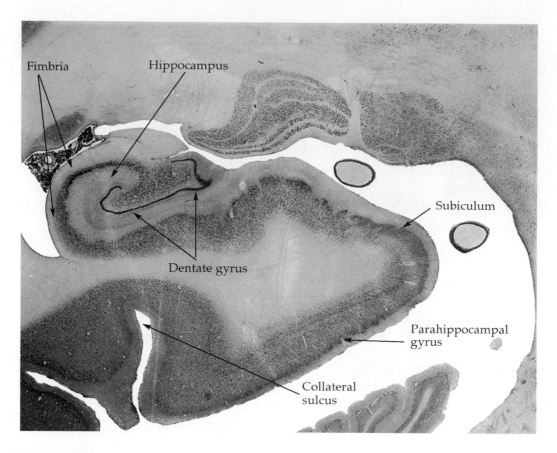

Figure 9   Illustration of a transverse section through the human hippocampal formation and parahippocampal gyrus. From "Structure of the Human Brain: A Photographic Atlas," 3rd ed. by S. J. DeArmond, M. M. Fusco, and M. M. Dewey, copyright 1974, 1976, 1989 by Oxford University Press, Inc. Used by permission of Oxford University Press, Inc.

fimbria, dentate gyrus, and subiculum, declarative memory impairment is less severe than when there is more radical loss of tissue.

Similar findings have been observed in nonhuman primates. When the hippocampal formation and its adjacent cortical region are lesioned, less severe declarative memory disturbance is observed than when the amygdala and its adjacent cortices are also involved. The most severe deficit is observed when the hippocampus, its adjacent cortical region, and the cortical region adjacent to the amygdala (i.e., the entorhinal and perirhinal cortices) are damaged. Damage to the amygdala, however, does not create any greater declarative memory deficit beyond what is caused by damage to the other three brain regions.

As discussed earlier, the amygdala is known to be important for processing sensory stimuli and information related to emotions. Studies show that the amygdala is important for remembering the emotional context of information. It is also implicated in certain types of nondeclarative memory, such as conditioning and evoking fear-related behaviors.

2. The Medial Diencephalon

The diencephalon is a region of several important nuclei located at the rostral part of the brain stem (Figs. 7 and 8). This region can be divided into four major areas: the epithalamus, thalamus, hypothalamus, and subthalamus. The divisions important to memory functioning include portions of the thalamus and hypothalamus. The thalamus is the largest subdivision of the diencephalon and is composed of several histopathologically distinct nuclei (Fig. 10). The hypothalamus lies below the thalamus and creates the floor of the third ventricle. It controls many autonomic, endocrine, and somatic functions and is composed of several distinct anatomical structures, including the mamillary bodies.

Severe amnesia results from damage to regions along the midline of the thalamus and hypothalamus.

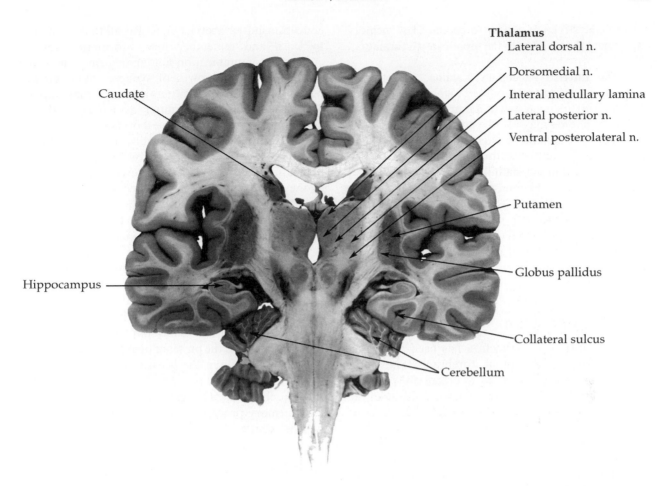

Figure 10 Coronal section of the brain at the level of the midbrain illustrating the thalamic nuclei. From "Structure of the Human Brain: A Photographic Atlas," 3rd ed. by S. J. DeArmond, M. M. Fusco, and M. M. Dewey, copyright 1974, 1976, 1989 by Oxford University Press, Inc. Used by permission of Oxford University Press, Inc.

There has been considerable controversy, however, concerning which of the many neuroanatomical structures and connections in this region must be damaged to cause memory dysfunction. The structures that have most often been implicated in diencephalic amnesia are the dorsomedial nucleus of the thalamus, the mamillary bodies of the hypothalamus, and the white matter (mamillothalamic) tract connecting these structures.

Patients who most commonly demonstrate diencephalic amnesia are individuals with Wernicke–Korsakoff syndrome. This disorder is caused by severe thiamine deficiency, often associated with chronic severe alcoholism. The first stage of this disorder involves an acute, global confusional state, oculomotor abnormalities, ataxia, and peripheral polyneuropathy. This stage is known as Wernicke's encephalopathy, during which the patient is in danger of suffering a potentially fatal midbrain hemorrhage unless treated immediately with thiamine. Approxi-

mately one-fourth of successfully treated patients regain the majority of their premorbid cognitive abilities. The remaining 75%, however, demonstrate severe, persistent anterograde and retrograde memory deficits.

a. The Mamillary Bodies and Dorsomedial Nucleus   The mamillary bodies and dorsomedial nucleus of the thalamus are both frequently damaged in Korsakoff syndrome. The few case studies in the literature of patients with naturally occurring lesions suggest that damage restricted to either the dorsomedial nucleus or the mamillary bodies is capable of interfering with memory.

In monkeys, lesions involving both the mamillary bodies and the dorsomedial thalamic nucleus result in memory deficits that are substantially more severe than those caused by lesions to either structure separately. Moreover, lesions to any single diencephalic structure appear to produce less memory impairment than lesions to the hippocampal formation.

b. The Internal Medullary Lamina A series of studies using an animal model of alcoholic Korsakoff syndrome in rats suggested that damage to the internal medullary lamina may also be critical in diencephalic amnesia. Diencephalic damage induced in rats via an experimentally controlled thiamine deficiency caused bilateral lesions in the mamillary bodies, dorsomedial nucleus of the thalamus, and internal medullary lamina of the thalamus. Rats with radio frequency-induced lesions to the internal medullary lamina demonstrated more similarities to rats with thiamine deficiency on measures of spatial memory than to rats with lesions to the mamillary bodies or midline thalamic nuclei.

3. The Basal Forebrain

Significant memory dysfunction has been associated with damage to the basal forebrain. The basal forebrain is a loose term used to describe the area of the brain superior to the optic chiasm. It includes the medial septal nuclei, nucleus accumbens, anterior hypothalamus, diagonal band of Broca, nucleus basalis of Meynert, and part of the prefrontal cortex (i.e., Brodmann's area 13). The structures within the basal forebrain project widely throughout the rest of the brain. The septal nuclei and nucleus basalis of Meynert (Fig. 8), for example, have extensive connections to and from the hippocampal formation, amygdala, and neocortex and are believed to be important to memory functioning.

Basal forebrain involvement in memory functioning is implicated primarily from the study of two patient groups: patients with ruptured aneurysm of the anterior communicating artery and patients with dementia due to Alzheimer's disease. The basal forebrain is perfused primarily by branches of the anterior communicating artery; thus, disturbances within this flow of circulation result in infarction and necrosis of basal forebrain tissue. Patients with stroke, hemorrhage, or damage to this area subsequent to aneurysm surgery often demonstrate declarative memory deficits.

Patients with Alzheimer's disease demonstrate marked degeneration within the basal forebrain as well as in the medial temporal lobes, as discussed earlier. The region of the basal forebrain most affected by Alzheimer's disease is the nucleus basalis of Meynert, a complex of neurons that produce the neurotransmitter acetylcholine. Recall that the ability to learn and remember new information reflects enhanced communication among neurons due to the development and growth of synapses. This growth occurs when neurotransmitters are in adequate supply. The primary neurotransmitter associated with the ability to encode and retain new declarative memories is acetylcholine. Thus, the depletion of acetylcholine in the brain caused by degeneration of neurons in the nucleus basalis of Meynert is believed to underlie part of the memory disorder associated with Alzheimer's disease.

In monkeys, combined lesions to the nucleus basalis of Meynert, medial septal nuclei, and diagonal band of Broca result in significant memory impairment. No significant memory impairment is noted, however, if each structure is lesioned separately. Thus, it appears that extensive damage to the basal forebrain, rather than specific damage to any given structure, is necessary to produce memory impairment. In light of these findings and the presence of extensive anatomical connections between the basal forebrain and medial temporal lobe structures, some have suggested that the basal forebrain most likely modulates medial temporal lobe memory processing but is not in and of itself a memory center.

4. The Prefrontal Cortex

Functional neuroimaging studies have found that activity in the anterior region of the prefrontal cortex (Figs. 6 and 7) increases when one attempts to retrieve previously learned information. Specifically, the prefrontal cortex is believed to play an important role in directing the attentional and organizational processes necessary for both encoding and retrieval of information. Disruption of these cognitive processes is associated with characteristic memory impairments, including source memory deficits, impaired temporal ordering, and confabulation.

Source memory and temporal ordering refer to the ability to recall the spatial and temporal contexts within which information was originally acquired. Patients with prefrontal cortical damage may recall factual information correctly, but they often have difficulty recalling where they learned the information. If they learned several pieces of information over a period of time, they may recall all the information adequately but be unable to report which information was learned first.

Another interesting behavioral consequence of prefrontal damage is the tendency to confabulate.

When patients with prefrontal damage cannot recall factual information, they often fabricate false information rather than indicate that they do not remember the correct information. This is different from lying because these patients have no desire or intent to deceive. Confabulation is believed to be a manifestation of source memory and temporal ordering deficits, coupled with poor self-monitoring abilities. When spatial and temporal contexts of information are missing it becomes very difficult to select accurate recollections from all the possible information that can be retrieved in a memory search. Patients with prefrontal damage, it is argued, simply choose one of the many alternatives retrieved from memory.

5. Subcortical Nuclei and White Matter

As illustrated in Figs. 8–10, two kinds of substances can be appreciated when the brain is cut—one light and one dark. The dark substance is known as gray matter and contains neuronal bodies, dendrites, and synapses. Gray matter covers the external surface of the brain (i.e., the cortex) and forms several discrete nuclei within the central portion of the brain (i.e., subcortical nuclei). The light substance separating the cortical and subcortical gray matter is known as white matter. White matter is made up of neuronal axons, the majority of which are covered in fatty sheaths known as myelin. It is the myelin that is responsible for the white appearance of these regions.

Information is processed and encoded in gray matter, whereas the white matter pathways provide the means by which information is transferred and communicated throughout the brain. Research suggests that the ability to search and retrieve information from long-term memory stores is a function of subcortical nuclei and white matter systems. These data derive primarily from studies of patients with basal ganglia diseases, such as Parkinson's disease and Huntington's disease, and from studies of patients with white matter diseases, such as multiple sclerosis. These patients tend to be slower when processing and learning information, and they demonstrate poor free recall. Their recognition memory, however, is usually equivalent to that of healthy controls, indicating a primary retrieval deficit.

B. A Model of Encoding and Memory Storage

Memory researchers believe that after sensory information is processed by the neocortex, it is sent along parallel pathways to the hippocampal cortices and medial diencephalon for memory processing. During encoding, associations are created among stimulus features. These associations serve as indices to the cortical sites where the information was originally processed. Input from the basal forebrain and prefrontal cortex modulates memory processing and tags the newly learned information with temporal and spatial information.

Once memories are formed, they must be stored in such a way as to be searched and accessed at a later time when the information is needed. One possibility is that long-term memories are stored in the same brain structures in which new memories are formed. Research on amnesic patients, however, suggests that this is unlikely. Patient H.M., for example, lost the ability to form new memories following bilateral removal of medial temporal lobe structures, but he was able to recall previously learned information normally. This suggests that after new memories are formed they are transferred elsewhere for long-term storage. Researchers believe that permanent memory storage develops in the neocortex; however, the exact nature of the stored information is not known. It remains unclear, for example, whether information is stored regionally or more diffusely throughout the brain and whether memories are stored as basic elemental forms or in more complex formats.

C. Neuroanatomical Correlates of Nondeclarative Memory

Nondeclarative memory is performance based and comprised of phenomena such as skill learning, conditioning, and priming. Unlike declarative memory, the formation of nondeclarative memories is not reliant on the medial temporal lobe/medial diencephalic system. Instead, memories underlying acquired skills or conditioned or primed responses are a function of the sensory and motor systems inherent in the involved behaviors.

1. Skill Learning and Memory

The ability to learn new motor skills and procedures is a function of the corticostriatal system and the cerebellum. The coroticostriatal system includes the basal ganglia and its projections from the neocortex. The basal ganglia are large subcortical nuclei that include the caudate nucleus, putamen, and globus pallidus (Figs. 8 and 10). The basal ganglia have extensive connections with the thalamus, subthalamic nucleus, amygdala, substantia nigra, and broad regions of the neocortex.

The basal ganglia are important for motor planning and programming. Patients with diseases causing dysfunction of the basal ganglia, such as Parkinson's disease and Huntington's disease, typically demonstrate impaired motor skill learning. Learning a new skill requires development and modification of accurate motor programs. As the skill is learned, appropriate movements are performed in the correct serial order and the correct temporal pattern within that order. A feedback system detects errors and generates new, more accurate movements as a result. Dysfunction of the basal ganglia interrupts complex motor and sensory circuits and thus interferes with the ability to generate and/or modify motor programs.

Skill learning that depends on integrating visual and motor information or that requires visual feedback to develop and refine the skill is believed to be a function of the cerebellum. Lesions to the cerebellum are associated with impairments of abilities such as learning and demonstrating the skill of tracing objects when looking at them in a mirror.

Learning visual perceptual skills that do not require motor responses, such as the ability to read text that is presented in reverse mirror-image, depends on the integrity of posterior cortical regions. During learning, the right parietal region becomes activated, presumably because of the need to process the visuospatial aspects of the information. Once the skill is acquired, however, this region becomes less active while activity in the left temporooccipital region increases. The left temporooccipital region is important to normal reading, suggesting that once the skill is learned, the need to decode the visuospatial aspects of the words diminishes and skilled reading occurs.

2. Conditioning

Animal studies indicate that the cerebellum is responsible for most types of conditioned learning. Electrophysiologic changes are observed in the cerebellum during conditioned learning, whereas lesions to the cerebellum disrupt learning. Electrophysiologic changes are also noted in the hippocampus during classical conditioning. Lesions to the hippocampus, however, do not inhibit conditioned learning, suggesting that the hippocampus reflects a parallel information processing system during conditioning but does not in and of itself mediate conditioned learning. In

humans, naturally occurring cerebellar lesions have been shown to interfere with conditioning, whereas lesions to the medial temporal lobes, medial diencephalon, or basal ganglia have no effect on conditioned learning.

The ability to condition a fear response by pairing a neutral stimulus, such as a light or tone, with an aversive unconditioned stimulus, such as electric shock, is a special case of classical conditioning and is a function of the amygdala. Ablation of the amygdala in a variety of mammalian species interferes with the animal's innate fear response and its ability to learn new fear responses. The site of storage for long-term fear-related memory, however, is believed to be outside the amygdala. When the amygdala is lesioned shortly after a new fear response is conditioned, the animal will not demonstrate the response; however, lesioning the amygdala several days after successful conditioning causes no disruption in the conditioned response. Brain areas that have been implicated as possible storage sites for fear memories include the insular cortex and the vermis of the cerebellum.

3. Priming

Patients with dysfunction of the medial temporal lobe, medial diencephalon, and basal ganglia demonstrate intact perceptual priming despite impaired declarative memory or skill learning. Therefore, perceptual priming does not appear to be dependent on these brain regions. Instead, perceptual priming is a function of the cortical regions necessary to process whatever information is primed. Brain imaging studies, for example, show that the right posterior cortex (i.e., the brain region responsible for processing physical features of visual stimuli) is necessary for perceptual priming of words. Patients with damage to this region do not demonstrate visual word priming despite the ability to remember the words on explicit recall tasks. Brain regions required for other forms of perceptual priming likely include cortical regions involved in processing the stimulus qualities and external demands inherent to the individual priming task. Conceptual priming, on the other hand, is believed to be a function of the left frontal cortex.

IV. SUMMARY

The past several decades have witnessed great progress in our understanding of cognitive, biological, and neuroanatomical processes underlying memory functioning. We have learned, for example, that there are two dissociable memory systems—one that is conscious and declarative in nature and another that is unconscious and expressed through performance rather than through conscious recollection. Each of these broad categories of memory is composed of several qualitatively different functions that can be defined along a variety of dimensions.

We have also learned that encoding and memory reflect changes in neuronal function in different brain structures. The medial temporal lobe structures and medial diencephalon, for example, are critical for the formation of new declarative memories but have little impact on memory for previously learned information or nondeclarative forms of learning and memory. On the other hand, basal ganglia dysfunction can disrupt some aspects of nondeclarative memory (i.e., skill learning) while sparing declarative memory. The cerebellum is essential to most forms of classical conditioning, whereas the amygdala plays a key role in conditioned learning of fear responses and emotional modulation of memory.

Despite our advances in knowledge, we still know relatively little about where and how memories are preserved in long-term storage. We know that this information is not stored in the brain structures in which they are created and we presume instead that they are stored in the neocortex. The exact location and format in which memories are preserved over long periods of time remain unclear.

See Also the Following Articles

ALZHEIMER'S DISEASE, NEUROPSYCHOLOGY OF • DEMENTIA • INFORMATION PROCESSING • INTELLIGENCE • MEMORY DISORDERS, ORGANIC • NEOCORTEX

Suggested Reading

Butters, N., Delis, D. C., and Lucas, J. A. (1995). Clinical assessment of memory disorders in amnesia and dementia. *Annu. Rev. Psychol.* **46,** 493–523.

Cermak, L. S. (1994). *Neuropsychological Explorations of Memory and Cognition: Essays in Honor of Nelson Butters.* Plenum, New York.

Crosson, B. (1992). *Subcortical Functions in Language and Memory.* Guilford, New York.

Gabrieli, J. D. E. (1998). Cognitive neuroscience of human memory. *Annu. Rev. Psychol.* **49,** 87–116.

Kandel, E. R. (1991). Nerve cells and behavior. In *Principles of Neural Science* (E. R. Kandel, J. H. Schwartz, and T. H. Jessell, Eds.), pp. 18–32. Appleton & Lange, Norwalk, CT.

Markowitsch, H. J. (2000). The anatomical bases of memory. In *The New Cognitive Neuroscience* (M. S. Gazzaniga, Ed.), pp. 781–796. MIT Press, Cambridge, MA.

Schachter, D. L., and Buckner, R. L. (1998). On the relations among priming, conscious recollection, and intentional retrieval: Evidence from neuroimaging research. *Neurobiol. Learning Memory* **70,** 284–303.

Scoville, W. B., and Milner, B. (1957). Loss of recent memory after bilateral hippocampal lesions. *J. Neurol. Neurosurg. Psychiatr.* **20,** 11–21.

Squire, L. R. (1987). *Memory and Brain.* Oxford Univ. Press, New York.